L. Cecconi, A. Pompili, F. Caroli
and E. Squillaci

MRI Atlas of Central Nervous System Tumors

In collaboration with M. Crecco

With a contribution by E. Tettamanti

Springer-Verlag Wien New York

Lucia Cecconi
Marcello Crecco
Service of Radiology and Diagnostic Imaging

Alfredo Pompili
Fabrizio Caroli
Division of Neurosurgery
Istituto Regina Elena
Rome, Italy

Ettore Squillaci
Institute of Radiology, Medical School
Università degli Studi di Roma 'Tor Vergata'
Rome, Italy

Enzo Tettamanti
Department of Physics, School of Science
Universitá degli Studi dell' Aquila
L'Aquila, Italy

Printed in Germany by Konrad Triltsch, D-W-8700 Würzburg
Printed on acid-free paper

With 236 Figures

ISBN 3-211-82304-2 Springer-Verlag Wien New York
ISBN 0-387-82304-2 Springer-Verlag New York Wien

FOREWORD

In early cancer research scientists peered through primitive microscopes at cell tumors they had transplanted into animals. They asked single questions about the life of the cancer cell. The 20th century has been characterized by a series of impressive discoveries in physical sciences and in biological sciences. Cancer research has benefit for both lines of investigations.

The understanding that the atom was not a single object but that it had orbiting electrons about a central nucleus made of other varieties of subatomic particles has led to the development of magnetic resonance imaging which makes the diagnosis of internal tumors possible at a much earlier stage and at a stage when some of them can be positively eradicated.

This volume is the result of a fruitful gathering of a group of neuroradiologists and neurosurgeons expert in oncology. The book addresses issues in the intriguing and fascinating field of tumors of the central nervous system, by combining in-depth clinical records, surgical contributions, gross pathology and histopathology. Very sharp photographs light the pages of the book, essentially devoted to neuroradiologists and neurosurgeons. The general oncologists will gain most browsing among the striking images.

The virtue of any such book, however, ultimately resides in the competence of the authors: their visible contribution is the published book, but of greater importance is their invisible hard work.

Antonio Caputo
Scientific Director, Istituto Regina Elena

FOREWORD

Magnetic resonance imaging (MRI) unquestionably is the newest and, in many respects, the most revolutionary neurodiagnostic procedure developed in the past few years. The procedure has grown at such a fast pace that, in a few years, image interpretation is no longer based on mere opinions but rather on certainties.

In introducing this book, we emphasize the painstaking efforts which were undertaken by our co-workers in the selection and study of the cases, as well as in the drafting of an atlas of central nervous system (CNS) oncology. We are indebted to them for their careful studies and scientifically rigorous data.

The atlas begins with an introductory chapter which elucidates the physical principles, the technical characteristics of the magnet and the phenomena which contribute to the detection of signals and formation of images. The individual chapters following it suggest some considerations which we regard as crucial in clinical practice.

Almost all the cases presented by the authors were validated by surgical and histologic findings. On this basis, it was possible to make accurate diagnoses and to show that, for the same oncotype, magnetic resonance (MR) images may be different, depending on various factors, such as regressive events and/or perilesional tissue reactions.

It is with pride that we can state that our co-workers have succeeded in translating their in-depth understanding of CNS anatomopathology and MRI into a study which epitomizes the day-to-day observation of the most typical cases diagnosed and operated on in our departments.

The atlas is obviously designed for neurosurgeons and neuroradiologists but it may also be extremely helpful for neurologists, radiologists, and any clinician who takes an interest in the complex issue of brain tumors.

Antonio Riccio
Head, Division of Neurosurgery,
Istituto Regina Elena

Saverio Squillaci
Head, Service of Radiology and Diagnostic Imaging,
Istituto Regina Elena

ACKNOWLEDGEMENTS

The authors thank radiology technicians Maurizio Abrugia, Sergio Dolzi, and, in particular, Marco Mattioli for their invaluable and continuing cooperation in the performance of the studies and in the acquisition of the images; all colleagues from the Division of Neurosurgery and from the Service of Radiology and Diagnostic Imaging, Istituto Regina Elena, and, in particular, Drs. Laura Raus and Francesco Calvosa for their review of our clinical series; Stefania Saraceni and Ennia Cucchiarelli for translating and editing the manuscript.

CONTENTS

LIST OF MAIN ACRONYMS

A.C.A. anterior cerebral artery
A.C.o.A. anterior communicating artery
ACTH adrenocorticotropin
AFP alpha-pheto-protein
A.I.C.A. antero-inferior cerebellar artery
AVM arterovenous malformation
B.A. basilar artery
BBB blood-brain-barrier
C.A. carotid artery
c.e. contrast enhancement
CNS central nervous system
CSF cerebrospinal fluid
CT computerized tomography
E.C.A. external carotid artery
FSH follicle-stimulating hormone
GH growth hormone
hCG chorionic gonadotropin
I.C.A. internal carotid artery
i.v. GD-DTPA intravenous gadolinium diethylenetriaminepentaacetic acid
LH luteinizing hormone
M.C.A. middle cerebral artery
MR magnetic resonance
MRI magnetic resonance imaging
P.C.A. posterior cerebral artery
P.I.C.A. postero-inferior cerebellar artery
PRL prolactin
RF radiofrequency
SC spinal cord
SR spin-echo
S.L.S. superior longitudinal sinus
SNR signal-to-noise-ratio
TE echo time
TI inversion time
TR repetition time
TSH thyroid-stimulating hormone
V.A. vertebral artery
WHO World Health Organization

CHAPTER I

Introduction to magnetic resonance imaging

Fundamentals

The uniqueness of MR images lies in the physical origin of the signal. In X-rays, the radiation (X) is "absorbed" more by bones and less by soft tissues. Consequently, in X-rays (negative), bones appear as the bright part of the image, whereas soft tissues are darker. The same applies to ultrasonography. Ultrasounds cross the tissues and are absorbed by them in differing degrees. The resulting image reflects the different level of ultrasound absorption by the tissues. In both cases, the image results from the interaction between the X radiation or ultrasounds and the electronic structure of matter.

In MRI, the process is different. The tissues which are placed in a magnetic field and irradiated by electromagnetic waves in the radiofrequency (RF) range are also sources of electromagnetic RF waves. It is the RF emitted by the tissues, i.e. the recorded and suitably processed MRI signal, that gives rise to the image. This schematic description clearly shows the difference existing between MR images and other images obtained with different techniques in the medical field. Unlike the above-mentioned X-ray and ultrasound techniques, MRI relies on the magnetic properties of matter and on the interaction of electromagnetic (RF) waves with nuclei and not with electrons.

The following paragraphs will qualitatively and descriptively discuss the principles which underlie this procedure, providing the fundamentals to understand the characteristics of MR images.

The physical bases of MRI

We will only refer to hydrogen nuclei, since they are more suitable for MRI: they are the most abundant among biological tissue nuclei and, density being equal, they generate the highest signals.

The nucleus of the hydrogen atom consists of the proton alone, to which a magnetic dipole moment is associated (i.e. it behaves like a small magnetic needle); this moment is called *nuclear magnetic moment* (μ).

In an external magnetic field, the nuclear magnetic moment may only take two directions with respect to the direction of this magnetic field: parallel (spin up) or antiparallel (spin down).

Quantum mechanical interpretation: energy levels

Consider a given volume of water and the hydrogen protons in it. Without external magnetic fields, the magnetic dipoles associated with the hydrogen protons may take any direction in space. Therefore, no magnetic moment will occur. If the same volume lies in a space with a homogeneous magnetic field (B_0), the magnetic dipoles may take only two directions, reflecting two different energy values. Two energy states will thus occur, corresponding to: the parallel direction, with the lower energy (E_1); and the antiparallel direction, with the higher energy (E_2). The energy difference between these two energy states or levels is equal to $\Delta E = \gamma\hbar\, B_0$, i.e. proportional to the applied magnetic field.

The N magnetic dipoles of the sample will distribute between these energy levels, obeying the Boltzmann statistics. A given number of them (n_1) will populate the lower energy level (parallel direction), whereas the others ($n_2 = N - n_1$) will populate the higher energy level (E_2) (antiparallel direction) *(Fig. 1)*.

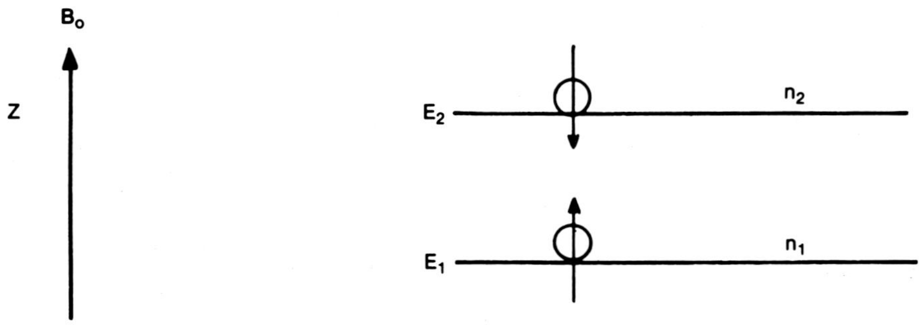

Fig. 1. Spin distribution over two energy levels: $E_2 > E_1$; $n_1 > n_2$.

Level E_1 will be more populated, since it has lower energy. Therefore, the sample under study will have a resulting magnetic moment M due to the difference $n_1 - n_2$. This resulting magnetic moment will be taken into account to understand the phenomenon of MRI. The above description or model is based on a quantum mechanical and statistical approach. The model may be used to understand MRI, in addition to the more common vectorial (traditional) model which is described below.

Traditional approach – vectorial model

The Larmor precession

In a magnetic field B_0, directed along the reference axis z, the dipole is subjected to a torque tending to align it parallel to the field. The torque, combined with the rotational motion of the proton on itself (spin), gives rise to a precession of the magnetic moment μ about the direction of B_0 *(Fig. 2)*. This motion, known as Larmor precession, occurs with the frequency:

$$\nu = \frac{1}{2\pi} \gamma \, B_0.$$

For the proton, $\gamma = 42.58$ MHz/Tesla; γ is termed gyromagnetic ratio.

This motion may be explained by referring to a spinning-top. If, while the spinning-top is rotating on itself, the upper end of its axis is pushed slightly towards the horizontal direction (torque), this axis will immediately start rotating (precess) about the vertical (direction of the gravitational force), forming a given angle with it. In this case, the gravitational field is the analog of the magnetic field. In the same analogy, the proton behaves in the magnetic field like a spinning-top. Therefore, out of the N protons which are present in the water sample, n_1 will precess so that each of them will have the component $+\mu z$ (parallel), and the remaining n_2 will have the component $-\mu z$. A resulting magnetic moment, $M = (n_1 - n_2) \times \mu z$, will occur along the direction of the B_0 field, which is assumed to coincide with the z direction.

Now, the resulting magnetic moment M should be considered as oriented along the direction of B_0 but rotating at the Larmor frequency *(Fig. 3)*.

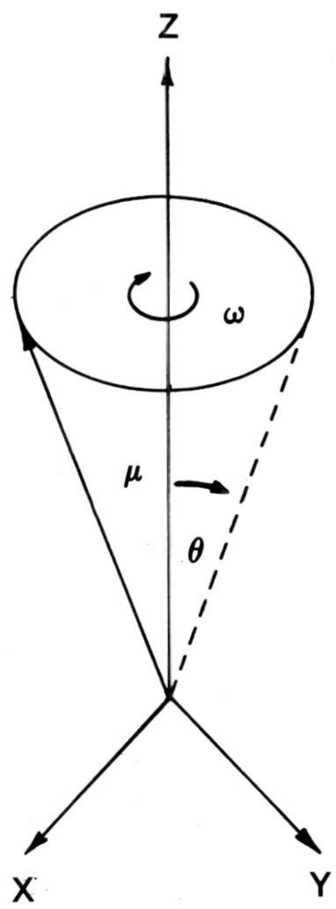

Fig. 2. In a magnetic field (B) in the z direction, the proton-associated magnetic moment (μ) precesses at the angular velocity $\omega = \gamma B$ about the B field direction and it forms an angle θ with it.

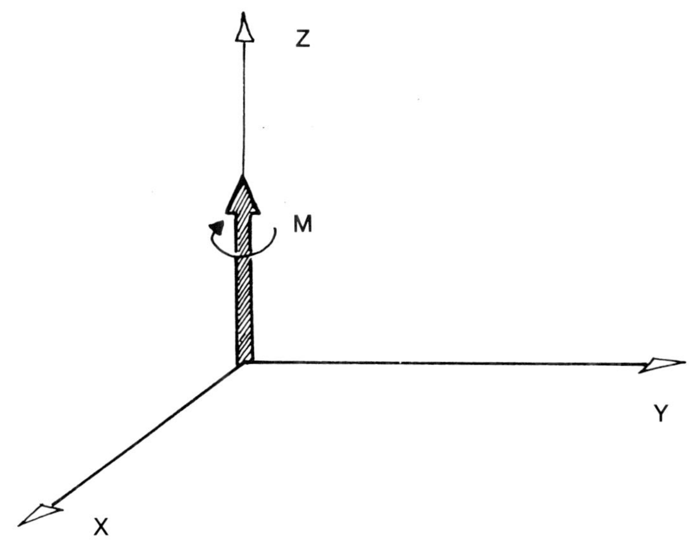

Fig. 3. In a magnetic field (B) in the z direction, the individual magnetic moments of the protons will have a component in this direction. The vector sum of these components generates the resulting magnetic moment (M) in the z direction which rotates at the angular velocity.

Nuclear magnetic resonance (NMR)

Through coil 1 *(Fig. 4)*, we generate a small sinusoidal magnetic field H_1 in the x direction. If the frequency of H_1 is equal to the Larmor frequency of the protons, the magnetic moment M (comparable to a bar magnet) will start tilting and continue to precess about the z direction. At the same time, at the ends of coil 2, an induced voltage will be observed. This voltage, which is sinusoidal at the Larmor frequency, reaches its maximum amplitude when M lies in the xy plane. If, at this time, we interrupt the current producing the H_1 field, the magnetic moment will precess in the xy plane. The H_1 field has been applied for such a long time (t) as to rotate the magnetic moment M by 90°. In this case, the applied pulse will be termed *90° pulse*. After this pulse, a sinusoidal (voltage) signal is induced at the ends of coil 2. The signal, called Free Induction Decay (FID), alternates at a frequency equal to the Larmor precession frequency. In this way, nuclear magnetism is evidenced by the signal that it induces in a coil.

This has been made possible only by the application of the H_1 field, oscillating at a frequency which is *exactly equal* to the Larmor frequency of the protons: this is the resonance condition.

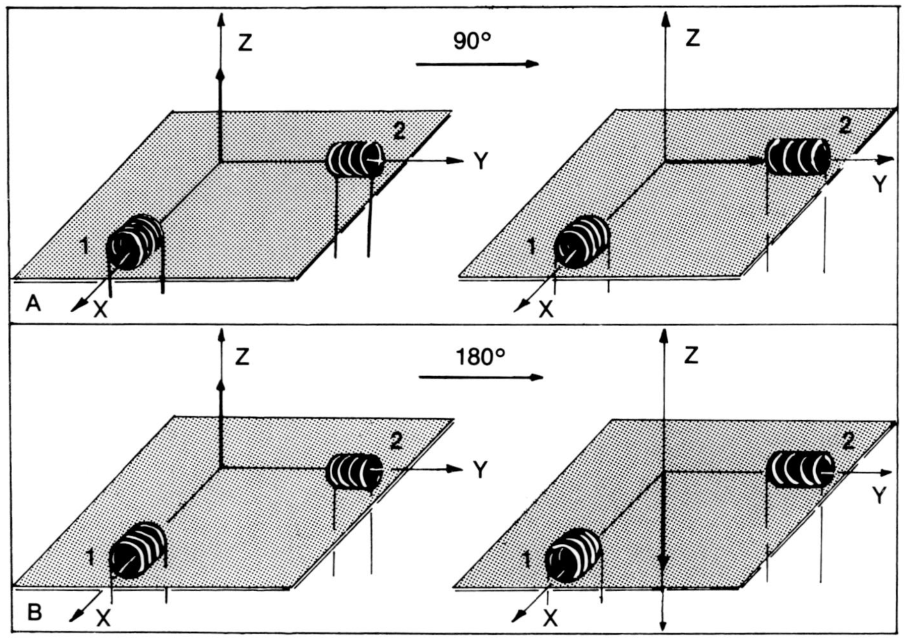

Fig. 4. Conceptual diagram showing the arrangement of coil 1, generating the RF (H_1 oscillating at the Larmor frequency) and of coil 2, receiving the RF signal, with respect to the direction of the B_0 magnetic field (z direction). The diagram also displays the effects of the 90° and 180° pulses on the magnetization vector (M).

Relaxation times and sequences

Transverse (spin-spin) relaxation (T_2)

The signal observed after the 90° pulse diminishes over time with a behavior which is given by the following equation:

$$A(t) = A_0 \exp(-t/T_2)$$

where $A(t)$ = signal recorded at the coil ends
T_2 = characteristic time constant of the substance under study.

This time constant T_2 is known as transverse or spin-spin relaxation time. It establishes the rate at which the signal decays to zero *(Fig. 5)*.

The signal decreases over time because the individual protons sense different "local" magnetic fields. Consequently, there are protons which precess at different rates. As time passes, elementary magnetic moments will scatter (dephase), producing a resulting magnetic moment which will fall off with time. When isotropic scattering takes place, the resulting magnetic moment will be zero, and the coil ends will no longer show induced voltage. This phenomenon is known as phase coherence loss.

Longitudinal (spin-lattice) relaxation (T_1)

We apply an RF pulse for such duration as to bring the magnetization M to the $-z$ direction. In this case, the applied pulse will be called 180° pulse. After this pulse, the spin system tends to go back to thermodynamic equilibrium. In the vectorial description of the phenomenon, this thermodynamic equilibrium corresponds to the orientation of M in the $+z$ direction. The rate at which the equilibrium is restored is governed by a time constant T_1, called longitudinal or spin-lattice relaxation time. The time behavior of the equilibrium recovery is given by the following equation:

$$M_z(t) = M_{z0} \cdot (1 - 2 \cdot e^{-t/T_1})$$

where M_{z0} is the value of the magnetization under equilibrium conditions.

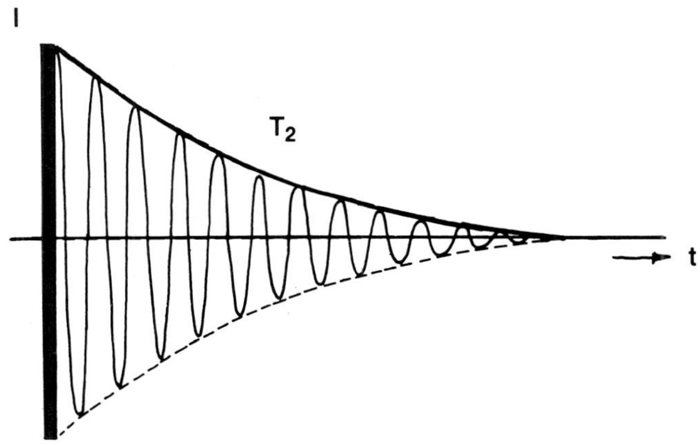

Fig. 5. Signal recorded at the end of the 90° pulse and its decay over time. The T_2 relaxation time is the one which would occur owing to the spin-spin interaction alone. In the real situation, given inhomogeneities of the static and RF fields, the decay is faster and governed by the relaxation time $T_2^* < T_2$.

To be detectable, the magnetization must precess in the xy plane in order to induce voltage in coil 2. Therefore, the following process is used. After a first 180° pulse, a 90° pulse is delivered to the system with a delay (t). The latter pulse brings the magnetization to the xy plane. The signal induced in the coil is proportional to the magnetization Mz of the system existing at time t. By repeating this process with different values of the time between the 180° and 90° pulses (Interpulse Time, TI), the return of the system to equilibrium can be followed through the signal amplitude induced in coil 2. A time $TR > 5\ T_1$ should be allowed between two subsequent excitations of the system (Repetition Time, TR) in order to enable it to go back to thermodynamic equilibrium before a new excitation.

The time behavior of this signal is given by the equation:

$$A(t) = A_0 (1 - 2e^{-TI/T_1}).$$

The return to equilibrium after the 180° pulse, also called Magnetization or Inversion Recovery, has the behavior shown in *Fig. 6*.

A set of multiple pulses makes up a sequence of pulses. The above two-pulse sequence is known as Inversion Recovery (IR) or 180° – TI – 90° sequence.

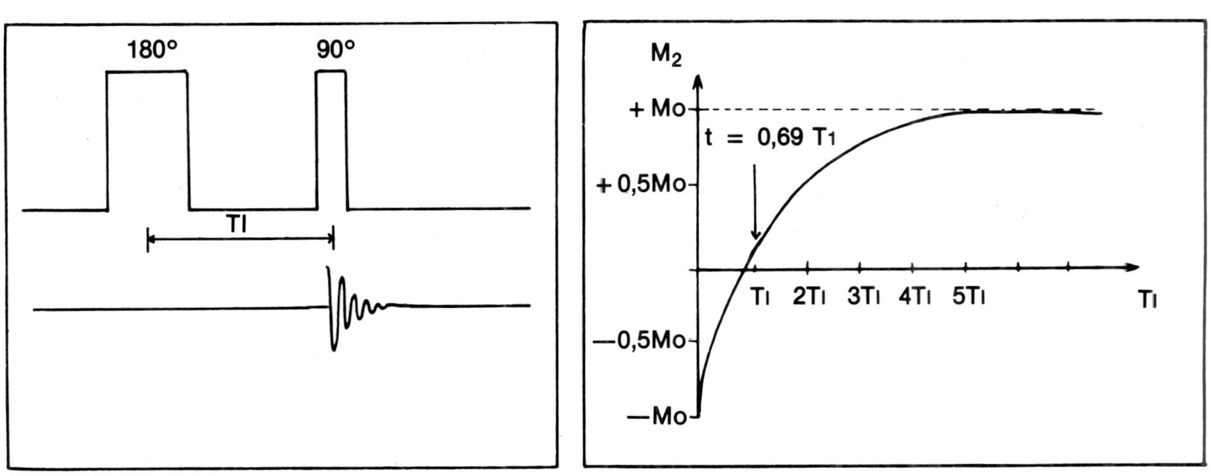

Fig. 6. Signal time behavior after magnetization inversion obtained with a 180° pulse. To sample the signal, a 90° pulse should be sent after a time interval, TI, in order to bring the magnetization Mz (TI) to the xy plane in order to be detected.

Spin-echo

Another interesting and fundamental phenomenon in MRI is the refocusing of magnetic moments. As previously pointed out, not all magnetic dipoles or spins sense the same value of the applied magnetic field B_0. The applied magnetic field B_0 is never completely homogeneous. In other terms, in the space occupied by the volume of the sample to be studied, the magnetic field will have different values from one point to the other. Suppose that this volume is divided into volume elements ΔV so small as to be considered to lie in a perfectly homogeneous magnetic field, but so large as to accommodate a high number of spins. In this situation, each volume element will have a value of the field B_i slightly different from the value of the applied external field. The Larmor precession inside the volume element, ΔV_i, will thus be $\omega_i = \gamma B_i$. The set of spins accommodated in the individual volume elements represents an *isochromatic group* of spins or an isochromat. To understand what happens after a 90° pulse, the phenomenon should be observed in an $x'y'z'$ reference system, rotating at the velocity $\omega_0 = \gamma B_0$ and where the observer is connected to the z' axis, coincident with z.

By feeding a 90° pulse to the system, the rotating observer will see the magnetization M passing to the y' axis. But the individual isochromats have different rotation velocities. Therefore, the faster ones will draw away from the y' axis in one direction, whereas the slower ones will draw away from it in the opposite direction *(Fig. 7)*. In other terms, the isochromats will scatter on the $x'y'$ plane, thereby reducing the magnetization in the y' direction. If, after a time interval τ, a 180° pulse is delivered to the system, all the isochromats will be flipped over by 180°, while they continue to precess. As shown in *Fig. 7,* after an interval τ has elapsed since the 180° pulse, the isochromats will be clustered (*refocused*) along the y' axis, producing the magnetization M. In other terms, at this

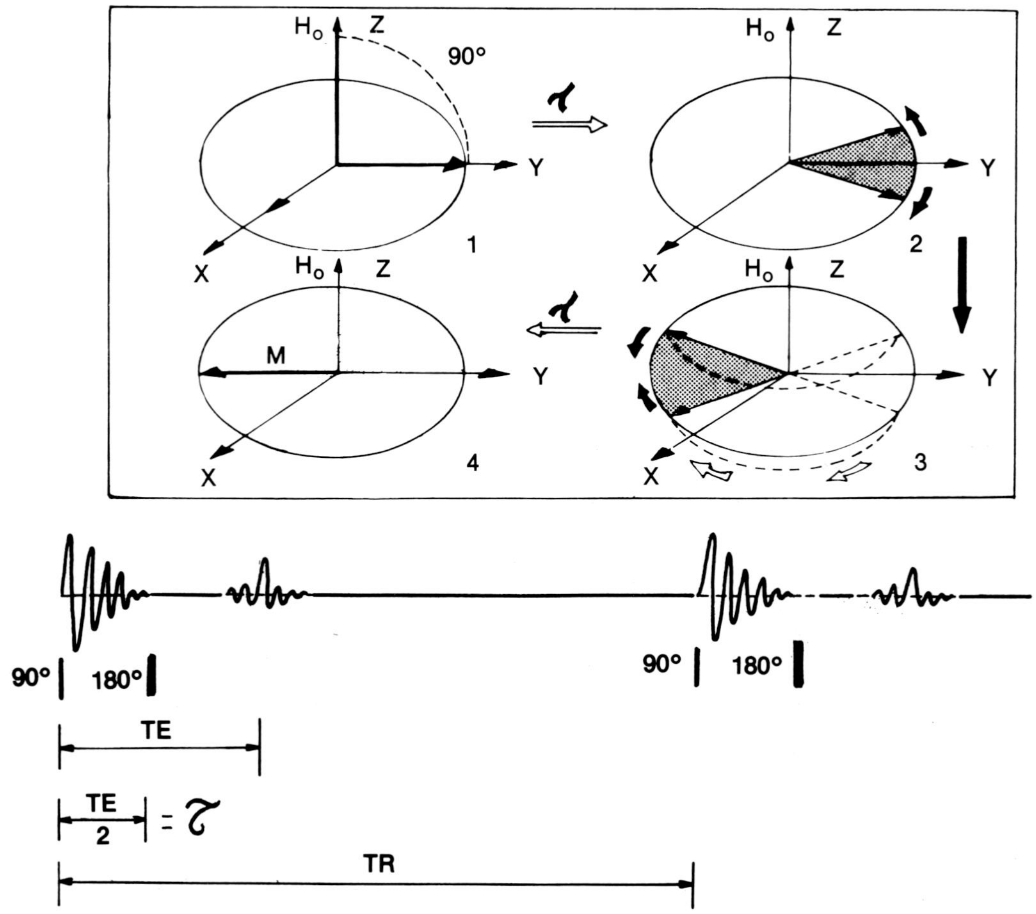

Fig. 7. Formation of the echo signal, seen in the rotating reference system. The small arrows indicate the direction of the motion of the isochromats in the rotating system, before and after the 180° pulse.

time point, by allowing an interval 2τ after the $90°$ pulse, the maximum signal will again be recorded in coil 2. This signal is called *echo*. The above description only considered the scattering of isochromats due to inhomogeneity of the applied magnetic field. This inhomogeneity does not change over time. Consequently, its effects are cancelled out by the process whereby the echo signal is formed. This implies that the echo signal should be equal to that observed at the end of the $90°$ pulse, whatever the time interval τ.

Actually, the amplitude of the echo signal decreases when τ increases, until it falls to zero. This decay stems from the fact that, at each time point, the individual spins reflect a "local" magnetic field which randomly changes over time. The dephasing (scattering) effects of this field cannot be removed by the $180°$ pulse-induced rephasing. This signal decay is governed by the parameter T_2, which depends on: substance under study, value of the magnetic field and temperature. Conversely, the signal decay observed after the $90°$ pulse alone originates from: inhomogeneities of the static magnetic field B_0 and local fields which randomly change in time and space. In this case, the decay is governed by the parameter T_2^*, with $T_2 > T_2^*$. The sequence consisting of one $90°$ pulse followed, after a time interval τ, by a $180°$ pulse, is called spin-echo sequence.

Spin-echo sequence

The previous description of the process whereby the echo signal is formed suggests that a single sequence may involve multiple echoes.

After the formation of the first echo, the isochromats start to scatter (to dephase) again. Hence, if a time interval 2τ is allowed after the first $180°$ pulse, and a series of $180°$ pulses with 2τ intervals is delivered, a series of echoes with 2τ intervals will be obtained *(Fig. 8)*. The signal amplitude of this series of echoes decreases according to the following time law:

$$A_n = A_1\, e^{-nTE/T_2}$$

where A_n = amplitude of the echo signal of order n
A_1 = amplitude of the first echo
n = order number of the echo signal
TE = Echo Time (time between $90°$ pulse and first echo).

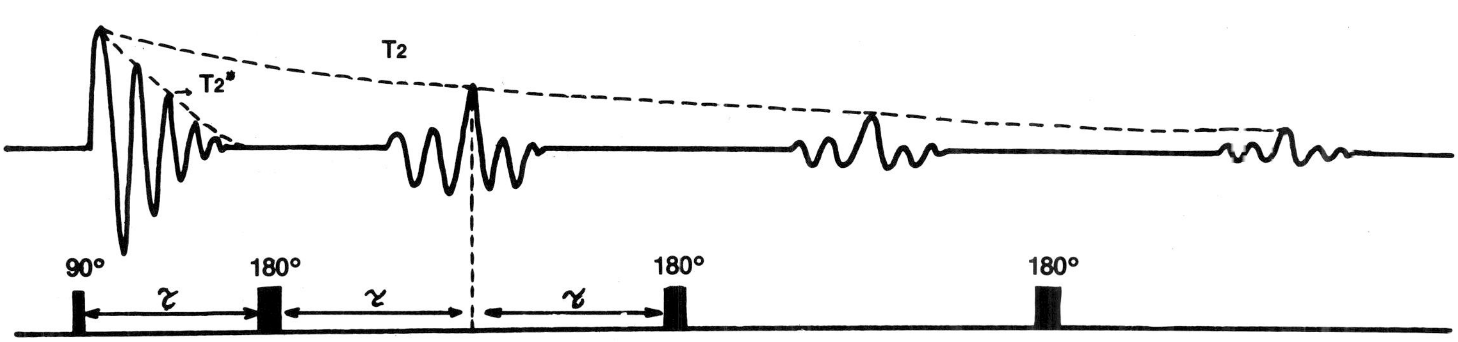

Fig. 8. Spin-echo signals on multi-echo sequence and sequence parameters. In this case, the echoes decay with the time constant T_2, since field inhomogeneity effects are cancelled out.

Saturation recovery (partial saturation)

Assume that two consecutive $90°$ pulses, with an interval TR, are delivered to the system initially under equilibrium conditions. If TR is very long vs. the T_1 of the sample under review ($TR > 5 \times T_1$), the second pulse will find the system completely relaxed. In other terms, the magnetization has had sufficient time to completely revert to the z direction. In this case, the two pulses are independent of each other. At the end of each of them, the maximum signal will occur, corresponding to the rotation of the magnetization M on the xy plane. If $TR < 5 \times T_1$ (usually $TR \simeq T_1$), the system has not had sufficient time to completely relax. Therefore, in the xy plane, the second pulse can rotate only the part of the magnetization which has returned to the z direction during the TR interval. Consequently, after the second pulse, the signal will be lower; its amplitude depends on the TR interval according to the following equation:

$$A\,(TR) = A_0 \cdot (1 - e^{-TR/T_1})$$

Clearly, the smaller the TR/T_1 ratio, the lower the signal recorded after the second 90° pulse, as shown in *Fig. 9*.

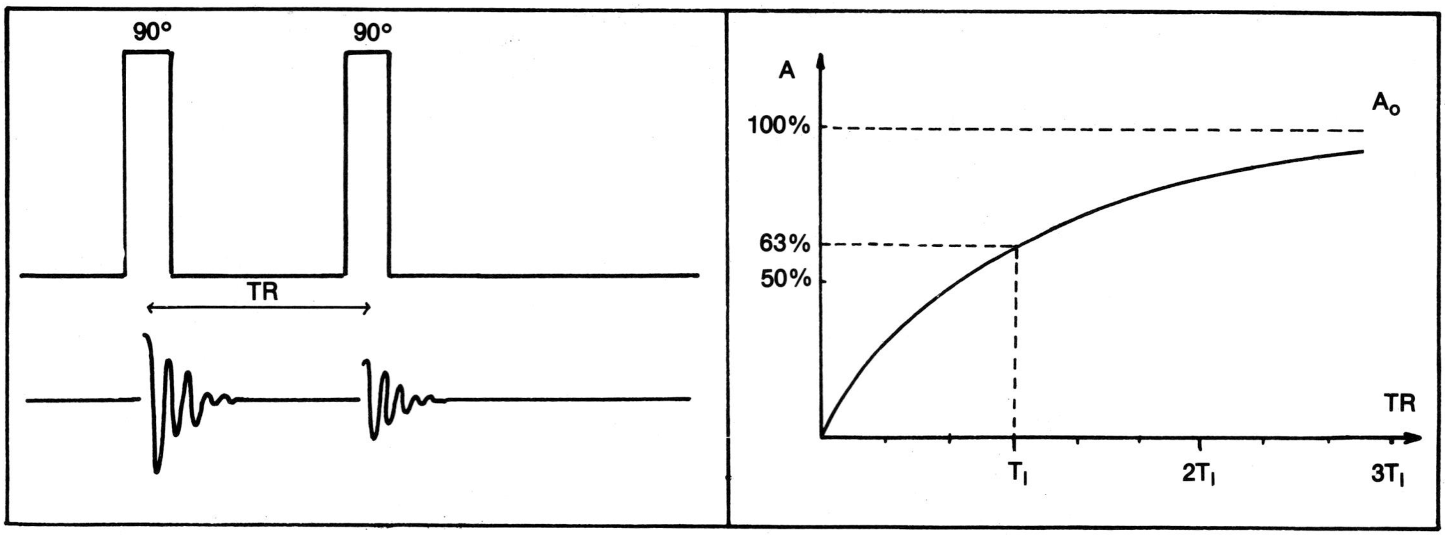

Fig. 9. Signal amplitude vs. pulse repetition time on the saturation recovery sequence.

Note, in practice, the signal used for the formation of the images is always an echo signal. This minimizes any inconvenience which may arise in signal acquisition and which would be chiefly due to the dead time of amplifiers. Therefore, all the sequences shown here include a 180° pulse, which is delivered after a TE/2 interval has elapsed since the 90° pulse. The 180° pulse is used to bring the magnetization to the xy plane in order to detect the signal.

Characteristics of the MR image

From the MR signal to the image

An adequate use of the MR signal can yield an image like the one in *Fig. 10*. The image consists of a set of adjacent volume elements, each of which is associated with a shade of gray. The shade of gray corresponds to a digit, expressing the intensity (Volts) of the MRI signal generated by the volume elements. The image can thus be considered as a mosaic whose tesserae are the individual volume elements (Voxels).

This schematic description infers that the formation of an image requires:

a) selection of the anatomical slice of interest
b) spatial encoding of the voxels in the slice.

This is achieved by superposing controlled inhomogeneities upon the static magnetic field. The inhomogeneities are linear magnetic field gradients which impart special characteristics to the MR signal. By subjecting the signal to appropriate mathematical operations, known as the Fourier transform (FT), the slice can be selected and divided into volume elements (Voxels), each of which has an associated signal intensity, hence producing the image.

Characteristics of the MR image

We have seen how we can spatially identify one volume element by simultaneously using adequate linear gradients and by applying the Fourier transform to the MRI signal.

The image of *Fig. 10* shows that the voxels containing different tissues have different intensities (shades of gray). The signal associated with each voxel depends on the material contained in it: proton density (protons per unit volume) and values of the relaxation times (T_1 and T_2) of the material. Furthermore, this intensity also depends on the scanning parameters: sequence used, TR and TE settings. The following paragraphs emphasize that each of the above parameters impact the appearance of the image and hence the intensity of the voxel signal.

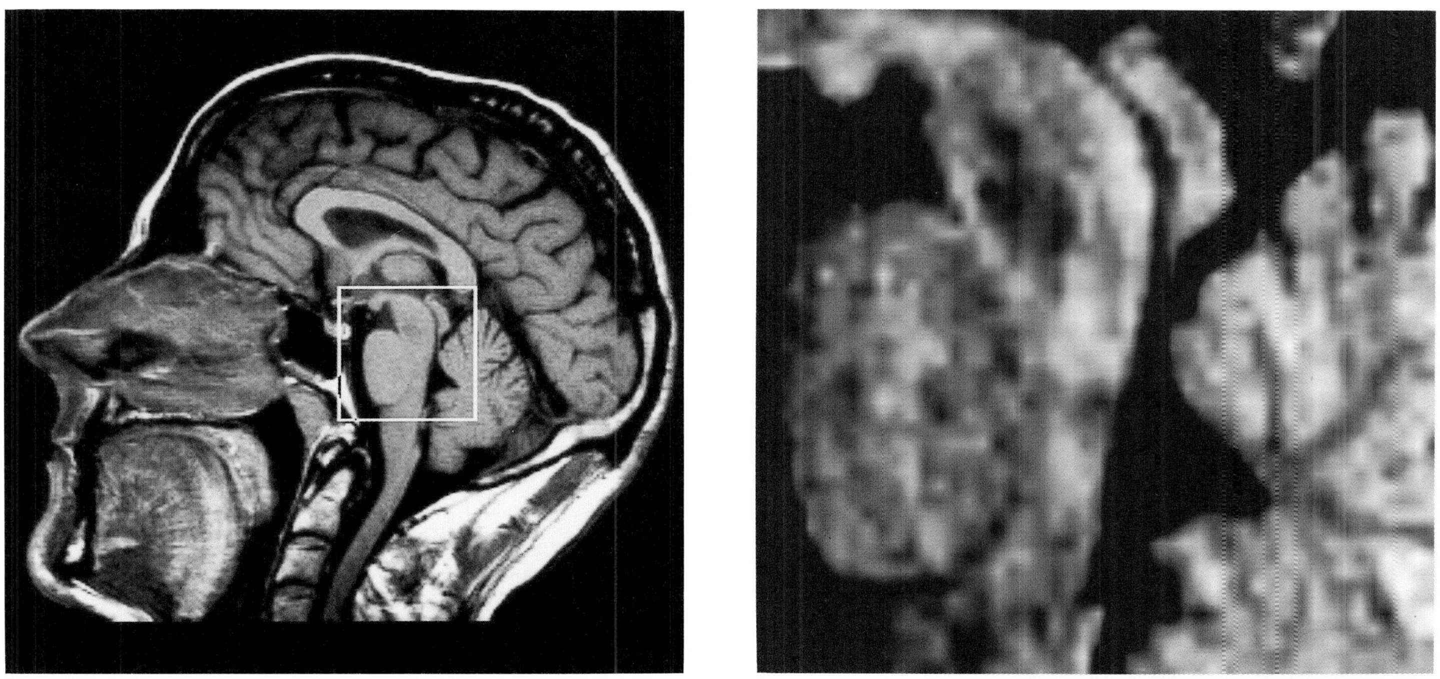

A B

Fig. 10. *Sagittal scan of the brain.* A – Image obtained with a sequence TR = 550 msec, TE = 15 msec, matrix = 256 × 256 and FOV = 30 cm (spatial resolution = 1.2 mm). B – Same image with magnification of the boxed area. The volume elements are visible.

Proton density (ϱ)

The proton density is the number of protons per unit volume (protons/cm^3) in the material under study. To discriminate between the intensities of two voxels containing materials with different ϱ, use is to be made of a sequence with a TR which is more than five times the longest T_1 relaxation time observed in this material. In this way, the system has sufficient time to go back to thermodynamic equilibrium before a subsequent excitation. The spin-echo (SE) sequence is to be used in this instance; its echo time (TE) should be as short as possible to prevent a possible contribution of the T_2 relaxation time to the signal decay. In this case, if the signal for two voxels is different, this is due to the fact that their proton content is different *(Fig. 11)*.

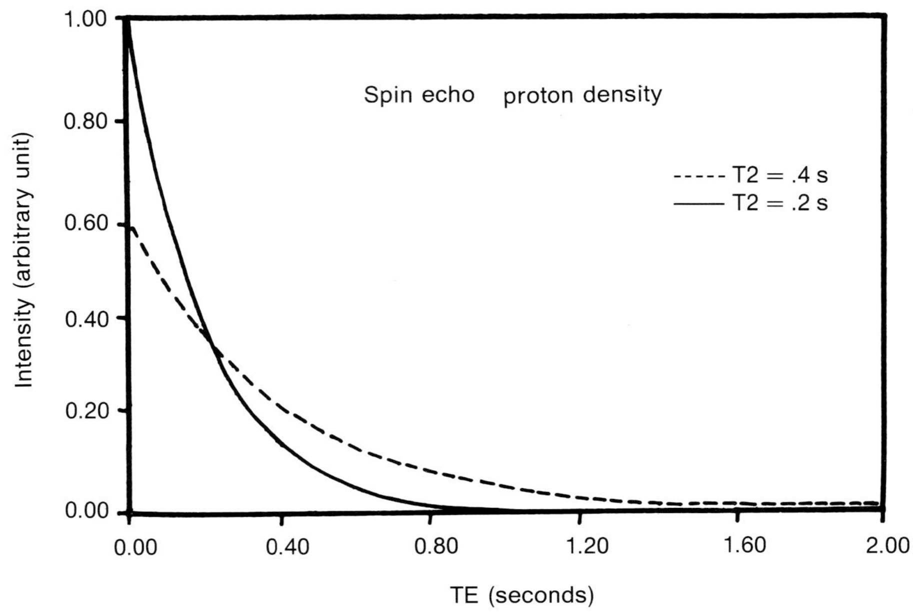

Fig. 11. *Decay of the echo signal vs. TE in two tissues with different proton densities and also different T_2s.* The proton-density characterization may be obtained by using a TR > 5 times the longest T_1 and the shortest possible TEs in order to minimize the influence of T_2 (anyhow, the TEs should be shorter than the time of crossover of the two curves).

T_2-characterized image (T_2-weighted image)

The SE sequence is the most suited for this characterization. As illustrated above, the echo signal decays over time according to a time law which is governed by the T_2 relaxation time. Assume that two voxels contain material having the same proton density and different T_1 and T_2 relaxation times. By using a TR $\simeq$ five times the longest T_1 relaxation time, a signal of equal intensity will be recorded when using the shortest possible TE. With longer TEs, the voxel having material with a shorter T_2 will be less intense than the other. Obviously, when TE increases, both signals decrease, but at different rates. This behavior is depicted in *Fig. 12.*

A special and interesting case for diagnostic purposes is the one where also the proton density is different.

In this case, the signals of the two voxels have different intensities at time zero (practically for a very small TE).

When TE increases, the two signals decrease at different rates, since the T_2 relaxation times are different. If the voxel with the lower proton density has a longer T_2, because of different steepness,

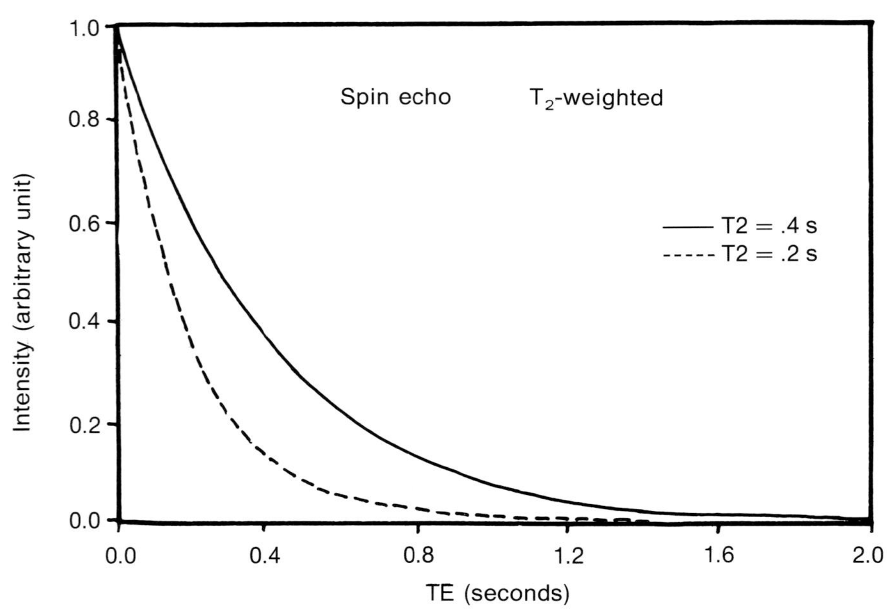

Fig. 12. *Amplitude of the echo signal vs. the echo time (TE) in two tissues with the same proton density and different T_2 relaxation times.* The signal intensity difference between the two tissues depends on the TE used.

the two decay curves may cross over before the two signals decay to noise level. As a result, for TE settings lower than the time corresponding to the crossover point, the voxel with the shorter T_2 will yield a more intense signal. The opposite occurs for TE settings greater than the time corresponding to the crossover point *(Fig. 11)*.

Once this phenomenon is understood, it can be used for diagnostic purposes. The signal inversion effect can be a useful tool in the study of the spine, in particular to obtain the myelographic effect, through which cerebrospinal fluid (CSF) is differentiated from bone marrow.

T_1-characterized image (T_1-weighted image)

Hypothesize that the material of the two voxels has the same proton density but different T_1 and T_2 values. By using an SE sequence with the shortest possible TE – to clear the effects due to T_2 – and a short TR (TR $\simeq T_1$ shorter than or intermediate between the two T_1s under review), the signal intensity of the two voxels depends on the corresponding T_1s. A higher signal will be produced by the voxel which has the material with the shorter T_1; for the selected TR, this voxel has had more time to relax. To understand this aspect, refer to *Fig. 13*, which exemplifies two tissues having T_1 relaxation times of 500 and 800 msec, respectively.

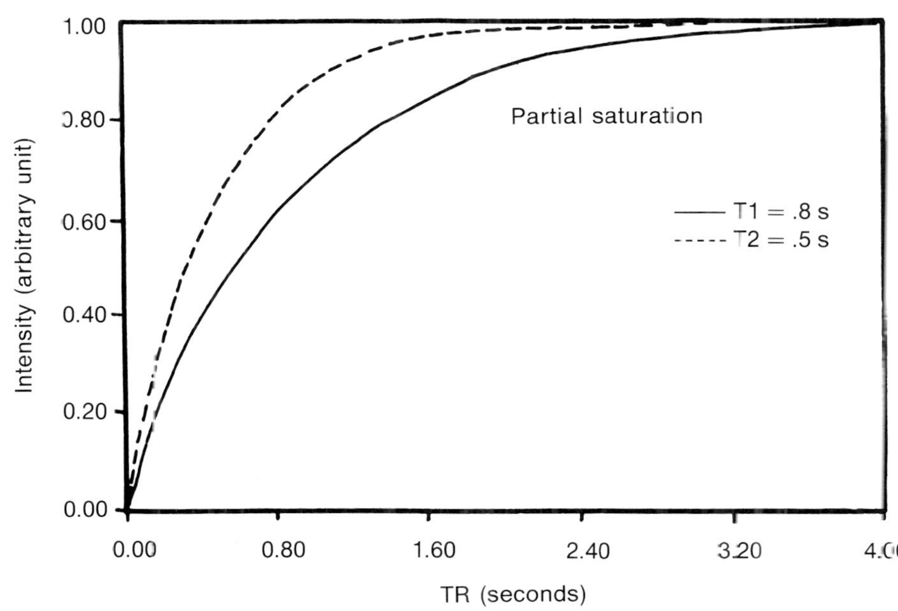

Fig. 13. The magnetization recovery has a different behavior for the two tissues. The tissue with the shorter T_1 returns more rapidly to equilibrium. As a result, for a given value of TR, the two tissues yield different signals and are thus distinguishable from each other. This differentiation is based on the different value of T_1; therefore, the resulting images will be called T_1-weighted.

T_1-weighted image with inversion recovery sequence

The sequence used is the Inversion Recovery one. The ensuing image is a purely T_1-weighted image, if use is made of a long TR ($> 5 \times T_1$) and of a short TE in order to compare the various tissues on the basis of differences in the T_1 relaxation time.

Assume – hopefully – that the MRI system allows to reconstruct the image by using the real part of the signal. For a selected TI, the voxels containing tissues with a T_1 such that the condition $TI = T_1 \times \ln 2$ is fulfilled will give a null signal. Their intensity is equal to the background one. Compared to the latter voxels, the voxels having material with a longer T_1 will have a negative signal and thus an intensity lower (darker) than the background. By contrast, their counterparts which contain tissues with a shorter T_1 will have a positive signal, thus brighter than the background *(Fig. 14)*.

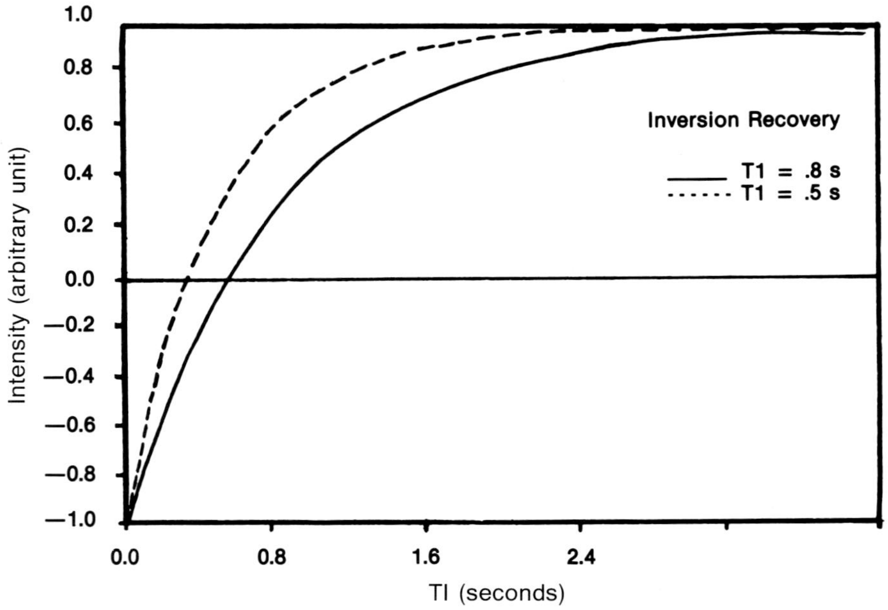

Fig. 14. *Magnetization recovery after a 180° pulse for two tissues having a different T_1 relaxation time.* For a given value of the time TI, the two signals are different, reflecting different tissues. Note the uniqueness of these curves which always have a null point at a time which depends on the corresponding T_1 relaxation time.

Image reconstruction via the signal module is more complex and also more misleading *(Fig. 15)*.

As displayed in the *Fig. 15*, tissues with different T_1s may have the same signal module intensity, making image interpretation difficult.

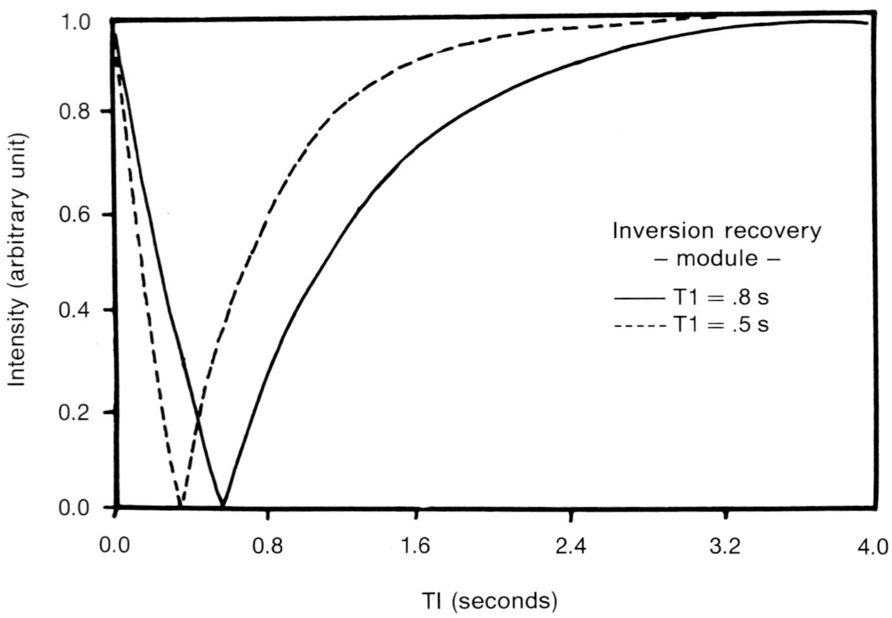

Fig. 15. *Signal time behavior on the IR sequence, using the signal module alone.* In other terms, it is impossible to discriminate positive values from negative ones. The behavior observed may give rise to difficulties of interpretation, since, for a given TI value, the same signal intensity may be associated with the two tissues, even if they have different T_1s.

Multislice acquisition

Consider a T_2-weighted SE sequence. This sequence uses a very long TR vs. the T_1 of the tissues under study in order to enable the protons of the excited slices to go back to equilibrium before repeating the sequence to encode the subsequent line. This time interval can be used to excite other slices of the volume under study. Hence, during the lag time which is needed for the first-slice spins to relax, other slices can be excited without wasting time *(Fig. 16)*.

In this scanning procedure, the TR is selected and a number of slices covering a volume equal to the thickness of the slice multiplied by the number of slices (plus the thickness due to the gap) is obtained. Generally, an interslice gap is recommended with a view to reducing interference between slices, which may cause an undesirable, partially T_1-weighted image.

Another procedure to minimize this interference and thus to have more closely-spaced (adjacent) slices consists in exciting the slices not sequentially but, for instance, in the following order:

slices:	1–2	3–4	5–6	7–8	9–10	11–12
order:	1.7	2.8	3.9	4.10	5.11	6.12

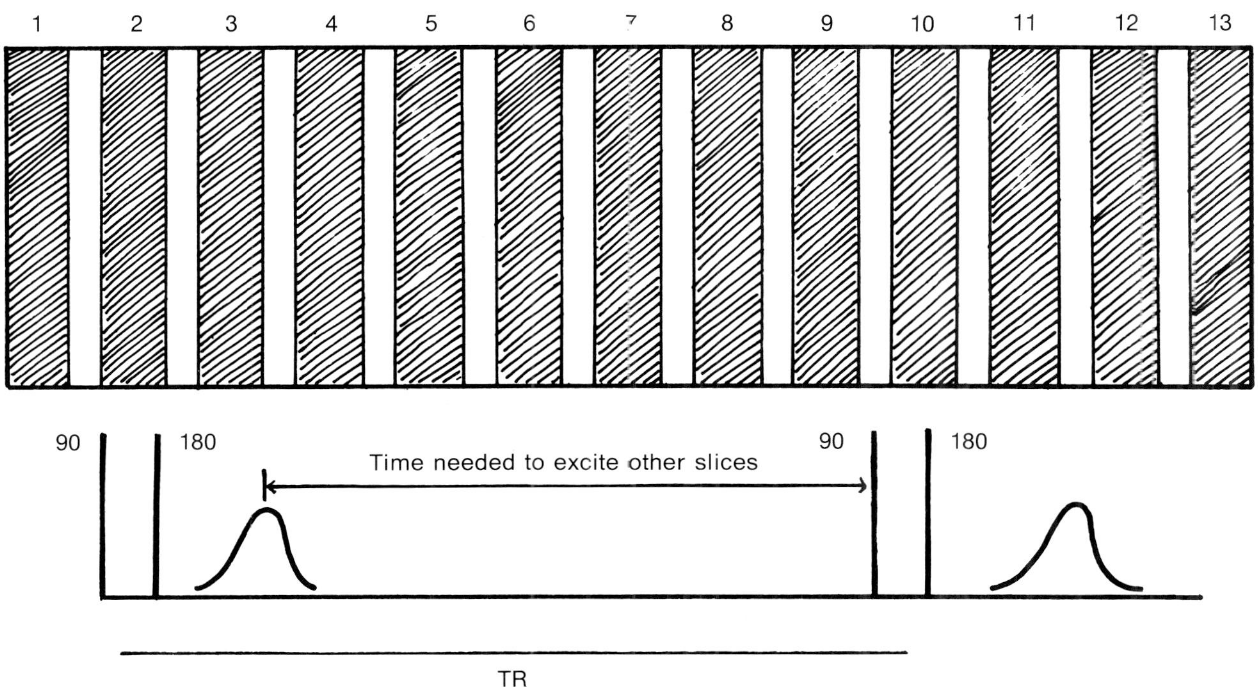

Fig. 16. *Diagram of the slices into which the volume under review was divided.* Whenever possible, it is advisable to leave an interslice gap, in order to avoid interferences due to overlapping (the slice never has a perfectly rectangular profile). 1 – Time needed to excite other slices.

Volume (3D) acquisition

This procedure relies on excitation and reception of the signal by the entire selected volume, as if it were a very thick slice. In order to be able to subsequently subdivide this volume into an N number of slices, use should be made of an additional gradient orthogonal to the slices, so as to encode the corresponding position. This gradient should be delivered by incrementing it as many times as the number of slices to be obtained (in this case N). Then the Fourier transform should be applied to the above direction. The total time to acquire the image thus rises by a factor N:

$$\text{Acquisition time} = N \times TR \times (\text{number of lines}) \times \text{Averages.}$$

The advantage of this procedure lies in the fact that the signal to be analyzed originates from the entire volume and not from the individual slice, subsequently obtained by computation. The ensuing increase in the signal-to-noise ratio (SNR) allows to break down the volume into slices which are thinner than those obtained through multislice acquisition. Obviously, as previously stressed, it takes time. In other terms, the duration of the procedure is generally very long.

Gradient echo

As previously explained, the echo signal can be achieved with an SE sequence (90° – TE/2 – 180°). An echo signal can be generated also without the 180° pulse. This is possible by subjecting the system at first to a positive gradient, so as to produce controlled spin dephasing, and subsequently to the same gradient with opposite sign. The second gradient gives rise to dephasing in the direction opposite to the first one and thus to spin refocusing or *gradient echo.*

Without the 180° pulse, much shorter TEs can be selected, thus increasing the SNR. Moreover, the procedure requires less RF power. Therefore, the RF amplifier system can work with very short TRs, thereby enabling the fast sequences discussed below. Note that the process leading to the gradient echo signal does not nullify the spin dephasing which is generated by nonuniformities of the B_0 field, unlike the SE sequence with the 180° pulse. Consequently, the signals will be much more dependent on such nonuniformities, including the local ones due to tissue discontinuities and to variations in magnetic susceptibility.

Fast sequences (fast imaging) – reduced flip angles (FAs)

As mentioned above, the generation of the echo signal without the 180° pulse, via gradient inversion, reduces the echo time TE and thus allows to get more intense echo signals. As observed for the sequences used to obtain T_1-weighted images, when TR diminishes, also the signal decreases. If TR is much lower than the T_1 of the tissue under study, the angle to which the magnetization is to be flipped to get the maximum signal is no longer equal to 90° but lower. In other terms, for a given tissue and thus for a given value of T_1, the FA producing the maximum signal depends on the selected TR value and is lower than 90°.

Short-TR sequences which use the gradient echo and an adequately reduced FA are called *Fast Imaging* Sequences.

Given their short TRs, these fast sequences afford volume (3D) acquisitions within reasonably short times, thus bypassing the drawback of the excessive duration of the procedure, typical of volume acquisition via a standard SE sequence.

Appearance of images of moving tissues

The previous paragraphs dealt with MR images of quiescent tissues. However, the body has voluntary and involuntary movements as well as moving fluids, such as blood and CSF. Let us see how movements impact the MR images. The topic will be covered in a simple and schematic way, referring the reader to more specific publications for greater understanding. We will review the case of flowing blood, since its images may provide clinical indications.

Other types of movements are sources of image artifacts which can be totally or partially eliminated by appropriate acquisition procedures.

Blood flow

The motion of the blood in a vessel can be laminar, turbulent or disturbed.

The flow is *laminar* if adjacent fluid layers flow upon each other without mixing. In this case, the velocity profile (velocity as a function of distance from the axis of the vessel) is parabolic. In other terms, the velocity is maximum near the axis and decreases with the square of the distance from the axis until it becomes zero along the walls *(Fig. 17)*. Under the same geometric conditions, if the velocity increases, the flow becomes turbulent.

In *turbulent* flow, adjacent layers of fluid mix with each other, since transverse components of velocity and vortical motion appear. In this case, the velocity profile is fairly rectangular rather than parabolic *(Fig. 17)*.

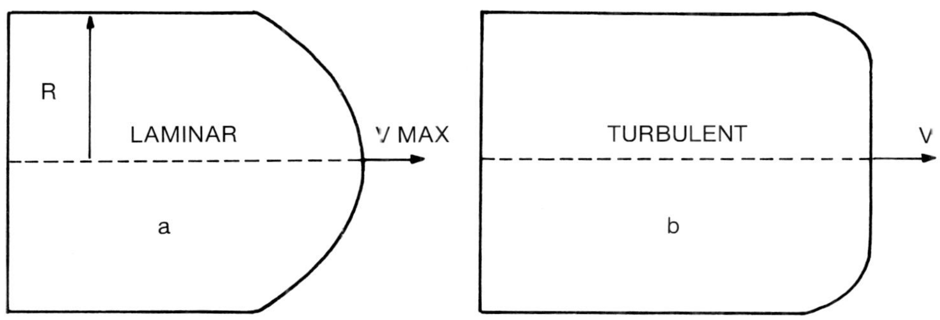

Fig. 17. Longitudinal section of a vessel, with velocity profile for laminar (a) and turbulent (b) flows.

The transition from laminar to turbulent flow does not only depend on the mean velocity of the flow (v_m) but also on the radius of the vessel (R_0) and on fluid characteristics (viscosity η and density ϱ). The product of these quantities is the Reynolds number:

$$Re = \frac{2 \cdot R_0 \cdot v_m \cdot \varrho}{\eta}$$

For $Re \geq 2000$, the flow is turbulent.
The flow is *disturbed,* if it is affected by pulsations.
Now, let us see how the motion affects the appearance of the images.

Slice crossing – time of flight

Assume that, through an SE sequence, a single slice of thickness D, whose plane coincides with the xy plane, is acquired and that a vessel crosses this slice orthogonally (the axis of the vessel is in the z direction) *(Fig. 18)*.

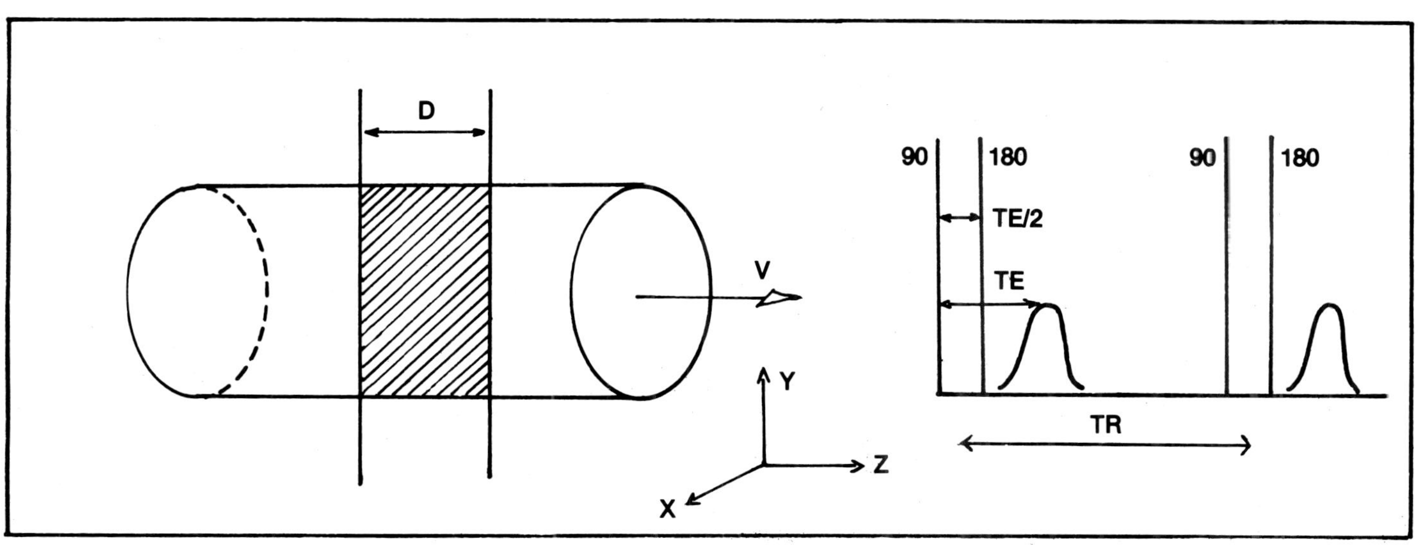

Fig. 18. *Diagram of a vessel which perpendicularly crosses the slice of thickness D.* The shaded area indicates the part of the vessel (and thus of the fluid) contained in the slice. Right, diagram of the SE sequence with parameters.

For TR $\geq 5T_1$ of the fluid, two cases may occur:

a) *slow flows*

In the TE/2 interval between the 90° and 180° pulses, some of the spins leave the slice. Since the replacement spins have not undergone the 90° pulse, they will not yield a signal. Consequently, with respect to the quiescent fluid, a signal reduction is observed.

b) *fast flows*

If the velocity of the fluid in the vessel is sufficiently high, the entire volume of the 90° pulse-excited fluid may have left the slice during the TE/2 interval. In this case, no signal is generated. This loss of signal is generally indicated as *high-velocity signal loss.*

For TR < 5 T_1, the phenomenon is more complex: also the spins replacing those which have left the slice during the TR interval will contribute to the signal. As the analytical treatment of the phenomenon is fairly complex, it will not be dealt with here. We will confine ourselves to underlining some fundamental aspects. These may serve as guidance for image interpretation or at least can suggest precautions in evaluations which involve moving fluids.

In the case of a short-TR (T_1-weighted) SE sequence, the phenomenon can be schematized in the following way:

- the 90° pulse will find the previously excited and relaxing spins (old spins) in the slice and new spins introduced into the slice by the flow;
- some of these spins leave the slice during the TE/2 interval and thus will not contribute to the echo signal.

For specified values of the slice thickness (D), of the repetition time (TR) and of the echo time (TE), the signal intensity vs. the flow velocity v will be a rather complex function of these parameters.

For some velocity values, the signal is higher than the one corresponding to the quiescent fluid. This phenomenon, known as *flow enhancement,* is caused by the contribution of fresh spins (introduced into the slice by the flow) to the signal.

Hence, the flow enhancement is related to the input of fresh spins into the slice. Nevertheless, the flow velocity should not be too high, otherwise high-velocity signal loss will prevail.

Flow-related spin dephasing (signal loss)

The distribution of velocity values inside a vessel (velocity profile) reduces the signal owing to the spin dephasing induced by the combination of flow and gradient. As this dephasing depends on the differences between velocities, these differences are clearly more significant in the proximity of the vessel walls. Therefore, a voxel placed in the vicinity of the vessel wall has spins with very different velocities. Consequently, significant spin dephasing takes place, which may make the signal null. If, instead, axial voxels are considered, where velocity is maximum but velocity differences are minimum, the dephasing is very small and therefore a signal may be generated.

Multi-echo sequences, even-echo rephasing

At constant flow velocities (without accelerations), the dephasing has a given value upon the first echo or any other echo of odd order. Conversely, no dephasing occurs upon the second echo or any other echo of even order. This phenomenon is known as *even-echo rephasing.*

The phenomenon implies that the signal inside a vessel may be more intense in the image obtained from the second echo than in the corresponding image from the first echo. This phenomenon occurs at constant flow velocities and with a magnetic field gradient in the direction of the flow.

When the flow is pulsatile, like in the arterial system, the spin dephasing is caused both by velocity and by accelerations. Acceleration produces dephasing which is not nullified in even echoes, thereby giving rise to loss of signal.

Practical considerations

The phenomenon of even-echo rephasing can be helpful in some instances. For example, to differentiate a slow flow from a thrombus, we may check whether the intravascular signal changes when passing from the first to the second echo. If this happens, it means that there is slow flow-induced rephasing. A similar analysis may be made on the basis of the effects of the velocity profile inside a vessel. Because of this profile, a black rim (for slices orthogonal to the vessel) is observed, which harbors an area with a more intense signal.

In Fast Imaging, blood usually generates an intense signal even when it is in motion (presence of flow). This derives from the fact that, in Fast Imaging, shorter echo times and TRs are used and that gradients remain active for a shorter time. Hence, with Fast Imaging, faster velocities are needed, in order to have a voxel signal loss similar to that of standard SE sequences.

Technical aspects

The previous paragraphs have focused on the physical aspects of the phenomenon with a view to making the image formation process understandable in logical terms. We will now give a schematic description of some more specific aspects, in order to understand how MRI systems work in practice.

Magnetic fields – magnets

Magnetic fields can be generated with systems, *magnets,* of different types.

Resistive magnets – electromagnets

They generally consist of air-core turns of a resistive conductor where an electric current of appropriate value flows. In the systems of this type used for MRI, the magnetic field is horizontal. These systems, however, have been dropped because of their high power supply requirements, excessive heat dissipation, insufficient stability and low magnetic field (max. .2 T).

Superconducting magnets

These magnets rely on the phenomenon of superconductivity, which occurs when some materials are kept at very low temperatures (liquid helium temperature). At these temperatures, the superconducting materials have zero electrical resistance; therefore, a high electric current can be circulated through them without any appreciable dissipation. This allows to generate high and very stable magnetic fields. The direction of the magnetic field produced by these magnets is horizontal. Cryogens (liquid helium and nitrogen) are needed to maintain conditions of superconductivity in the winding where the electric current generating the magnetic field flows. Once the system is activated, it no longer needs electric power since, thanks to superconductivity, the current circulates through the winding without power dissipation. In other terms, the electric current continues to flow in these turns for a theoretically infinite time. It follows that the magnetic field is always ON, since the magnet can be only "turned off" through complex and costly operations. Note that cryogen consumption affects operating costs (liquid helium is very expensive).

Permanent magnets

These systems use materials which, after being magnetized, permanently generate a magnetic field. The magnet is designed in such a way as to produce a field in the vertical direction. This fact allows the use of solenoidal coils, having higher efficiency than those having a different geometry (this applies only to low frequencies).

In this way, we can partially offset the disadvantage due to the lower MRI signal which can be induced at low fields. In effect, the magnetic field generated by the present systems of this type does not exceed .2T.

RF coils

As previously stated, the RF magnetic field which is required for resonance should be normal to the static magnetic field B_0. As a result, since the patient is to be placed in this field, the RF coils are designed according to a fixed geometry.

In the case of resistive and superconducting magnets, the B_0 field is horizontal; hence, solenoidal coils cannot be used. Instead, use is generally made of "saddle-type" coils, generating a B_1 field normal to B_0 and capable of accommodating the patient *(Fig. 19)*.

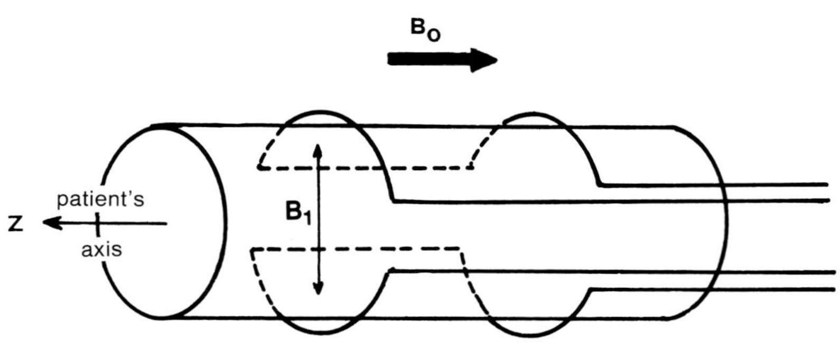

Fig. 19. *Diagram of the geometry of a saddle coil: z is the direction of the static magnetic field (B_0) generated by the magnet.* The patient is placed with his longitudinal axis along the z direction.

As permanent magnets generate a vertical field (B_0), their coils are solenoids where the patient or anatomical parts can be easily fitted *(Fig. 20)*. These coils generally have better efficiency than those with a different geometry, at least at some values of the operating frequency of the system, in particular at the field values generated by permanent magnets.

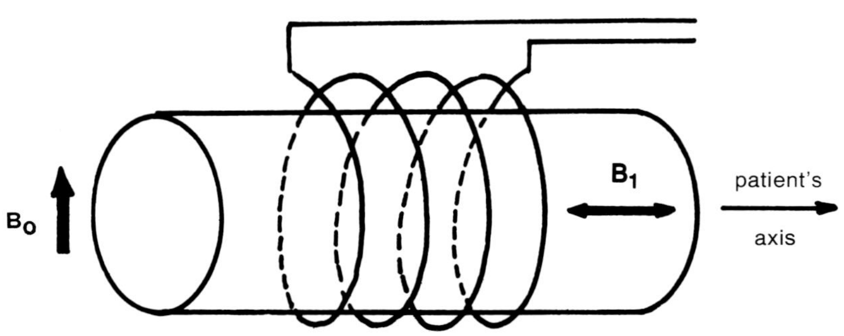

Fig. 20. *Diagram of a solenoidal coil whose axis is normal to the direction of the static magnetic field (B_0) (in this case vertical).* The patient is placed horizontally inside the coil.

Coils for gradient generation

These coils are used to generate the linear magnetic field gradients which are needed for spatial encoding of the MRI signal. They are housed inside the hole of the magnet (gantry) and have

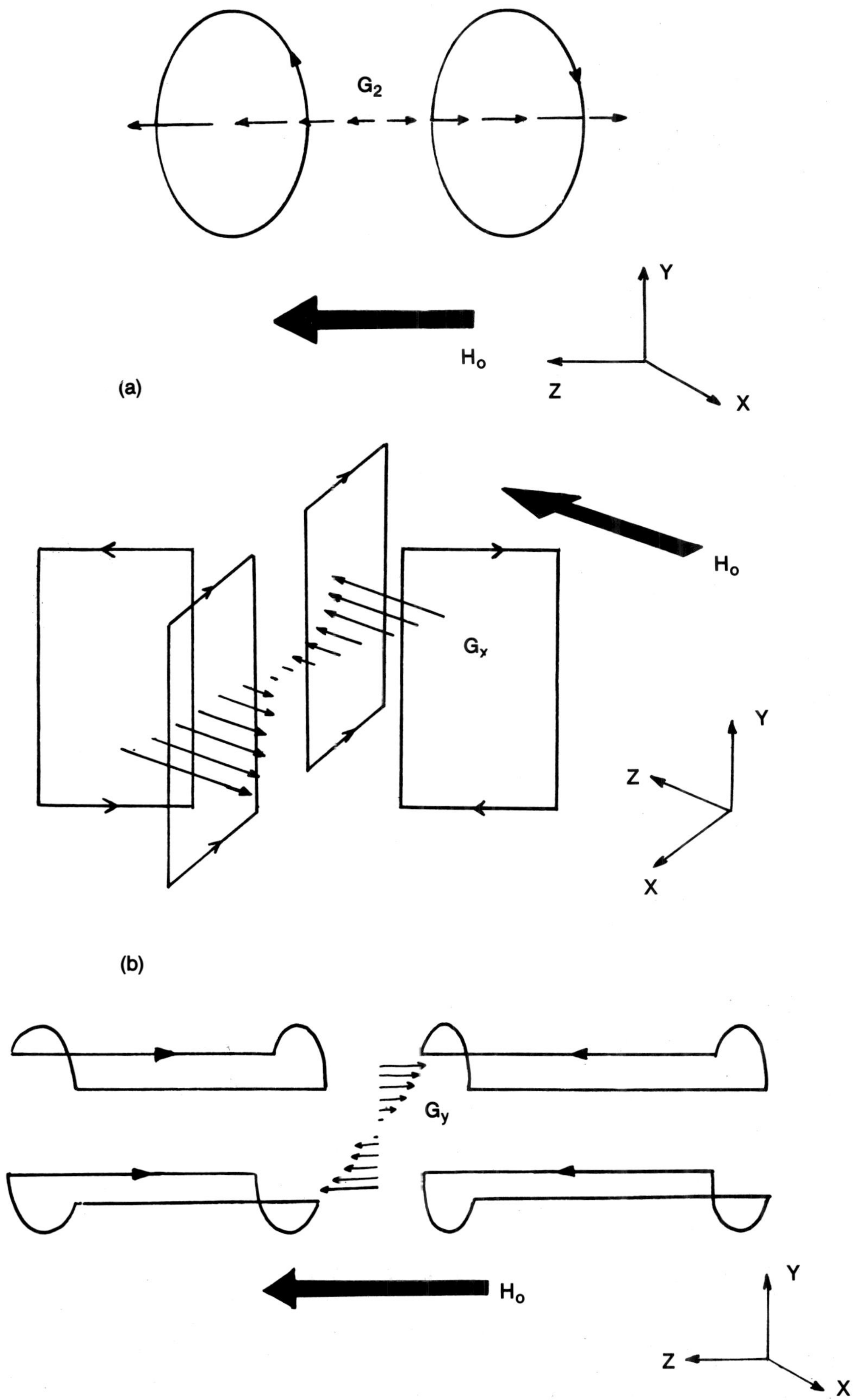

Fig. 21. *Geometry of three coil systems for gradient generation.* These coils are housed inside the gantry. Fairly high current pulses flow in these coils. During these pulses, the coils are subjected to magnetic forces. The resulting vibrations are the source of the typical noise which is heard during scanning.

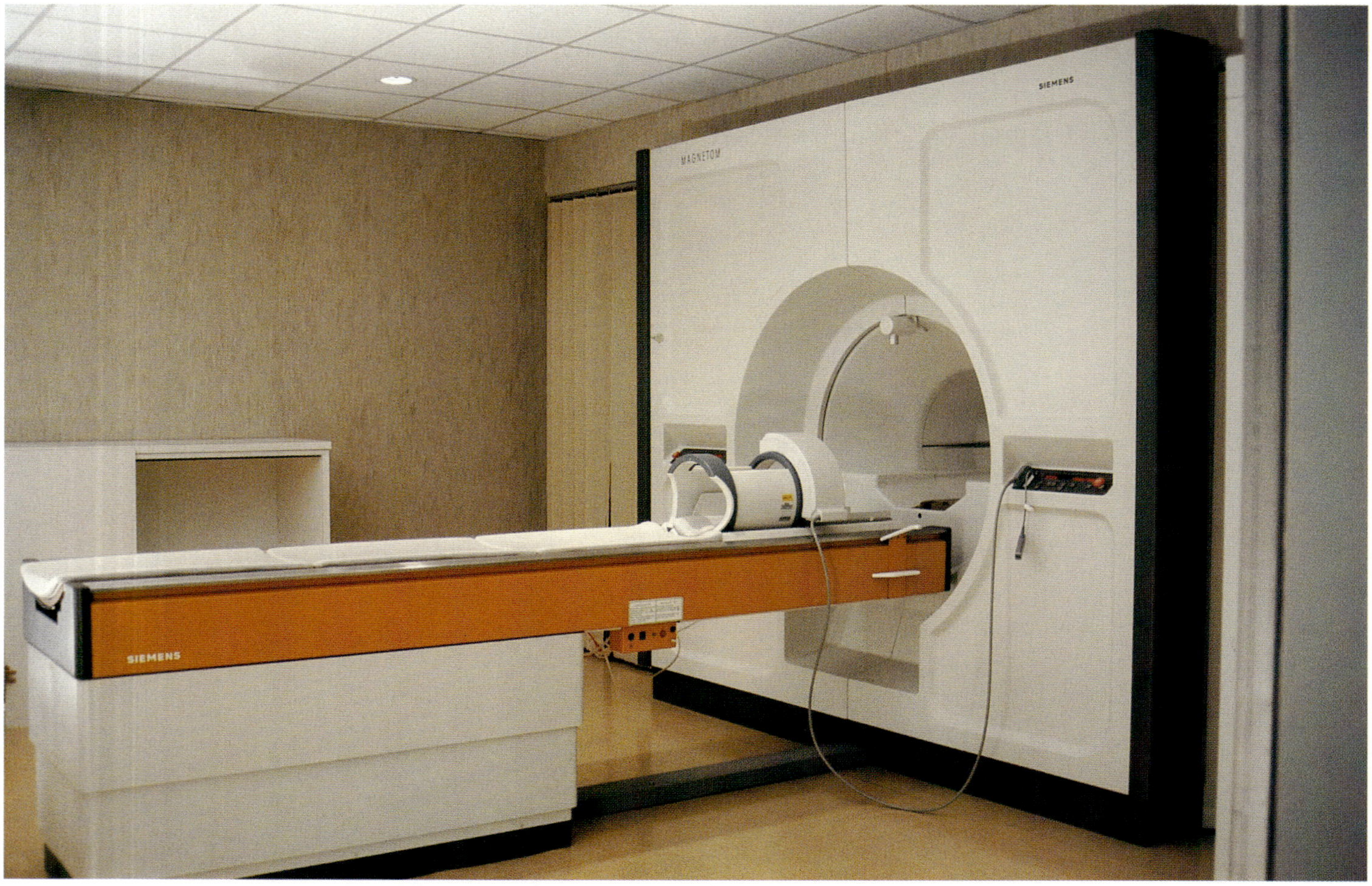

Fig. 22. *1.5 Tesla "Magnetom 63" MR tomograph* used by Radiology and Diagnostic Imaging, Istituto Regina Elena, Rome.

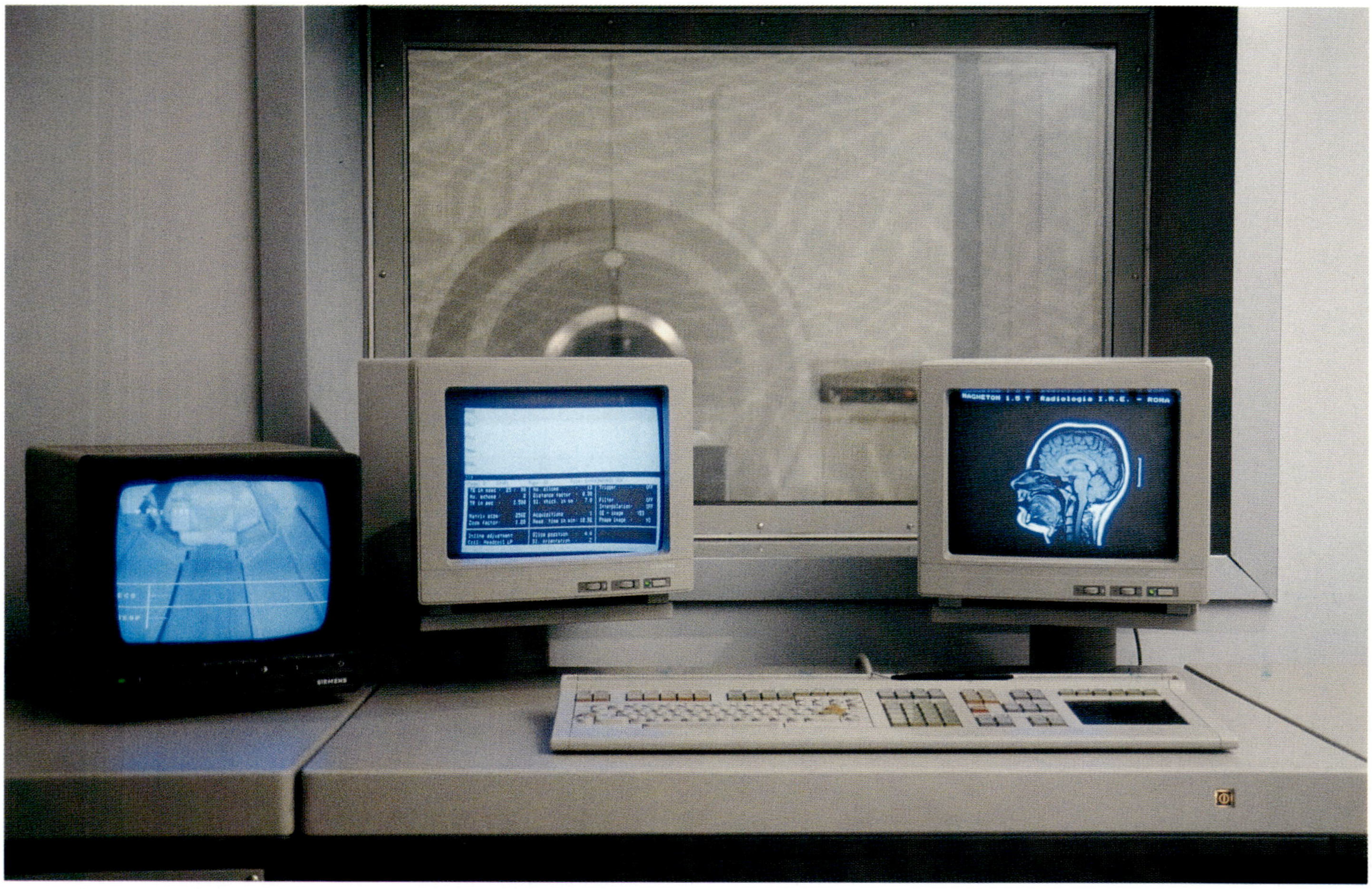

Fig. 23. Control console.

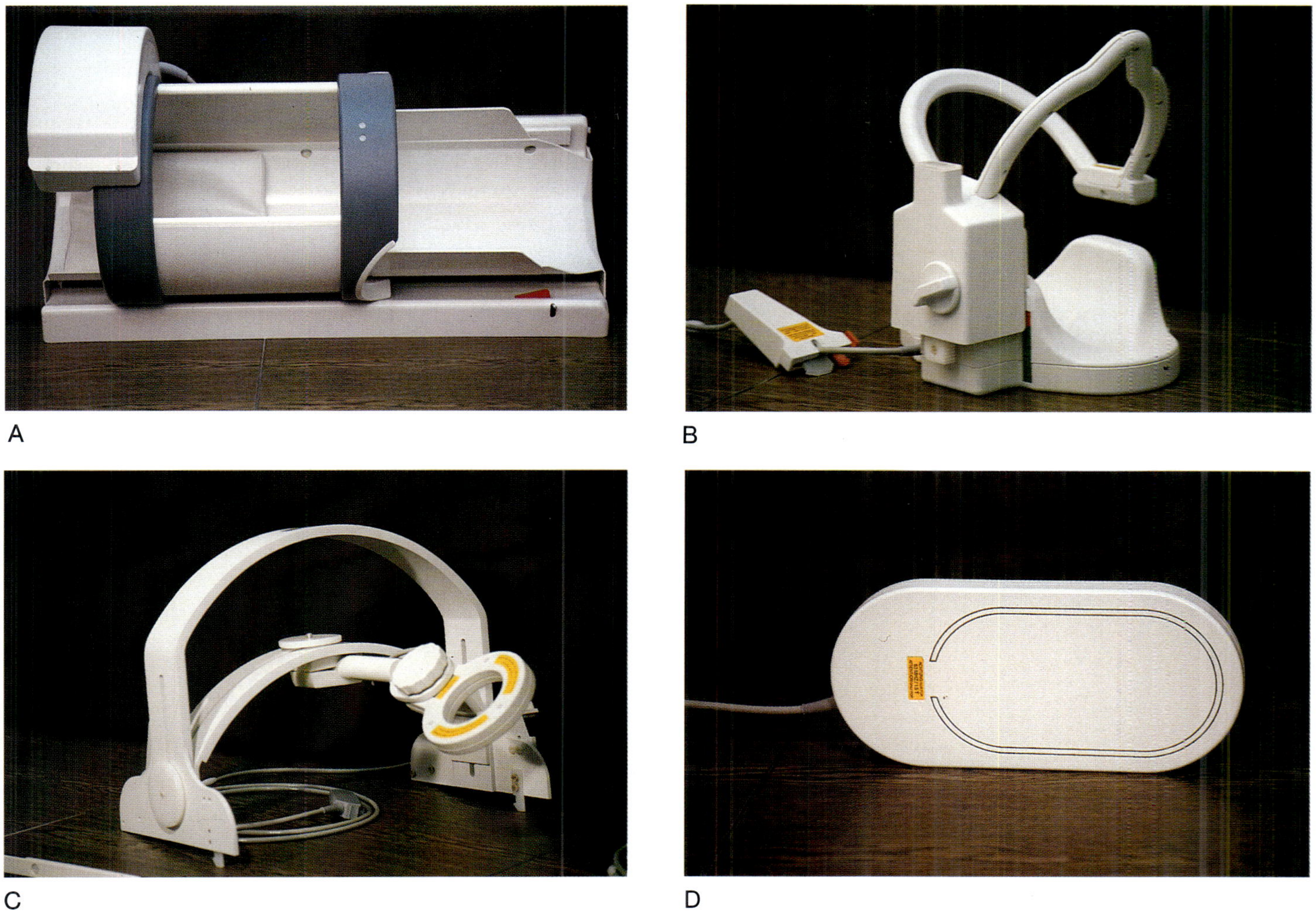

Fig. 24. *Surface coils:*
A – circular polarization transmitting/receiving coil for the study of the head;
B – Helmholtz coil for the study of the cervical region;
C – coil for the study of the orbit and of the petrous bone;
D – elliptical coil for the study of the spine and of the spinal cord.

different shapes depending on the direction of the gradient to be produced. There are three types of gradient coils, for the directions x, y and z, respectively *(Fig. 21)*.

Surface coils

These coils are designed to be placed in the immediate vicinity of the anatomical system or feature to be studied. They may have different shapes, depending on the study to be carried out. They allow to use smaller fields of view (FOVs) and thus to achieve higher spatial resolution. They should be adequately positioned, in order to prevent their plane (for instance a circular antenna) from being normal to B_0, otherwise no MRI signal would be produced. Usually, these coils are receiving coils only: they are electronically conceived to pick up the RF signal emitted by the tissues, which are excited via another coil. *Fig. 23* shows some examples of these surface coils.

Given its generally plane geometry, the signal decays very quickly with distance from the coil. Therefore, these coils are only suitable for the study of shallow anatomical features.

References

1. Abragam A (1970) The principles of nuclear magnetism. Oxford University Press, Oxford
2. Mansfield P, Morris PG (1982) NMR imaging in biomedicine. Adv Magn Reson [Suppl 2]
3. Partein CL, James AG et al. (1984) Nuclear magnetic resonance (NMR) imaging. W. B. Saunders Co, Philadelphia
4. Kressel HY (1985) Magnetic resonance annual 1985. Raven Press, New York
5. Morris PG (1986) Nuclear magnetic resonance imaging in medicine and biology. Oxford Sciences Publication, Oxford
6. Foster MA, Hutchinson JMS (1987) Practical NMR imaging; IRL Press, Oxford
7. Higgins GB, Hricak H (1987) Magnetic resonance imaging of the body. Raven Press, New York
8. Brant-Zawadzki M, Norman D (1987) Magnetic resonance imaging of the central nervous system. Raven Press, New York
9. Stuart Young W (1988) Magnetic resonance imaging, basic principles. Raven Press, New York
10. Kressel HY (1988) Magnetic resonance annual 1988. Raven Press, New York
11. Runge VM (1989) Enhanced magnetic resonance imaging. C. V. Mosby Co, St. Louis
12. Pomeranz SJ (1989) Craniospinal magnetic resonance imaging. W. B. Saunders Co, Philadelphia

CHAPTER II

MRI brain anatomy

Image formation

A correct understanding of magnetic resonance (MR) images requires knowledge of the parameters which contribute to their formation.

First of all, unlike other imaging techniques, the MRI signal intensity is a function of multiple tissue-specific parameters, the most important being spin-lattice relaxation time (T_1), spin-spin relaxation time (T_2), proton density and flow. The wide variability of these parameters in both normal and pathologic tissues, in particular of T_1 and T_2, explains the high image contrast which is typical of this technique.

Furthermore, the operator can select the technical parameters for the sequences, such as type of RF (radiofrequency) pulses (90°, 180°, >90°) and their succession, values of repetition time (TR), echo time (TE) and inversion time (TI). Consequently, he can critically affect the contribution of the different parameters to the formation of the signal, often enhancing tissue contrast.

By adjusting the technical parameters for the programming of sequences, we can obtain images whose contrast will be predominantly affected by T_1, T_2, proton density or, finally, by blood flow characteristics. In clinical practice, the possibility of identifying and characterizing a wider range of normal or pathologic tissues relies on the comparative analysis of the images obtained with different weightings.

At present, the sequence which best responds to these diagnostic requirements is the spin-echo (SE) sequence. Over short time intervals (15–20′), this sequence provides T_1-, T_2- and proton density-weighted images.

The images acquired with short TR and TE settings (TR 550 msec; TE 15 msec) highlight the variations in the T_1 relaxation times of the different tissues. In effect, high signal density foci reflect short T_1 structures; low signal density foci, instead, reflect long T_1 structures.

On the images obtained with this sequence, the intraorbital and subcutaneous fat, as well as the fat in the cancellous bone of the diploe and of the skull base, appear as hyperintense, whereas the signal of the cerebrospinal fluid (CSF), meningeal sheaths and of compact bone is clearly hypointense. The brain tissue has an intermediate signal density, in which the darker gray matter can be discriminated from the white matter thanks to its higher water content and lower lipid component. Finally, the intrasinusal air and the high-flow vessels appear as very dark areas owing to signal loss.

The T_1-weighted images require short acquisition times. Therefore, they are scarcely affected by background noise and provide excellent anatomical detail. They are particularly suitable for the study of regions with high natural contrast between CSF and nervous tissue.

Long-TR (2500 msec) and short-TE (15–20 msec) images are mainly dependent on proton density. However, for very short TEs, they are affected by T_1, too, albeit to a lesser extent

In proton density, the contrast ratio between gray matter and white matter reverses. The white matter has a much lower signal intensity and can be better distinguished not only from the cortex but above all from the basal ganglia. On these images, the CSF signal has not yet reached the T_2 curve inversion point (see Chap. I, p. 19). Therefore, it still appears as hypointense with the brain tissue, but to a much lesser extent than on short-TR sequences. Air, compact bone, dura and vessels also maintain a low signal on these images, whereas fat tissue has an initial reduction in brightness.

Long-TR and -TE (TR 2500 msec, TE 90 msec) images are called T_2-weighted, since they depend on the spin-spin relaxation time. On them, higher signal density districts correspond to long-T_2 elements. Owing to the above-mentioned contrast inversion phenomenon, the CSF signal shifts to highly hyperintense (cisternographic and myelographic effect) with respect to nervous tissue. In effect, since the signal of this tissue is highly degraded, it creates contrast in CSF spaces which demonstrates the normal vascular and nervous structures contained therein.

On T_2-weighted images and especially at high magnetic fields (1.5 T), the basal ganglia (globus pallidus and putamen), the nuclei of the midbrain (red nucleus, substantia nigra) and the cerebellar dentate nucleus appear as markedly hypointense areas. This reduction in signal intensity was correlated with iron content in such structures.

Long echo times induce a progressive decline in the fat tissue signal, whereas compact bone, air-filled structures and vessels remain markedly hypointense due to a nearly complete signal loss.

Even if these long-TR and long echo time sequences are degraded by background noise and motion artifacts, they are the sequences mostly used for diagnostic purposes. In effect, they are the most responsive to pathologic alterations of secondary tissues and to variations in water and protein content, to alterations of myelin or to paramagnetic contrast agents.

Their use is thus a "must" for a correct diagnostic interpretation of CNS diseases, whether neoplastic, degenerative or inflammatory. They allow alterations of the T_2-weighted image signal to be correlated with the corresponding proton density images.

The uniqueness of MRI lies in the fact that its semeiology is based on the integrated evaluation of multiple images, acquired with adequate sequences: this generates complexity but also greater diagnostic potential.

Anatomy

Given the complexity of MRI, the chapters on pathologies will be preceded by illustrations of the normal MRI brain anatomy correlated with anatomical sections. Identification of the various structures will be facilitated by explanatory schematic drawings.

We have tried to reproduce the anatomical sections which are mostly used in practice, giving priority to the axial and coronal scans, since they are more complex and provide a wider array of anatomical relationships.

We are indebted to Augusto Casagrande, M.D., Institute of Pathology, Medical School of the University of Rome "La Sapienza", for his invaluable help in the drafting of this Chapter and for his guidance in the selection of the most suitable section planes and in the preparation of the anatomical sections.

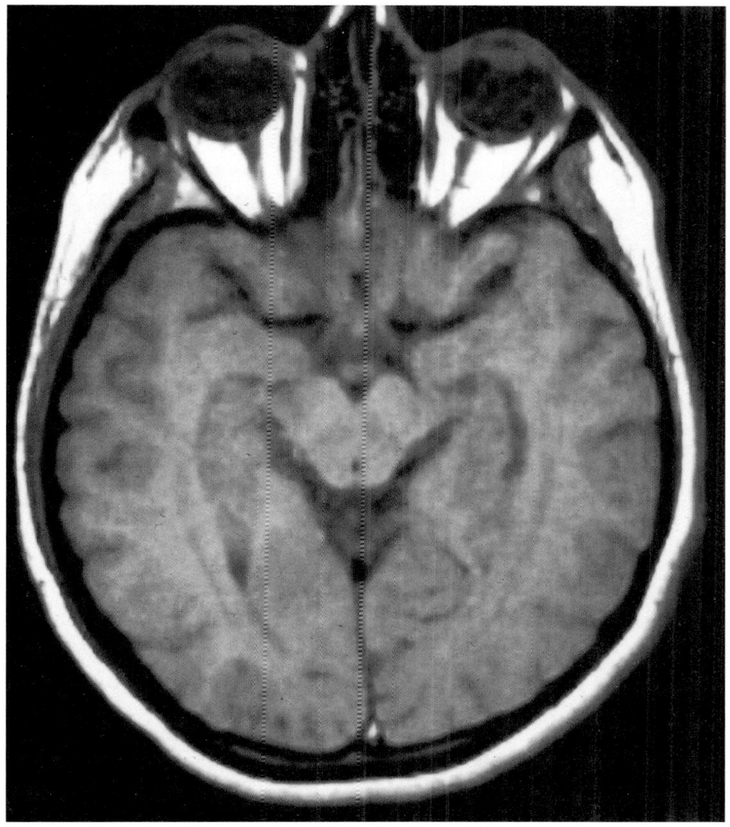

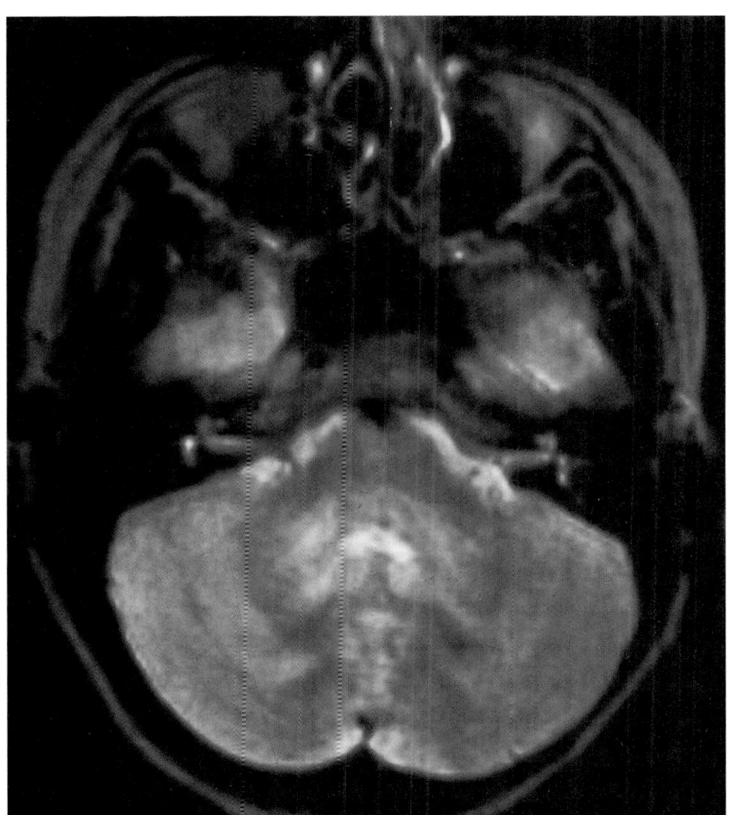

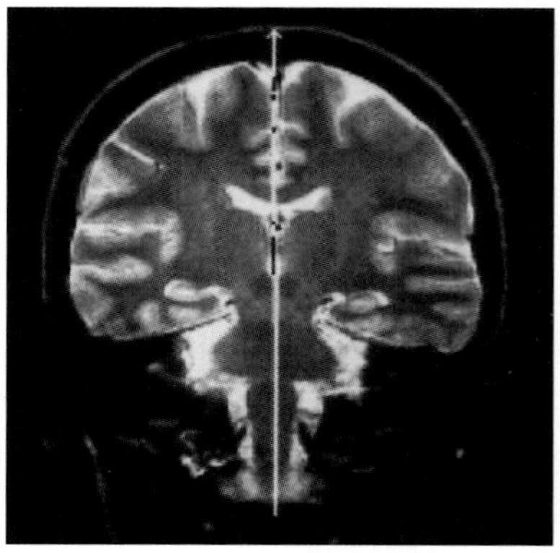

Fig. 1
1) genu of the corpus callosum
2) cingulate gyrus
3) splenium of the corpus callosum
4) Galen's vein
5) massa intermedia
6) lateral ventricle
7) fornix
8) 3rd ventricle
9) optic tract
10) pituitary stalk
11) pituitary gland
12) sphenoid sinus
13) basilar artery
14) pons
15) red nucleus of the midbrain
16) pineal gland
17) quadrigeminal plate
18) aqueduct
19) 4th ventricle
20) cerebellar vermis
21) bulb
22) tentorium

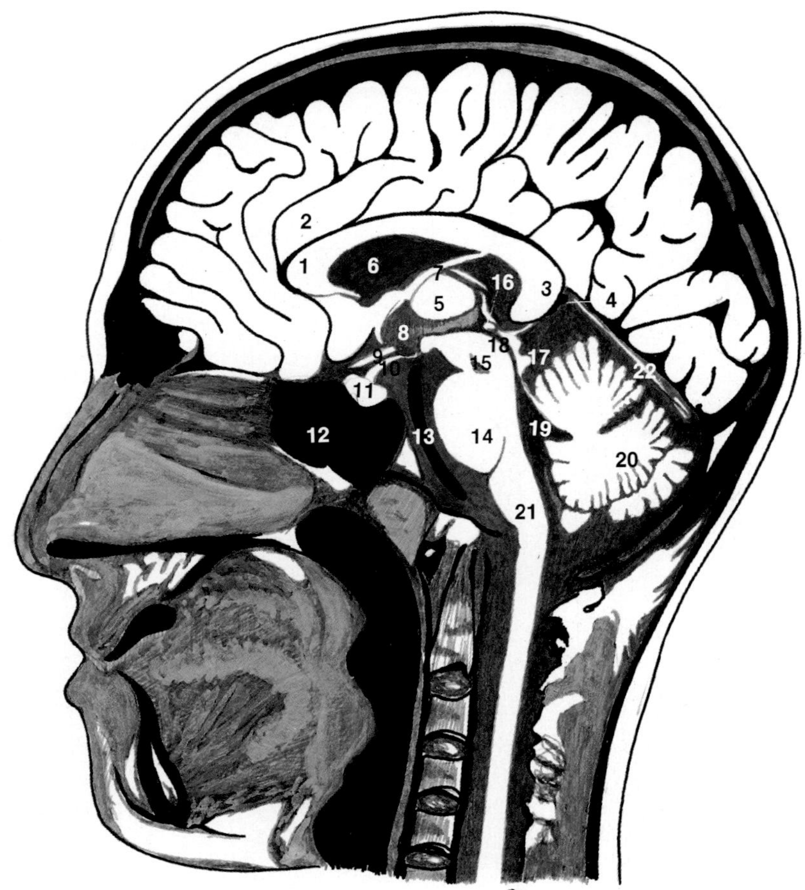

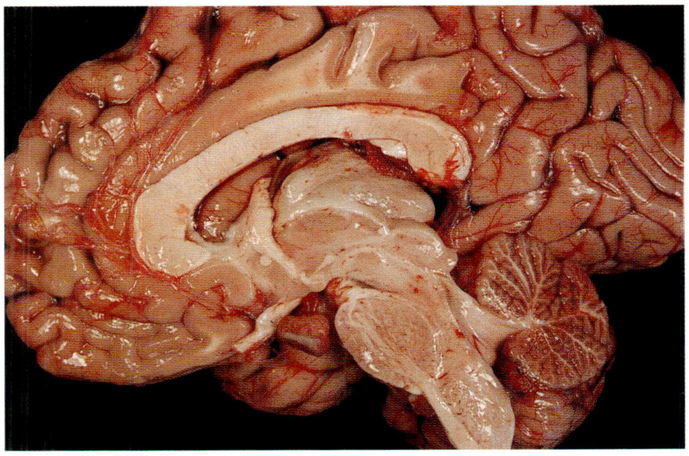

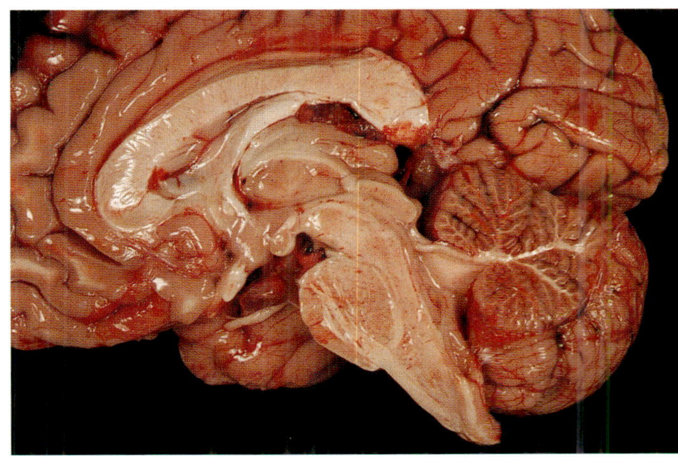

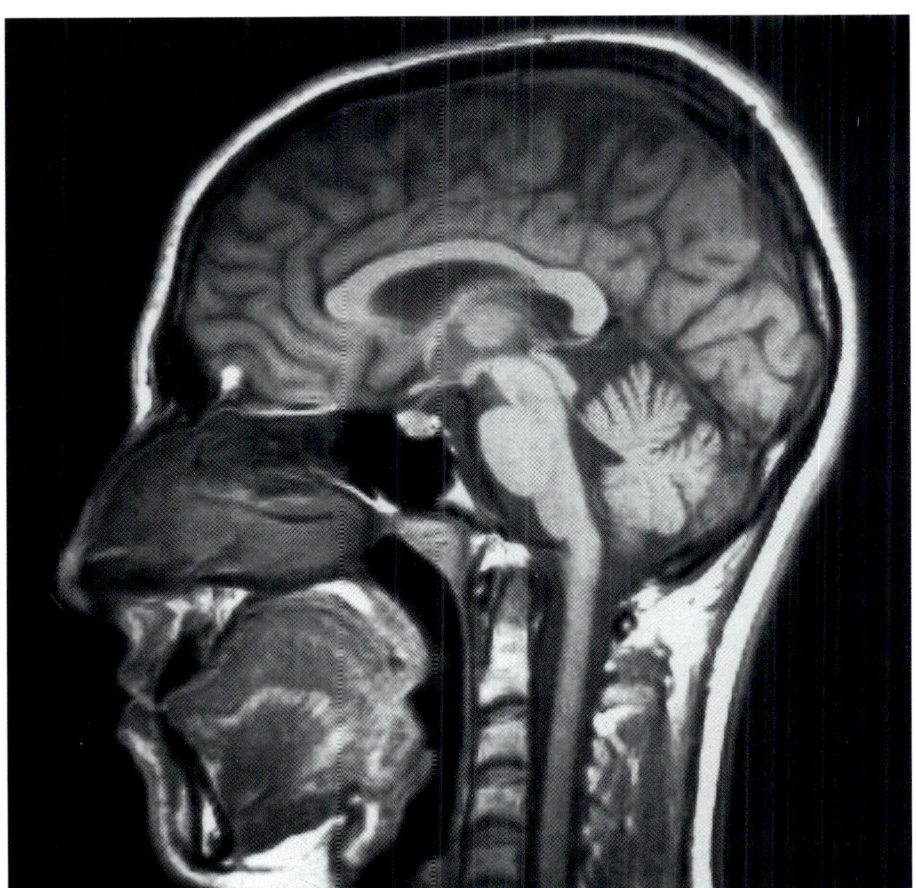

TR = 550 msec
TE = 15 msec

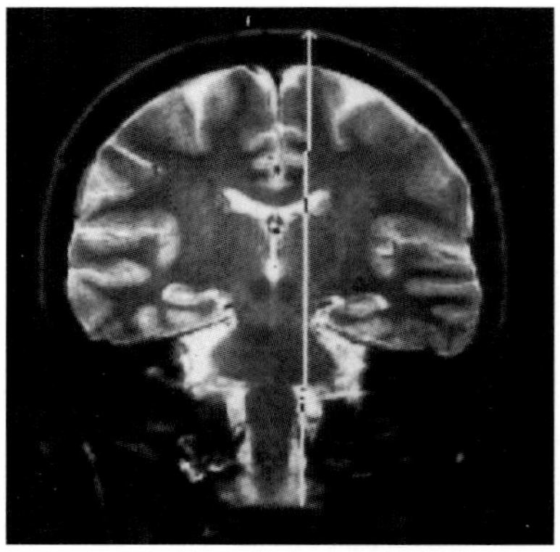

Fig. 2
1) corpus callosum
2) lateral ventricle
3) thalamus
4) cerebral peduncle
5) head of the caudate nucleus
6) brainstem
7) cerebellar peduncle
8) cerebellum
9) cerebellar tonsil
10) fissure of Rolando
11) marginal branch of the cingulate sulcus
12) parietooccipital sulcus
13) gyrus rectus

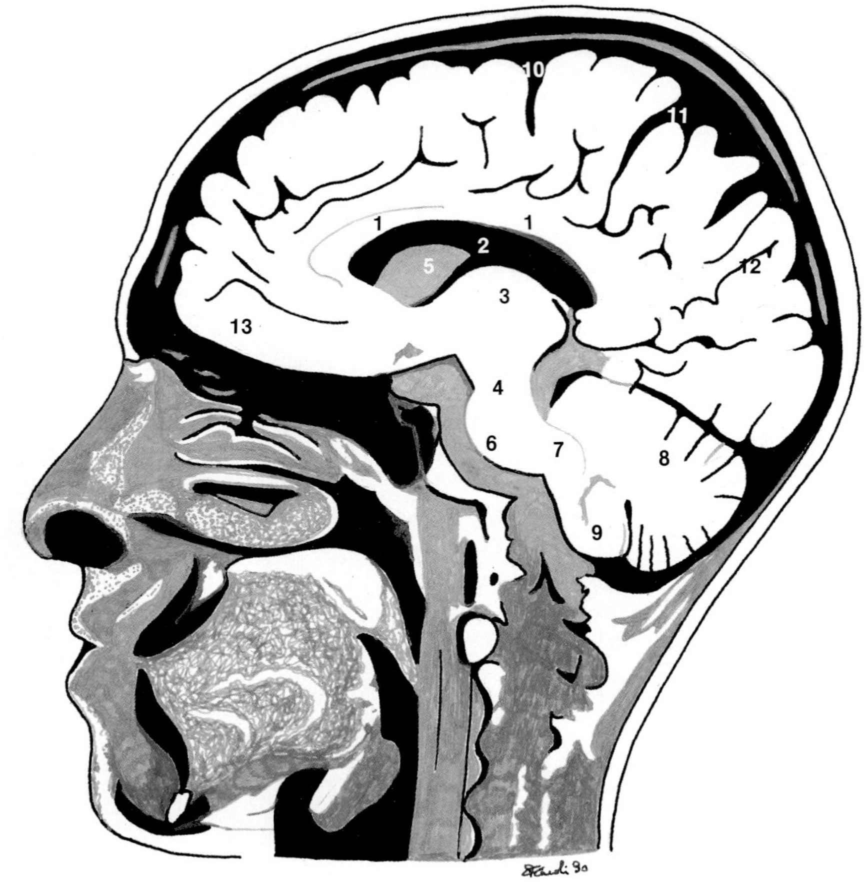

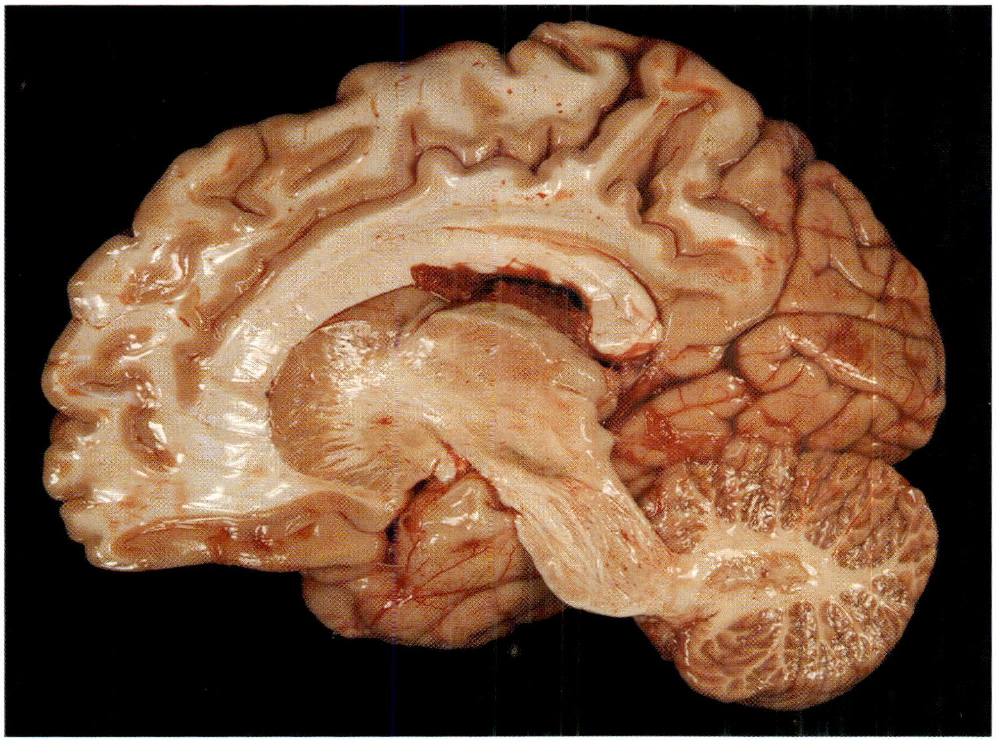

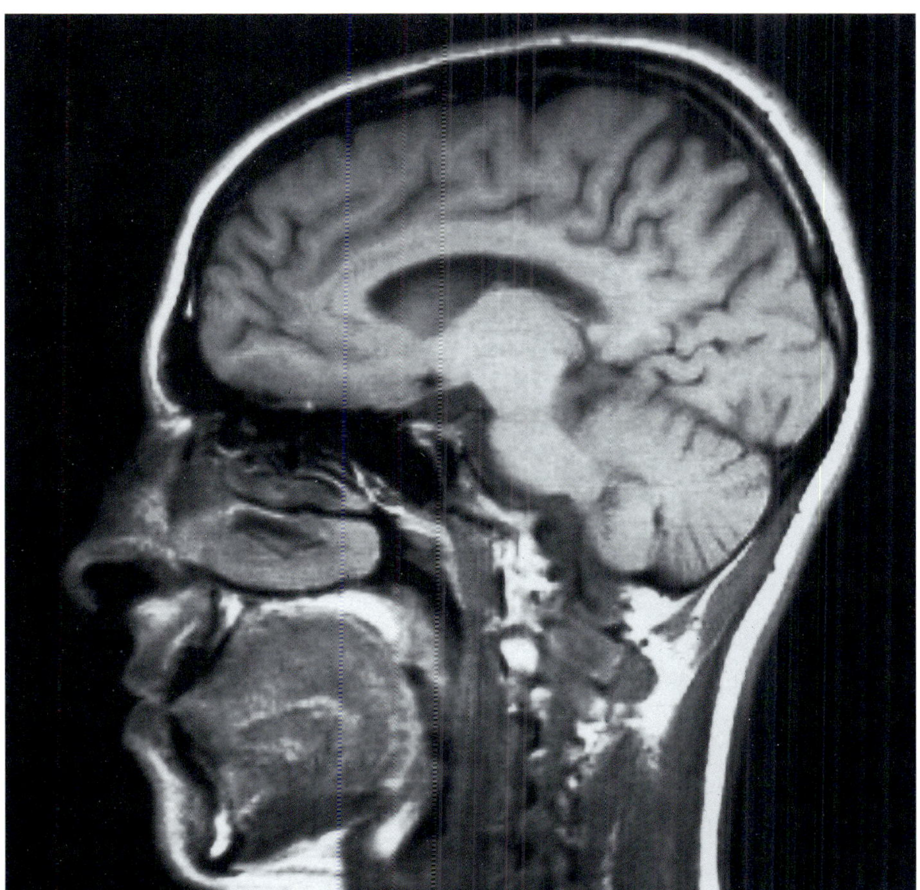

TR = 550 msec
TE = 15 msec

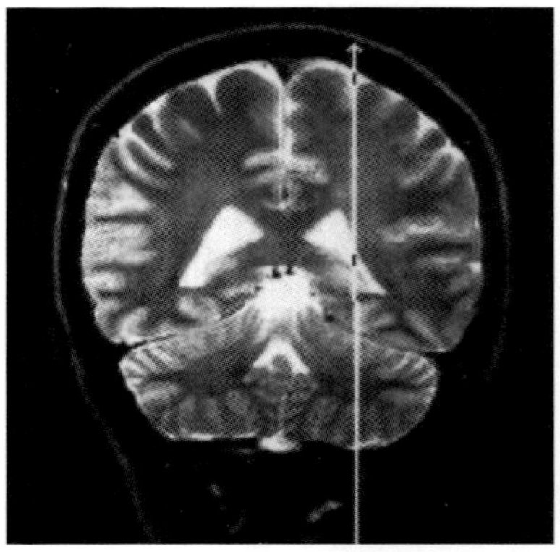

Fig. 3
1) anterior horn of the lateral ventricle
2) trigonum of the lateral ventricle
3) putamen
4) globus pallidus
5) thalamus
6) temporal horn of the lateral ventricle
7) hippocampus
8) sulcus of the middle cerebral artery
9) parietoocipital sulcus
10) cerebellar hemisphere

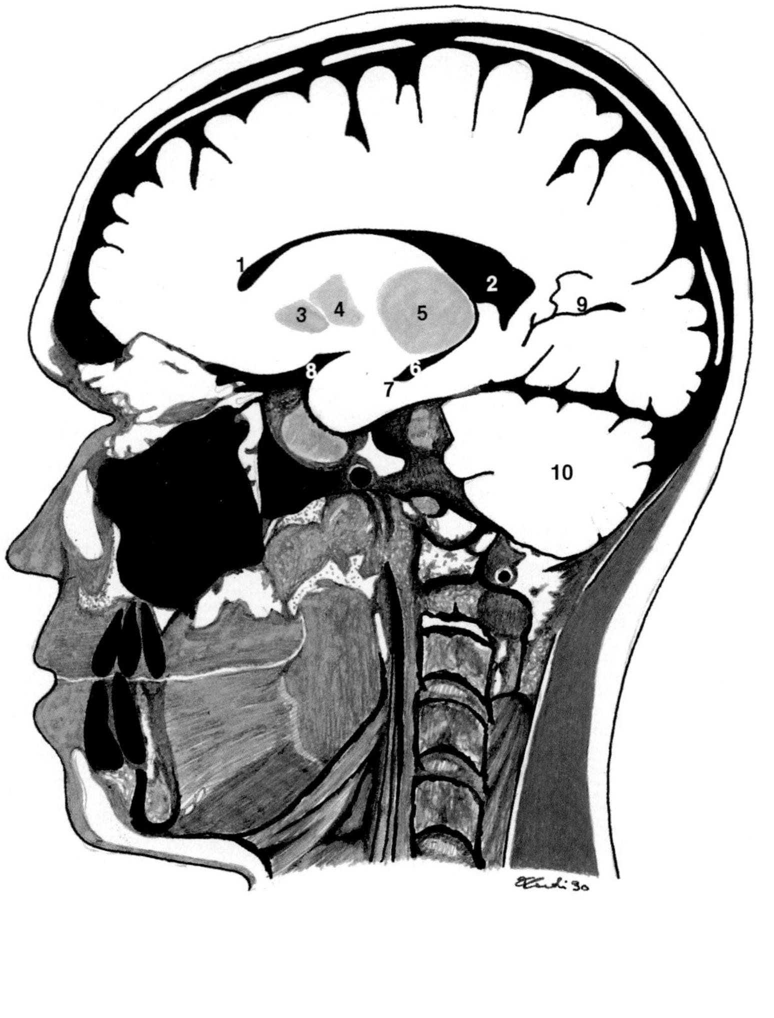

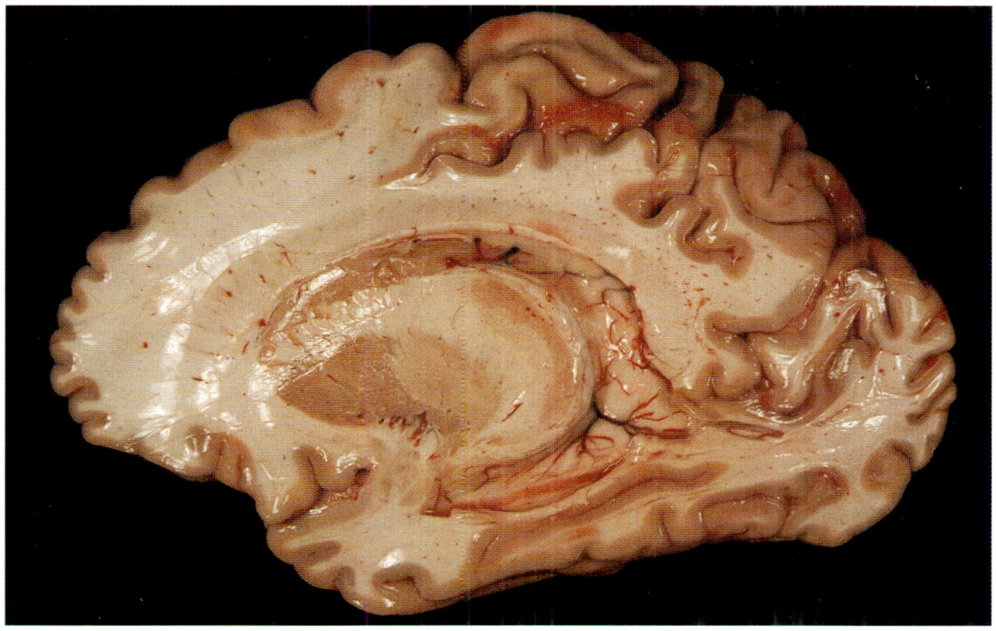

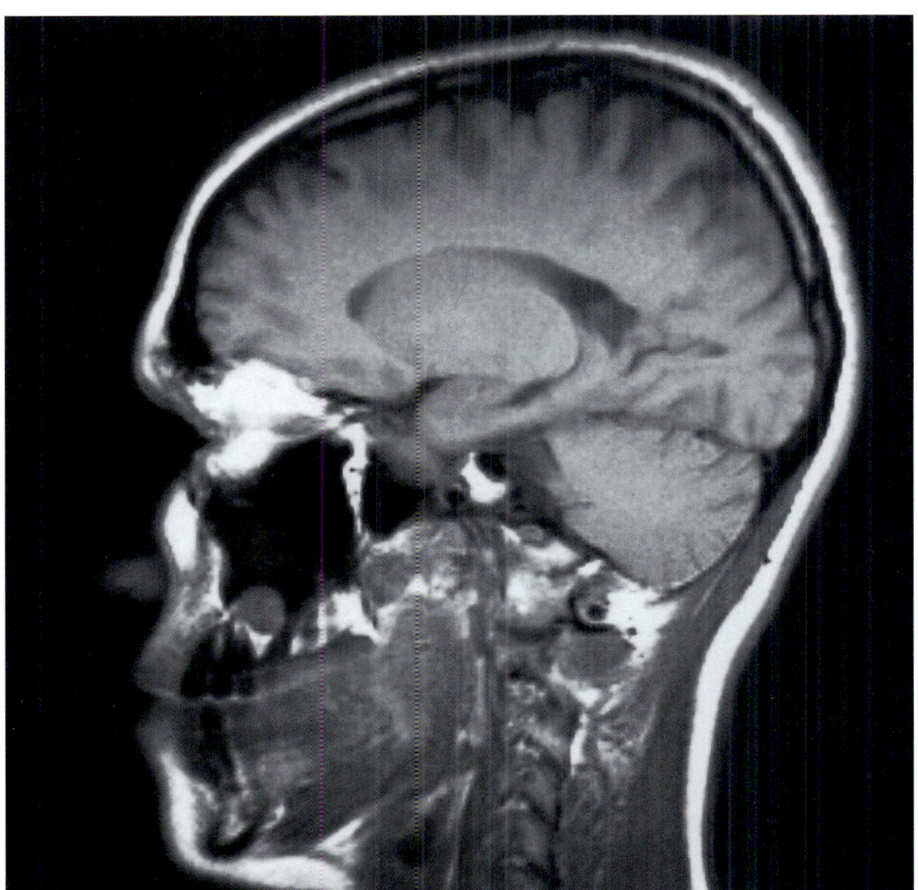

TR = 550 msec
TE = 15 msec

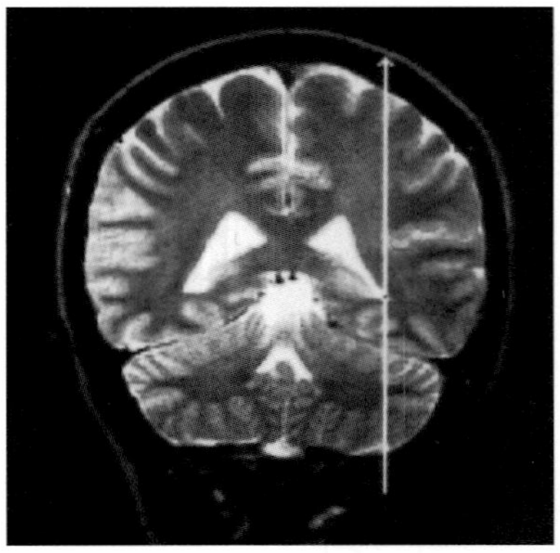

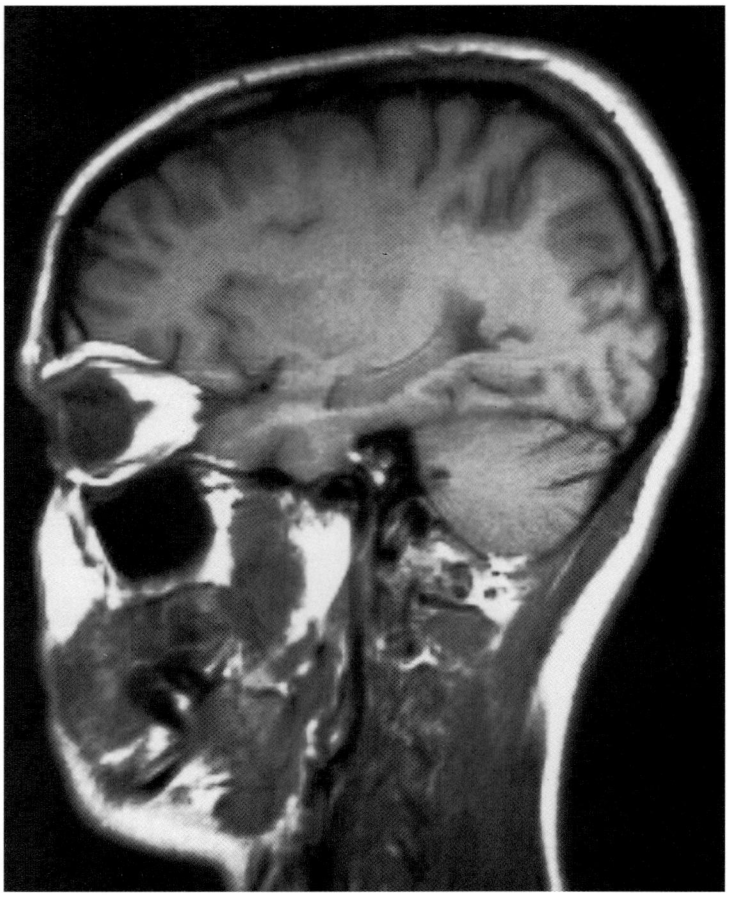

TR = 550 msec
TE = 15 msec

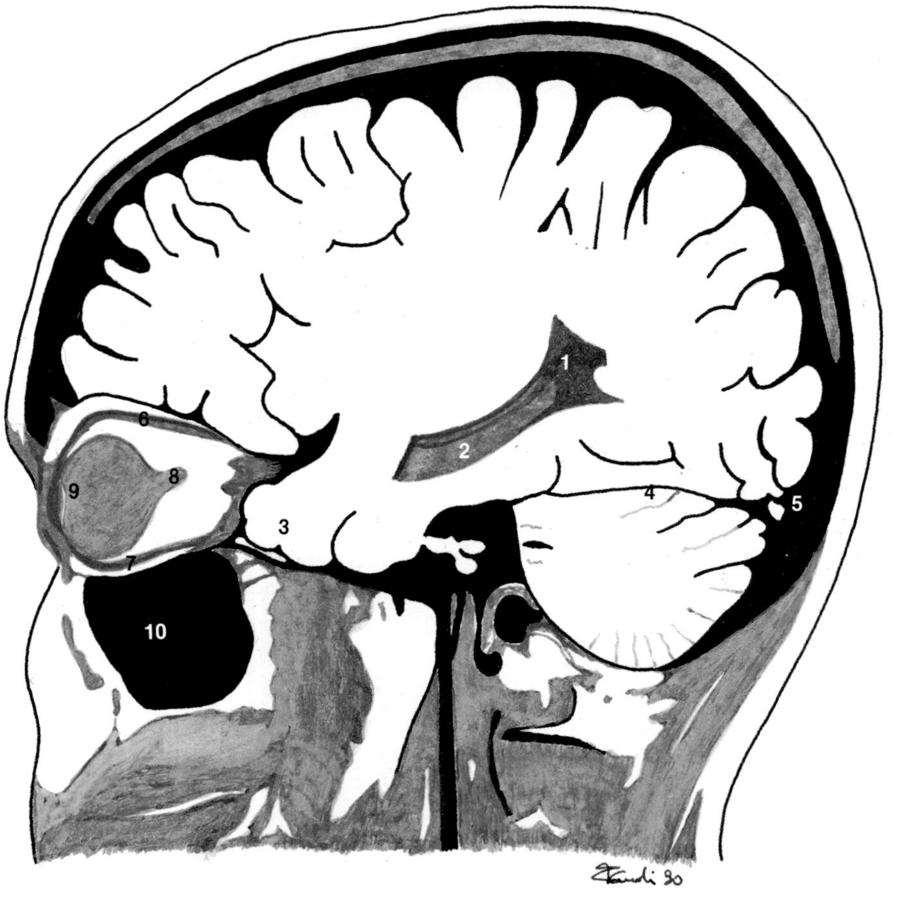

Fig. 4
1) trigonum of the lateral ventricle
2) hippocampus
3) pole of the temporal lobe
4) tentorium
5) transverse sinus
6) superior rectus muscle
7) inferior rectus muscle
8) optic nerve
9) globe
10) maxillary sinus

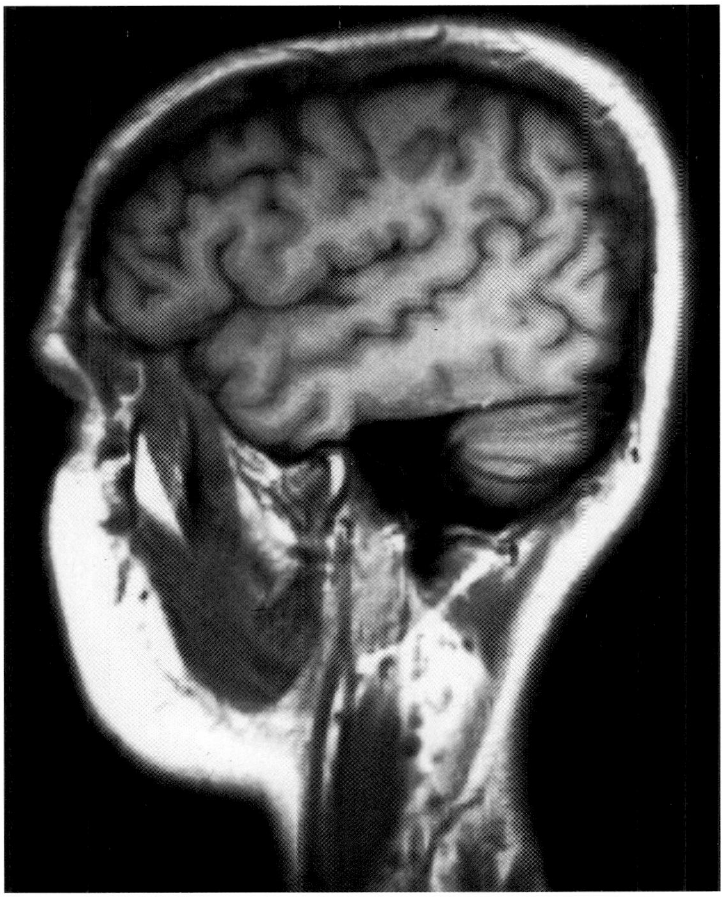

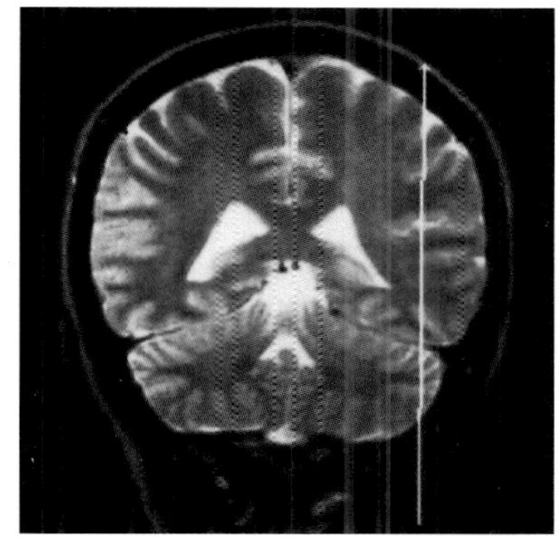

TR = 550 msec
TE = 15 msec

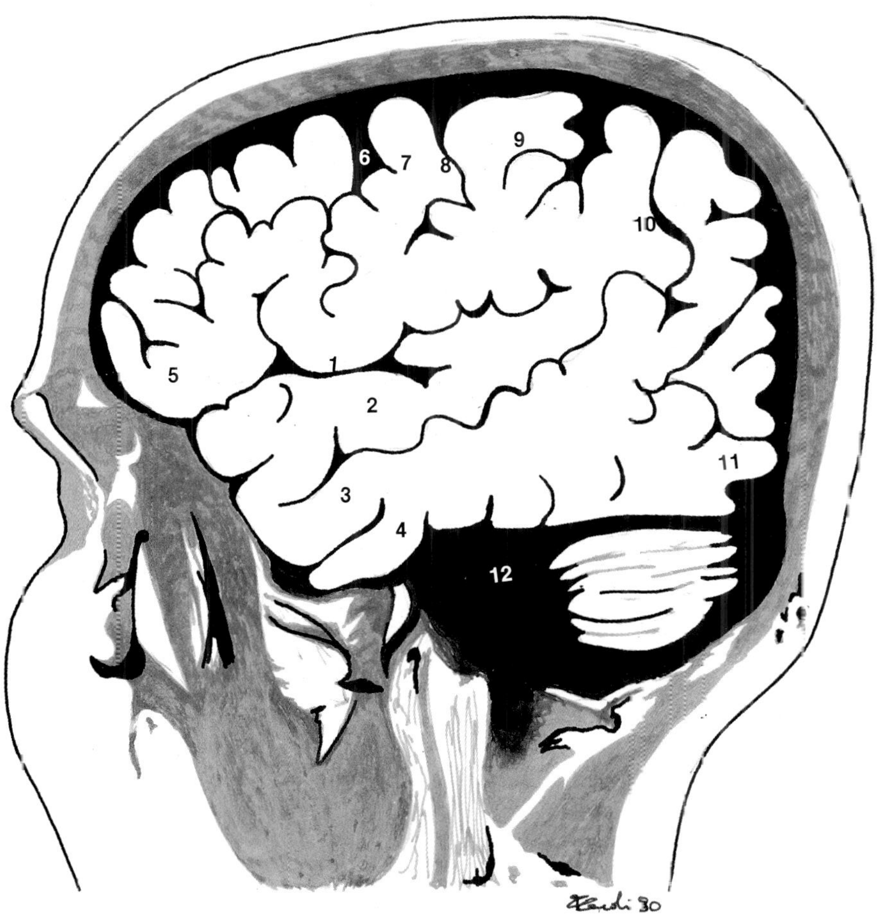

Fig. 5
1) Sylvian fissure
2) superior temporal gyrus
3) middle temporal gyrus
4) inferior temporal gyrus
5) frontal pole
6) precentral sulcus
7) prerolandic gyrus
8) fissure of Rolando
9) postrolandic gyrus
10) intraparietal sulcus
11) occipital pole
12) temporal bone

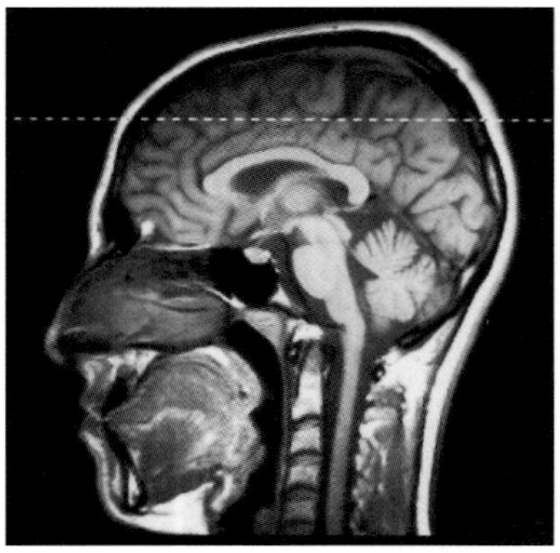

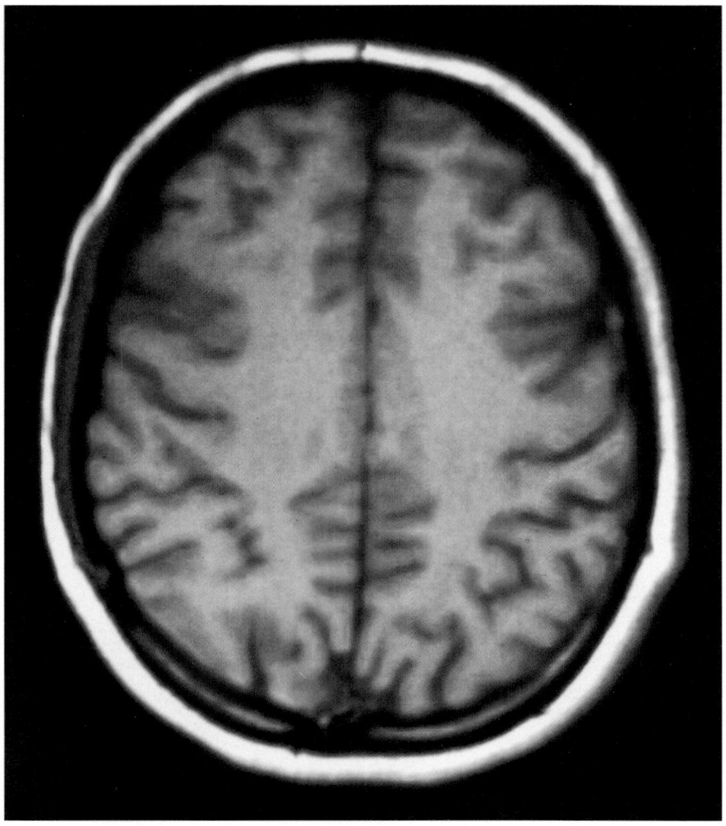

TR = 550 msec, TE = 15 msec

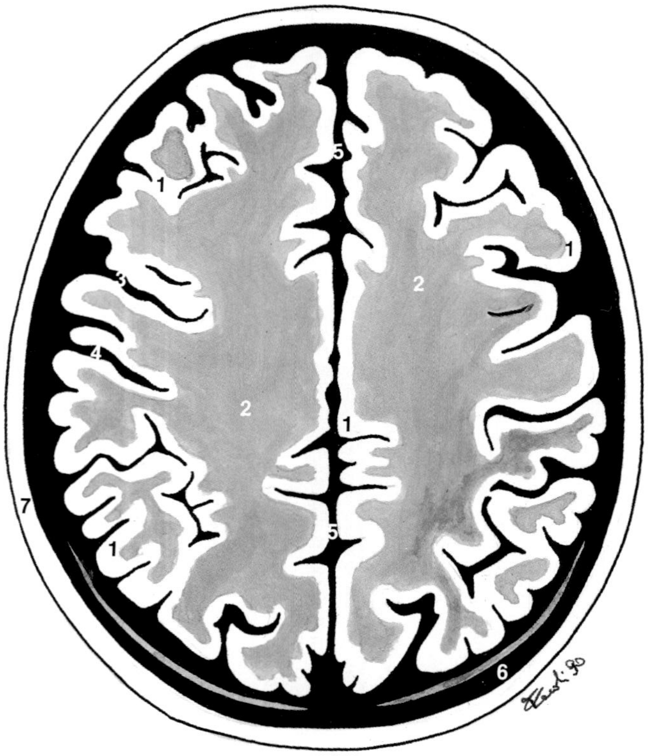

Fig. 6
1) cortical grey matter
2) white matter
3) precentral sulcus
4) fissure of Rolando
5) interhemispheric fissure
6) cranial vault

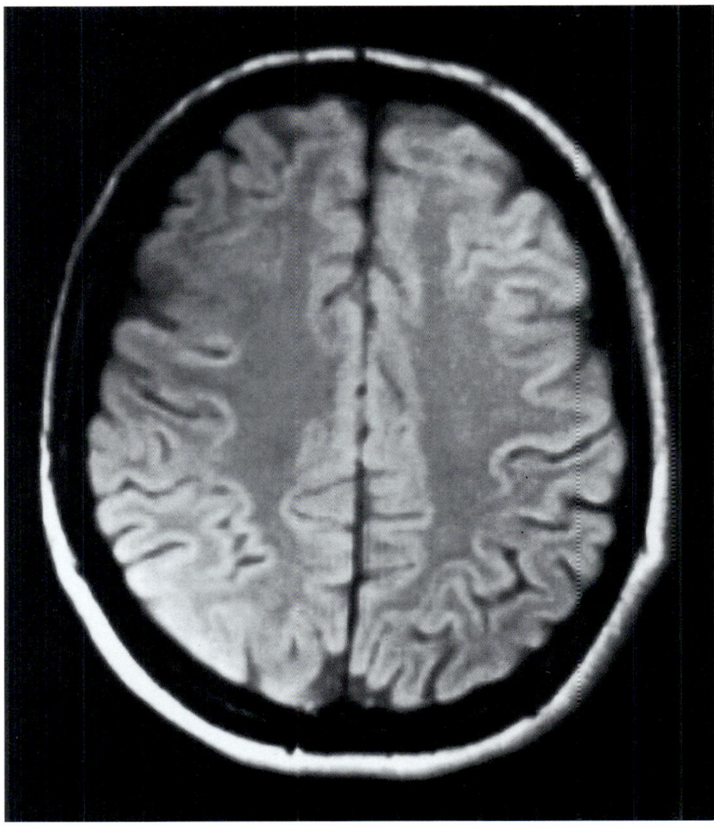

TR = 2,500 msec, TE = 15 msec

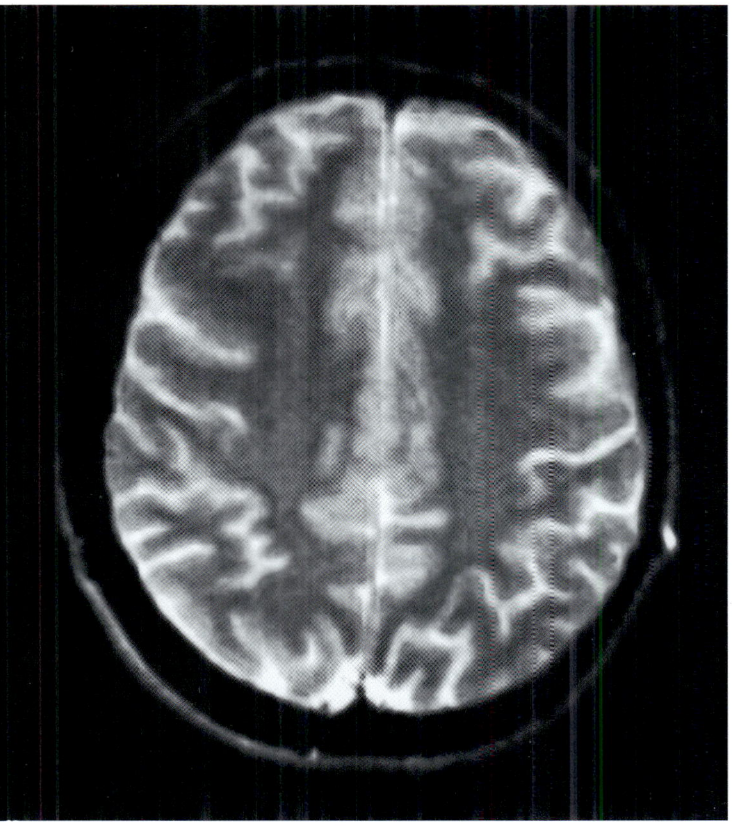

TR = 2,500 msec, TE = 90 msec

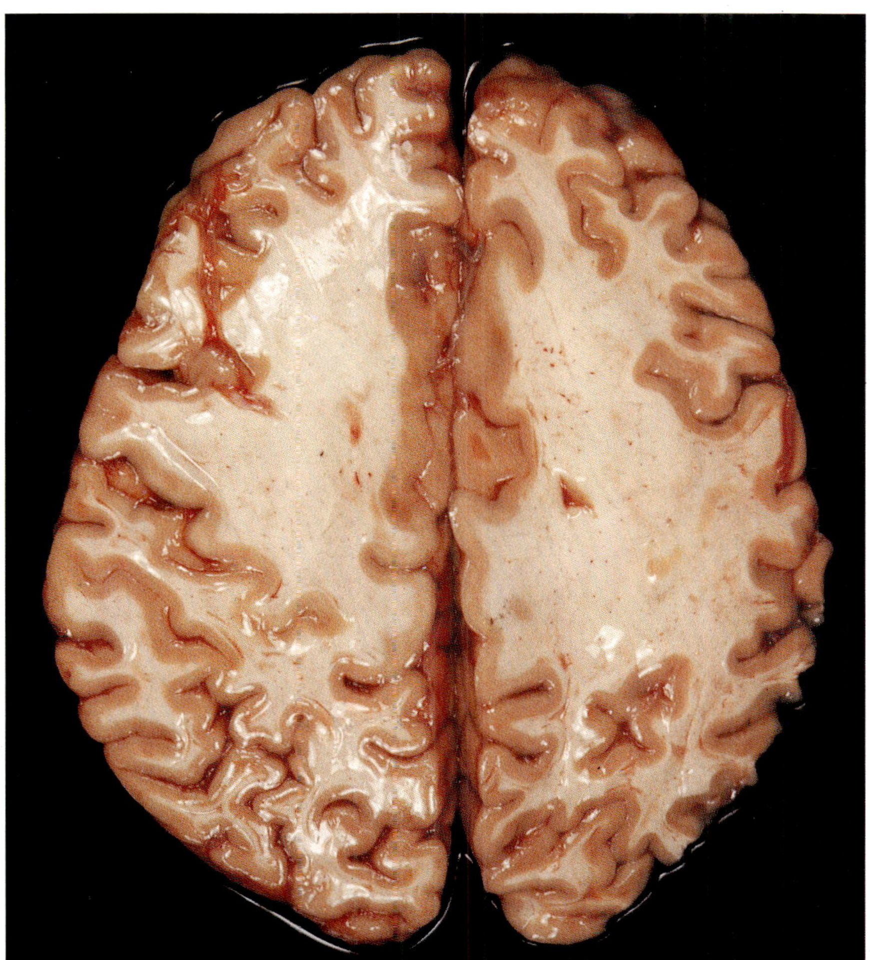

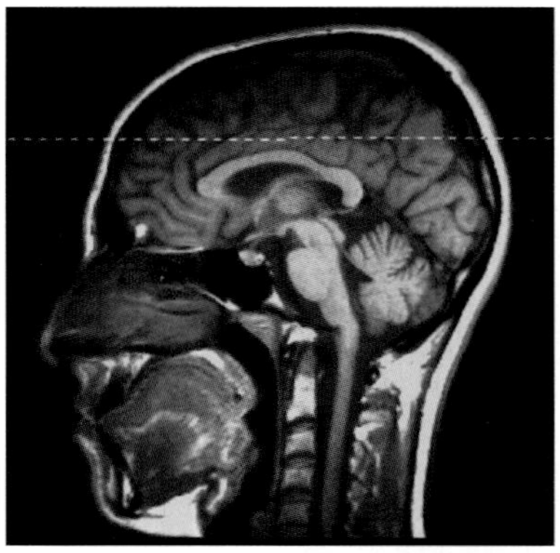

Fig. 7
1) lateral ventricle
2) corpus callosum
3) corona radiata
4) interhemispheric fissure
5) body of the caudate nucleus
6) grey matter
7) diploe

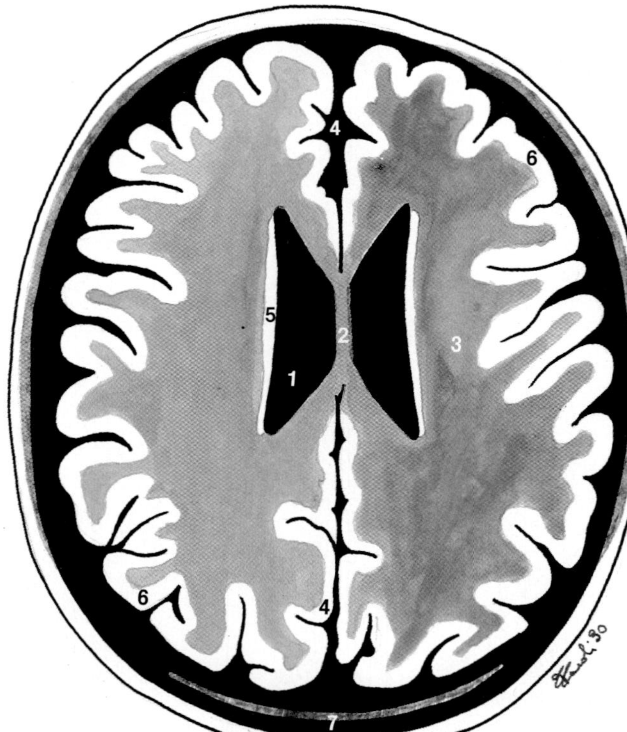

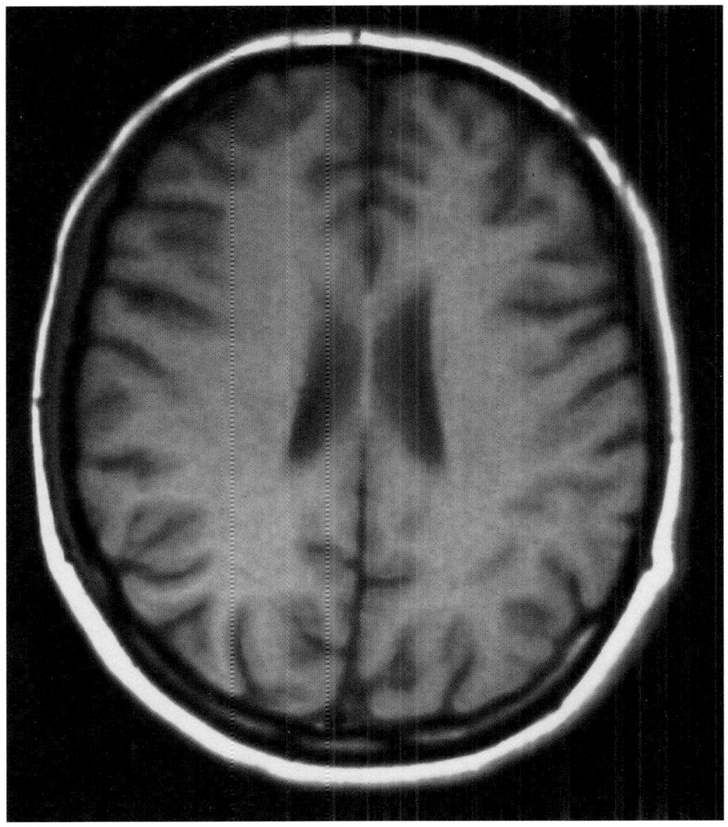

TR = 550 msec, TE = 15 msec

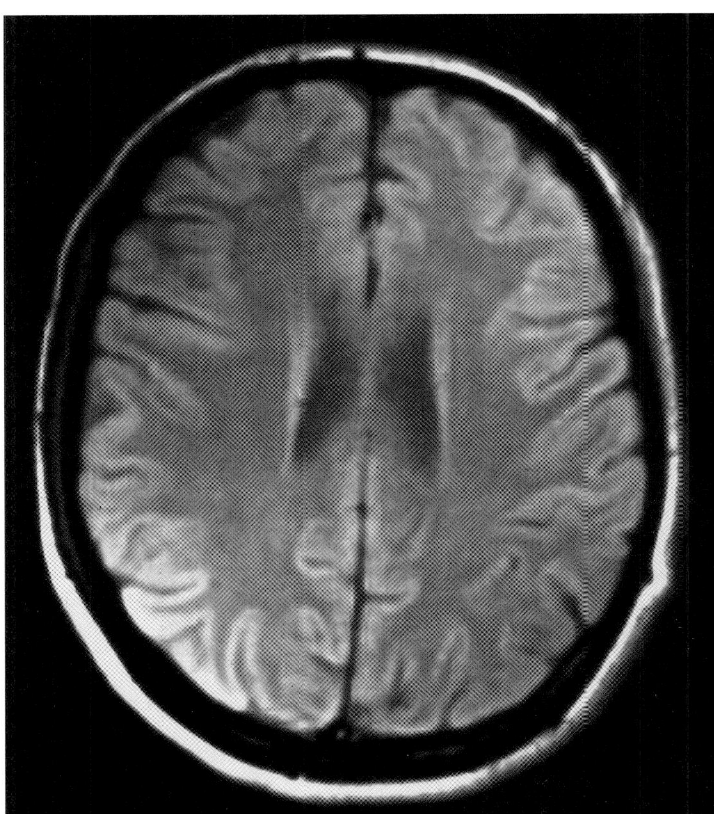

TR = 2,500 msec, TE = 15 msec

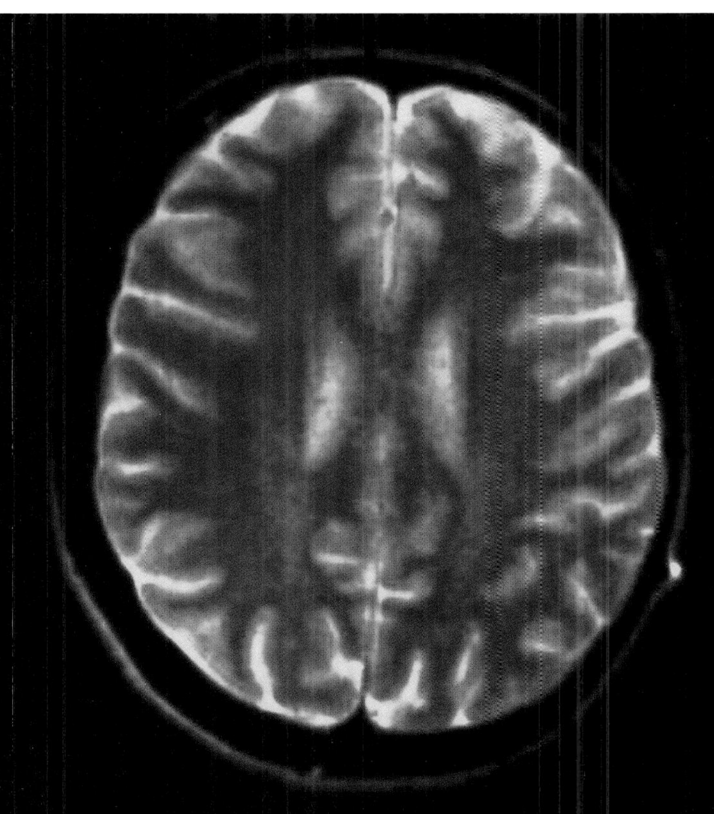

TR = 2,500 msec, TE = 90 msec

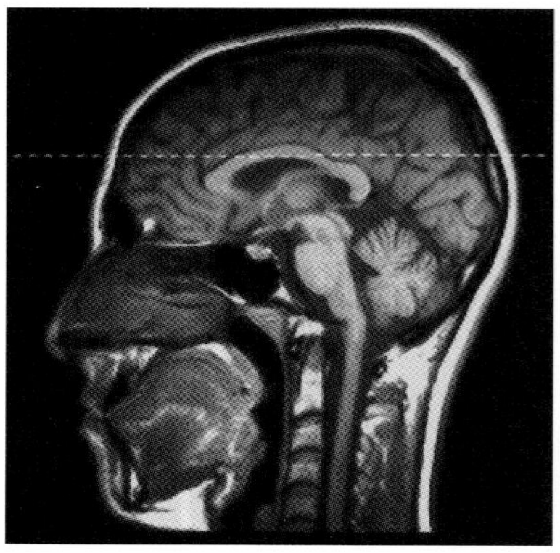

Fig. 8
1) genu of the corpus callosum
2) splenium of the corpus callosum
3) head of the caudate nucleus
4) septum pellucidum
5) fornix
6) columns of the fornix
7) choroid plexus
8) cingulate sulcus
9) pericallosal artery

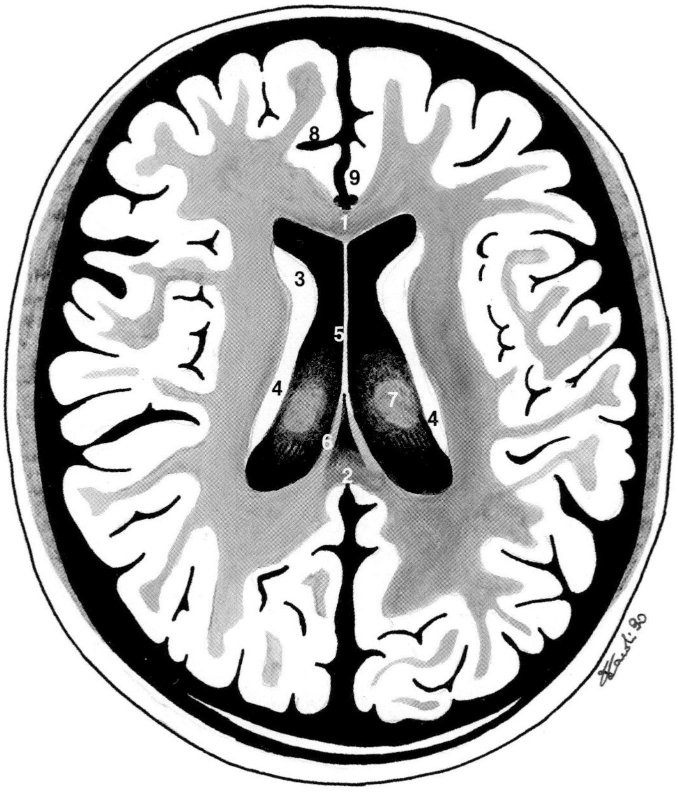

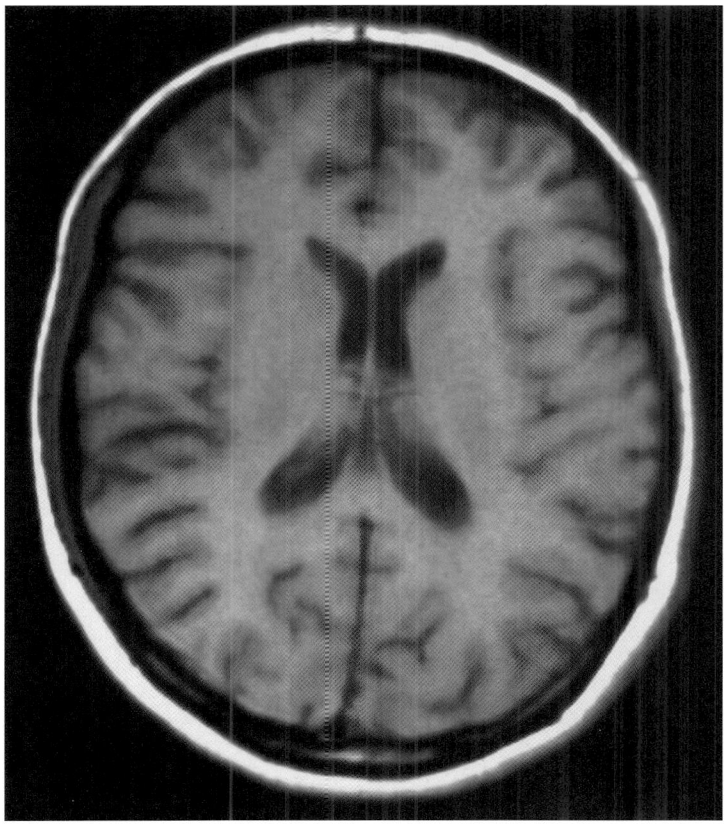

TR = 550 msec, TE = 15 msec

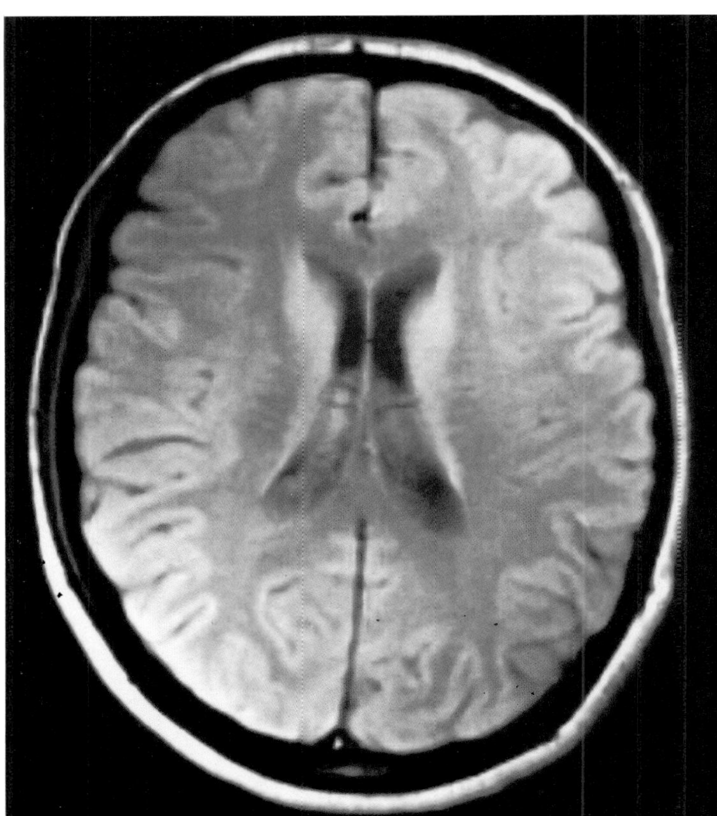

TR = 2,500 msec, TE = 15 msec

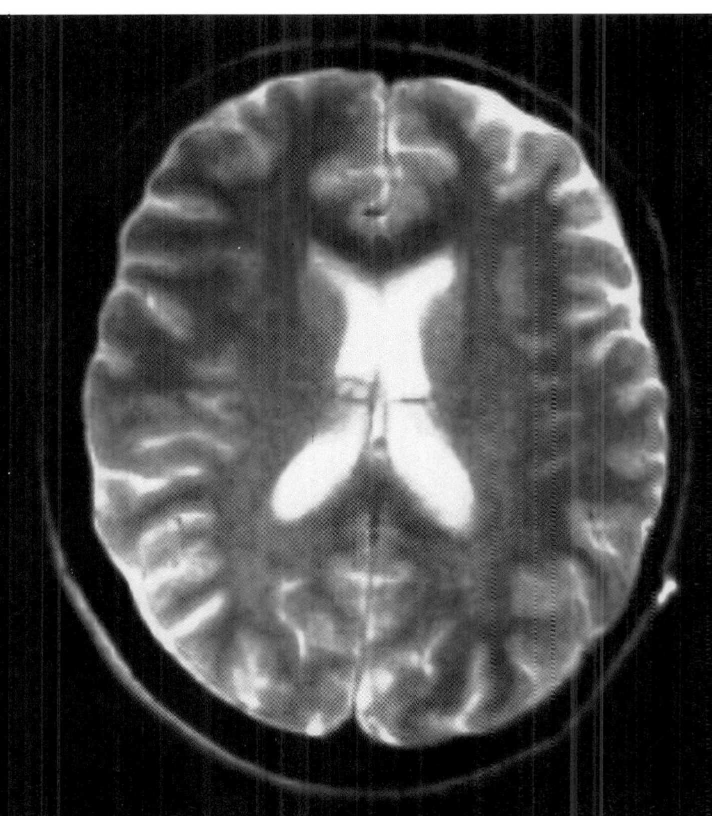

TR = 2,500 msec, TE = 90 msec

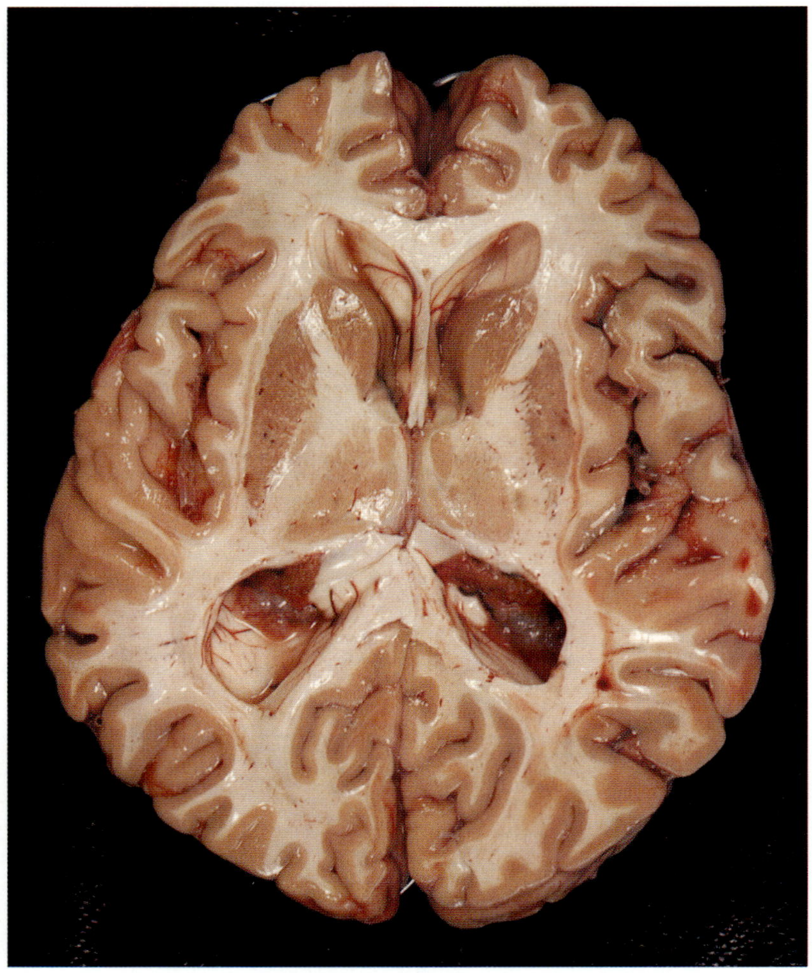

Fig. 9 A. Axial section. Lower surface of anatomic preparation; *Fig. 9 B* shows the upper surface. This image shows: corpus callosum, septum pellucidum, head of the caudate nucleus, putamen, a small portion of globus pallidus (left), internal capsule, external capsule, thalamus and choroid plexa.

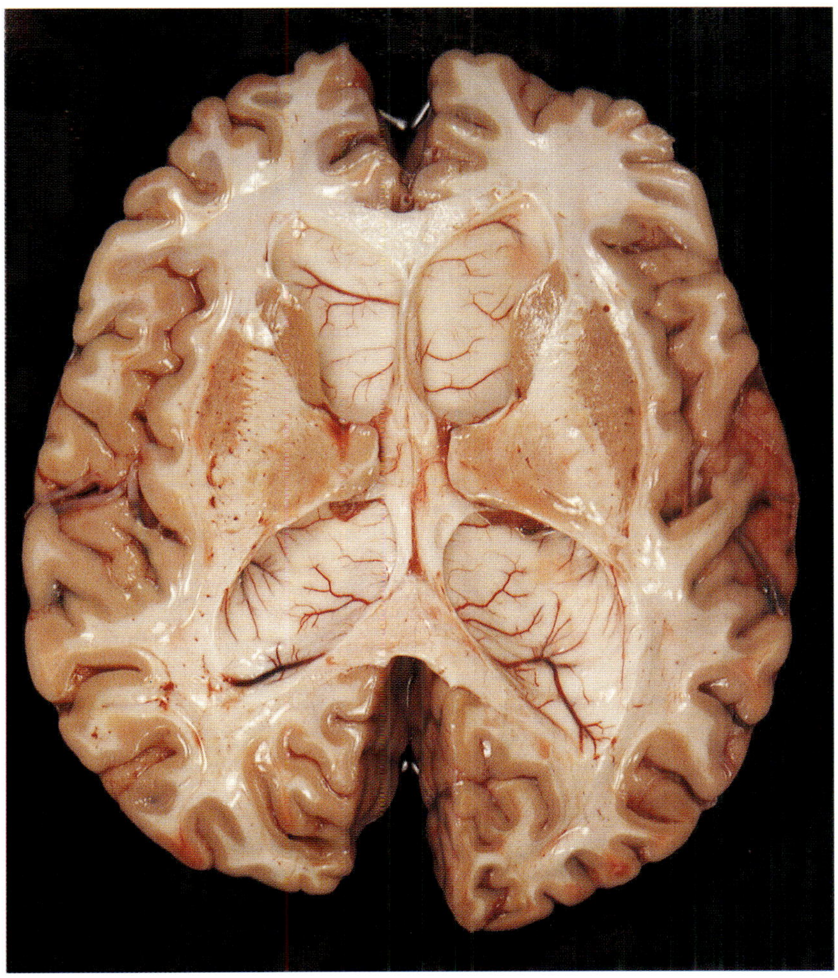

Fig. 9 B. This image better shows the ependymal vessels and the splenium of the corpus callosum.

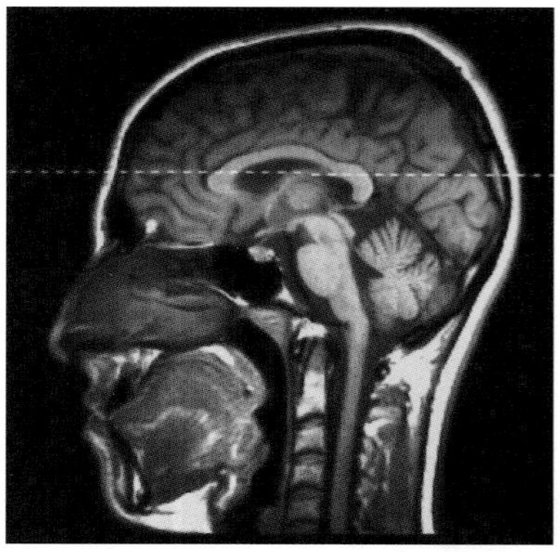

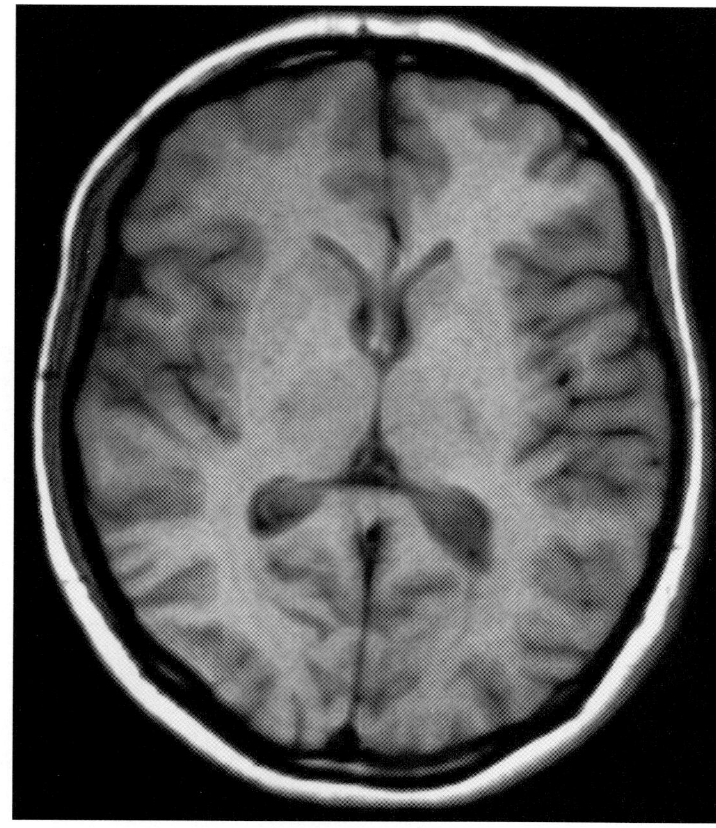

TR = 550 msec, TE = 15 msec

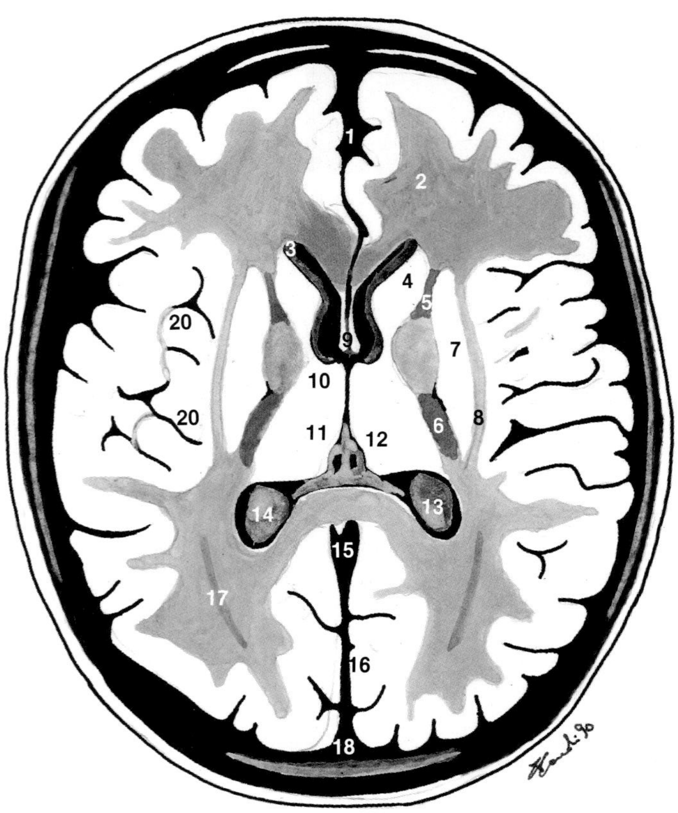

Fig. 10

1) falx and interhemispheric fissure
2) white matter
3) frontal horn of the lateral ventricle
4) head of the caudate nucleus
5) anterior arm of the internal capsule
6) posterior arm of the internal capsule
7) putamen
8) external capsule
9) fornix
10) Monro's foramen
11) thalamus
12) internal cerebral veins
13) trigonum
14) choroid plexus
15) Galen's vein
16) interhemispheric fissure
17) optic radiations
18) superior longitudinal sinus
19) globus pallidus
20) insula

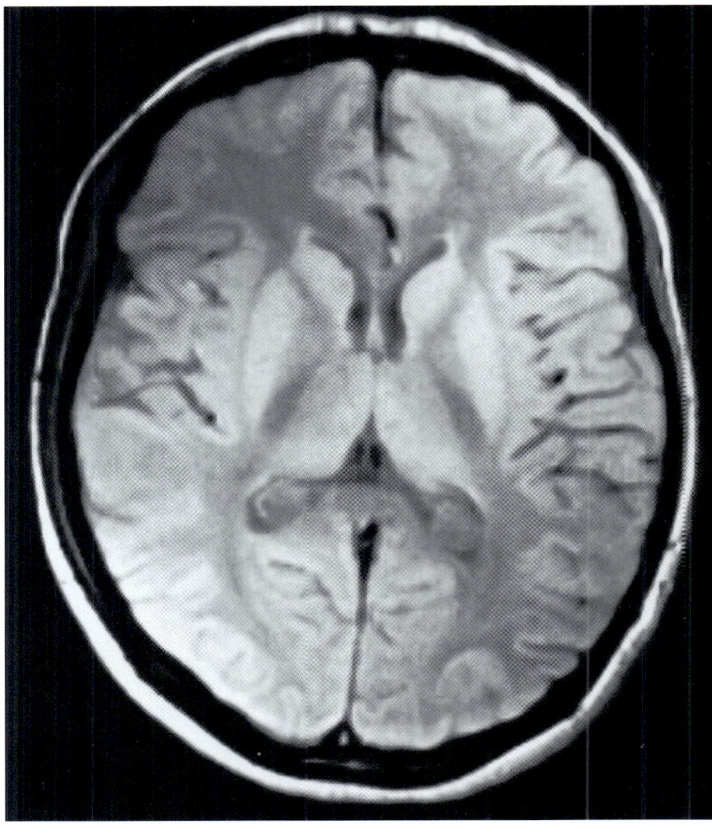

TR = 2,500 msec, TE = 15 msec

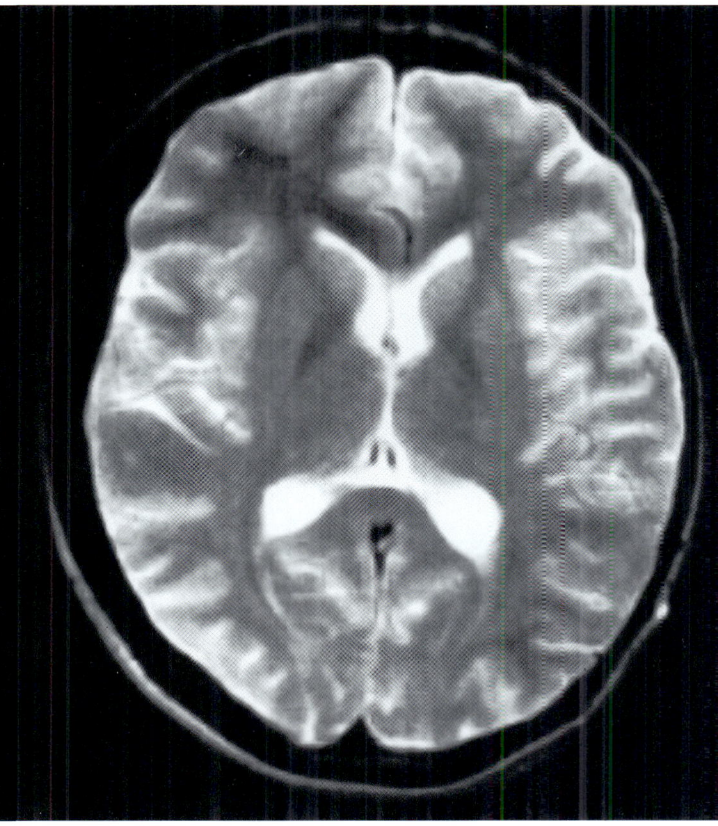

TR = 2,500 msec, TE = 90 msec

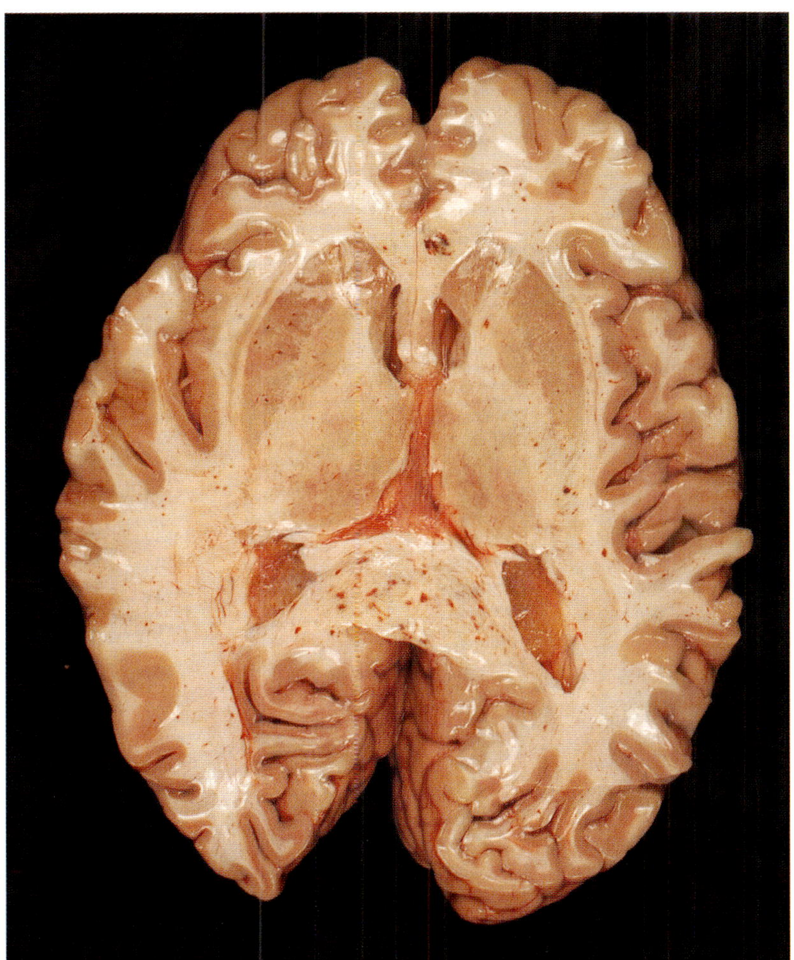

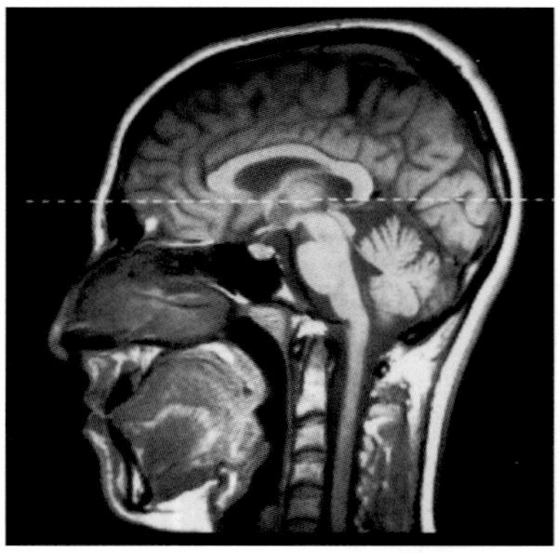

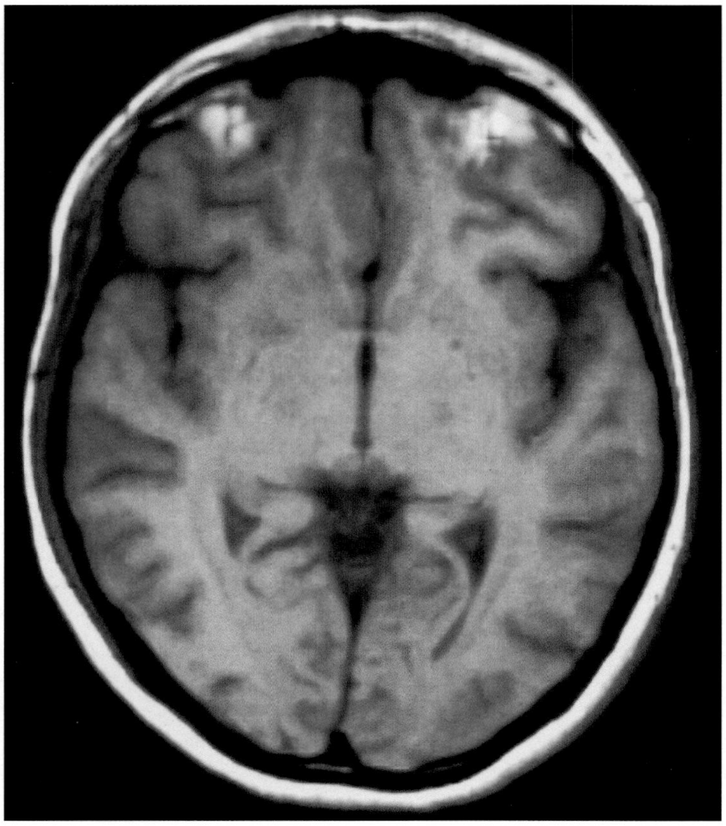

TR = 550 msec, TE = 15 msec

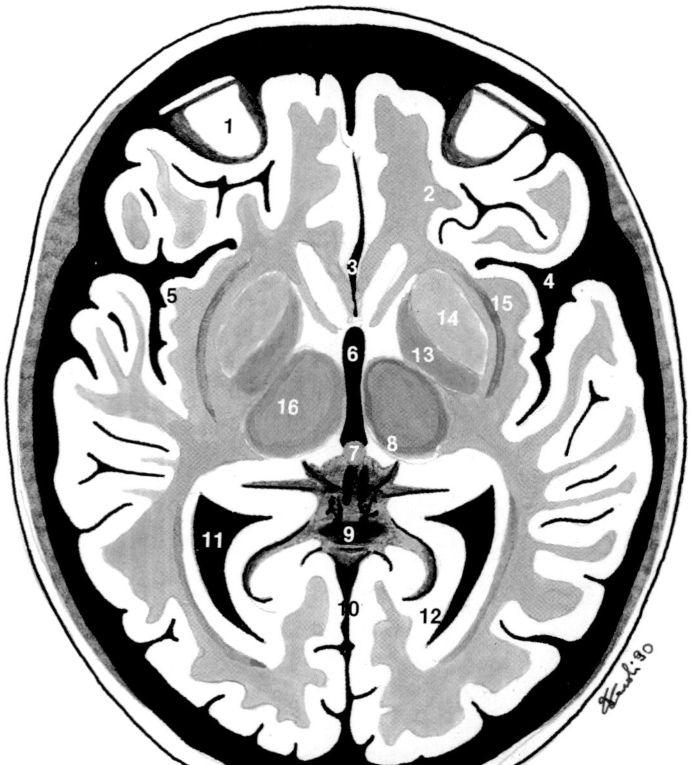

Fig. 11

1) roof of the orbit
2) white matter
3) pericallosal arteries
4) Sylvian cistern
5) insula
6) 3rd ventricle
7) pineal gland
8) internal cerebral veins
9) quadrigeminal plate cistern
10) straight sinus
11) trigonum
12) occipital horn of the lateral ventricle
13) globus pallidus
14) putamen
15) claustrum

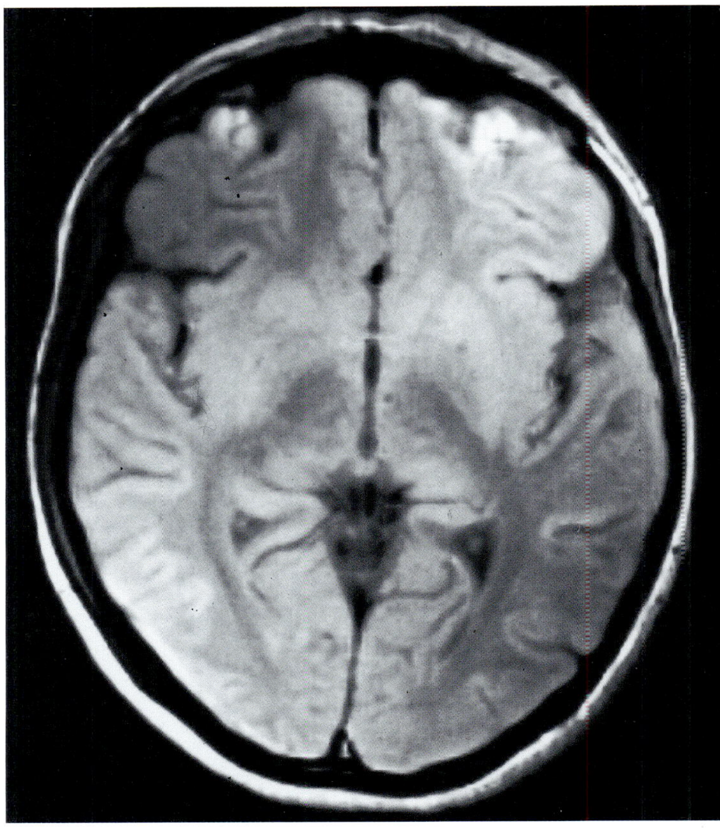

TR = 2,500 msec, TE = 15 msec

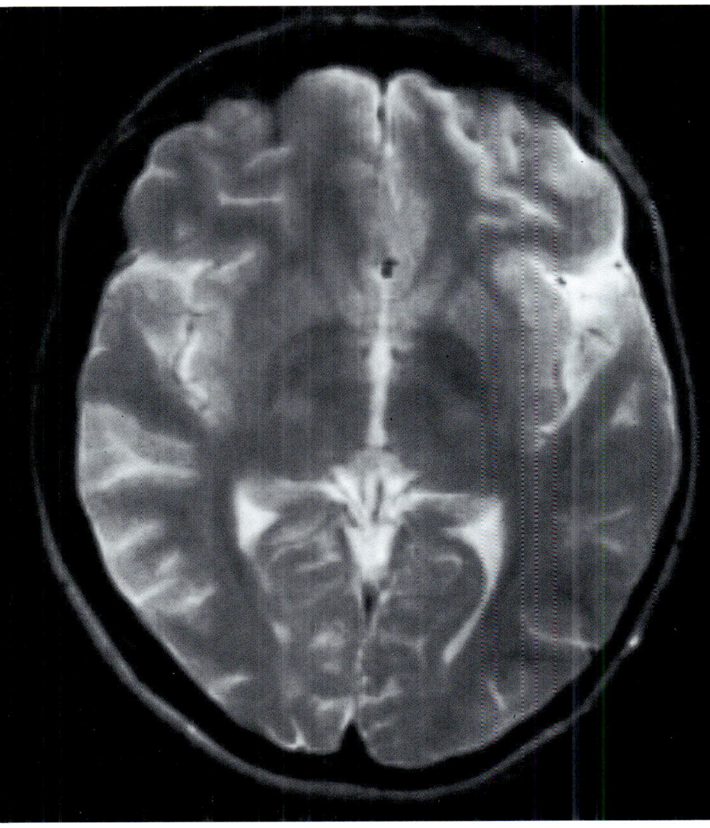

TR = 2,500 msec, TE = 90 msec

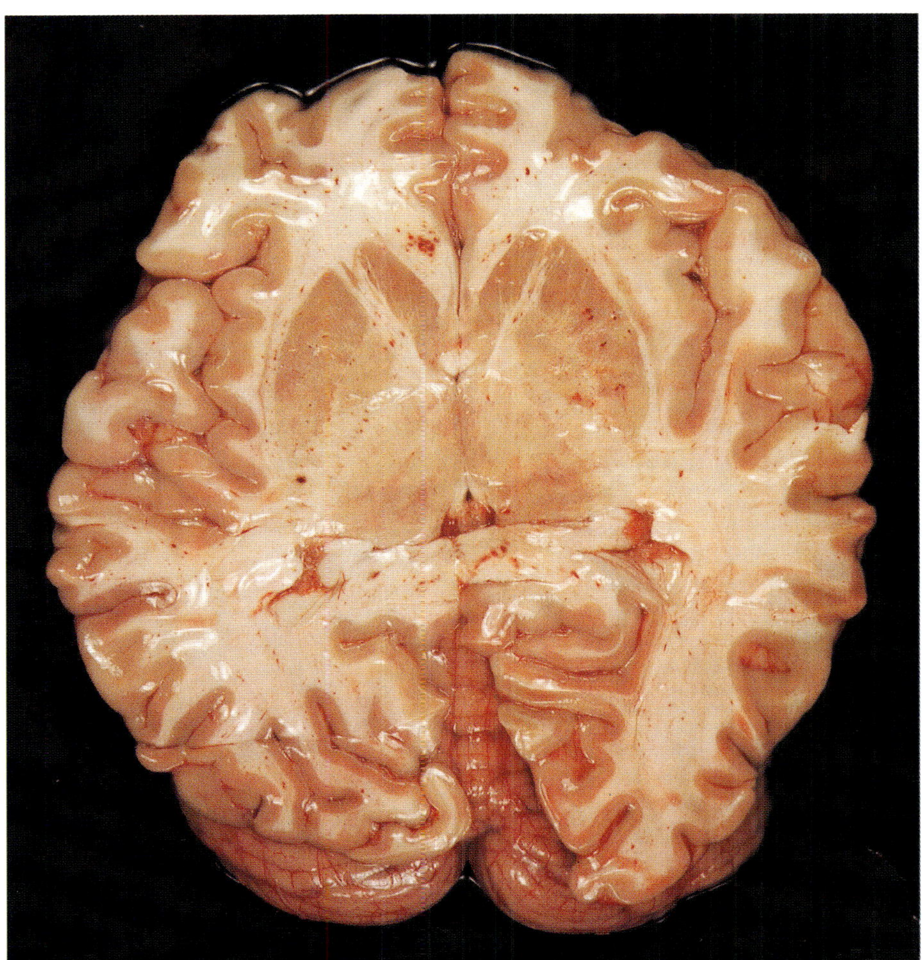

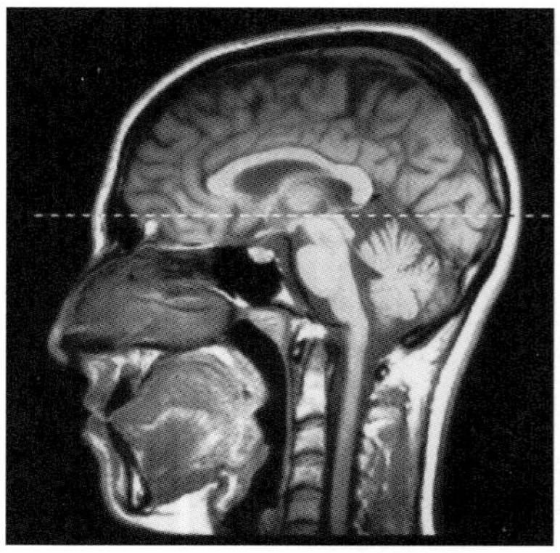

Fig. 12
1) gyrus rectus
2) middle cerebral artery
3) optic tract
4) mammillary bodies
5) midbrain
6) Sylvian aqueduct
7) cisterna ambiens
8) upper cerebellar vermis
9) straight sinus
10) torcular

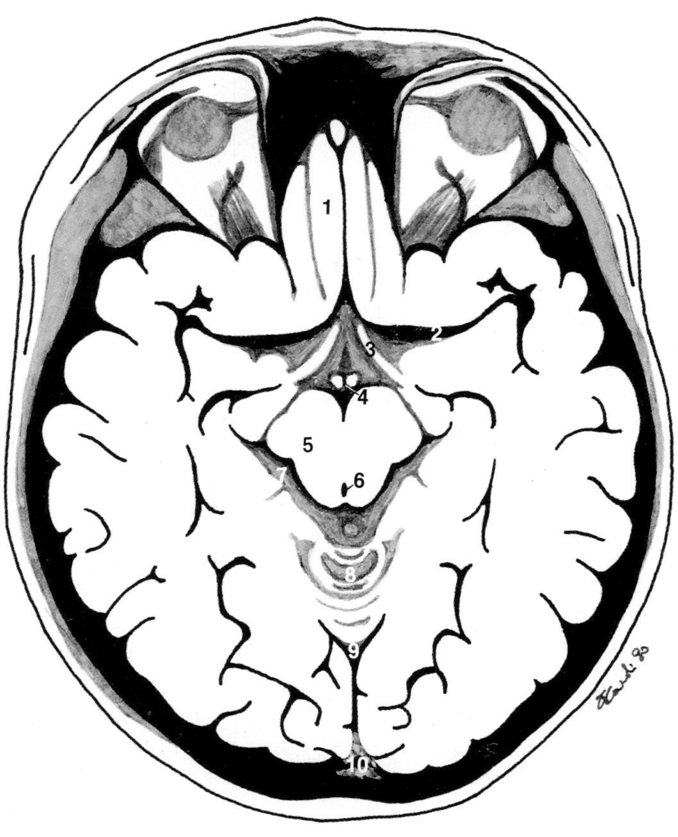

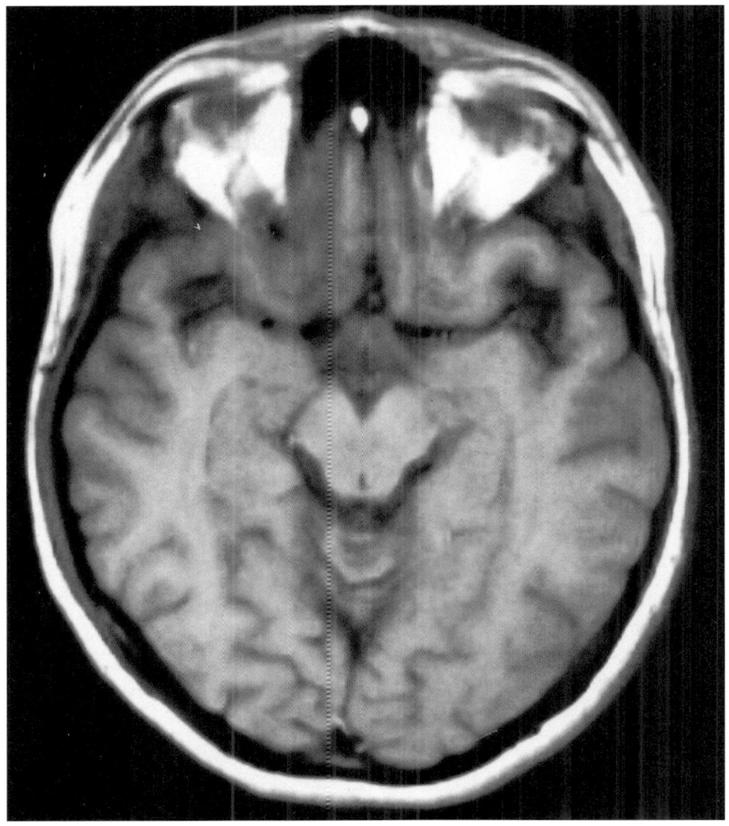

TR = 550 msec, TE = 15 msec

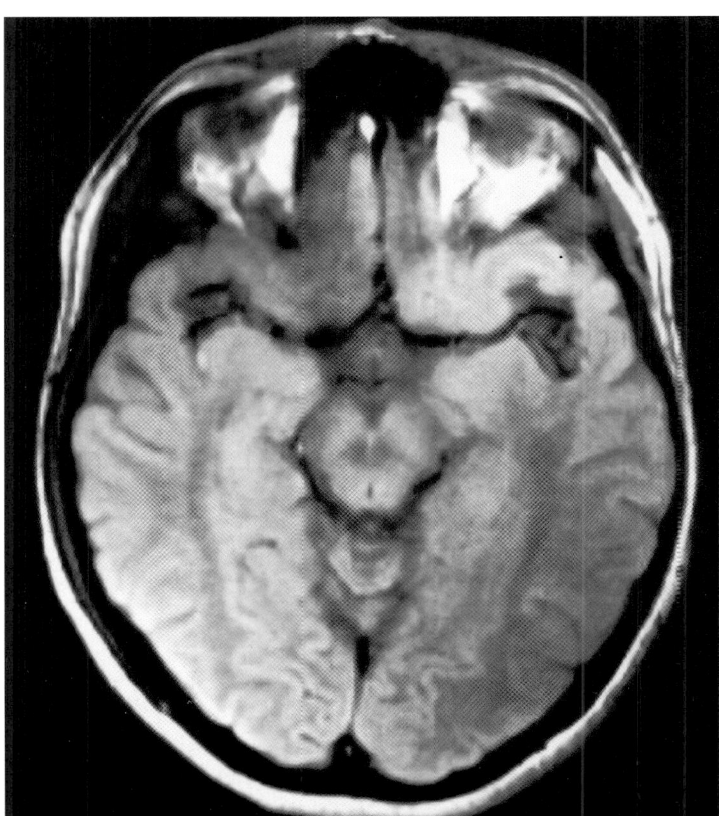

TR = 2,500 msec, TE = 15 msec

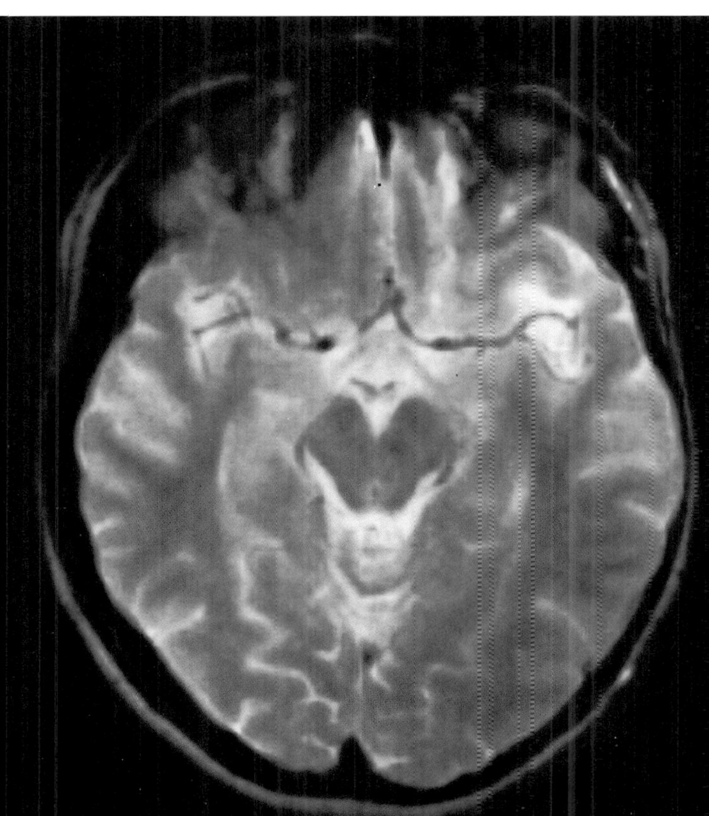

TR = 2,500 msec, TE = 90 msec

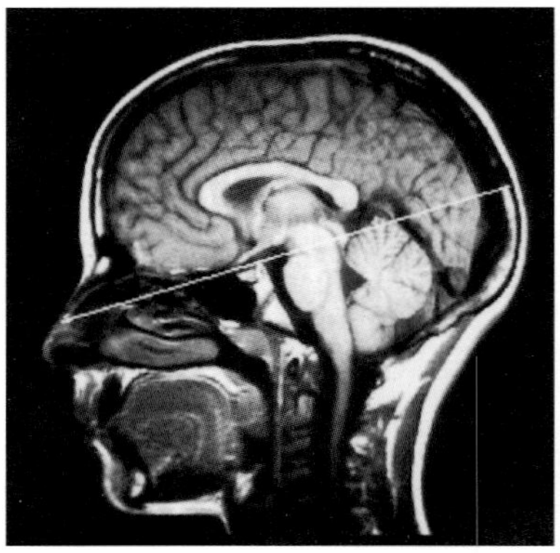

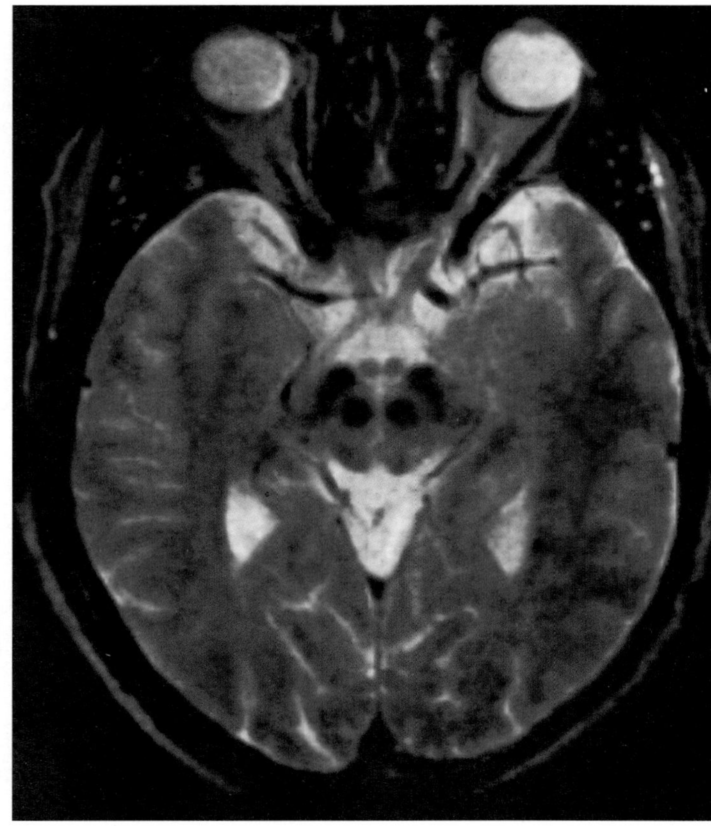

TR = 2,500 msec, TE = 90 msec

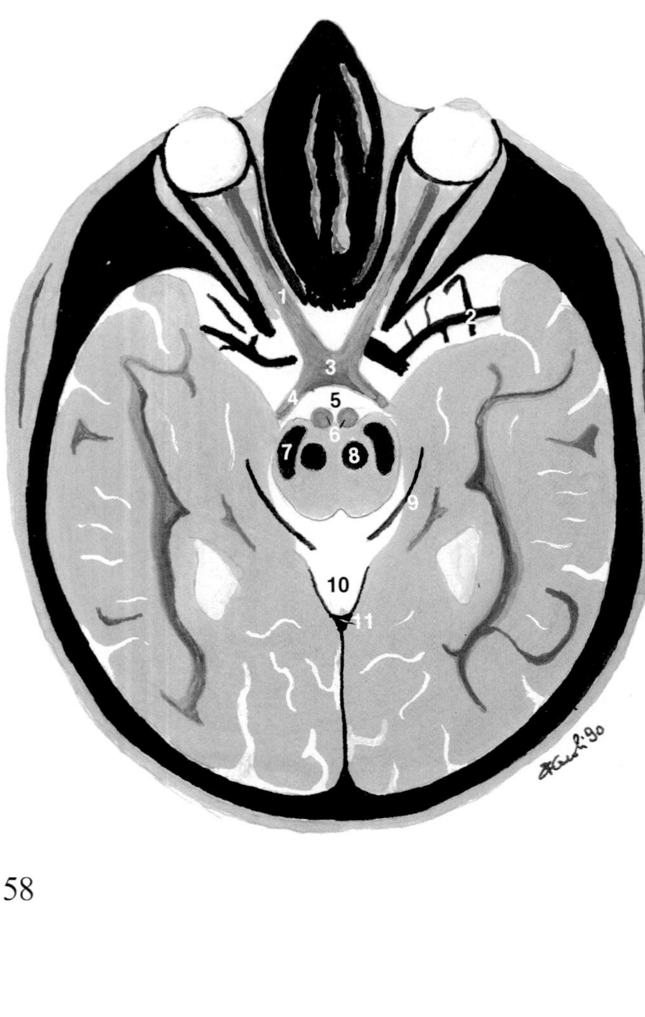

Fig. 13
1) optic nerve
2) middle cerebral artery
3) optic chiasm
4) optic tract
5) chiasmatic cistern
6) mammillary bodies
7) substantia nigra
8) red nucleus
9) tentorium
10) quadrigeminal plate cistern
11) Galen's vein

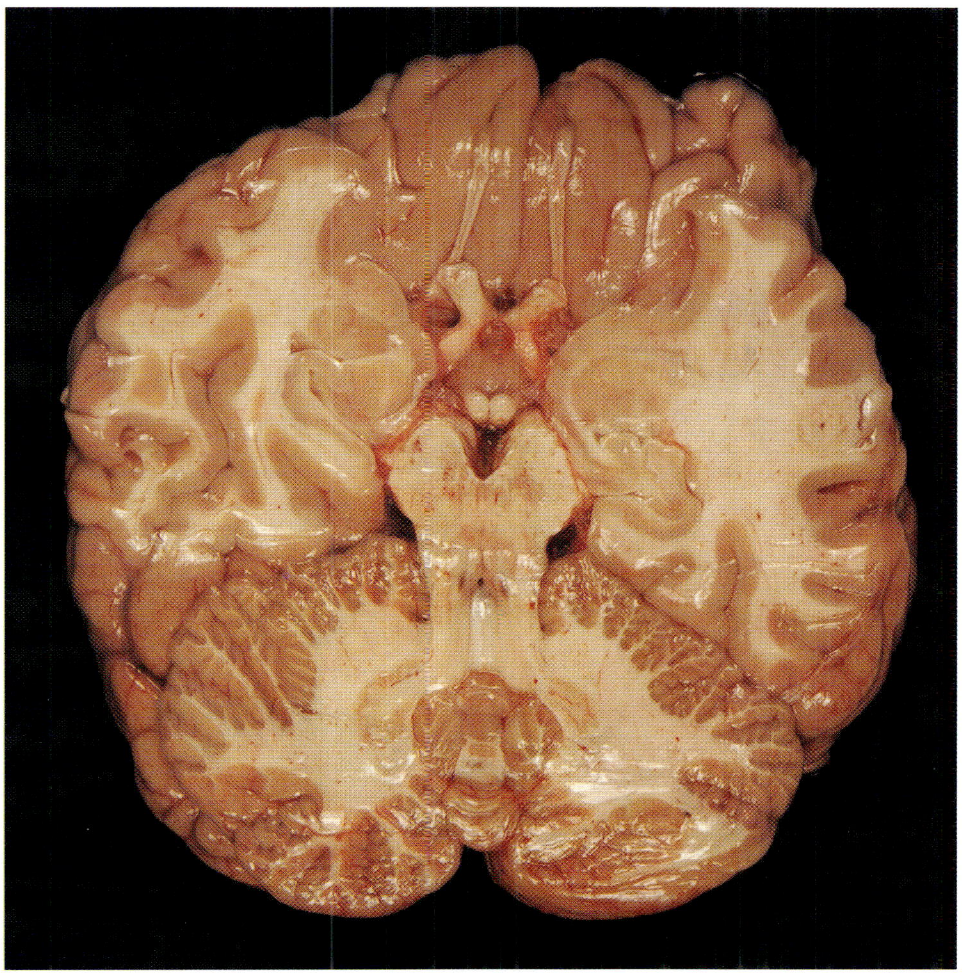

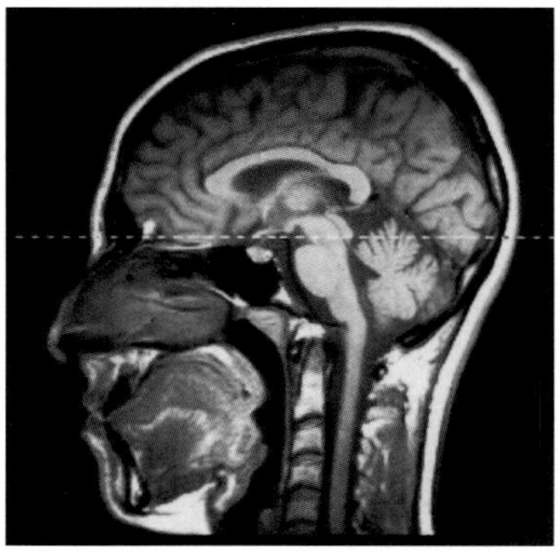

Fig. 14
1) globe
2) medial rectus muscle
3) optic nerve
4) lateral rectus muscle
5) pituitary gland
6) basilar artery
7) temporal horn of the lateral ventricle
8) prepontine cistern
9) lateral dura of the cavernous sinus
10) pons
11) medial longitudinal bundle
12) 4th ventricle
13) cerebellar vermis
14) confluence of straight sinus into the torcular

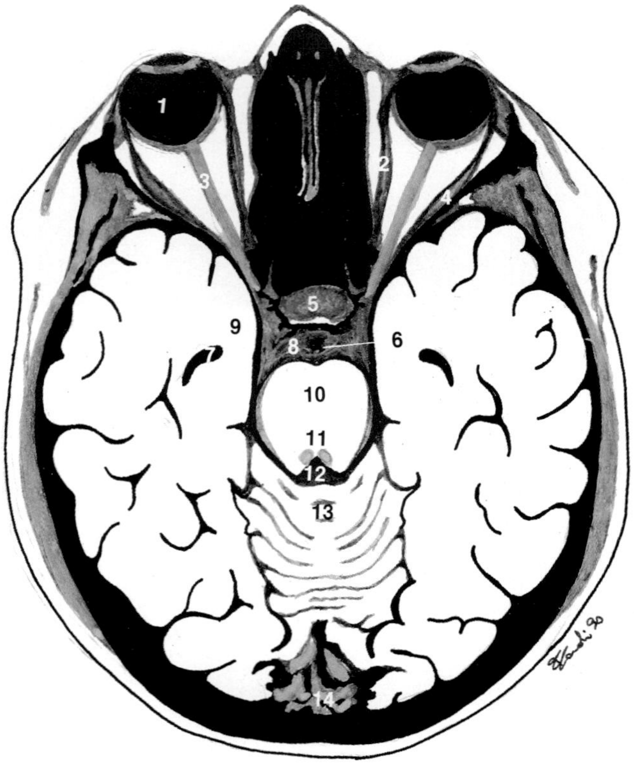

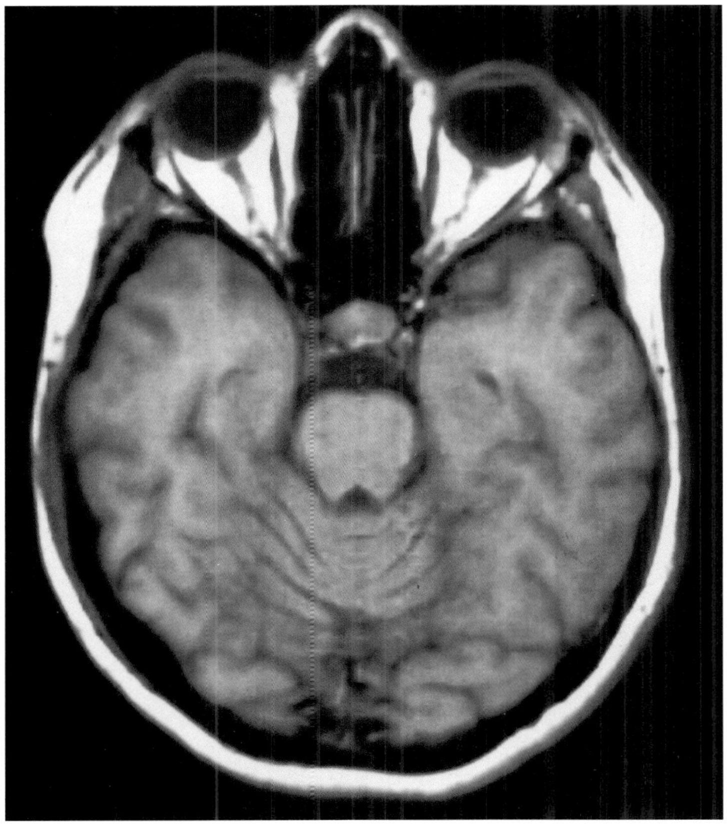

TR = 550 msec, TE = 15 msec

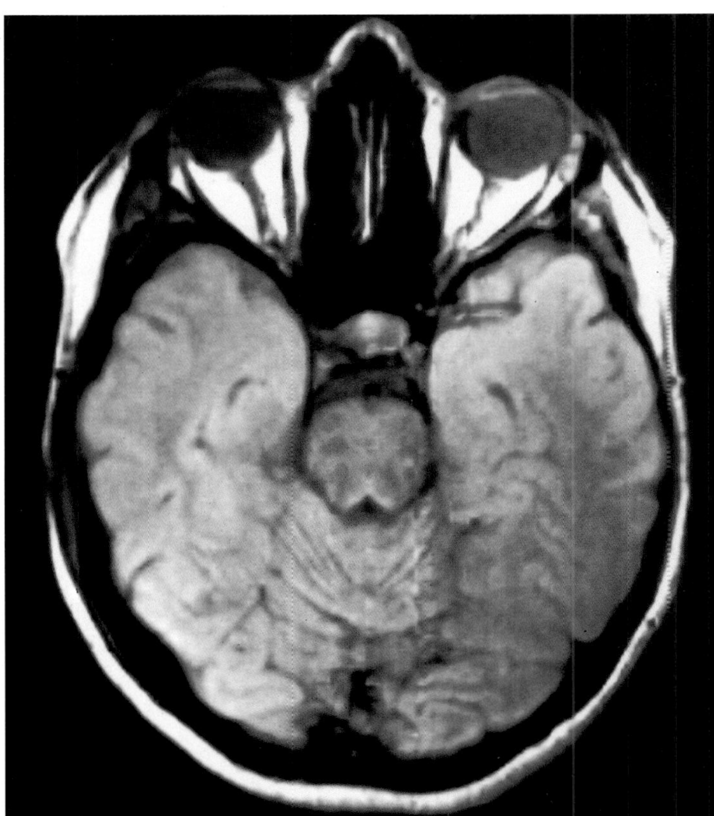

TR = 2,500 msec, TE = 15 msec

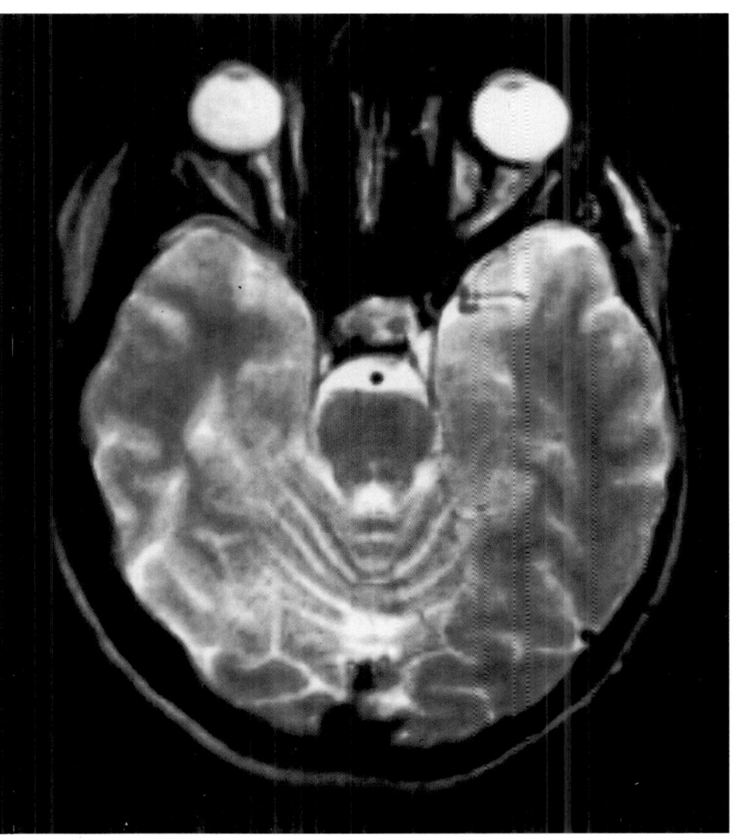

TR = 2,500 msec, TE = 90 msec

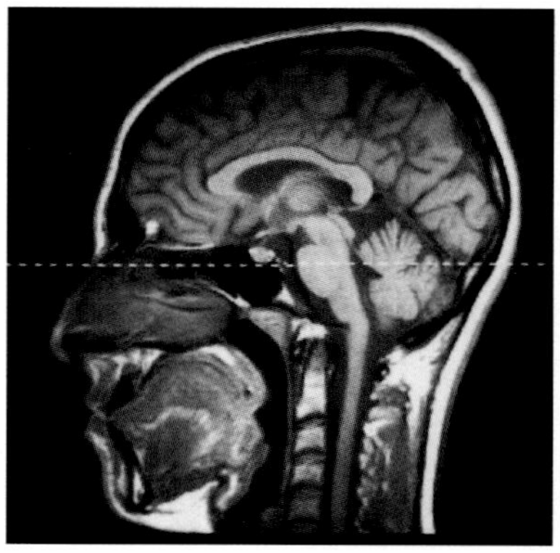

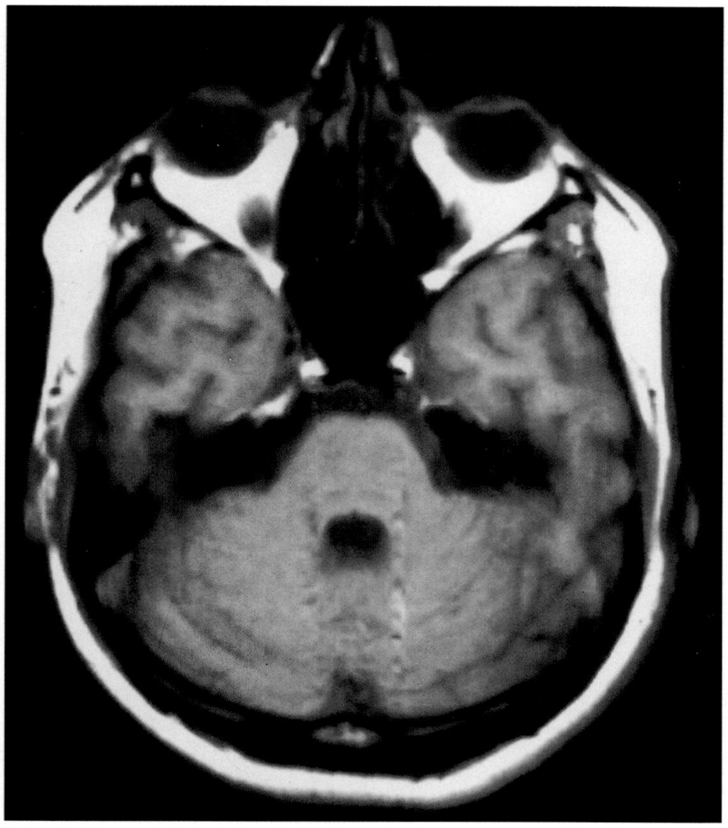

TR = 550 msec, TE = 15 msec

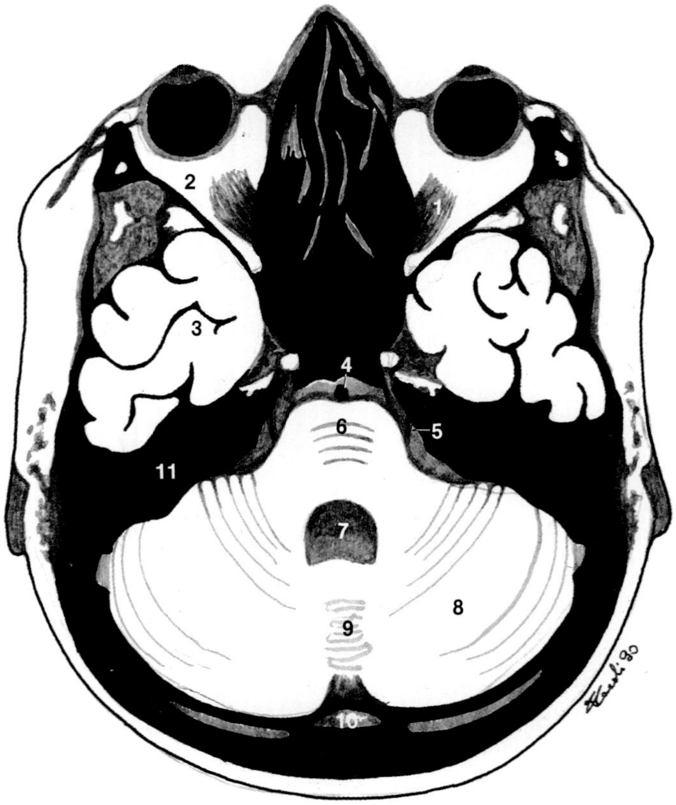

Fig. 15

1) inferior rectus muscle
2) intraorbital fat
3) temporal lobe
4) basilar artery
5) 5th cranial nerve
6) pons
7) 4th ventricle
8) cerebellum
9) cerebellar vermis
10) diploe of the internal occipital crest
11) petrous bone

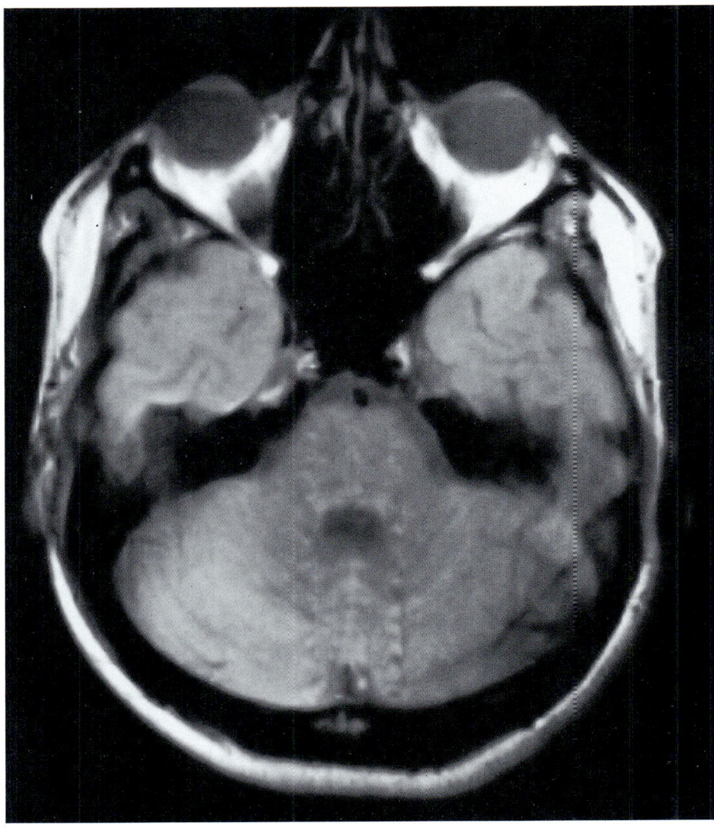

TR = 2,500 msec, TE = 15 msec

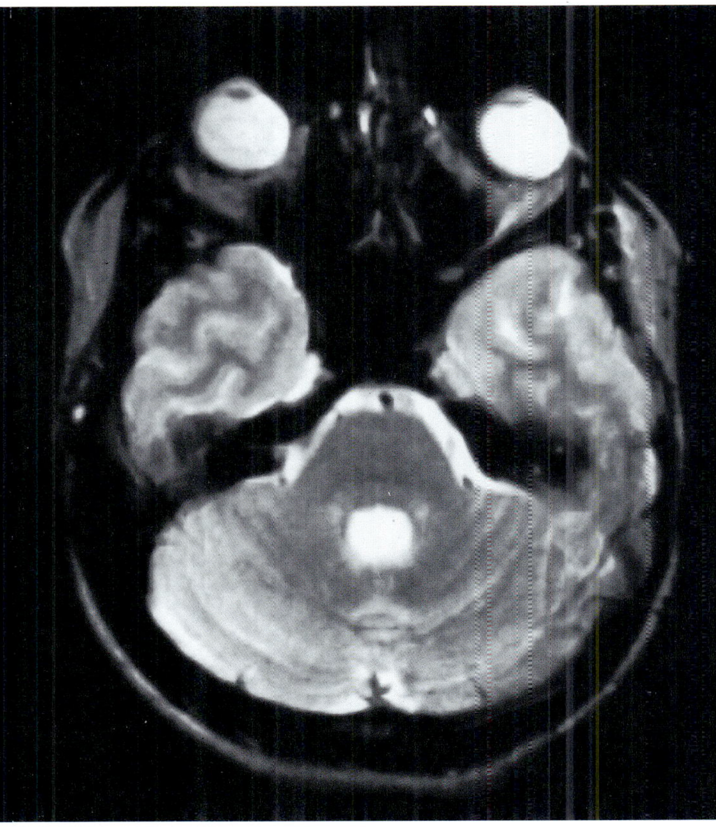

TR = 2,500 msec, TE = 15 msec

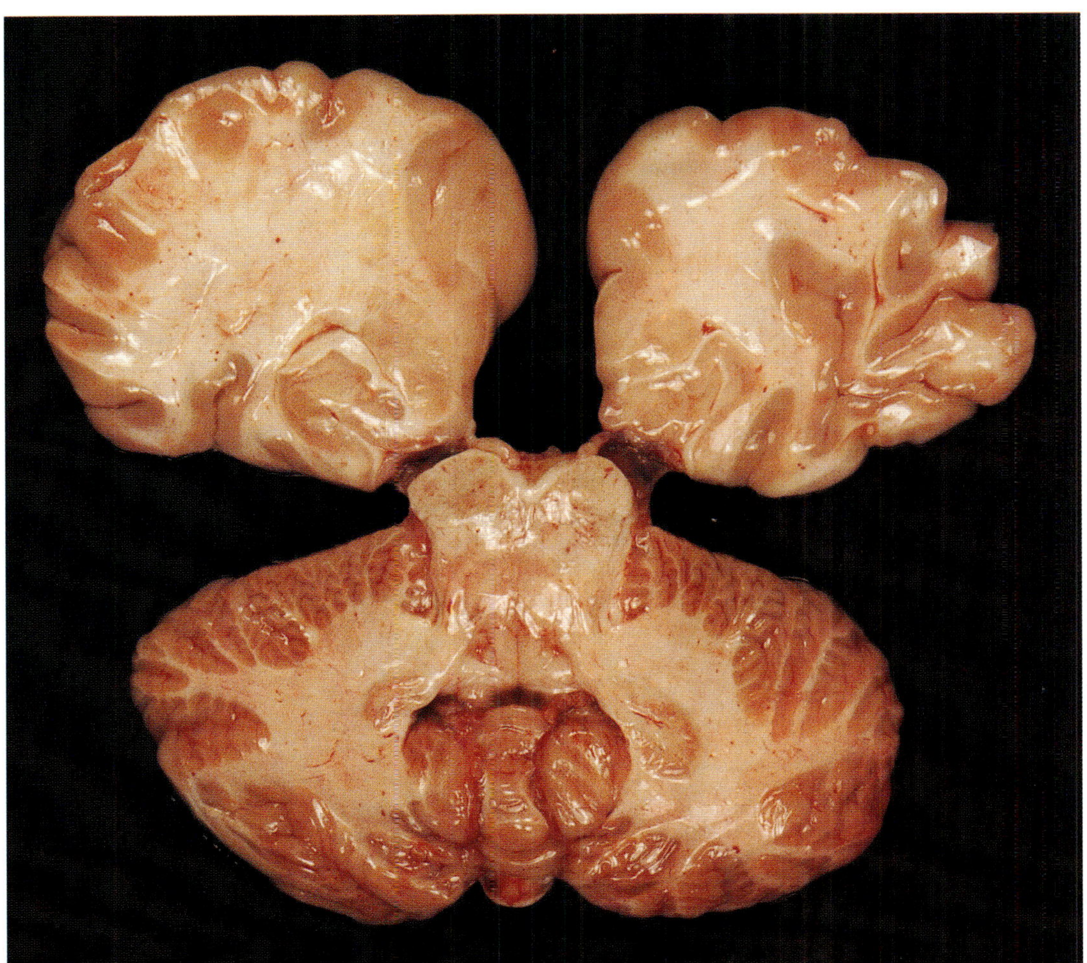

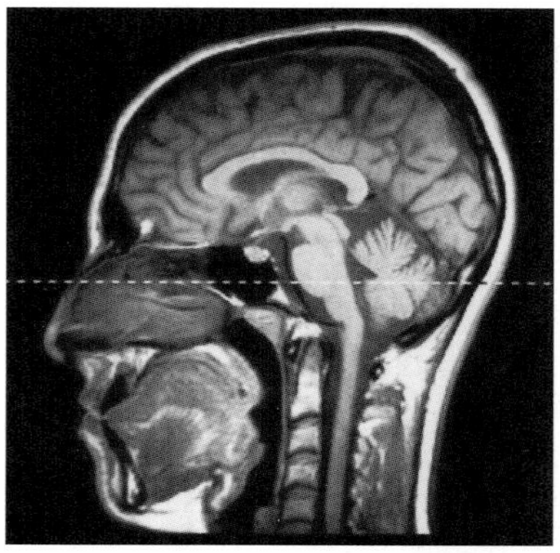

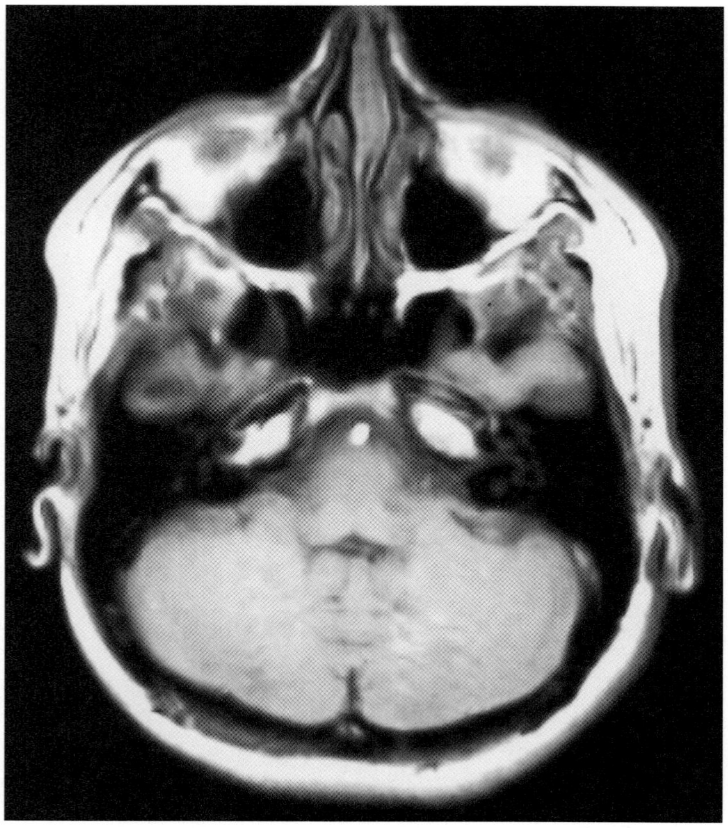

TR = 550 msec, TE = 15 msec

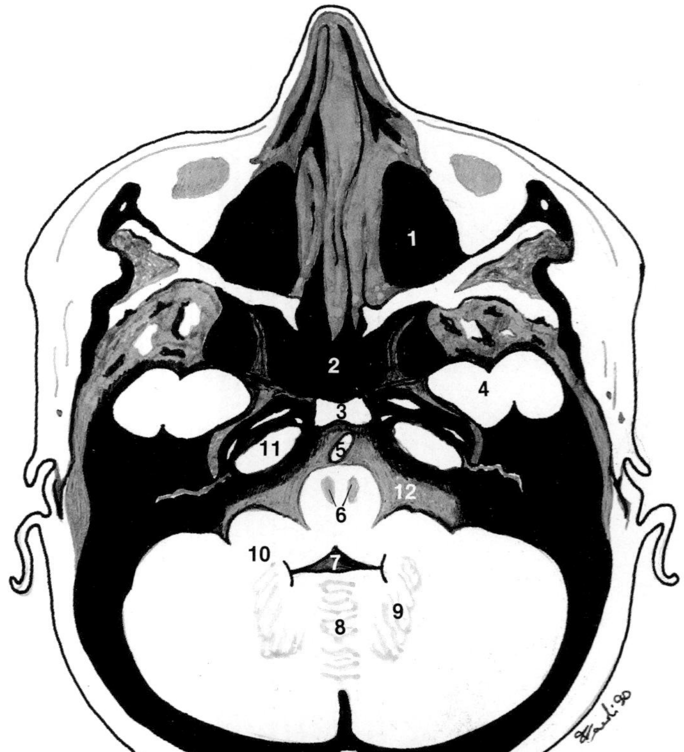

Fig. 16

1) maxillary sinus
2) sphenoid sinus
3) clivus
4) temporal lobe
5) basilar artery
6) lemniscus medialis
7) 4th ventricle
8) cerebellar vermis
9) dentate nucleus
10) lower cerebellar peduncle
11) intrapetrosal portion of the internal carotid artery
12) cistern of the cerebellopontine angle

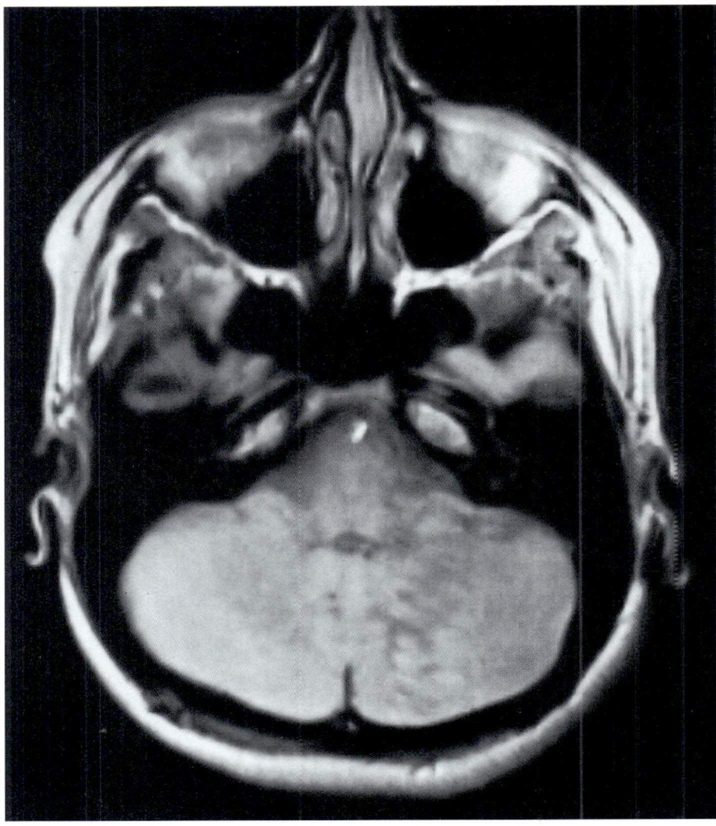

TR = 2,500 msec, TE = 15 msec

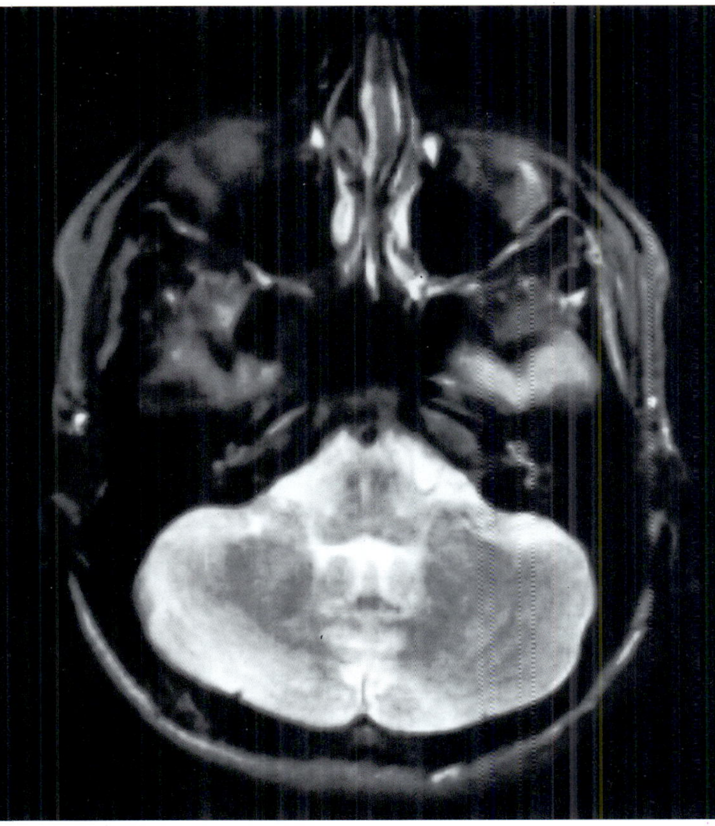

TR = 2,500 msec, TE = 90 msec

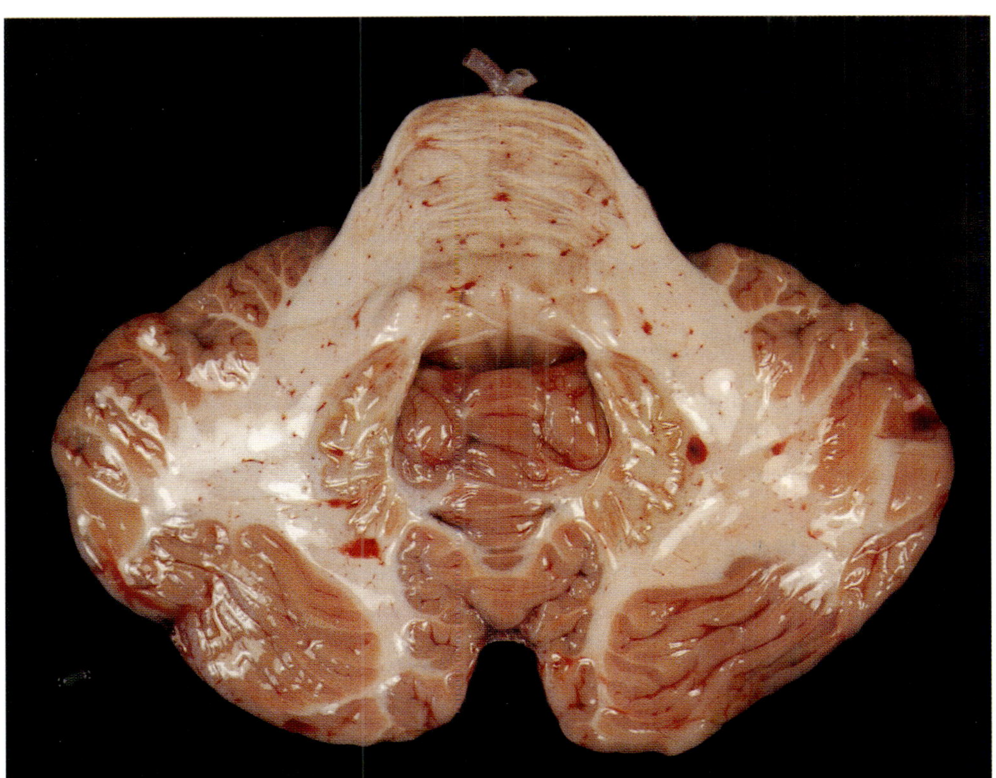

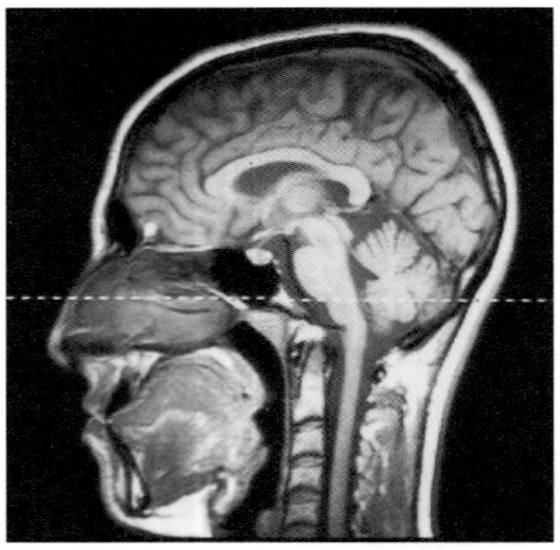

Fig. 17
1) maxillary sinus
2) condyle of the mandible
3) basilar artery
4) vertebral artery
5) medulla oblongata
6) cerebellar tonsils
7) lower cerebellar vermis

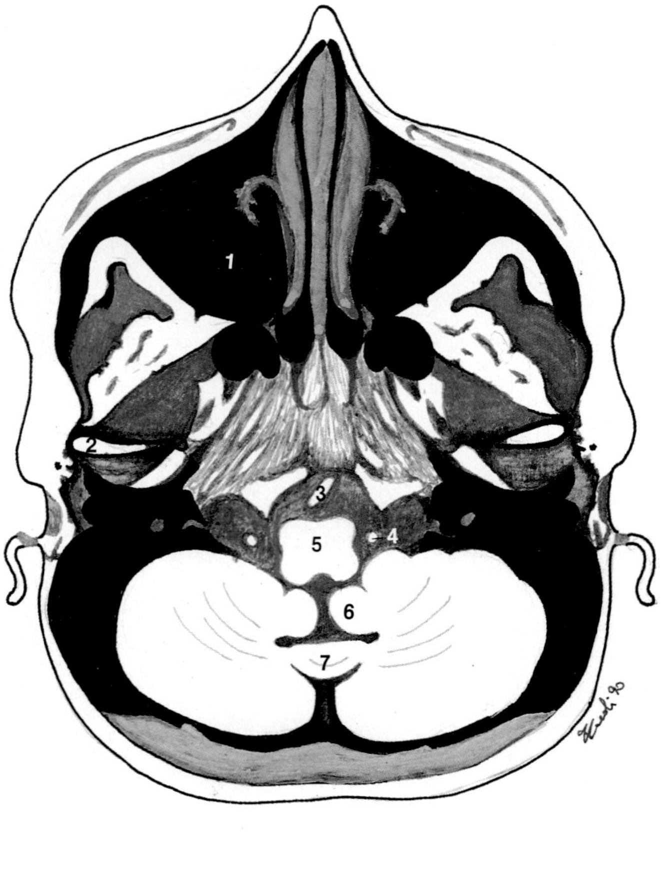

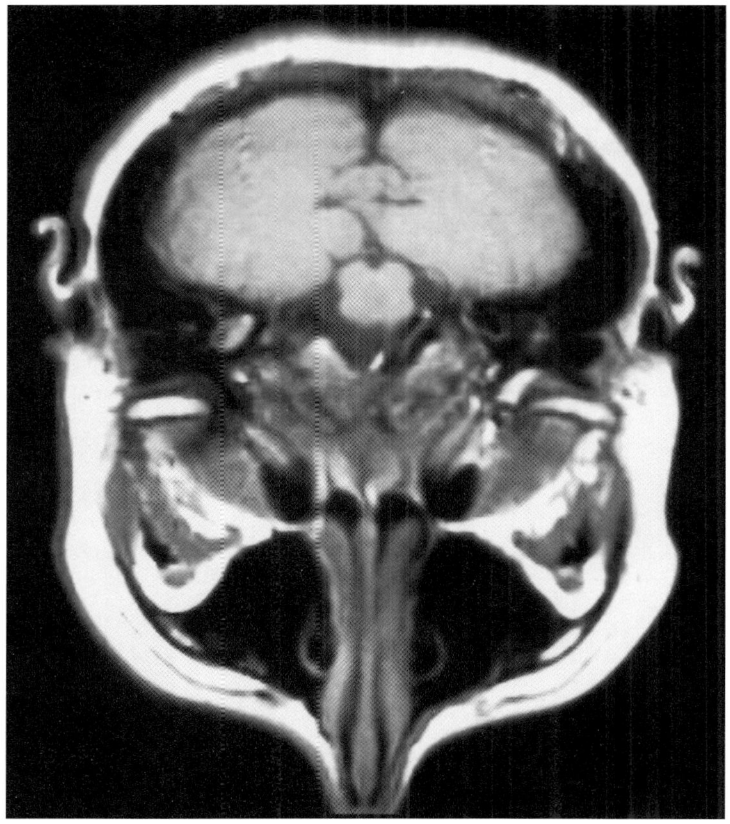

TR = 550 msec, TE = 15 msec

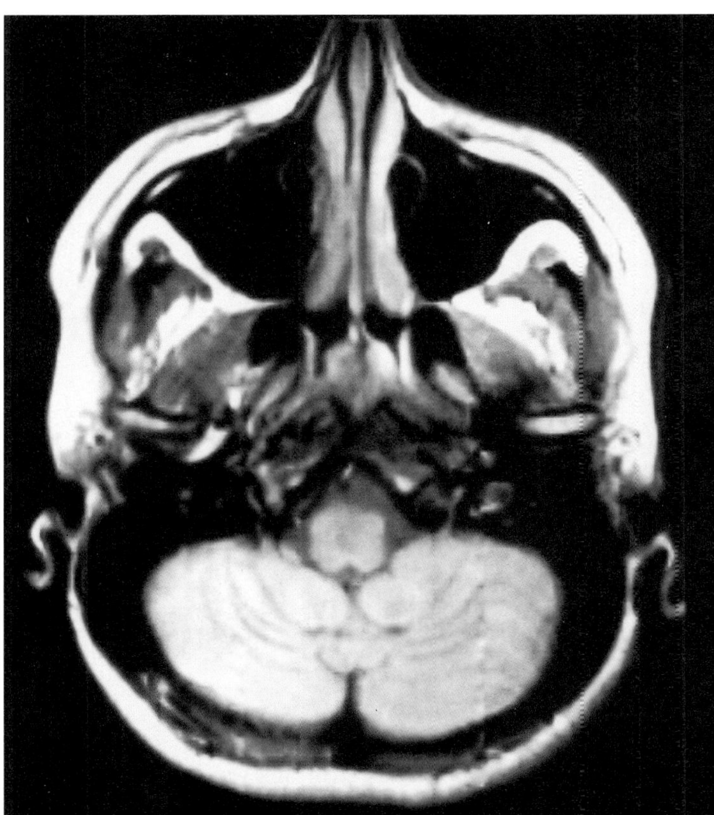

TR = 2,500 msec, TE = 15 msec

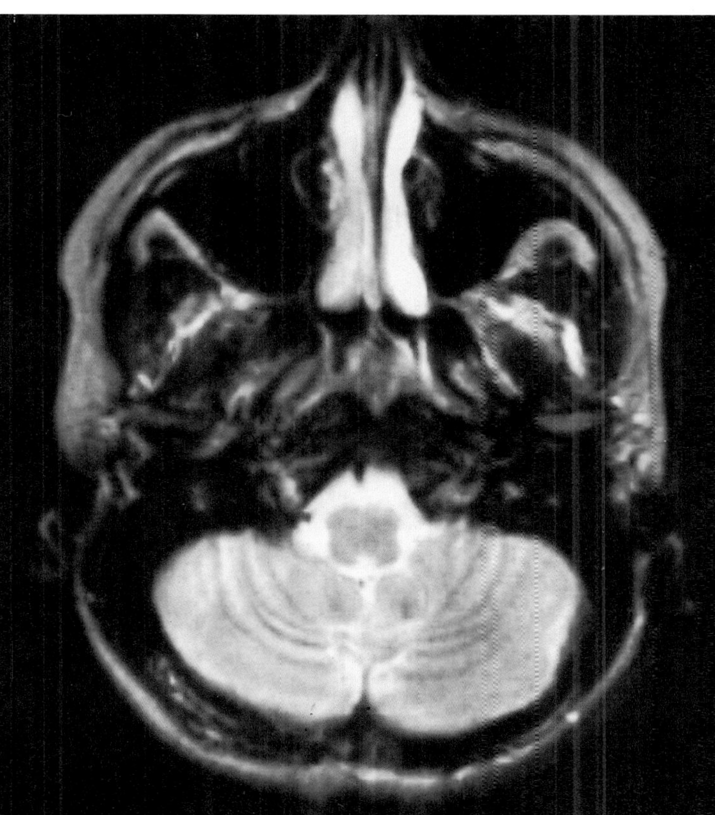

TR = 2,500 msec, TE = 90 msec

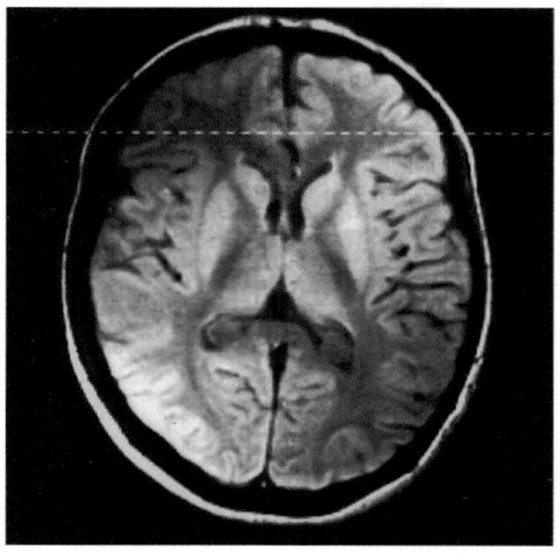

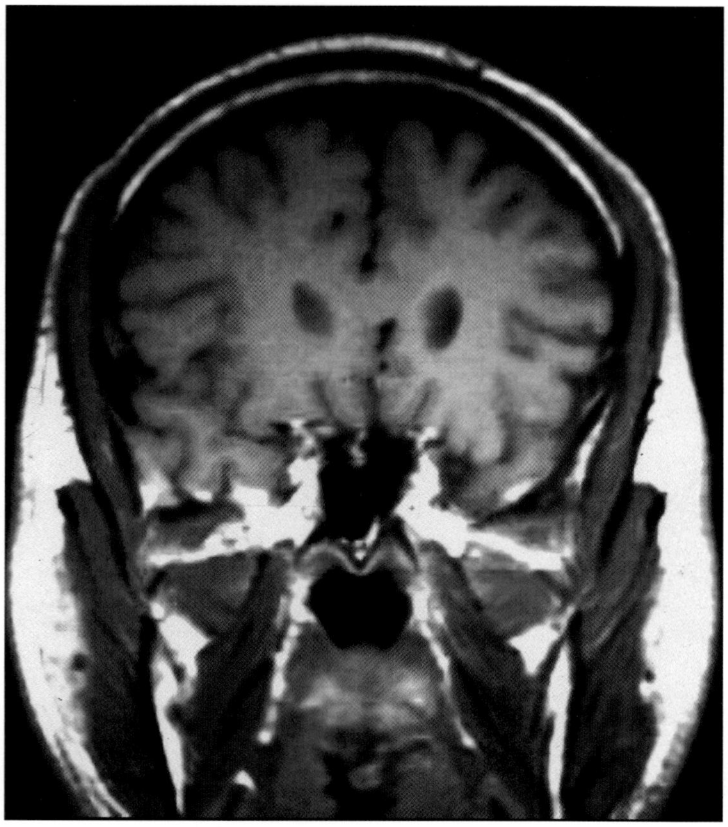

TR = 550 msec, TE = 15 msec

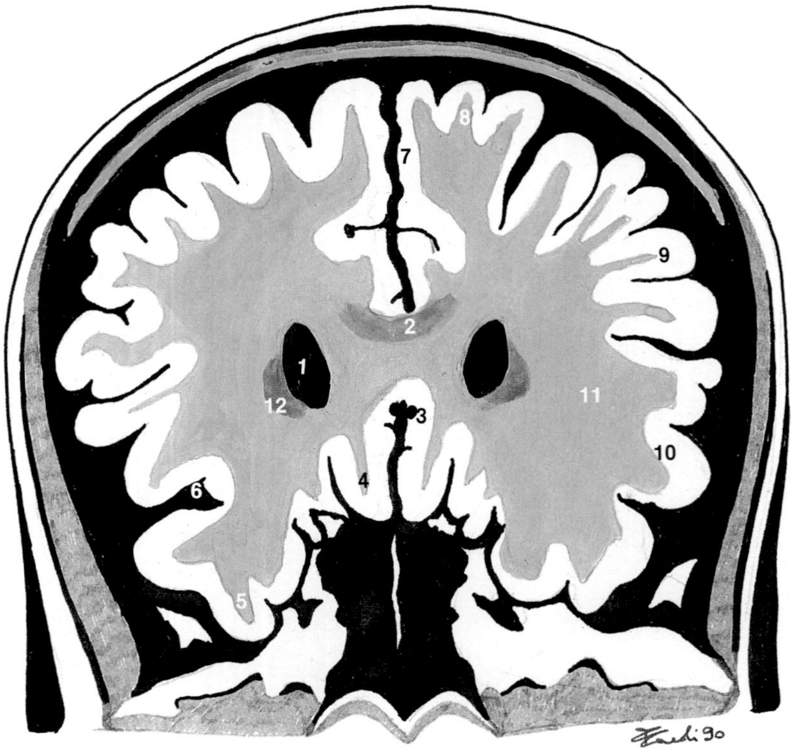

Fig. 18
1) frontal horn of the lateral ventricles
2) corpus callosum
3) anterior cerebral artery
4) gyrus rectus
5) pole of the temporal lobe
6) Sylvian fissure
7) interhemispheric fissure
8) superior frontal gyrus
9) medial frontal gyrus
10) inferior frontal gyrus
11) white matter
12) head of the caudate nucleus

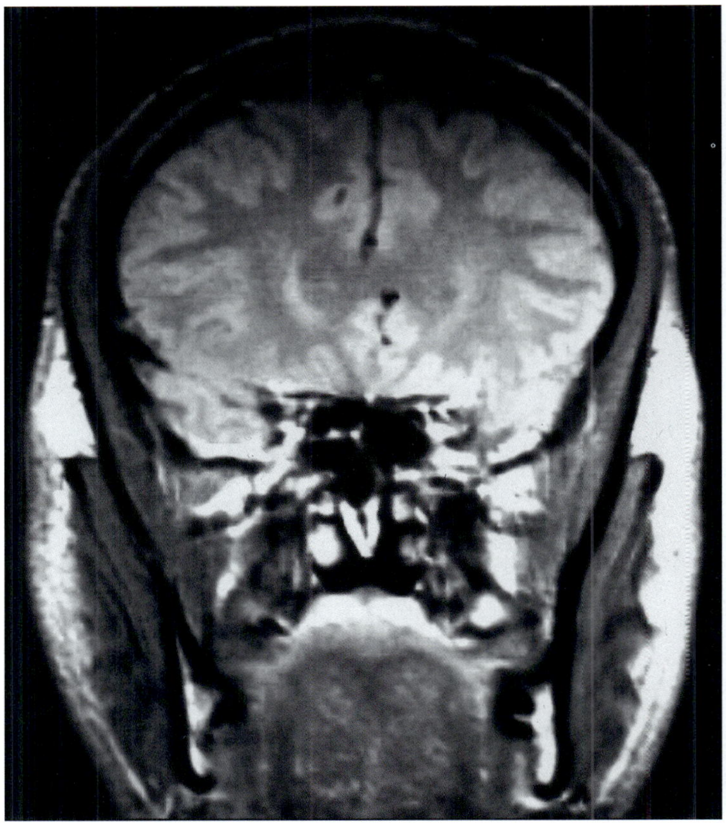

TR = 2,500 msec, TE = 15 msec

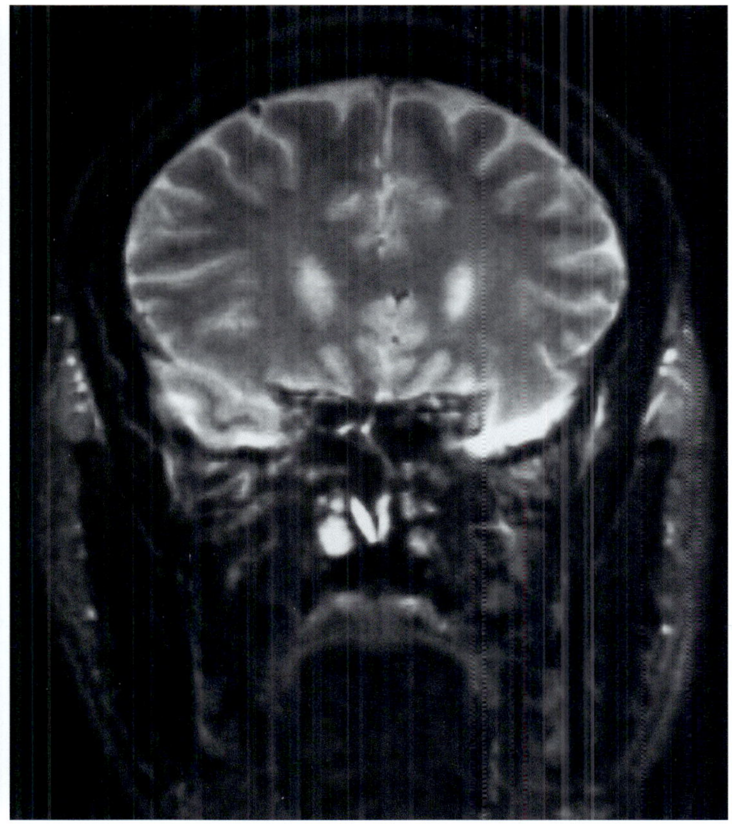

TR = 2,500 msec, TE = 90 msec

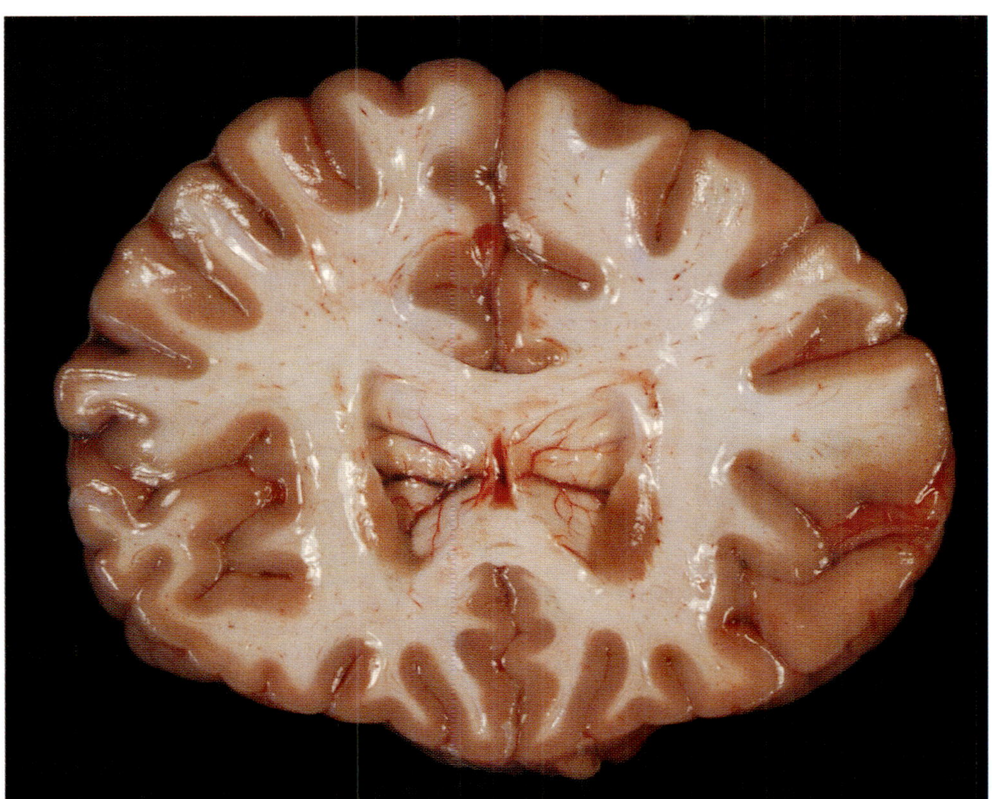

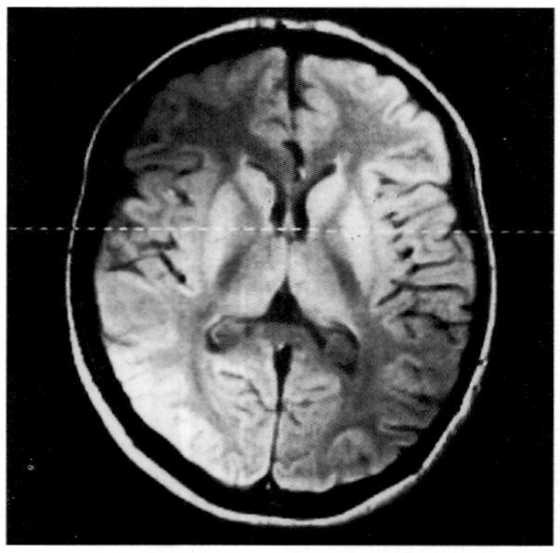

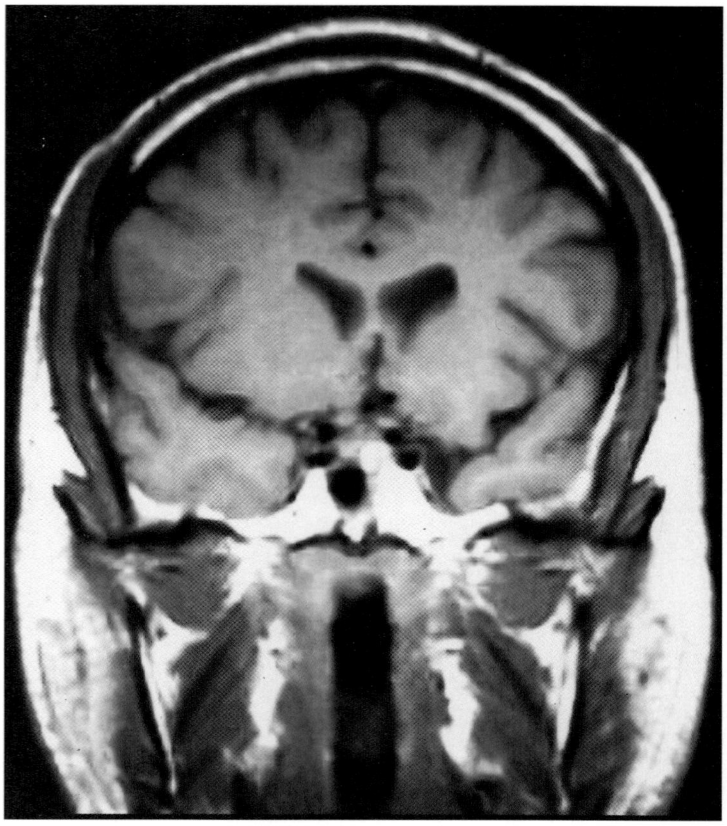

TR = 550 msec, TE = 15 msec

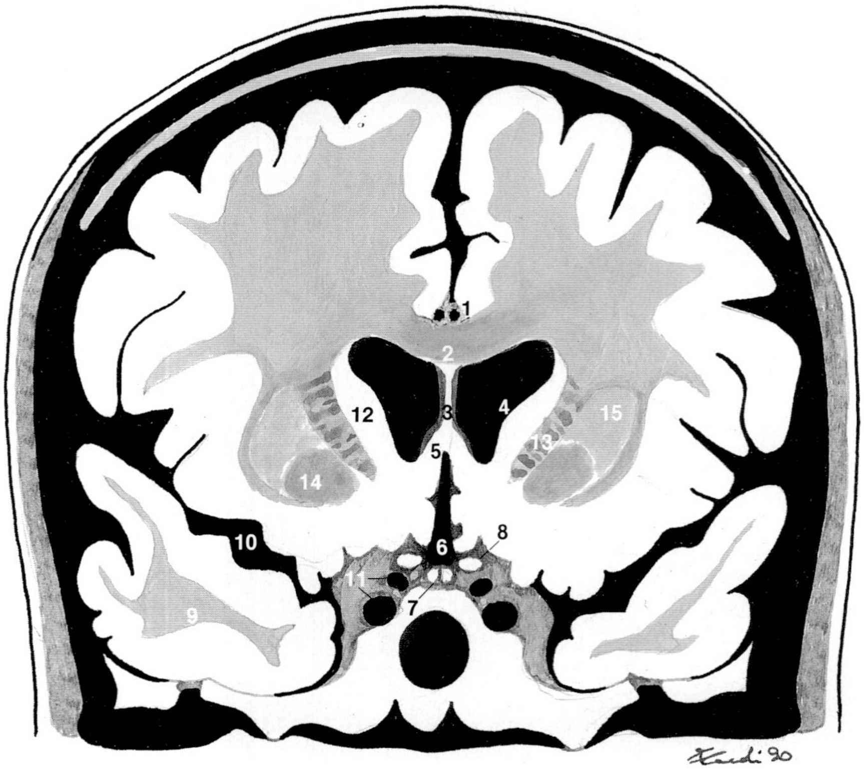

Fig. 19
1) pericallosal artery
2) corpus callosum
3) septum pellucidum
4) frontal horn of the lateral ventricle
5) fornix
6) anteroinferior part of the 3rd ventricle
7) olfactory nerve
8) optic nerve (T_1) – chiasm (T_2)
9) temporal lobe
10) Sylvian fissure
11) intracavernous portion of the internal carotid artery
12) head of the caudate nucleus
13) anterior arm of the internal capsule
14) globus pallidus
15) putamen

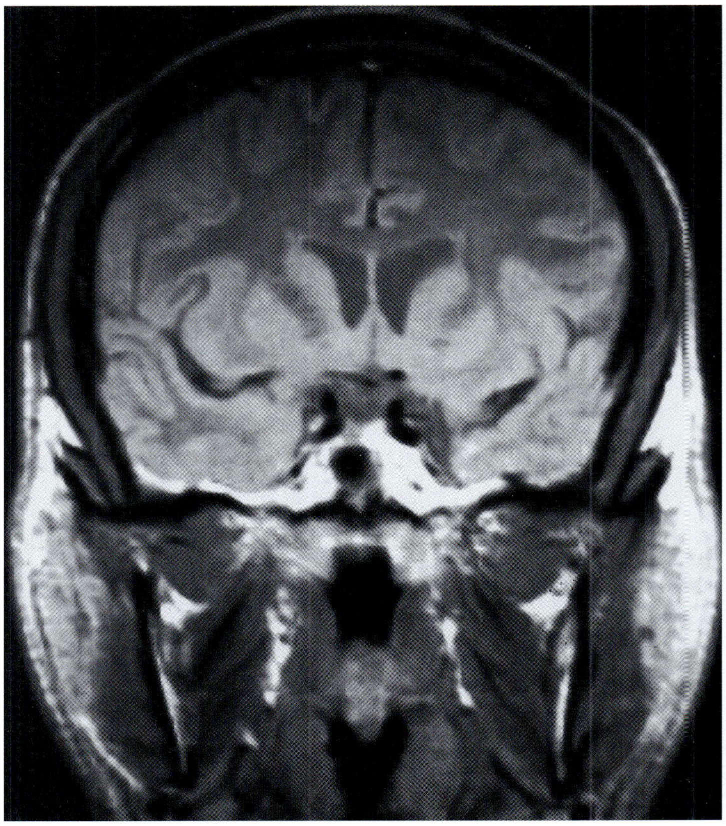

TR = 2,500 msec, TE = 15 msec

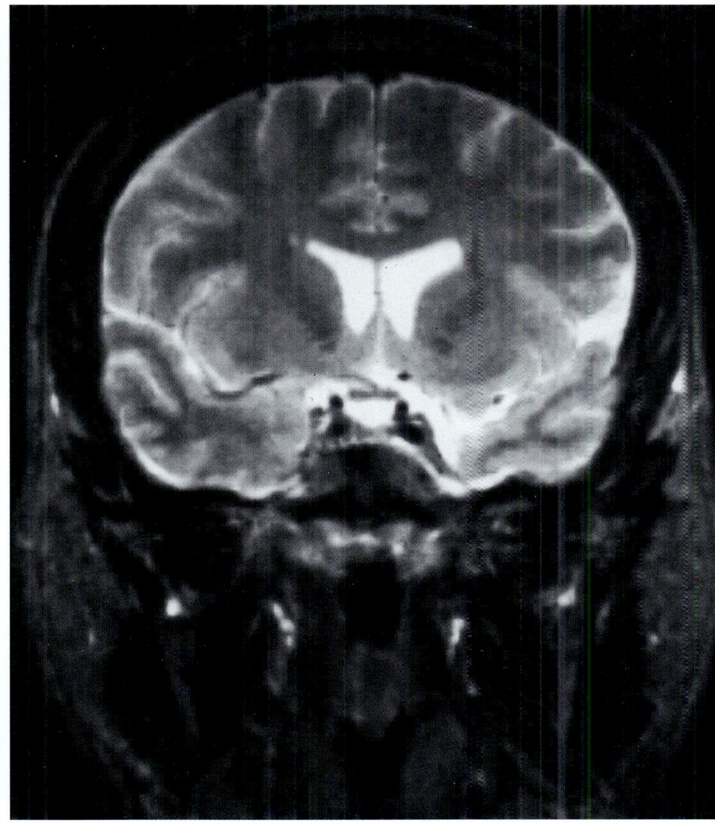

TR = 2,500 msec, TE = 90 msec

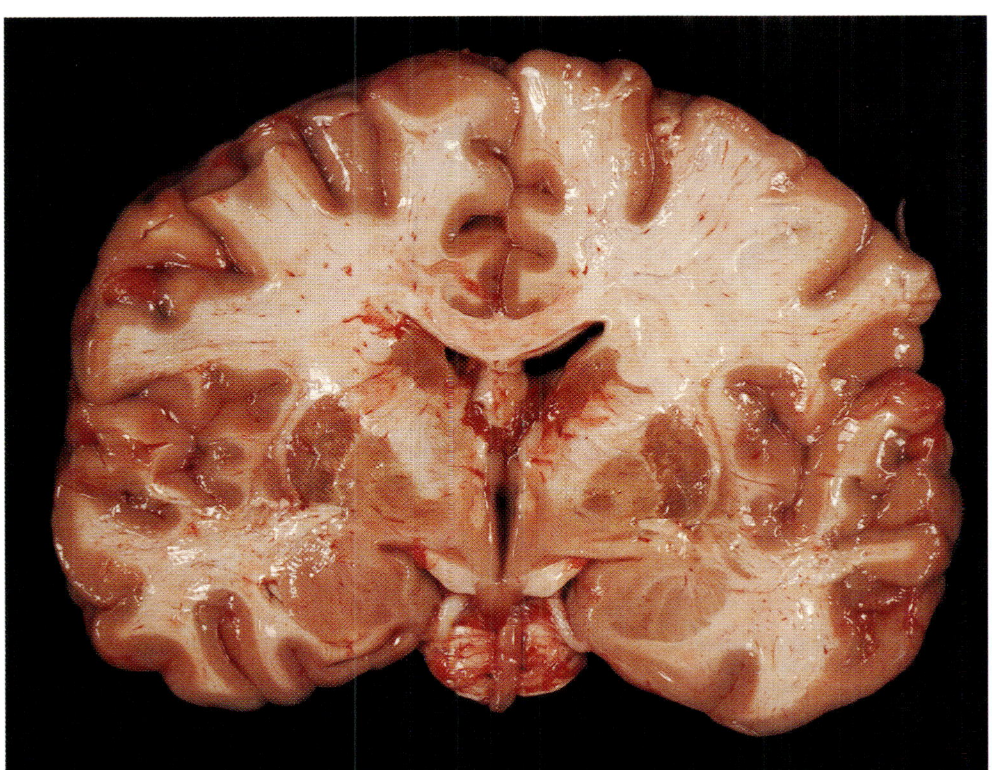

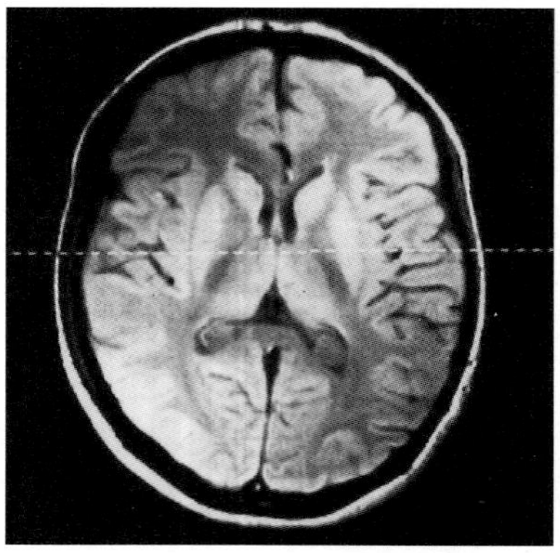

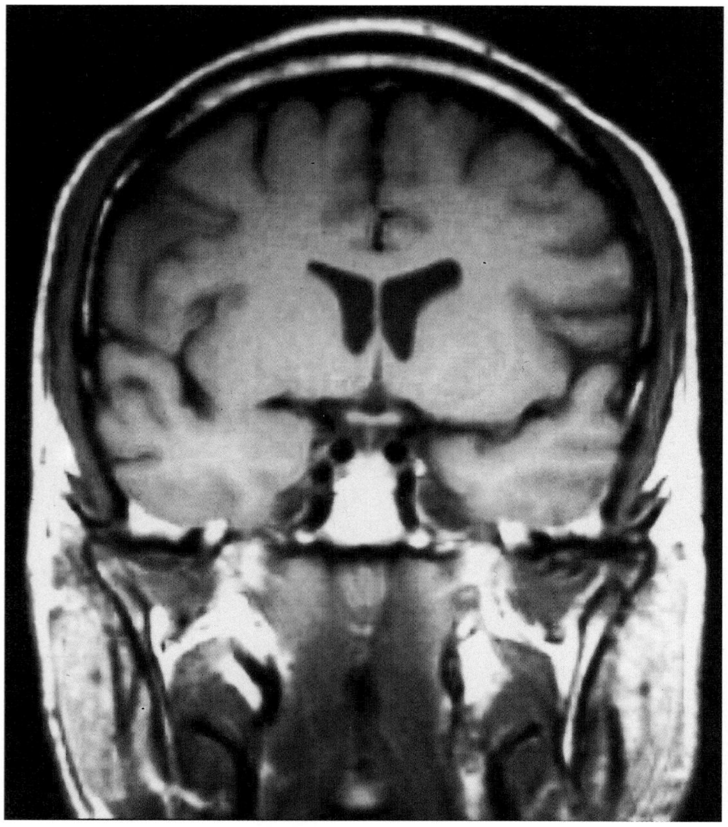

TR = 550 msec, TE = 15 msec

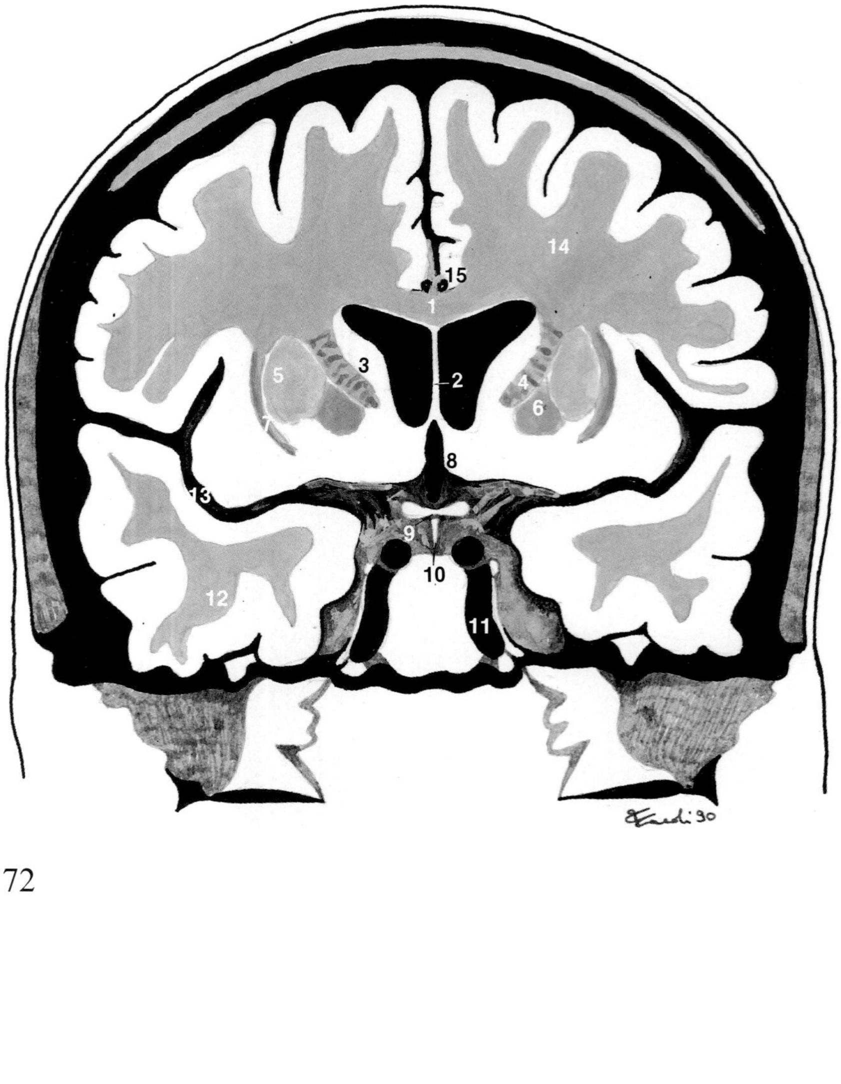

Fig. 20

1) corpus callosum
2) septum pellucidum
3) body of the caudate nucleus
4) knee of the internal capsule
5) putamen
6) globus pallidus
7) external capsule
8) hippocampus
9) chiasm (T_1) – optic tracts (T_2)
10) pituitary stalk
11) intrapetrosal portion of the internal carotid artery
12) temporal lobe
13) Sylvian fissure with the middle cerebral artery
14) corona radiata
15) pericallosal arteries

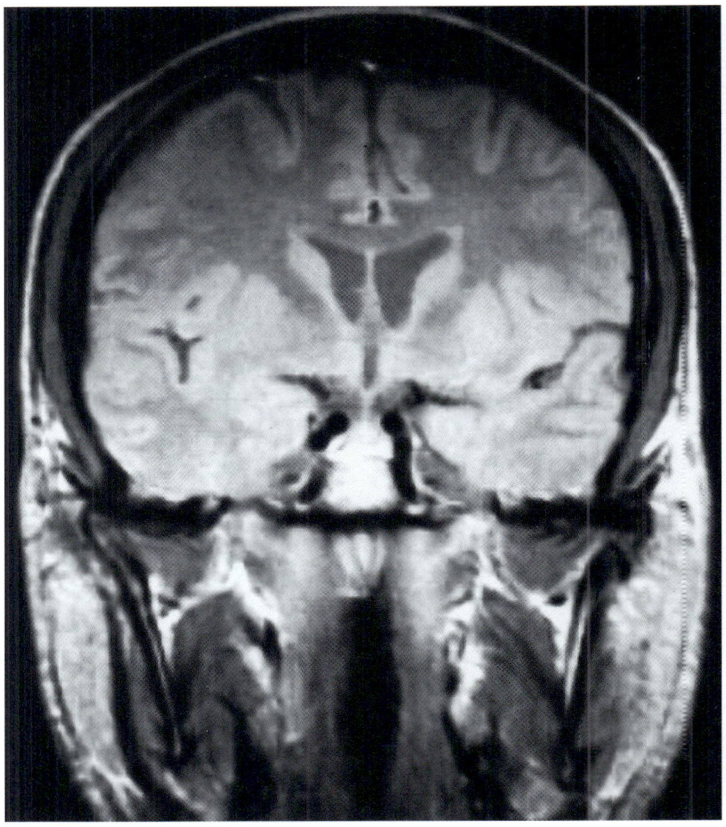

TR = 2,500 msec, TE = 15 msec

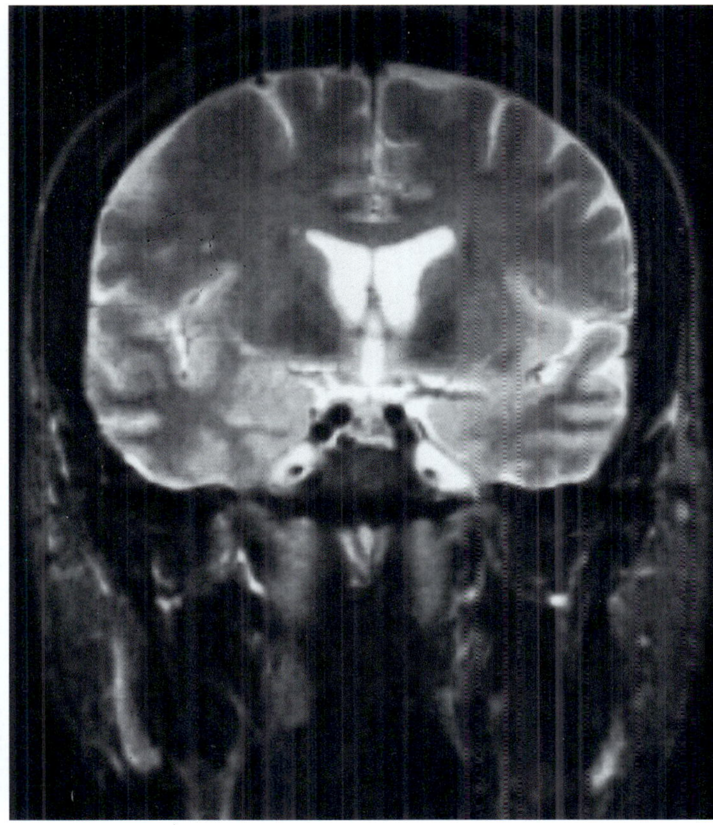

TR = 2,500 msec, TE = 90 msec

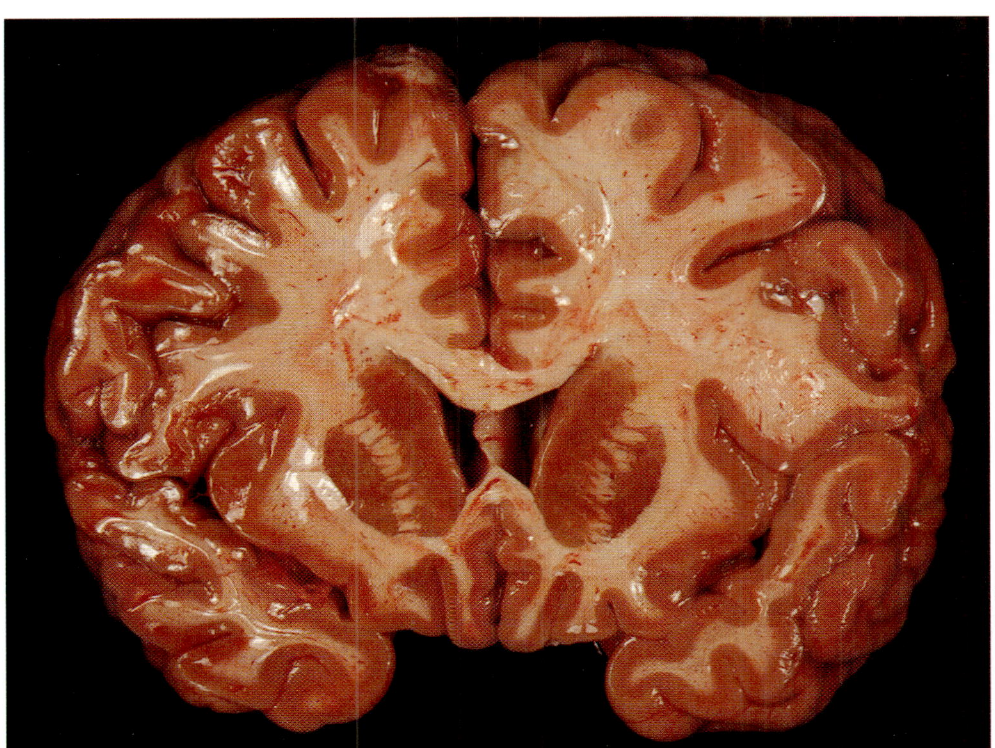

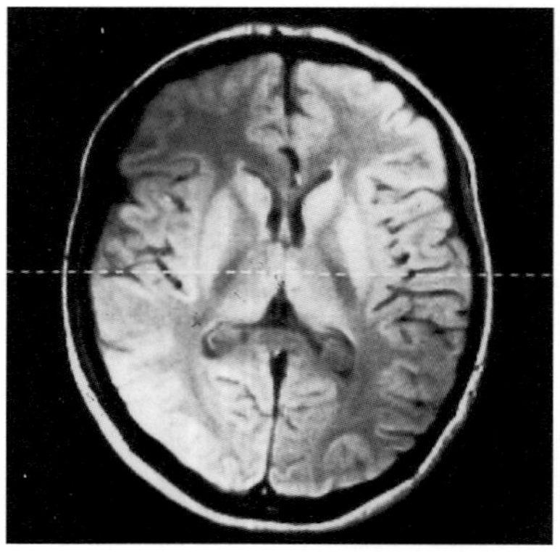

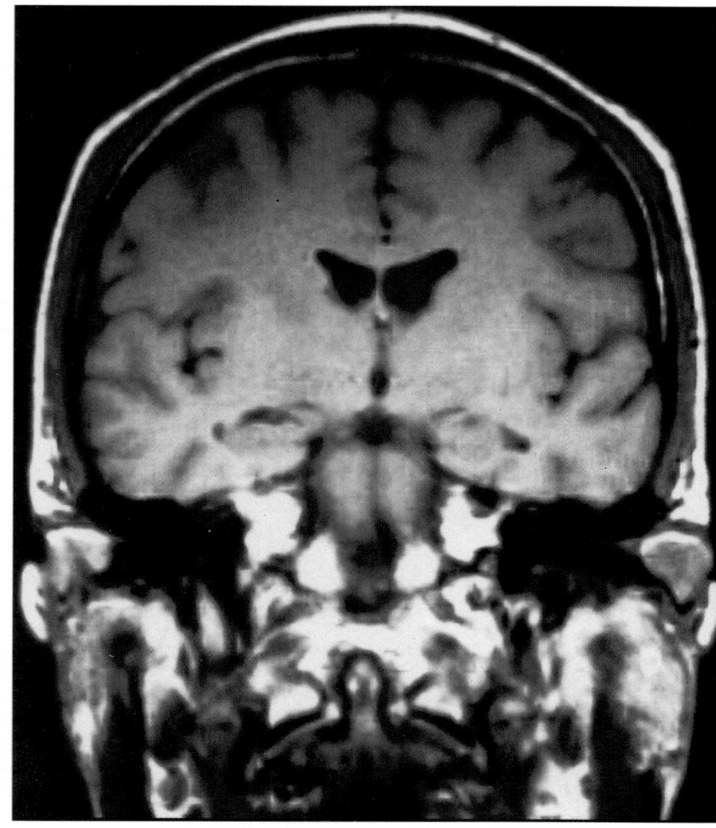

TR = 550 msec, TE = 15 msec

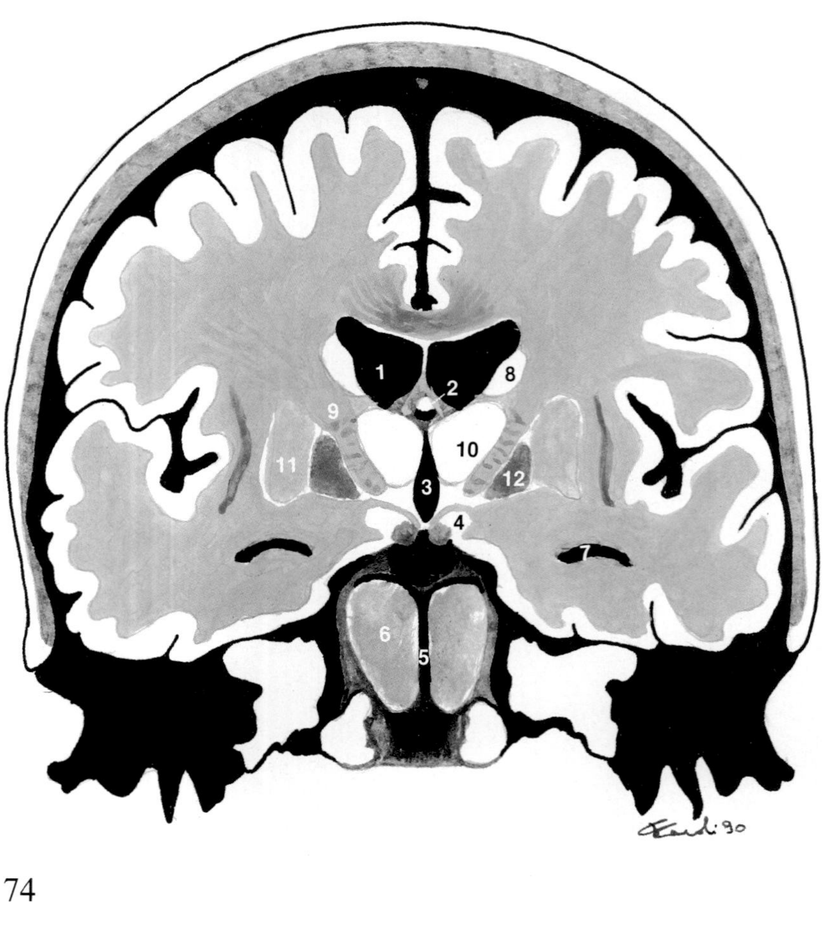

Fig. 21

1) lateral ventricle
2) fornix
3) 3rd ventricle
4) mammillary bodies
5) basilar artery and posterior cerebral arteries
6) pons
7) temporal horn of the lateral ventricle
8) tail of the caudate nucleus
9) internal capsule
10) thalamus
11) putamen
12) globus pallidus

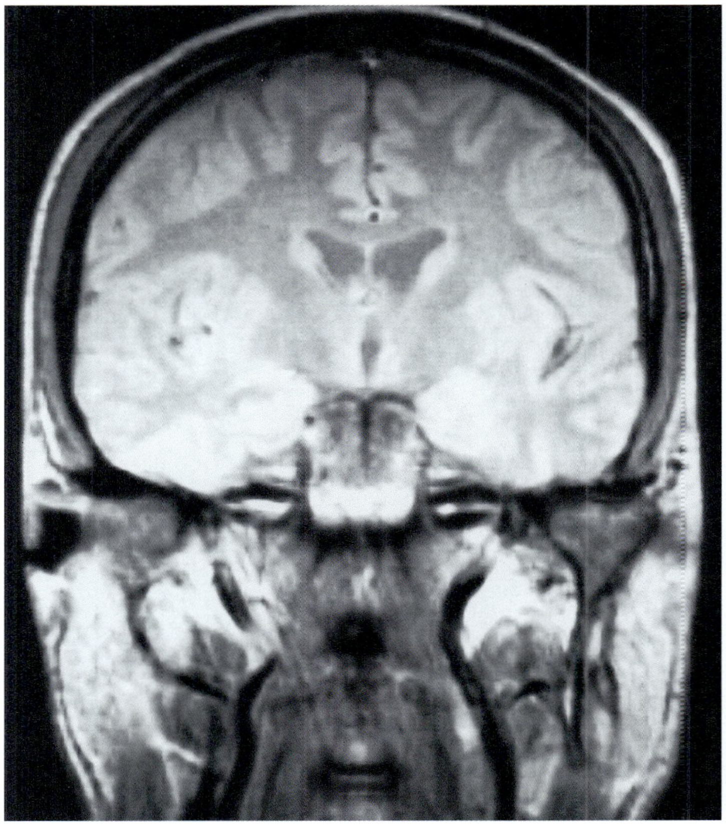

TR = 2,500 msec, TE = 15 msec

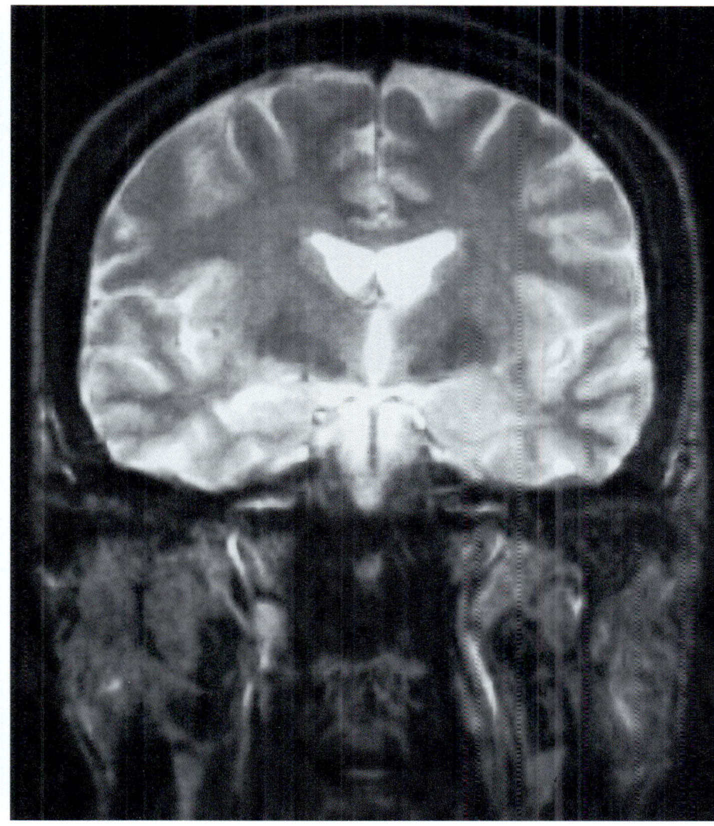

TR = 2,500 msec, TE = 90 msec

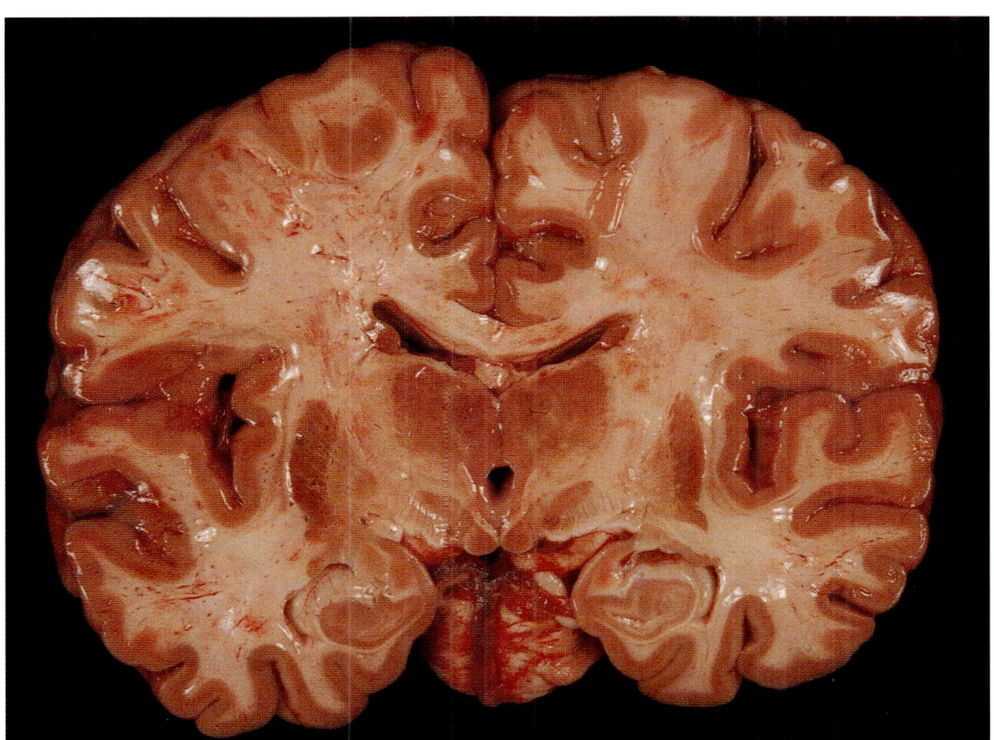

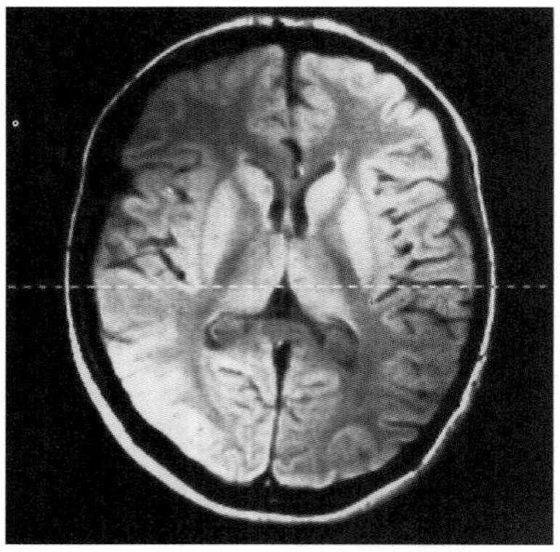

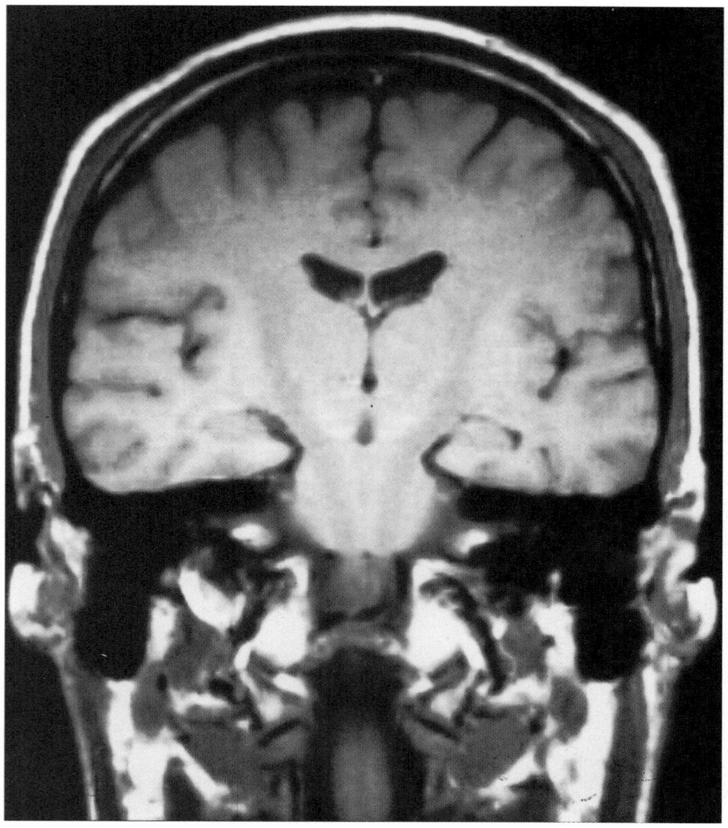

TR = 550 msec, TE = 15 msec

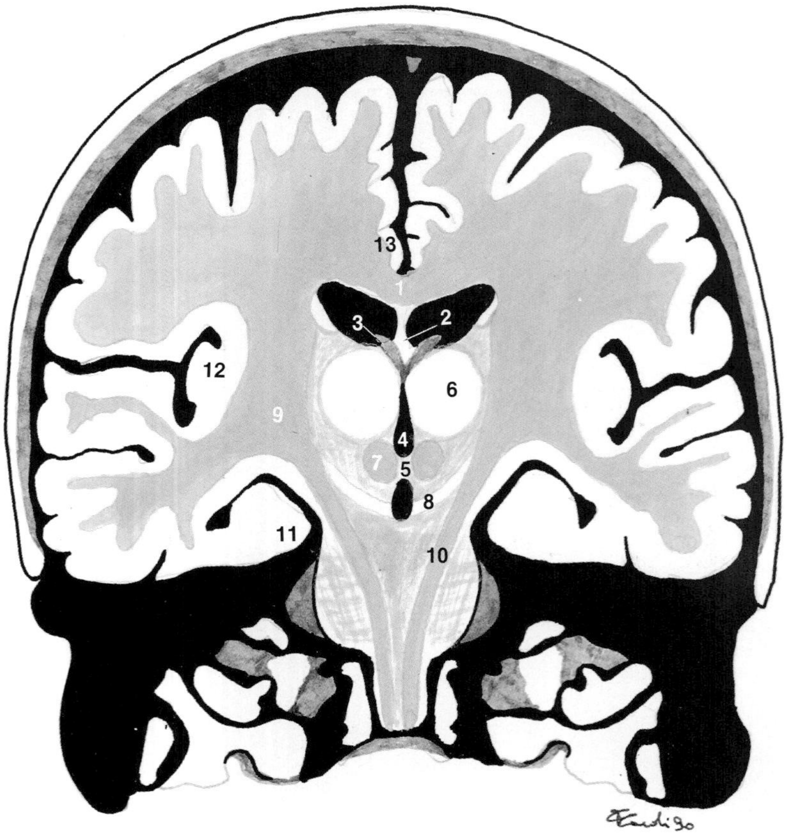

Fig. 22

1) corpus callosum
2) fornix
3) Monro's foramina
4) 3rd ventricle
5) massa intermedia
6) thalamus
7) red nucleus
8) substantia nigra
9) posterior arm of the internal capsule
10) cerebral peduncle – pyramidal tract
11) uncus hippocampi
12) insula
13) cingulate gyrus

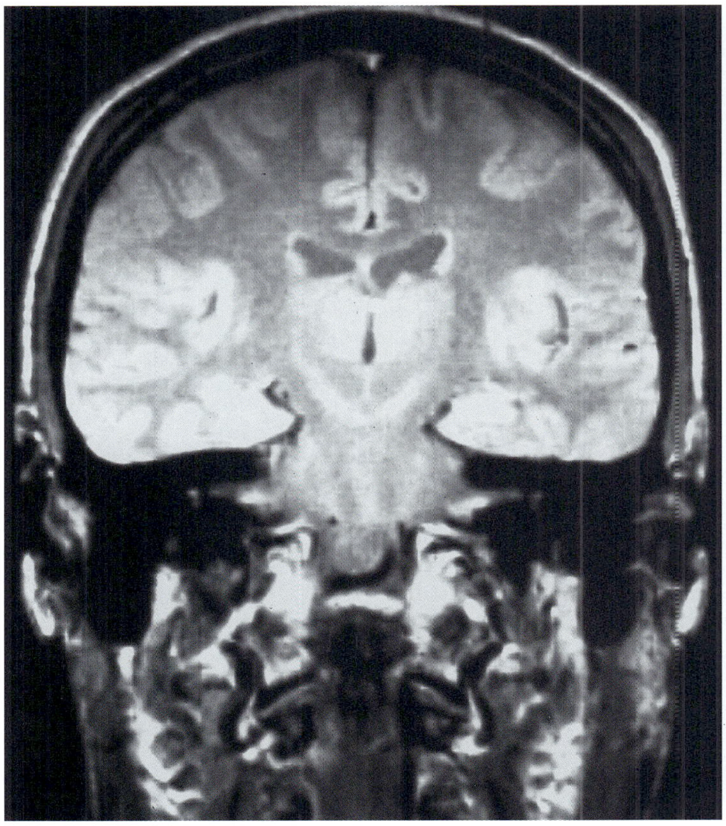

TR = 2,500 msec, TE = 15 msec

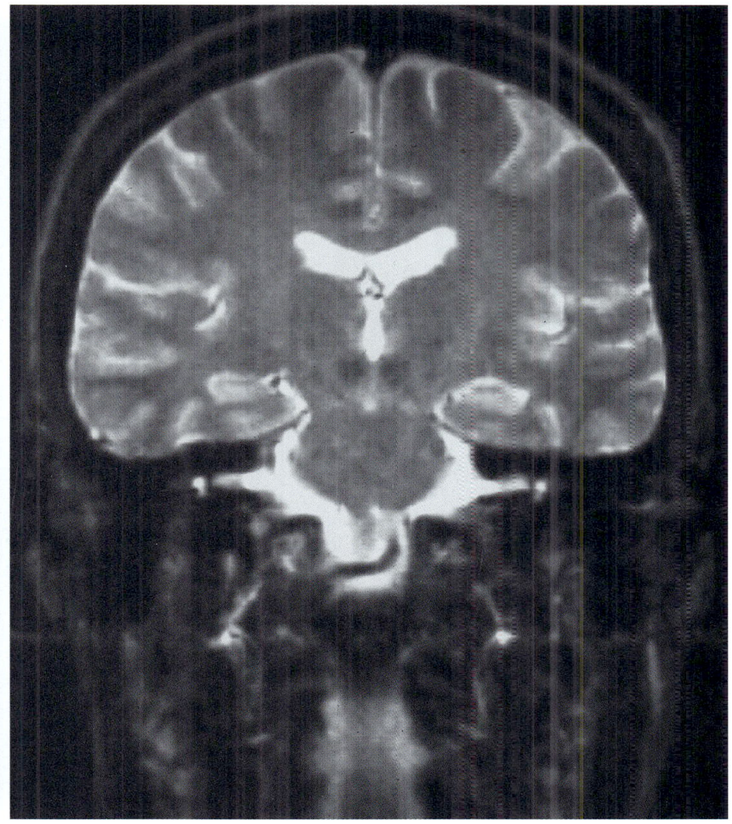

TR = 2,500 msec, TE = 90 msec

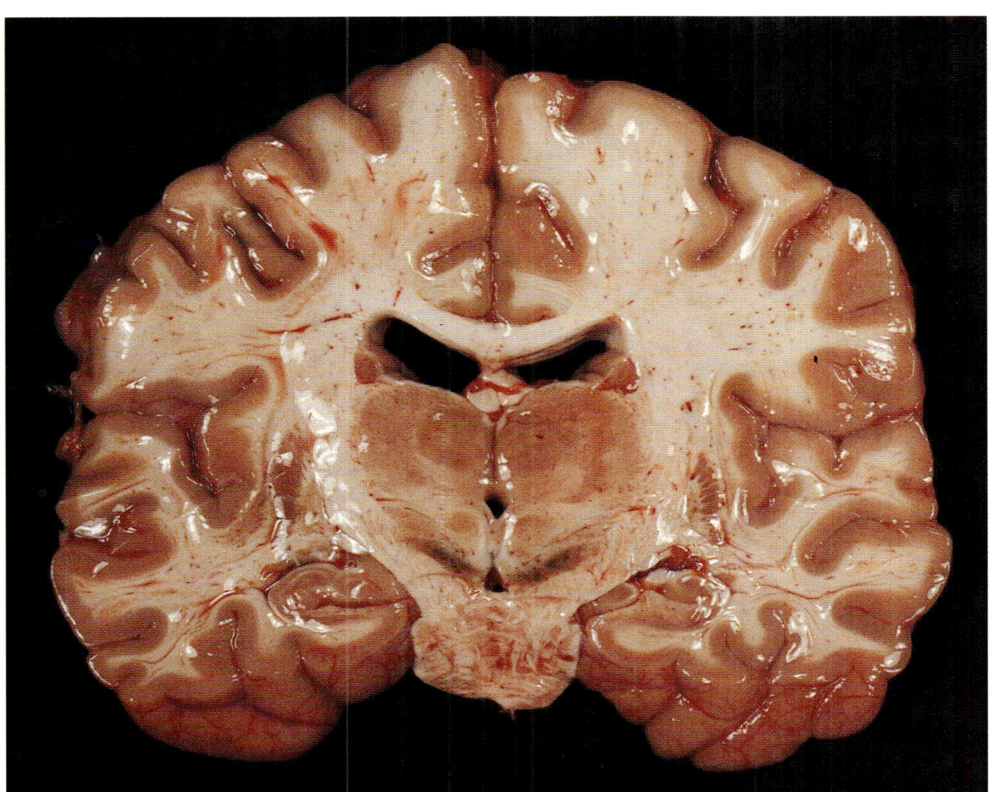

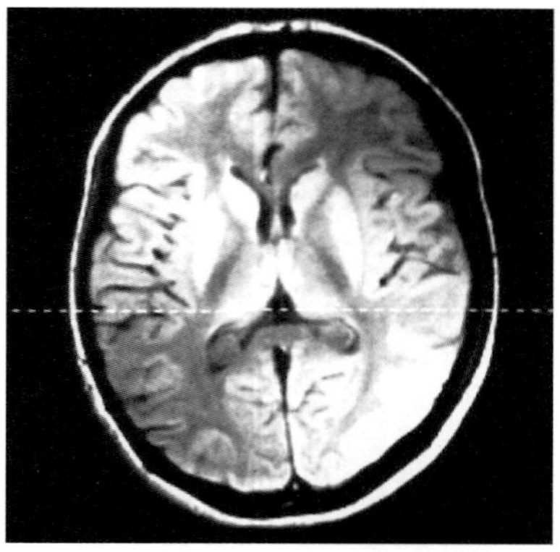

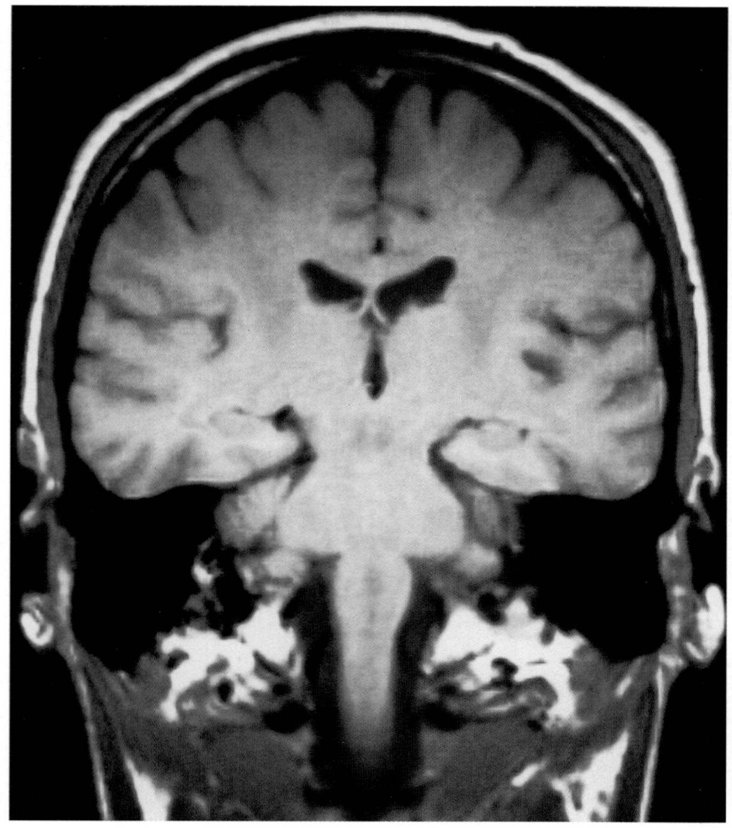

TR = 550 msec, TE = 15 msec

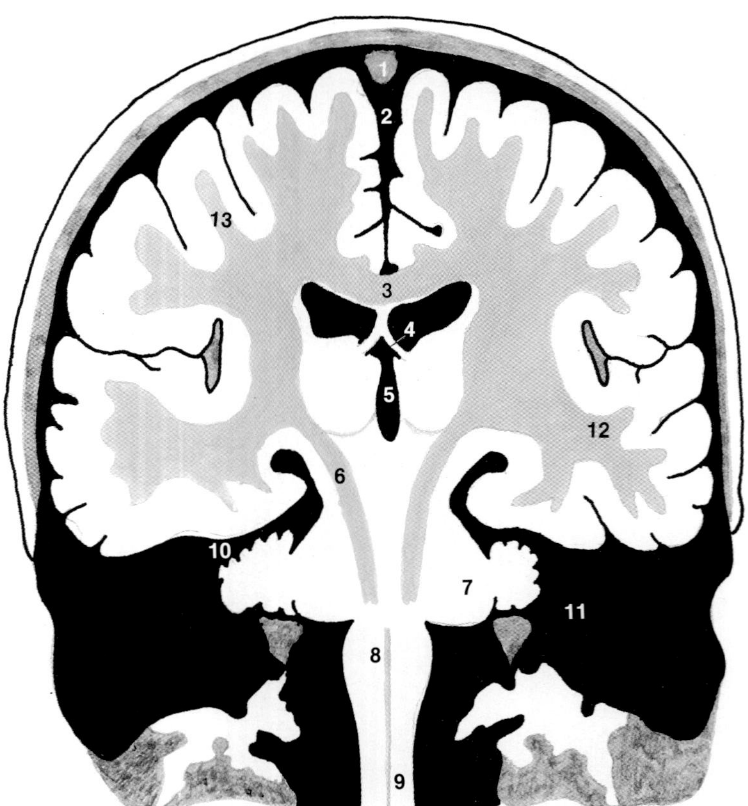

Fig. 23
1) superior sagittal sinus
2) interhemispheric fissure
3) corpus callosum
4) fornix
5) 3rd ventricle
6) cerebral peduncle
7) pons
8) bulb
9) ependymal canal
10) tentorium
11) petrous bone
12) posterior horn of the temporal lobe
13) parietal lobe

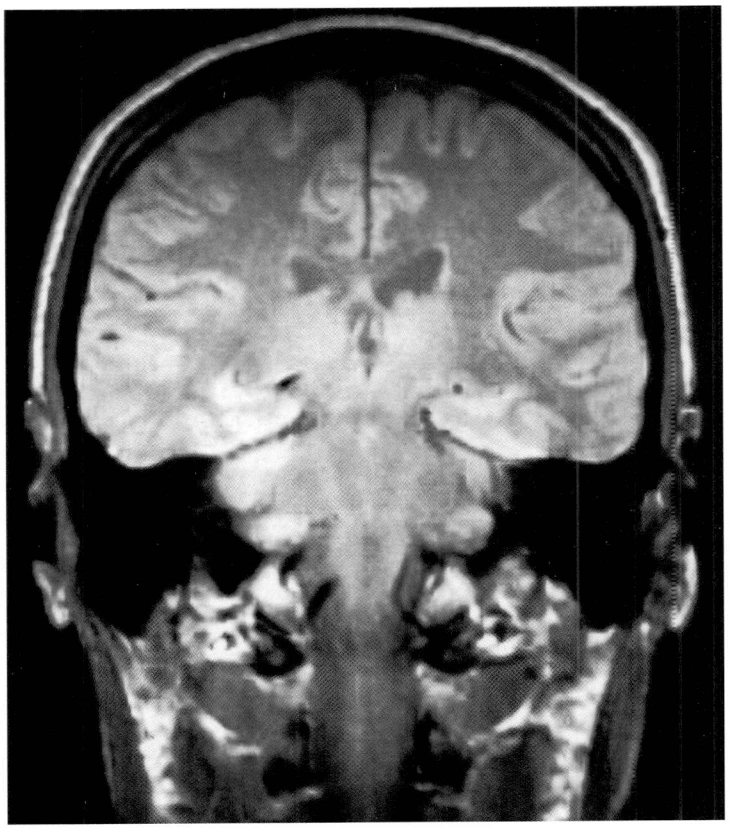

TR = 2,500 msec, TE = 15 msec

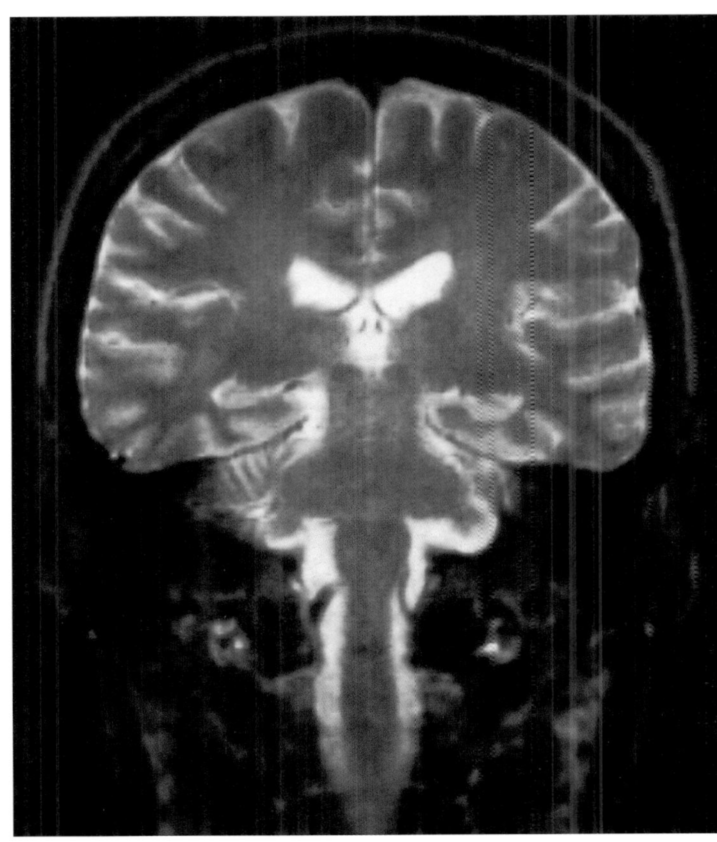

TR = 2,500 msec, TE = 90 msec

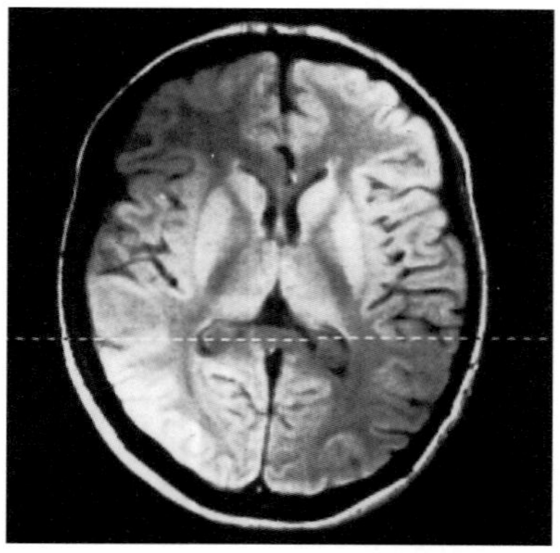

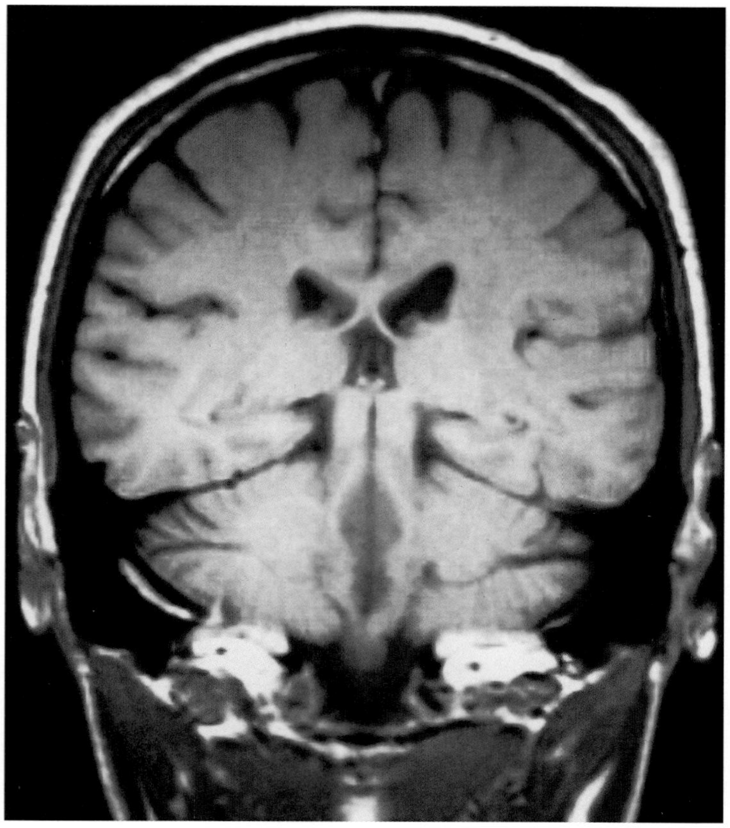

TR = 550 msec, TE = 15 msec

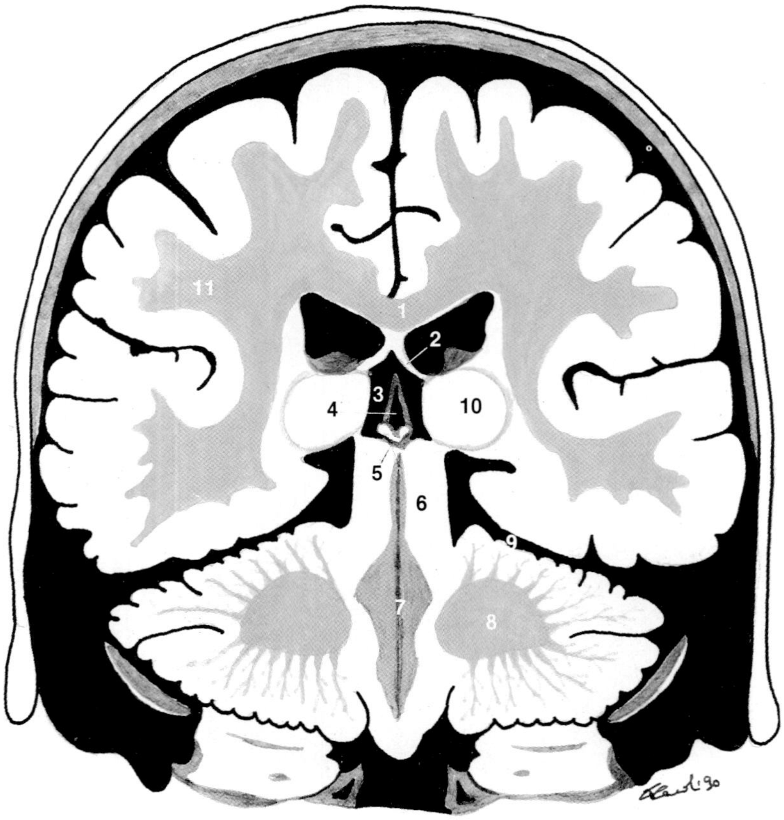

Fig. 24

1) splenium of the corpus callosum
2) fornix
3) posterior part of the 3rd ventricle
4) Galen's vein
5) pineal gland
6) Sylvian aqueduct
7) 4th ventricle
8) cerebellar lobes
9) tentorium
10) pulvinar
11) parietal lobe

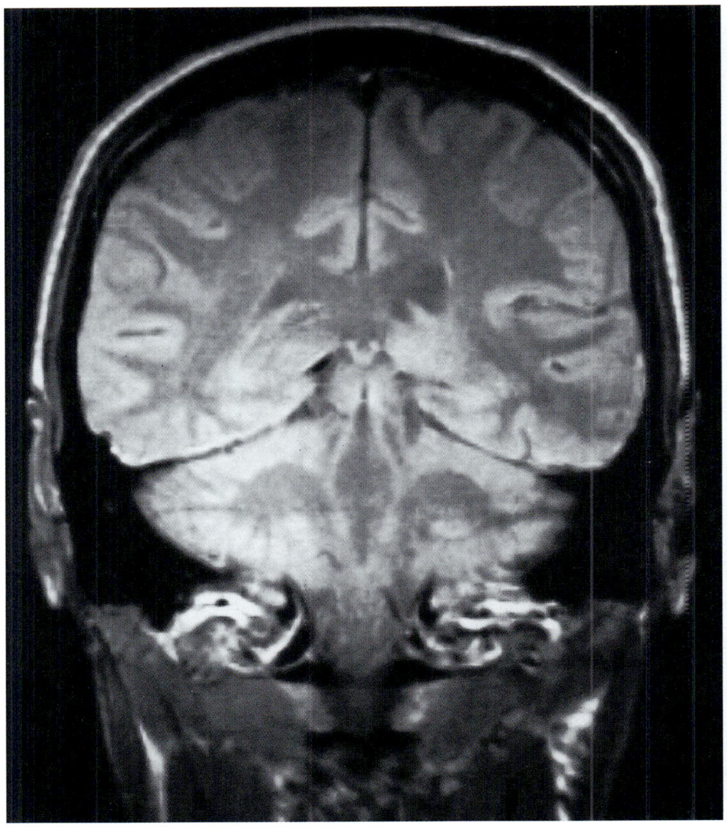

TR = 2,500 msec, TE = 15 msec

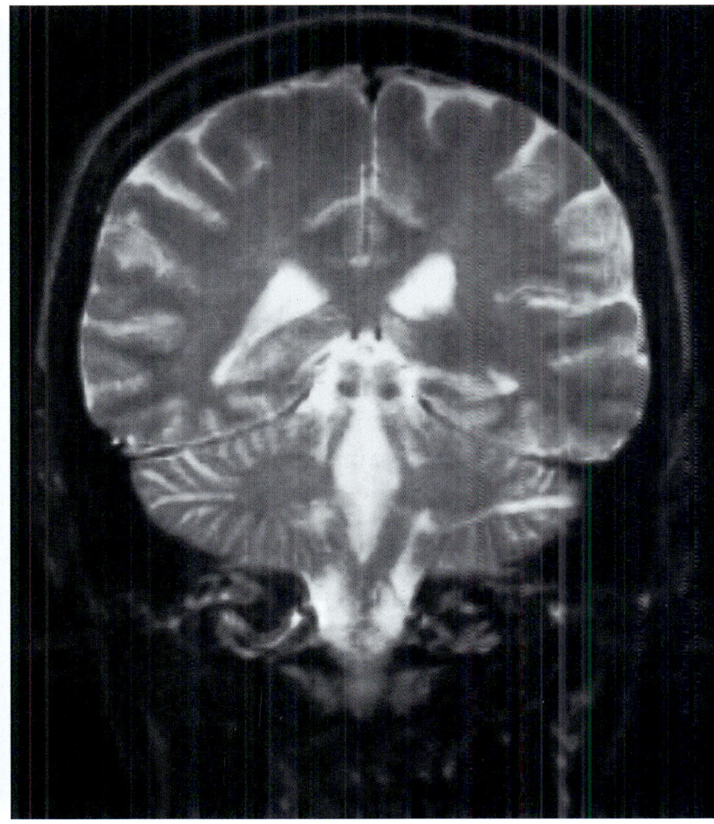

TR = 2,500 msec, TE = 90 msec

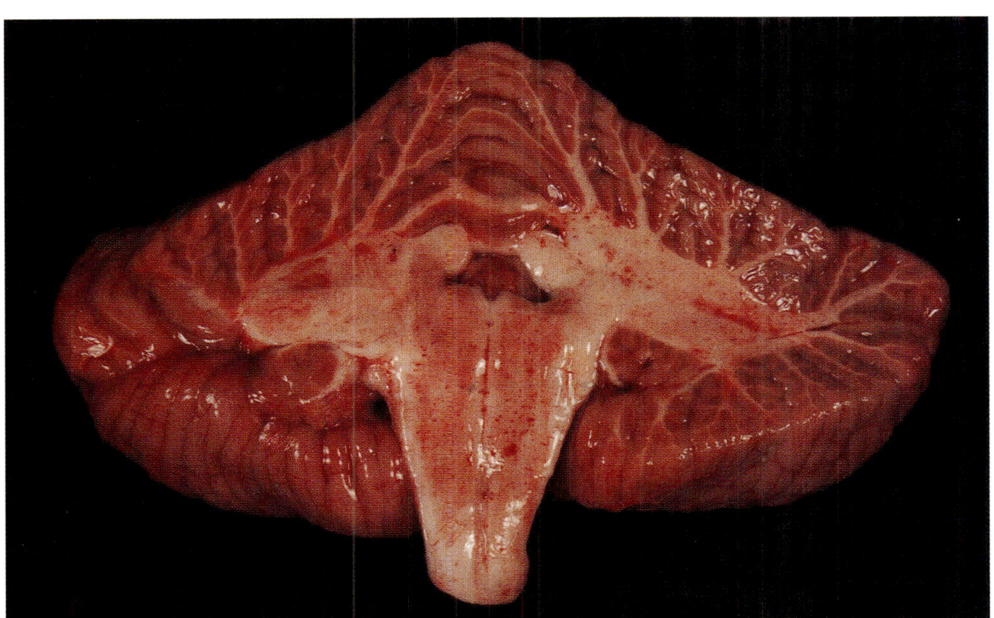

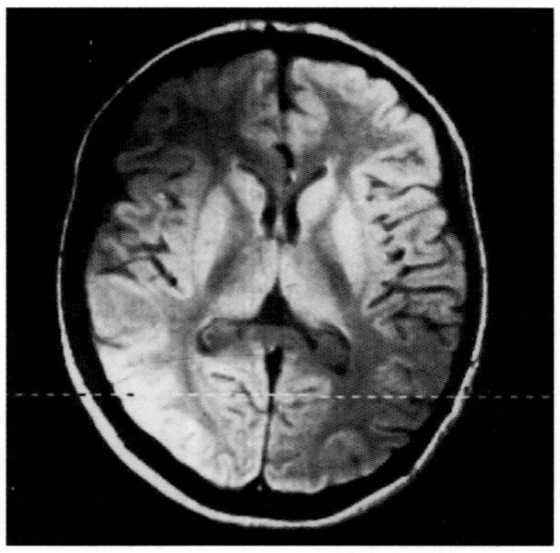

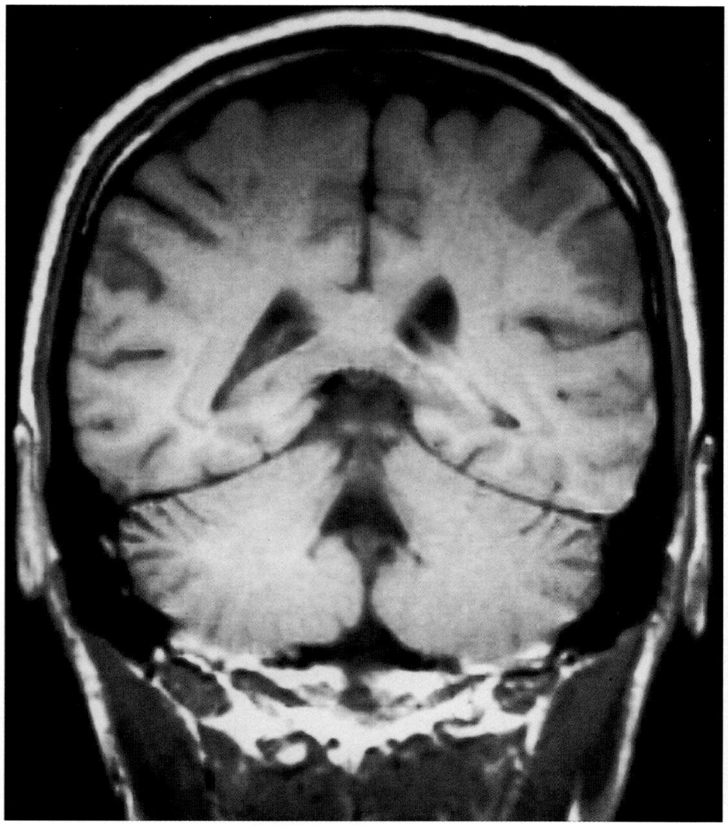

TR = 550 msec, TE = 15 msec

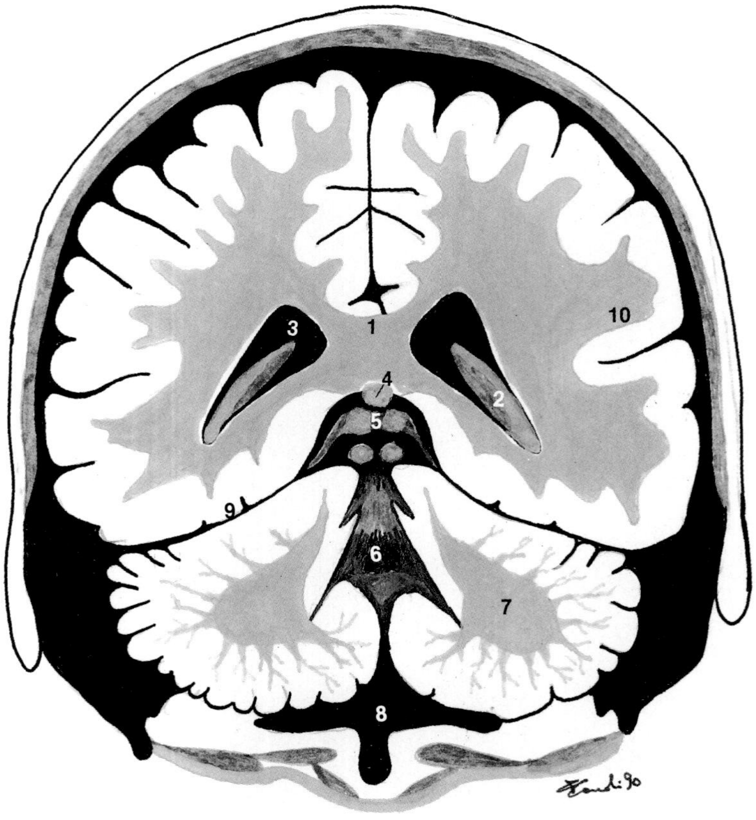

Fig. 25
1) splenium of the corpus callosum
2) choroid plexus
3) trigonum
4) pineal gland
5) quadrigeminal plate
6) 4th ventricle
7) cerebellar lobe
8) cisterna magna
9) tentorium
10) parietal lobe

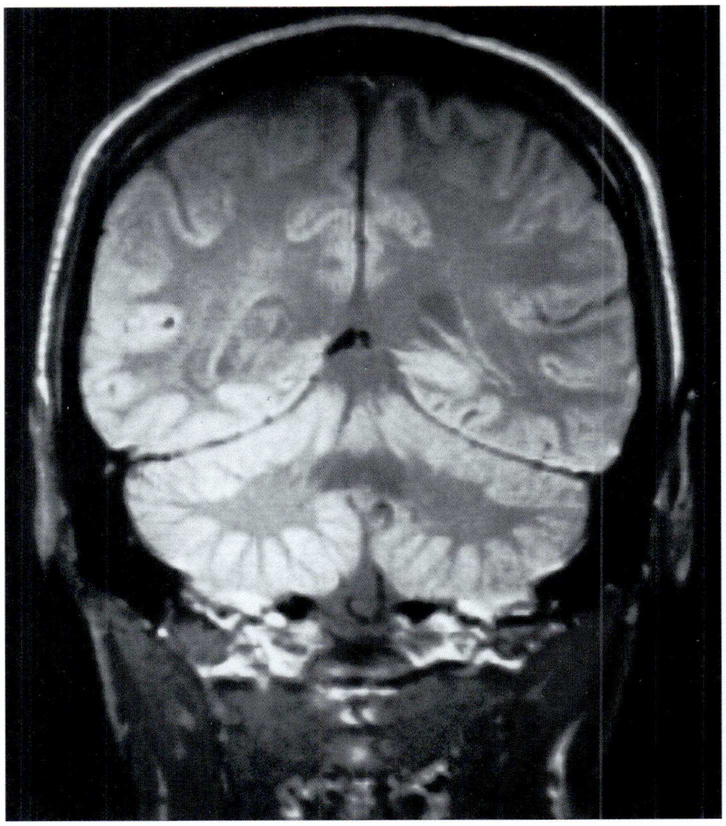

TR = 2,500 msec, TE = 15 msec

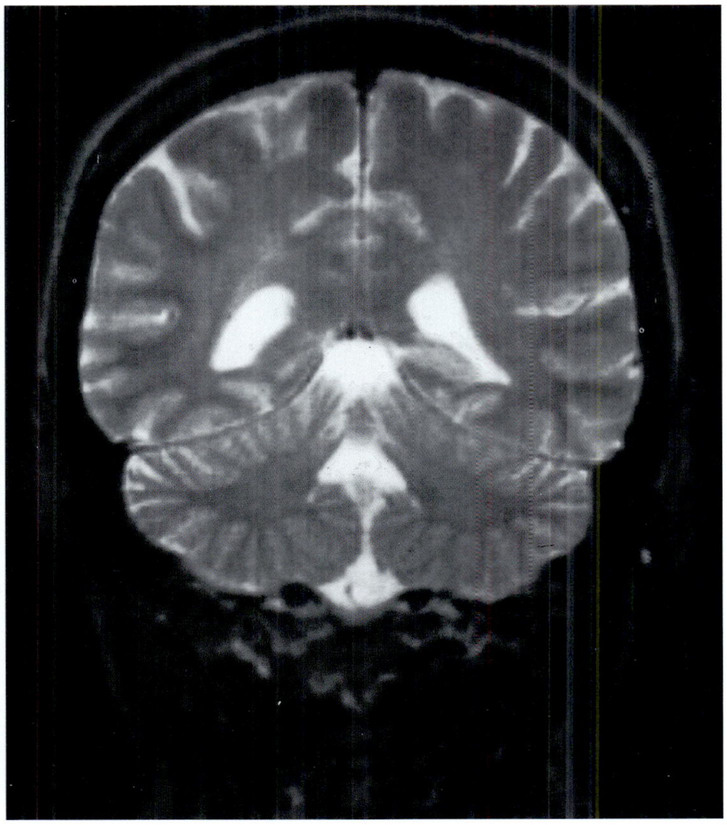

TR = 2,500 msec, TE = 90 msec

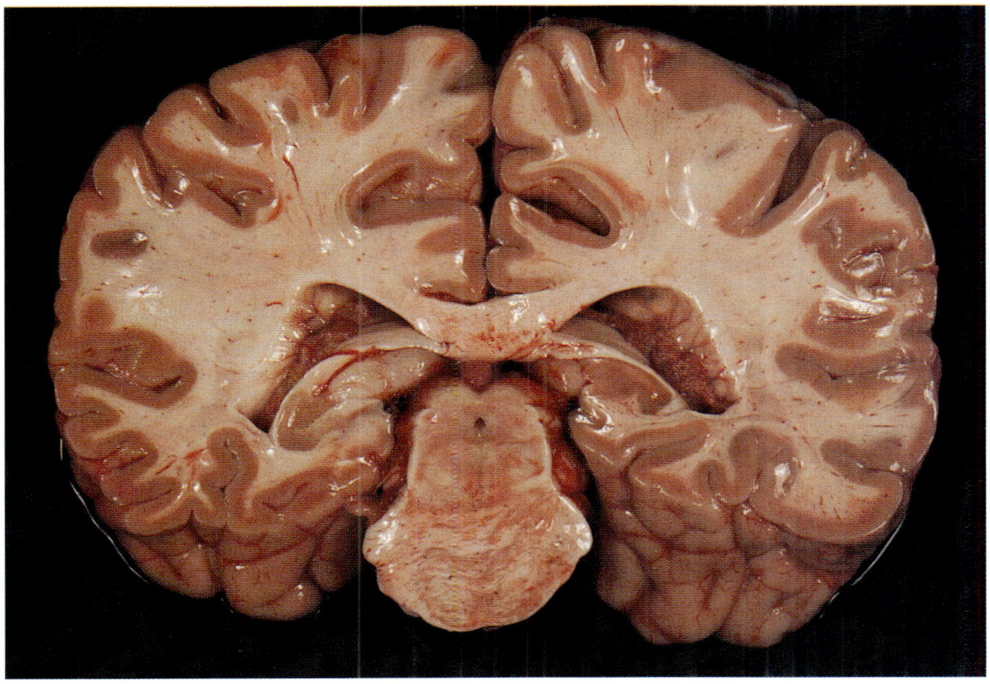

CHAPTER III

Classification of CNS tumors

The need for classifying CNS tumors in a standard way led WHO to set up study groups for tumor characterization. The resulting classification is based on the microscopic characteristics of oncotypes.

The difficulty in assigning these tumors to malignancy scales lies in the fact that their growth in a confined space causes fatal events, regardless of their characteristics. This involves malignancy which is more clinical than histological. These events range from compression of vital structures to obstruction of the CSF flow with ensuing hypertensive hydrocephalus. The criteria applicable to oncotypes in other locations, such as tumor growth and metastasizing capability, are thus inapplicable to brain diseases. As a result, in addition to simple histologic and cytologic data, other factors were considered.

A retrospective analysis of the prognosis of some oncotypes allowed the malignancy findings, such as increased cellularity, mitosis, pleomorphism of tumor cells or of supporting tissues, necrosis, stromal reaction and presence of pathologic vessels to be substantiated or invalidated.

Nevertheless, some of these findings, especially in the group of neuroepithelial tumors, are not associated with malignancy. Absence of clear demarcation owing to invasion of the surrounding tissue is not always combined with cellular anaplasia and clinical malignancy (e.g. fibrillary astrocytoma). Infiltration of the leptomeninges may be present, without however signalling malignancy, such as in pilocytic astrocytomas. Metastases via the CSF pathway, which are often associated with malignant tumors (medulloblastoma), may be found in some cases of oligodendroglioma. Let us refer to the WHO CNS tumor classification, to which we will add some short explanatory notes for greater understanding, referring the readers to specific texts of neuropathology for the study of the individual oncotypes and in part to the introductory sections of the following chapters.

For neuroepithelial tumors, the term anaplasia includes findings of malignant biological behavior, such as increased cellularity, mitosis, absence of cellular differentiation, vascular proliferation. This malignant behavior translates into rapid growth, invasion of the parenchyma and possibility of metastases.

As to astrocytomas, the first three (fibrillary, protoplasmic and gemistocytic) correspond to Grade II of the old Kernohan classification. The gemistocytic astrocytoma is the one which most frequently shows areas of anaplasia. The pilocytic astrocytoma (Grade I) encompasses the juvenile pilocytic astrocytoma, the so-called "glioma" of the optic nerve and the cerebellar (cystic or solid) astrocytoma. The term "primary polar spongioblastoma", which was previously used to indicate pilocytic astrocytomas, is used in the present classification to identify a very rare tumor occurring in childhood and adolescence, characterized by uni- or bipolar cells and histologically corresponding to Grade IV.

Oligodendrogliomas of the "pure" variety correspond to Grade I, but more frequently to Grade II, such as the "mixed" oligoastrocytoma variety; the anaplastic type is equivalent to Grade III.

Among ependymomas, the mixopapillary, papillary and subependymoma types correspond to Grade I, the anaplastic type to Grades III–IV. Among other tumor types, the papilloma of the choroid plexus and the gangliocytoma belong to Grade I.

It is worth pointing out that the neuroepithelial tumor classification defines the basic oncotype according to its dominant cell type. Therefore, within the same tumor, combinations of different cell types can be found.

In the group of meningeal tumors, the hemangiopericytic and papillary meningiomas are malignant due to their faster growth and more frequent early recurrences.

The class of malignant primary tumors also includes lymphomas, microgliomas, reticulosarcomas, diffuse periadventitial sarcomas and other types of brain lymphomas.

The hemangioblastoma, a vascular tumor, can be differentiated microscopically from the hemangioblastic meningioma only through its location: the former is located in the cerebellum, brainstem and spine, while the latter occurs in the supratentorial compartment.

The less frequent tumors will be dealt with in the corresponding chapter (Chapter XI) together with nontumoral space-occupying lesions.

In childhood and adolescence, neuroepithelial tumors account for the majority of intracranial tumors and the subtentorial compartment is the most favorite location. In this region, the most common oncotypes are pilocytic astrocytomas and medulloblastomas, while less frequent tumors are ependymomas and papillomas of the choroid plexus. In childhood, midline gliomas (of the third ventricle and of the chiasm) and astrocytomas of the midbrain and of the pons cerebelli are reported.

In the first and second decades of life, other midline neoplasms are observed, such as teratomas, craniopharyngiomas and germinomas. In adulthood, astrocytomas and brain hemisphere oligodendrogliomas are more frequent. In this period of life, the subtentorial compartment may present hemangioblastomas and desmoplastic medulloblastomas. Glioblastomas have greater incidence in subsequent periods. In the last decades of life, metastases, meningiomas and neurinomas are also frequent. Unlike in adolescence, supratentorial tumors are more frequent in adults and in the aged.

As to location, some oncotypes have specific sites; others have favorite sites or are ubiquitous. Adenomas, pineocytomas and craniopharyngiomas, for instance, are recorded in a single site, whereas neurinomas have a predilection for the eighth pair of the cranial nerves. For favorite sites, the reader may refer to Table 2. Table 1, instead, compares ours with two of the leading brain tumor series reported in the literature.

In the Olivecrona series (5,250 cases), the term astrocytoma includes all neuroectodermal tumors, excluding the papillomas of the choroid plexus and neurinomas.

In the Zülch series, the class "other tumors" also encompasses nontumoral lesions and masses deriving from systemic diseases (arachnoidites, ependymites, parasitoses, myelomas, Hand-Schüller-Christian disease, etc.)

The high number of metastases in our cases is due to the type of hospital (cancer hospital) where our neurosurgical department operates.

A definition of the most frequent regressive events of CNS tumors completes this presentation. By evidencing these phenomena, MRI might add another piece to the spectrum of imaging techniques, which are drawing closer and closer to the characterization of oncotypes.

Necroses are due to abrupt vascular occlusions and are more frequent in malignant neuroepithelial tumors (glioblastomas). Small necrotic areas may be found also in oligodendrogliomas, whereas in other benign gliomas, cysts are more common.

Cysts arise from a process of mucoid degeneration. In some cases (cerebellar pilocytic astrocytoma and hemangioblastoma), the solid nodule is small if compared to the fluid component.

The cyst content changes with type of tumor. In craniopharyngiomas, for instance, it is dense, oily, brown-blackish with small cholesterin crystals. In hemangioblastomas, it is hemorrhagic and, after drainage punctures, it is resupplied by transudation. Cysts are therefore oncotype-specific and independent of tumor site (spinal, encephalic, intraventricular).

Calcification is a fairly frequent regressive event in CNS tumors. In oligodendrogliomas, calcifications are observed in the surrounding brain tissue, inside the tumor and in the capillary system of the cortex, because the calcification occurs inside the vessels. Other tumors with reported calcifications are gangliocytomas and ependymomas. In meningiomas, psammomatous masses are found: these are calcareous incrustations of cell nests.

Table 1. Surgical series of the Division of Neurosurgery, Istituto Regina Elena, Rome, and comparison with two of the major series in the literature.

	Olivecrona (5250 cases)	Zülch (6000 cases)		Isto. Reg. Elena (1417 cases)	
ASTROCYTOMAS	46.5	381	6.4	245	17.3
PILOCYTIC ASTROCYTOMAS		419	7.0	74	5.2
OLIGODENDROGLIOMAS		490	8.2	31	2.2
EPENDYMOMAS		259	4.3	24	1.7
PAPILLOMAS OF THE CHOROID PLEXUS	0.3	30	0.5	2	0.1
PINEALOMAS		25	0.4	15	0.4
GANGLIOCYTOMAS		27	0.4	3	0.2
GLIOBLASTOMAS		738	12.3	168	11.9
MEDULLOBLASTOMAS		230	3.8	60	4.2
NEURINOMAS	8.0	451	7.6	37	2.6
MENINGIOMAS	19.2	1079	18.0	221	15.6
SARCOMAS		162	2.7	8	0.6
HEMANGIOBLASTOMAS	2.4	78	1.3	11	0.8
GERMINOMAS				6	0.4
TERATOMAS	0.3	14	0.2	2	0.1
CRANIOPHARYNGIOMAS	1.7	150	2.5	38	2.7
DERMOIDS AND EPIDERMOIDS	0.7	104	1.9	34	2.4
COLLOID CYSTS				5	0.4
LIPOMAS				4	0.3
CAVERNOUS ANGIOMAS				9	0.6
ANGIOMAS AND GIANT ANEURYSMS	7.0	151	2.5	56	4.0
PITUITARY ADENOMAS	8.5	478	8.0	84	5.9
CHORDOMAS				4	0.3
OSTEOMAS		4	0.1	6	0.4
METASTASES	3.4	242	4.0	201	14.2
UNCLASSIFIED AND OTHER TUMORS	2.0	459	7.6	79	5.5
TOTAL	100%	100%		100%	

Fat degeneration is typical of neurinomas and occurs as a result of necrobiosis of the tissue: it is recorded also in glioblastomas, at the boundaries of necrotic areas.

Massive intratumoral hemorrhages take place in glioblastomas and oligodendrogliomas. Also pituitary adenomas may show hemorrhages which occurred at different times. These events, which may often induce fast clinical deterioration, are due to the pathologic structure of the vessels.

MR images undoubtedly contribute to the pre-operative diagnosis of CNS tumors but may still be inconclusive. This is why Table 2 provides a grouping of the main oncotypes of the intracranial district, associating the data on signal intensity and on behavior after GD-DTPA with general characteristics, such as age, site, regressive processes, etc. The table is a prompt reference for the reader who needs an overall picture for diagnostic evaluation of CNS tumors.

Table 2. Guidelines for the differential diagnosis of the most frequent intracranial tumors

Oncotype	**Age of decades**	**Favorite sites**	**Characteristics of signal** T_1**-weighted sequence**	T_2**-weighted sequence**
LOW-GRADE ASTROCYTOMA	3rd–5th	Frontal lobes Temporal lobes	Hypo/isointensity	Hyperintensity
PILOCYTIC ASTROCYTOMA	1st–2nd	Cerebellum brainstem Chiasm hypothalamus Temporal lobe	Hypo/isointensity	Hyperintensity
ANAPLASTIC ASTROCYTOMA	3rd–5th	Supratentorial	Hypo/isointensity	Hyperintensity
GLIOBLASTOMA MULTIFORME	4th–6th	Supratentorial	Inhomogeneity	Inhomogeneity
OLIGODENDRIOGLIOMA	3rd–4th	Frontal lobes	Hypo/isointensity	Relative hyperintensity
MEDULLOBLASTOMA	1st–2nd	Cerebellar vermis	Hypointensity	Relative hyperintensity
EPENDYMOMA	1st–4th	Lateral ventricles	Hypointensity	Hyperintensity
MENINGIOMA	4th–7th	Falx Convexity Skull base	Iso/hypointensity Iso/hypointensity	Relative hyperintensity
NEURINOMA	3rd–4th	Cerebellopontine angle Meckel's cave	Iso/hypointensity	Iso/hyperintensity
PITUITARY ADENOMA	2nd–5th	Pituitary (microadenoma) Sellar region (macroadenoma)	Hypo/isointensity	Iso/hyperintensity
CRANIOPHARYNGIOMA solid-cystic	1st–4th	Sellar region Hypothalamus	Hyperintensity Inhomogeneity	Hyperintensity Inhomogeneity
CAVERNOUS ANGIOMA	2nd–4th	Supratentorial	Hyperintensity	Inhomogeneous hyperintensity Hypointense rim
METASTASES	5th–6th	Cortical-subcortical (single metastases) All sites (multiple metastases)	Iso/hypointensity Hyperintensity (lung adenocarcinoma melanoma, hemorrhagic lesions	Iso/hypointensity Hypointensity (melanoma, hemorrhagic lesions)

Signal changes after GD-DTPA (T_1-weighted sequence)	**Regressive processes**	**Edema**	**Other characteristics**
None	Microcysts (rare)	Absent Moderate	Regular contours
Hyperintensity (of varying degree)	Cysts Microcysts	Absent Moderate	Mural nodules in cystic lesions Sharp and regular contours
Irregular hyperintensity	Necrosis Hemorrhages	Present	Infiltrating
High hyperintensity (viable portions of tumor)	Necrosis Hemorrhages Cysts	Present	Infiltrating
None (low-grade) Hyperintensity (high-grade)	Calcifications Hemorrhages	Absent (low-grade) Present (high-grade)	Cortical-subcortical site Surface spread
Hyperintensity (of varying degree)	Cysts Hemorrhages Calcifications	Absent Moderate	CSF-mediated metastases
Hyperintensity (of varying degree)	Cysts Hemorrhages Calcifications	Absent Moderate	CSF-mediated metastases (in malignant lesions)
High hyperintensity	Calcifications Cysts Hemorrhages Necroses (rare)	Present	Extraparenchymal spread CSF watershed and/or presence of pseudocapsule
Hyperintensity	Hyaline degeneration Microcysts	Absent	Extraparenchymal spread Widening of acoustic canal Recklinghausen's disease
Hypointensity Occasional hyperintensity	Necroses Hemorrhages	Absent	Endocrinopathies Compression of optic pathways
None	Cysts Calcifications	Absent	Typical appearance
None	Hemorrhages	Absent	Typical appearance
Hyperintensity	Necroses Hemorrhages	Present	Frequent multiple locations

NEUROEPITHELIAL TUMORS

TUMORS OF THE ASTROCYTIC SERIES

ASTROCYTOMA

- fibrillary
- protoplasmic
- gemistocytic

PILOCYTIC ASTROCYTOMA

GIANT-CELL SUBEPENDYMOMA

ASTROBLASTOMA

ANAPLASTIC ASTROCYTOMA

TUMORS OF THE OLIGODENDROGLIAL SERIES

OLIGODENDROGLIOMA

MIXED OLIGO-ASTROCYTOMA

ANAPLASTIC OLIGODENDROGLIOMA

EPENDYMAL AND CHOROID-PLEXUS TUMORS

EPENDYMOMAS

- mixopapillary
- papillary
- subependymoma

ANAPLASTIC EPENDYMOMA

PAPILLOMA OF THE CHOROID PLEXUS

ANAPLASTIC PAPILLOMA OF THE CHOROID PLEXUS

PINEAL TUMORS

PINEOCYTOMA (pinealocytoma)

PINEOBLASTOMA (pinealoblastoma)

NEURONAL TUMORS

GANGLIOCYTOMA

GANGLIOGLIOMA

GANGLIONEUROBLASTOMA

ANAPLASTIC GANGLIOMA AND GANGLIOCYTOMA

NEUROBLASTOMA

EMBRYONIC TUMORS OF NEUROEPITHELIAL ORIGIN

GLIOBLASTOMA

- with sarcomatous component
- giant-cell

MEDULLOBLASTOMA

- desmoplasmic
- medullomyoblastoma

MEDULLOEPITHELIOMA

SPONGIOBLASTOMA

CEREBRAL GLIOMATOSIS

NERVE SHEATH TUMORS

NEURILEMMOMA (schwannoma, neurinoma)

ANAPLASTIC NEURILEMMOMA

NEUROFIBROMA

ANAPLASTIC NEUROFIBROMA (neurofibrosarcoma, neurogenic sarcoma)

MENINGEAL ENVELOPE TUMORS

MENINGIOMAS

- meningotheliomatous (endotheliomatous, syncytial, arachnotheliomatous)
- fibrous (fibroblastic)
- transitional (mixed)
- psammomatous
- angiomatous
- hemangioblastic
- hemangiopericytic
- papillary
- anaplastic meningioma (malignant)

MENINGEAL SARCOMAS

- fibrosarcoma
- polymorphous-cell sarcoma
- primary meningeal sarcomatosis

XANTHOMATOUS TUMORS

- fibroxanthoma
- xanthosarcoma (malignant fibroxanthoma)

PRIMARY MELANOCYTIC TUMORS

- melanoma
- meningeal melanomatosis

VASCULAR TUMORS

HEMANGIOBLASTOMA (capillary hemangioblastoma)

MONSTROCELLULAR SARCOMA

GERM-CELL TUMORS

GERMINOMA

EMBRYONIC CARCINOMA

CHORIOCARCINOMA

TERATOMA

MALFORMATIONS AND TUMOR-LIKE LESIONS

CRANIOPHARYNGIOMA

CYST OF RATHKE'S POUCH

EPIDERMOID CYST

DERMOID CYST

COLLOID CYST OF THE 3RD VENTRICLE

ENTEROGENOUS CYST

OTHER CYSTS

LIPOMA

CHORISTOMA (granular-cell myoblastoma, pituicytoma)

HYPOTHALAMIC NEURONAL HAMARTHOMA

NASAL GLIAL HETEROTOPY (nasal glioma)

VASCULAR MALFORMATIONS

CAPILLARY TELANGIECTASIA

CAVERNOUS ANGIOMA

ARTEROVENOUS MALFORMATIONS

VENOUS MALFORMATIONS

STURGE-WEBER DISEASE

PITUITARY TUMORS

PITUITARY ADENOMAS

- acidophilic (PRL-GH)
- basophilic (ACTH-TSH-FSH)
- mixed acidophilic-basophilic
- chromophobic (non-PRL-GH-secreting)

INTRA-EXTRACRANIAL TUMORS

TUMOR OF THE JUGULAR GLOME (chemodectoma, paraganglioma)

CHORDOMA

CHONDROMA

CHONDROSARCOMA

OLFACTORY NEUROBLASTOMA (esthesioneuroblastoma)

CYSTIC ADENOCARCINOMA (cylindroma)

OTHERS

METASTATIC TUMORS – PRIMARY MALIGNANT TUMORS – UNCLASSIFIED TUMORS

References

1. Bailey P, Cushing HA (1926) A Classification of the Tumours of the Glioma Group on a Histogenetic Basis with a Correlated Study of Prognosis. J. B. Lippincott Co, Philadelphia
2. Becker L, Hinton D (1983) Primitive neuroectodermal tumor of the central nervous system. Hum Pathol 14:538–550
3. Boetz MI (1974) Frontal lobe tumors. In: Vinken PJ, Bruyn GW (eds) Handbook of Clinical Neurology, Vol 17. Tumors of the Brain and Skull, Part II. North-Holland, Amsterdam, 234–280
4. Bronen RA, Sze G (1990) Magnetic resonance contrast agents: theory and application to the central nervous system. J Neurosurg 73:820–840
5. Burger PC, Vogel FS, Green SB et al. (1985) Glioblastoma multiforme and anaplastic astrocytoma. Pathological criteria and prognostic implications. Cancer 56:1106–1111
6. Burger PC (1985) Gliomas: Pathology. In: Wilkins RH, Rengachary SS (eds) Neurosurgery, Vol 1. McGraw-Hill, New York, 553–563
7. Burger PC (1986) Malignant astrocytic neoplasms: Classification, pathologic anatomy and response to treatment. Semin Oncol 13:16–26
8. Chou SM, Miles JM (1991) The pathology of meningiomas. In: Al-Mefty O (ed) Meningiomas. Raven Press, New York, 37–57
9. Clark GB, Henry JM, Mc Keever PE (1985) Cerebral pilocytic astrocytoma. Cancer 56:1128–1133
10. Cushing H, Eisenhardt L (1938) Meningiomas: Their Classification, Regional Behaviour, Life History, and Surgical End Results. Charles C. Thomas, Springfield, Illinois
11. Davis RL (1987) Pathological lesions of the third ventricle and adjacent structures. In: Apuzzo MLJ (ed) Surgery of the third ventricle. Williams & Wilkins, Baltimore, 235–252
12. Kernohan JW, Sayre GP (1952) Tumours of the Central Nervous System. Armed Forces Fascicles of Pathology, Washington
13. Mork SJ, Halvorsen TB, Lindegaard KF et al. (1986) Oligodendroglioma. Histologic evaluation and prognosis. J Neuropathol Exp Neurol 45:65–73
14. Shapiro JR (1986) Biology of gliomas: Heterogeneity, oncogenes, and growth factor. Semin Oncol 13:4–15
15. Rorke LB, Gilles FM, Davis RL, Becker LE (1985) Revision of the WHO classification of brain tumors for childhood brain tumors. Cancer 56:1869–1886
16. Rubinstein LJ (1972) Tumors of the central nervous system. In: Rubinstein LJ (ed) Atlas of Tumor Pathology, Series 2, Fascicle 6. Armed Forces Institute of Pathology, Washington, DC, 269–284
17. Russel DS, Rubinstein LJ (1977) Pathology of Tumors of the Nervous System. Williams & Wilkins, Baltimore
18. Strobos RJ (1974) Temporal Lobe Tumors. In: Vinken PJ, Bruyn GW (eds) Handbook of Clinical Neurology, Vol 16, Tumors of the Brain and Skull, Part I. North-Holland, Amsterdam, 281–295
19. Weber G (1974) Midbrain tumors. In: Vinken PJ, Bruyn GW (eds) Handbook of Clinical Neurology, Vol 16. Tumors of the Brain and Skull, Part II. North-Holland, Amsterdam, 620–647
20. Zulch KJ, Christensen E (1956) Pathologische Anatomie der raumbeengenden intrakraniellen Prozesse. In: Olivecrona H, Toennis W (Hrsg) Handbuch der Neurochirurgie, Bd III. Springer, Berlin, Heidelberg
21. Zulch KJ, Mennel HD, Zimmermann V (1974) Intracranial hypertension. In: Vinken PJ, Bruyn GW (eds) Handbook of Clinical Neurology, Vol 16. Tumors of the Brain and Skull, Part I. North-Holland, Amsterdam, 89–149
22. Zulch KJ (1980) Principles of the new World Health Organization (WHO) classification of brain tumors. Neuroradiology 19:59–66
23. Zulch KJ (1986) Brain tumors: Their Biology and Pathology, 3rd edn. Springer, New York

CHAPTER IV

Neuroepithelial tumors

Taken globally, neuroepithelial tumors are the most common tumors of the CNS. They may arise from both neuronal cells, such as gangliogliomas which however are very rare, or from glial cells, as is the case with the more frequently reported gliomas. Others, like medulloblastoma, derive from the cells of the early neuroepithelium.

For a classification of these tumors, reference can be made to Chapter III. It is worth mentioning here, however, that neuroepithelial tumors are a very heterogeneous group including neoplasms that are biologically benign or malignant and whose clinical behavior is often influenced by site. The most frequent tumors deriving from the neuroepithelium are the astrocytic neoplasms which can be distinguished into low-malignant *(Figs. 1, 2, 3, 27)*, intermediate- and high-malignant *(Figs. 4, 5, 6, 7, 8, 9)*; the glioblastoma multiforme is the most dedifferentiated and aggressive type of glioma *(Figs. 10, 11, 12, 13, 14, 15)*. There are various subgroups of astrocytomas: fibrillary, pilocytic, gemistocytic, etc. Except for the pilocytic astrocytoma, the other types all tend to infiltrate the surrounding tissue so deeply and finely that modern diagnostic imaging techniques are unable to detect them. This means that, for the time being, total removal "*en bloc*" of these tumors is an unfeasible option. Nonetheless, in recent years, thanks to diagnostic imaging techniques and to innovative surgical approaches, many glial neoplasms that had hitherto been considered inoperable are now successfully treated with surgery. Symptomatology varies widely and depends on the site of the tumor. Convulsion episodes, sensorimotor disorders and psychic symptoms are frequently reported. Intracranial hypertension is no longer a common finding because, since the appearance of CT and MRI on the diagnostic scene, these tumors have been detected in their early stages.

If the tumor is in a favorable site, as is the case of tumors restricted to one lobe of the non-dominant hemisphere *(Figs. 14, 27)*, surgical resection of the mass up to the macroscopically healthy tissue is possible and, where combined with radiation therapy, fairly long survival, in good conditions, is secured. If access to the site is difficult *(Figs. 4, 9, 8, 10)* or if the tumor is multicentric *(Fig. 15)*, it may be worthwhile taking only a biopsy using the stereotactic technique so as to characterize the neoplasm. It must however be recalled that, even after surgery and radiation therapy, malignant astrocytomas and glioblastomas seldom allow survivals of over two years. On the contrary, benign astrocytomas often allow survival for a few decades even without therapy. It must also be pointed out that gliomas, and astrocytomas in particular, are often polymorphic. Therefore, non-malignant areas may often border on islands of more dedifferentiated tissue and astrocytomas that are benign in their early stages tend to become more aggressive with time.

Special mention must be made of pilocytic astrocytomas, or spongioblastomas according to a former classification, which are also called juvenile astrocytomas. These are absolutely non-malignant and they mostly affect children and young adults; they are often cystic and well demarcated from the surrounding tissue. The sites where they most commonly occur are the cerebellum *(Figs. 16, 18)*, the hypothalamus *(Figs. 21, 22, 23)*, the temporal lobe and the brainstem *(Figs. 17, 19, 20)*, the optic nerve and the chiasm *(Figs. 24, 25, 26)*. While astrocytomas of the cerebellum and temporal lobe can be easily removed and offer substantial probabilities of biological cure, those involving other sites may present some problems for surgery and so they virtually turn into clinically malignant tumors even though with long survival rates. The gliomas of the optical pathways are found to have a different clinical behavior depending on whether they involve the optic nerve, the optic nerve plus the chiasm or the chiasm and the hypothalamus. In particular, the tumors of the optic nerve evolve slowly, have good prognosis *(Fig. 24)* and their surgical resection leads to clinical cure. If during surgery the tumor is found to have infiltrated the chiasm *(Figs. 25, 26)*, the biopsy is followed by a cycle of radiation therapy.

In spite of surgery and radiation therapy, gliomas of the chiasm with hypothalamic involvement have poor prognosis.

Oligodendrogliomas derive from oligodendroglia; they are common in adults and are located in the brain hemispheres. They are seldom found elsewhere. Clinically, they are often accompanied by convulsion symptomatology. They are infiltrating tumors even though they are generally histologically benign. They may be small in size *(Figs. 28, 29)* or they may involve both hemispheres *(Fig. 30)* and they may be found inside the ventricles *(Fig. 31)*. If they are small and in a site where access is easy *(Fig. 32)*, surgery plus radiation therapy may secure many years of survival and even complete cure. If located in difficult sites, they cause deficits and lead to death within a short time, especially if, as is sometimes the case, areas consisting of mature oligodendrocytes alternate with areas of immature cells or cells that are similar to malignant astrocytomas or to glioblastoma multiforme *(Fig. 30)*.

Cell pleomorphism of malignant gliomas influences the macroscopic appearance and density of the neoplasm. Abundantly vascularized areas thus alternate with areas of hyaline necrosis containing micro and macro cysts. Generally, the borders of the gliomas consist of more viable cells with respect to the center of the tumor which is often necrotic (they have a cyst-like appearance on CT and MRI scans). Oligodendrogliomas have typically microcalcified areas *(Fig. 32)*. Cleavage with the surrounding tissue is not sharp and the neoplasm tends to merge with the edema and with the peritumoral reactive gliosis, which makes it difficult to define the boundaries of the tissue to be resected.

Ependymomas derive from the cells lining the ependyma of the ventricles. Fourth ventricle ependymomas are the types most frequently found in children. Supratentorial types may occur in adults. These are generally benign, but aggressive and/or immature varieties may occur. They may be cystic. Ependymomas of the lateral ventricles may reach appreciable sizes and do not always cause hydrocephalus at an early stage *(Fig. 33)*. Instead, fourth and third ventricle ependymomas *(Figs. 34, 35)* do cause early hydrocephalus because they obstruct the CSF pathways with a clinical picture of intracranial hypertension. Except for those which have their base on the ependyma of the third and fourth ventricle and on the medial wall of the lateral ventricle, ependymomas can be easily removed. With respect to other gliomas, the surgical procedure may be more difficult, but their prognosis is better because these tumors are fairly radiation-sensitive.

Medulloblastomas derive from the early neuroepithelium and occur mainly in children and in young adults. They are located along the midline of the cerebellum *(Figs. 36, 37, 38)* at the roof of the fourth ventricle. They cause gait disorders and an early intracranial hypertension syndrome owing to obstruction of the fourth ventricle and/or of the aqueduct of Sylvius. These tumors are decidedly malignant but surgical treatment combined with radiation therapy, to which medulloblastoma is very sensitive, may offer long periods of well-being. Relapses, both local *(Fig. 39)* and in the form of metastases via the CSF pathway along the neuraxis, are frequent (Chap. XII, *Figs. 21, 22, 23*).

In studying encephalic glial neoplasms, MRI affords diagnostic elements that are far better than any other neuroradiological investigation and even better than CT scans. Indeed, not only does it offer a better defined anatomical picture of the tumor site thanks to its multiplanar scans and to absence of bone-related artifacts, but it also allows for altered tissue components to be clearly distinguished by adjusting signal intensity, at times even before morphological changes have set in. Given the morphological and structural complexity of encephalic gliomas, the gathering of as many diagnostic elements as possible requires the use of a suitable and exhaustive evaluation technique: SE T_1-, proton density- and T_2-weighted sequences at least along two orthogonal planes; if necessary, multi-echo sequences of selected slices may be followed by another set of T_1 sequences after administering an i.v. paramagnetic contrast medium.

Neoplasms usually have longer T_1 and T_2 relaxation times, mainly due to greater water and protein content. Therefore, on short-TR sequences *(Figs. 23, 27)*, the signal is weak, while for long TRs, the signal is more intense *(Figs. 2, 3, 5, 7, 20, 22)*. These signal characteristics are typical of solid and homogeneous neoplasms. However, the presence of structural inhomogeneities (necroses, cysts, hemorrhages, calcium deposits) substantially modifies the dominant water signal, thus producing complex morphologies, which at times are useful for making a differential diagnosis among the various types of gliomas. Some gliomas may have a true cystic appearance *(Fig. 18)*, whereas pseudocystic components may be found in tumor tissues due to hemorrhage, necrosis and entrapment of neighboring CSF spaces. Generally, cystic neoplasms have irregular walls and are often multiloculated; the MRI signal differs from that of the CSF as the T_1, T_2 values are longer, and at times the fluid content differs in density owing to the presence of cell degradation material. All of these elements are reflected by signal changes, which can be enhanced by multi-echo sequences *(Fig. 22)*. At times, MRI can hardly discriminate between a solid, highly cellular and clearly delimited tumor, such as a pilocytic astrocytoma *(Fig. 16)*, and a protein-dense cystic component. In these cases, i.v. GD-DTPA may help, since solid tumors and the walls of their cystic components will become selectively perfused.

Bleeding inside the tumor tissue due to rupture of tumoral vessels is frequently reported. These are mainly clinically silent hemorrhagic foci which involve delimited areas of the neoplastic mass. These foci are more easily detected by MRI than by CT, because with the former technique the presence of methemoglobin and hemosiderin is traced for a longer period of time *(Figs. 11, 12, 28, 33)*.

As occurs with intraparenchymal hematomas, three typical stages can be identified in the MRI signal evolution portraying hemorrhagic foci: stage 1 (recent bleeding) characterized by iso- or hypointense, short-TR sequences and hypointense, long-TR sequences; stage 2 (subacute hemorrhage) characterized by a high intensity signal on both short- and long-TR sequences without clear evidence of hemosiderin; stage 3 (chronic phase) characterized by areas of high signal intensity which are clearly bounded by a low intensity ring (hemosiderin) on long-TR sequences. All of these three aspects may be observed concurrently in neoplastic tissue as a result of recurrent bleeding.

Paramagnetic contrast medium (GD-DTPA) delivered i.v. in MRI studies of neuroepithelial neoplasms proved to be useful and at times absolutely necessary. On the basis of signal changes after i.v. GD-DTPA, a distinction can be made between neoplasms for which there is no signal alteration, such as low-malignant gliomas, and neoplasms for which the signal on the T_1-weighted sequences is strongly enhanced. This occurs because of the greater perfusion of paramagnetic contrast media in viable neoplastic tissue, as occurs with dedifferentiated neoplasms. This different behavior is dependent on differing degrees of alteration of the Blood-Brain Barrier (BBB). In low-malignant neoplasms, changes in vascular permeability allow for the passage of only water and protein molecules having the size of albumin, but not for the passage of more complex molecules, such as those of contrast media *(Figs. 2, 8)*. In addition and amongst other things, GD-DTPA: i) helps discriminate between the viable and necrotic portions of the tumor tissue *(Figs. 4, 10, 14, 17)*; ii) facilitates the study of cystic tumor walls, easily detecting neoplastic nodules; iii) helps better define the boundaries between neoplasm and edema *(Figs. 14, 15)*; and, finally, iv) helps identify small foci in multifocal tumors. Paramagnetic media are also necessary for the post-surgical evaluation of tumor remnants or of relapses, as well as in the follow-up of tumors with metastases via the CSF pathway.

In the latter case, it is possible to rapidly carry out an examination of both brain and spinal cord (SC) and thus to identify otherwise undetectable, small meningeal foci.

The diagnostic advantages of MRI for this type of pathology are manifold and can thus be summarized: greater sensitivity in identifying the neoplasm, hence allowing for earlier diagnosis; excellent delineation of the lesion, thus affording a more accurate evaluation of the surgical approach or a more careful selection of alternative therapies; more accurate analysis of alterations within the tumoral tissue and the surrounding cerebral parenchyma; good evaluation of preferential routes of growth, especially in terms of spread to the white matter and of involvement of the corpus callosum. Unfortunately, as with any other imaging technique, MRI performs poorly when it comes to characterizing the tumors and determining tissue specificity. But knowledge of the clinical picture and of the physiopathology of the neoplastic processes combined with diagnostic imaging will help make a differential diagnosis of the tumor, while the histological definition of the lesion can be left to stereotactic or open surgical biopsy (Chap. III, Table 2).

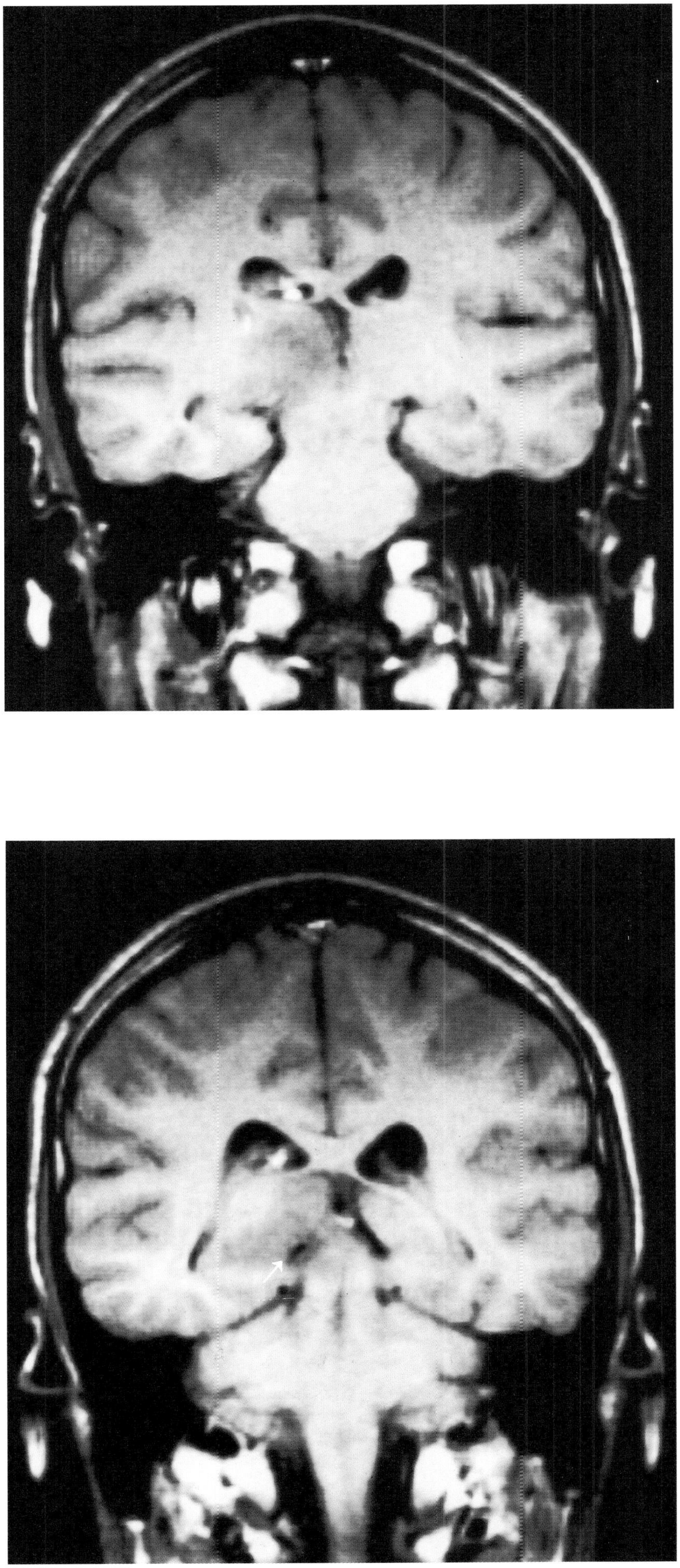

Fig. 1. *Right thalamic fibrillary astrocytoma.* T_1-weighted coronal images. The right thalamus is swollen by a hypointense and homogeneous neoplasm: posteriorly, it extends to the pulvinar (↗) and to the cerebral peduncle; anteriorly, it involves the fornix; medially, it deforms the third ventricle.

Fig. 2. *Right frontotemporal low-grade astrocytoma.* 20-year-old woman with history of seizures. A – Post-contrast CT shows deep frontal hypodensity on the right, with mild compression on the frontal horn of the lateral ventricle. B – Post-i.v. GD-DTPA T_1-weighted coronal views better document the spread of the lesion. The hypointense, non-enhancing lesion encases the Sylvian fissure. On the T_2-weighted images (C), the different signal intensity between the neoplasm and the surrounding tissue is well outlined. Also the subcortical location and the integrity of the grey matter are better visualized. This finding, together with the absence of edema, is consistent with low-grade astrocytomas.

A

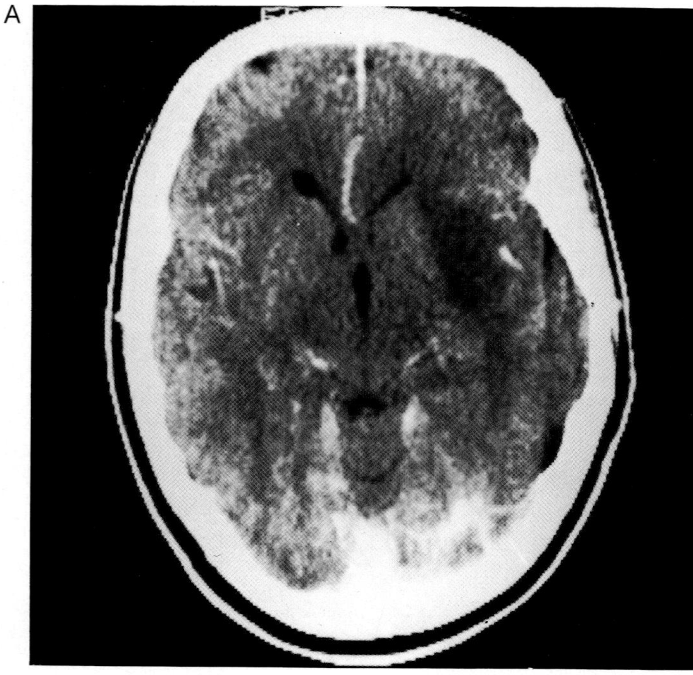

B

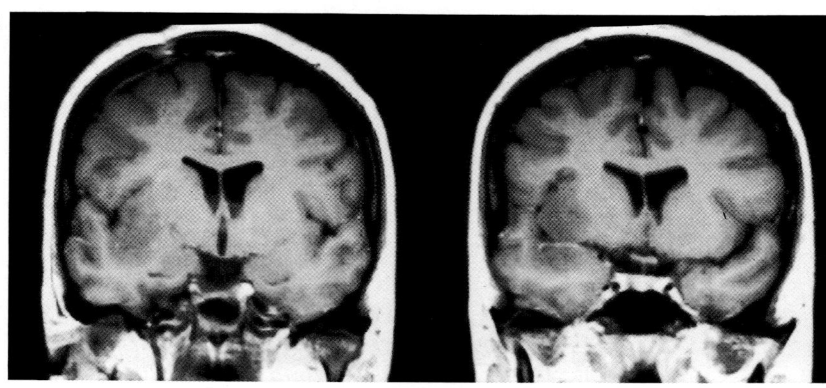

C

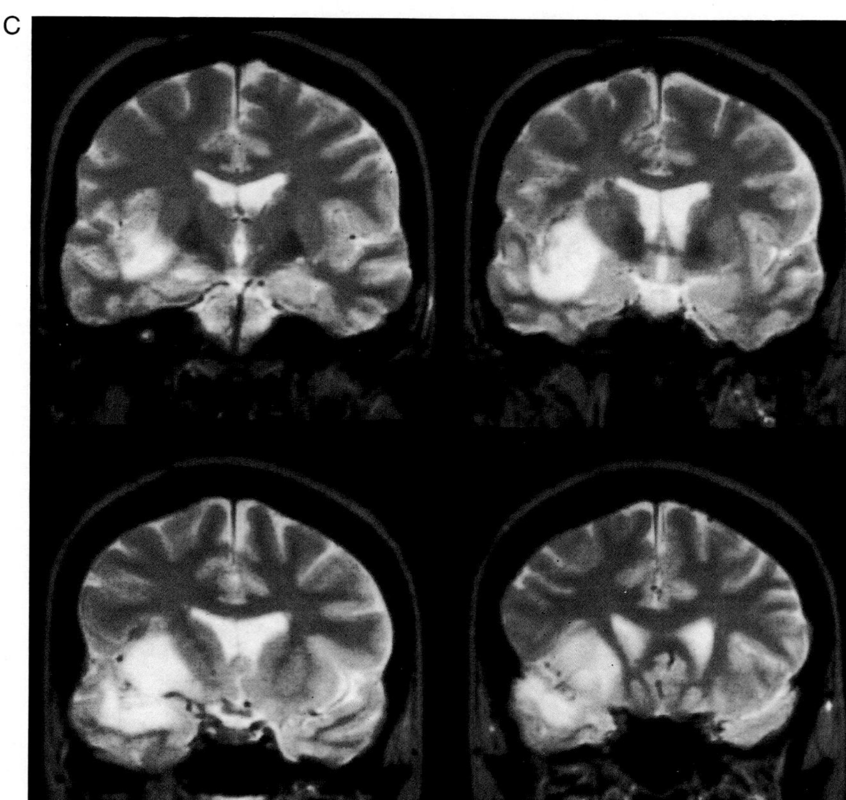

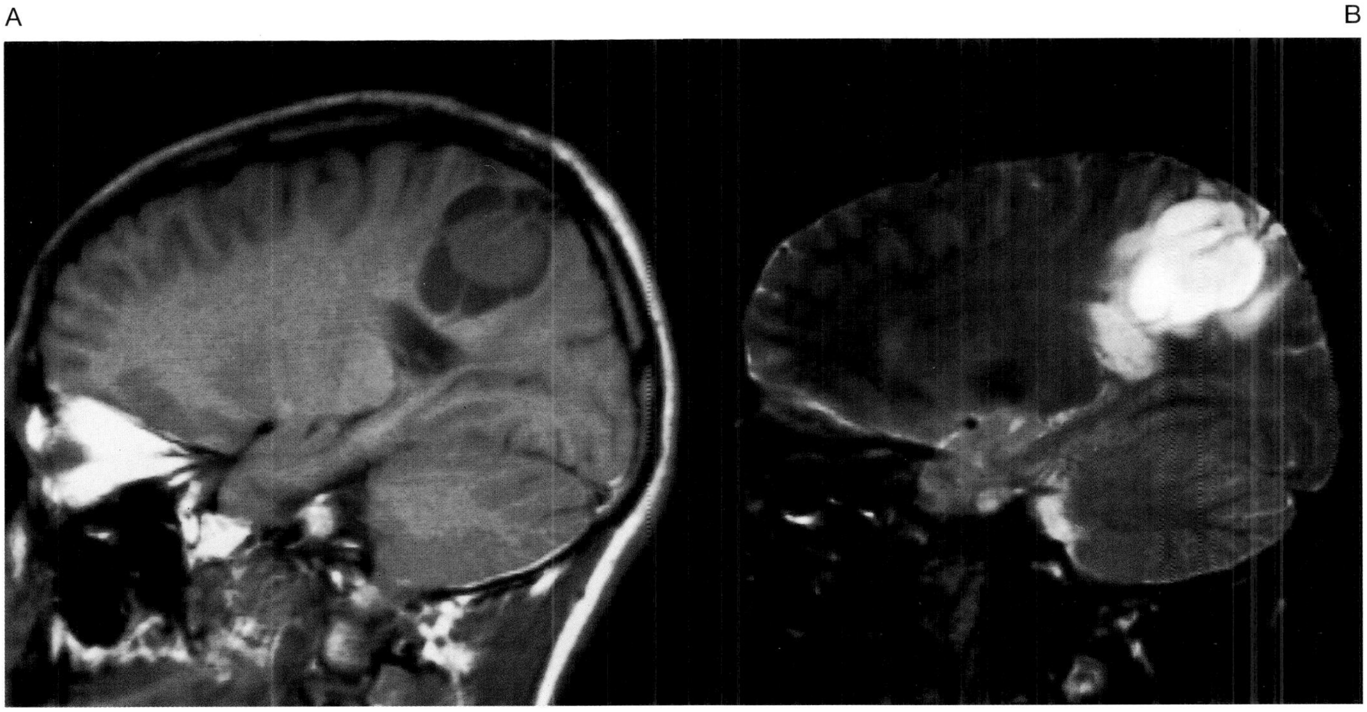

Fig. 3. *Recurrent left parietal low-grade astrocytoma.* T_1- (A) and T_2- (B) weighted sagittal cuts revealing a solid mass, isointense on A and hyperintense on B. The mass is suspended inside the remnant cavity from the previous surgical resection by scar tissue, which delimits some CSF collections. The T_2-weighted sequence better reflects the perilesional edema.

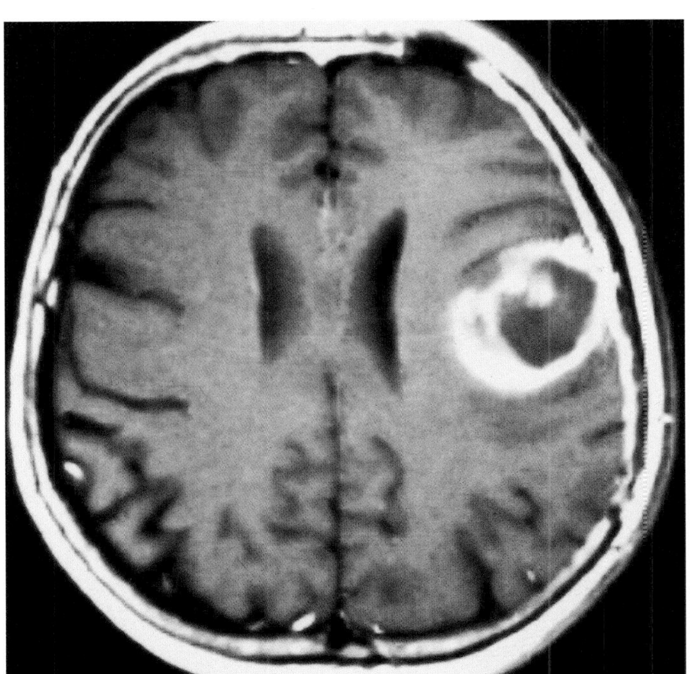

Fig. 4. *Left posterior frontal anaplastic astrocytoma.* Post-GD-DTPA T_1-weighted axial image. The solid component of the neoplasm is enhanced, whereas the necrotic-cystic core remains hypointense. There is a mild edema posterior to the mass.

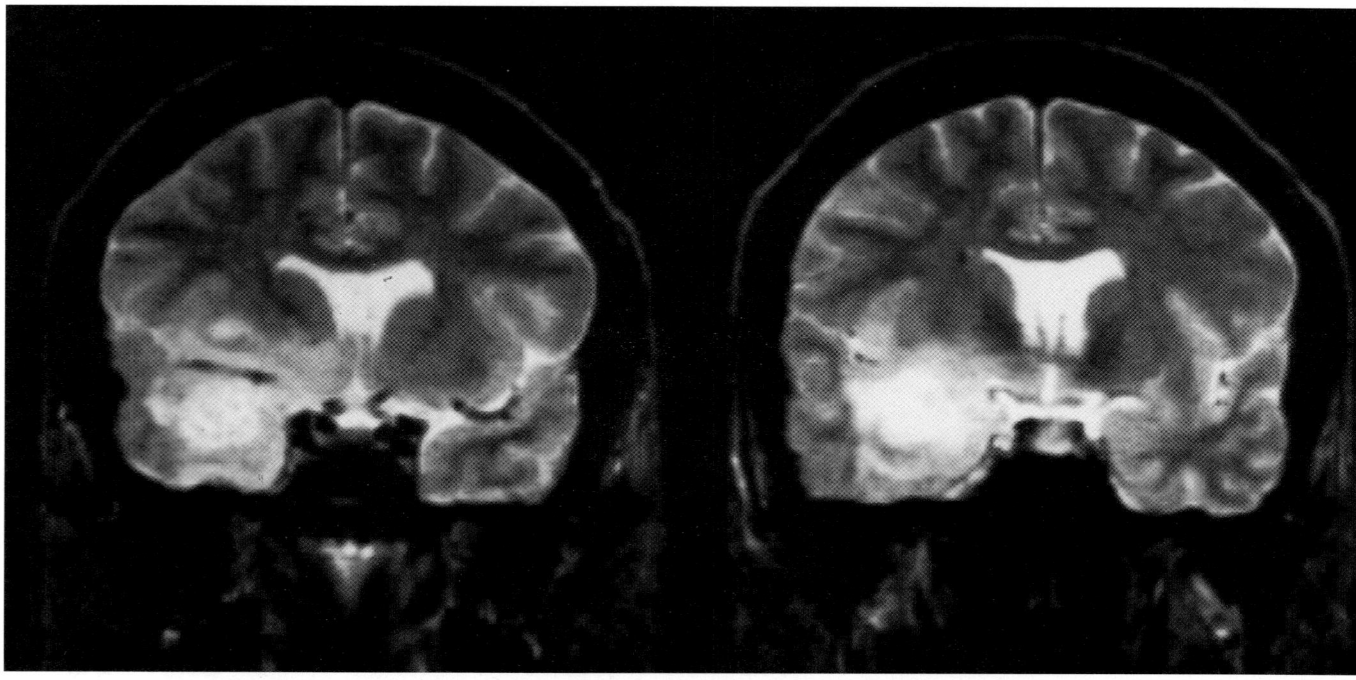

A

B

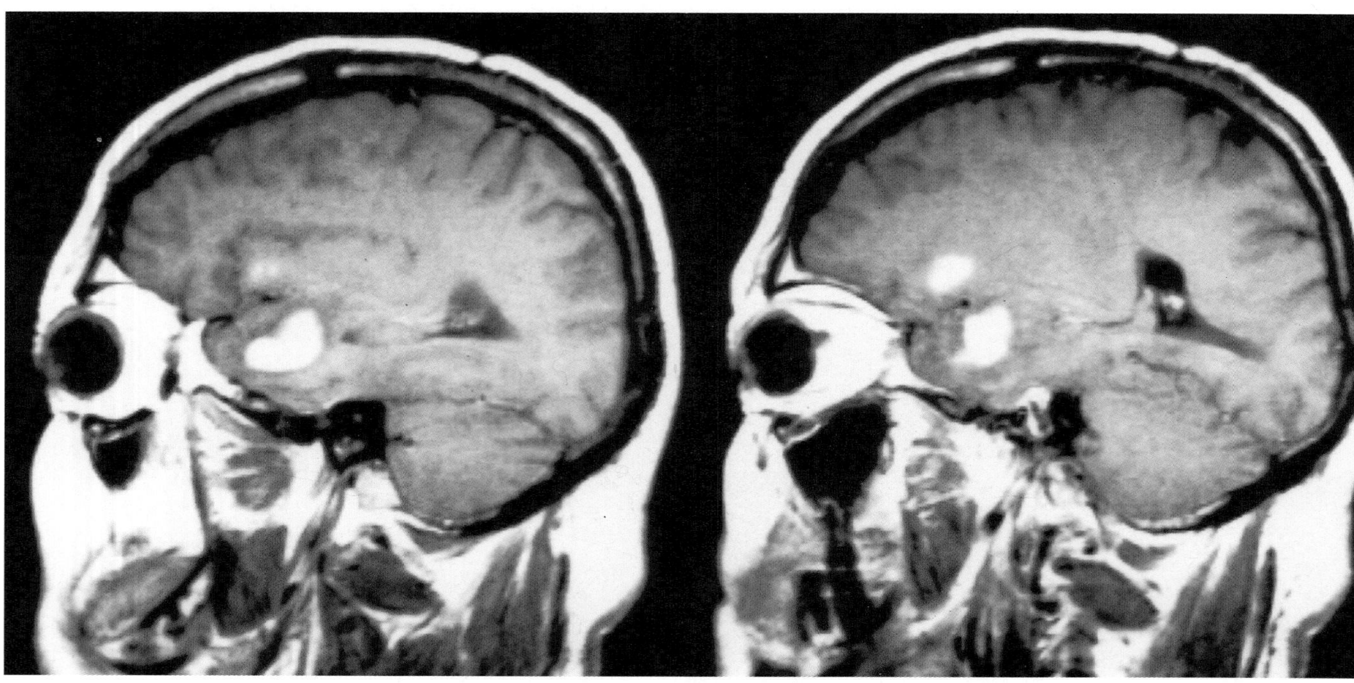

Fig. 5. *Right frontotemporal high-grade or anaplastic astrocytoma*. Compared with the previous case, the cortical structure and especially the medial gyri of the temporal lobe are deranged. On the T_2-weighted images (A), the lesion is nonhomogeneous and infiltrates the Sylvian fissure. GD-DTPA (B) enhances two capillary-laden foci with altered BBB.

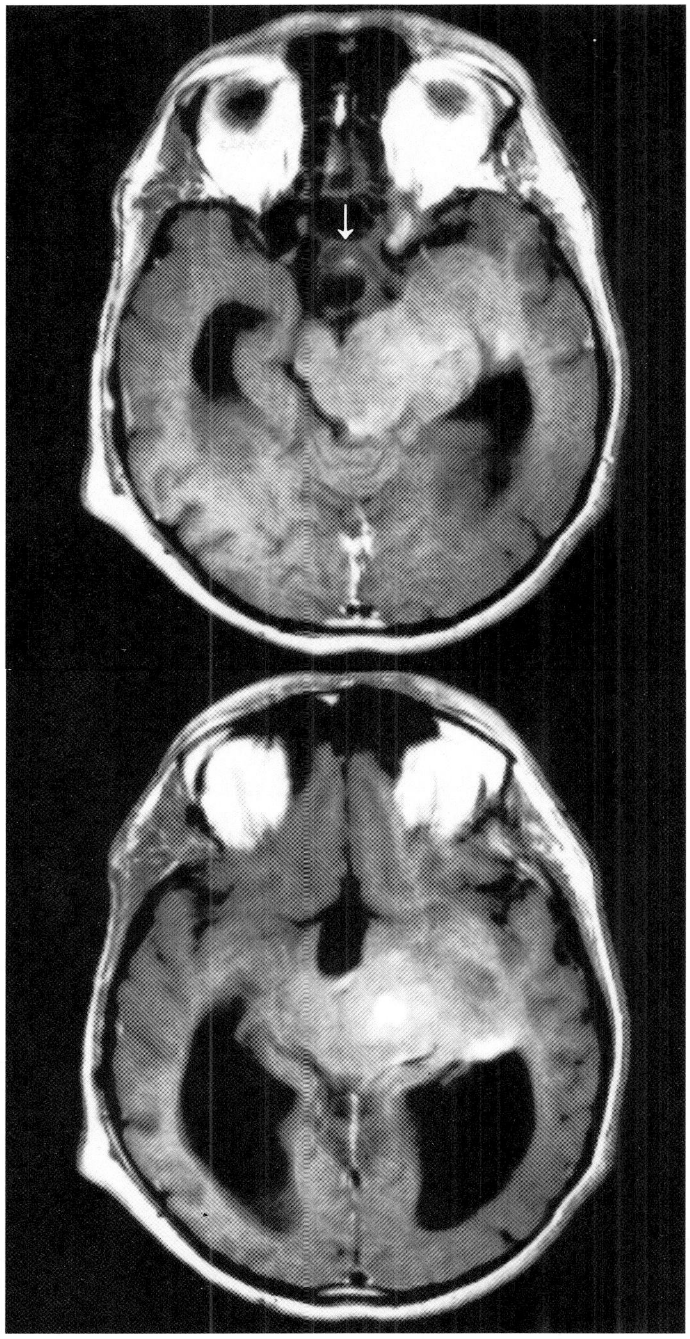

Fig. 6. *Left deep temporal anaplastic astrocytoma.* Patient with Recklinghausen's disease and aqueductal stenosis, treated 16 years ago with Torkildsen intrathecal shunt. Post-GD-DTPA T_1-weighted images. Massive infiltrating neoplasm which originates from the temporal lobe, crosses the thalamus and the cerebral peduncle and involves the midbrain. The neoplasm is inhomogeneous with more contrast-enhanced foci. This appearance suggests supratentorial hydrocephalus and extreme dilatation of the third ventricle, in front of which the chiasm (↓) and the pituitary stalk are visible.

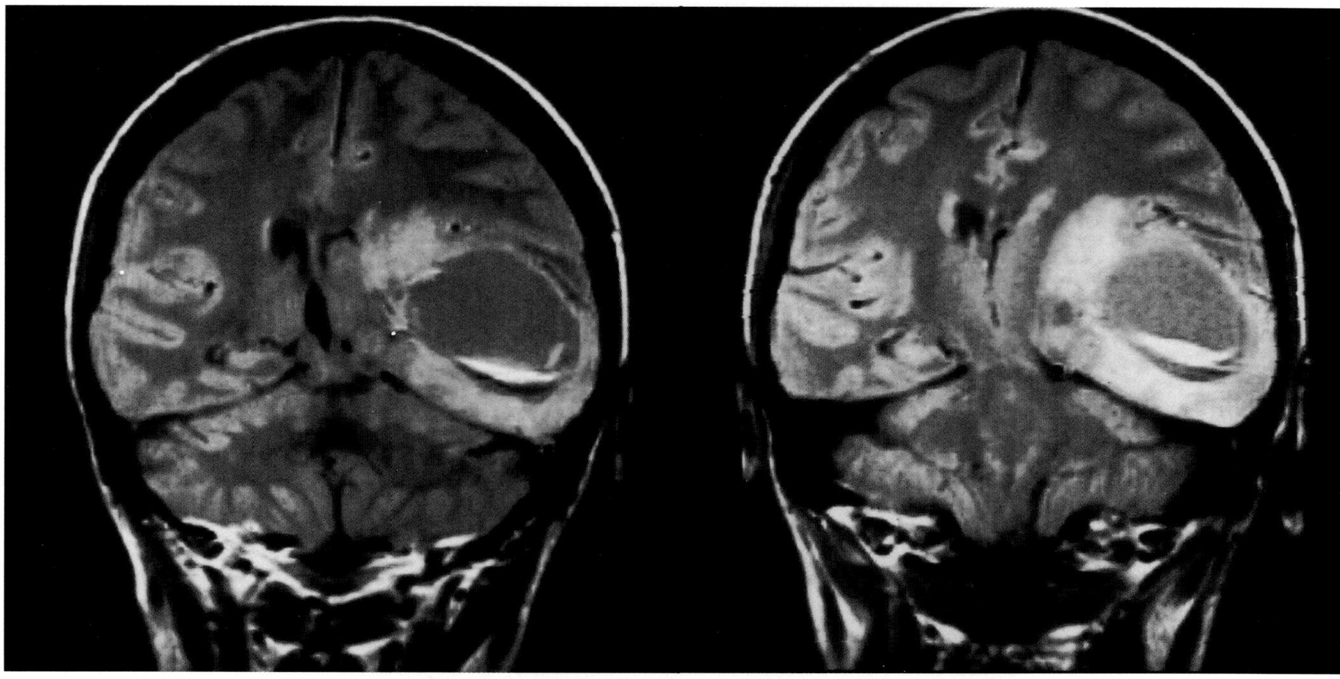

Fig. 7. *Left posterior temporal cystic anaplastic astrocytoma.* Patient with intracranial hypertension, phasic disorders and right-sided hemiparesis. Proton density-weighted coronal images: the tumor has a medial solid component within the edematous tissue and a huge cystic focus, containing remnants of recent (hyperintensity) and old (hypointensity) hemorrhages. Note the significant distortion of the median structures.

A B

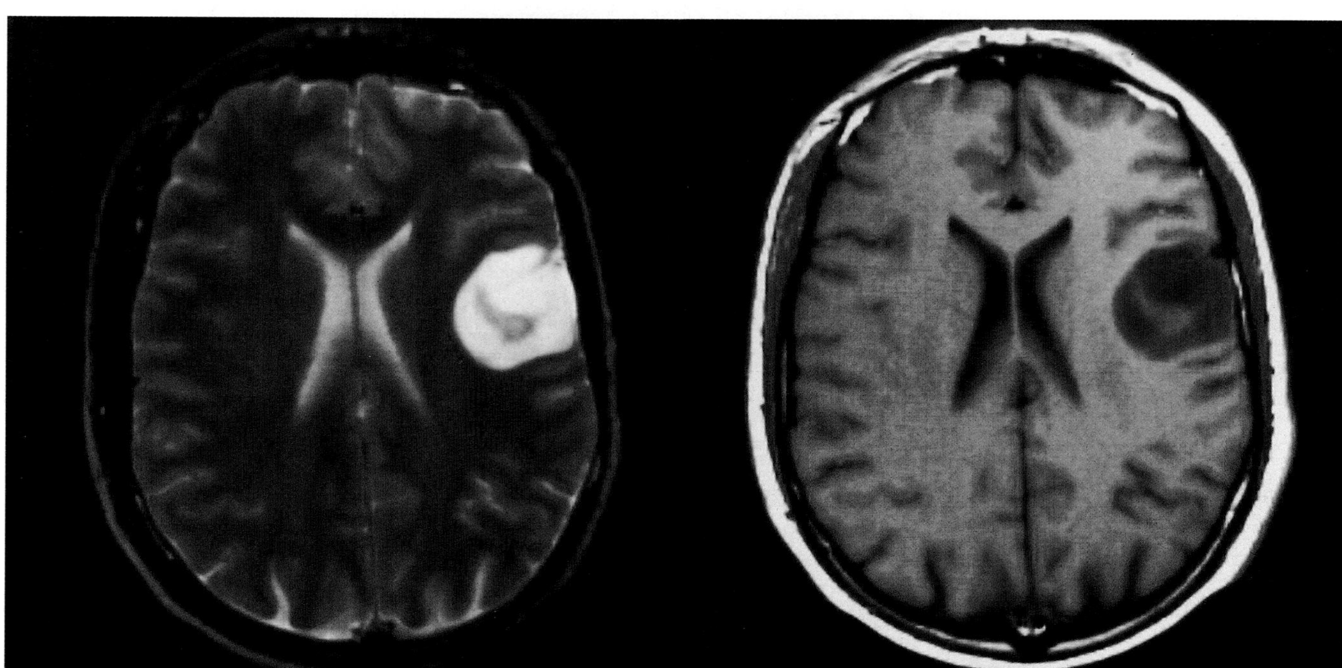

Fig. 8. *Intermediate-malignant astrocytoma.* 37-year-old man with seizures. In the left posterior frontal region, there is a non-edematogenic tumor, markedly hyperintense on the T_2-weighted sequence (A) and hypointense on the T_1-weighted one and without enhancement after GD-DTPA (B). These findings suggested the diagnosis of cystic astrocytoma. At surgery, a solid tumor was found and excised.

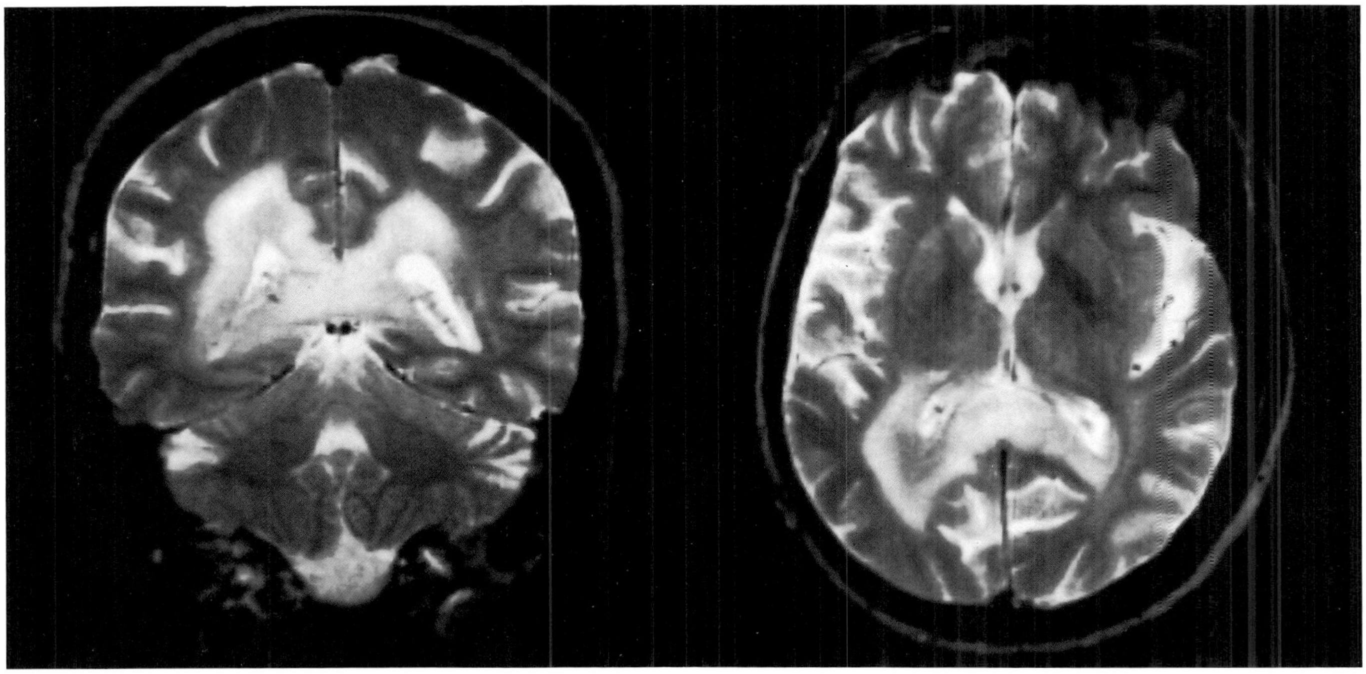

Fig. 9. *Intermediate-malignant astrocytoma (Grade II–III according to Kernohan) of the splenium of the corpus callosum.* T_2-weighted coronal and axial views. The neoplasm originates from the splenium of the corpus callosum and spreads in a butterfly fashion around the occipital horns; its signal intensity is high and partly inhomogeneous. The infiltrating nature of the neoplasm explains the non-compression of the neighboring structures.

A B

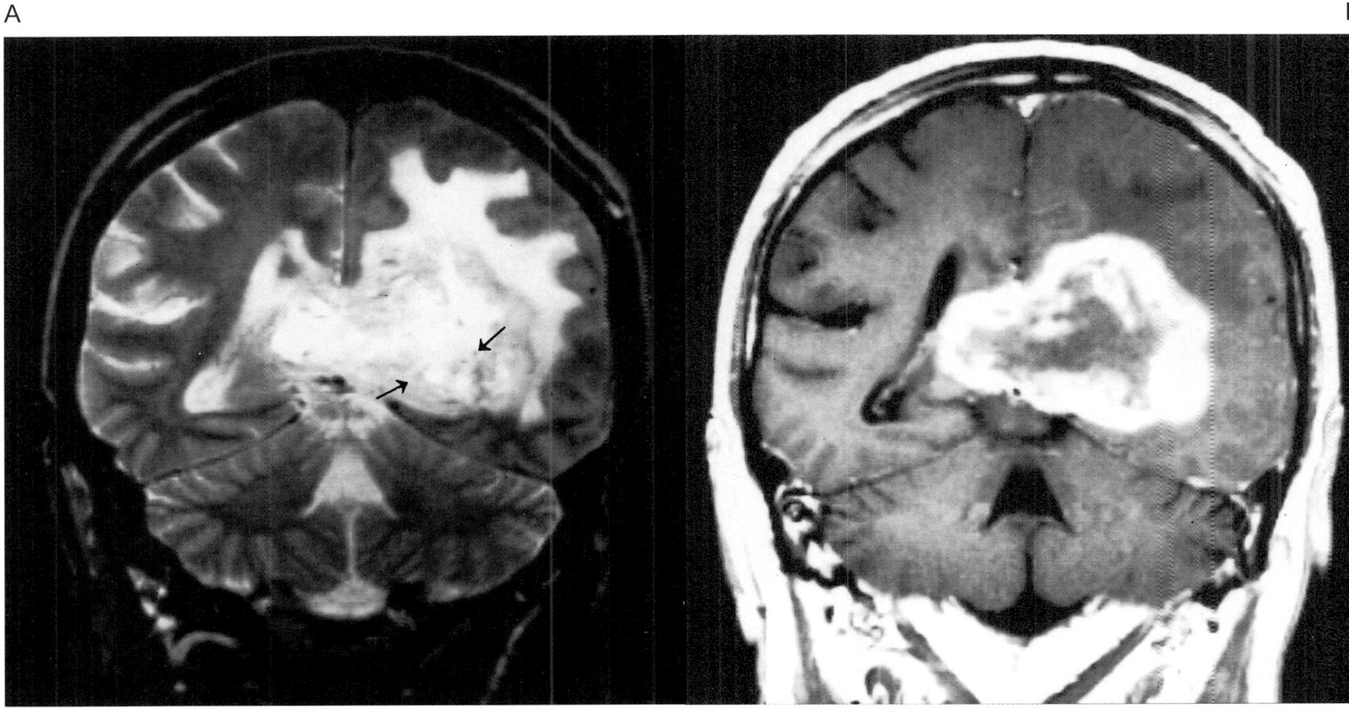

Fig. 10. *Glioblastoma multiforme of the splenium of the corpus callosum.* The site of the tumor is similar to the previous case. However, its morphology is typical for high-malignant neoplasms: marked compression (obliteration of the left lateral ventricle) and extremely inhomogeneous signal. The T_2-weighted sequence (A) reveals: hyperintense, wide, central necrotic core; viable neoplastic tissue with vascular structures (↙); and intense edema. The post-GD-DTPA T_1-weighted image (B) better delimits the viable tumoral component from the necrotic one.

A

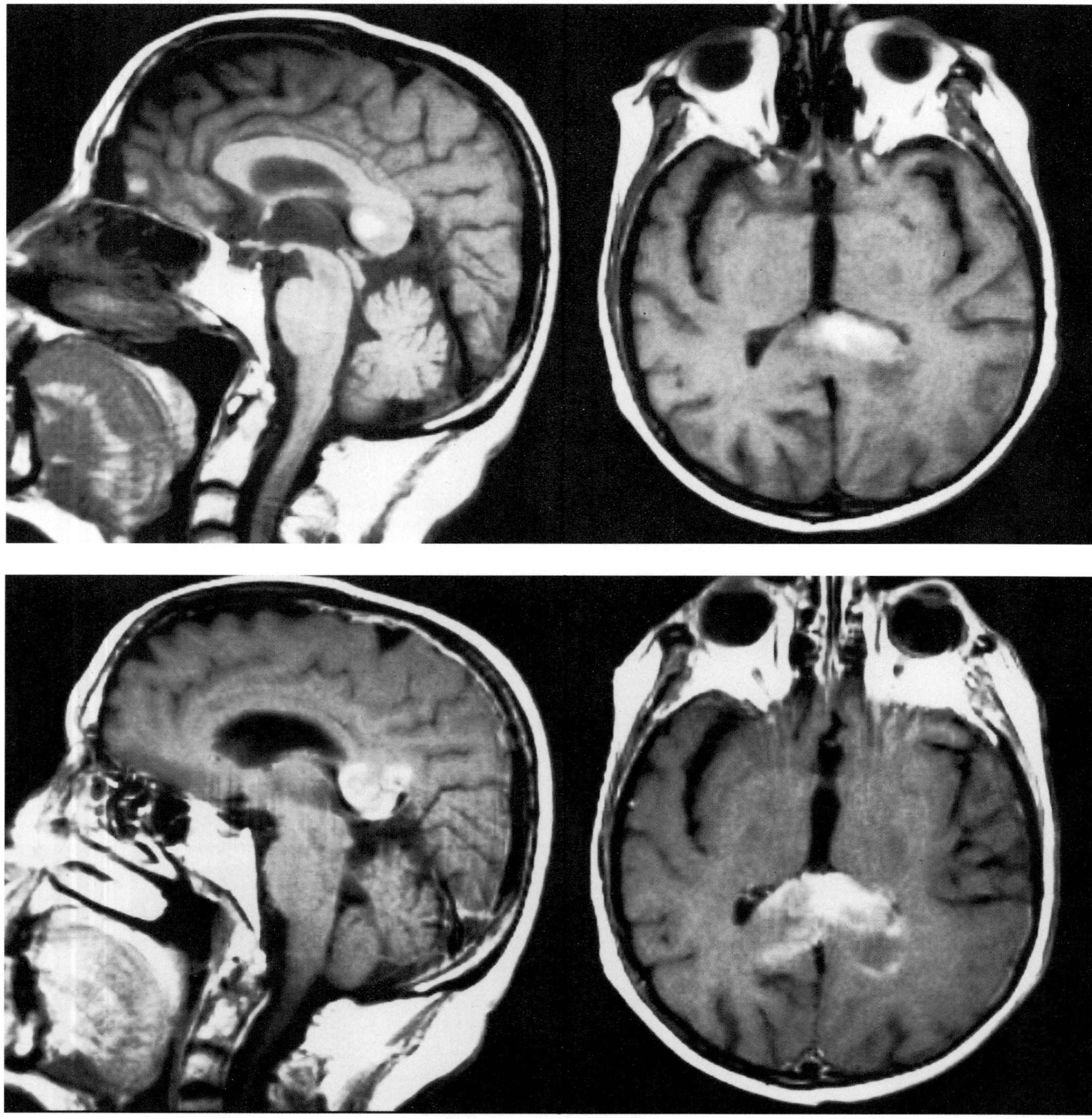

B

Fig. 11. *Glioblastoma multiforme of the splenium of the corpus callosum.* A – T_1-weighted sagittal and axial cuts: the neoplasm enlarges the splenium of the corpus callosum and has a hyperintense focus due to subacute hemorrhage. B – Same sequence after i.v. GD-DTPA. The neoplasm spreads bilaterally in a butterfly fashion. Compression of the left occipital horn.

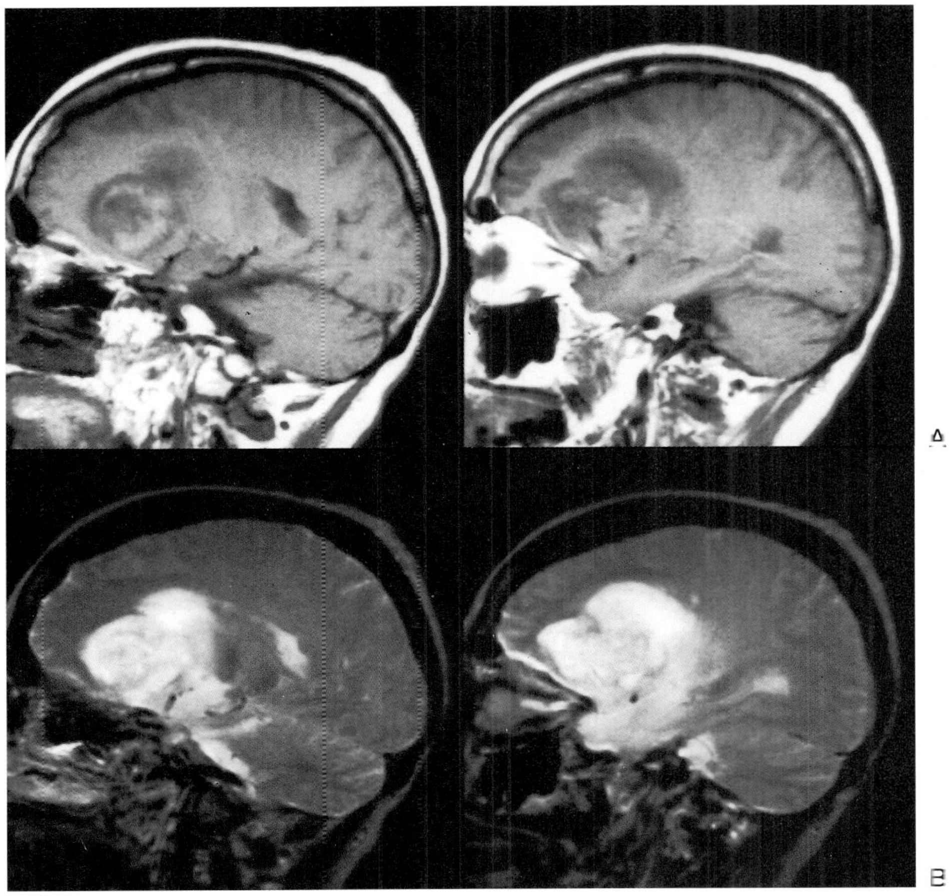

Fig. 12. *Left posterior frontal glioblastoma multiforme.* The tumor has a small necrotic component but large hemorrhagic foci with high signal on both T_1- (A) and T_2- (B) weighted images. The boundary is ill-demarcated and blends with the surrounding edema.

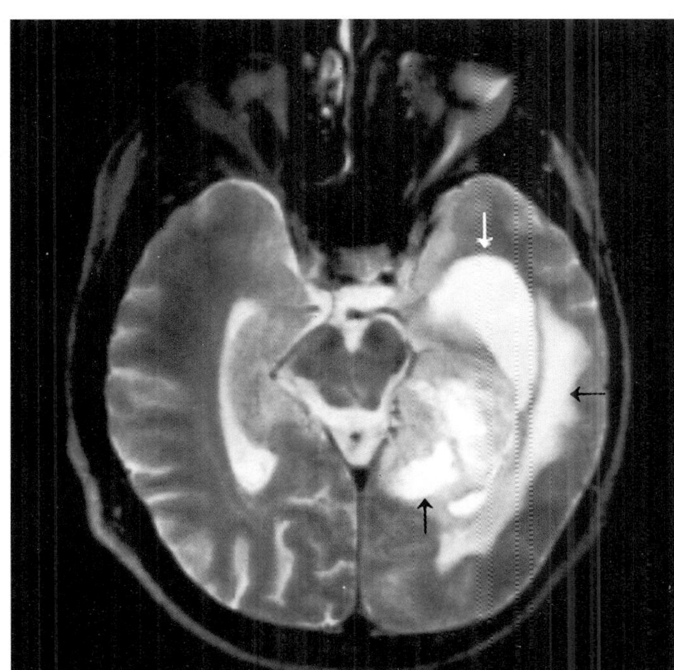

Fig. 13. *Left temporooccipital glioblastoma multiforme.* SE sequence (TR 2,500 msec, TE 90 msec). The necrotic and viable components of the neoplasm are evident. Observe the dilatation of the excluded temporal horn of the lateral ventricle and, medially, the compression of the cisterna ambiens and of the brainstem. The decreasing signal intensity of the necrosis (↑), of the CSF (↓) and of the edema (←) are well shown.

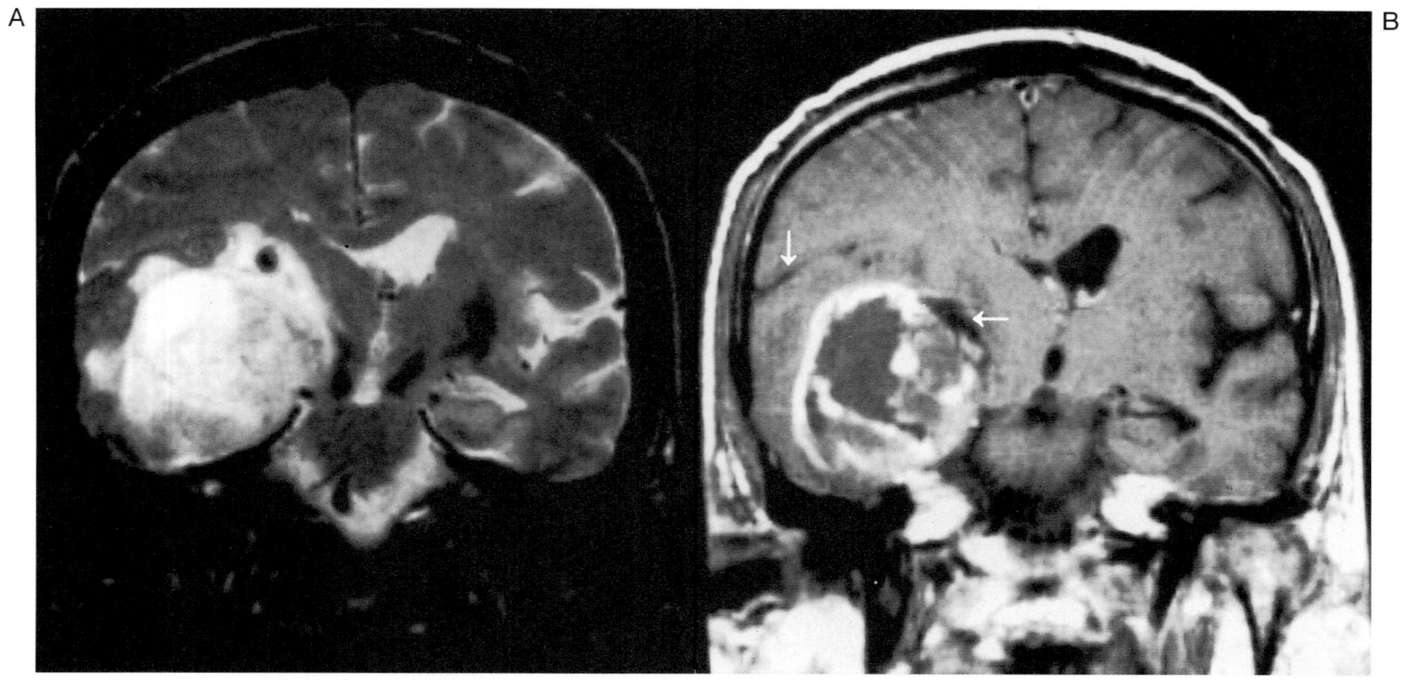

Fig. 14. *Right temporal glioblastoma multiforme.* The tumor is confined to the temporal lobe; it is located below and externally to the temporal horn (←) and under the posterior aspect of the Sylvian fissure (↓); macroscopically radical surgery is feasible. Both T_2-weighted (A) and post-GD-DTPA (B) images discriminate viable tumoral components from necrotic ones. Major distortion of the median structures and of the basal nuclei; these are markedly hypointense on T_2-weighted views owing to their high iron content.

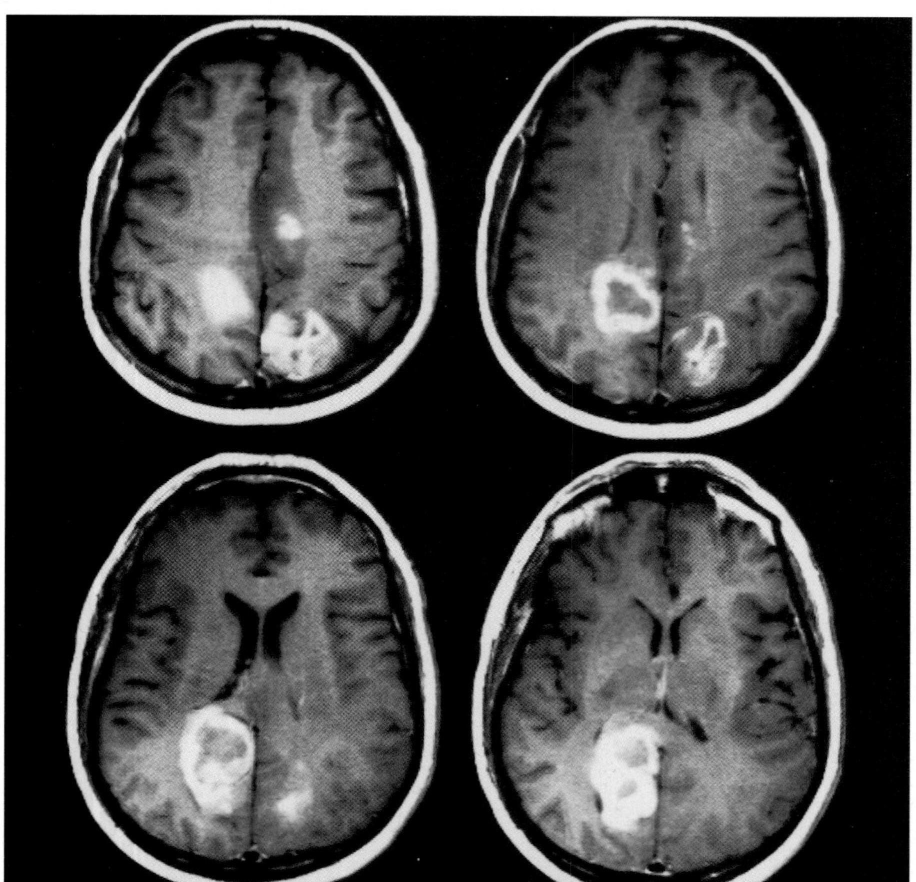

Fig. 15. *Multifocal glioblastoma multiforme.* T_1-weighted images obtained after i.v. GD-DTPA: the lesions elicit high signal owing to intense perfusion of paramagnetic contrast medium; their structure is inhomogeneous due to central necrosis. The largest lesion has a right-sided deep parietal location and spreads to the splenium of the corpus callosum.

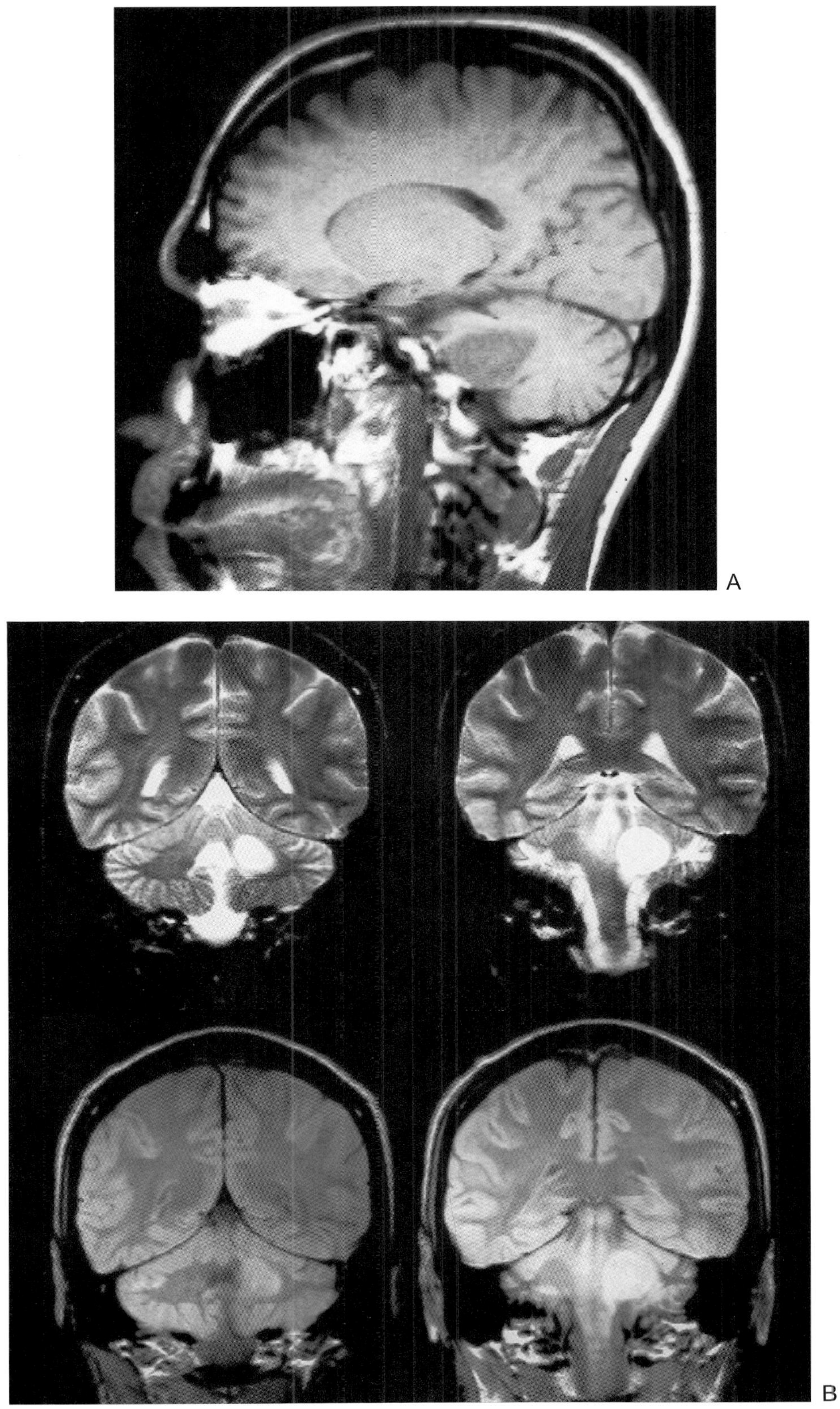

Fig. 16. *Left cerebellar solid pilocytic astrocytoma.* 24-year-old man with cerebellar hemisyndrome. A – Left paramedian sagittal scan (TR 550 msec, TE 15 msec). The cerebral peduncle exhibits a well-demarcated, low-signal area but with intensity values higher than the CSF. B – Coronal scan (TR 2,500 msec, TE 30, 90 msec). The lesion emits a homogeneous signal, whose intensity grows with TE elongation; its appearance is similar to a cystic neoplasm. The poor stromal component of this highly cellular tumor may explain the behavior of the signal.

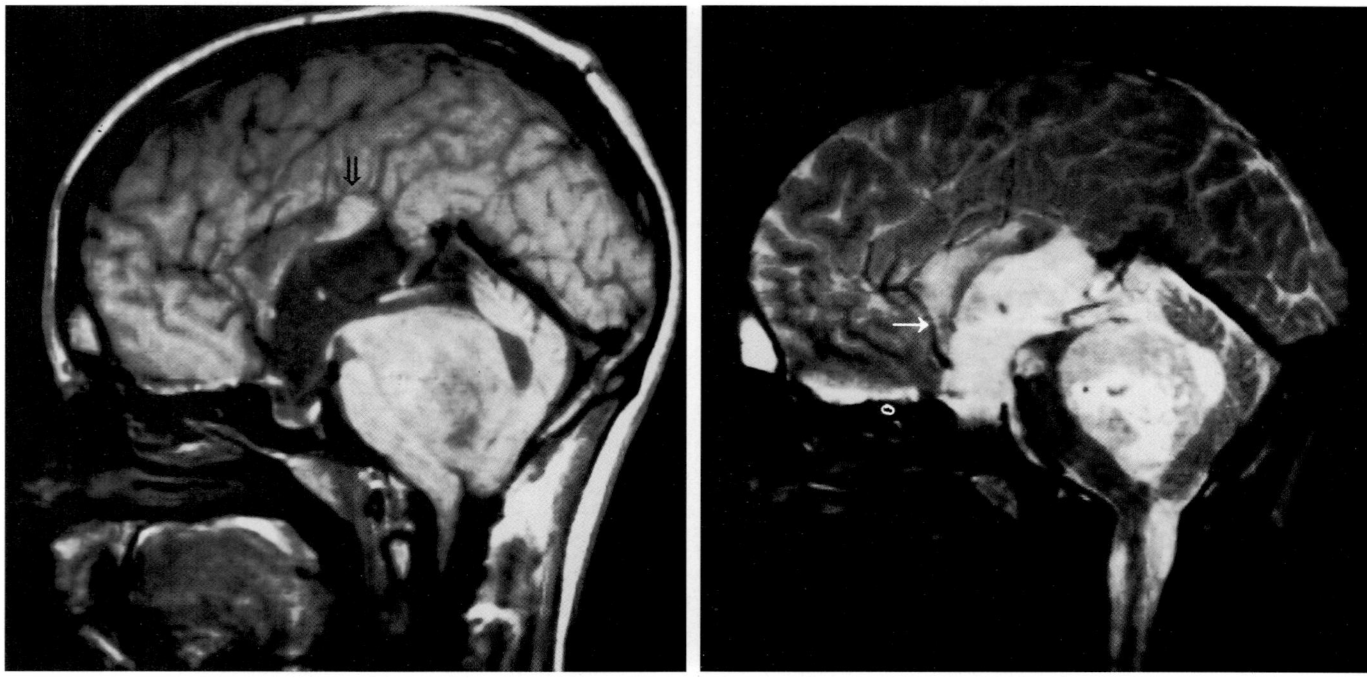

A

B

C

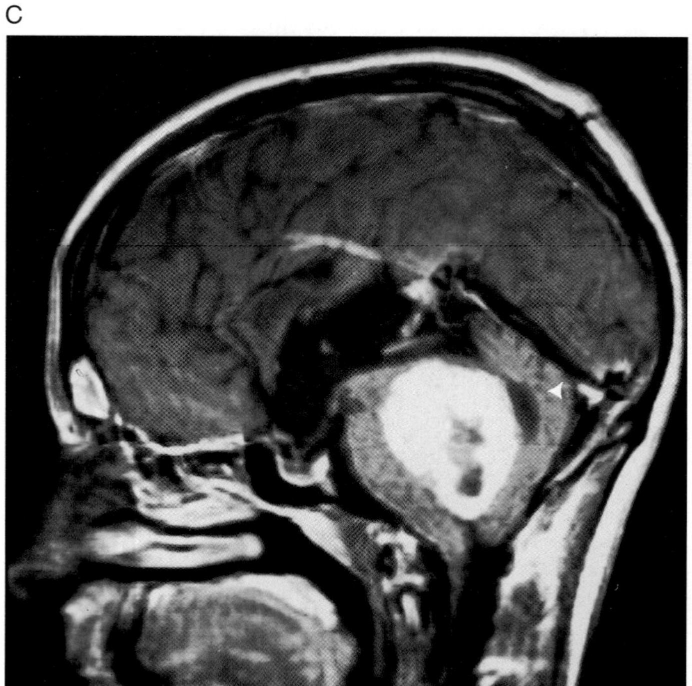

Fig. 17. *Pilocytic astrocytoma of the floor of the fourth ventricle.* 16-year-old boy with ataxia and recent onset of phonation disorders. The T_1- (A) and T_2- (B) weighted and post-GD-DTPA (C) sagittal images show a huge (5 × 6 cm) neoplasm with central necrosis; the neoplasm fills the fourth ventricle almost entirely and compresses the brainstem. The third ventricle is dilated with associated empty sella; there is also an independent agenesis of most of the corpus callosum, of which only the central component is left (⇓). The A.C.A. (→) has a slightly abnormal course. The roof of the midbrain has a reversed obliquity and overlies a dilated aqueduct. D – The post-GD-DTPA axial image documents the spread of the neoplasm, which crosses the left Luschka's foramen and occupies the cerebellopontine angle. The mass does not affect the right posterior (↑) and lateral (←) aspect of the fourth ventricle, suggesting that it originates from the left lateral recess. These morphological data were not clearly demonstrated by CT (E). Post-GD-DTPA coronal sections better document the tumor communication with the aqueduct (→), which is patent but displaced to the right and which encircles the tumor. This finding, together with the agenesis of the corpus callosum, is more typical of malformative than of hypertensive-obstructive hydrocephalus.

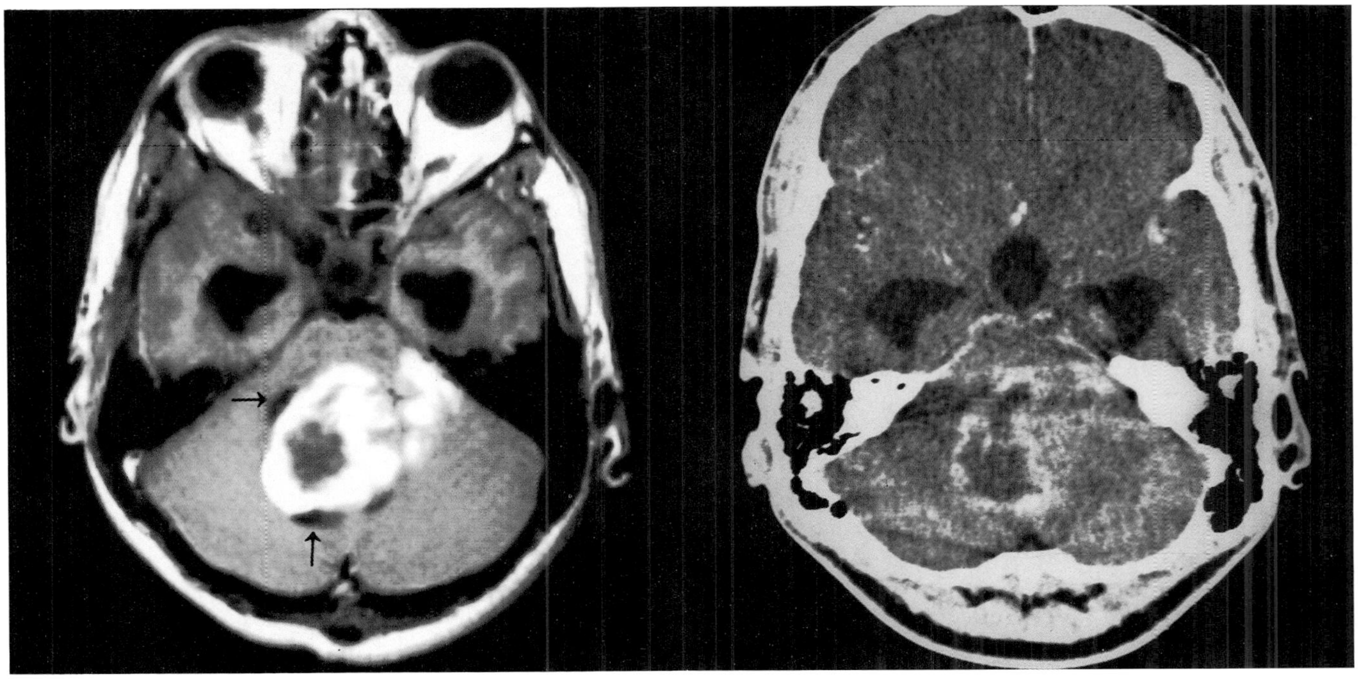

D E

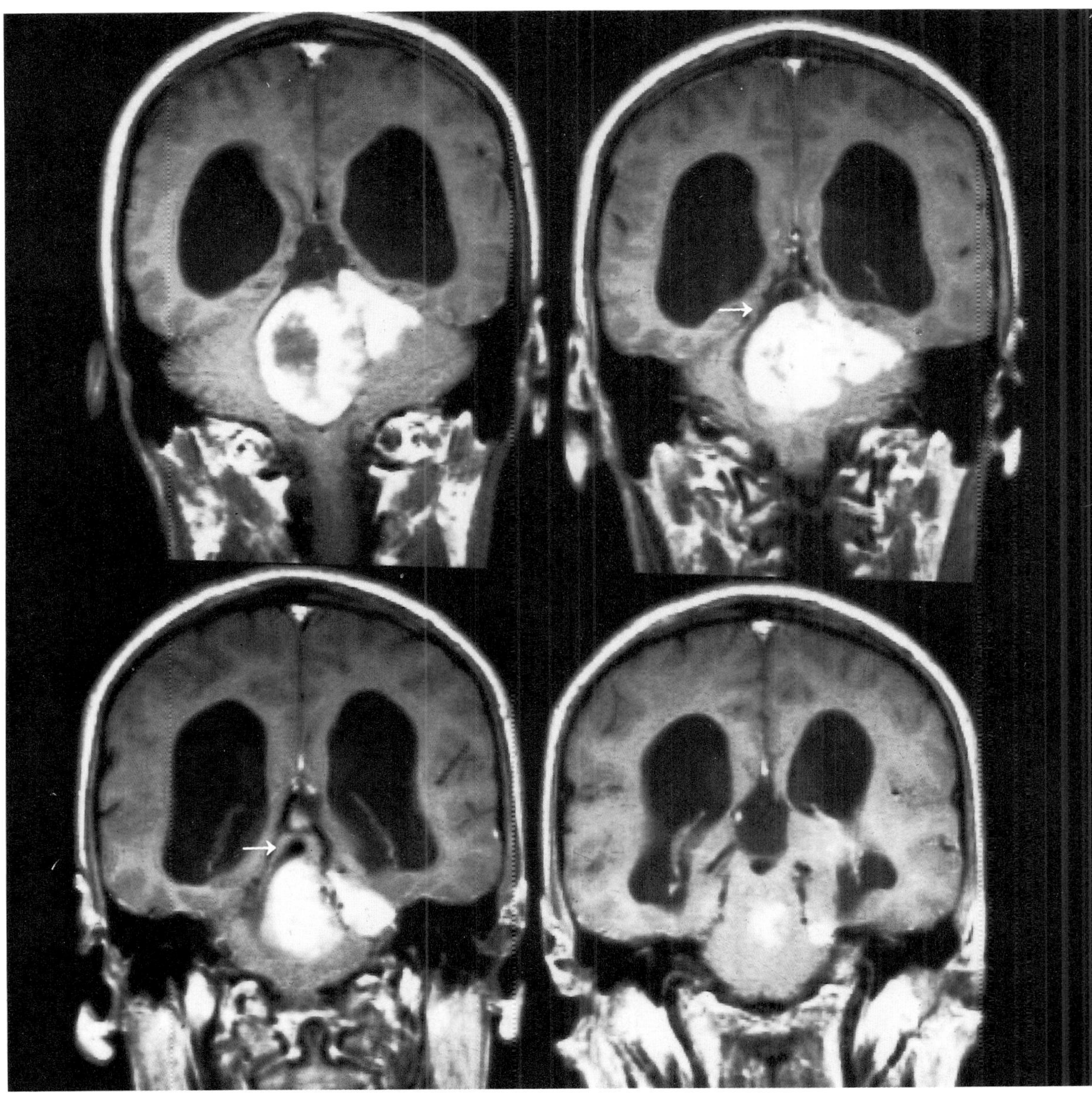

F

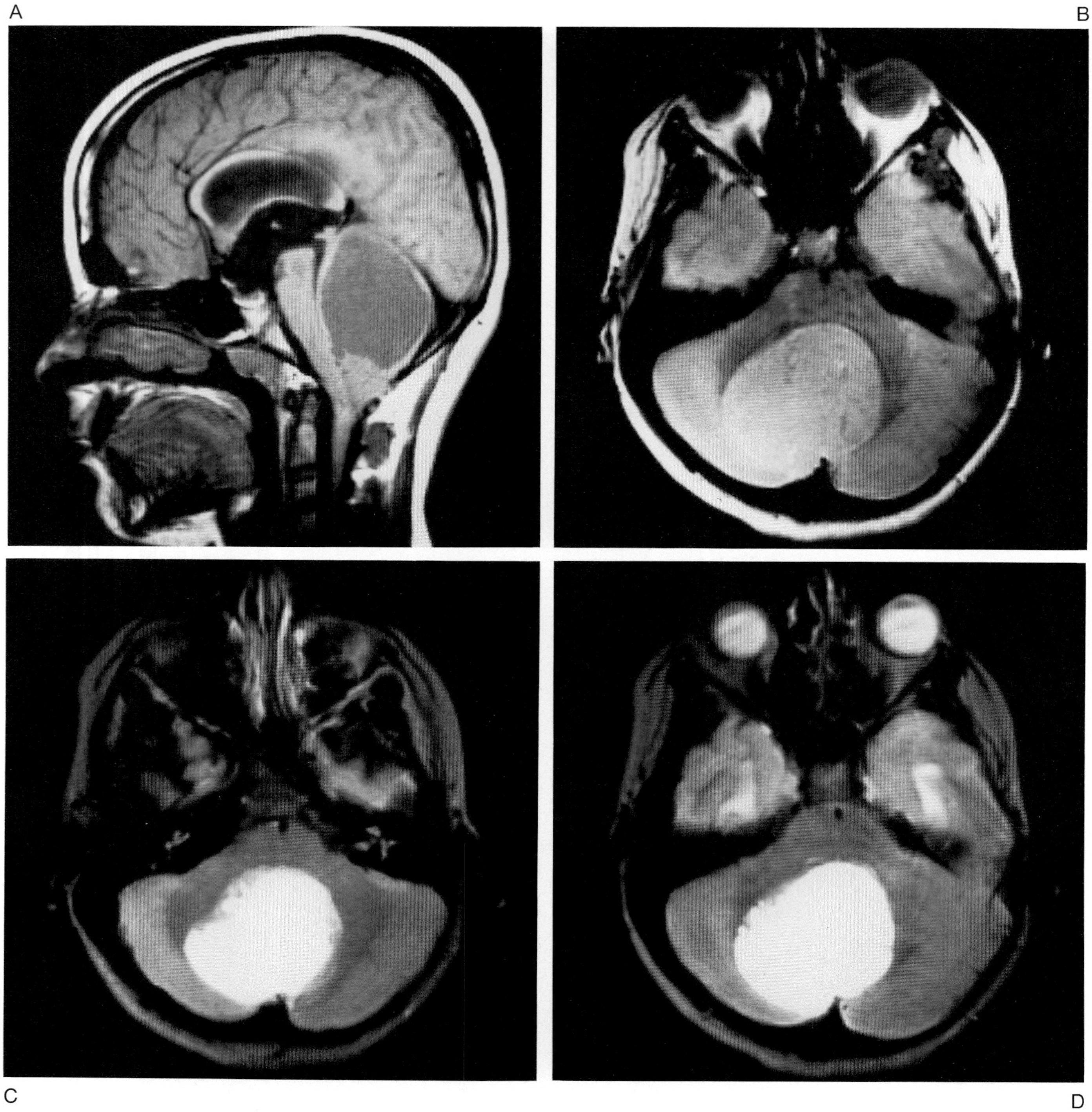

Fig. 18. *Cerebellar cystic astrocytoma.* 11-year-old girl with ataxic syndrome and intracranial hypertension. A – T_1-weighted sagittal section: huge cystic tumor in the vermis, which compresses and deforms the brainstem, effacing the fourth ventricle cavity. Dilated aqueduct and third ventricle. B – Proton density-weighted axial image: the lesion has a hypointense demarcation wall; its content has a signal intensity higher than the CSF. C, D – T_2-weighted axial images: better demarcation of the cystic component from the cerebellar tissue.

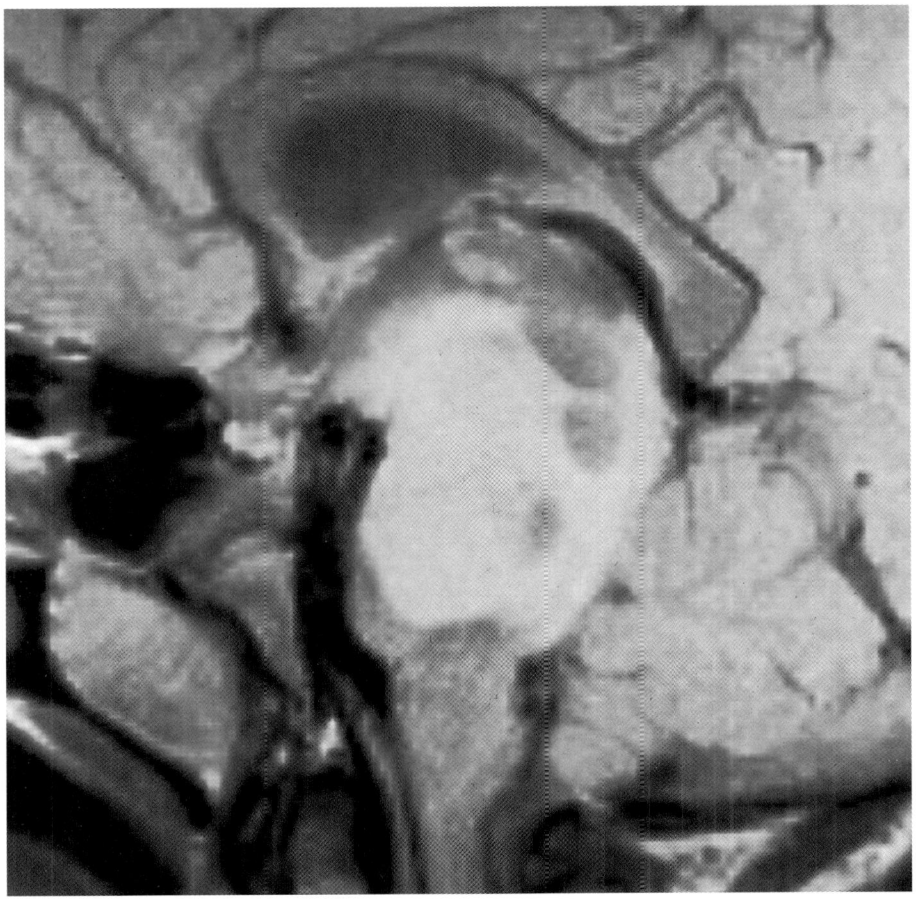
A

Fig. 19. *Pontine-midbrain pilocytic astrocytoma.* 7-year-old boy with right hemiparesis. A – The proton density-weighted sagittal scan shows the craniocaudal spread of the tumor. Major distension of the midbrain and of the superior aspect of the pons. The neoplasm elicits a high signal and is predominantly solid, with small cystic foci inferiorly. The cerebellum is displaced posteriorly. The third ventricle is partially obliterated. The anatomy of the quadrigeminal plate and of the pineal region is altered. B – T_1-weighted axial scan through the chiasm and the quadrigeminal plate: the mass also involves the left optic tract. The signal from the posterior portion of the cyst is more hypointense.

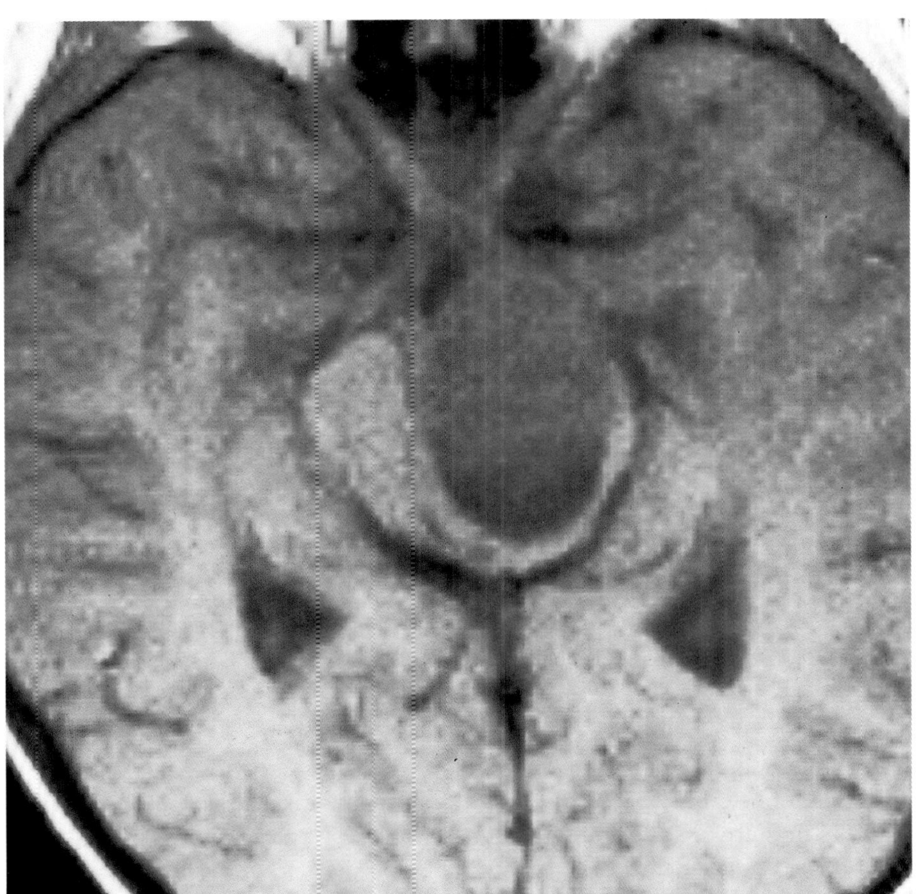
B

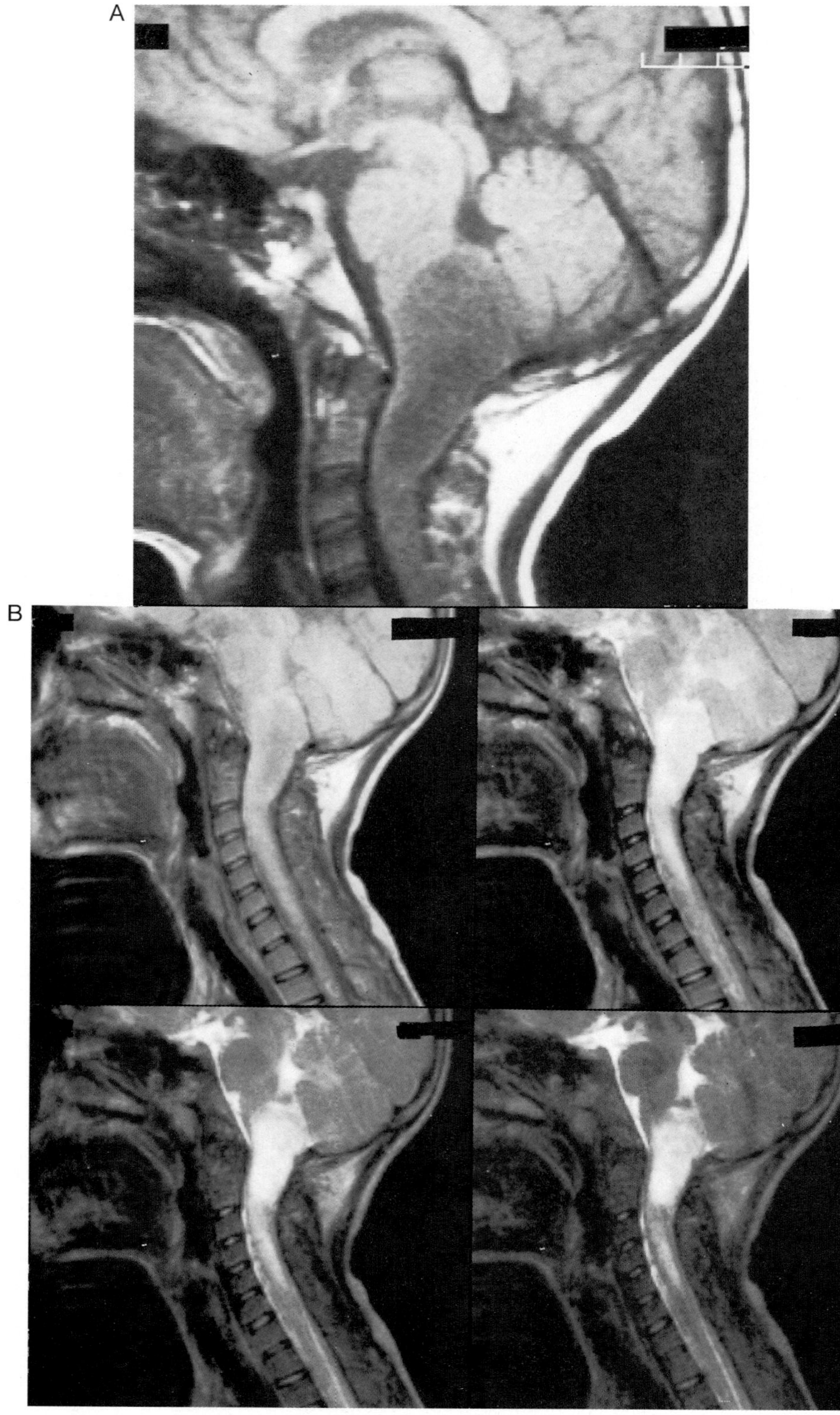

Fig. 20. *Bulbomedullary pilocytic astrocytoma.* 16-year-old boy. A – median T_1-weighted sagittal image. Bulging of the upper cervical spine, secondary to the hypointense neoplasm. The well-circumscribed hypointense tumor uplifts and deforms the fourth ventricle. The cisterna magna is obliterated. On multi-echoes (B), the tumor progressively increases its signal, hence its cervical growth can be better appreciated.

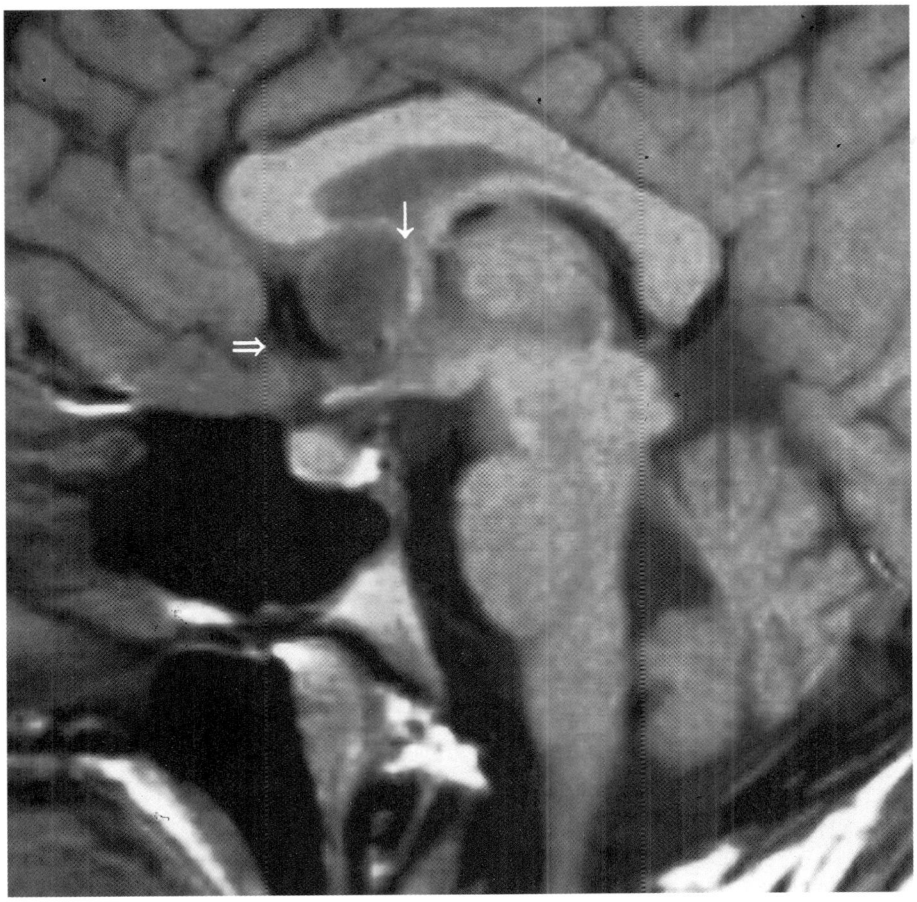

A

Fig. 21. *Hypothalamic pilocytic astrocytoma.* 22-year-old woman with diabetes insipidus. The T_1-weighted sagittal view (A) shows a hyperintense neoplasm which obliterates the anterior aspect of the third ventricle; however, the ventricle wall does not appear to be involved (↓). The hypothalamic origin of the tumor is inferred from the anterior displacement of the A_2 portions of the A.C.A. (⇒). The structure is homogeneous and on the T_2-weighted sequence (B) the signal is highly hyperintense. On the coronal view (B), note the thickening of the pituitary stalk (↘).

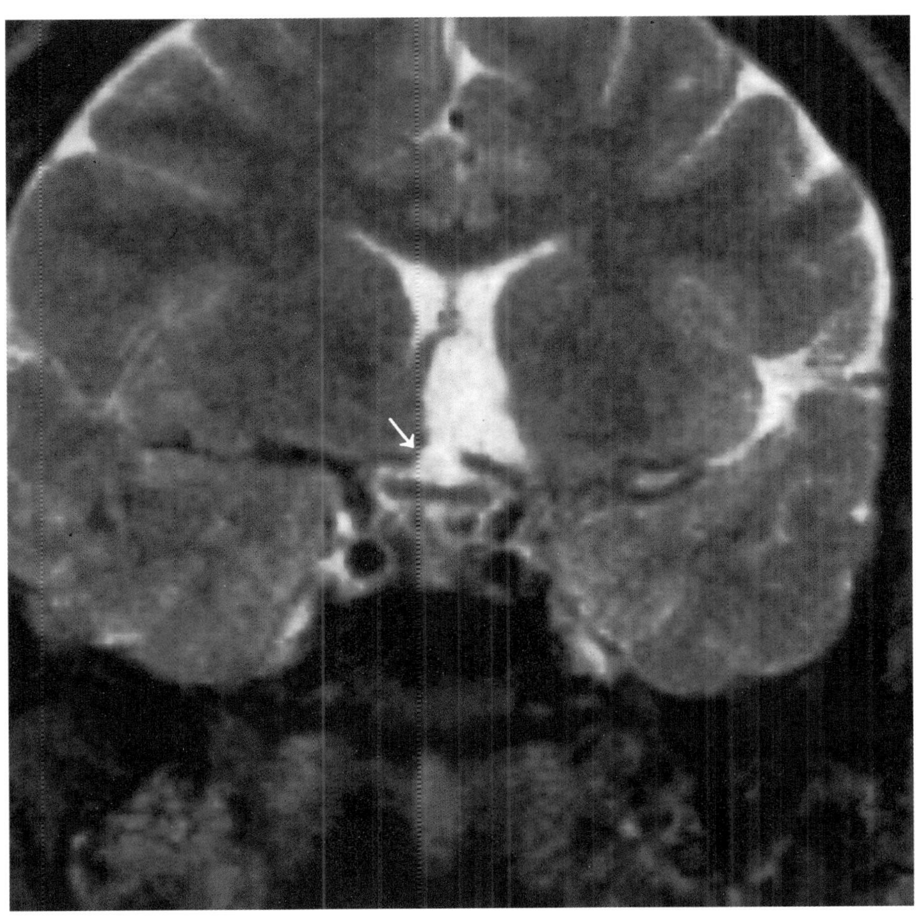

B

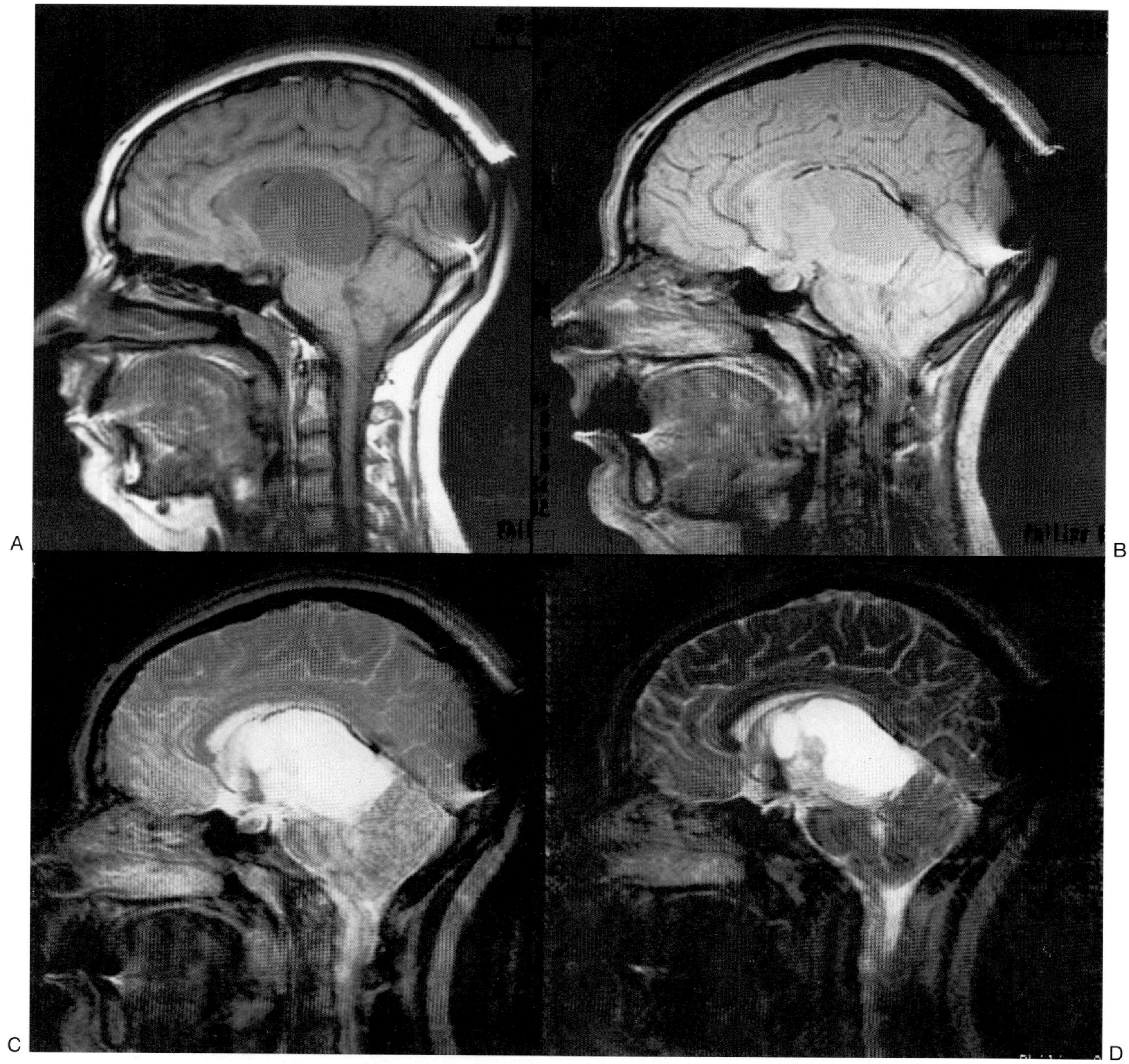

Fig. 22. *Hypothalamic cystic pilocytic astrocytoma.* 24-year-old woman. History of prior CSF shunt surgery owing to obstructive hydrocephalus, sudden onset of coma, vertical gaze palsy and bradycardia. T_1-weighted median sagittal spin-echo (A) and multi-echo (B) sequences, TE = 30, 90, 180 msec (B, C, D). There is a predominantly cystic neoplasm; the solid component is located in the hypothalamus; the cystic component occupies the third ventricle and the pineal region and compresses the quadrigeminal plate and the midbrain. On the T_1-weighted sequence (A), the solid tumor appears as isointense; the cystic component has a signal similar to the CSF. By elongating the echo times, a better differentiation is obtained, evidencing signs of septations inside the tumor.

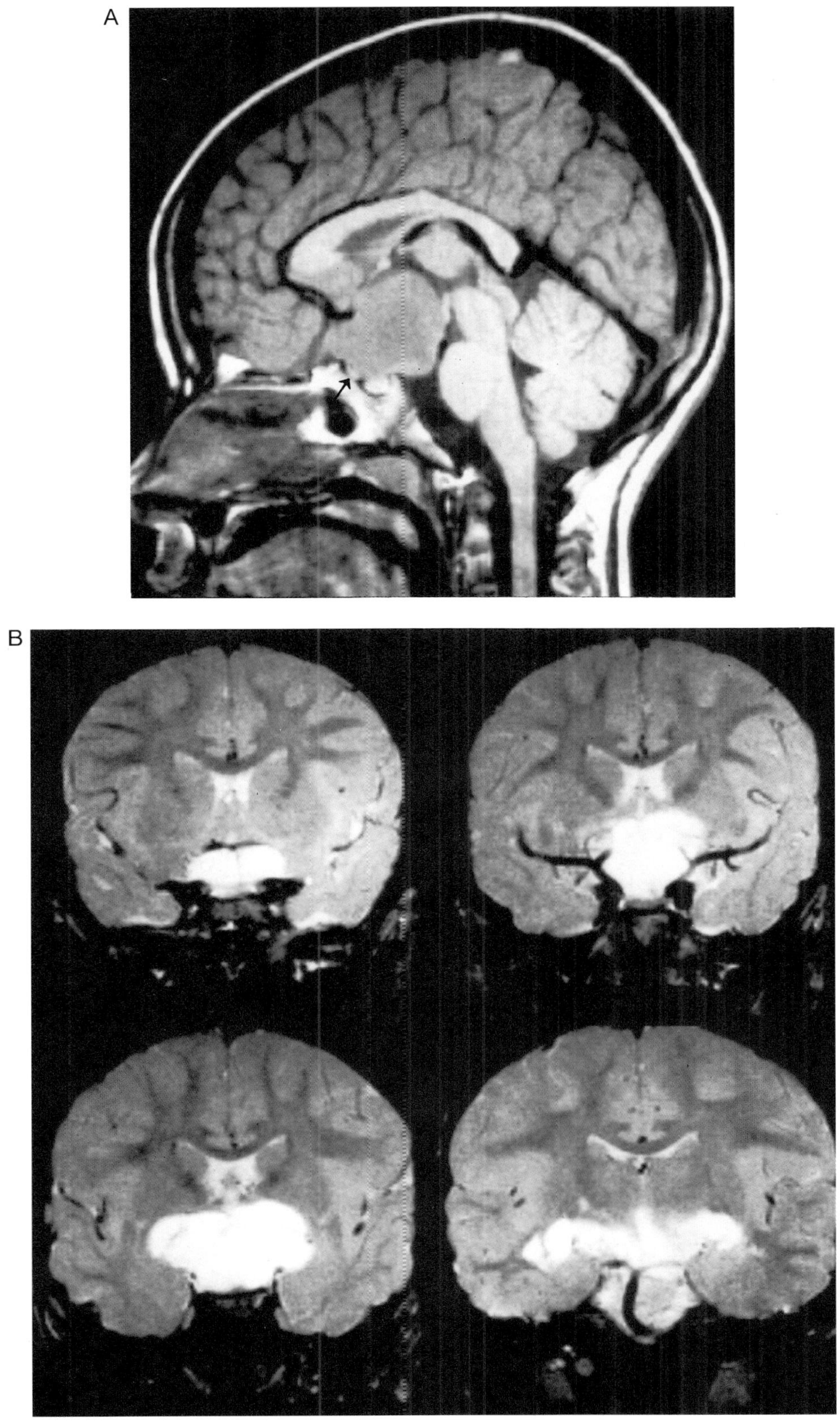

Fig. 23. *Chiasm-hypothalamic solid pilocytic astrocytoma.* 9-year-old girl with severe somatic hypoevolutism. A – The T_1-weighted mid-sagittal image outlines a huge, homogeneous, hypothalamic neoplasm adhering to the chiasm (↗); it occupies the third ventricle, displaces part of the hypothalamic nuclei posteriorly, and verticalizes the brainstem. No hydrocephalus is observed, since Monro's foramina are patent. The T_2-weighted images (B) visualize the partly infiltrating character of this pilocytic astrocytoma, presumably spreading to the white matter of the temporal lobes. Note the relationships between the mass and the vessels of the circle of Willis.

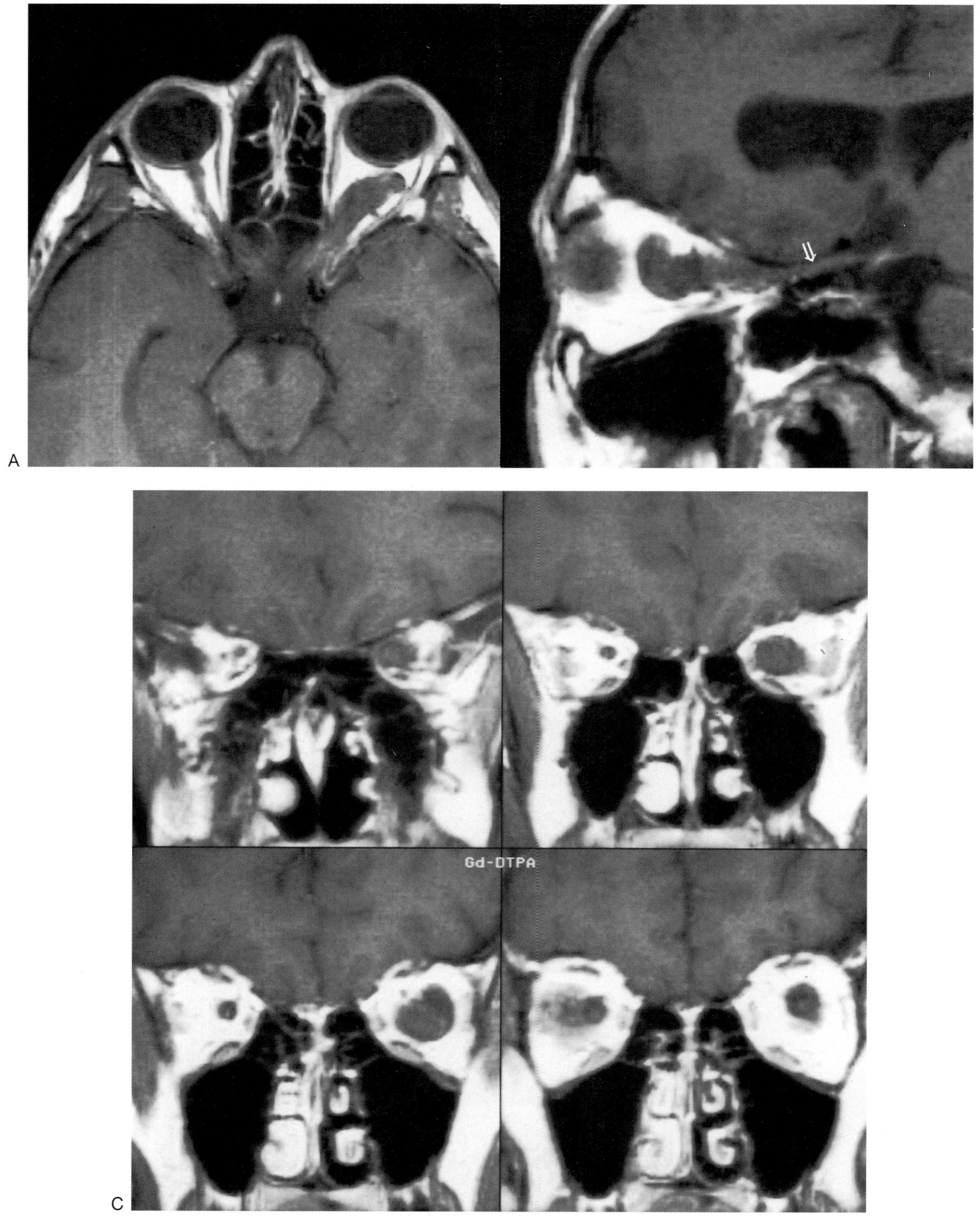

Fig. 24. *Left optic nerve glioma.* 11-year-old boy with mild exophthalmos and visual loss. Examination after i.v. GD-DTPA with T_1-weighted sequence. A – The axial image documents the enlargement of the intraorbital and intracanalar portions of the optic nerve. B – The oblique paraaxial image confirms that the chiasm and the optic tract (⇓) are disease-free. C – Coronal image showing the distension of the nerve from the orbital apex to its retrobulbar portion.

A

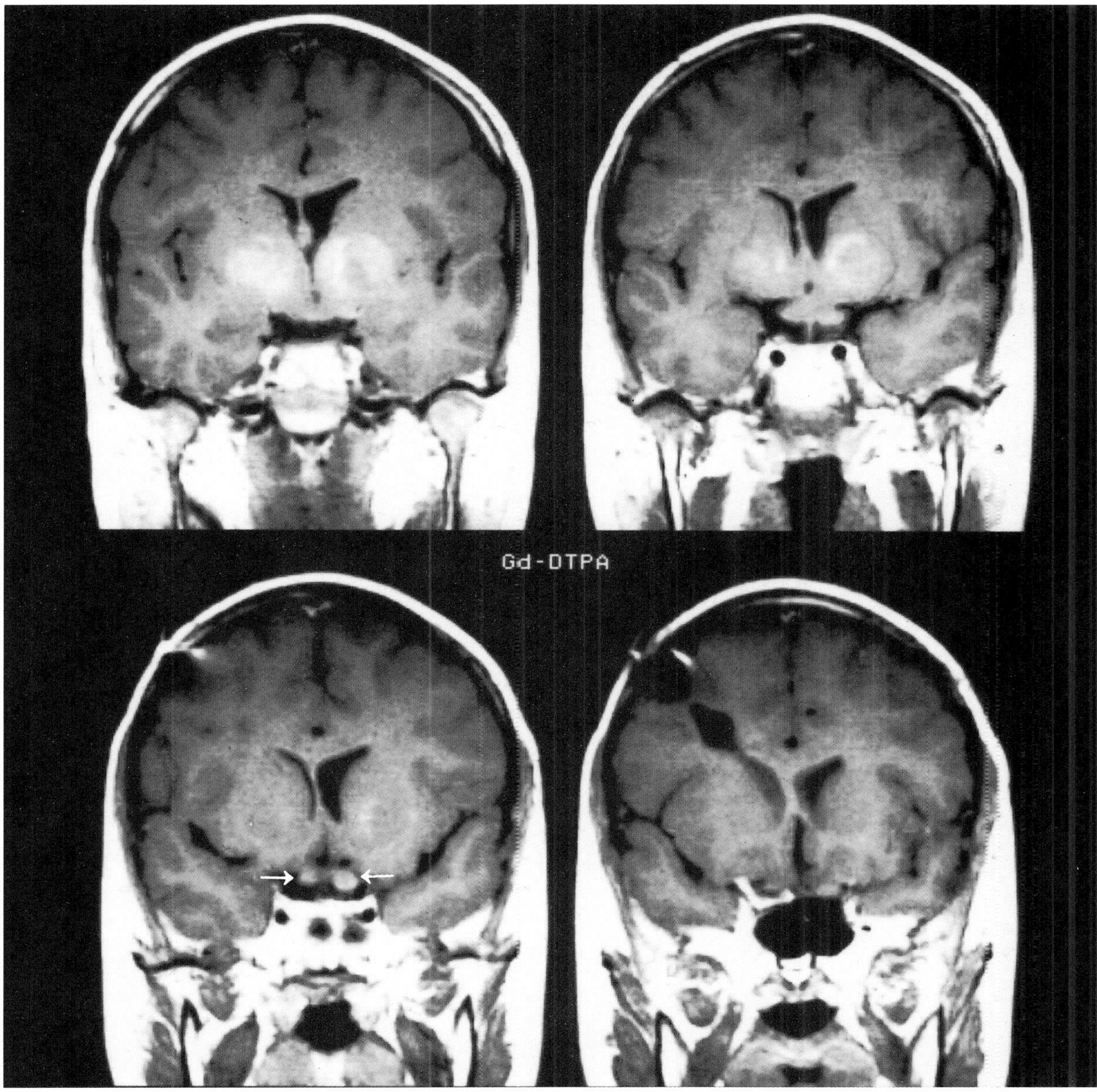

B

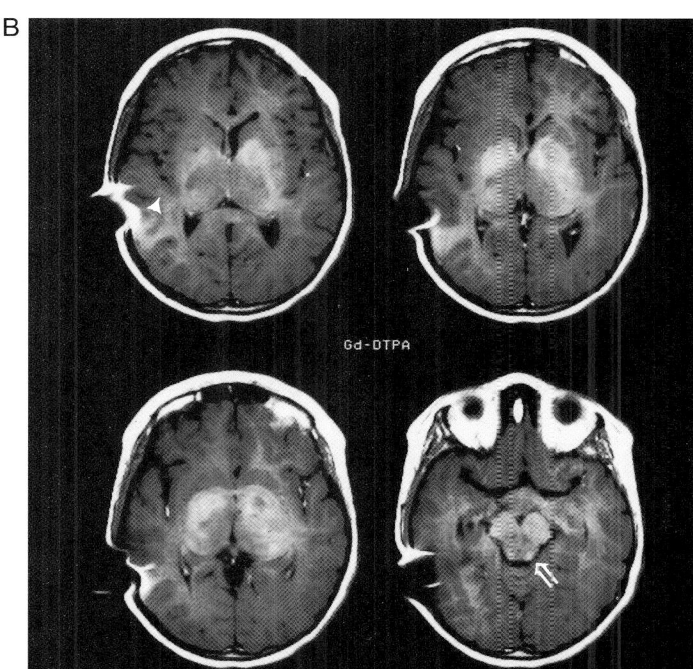

Fig. 25. *Opto-chiasmatic glioma.* 10-year-old girl with a history of ventricular-peritoneal CSF shunt surgery owing to aqueductal stenosis, secondary to Recklinghausen's disease. At present, mild left-eye visual impairment and moderate mental hypoevolutism. A – T_1-weighted coronal images after i.v. GD-DTPA. Note the enlargement of the chiasm and the neoplasm inside its left portion. The intradural optic nerves in the intracranial region (←) are enlarged and hyperintense owing to c.e. The hyperintensity of the basal ganglia with apparent sparing (B) of the thalami and of the caudate nuclei is an unusual finding, likely to be ascribed to dysplastic gliosis secondary to Recklinghausen's disease. The brainstem exhibits minor fibromas (⇑). The superficial artifacts (◂) are due to the CSF shunt.

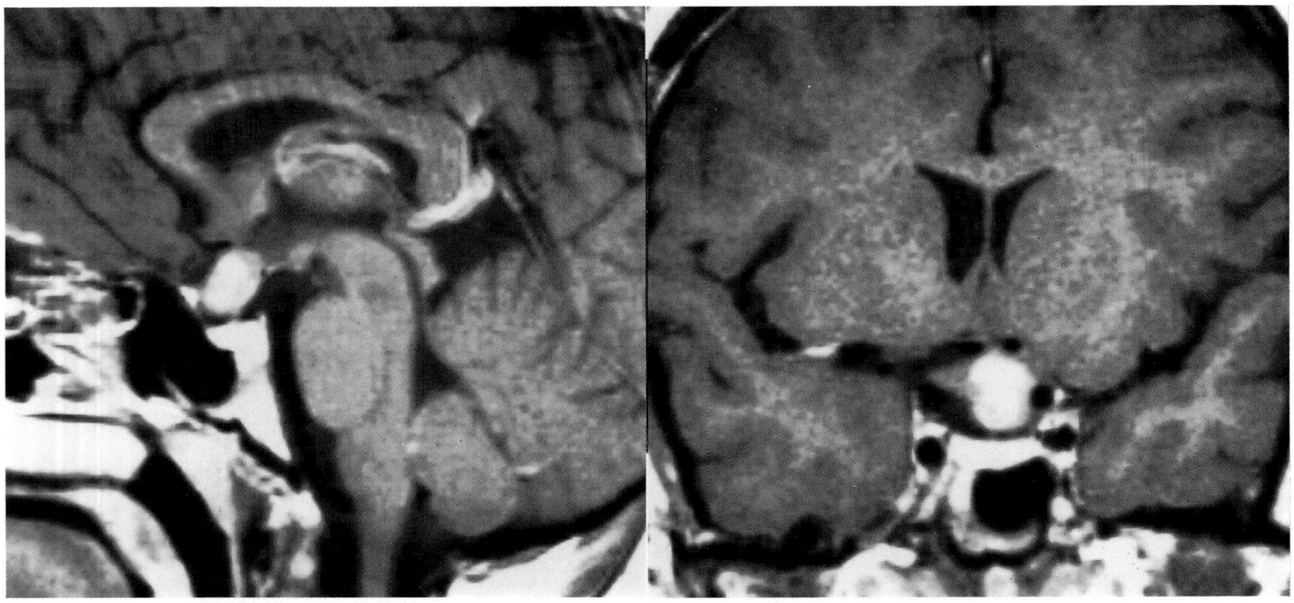

Fig. 26. *Chiasmatic glioma.* 18-year-old woman with severe left-eye visual impairment. The examination after i.v. GD-DTPA well depicts the spread of the neoplasm, which fills the left part of the chiasm and the ipsilateral optic tract.

A
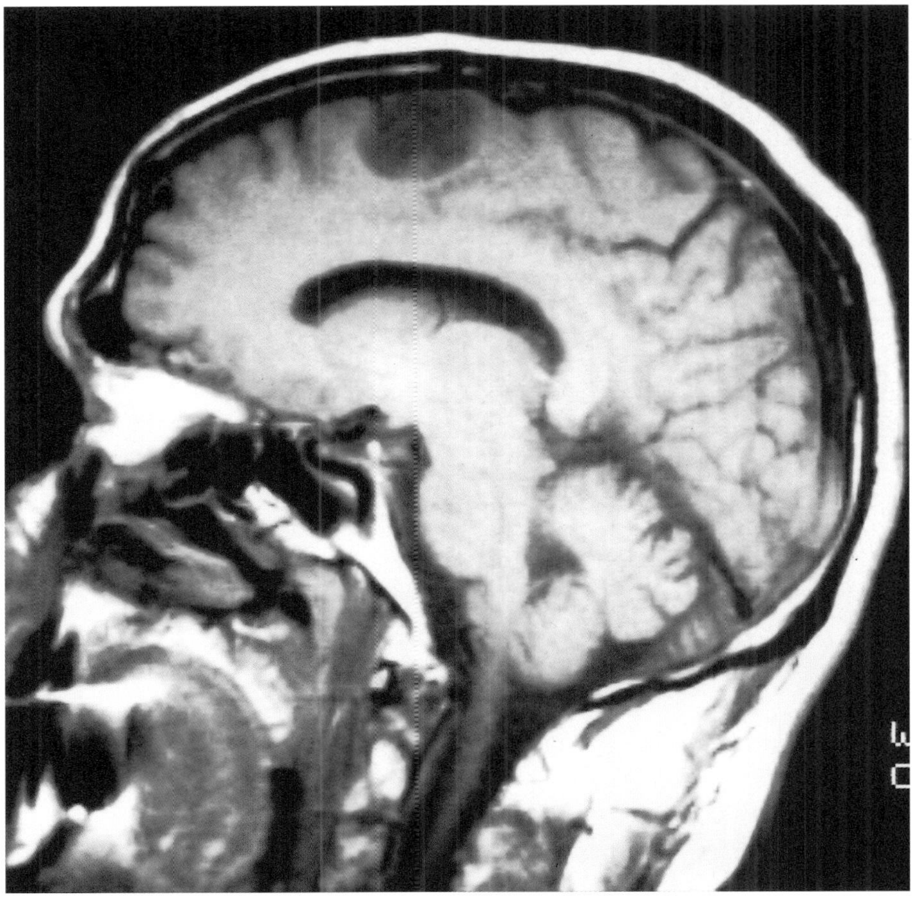

B
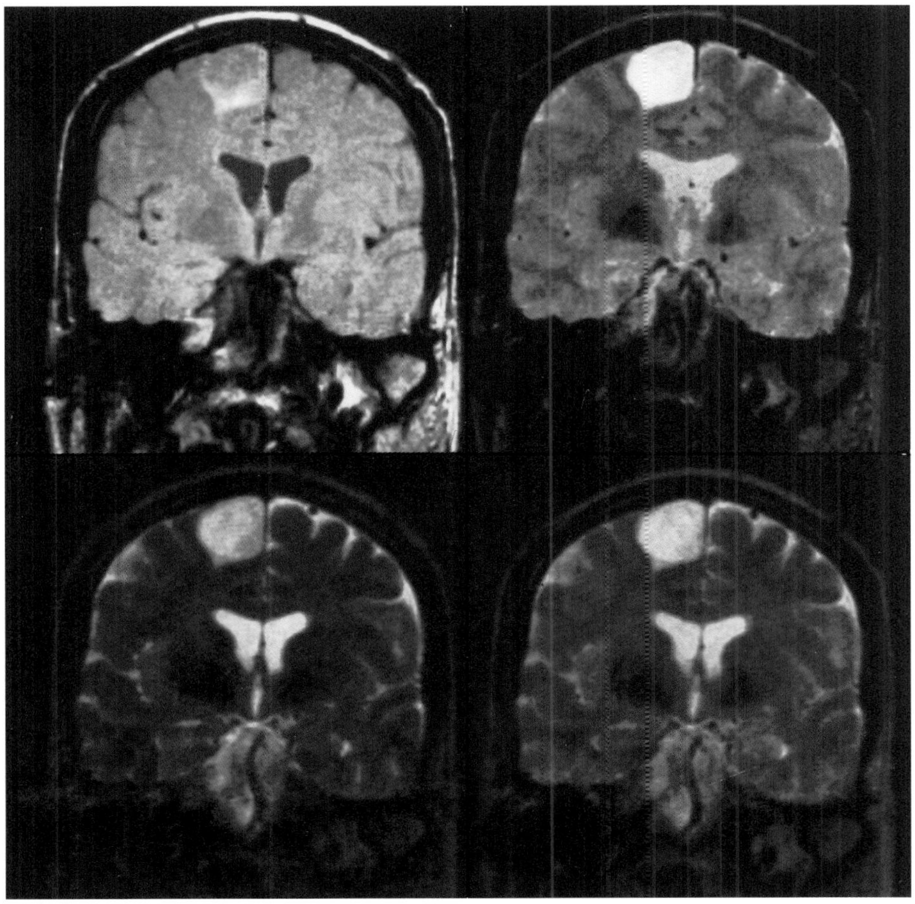

Fig. 27. *Right parasagittal prerolandic low-grade astrocytoma.* (A) – T_1-weighted sagittal image showing a rounded lesion (3 cm) with CSF-like signal. The medial gyri appear to be compressed as if by an extraaxial tumor. The coronal multi-echo sequence (B) specifies the solid nature of the lesion; early echoes show mild perilesional edema; late echoes show slight signal inhomogeneity.

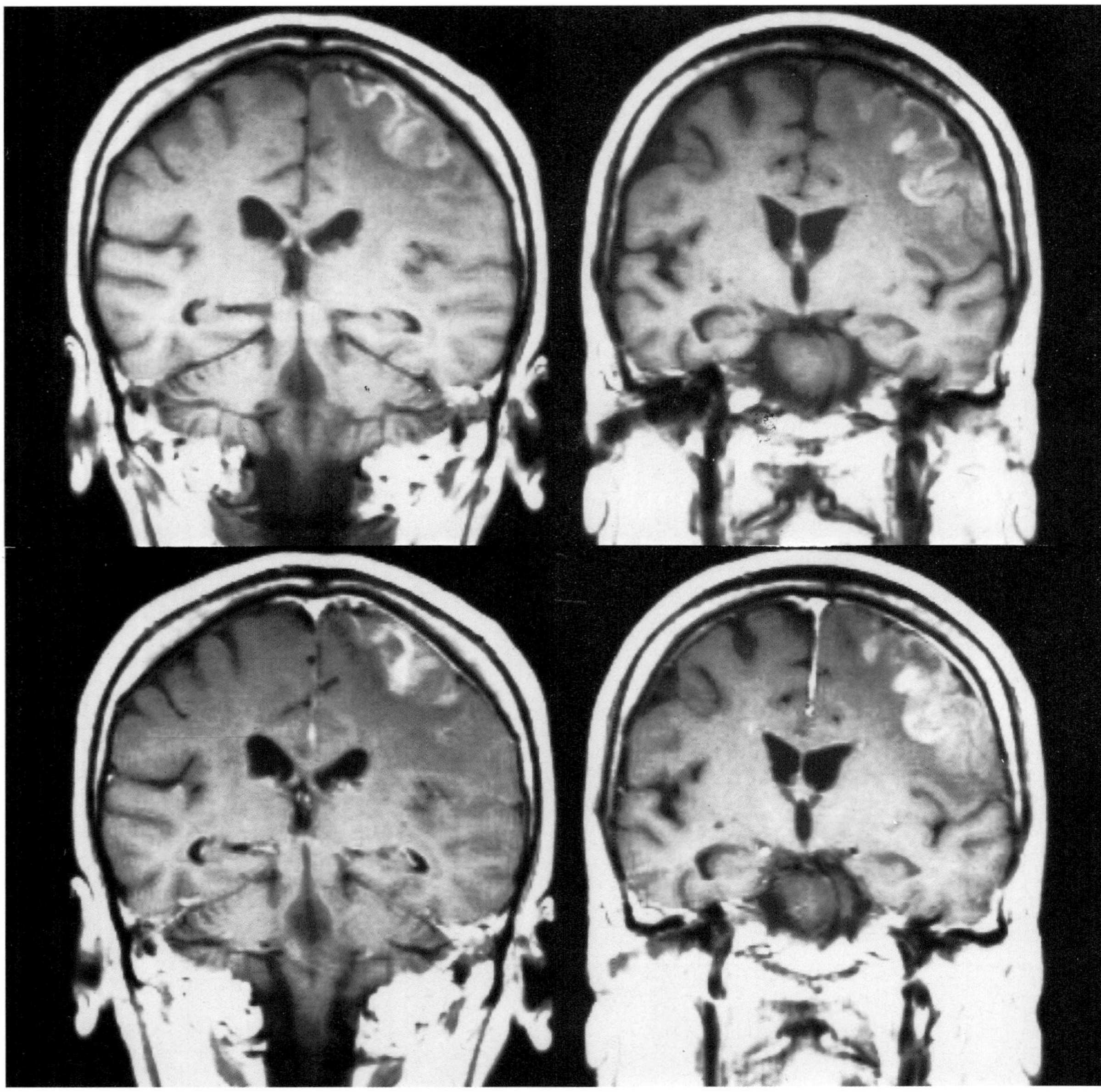

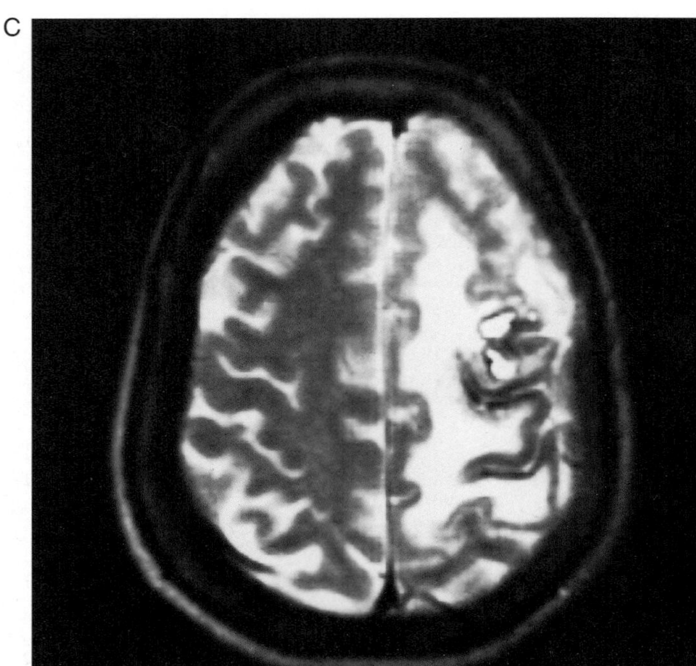

Fig. 28. *Left frontoparietal oligodendroglioma.* 50-year-old woman with right hemiplegia and aphasia. Pre- (A) and post- (B) GD-DTPA T_1-weighted images demonstrate an infiltrating tumor. This follows the course of the gyri, which appear to be drawn by a recent hemorrhagic effusion. The tissue significantly enhances after GD-DTPA; within it, the minute low-signal images can be ascribed to typical punctiform calcifications. Observe the edema of the white matter. C – The T_2-weighted axial image better shows the perilesional edema and the foci of hemorrhagic infarction, encircled by hemosiderin.

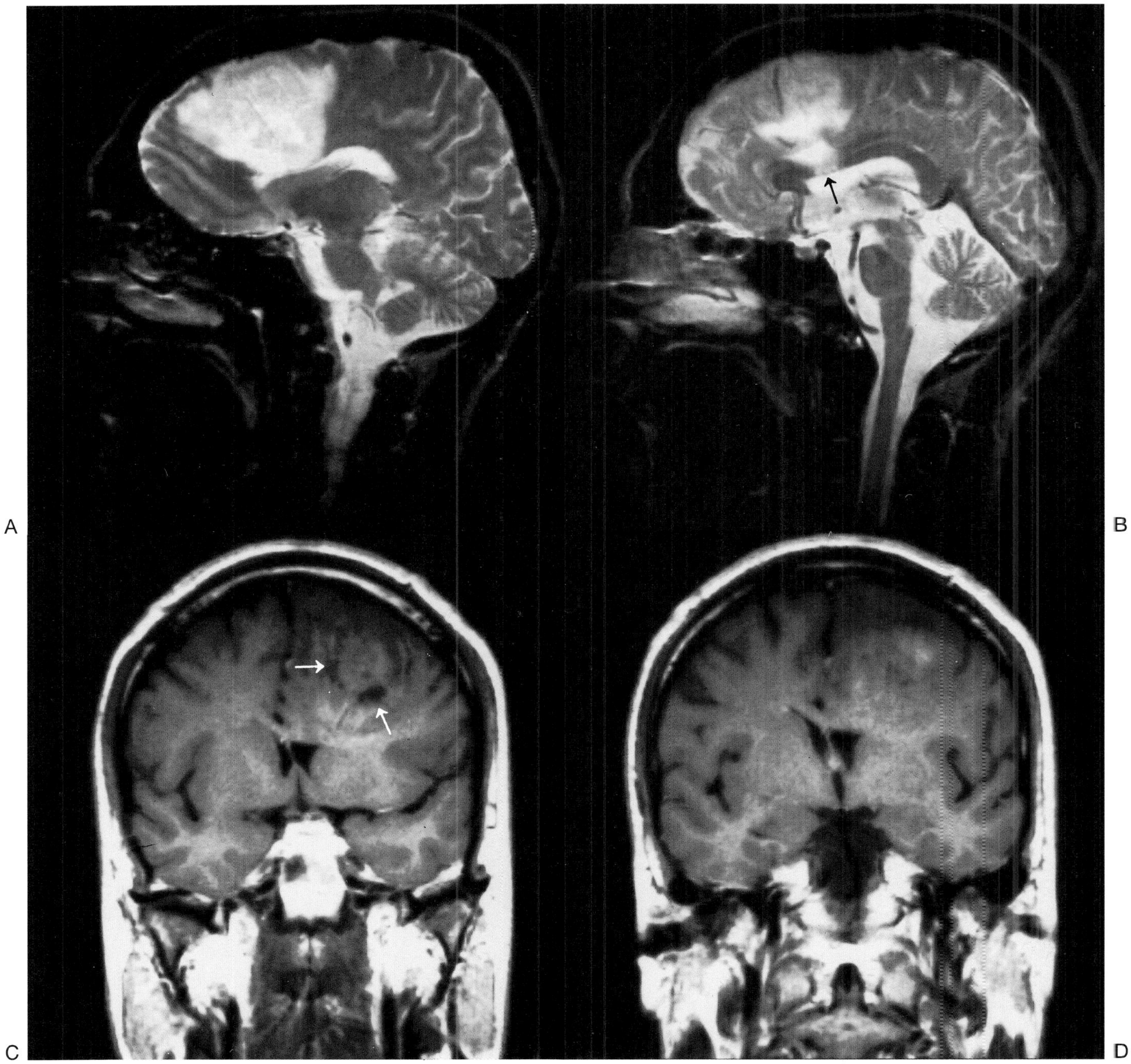

Fig. 29. *Left posterior frontal oligodendroglioma.* 25-year-old man with recent seizures. A, B – T_2-weighted sagittal images: hyperintense, moderately inhomogeneous, rounded neoplasm anteriorly to the ascending frontal gyrus. The edema makes the tumor image brighter. Note the compression of the corpus callosum, damaged by the edema (↖). C, D – T_1-weighted coronal images after GD-DTPA: note the calcifications (→ ↖) and the poor and inhomogeneous c.e.

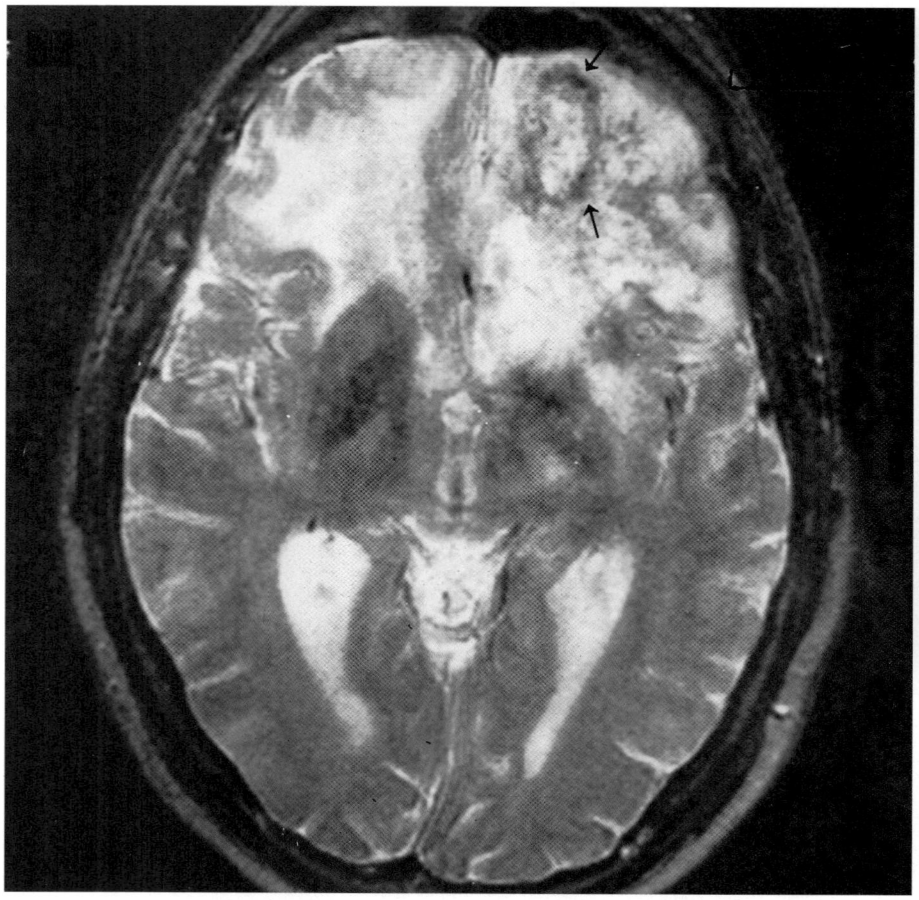

A

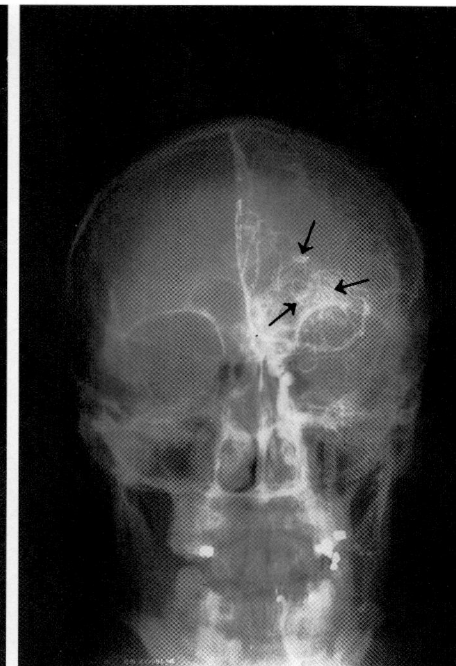

C

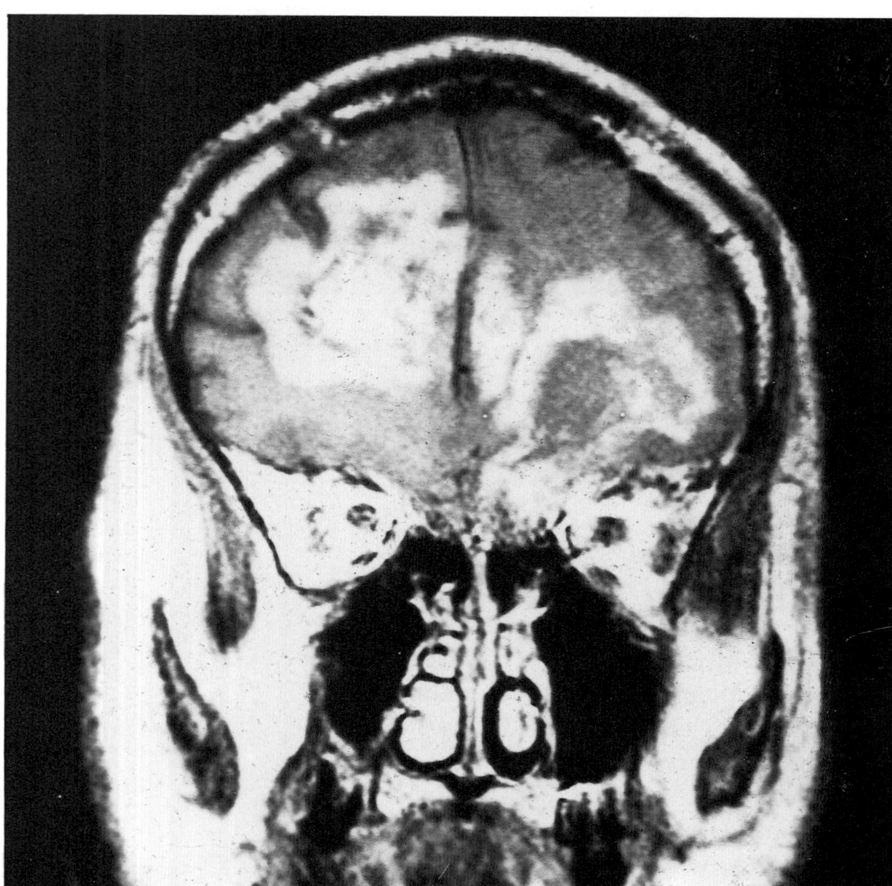

B

Fig. 30. *Bifrontal anaplastic oligodendroglioma with glioblastoma multiforme foci.* The T_2-weighted axial image evidences a largely inhomogeneous mass occupying the base of both frontal lobes. The left neoplastic component is more calcified (↙ ↖) and more inhomogeneous, suggesting a high-malignant neoplasm. After GD-DTPA (B), the image is enhanced and the tumor is better delimited from the edema. Note the left frontal necrotic component whose appearance is similar to the glioblastoma multiforme. This assumption is corroborated by angiography (C), showing a typical tumoral blush with early arterovenous shunts and "corkscrew" vessels.

Fig. 31. *Third-ventricle oligodendroglioma.* 16-year-old girl with severe intracranial hypertension. The proton-density coronal SE image portrays a high-signal neoplasm which totally occupies the third ventricle (←). Through Monro's foramen, the neoplasm extends to the left lateral ventricle, which is dilated and deviates the septum pellucidum. The right lateral ventricle and the temporal horns are less dilated. Observe the displacement of the internal cerebral veins (↗) and of the left thalamostriated vein.

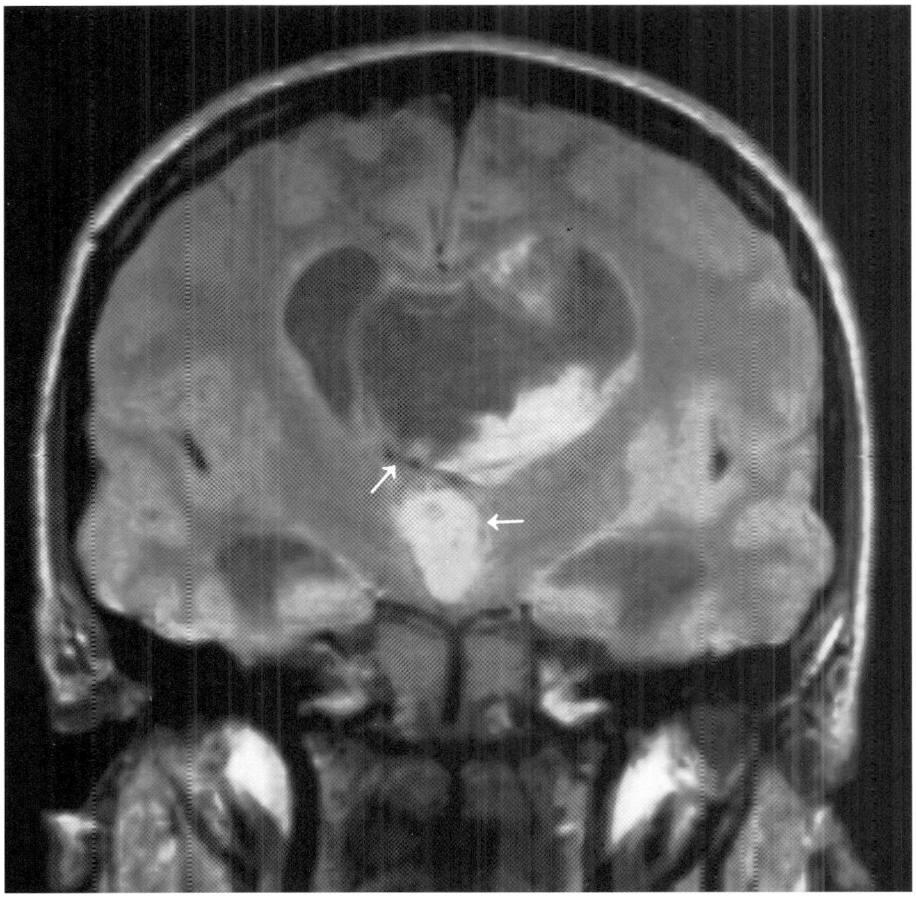

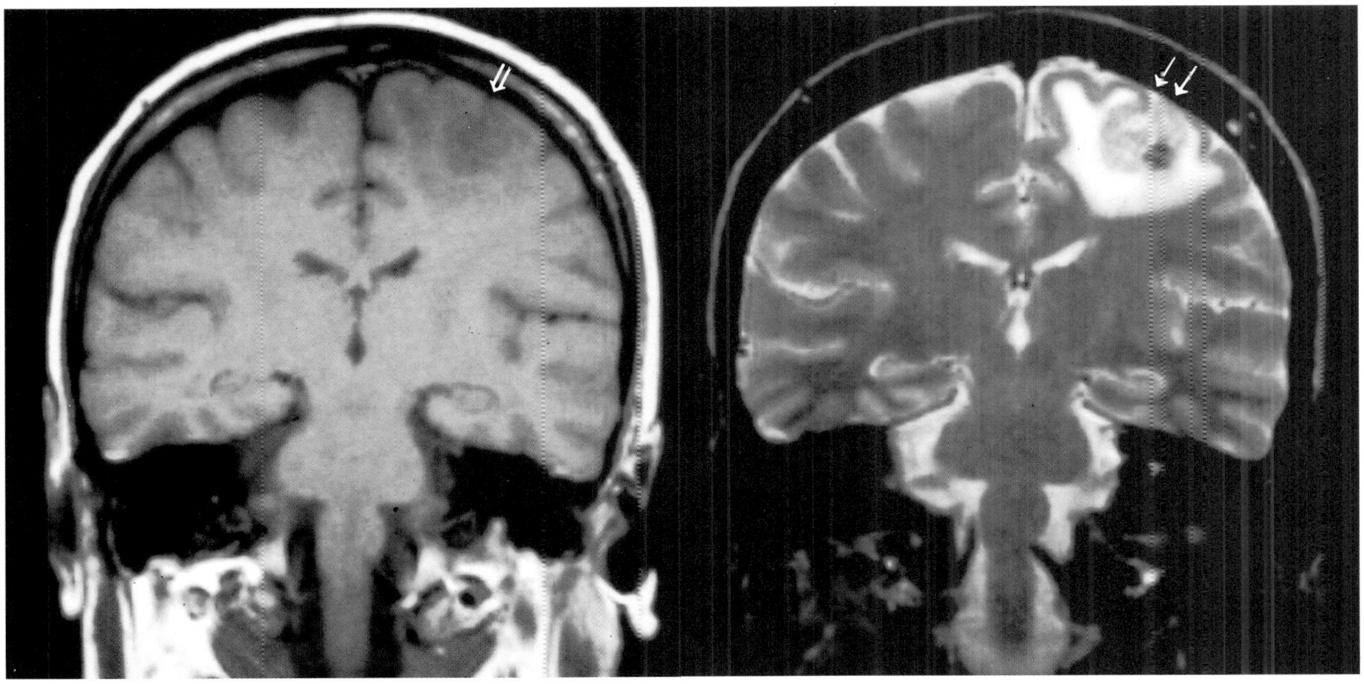

Fig. 32. *Left posterior frontal oligodendroglioma.* Small subcortical tumoral nodule highlighted by the surrounding edema. The T_1-weighted image shows an isointense tumor (⇓). The T_2-weighted image better depicts the edema, the calcification, and the neoplasm which is slightly hyperintense with the cerebral tissue. GD-DTPA administration did not give rise to signal enhancement

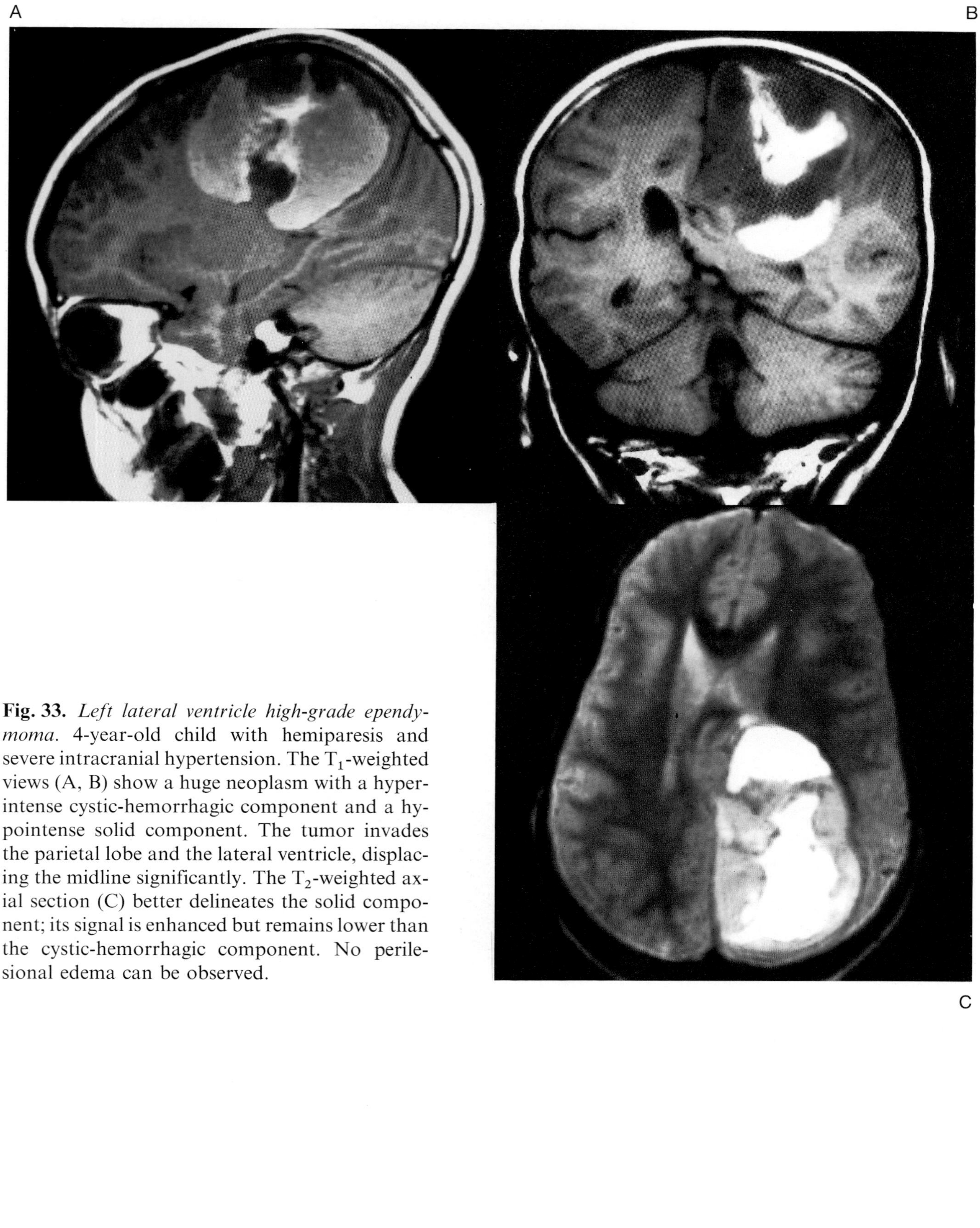

Fig. 33. *Left lateral ventricle high-grade ependymoma.* 4-year-old child with hemiparesis and severe intracranial hypertension. The T_1-weighted views (A, B) show a huge neoplasm with a hyperintense cystic-hemorrhagic component and a hypointense solid component. The tumor invades the parietal lobe and the lateral ventricle, displacing the midline significantly. The T_2-weighted axial section (C) better delineates the solid component; its signal is enhanced but remains lower than the cystic-hemorrhagic component. No perilesional edema can be observed.

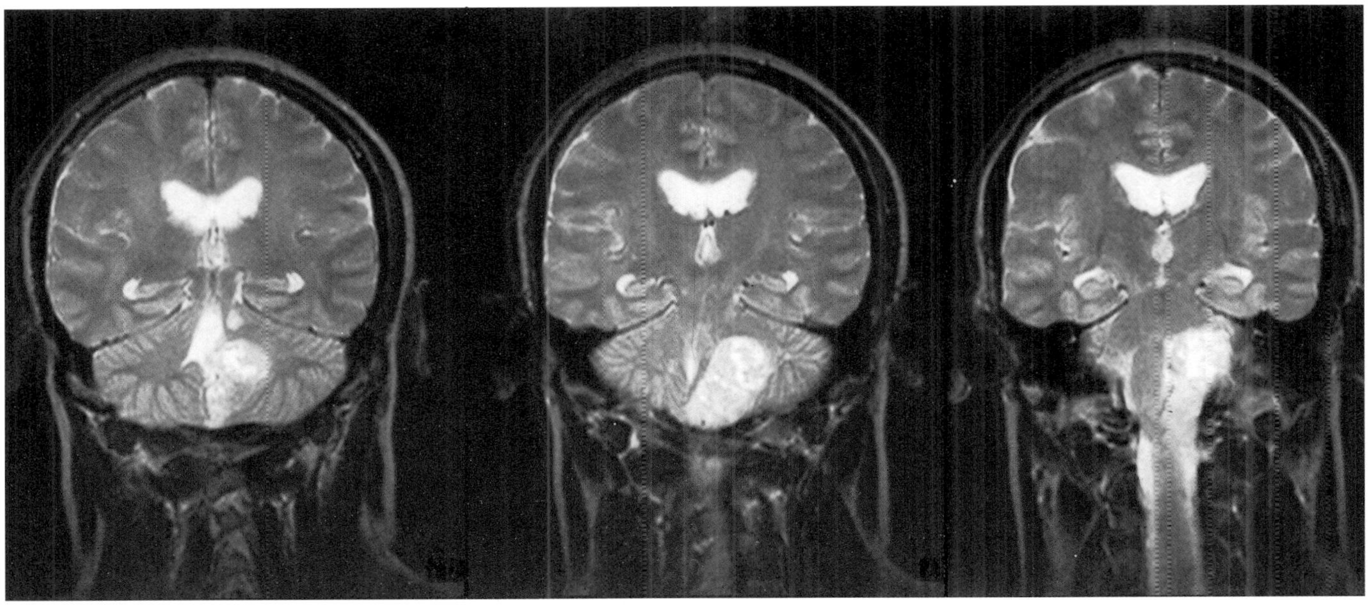

A

B

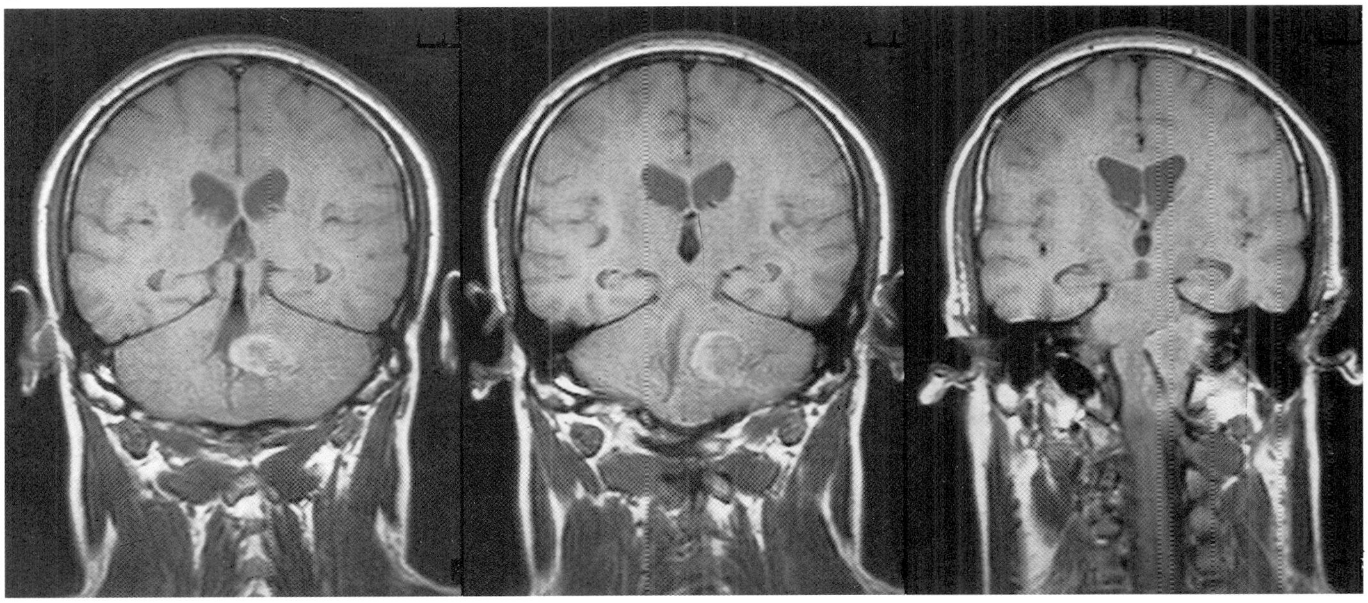

Fig. 34. *Fourth ventricle left lateral recess ependymoma.* (A) – T_2-weighted scans demonstrate a fairly inhomogeneous, hyperintense neoplasm: it originates from the lateral recess, passes through Luschka's foramen and grows into the spinal canal as far as C2. (B) – GD-DTPA enhances the tumor, delimiting it from the surrounding tissue. The extraaxial component medializes the V.A. and distorts the bulbopontine junction.

A B

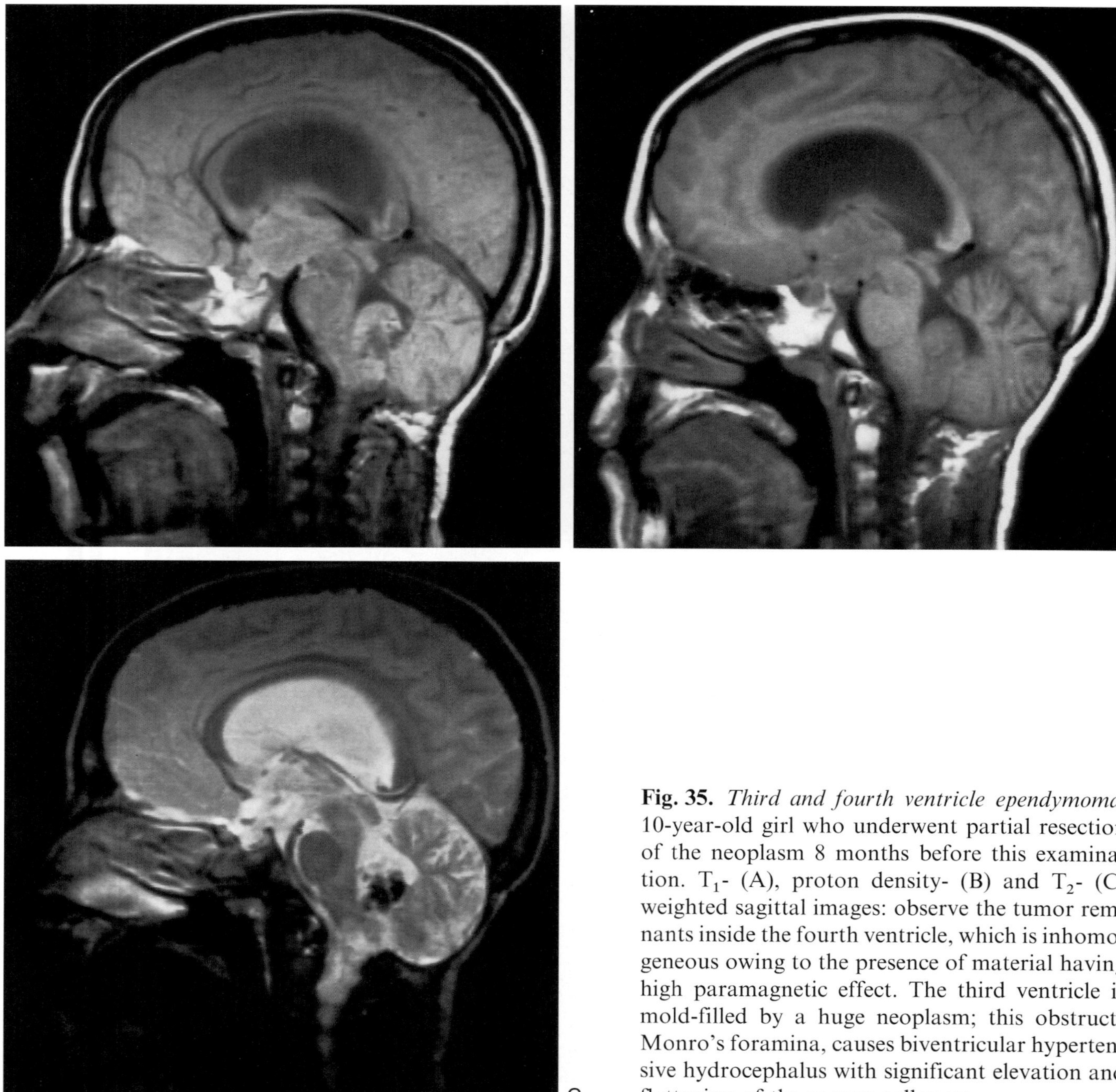

C

Fig. 35. *Third and fourth ventricle ependymoma.* 10-year-old girl who underwent partial resection of the neoplasm 8 months before this examination. T_1- (A), proton density- (B) and T_2- (C) weighted sagittal images: observe the tumor remnants inside the fourth ventricle, which is inhomogeneous owing to the presence of material having high paramagnetic effect. The third ventricle is mold-filled by a huge neoplasm; this obstructs Monro's foramina, causes biventricular hypertensive hydrocephalus with significant elevation and flattening of the corpus callosum.

A

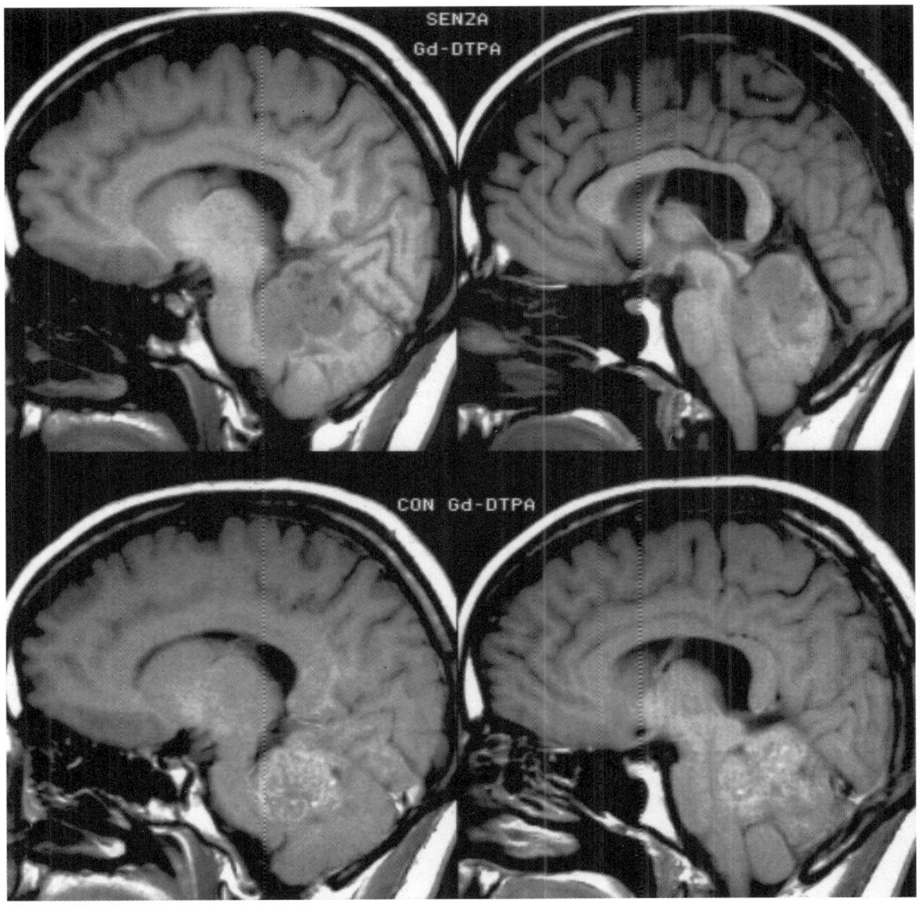

B

C

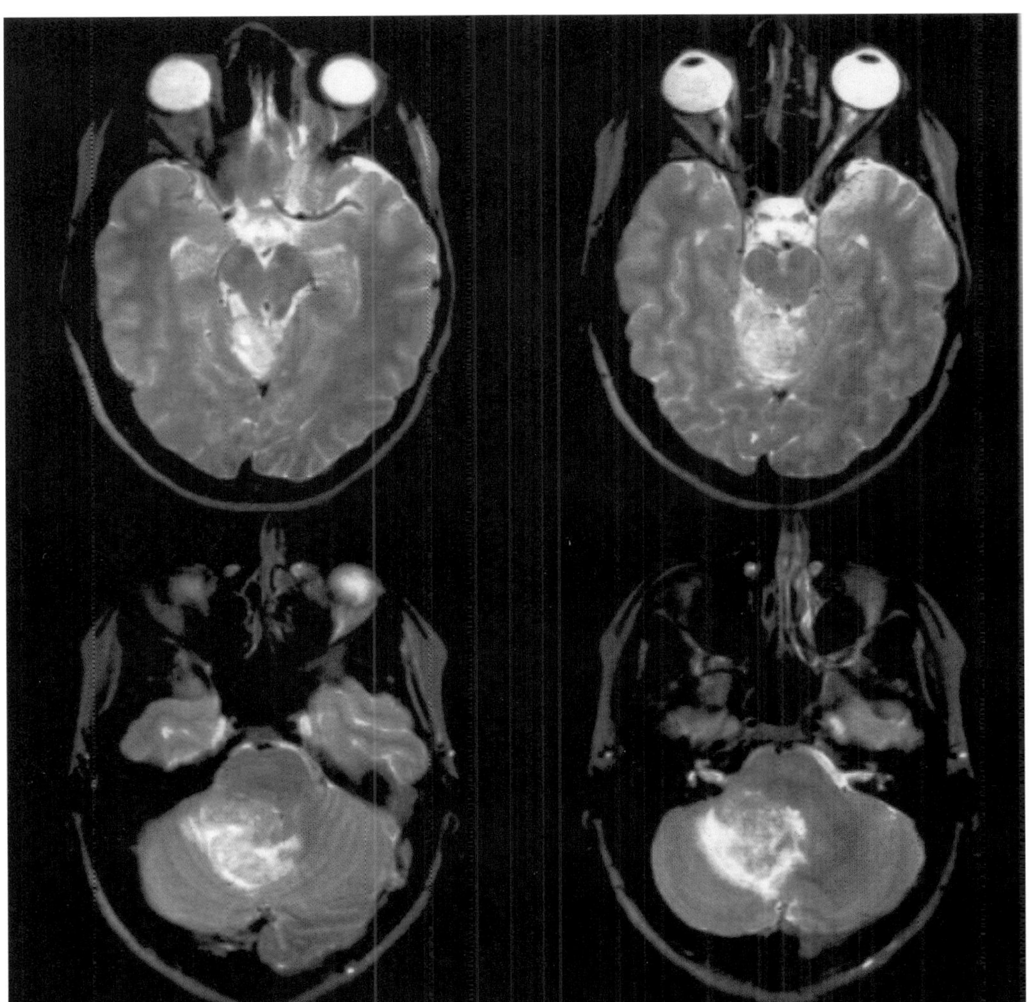

Fig. 36. *Medulloblastoma.* 20-year-old woman with gait disorders and vomiting. The T_1-weighted sagittal images before (A) and after (B) GD-DTPA show a hypointense neoplasm starting from the upper vermis and eccentrically growing into the right cerebellar lobe. Vascular structures can be observed which become hyperintense after GD-DTPA administration. The signal is enhanced after GD-DTPA. Note the compression of the posterior aspect of the pons and the absence of hydrocephalus. C – The T_2-weighted images demonstrate the edema of the cerebellar hemisphere, a subtle structural inhomogeneity of the neoplasm and its spread towards the tentorial notch and the pineal region.

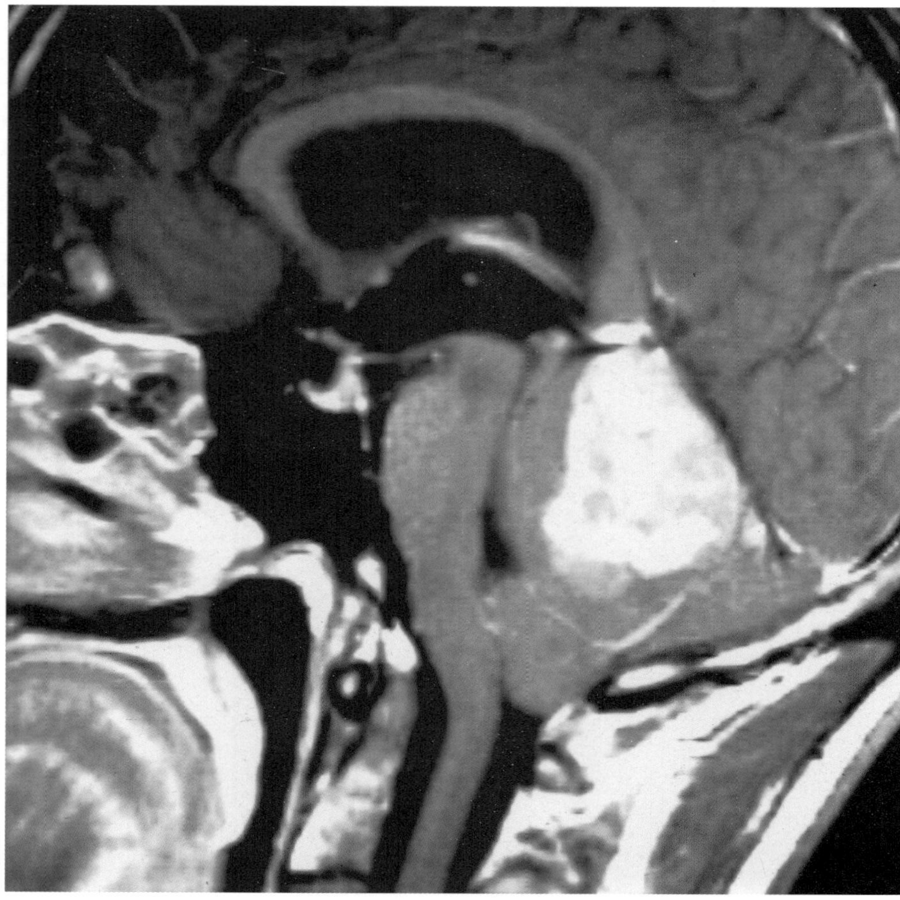

A

B

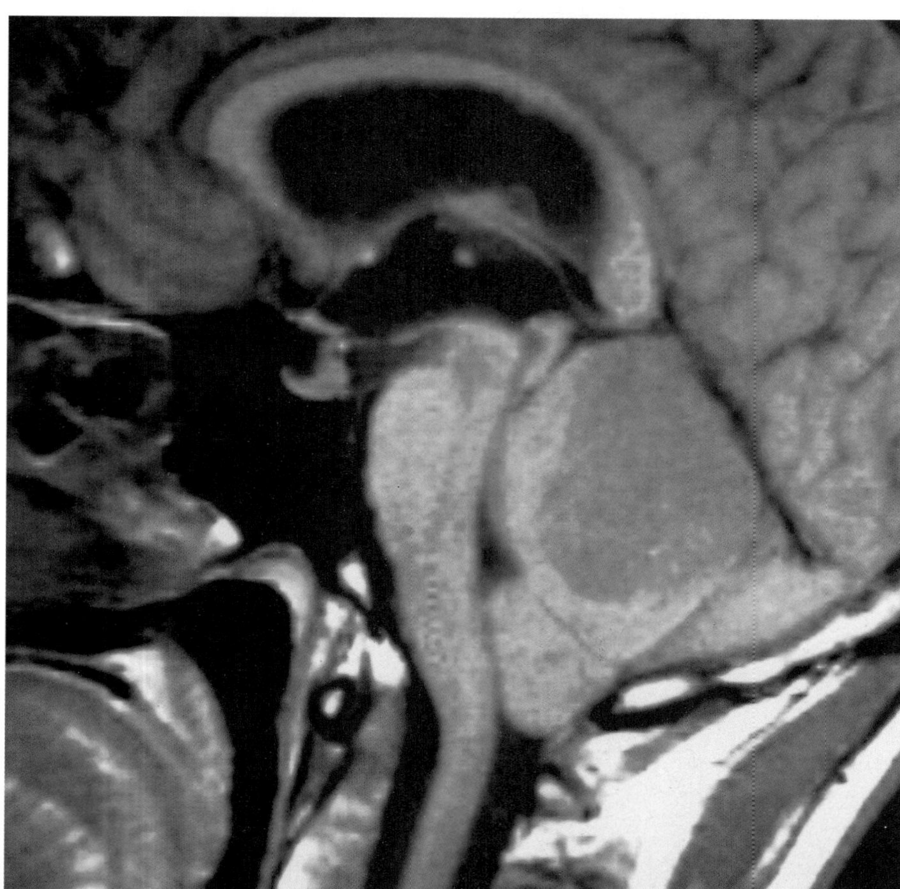

Fig. 37. *Upper vermis medulloblastoma.* T_1-weighted views before (A) and after (B) GD-DTPA. The tumor is more contrast-enhanced than in the previous case. Its structure is more uniform. The compression of the Sylvian aqueduct causes triventricular hydrocephalus. The fourth ventricle is displaced but not occupied by the tumor. Note the herniation of the cerebellar tonsil in the occipital foramen and the P.I.C.A. with lowered choroidal point.

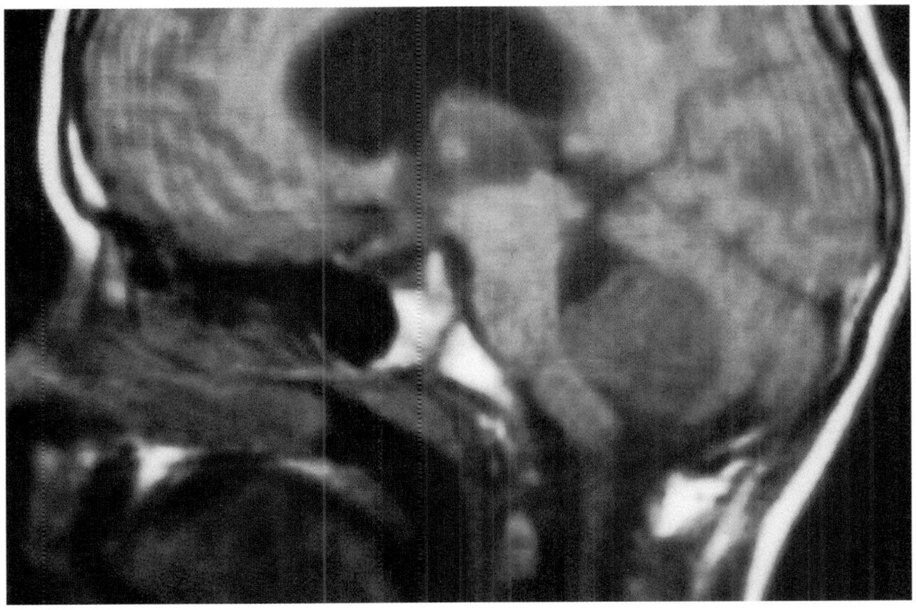

Fig. 38. *Medulloblastoma of the lower vermis.* 11-year-old boy with severe intracranial hypertension and gait disturbances. T_1-weighted sagittal view: hypointense mass occupying the lower half of the fourth ventricle and displacing the brainstem anteriorly and the cerebellum posteriorly. The hydrocephalus is caused by the obliteration of the fourth ventricle.

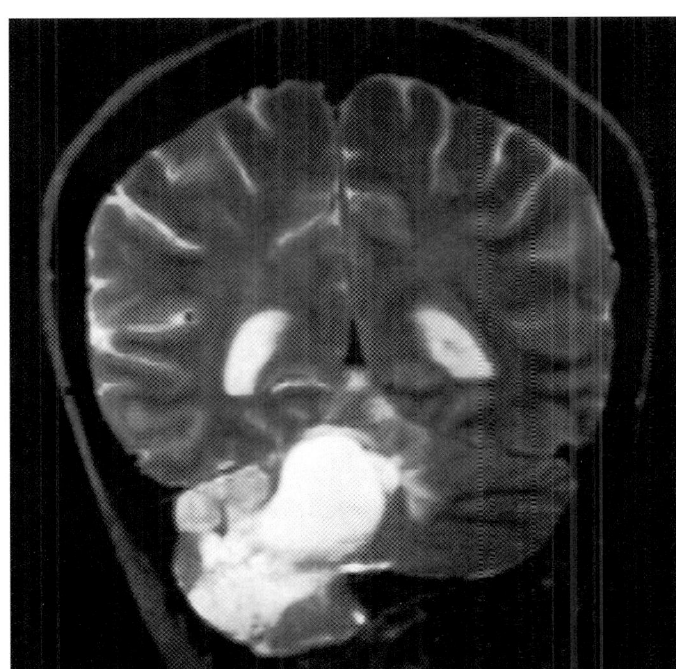

Fig. 39. *Recurrent medulloblastoma.* T_2-weighted coronal section: the surgical cavity is occupied by a markedly hyperintense CSF. At the level of the right cerebellar convexity, adjacent to the tentorium, two relatively hyperintense neoplastic nodules are evident.

References

1. Afea D, Muller W, Slowik F et al. (1983) Supratentorial lobar ependymomas: report on the grading and surgical periods in 80 cases, including 46 recurrences. Acta Neurochir 69:243–251
2. Albert A, Lee BCP, Saint-Louis L et al. (1986) MRI of optic chiasm and optic pathways. AJNR 7:255–258
3. Albright AL, Price RA, Guthkelch NA (1983) Brain stem gliomas of children: A clinicopathological study. Cancer 52:2313–2319
4. Allen JC, Epstein F (1982) Medulloblastoma and other primary malignant neuroectodermal tumours of CNS. The effect of patient's age and extent of disease on prognosis. J Neurosurg 57:446–451
5. Ammirati M, Vick N, Liao Y et al. (1987) Effect of extent of surgical resection on survival and quality of life in patients with supratentorial glioblastoma and anaplastic astrocytomas. Neurosurgery 21:201–206
6. Apuzzo MLJ, Chondrorome PT, Cohen D et al. (1987) Computed imaging stereotaxi: experience and perspective related to 500 procedures applied to brain masses. Neurosurgery 20:930–937
7. Atlas SW, Grossman RI, Gomori JM et al. (1987) Hemorrhagic intracranial malignant neoplasms: spin-echo MR imaging. Radiology 164:71–77
8. Azar-Kia B, Naheedy MH, Elias DA et al. (1987) Optic nerve tumors: role of magnetic resonance imaging and computed tomography. Radiol Clin North Am 25:561–581
9. Ball WS Jr, Towbin RB (1989) MRI of pediatric central nervous system neoplasms. In: Pomeranz SJ (ed) Craniospinal Magnetic Resonance Imaging. W. B. Saunders Co, Philadelphia, 177–207
10. Bognanno JR, Edwards MK, Lee TA et al. (1988) Cranial MR imaging in neurofibromatosis. AJNR 9:461–468
11. Brant-Zawadzki M, Norman D, Newton TH et al. (1984) Magnetic resonance of the brain: the optimal screening technique. Radiology 152:71–77
12. Brant-Zawadski M, Badami JP, Mills CM et al. (1984) Primary intracranial tumor imaging. A comparison of magnetic resonance and CT. Radiology 150:435–440
13. Brant-Zawadzki M, Berry I, Osaki L et al. (1986) Gd-DTPA in clinical MR of the brain. 1. Intraaxial lesions. AJR 147:1223–1230
14. Bronen RA, Sze G (1990) Magnetic resonance contrast agents: theory and application to the central nervous system. J Neurosurg 73:820–840
15. Bruce DA, Shut L, Sutton LN (1990) Supratentorial brain tumors in children. In: Youmans JR (ed) Neurological Surgery, 3rd edn. W. B. Saunders Co, Philadelphia, 3000–3016
16. Bryan P (1974) CSF seeding of intra-cranial tumours: A study of 96 cases. Clin Radiol 25:355–360
17. Burger PC (1985) Gliomas: pathology. In: Wilkins RH, Rengachary SS (eds) Neurosurgery, Vol 1., McGraw-Hill, New York, 553–563
18. Burger PC (1986) Malignant astrocytic neoplasms: Classification, pathologic anatomy and response to treatment. Semin Oncol 13:16–26
19. Chadduck WM, Roycroft D, Brown MW (1983) Multicentric glioma as a cause of multiple cerebral lesions. Neurosurgery 13:170–175
20. Ciric I, Vick NA, Mikhael MA et al. (1990) Aggressive surgery for malignant supratentorial gliomas. Clin Neurosurg 36:375–383
21. Clark GB, Henry JM, Mc Keever PE (1985) Cerebral pilocytic astrocytoma. Cancer 56:1128–1133
22. Claussen C, Laniado M, Shorner W et al. (1985) Gadolinium-DTPA in MR imaging of glioblastomas and intracranial metastases. AJNR 6:669–674
23. Cushing H (1931) Experience with the cerebellar astrocytoma. A critical review of 76 cases. Surg Gynecol Obstet 52:129–191
24. De Sousa AL, Kalsbeck IE, Mealey J, Fitzgerald J (1979) Diencephalic syndrome and its relation to optico-chiasmatic glioma. Review of twelve cases. Neurosurgery 4:207–209
25. Destian S, Sze G, Krol G et al. (1988) MR imaging of hemorrhagic intracranial neoplasms. AJNR 9:1115–1122
26. Epstein F, Mc Cleary EL (1986) Intrinsic brain stem tumors of childhood; surgical indications. J Neurosurg 64:11–16
27. Felix R, Shorner W, Laniado M et al. (1985) Brain tumors: MR imaging with gadolinium-DTPA. Radiology 156:681–688
28. Fokes EC Jr, Earle KM (1969) Ependymomas: Clinical and pathological aspects. J Neurosurg 30:585–594
29. Gadian DG, Payne JA, Bryant DJ et al. (1985) Gadolinium-DTPA as a contrast agent in MR imaging: theoretical projections and practical observations. J Comput Assist Tomogr 9:242–251
30. Gjerris F, Klinken L (1978) Long-term prognosis in children with benign cerebellar astrocytoma. J Neurosurg 49:179–184
31. Greig NH (1989) Brain tumors and the blood-tumor barrier. In: Neuwelt EA (ed) Implications of the Blood-Brain Barrier and its Manipulation, Vol 2. Clinical Aspects. Plenum Press, New York, 77–106

32. Harms SE (1989) Orbital magnetic resonance. In: Pomeranz SJ (ed) Craniospinal Magnetic Resonance Imaging. W. B. Saunders Co, Philadelphia, 587–634
33. Harsh GR IV, Wilson CB (1990) Neuroepithelial tumors of the adult brain. In: Youmans JR (ed) Neurological Surgery, 3rd edn. W. B. Saunders Co, Philadelphia, 3040–3136
34. Hoffmann HJ, Henrich EB, Humphreys RP (1976) Metastasis via ventriculoperitoneal shunt in patients with medulloblastoma. J Neurosurg 44:562–566
35. Hoffman HJ, Goumnerova L (1990) Pediatric brain stem gliomas. In: Wilkins RH, Rengachary SS (eds) Neurosurgery Update II. McGraw-Hill, New York, 326–335
36. Horwich A, Bloom HJG (1985) Optic gliomas: Radiation therapy and prognosis. Int J Radiat Oncol Biol Phys 11:1067–1079
37. Hughes PG (1984) Cerebellar medulloblastoma in adults. J Neurosurg 60:994–997
38. Just M, Thelen M (1988) Tissue characterization with T1, T2, and proton density values: results in 160 patients with brain tumors. Radiology 169:779–785
39. Kelly PJ (1987) Stereotactic technology in tumor surgery. Clin Neurosurg 35:215–253
40. Kent DL, Larson EB (1988) Magnetic resonance imaging of the brain and spine: is clinical efficacy established after the first decade? Ann Intern Med 107:402–424
41. Kets E (1974) Brain tumors and epilepsy. In: Vinken PJ, Bruyn GW (eds) Handbook of Clinical Neurology, Vol 16. Tumors of the Brain and Skull, Part I. North-Holland, Amsterdam, 254–269
42. Kjos BO, Brant-Zawadzki M, Kucharczyk W et al. (1985) Cystic intracranial lesions: magnetic resonance imaging. Radiology 155:363–369
43. Koos WT, Miller MH (1971) Intracranial tumors of infants and children. Mosby, St. Louis
44. Kwan E, Wolpert SM, Smith SP, Modic MT (1987) Radiology of third ventricular lesions. In: Apuzzo MLJ (ed) Surgery of the third ventricle. Williams & Wilkins, Baltimore, 262–300
45. Laws ER, Taylor WF, Clifton MB, Okazaki H (1984) Neurosurgical management of low grade astrocytomas of the cerebral hemispheres. J Neurosurg 61:667–673
46. Loftus CM, Copeland BR, Carmel PW (1985) Cystic supratentorial gliomas: Natural history and evaluation of modes of surgical therapy. Neurosurgery 17:19–24
47. Mac Carthy CS, Boyd AS, Childs DS (1970) Tumors of the optic nerve. J Neurosurg 33:439–444
48. Matson DD (1956) Cerebellar astrocytoma in childhood. Pediatrics 18:150–158
49. Modic MT, Beale SM (1990) Magnetic resonance imaging of supratentorial neoplasms. In: Wilkins RH, Rengachary SS (eds) Neurosurgery. McGraw-Hill, New York, 12–29
50. Nazzaro JM, Neuwelt EA (1990) The role of Surgery in the management of supratentorial intermediate and high-grade astrocytomas in adults. J Neurosurg 73:331–334
51. Packer RJ, Savino PJ, Bilamink LT (1983) Chiasmatic gliomas of childhood: A repraisal of natural history and effectiveness of cranial irradiation. Child's Brain 10:393–403
52. Packer RJ, Batzinski S, Cohen ME (1985) Magnetic Resonance imaging in the evaluation of intracranial tumors of childhood. Ann Neurol 18:217–277
53. Packer RJ, Zimmermann RA, Cenrson T et al. (1985) Nuclear magnetic resonance in the evaluation of brain stem gliomas of childhood. Neurology 35:397–401
54. Packer RJ, Shut L, Sutton LN, Bruce DA (1990) Brain tumors of the posterior cranial fossa in infants and children. In: Youmans JR (ed) Neurological Surgery, 3rd edn. W. B. Saunders Co, Philadelphia, 3017–3039
55. Parizel PM, Degryse HL, Gheuens J et al. (1989) Gadolinium-DTPA enhanced MR imaging of intracranial lesions. Comput Assist Tomogr 13:378–385
56. Park TS, Hoffmann HJ, Hendrich EB et al. (1983) Medulloblastoma, clinical presentation and management. Experiences at the Hospital for Sick Children, Toronto, 1950–1980. J Neurosurg 58:543–552
57. Pierre-Kalm A, Hirsch JF, Roux FX et al. (1983) Intracranial ependymomas in childhood – surgical and function results of 47 cases. Child's Brain 10:145–156
58. Pomeranz SJ (1989) MR of supratentorial neoplasia. In: Pomeranz SJ (ed) Craniospinal Magnetic Resonance Imaging. W. B. Saunders Co, Philadelphia, 208–247
59. Pomeranz SJ (1989) Posterior fossa, skull base, craniocervical junction. In: Pomeranz SJ (ed) Craniospinal Magnetic Resonance Imaging. W. B. Saunders Co, Philadelphia, 248–274
60. Powers TA, Partian CL, Kessler RM et al. (1988) Central nervous system lesions in pediatric patients: Gd-DTPA enhancing MR imaging. Radiology 169:723–726
61. Raimondi AJ, Tomita T (1983) Brain tumors during the first year of life. Child's Brain 10:193–207
62. Ransohoff J, Kelly PJ, Laws ER Jr (1986) The role of intracranial surgery for the treatment of malignant gliomas. Semin Oncol 13:27–37
63. Salcman M (1985) Supratentorial gliomas: clinical features and surgical therapy. In: Wilkins RH, Rengachary SS (eds) Neurosurgery. McGraw-Hill, New York, 579–590

64. Schenwirth RM (1974) Parietal lobe tumors. In: Vinken PJ, Bruyn GW (eds) Handbook of Clinical Neurology, Vol 16. Tumors of the Brain and Skull, Part I. North-Holland, Amsterdam, 296–309
65. Shapiro JR (1986) Biology of gliomas: Heterogeneity, oncogenes, and growth factor. Semin Oncol 13:4–15
66. Smith MT, Ludwig MT, Armbrustmacher VW (1986) A clinicopathologic study of 323 patients with oligodendrogliomas. Ann Neurol 19:15–21
67. Tomita T, Mc Lone DG (1986) Medulloblastoma in childhood: Results of radical resection and low-dose neuraxis radiation therapy. J Neurosurg 64:238–242
68. Waluch V, Dyck P (1990) Magnetic resonance imaging of posterior fossa masses. In: Wilkins RH, Rengachary SS (eds) Neurosurgery Update I. McGraw-Hill, New York, 30–46

CHAPTER V

Tumors of the pineal region

The tumors originating in this site make up a heterogeneous group of neoplasms and account for approximately 1% of all intracranial tumors. Some derive from the parenchymal cells of the pineal gland: pineocytoma and pineoblastoma; others originate from the supporting tissues: tumors of glial origin; additionally, with greater incidence, others may originate from embryonic cell nests which do not belong to the pineal gland: germinomas and teratomas. In this site, papillomas of the choroid plexus and meningiomas are less frequent. Nontumoral space-occupying processes of the pineal gland, mostly arachnoid and parasitic cysts, will be discussed in a separate chapter.

Clinically, these tumors may occur with intracranial hypertension secondary to triventricular hydrocephalus, due to occlusion of the Sylvian aqueduct and, when the superior collicula and the pretectal area are involved, with typical ocular signs: palsy of vertical gaze (Parinaud's syndrome) and of convergence, abnormalities in pupillary reactivity and retraction nystagmus. A rare and hardly understandable symptom is precocious puberty in children suffering from space-occupying lesions in this region.

Pineal-cell neoplasms account for roughly 20% of the tumors in this region. Macroscopically, they cannot be differentiated from other histotypes, since they may be circumscribed, when they are benign, or infiltrating and with frequent metastases via the CSF pathway, when they are malignant. Pineocytoma *(Fig. 1)* is the benign type (neuronal or neuronal-astrocytic), which remains circumscribed and has slow growth. Pineoblastoma is similar, macroscopically and behaviorally, to medulloblastoma. The retinoblastomatous variety which is occasionally reported is not surprising, since the pineal gland derives from a neurosensory photoreceptor system.

Glial tumors in this region derive both from astrocytes and from elements of the surrounding brain formations: astroblastomas, astrocytomas, glioblastomas, ependymomas, oligodendrogliomas *(Figs. 2, 3)*. In their macroscopic appearance and behavior, they are similar to the tumors in other sites.

Germinomas are the most frequent neoplasms of the pineal region, since they represent approximately 50% of lesions. They are highly malignant and have rapid growth but are also extremely radiation-sensitive. They appear as ill-delimited lesions, sometimes connected with a suprasellar mass owing to invasion of the third ventricle walls *(Figs. 4, 5)*. They are generally grayish and solid; inside them, hemorrhages, necroses, cystic degenerations may occur, albeit rarely. Frequent metastases develop via the CSF pathway, sometimes facilitated by CSF diversion procedures.

Teratomas are tumors containing structures which derive from the three embryonic sheets. They are more frequent in males and well circumscribed. They cause compression on the surrounding structures and may contain fragments of bone, cartilage and even teeth. Cysts, which are a frequent finding, harbor air or keratinous material. Their fissures may cause irritating material to flow into the CSF compartment. Other embryonic-cell neoplasms are seldom encountered: embryonic carcinoma, intradermal sinus tumor and choriocarcinoma. They represent a group of very malignant infiltrating neoplasms, often with metastases along the CSF pathway.

Axial, sagittal and coronal MRI scans offer an excellent anatomical evaluation of the pineal region as well as an exhaustive demonstration of the nidus of the lesion and of its relations to adjacent structures: roof of midbrain, posterior part of the third ventricle, splenium, deep venous system and Galen's vein.

Based on our experience and on the literature, the signal characteristics are not such as to differentiate among the various neoplastic types, except for teratomas and choriocarcinomas. The former produce a highly inhomogeneous signal owing to the presence of different tissues; the latter give a T_1 and T_2 hyperintense signal due to hemorrhagic events. As is known, it is more difficult for MRI than for CT to identify intratumoral calcifications, a diagnostic element which may be important in the characterization of pineocytomas. A greater sensitivity in detecting calcifications is achieved by T_2-weighted fast imaging.

In this pathology, paramagnetic contrast agents are absolutely necessary to diagnose malignant oncotypes and to better delineate long-term CSF-mediated metastases, whether cerebral or spinal.

After diagnosis via open or CT-guided stereotactic biopsy and alpha-fetoprotein (AFP) and chorionic gonadotropin (hCG) assays, the treatment of germinomas consists in conventional radiation therapy limited to the brain or extended to the entire neuraxis in case of positive cytologic CSF findings. Metastases via the CSF pathway, like suprasellar ectopic lesions, respond to chemotherapy *(Fig. 4)*. This treatment is also beneficial in other germ-cell tumors, when cytologic CSF findings point to the presence of malignant cells or when CSF-mediated metastases or increases in tumor markers are observed. Surgery is used when diagnostic studies predict a benign lesion, when the tumor has not been characterized, or in patients treated with extrathecal shunting and radiation therapy alone and when the patient's symptoms worsen.

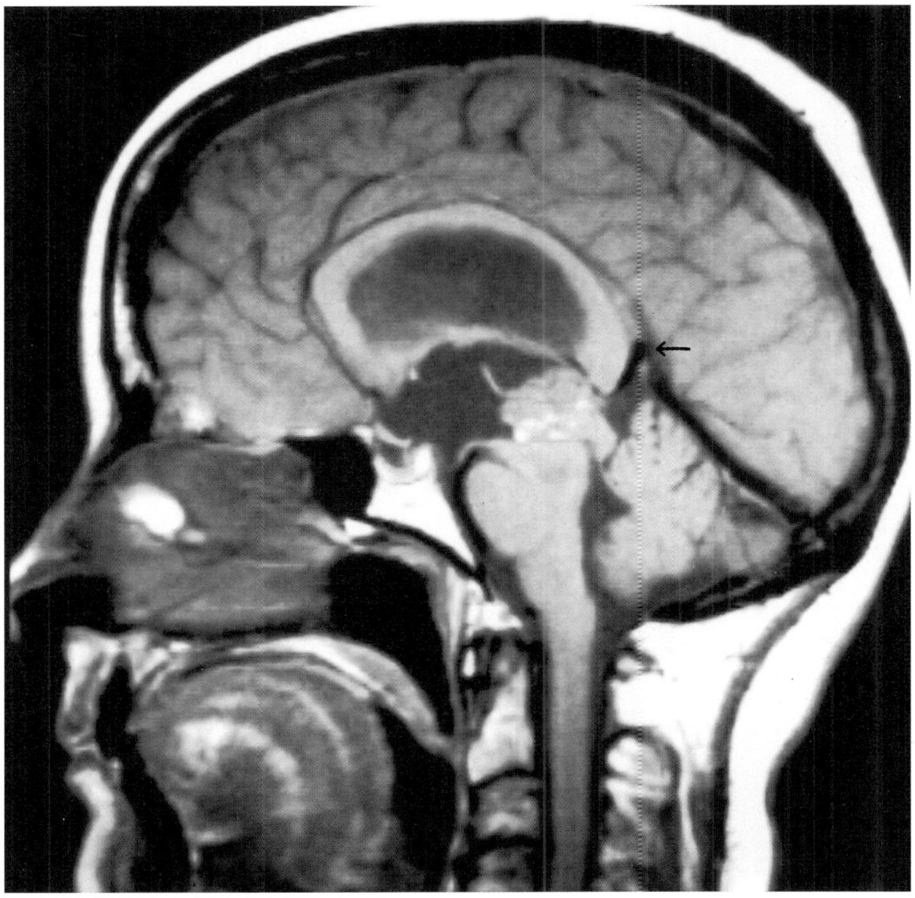

A

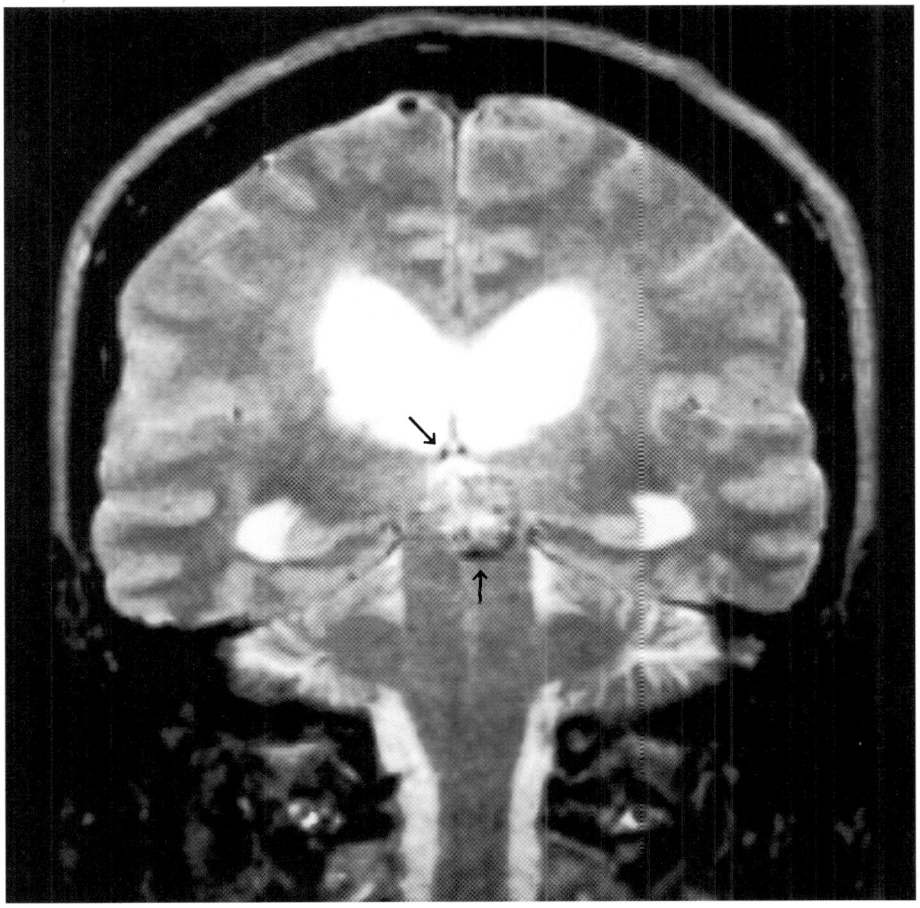

B

Fig. 1. *Pineocytoma.* 46-year-old woman: about 6 months of gait disorders with lateropulsion, progressive frontal headache, swallowing problems, visual loss and accommodation impairment. CT showed a 1.5–2 cm, pineal space-occupying lesion with calcium deposits and triventricular hydrocephalus. A – T_1-weighted sagittal view: in the posterior aspect of the third ventricle and pineal region, there is a tiny, isointense, berry-like mass containing small, hyperintense foci. This tumor causes stenosis of the aqueduct, dilatation of the third ventricle and secondary empty sella. The fourth ventricle has normal morphology; Galen's vein is visible (←). B – T_2-weighted coronal view: note the supratentorial hydrocephalus with dilatation of the lateral ventricles and temporal horns. A small portion of the third ventricle is free above the mass; the internal cerebral veins are well outlined (↘). The neoplasm has inhomogeneous intensity with hypointense calcific foci (↑).

A

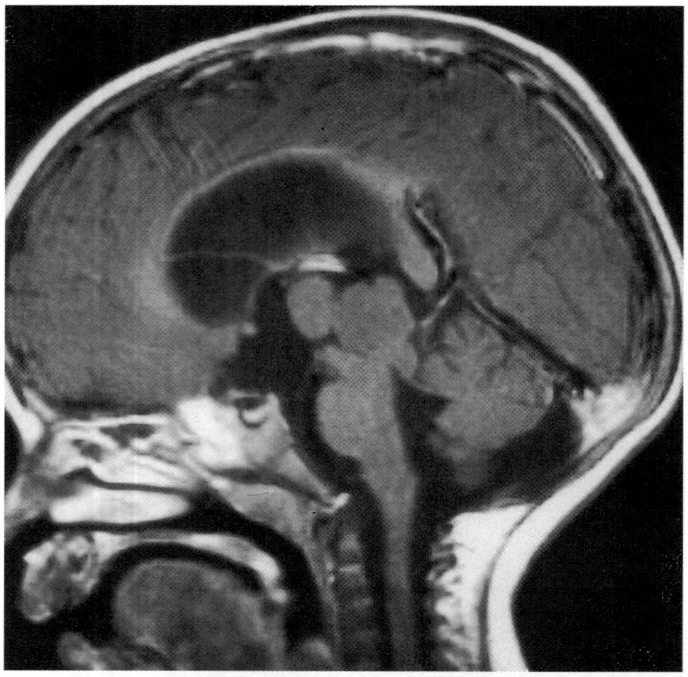

Fig. 2. *Low-grade astrocytoma of the pineal region.* 18-month-old child with motor retardation. (A) – T_1-weighted sagittal view after GD-DTPA (TR 560 msec, TE 15 msec): evidence of triventricular hydrocephalus owing to a non-enhancing, hypointense mass that compresses the quadrigeminal plate and obstructs the aqueduct. Note the flattening of the corpus callosum. (B) – Multiecho axial view (TE 60–90–120–180 msec): severe hydrocephalus with transependymal reabsorption. The lesion seems to be solid. Its signal is moderately hyperintense with the tissue and definitely hypointense with the CSF on the late echoes.

B

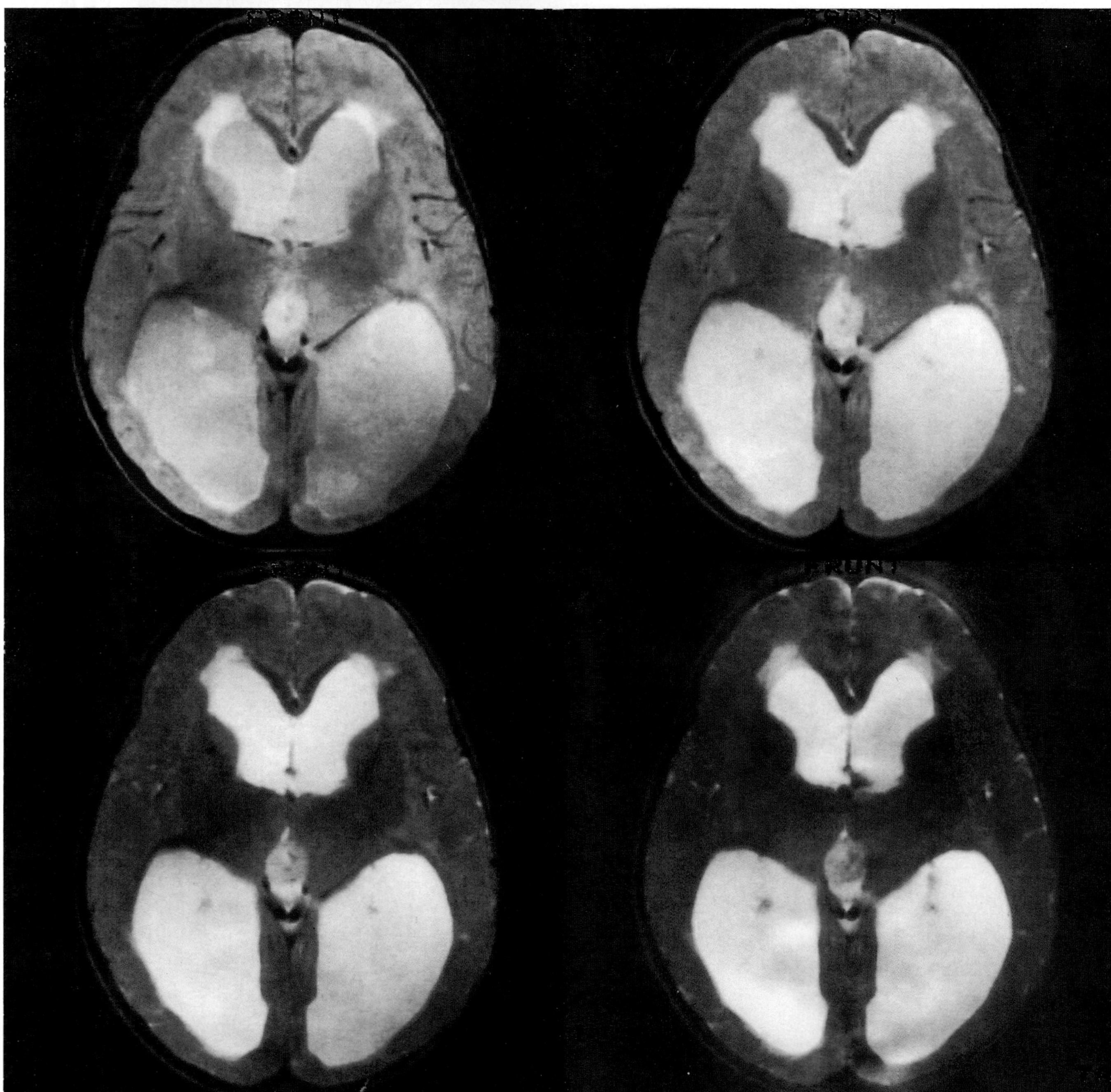

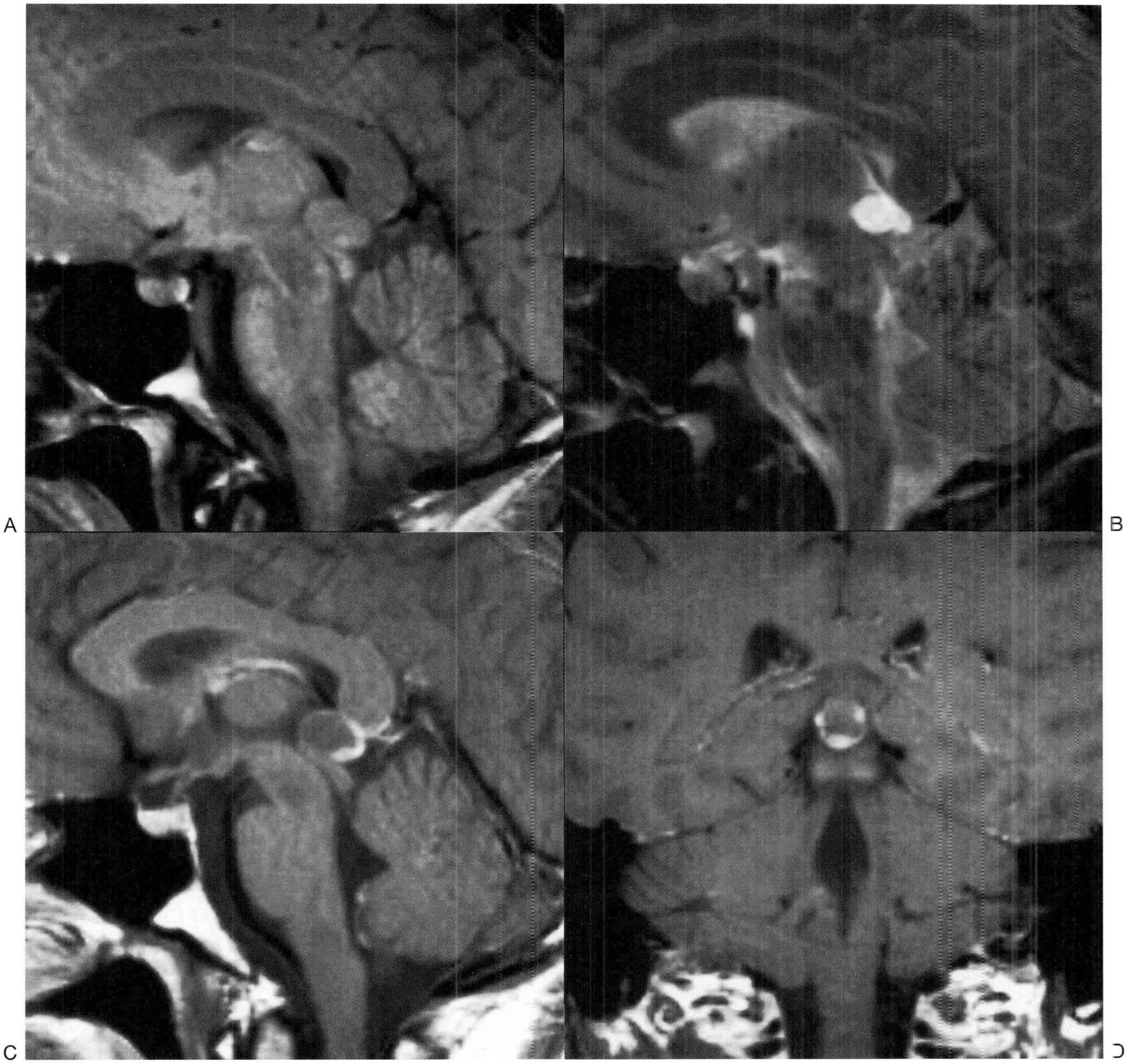

Fig. 3. *Cystic astrocytoma of the pineal region.* 20-year-old man referred to our department with a diagnosis of spinal astrocytoma (Chap. XII, *Fig. 25*). In addition to tetraparesis, the patient had upward gaze palsy. A small rounded tumor was found to overlie the quadrigeminal plate and to partially obstruct the Sylvian aquaeduct. The cystic nature of the lesion is well demonstrated by peripheral enhancement after GD-DTPA (C, D). The standard T_1- (A) and T_2- (B) weighted images are not capable of demonstrating the fluid component with certainty.

A A

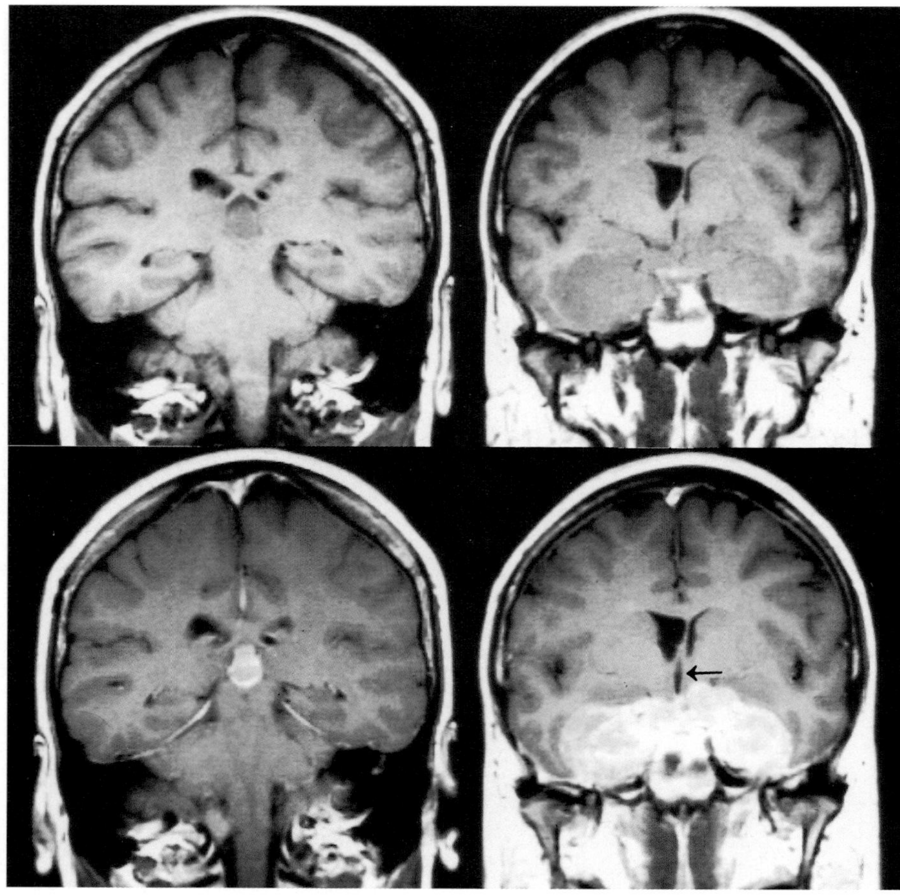

B B

C D

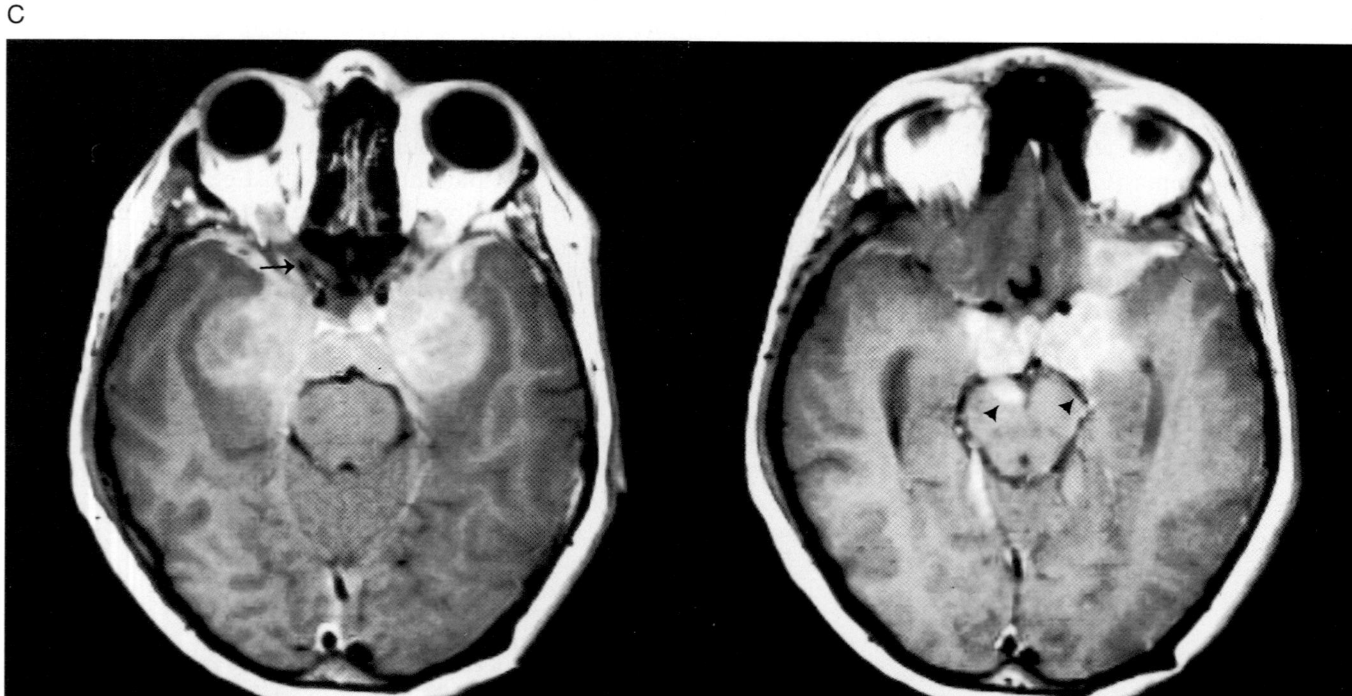

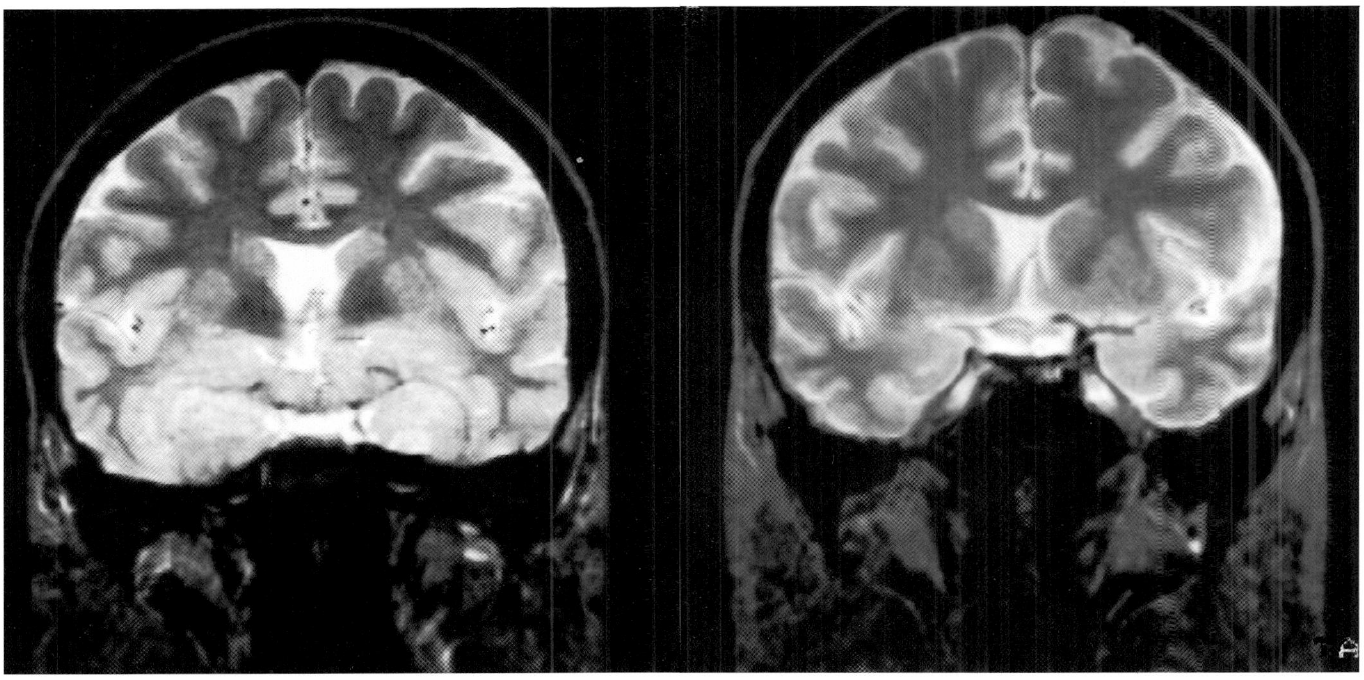

E F

Fig. 4. *Germinoma of the pineal region: temporal basal spread and infiltration of the cerebral peduncle at follow-up examination.* A – T_1-weighted coronal cuts: the germinoma recurrence and the temporal basal spread are moderately hypointense. B – Similar images after GD-DTPA. The intense c.e. highlights the alterations; the chiasmatic-retrochiasmatic component; and the relationships with the third ventricle (←). C – Axial view after GD-DTPA: bilateral extension of the basal mass; on the left, it reaches the temporal lobe; on the right, it occupies the cisterna ambiens, whereas the prepontine cistern appears to be free. Observe the carotid siphons and the optic nerves inside the orbit and the orbital canal (→). D – Upper level image: M.C.A.s, B.A., P.C.A.s (←). Towards the left, the mass reaches the basal part of the frontal lobe whereas, on the right, it infiltrates the cerebral peduncle posteriorly. E – T_2-weighted coronal scan: the temporal spread of the tumor has a more intense signal than the cerebral tissue. F – T_2-weighted coronal image of the same level as E after chemotherapy: morphological repair of the temporal lobes and insula bilaterally. At present, there is no sign of other secondary localization.

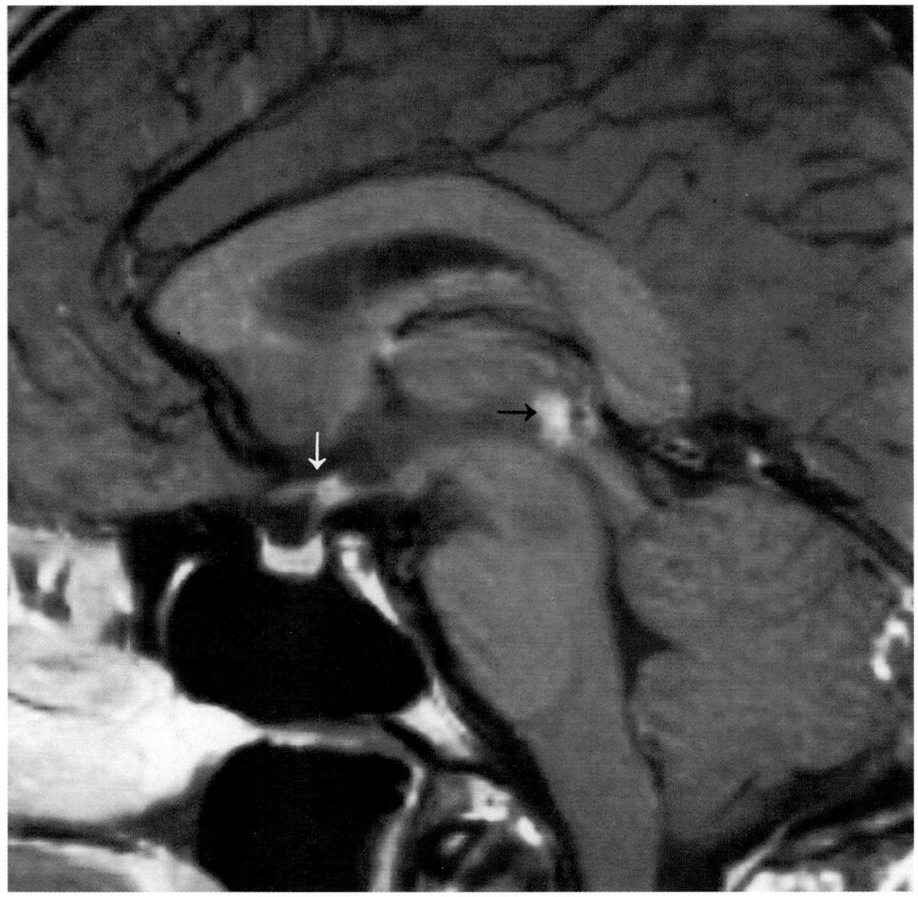

A

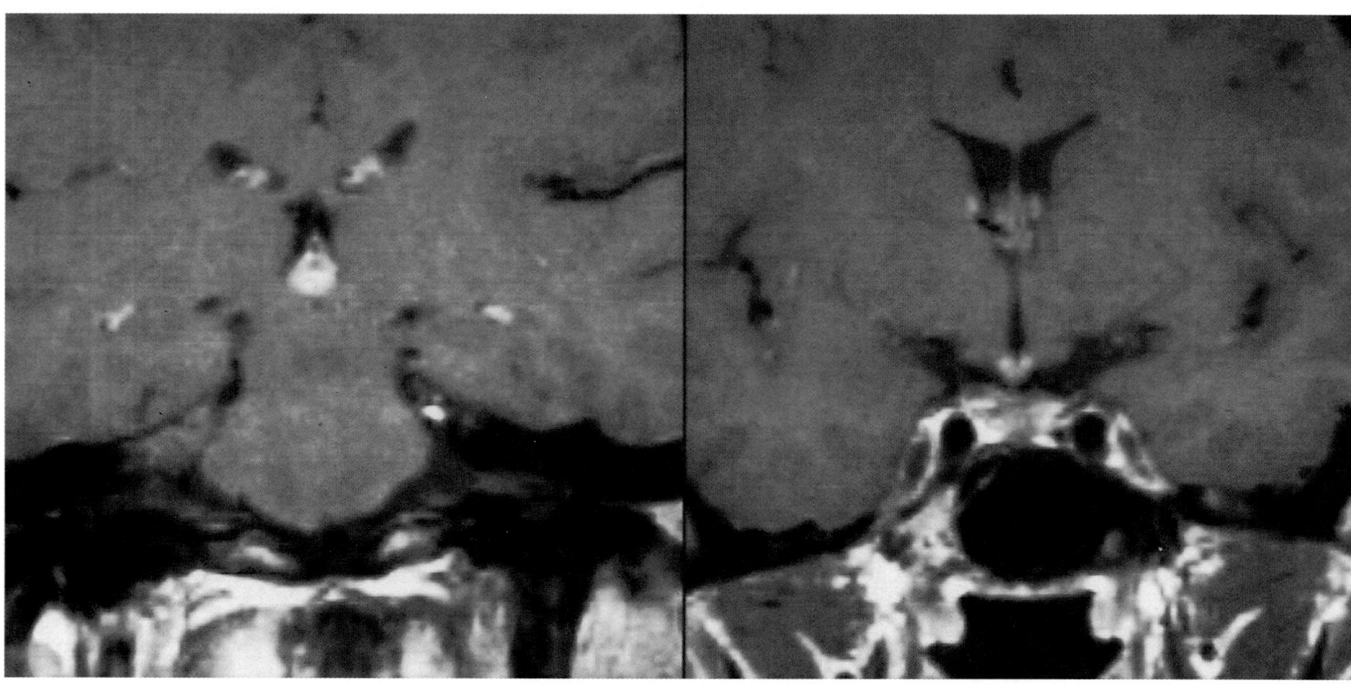

B

Fig. 5. *Germinoma of the pineal gland and of the infundibulum.* 24-year-old man with diabetes inspidus. The T_1-weighted sagittal image after GD-DTPA (A) shows two markedly enhanced small lesions, one of the pineal gland (→) and the other of the infundibulum (↓). The coronal images (B) validate the site and the small size of the lesions.

References

1. Ball WS Jr, Towbin RB (1988) MRI of pediatric central nervous system neoplasms. In: Craniospinal magnetic resonance imaging. In: Pomeranz SJ (ed) Craniospinal Magnetic Resonance Imaging. W. B. Saunders Co, Philadelphia, 177–207
2. Brant-Zawadski M, Badami JP, Mills CM et al. (1984) Primary intracranial tumor imaging. A comparison of magnetic resonance and CT. Radiology 150:435–440
3. Bronen RA, Sze G (1990) Magnetic resonance contrast agents: theory and application to the central nervous system. J Neurosurg 73:820–840
4. Bruce JN, Fetell MR (1990) Surgical approaches to pineal tumors. In: Wilkins RH, Rengachary SS (eds) Neurosurgery. McGraw-Hill, New York, 389–398
5. Bryan P (1974) CSF seeding of intra-cranial tumours: A study of 96 cases. Clin Radiol 25:355–360
6. Danoff B, Sheline GE (1984) Radiotherapy of pineal tumours. In: Neuwelt EA (ed) Diagnosis and Treatment of Pineal Region Tumours. Williams & Wilkins, Baltimore, 300–308
7. Gadian DG, Payne JA, Bryant DJ et al. (1985) Gadolinium-DTPA as a contrast agent in MR imaging: theoretical projections and practical observations. J Comput Assist Tomogr 9:242–251
8. Jennings MT, Gelman R, Hochberg F (1984) Intracranial germ cell tumours: Natural history and pathogenesis. In: Neuwelt EA (ed) Diagnosis and Treatment of Pineal Region Tumours. Williams & Wilkins, Baltimore, 116–138
9. Jooma R, Kendall BE (1983) Diagnosis and management of pineal tumors. J Neurosurg 58:654–665
10. Koos WT, Miller MH (1971) Intracranial tumors of infants and children. Mosby, St Louis
11. Kwan E, Wolpert SM, Smith SP, Modic MT (1987) Radiology of third ventricular lesions. In Apuzzo MLJ (ed) Surgery of the Third Ventricle. Williams & Wilkins, Baltimore, 262–300
12. Lapras C, Patet JD (1987) Controversies, techniques, and strategies for pineal tumor surgery. In: Apuzzo MLJ (ed) Surgery of the Third Ventricle. Williams & Wilkins, Baltimore, 649–662
13. Modic MT, Beale SM (1990) Magnetic resonance imaging of supratentorial neoplasms. In: Wilkins RH, Rengachary SS (eds) Neurosurgery. McGraw-Hill, New York, 12–29
14. Muller-Forell W, Schroth G, Egan PJ (1988) MR Imaging in tumors of the pineal region. Neuroradiology 30:224–231
15. Neuhold A, Fezoulidis I, Fruhwald F et al. (1989) Space-occupying lesions of the pineal region in Magnetic Resonance Tomography. ROFO 151:210–215
16. Neuwelt EA, Glasberg M, Frenkel E et al. (1979) Malignant pineal region tumours. A clinico-pathological study. J Neurosurg 51:597–607
17. Packer RJ, Batzinski S, Cohen ME (1985) Magnetic resonance imaging in the evaluation of intracranial tumors of childhood. Ann Neurol 18:217–277
18. Parizel PM, Degryse HL, Gheuens J et al. (1989) Gadolinium-DTPA enhanced MR imaging of intracranial lesions. Comput Assist Tomogr 13:378–385
19. Pomeranz SJ (1989) MR of supratentorial neoplasia. In: Pomeranz SJ (ed) Craniospinal Magnetic Resonance Imaging. W. B. Saunders Co, Philadelphia, 208–247
20. Rippe DJ, Boiko OB, Friedman HS et al. (1990) Gd-DTPA-enhanced MR Imaging of leptomeningeal spread of primary intracranial CNS tumors in children. AJNR 11:329–332
21. Sano K (1987) Pineal region and posterior third ventricular tumors: A surgical overview. In: Apuzzo MLJ (ed) Surgery of the Third Ventricle. Williams & Wilkins, Baltimore, 663–683
22. Tien RD, Barkovich AJ, Edwards MS (1990) MR Imaging of pineal tumors. AJNR 11:557–565
23. Zee CS, Segall H, Apuzzo MLJ et al. (1991) MR Imaging of pineal region neoplasms. J Comput Assist Tomogr 15:56–63

CHAPTER VI

Meningiomas

Meningiomas (m.) are tumors of adulthood with a predilection for the female sex, especially the spinal ones. They are mesodermal tumors which originate from the outer sheet of the arachnoid. According to their staminal mesodermal cell, they may differentiate as fibroblastic, chondroblastic, etc. They vary in histologic type depending on the amount of fibroblasts (transitional and fibroblastic m.), of calcium deposits (psammomatous m.), and on the content of meningeal cells grouped in the syncytial structures, which are poor in connective fibers (syncytial or meningothelial m.). Less common types are the angioblastic, xanthomatous, papillary and atypical m. The latter tumor, with mitoses and cell atypias, behaves like a sarcoma and generally has local malignancy.

Except for the atypical variety, m. are benign and grow slowly, displacing the vasculo-nervous structures without invading them *(Fig. 5)*. However, in growing they may encase vessels and nerves *(Fig. 6)*, which makes their removal difficult. The bone close to the tumor may show a significant inflammatory reaction, evidenced by hyperostosis. Occasionally, especially in "*en plaque*" m. of the sphenoid wing, the hyperostotic bone is infiltrated by the tumor which, at any rate, remains histologically benign *(Fig. 4)*.

M. are usually highly vascularized: the tumor is mostly supplied by the meningeal branches of the E.C.A.. Sometimes, they receive blood also from the branches of the I.C.A. and of the ophthalmic artery. Angiography is thus an important complementary diagnostic procedure *(Figs. 3, 10, 15)*, even if MR angiography may be very demonstrative *(Fig. 15)*.

M. may progress into extensive calcifications *(Figs. 8, 9)* or have regressive processes *(Fig. 16)*. At times, satellite CSF cysts are observed which are due to CSF entrapped in the arachnoid space *(Figs. 12, 13, 17)*.

Regardless of their histotype, they may cause severe edema in the surrounding brain *(Fig. 5)*. These neoplasms grow very slowly and the brain tends to adjust to the new anatomical status; this is the reason why the ones which are located in the so-called "mute" areas often reach remarkable proportions *(Fig. 3)*.

M. are practically ubiquitous in the intracranial compartment and except for the rare cases of intraventricular location, they constantly have a dural implantation, which may be adjacent to or involve important meningeal structures, such as the dural venous sinuses *(Figs. 4, 14)* or the dura of the basal foramina. Occasionally, they may be multifocal *(Fig. 17)*.

Clinically, they appear with focal symptoms, depending on their site and/or general dysfunction, such as epilepsy and intracranial hypertension.

The diagnosis of m., sometimes based on massive calcifications *(Fig. 8)* or hyperostotic bone reactions evidenced by standard radiograms alone, has been simplified in recent decades by the routine use of CT. The CT appearance of m. is typical: well-defined, relatively hyperdense areas in basal conditions, often with calcifications and with typical high enhancement after administration of iodinated contrast media.

MRI detection of m. is less straightforward, especially when they are small-sized, owing to the weak difference in signal between the meningiomatous tissue and the neighboring brain tissue *(Fig. 1)*. In most cases, high field magnets reveal moderately hypointense tumors on T_1-weighted images and equally moderately hyperintense tumors on T_2-weighted images with respect to the brain tissue. The signal intensity variation and the degree of diagnostic sensitivity of MRI for this tumor cannot compare with those for glial tumors. Before the introduction of paramagnetic contrast agents, the percentage of unnoticed m. was significant (5–10%). This fact questioned the suitability of MRI as a first diagnostic modality. At present, the use of GD-DTPA has substantially changed the diagnostic sensitivity of MRI, which may reach 100%. Paramagnetic contrast media facilitate and characterize the diagnosis of m., similarly to iodinated contrast media in CT. These media allow a diagnosis to be formulated even in the presence of tumors of small size and located in difficult sites: base of the skull *(Figs. 18, 19)*, occipital foramen *(Fig. 20)*. Perfusion of the tumor mass is generally: – intense, with signal enhancement on T_1-weighted sequences of up to 180%; – homogeneous; – early (3–5 min after i.v. injection); and – persistent (1 h) and with slow decline over time. The intense perfusion of these neoplasms is related to their rich vascularization and to absence of the BBB.

MRI has intrinsic advantages in the evaluation of m. Thanks to multiplanar scans and to greater contrast resolution, MRI better demonstrates their extraparenchymal location, often displaying a CSF and/or vascular interface between tumor and brain tissue *(Figs. 10, 11)*. Furthermore, it better shows the possible implantation of the tumor in the dura, its compressive and non-infiltrating effects on neighboring structures and above all vascular alterations, such as displacement and incorporation of arterial vessels *(Figs. 5, 6, 16)*, infiltration and/or thrombosis of venous sinuses *(Fig. 4)*.

MRI has proved to be a very sensitive procedure in demonstrating the involvement of venous sinuses, often surpassing the diagnostic capabilities of angiography in cases of partial infiltration. When the flow slows down or when the venous sinus is obstructed, the typical void image is replaced (on T_1 images) by signal enhancement due to static flow. Finally, to evaluate vessel patency, fast imaging sequences with flow compensation (FLASH V12, TR 0.115; TE 10; FRA 30°) *(Fig. 15)* are very helpful. MRI is certainly inferior to CT and to conventional radiography in delineating reactive bone alterations or calcifications within a given mass. Nevertheless, it can paradoxically visualize a neoplastic involvement of the bone which is not associated with bone density or thickness variations, as the cases of tumor invasion along the Haversian canals *(Fig. 4)*.

The treatment of m. is surgical and can be relatively simple if they are located in the cerebral convexity or in the cerebellar hemispheres and if they are not connected with major vasculo-nervous or meningeal structures. Much more challenging is the removal of m. which originate from the base of the skull and which are close to the circle of Willis *(Figs. 6, 7)*, to the cavernous sinus *(Fig. 18)*, to the optic nerves *(Figs. 21, 22)*, to the structures of the cerebello-pontine angle *(Fig. 19)*, or which infiltrate the dura mater of the venous sinuses. Even more difficult is the resection of m. of the tentorium and of the clivus, which grow in the interpeduncular cistern close to the anterior aspect of the brainstem *(Fig. 20)*. In the above instances, the surgical procedure is carried out with the operating microscope. Occasionally, if the risks of impairing vital structures are deemed to be excessive, it may be appropriate to remove only a portion of the tumor, given its slow growth. Removal of m. of the falx and/or of the floor of the anterior cranial fossa is of intermediate difficulty.

The therapeutical results are currently very good. Over the past few years, mortality has dropped below 5%; cases of major morbidity, with severe permanent deficits, are very rare. This result has been achieved via more sophisticated surgical procedures and thanks to the current opportunities for an earlier and more careful diagnosis.

A B

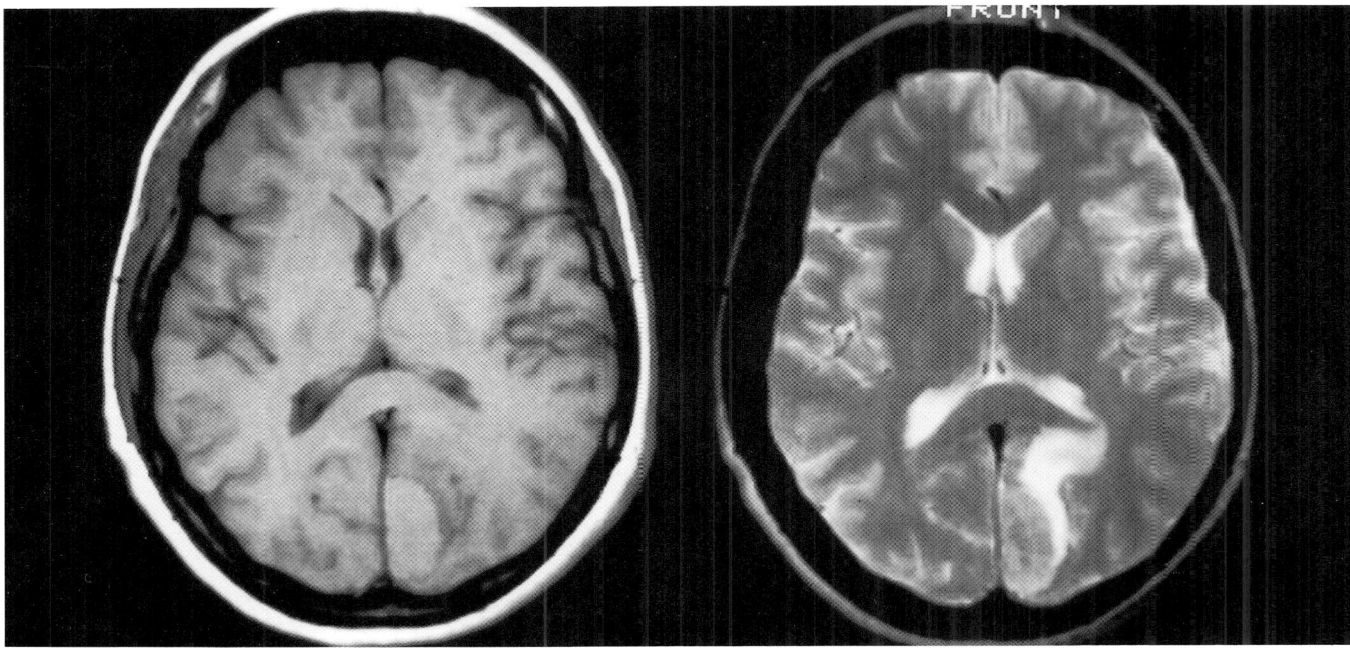

Fig. 1. *Small meningiothelial meningioma of the posterior third of the falx.* On the T_1-weighted sequence (A), the meningioma is hardly identifiable, being almost isointense with the cerebral tissue. On the T_2-weighted sequence (B), the neoplasm becomes better evidenced by the perilesional edema.

A B

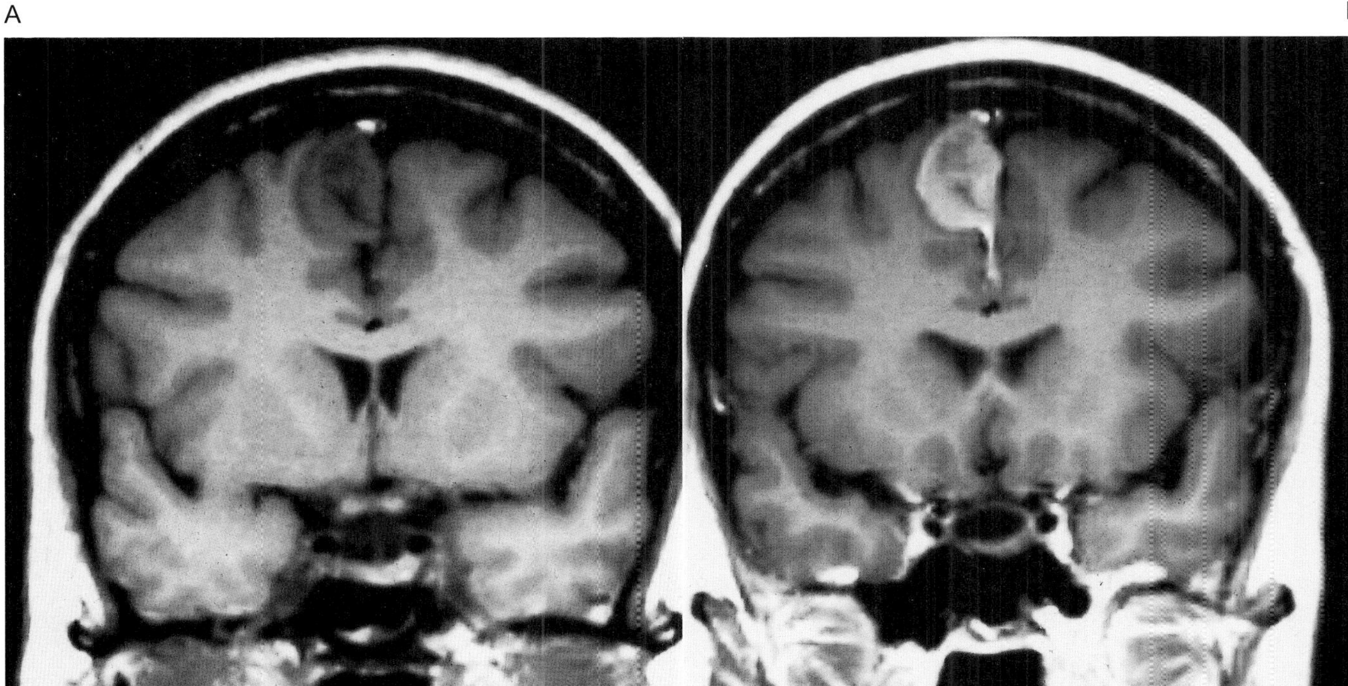

Fig. 2. *Meningioma of the falx.* 44-year-old woman with mild headache. T_1-weighted scan before (A) and after GD-DTPA (B). On A, the mass adhering to the falx has the same intensity as the grey matter; a low signal inside the mass suggests the presence of calcium. I.v. GD-DTPA optimally visualizes the soft part of the tumor.

A

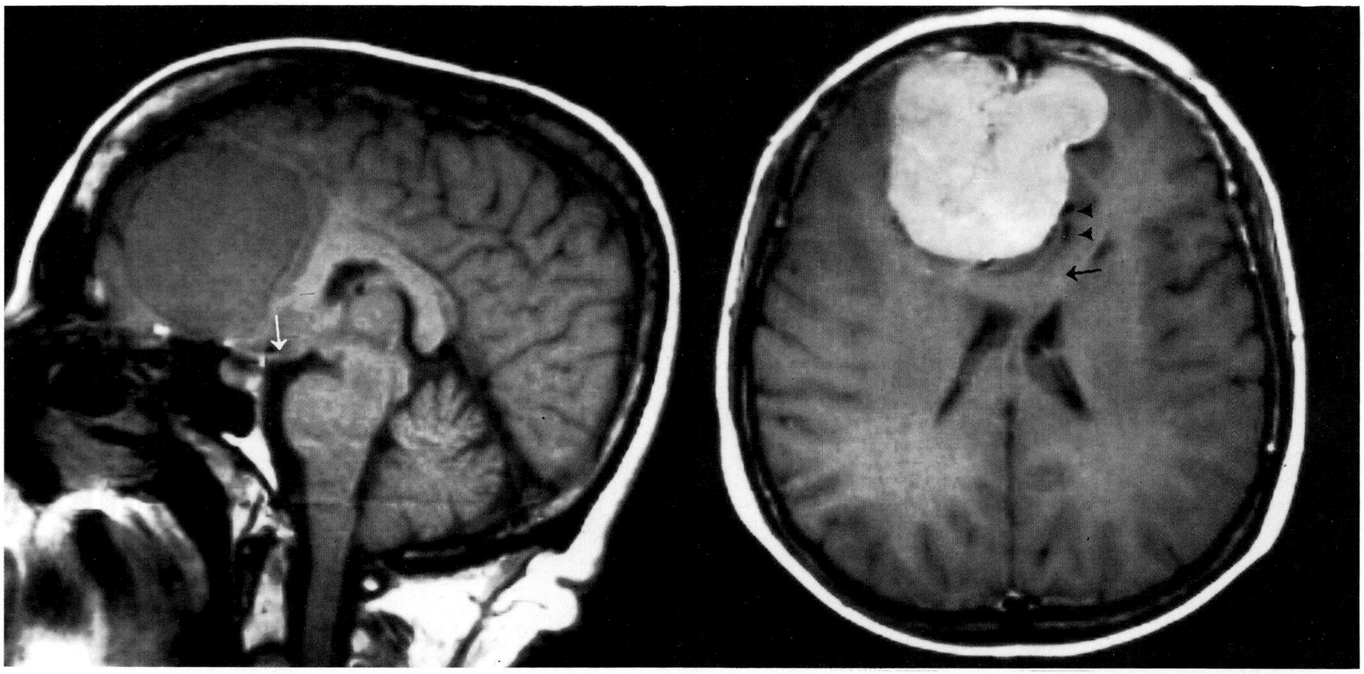

B

C

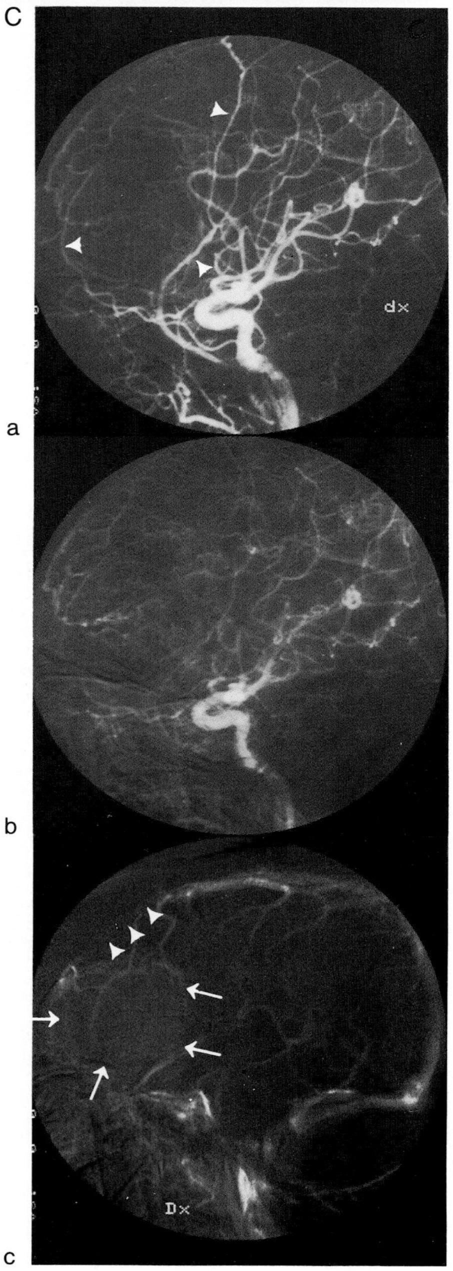

a

b

c

Fig. 3. *Bilaterally-expanding fibroblastic meningioma of the falx*. 64-year-old woman with severe psychoorganic syndrome. A – TR = 550; TE = 15; the mid-sagittal image shows a huge meningioma with signal intensity similar to cerebral tissue. The tumor compresses the genu of the corpus callosum and displaces the chiasm downwards (↓), giving it a hammock shape. B – Same sequence after GD-DTPA; the axial view confirms distortion of the corpus callosum and posterior displacement of the ventricular system. The A.C.A.s (←) are both displaced to the left (←). C – Right carotid angiogram. In the early arterial phase (a), posterior displacement of the A.C.A. and compression of the carotid siphon. Two meningeal branches of the E.C.A. are hypertrophic (←). In the late arterial phase (b), a tumoral blush is visible, which is mostly supplied by the frontal branch of the middle meningeal artery. In the venous phase (c), there is persistence of the blush, which depicts the neoplasm (→) and the thrombosis of the anterior third of the S.L.S. (←).

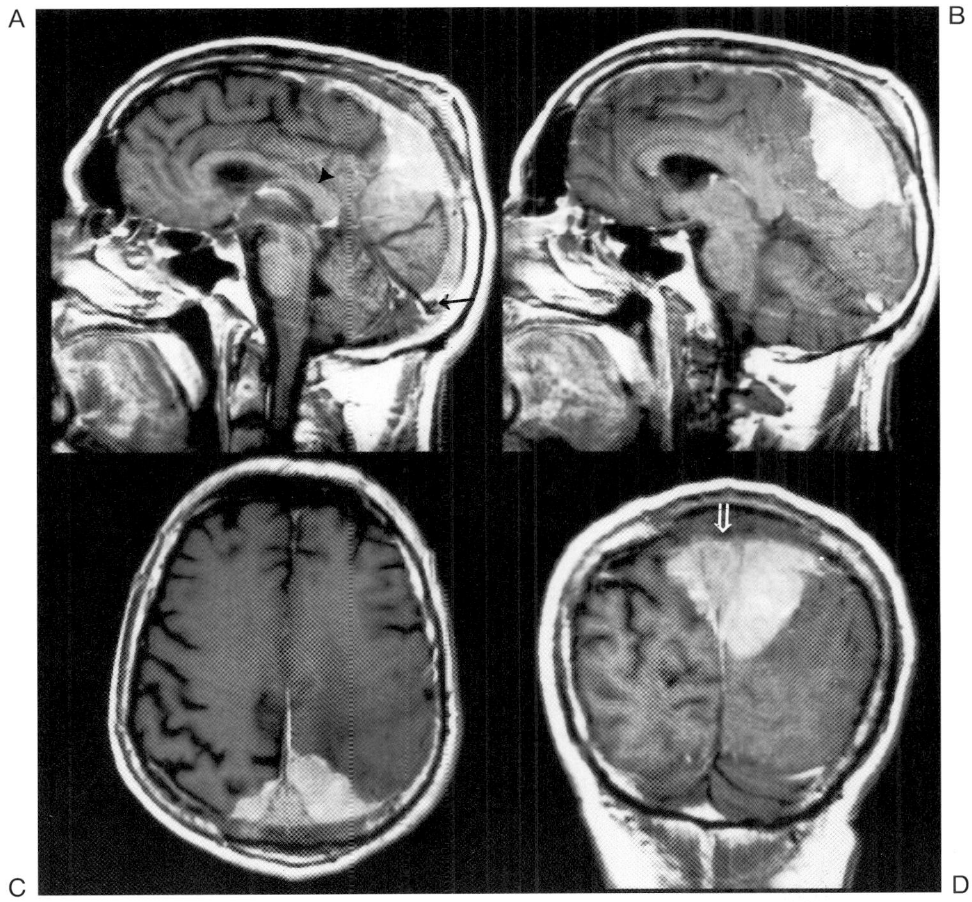

Fig. 4. *Meningothelial meningioma of the posterior third of the falx.* 67-year-old man whose dominant symptom was an extracranial tumefaction. T_1-weighted sagittal images after GD-DTPA (A, B): evidence of neoplasm with intense and homogeneous perfusion, that extensively infiltrates the S.L.S., from the middle third to the torcular (←) and displaces the splenium anteriorly (◂). A small tumoral component is found in the extrathecal tissues, reached through the Haversian canals. The bone, whose internal and external layers seem unaffected, gives an altered signal (hypointensity) owing to reduced marrow content in the dipole. The axial (C) and coronal (D) scans validate the finding of invasion of the S.L.S. (⇓).

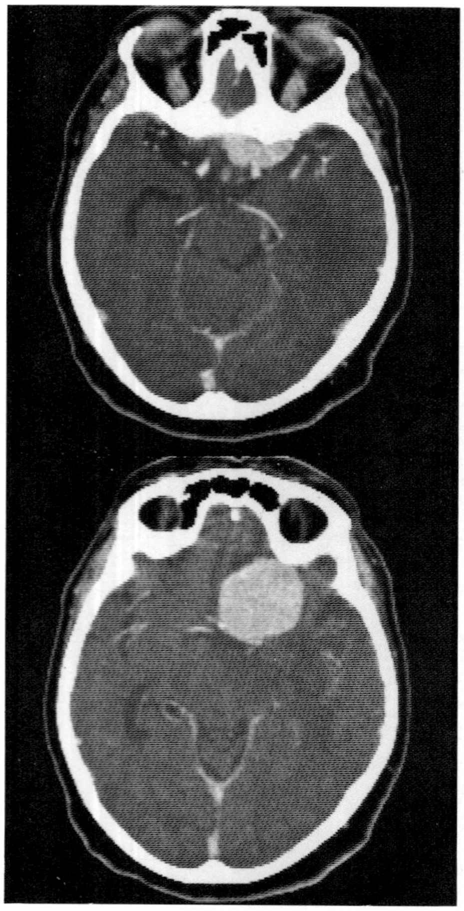

A

Fig. 5. *Right clinoid transitional meningioma.* 74-year-old woman with severe demential syndrome. A – CT after c.e.: meningioma with an extensive base on the internal third of the sphenoid wing and on the right clinoid. The lesion has intense and uniform enhancement. The supraclinoid tract of the I.C.A. is surrounded by the tumor; the A1 tract of the A.C.A. is flattened and displaced. B – MRI: T_2-weighted coronal section: the tumor is less homogeneous than on CT and the I.C.A. is only displaced downwards. Note the carotid branching (↓) with the A1 tract (⇑) and the M.C.A. (↑). The tumor grows above all in the right frontal lobe that is so edematous as to give rise to transfalcal cerebral herniation (→).

B

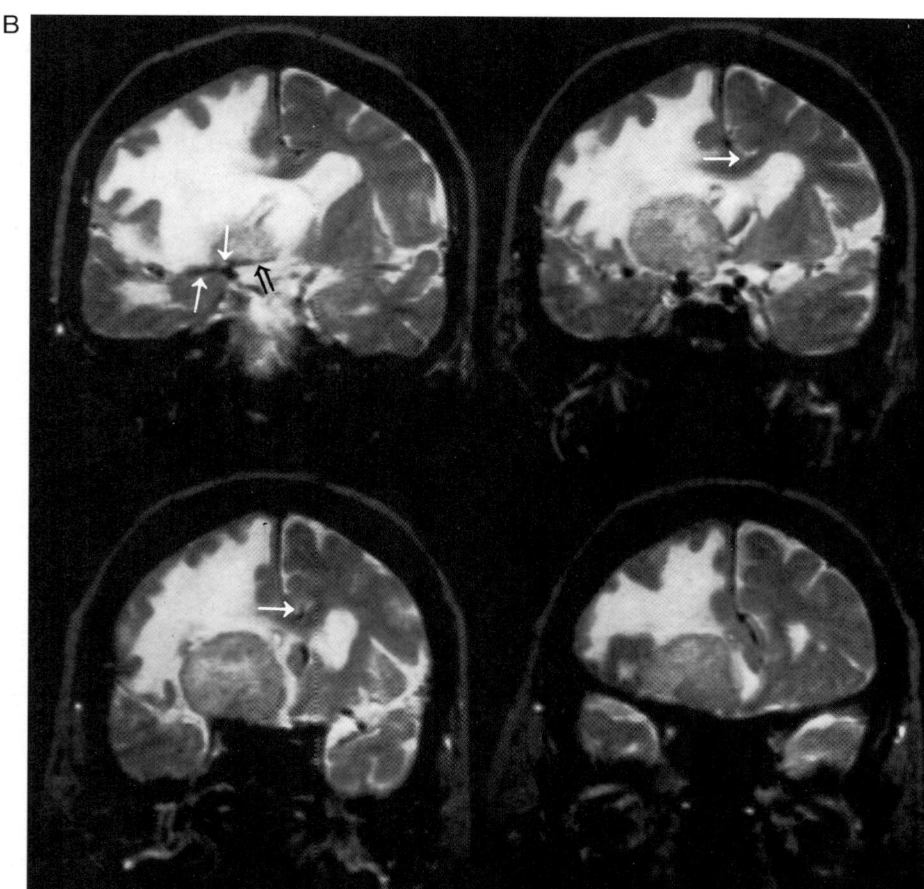

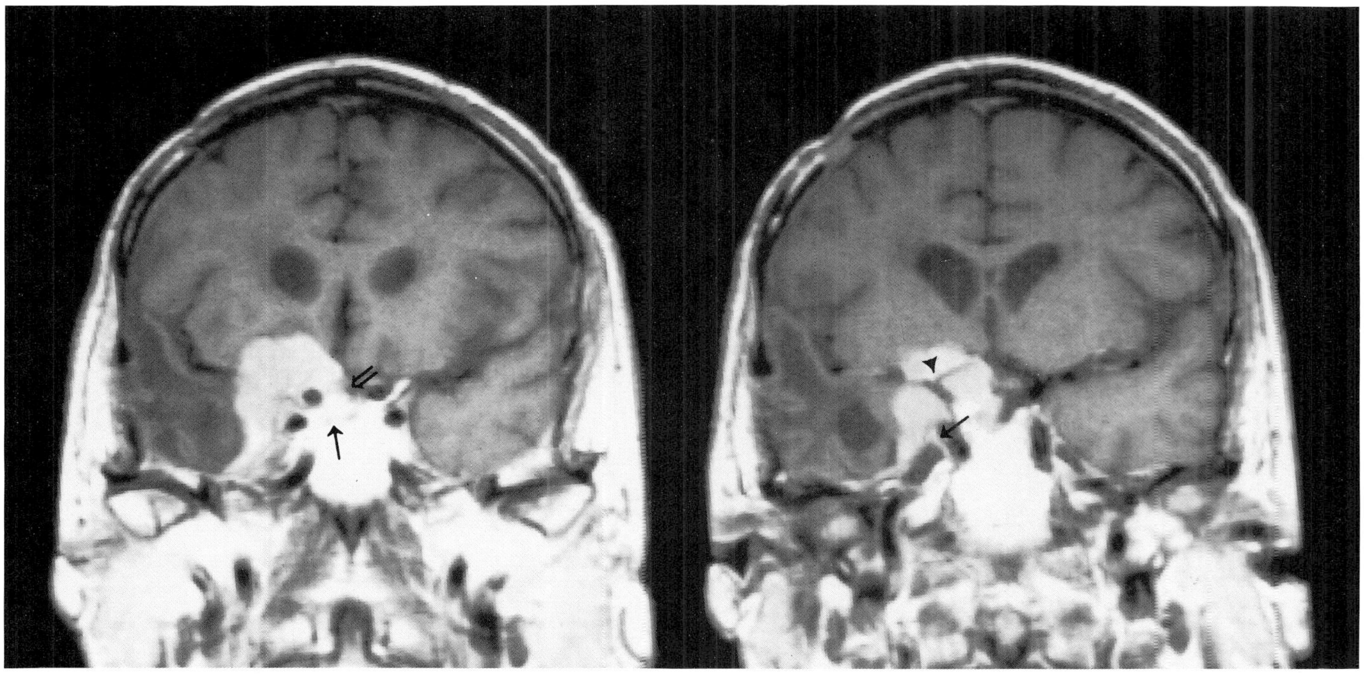

Fig. 6. *Remnant of right clinoid meningothelial meningioma after partial resection.* Patient with grand-mal seizures and inability to understand road signs. T_1-weighted coronal scan after GD-DTPA: the tumor grows around vital vasculonervous structures, such as the supraclinoid I.C.A., its branches (←) and the optic nerve (⇐), infiltrating the cavernous sinus (↙). In any oligosymptomatic patient, these findings counterindicate radical surgery. In the case in point, note the extension of the tumor to the right half of the sellar cavity (↑).

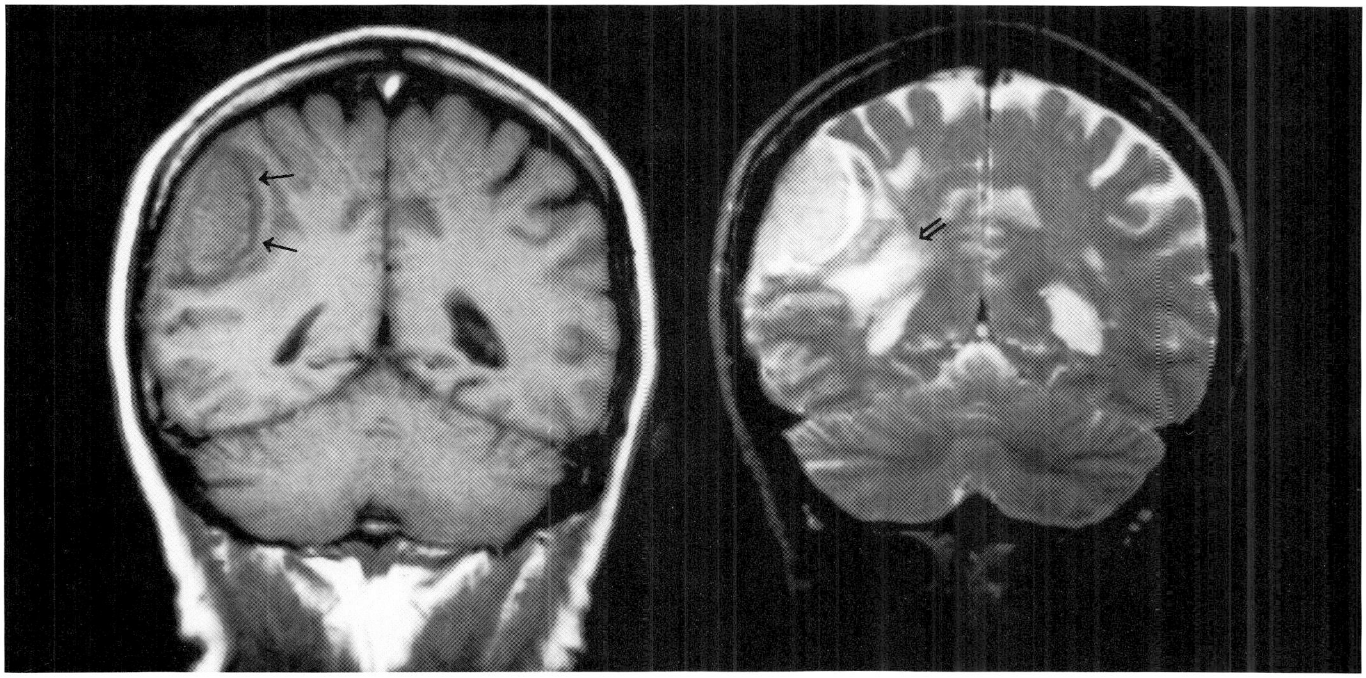

Fig. 7. *Right parietal convexity meningothelial meningioma.* 52-year-old man with seizures. The T_1-weighted MRI scan gives a clear visualization of the mass thanks to the CSF tumor-tissue interface, even though its signal intensity is similar to that of the tissue (←). This finding is validated by the T_2 sequence, which also shows edema (⇓).

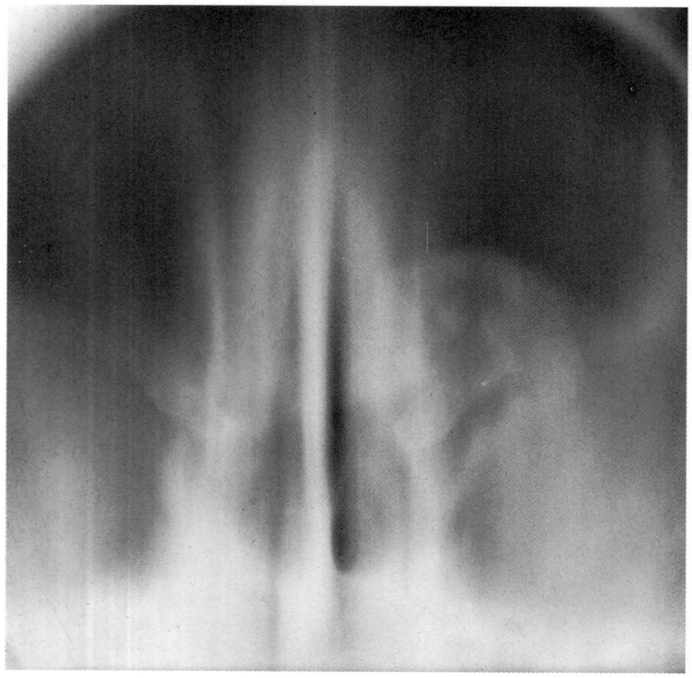

A

Fig. 8. *Extensively calcified left clinoid meningioma.* 54-year-old man who underwent X-ray after mild cranial trauma. Plain radiogram and laminography (A) show a calcific mass starting from the left anterior clinoid with bone involvement at the margins of the superior sphenoid fissure. MRI: The T_1- (B) and T_2- (C) weighted scans show the inhomogeneity of the lesion. Note the central focus with higher signal on the long-TR sequences, which represents the soft part of the neoplasm, and the calcium deposits which are increasingly visible with TR and TE elongation.

B

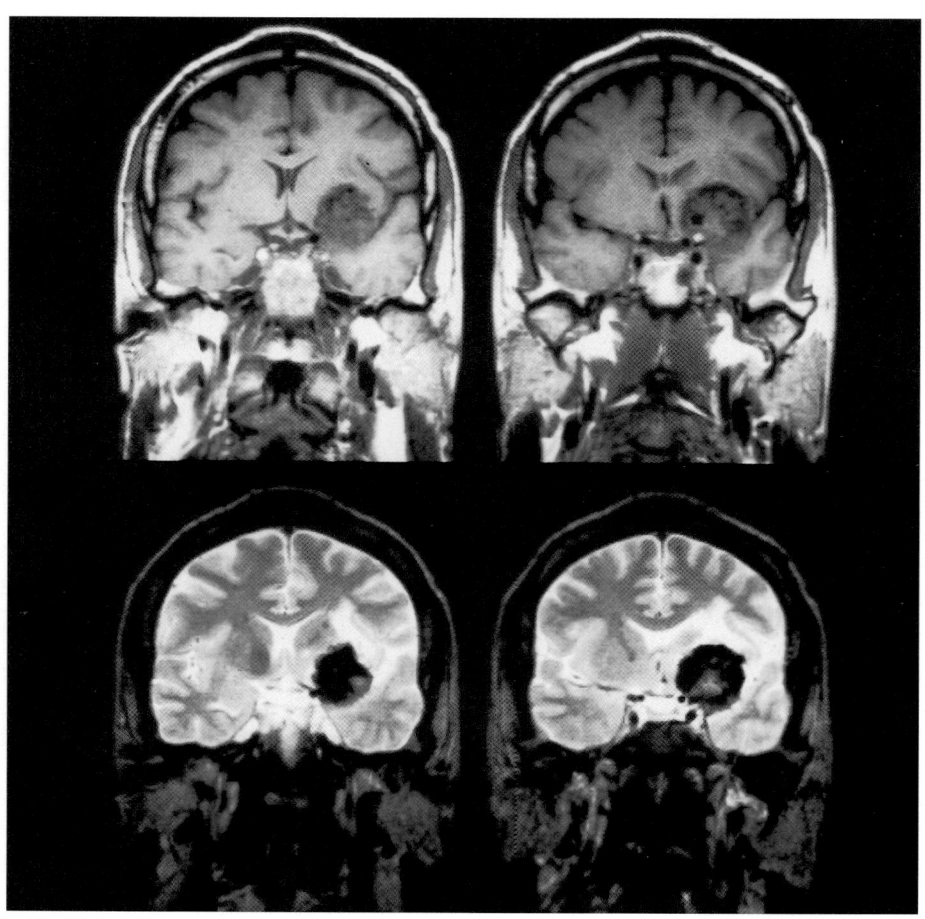

C

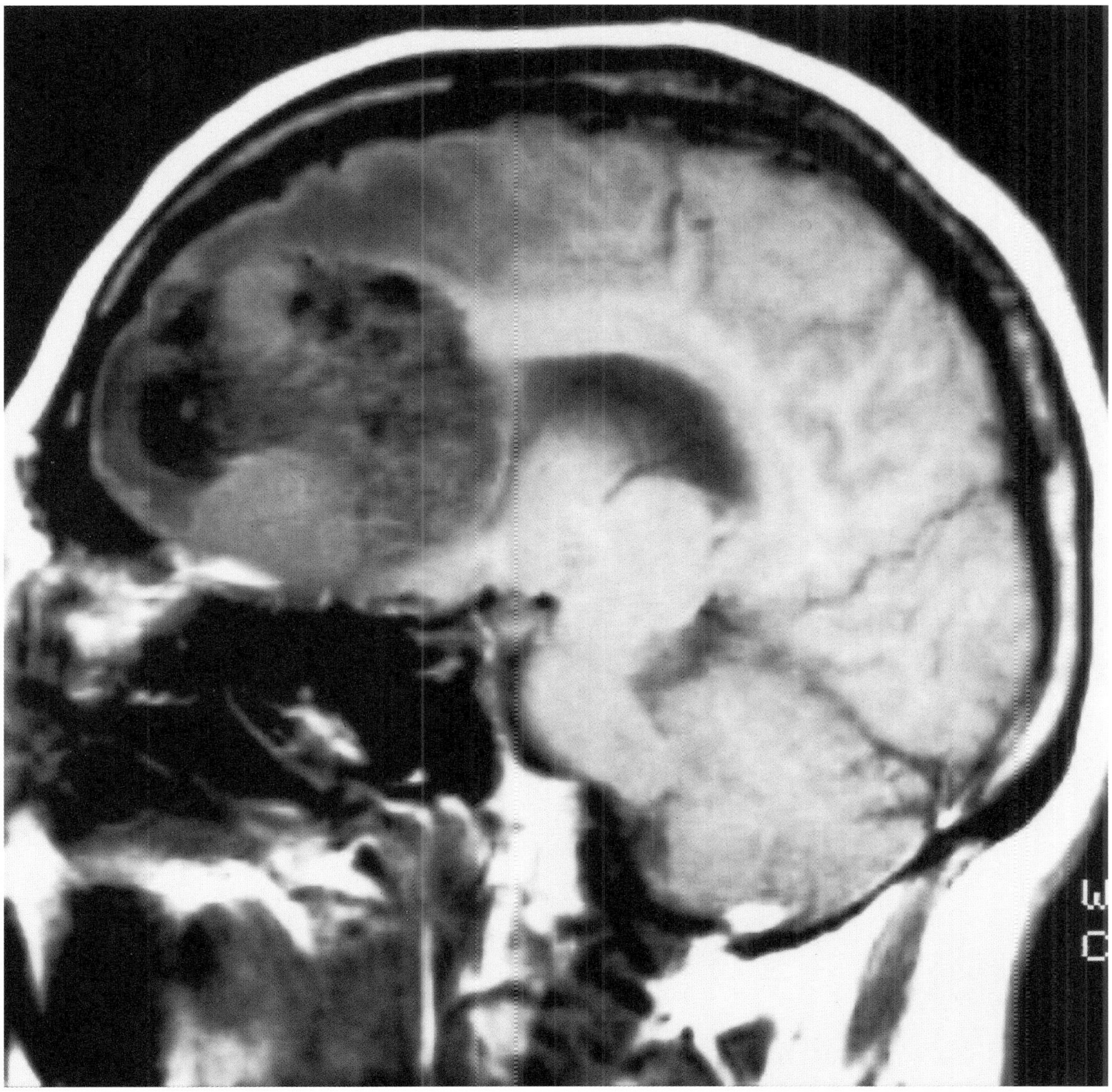

Fig. 9. *Right frontobasal meningioma.* Paramedian right-sided sagittal T_1-weighted scan. Round-shaped mass originating from the olfactory groove, with multiple hypointense foci due to calcifications. The cellular components of the tumor are isointense with the brain tissue. A mild edema of the frontal lobe (hypointense signal) and major deformation of the corpus callosum and of the frontal horn of the lateral ventricle can be seen. Note the posterior displacement of the midbrain.

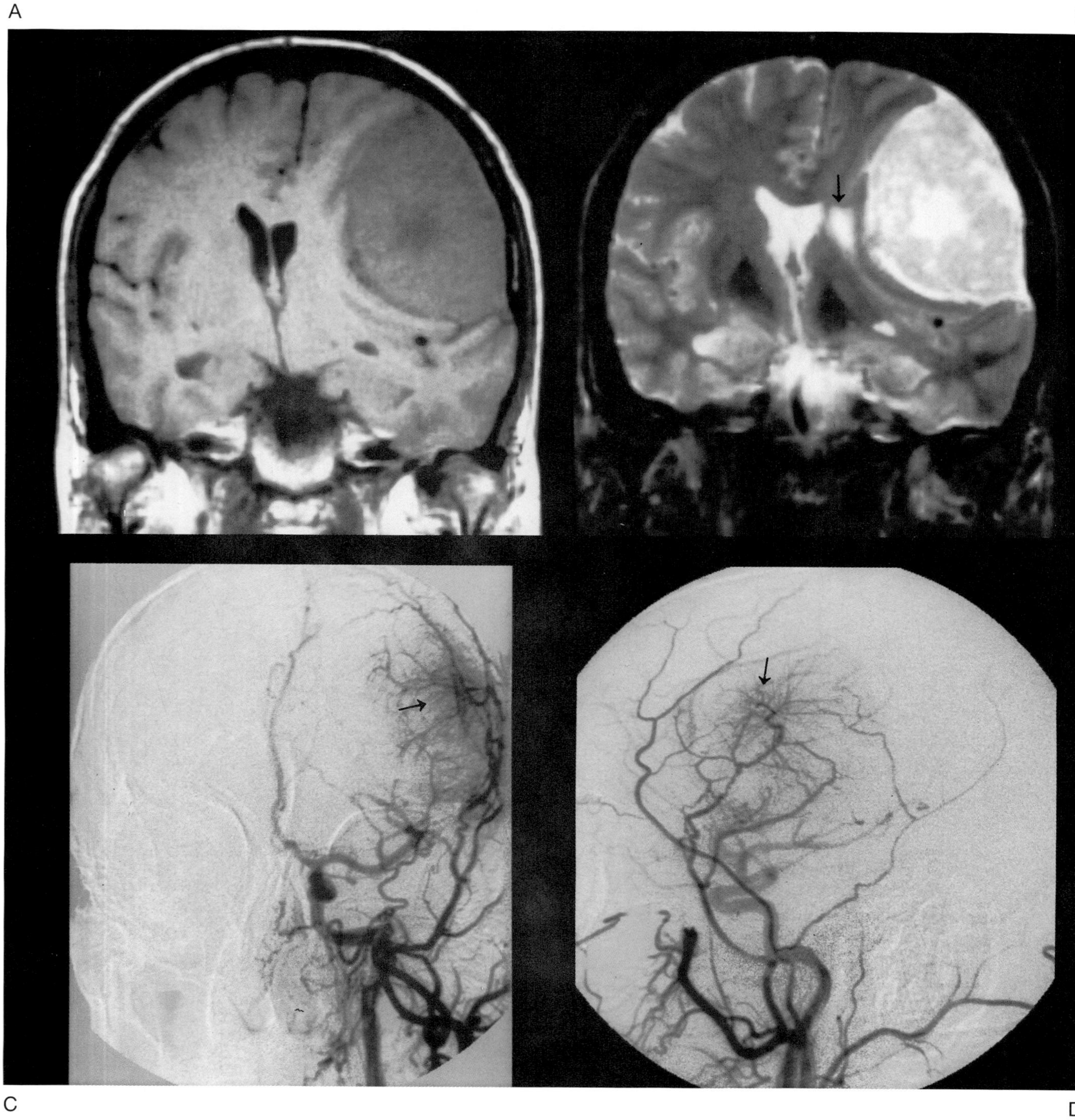

Fig. 10. *Left posterior frontal meningothelial meningioma.* 42-year-old man with right adversative seizures accompanied by transient aphasia. A – T_1-weighted coronal scan: suprasylvian hypointense rounded mass with core of xanthomatous degeneration; the core is hyperintense and the mass which is well bounded by a CSF watershed. B – T_2-weighted image showing the degenerated area as a high-signal focus and the CSF watershed tumor-tissue delimiting boundary as a hyperintense rim. Compression of the cerebral tissue and mild edema (↓). The CSF has a signal intensity higher than the edema. Left carotid angiogram in A-P (C) and lateral (D): lowering of the Sylvian vessels suggesting suprafissural tumor and blush (→). The predominant opacification of the E.C.A. shows a radial blush (↓), typical of meningioma and supplied by a manifestly hypertrophic middle meningeal artery.

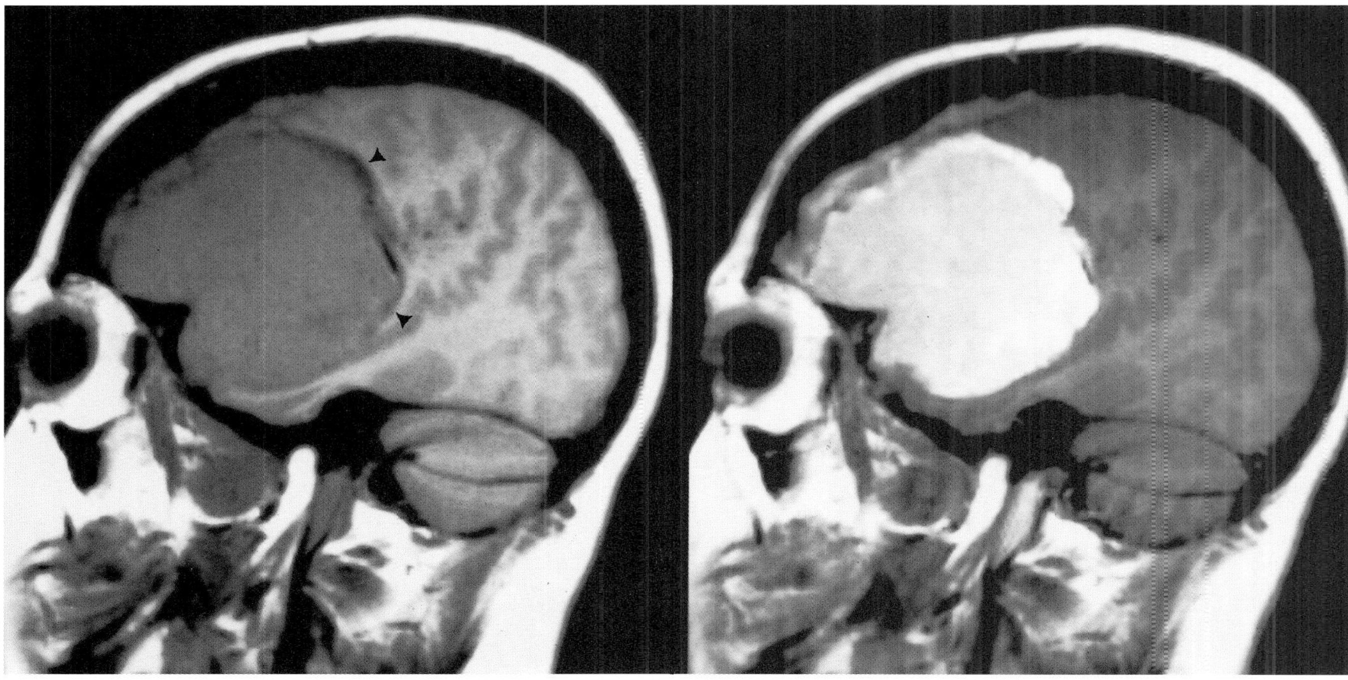

Fig. 11. *Right frontotemporal meningothelial meningioma.* The T_1-weighted sections before and after GD-DTPA indicate a fairly homogeneous structure with evident peripheral margins; in this case, these margins are due to an intensely vascularized capsule (←).

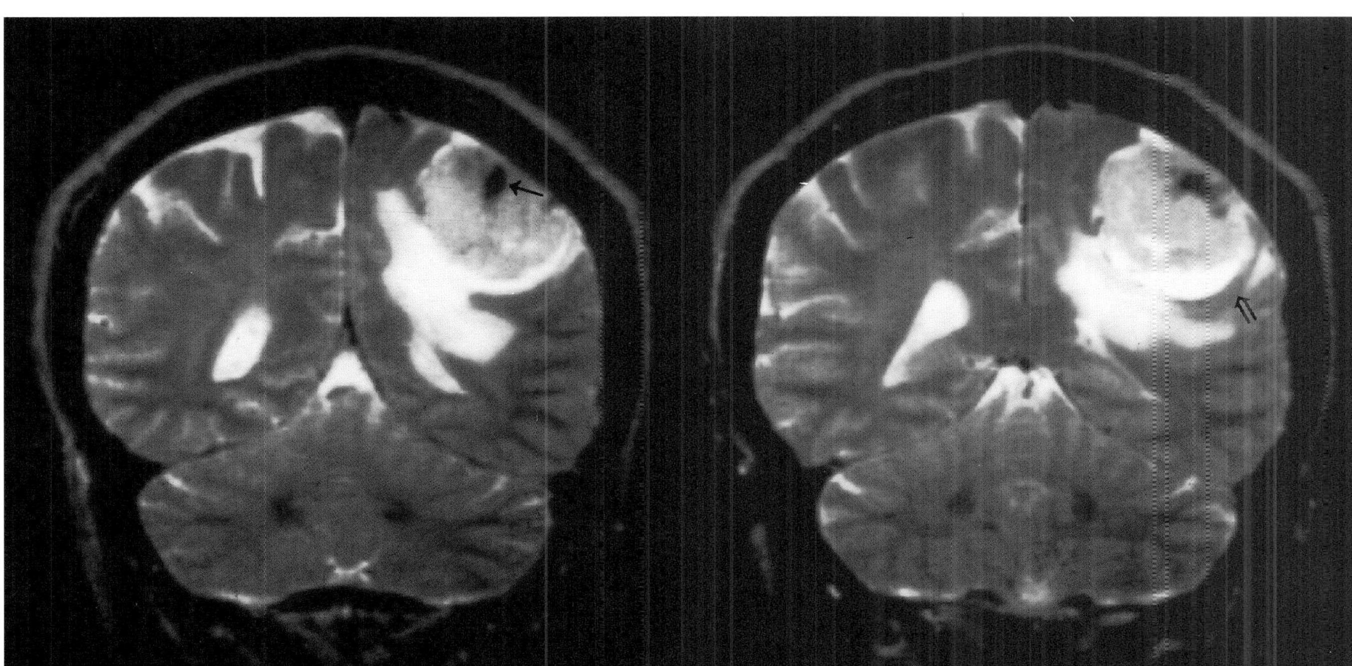

Fig. 12. *Left posterior parietal convexity meningothelial meningioma.* T_1-weighted coronal sections: well-outlined calcifications (←); the signal from the peritumoral CSF watershed (⇑) is more intense than the edema. In some spots, the CSF collection has a pseudo-cystic appearance.

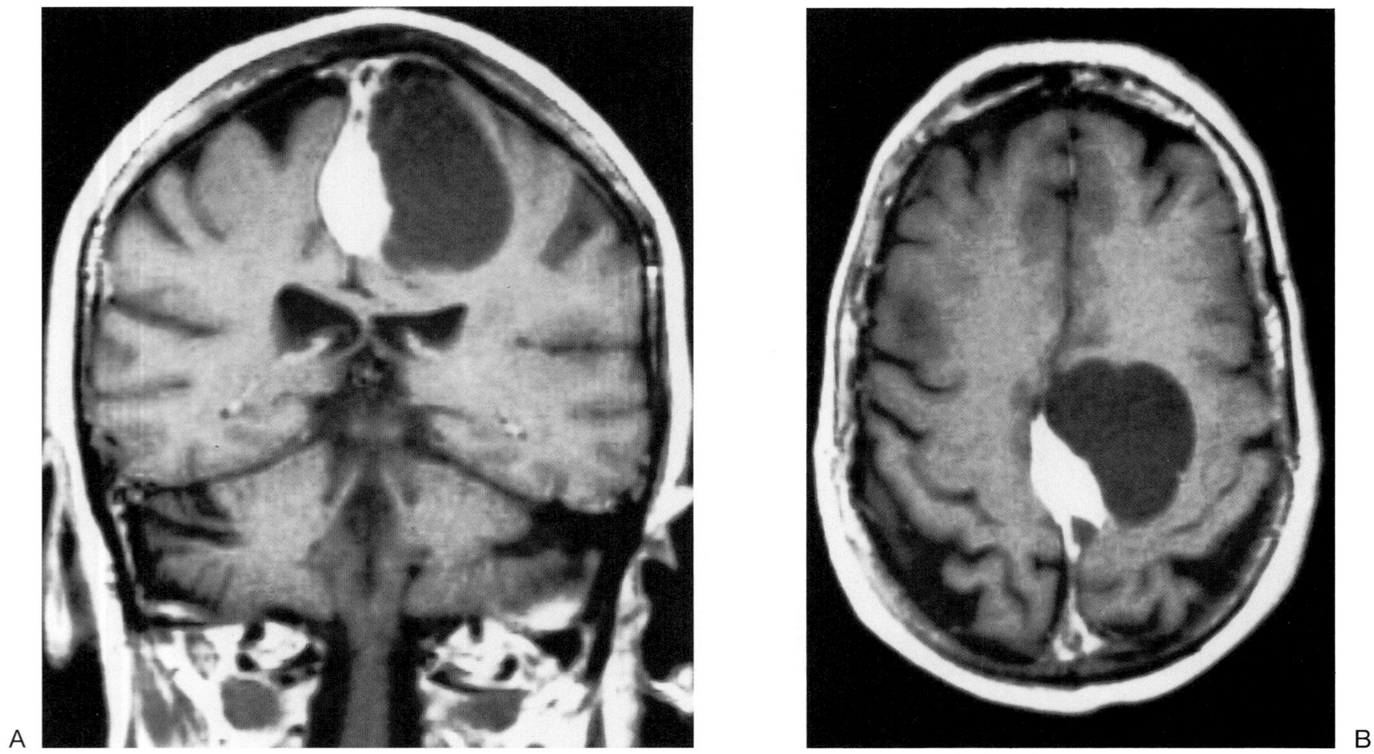

Fig. 13. *Cystic left parasagittal parietal meningioma.* T_1-weighted images after GD-DTPA: coronal (A) and axial (B) scans. The solid component is entirely medial, since the tumor originates from the falx, which is affected up to the S.L.S. The cyst has no wall and is full of apparently sequestrated CSF.

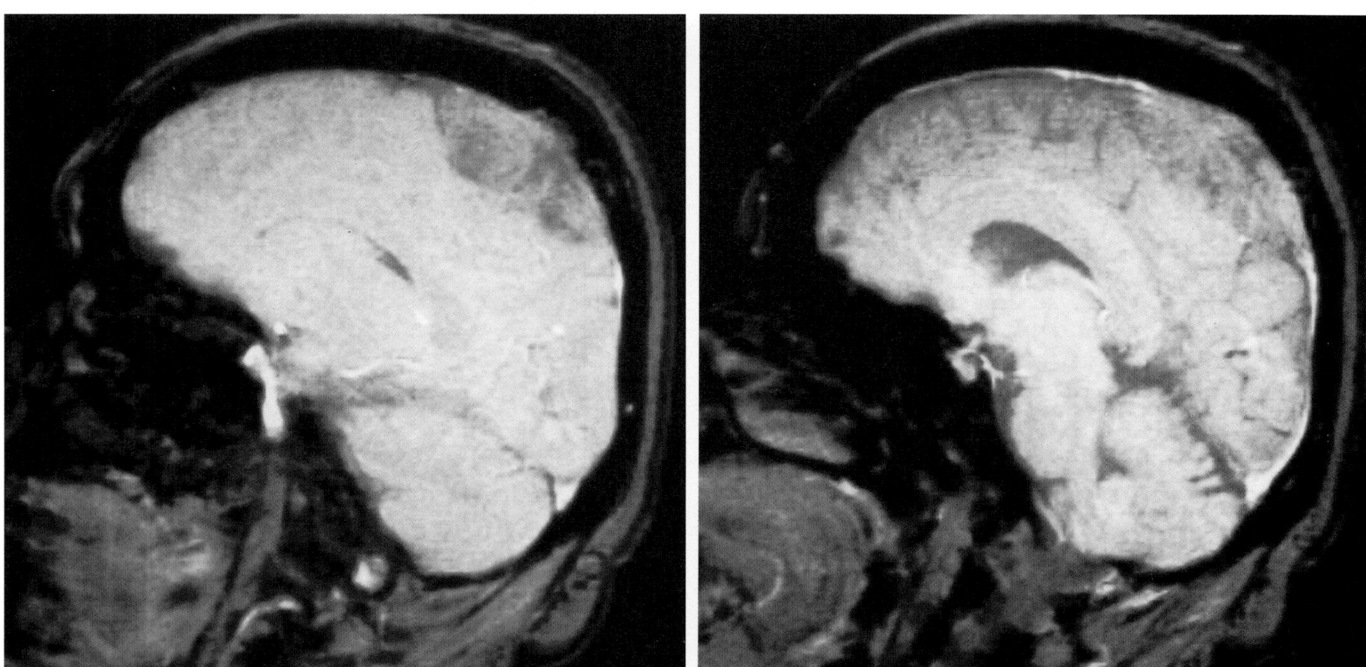

Fig. 14. *Meningioma of the middle third of the S.L.S.* Sagittal gradient-echo images (Flash TR 100 msec, TE 10 msec, FA 20°). This method yields flow-velocity-dependent images; therefore, the vessels have high signal. In this case, MRI visualizes the absence of flow in the sinus throughout the extension of the neoplasm.

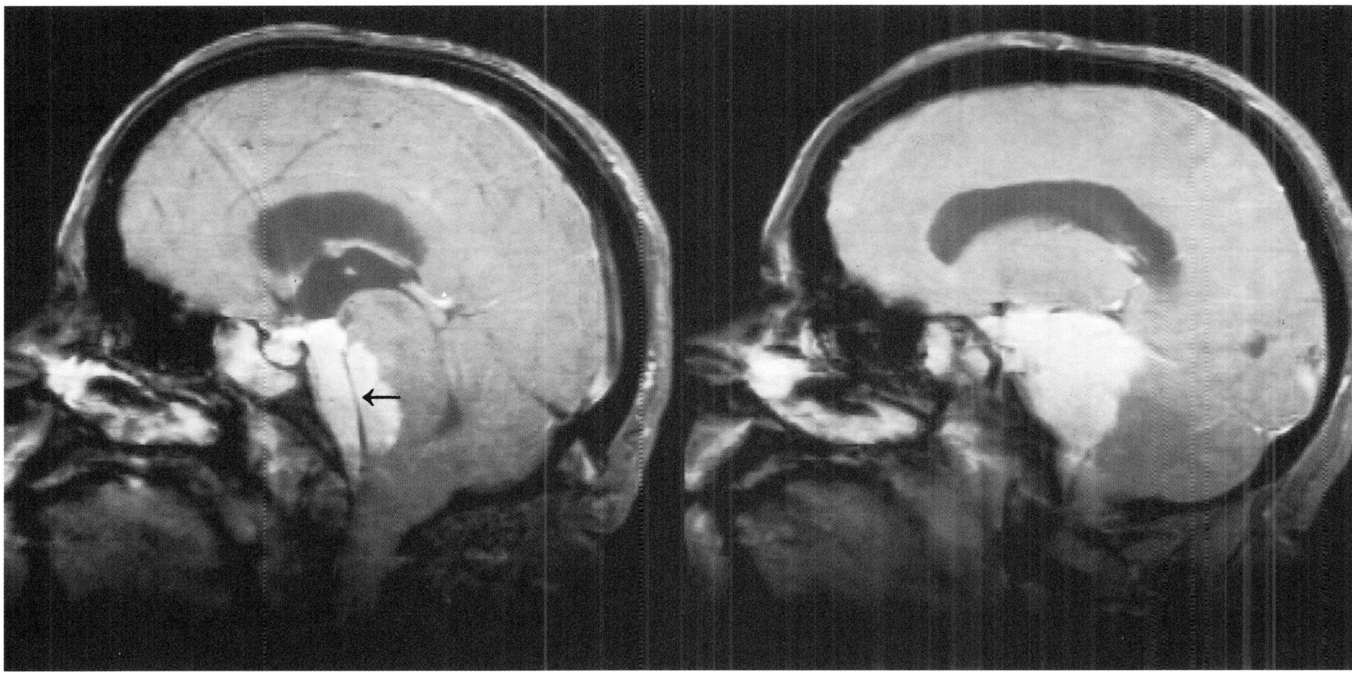

A

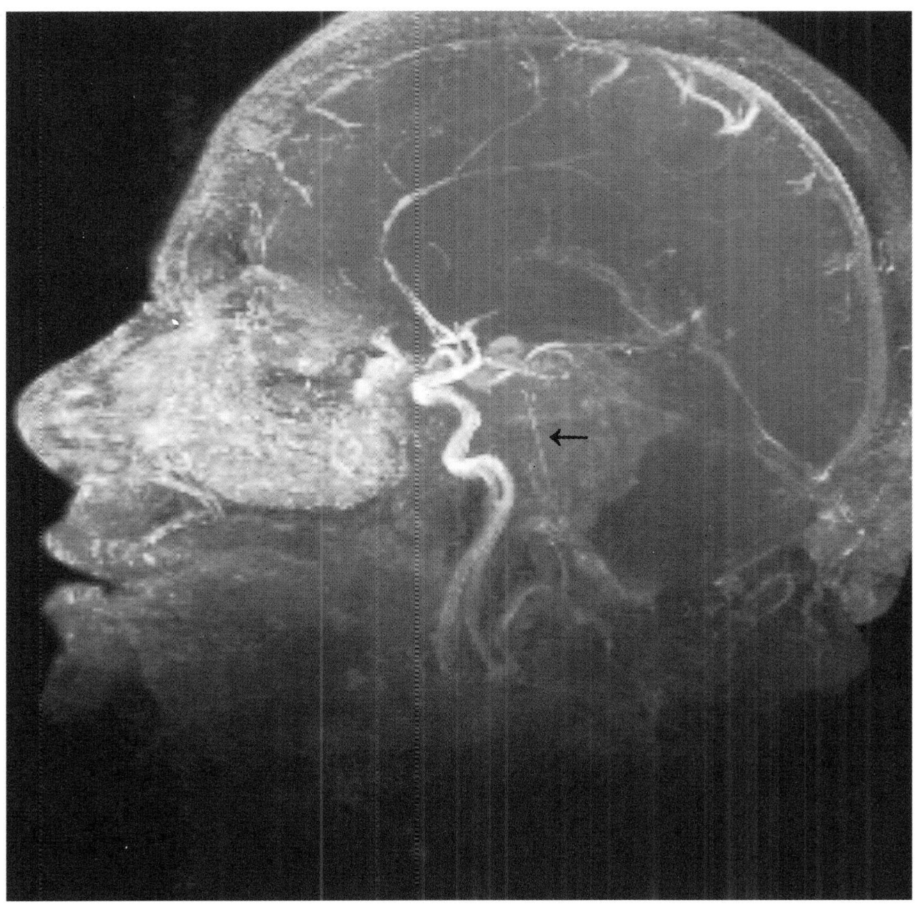

B

Fig. 15. *Left petroclival meningioma.* 58-year-old woman without major clinical symptoms. A – The gradient-echo sagittal views after GD-DTPA show: the considerably spread of the neoplasm, which starts from the clivus, encases the B.A. (←) and the cavernous sinus and invades the sella turcica and the sphenoid sinus. This sequence well portrays the integrity of the bone structures of the clivus and of the sellar floor. B – Vascular MRI after GD-DTPA simultaneously shows enhancement of the venous and arterial vasculature and of the neoplasm.

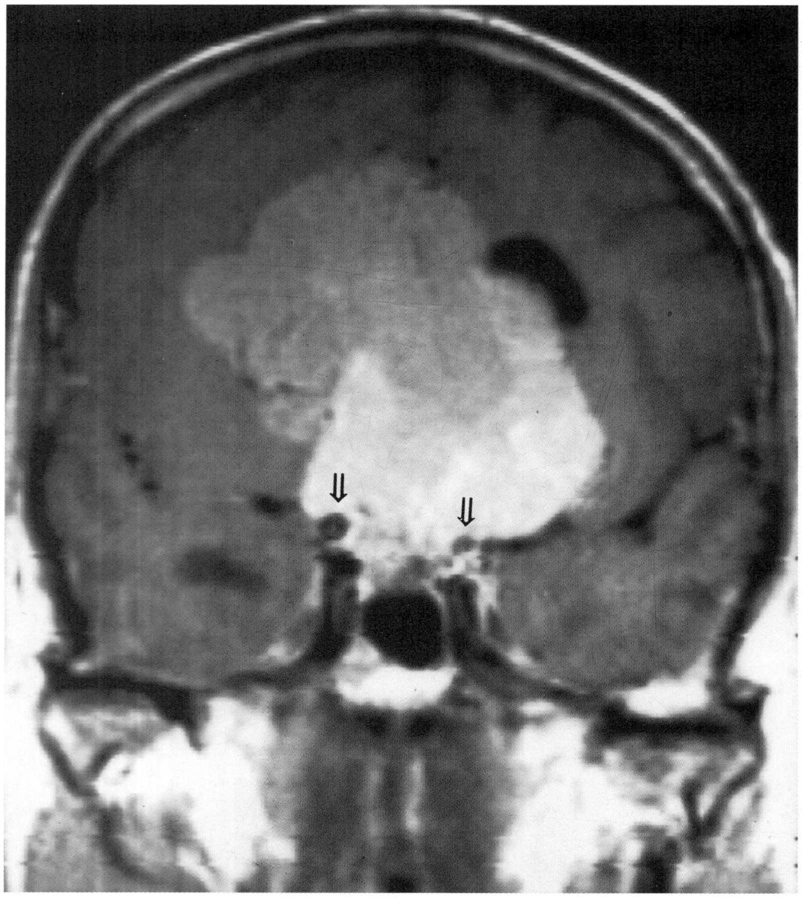

Fig. 16. *Giant meningioma of the sphenoid plane*. Patient with severe consciousness impairment and tetraparesis. The neoplasm grows caudocranially, occupying the third ventricle and the lateral ventricles and it partially embeds both I.C.A.s (⇓). The T_1-weighted image obtained after GD-DTPA shows the digitated shape of the mass and its inhomogeneity, which is due to a more vascularized basal component with greater consistency and to a superior component which proved to be degenerated and soft at surgery.

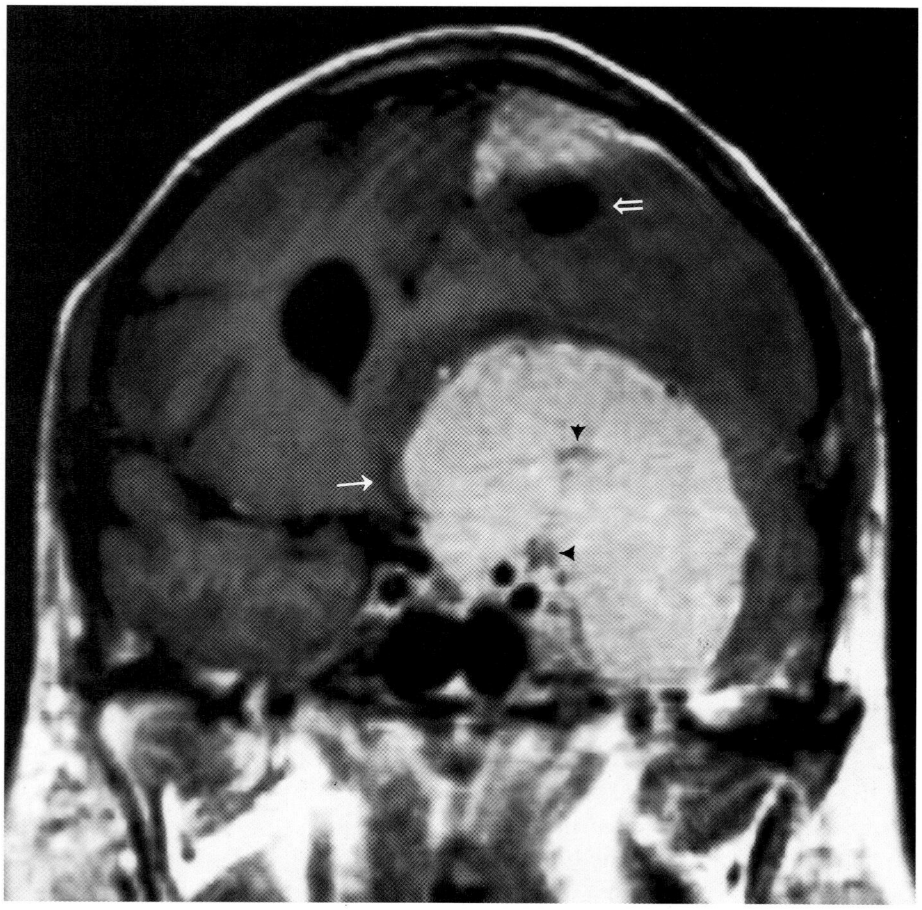

Fig. 17. *Multiple meningiomas of the falx and of the sphenoid wing*. T_1-weighted coronal view after i.v. GD-DTPA. The meningioma of the falx with its adjacent CSF cyst (⇐) is an occasional finding in this 69-year-old patient with severe demential syndrome and left-eye blindness. Observe the intense perfusion of both neoplasms, their relationships with the I.C.A. and the A.C.A. (→) and the small low-signal foci. The foci correspond to sprinkled calcifications (◀) which are typical of this psammomatous meningioma.

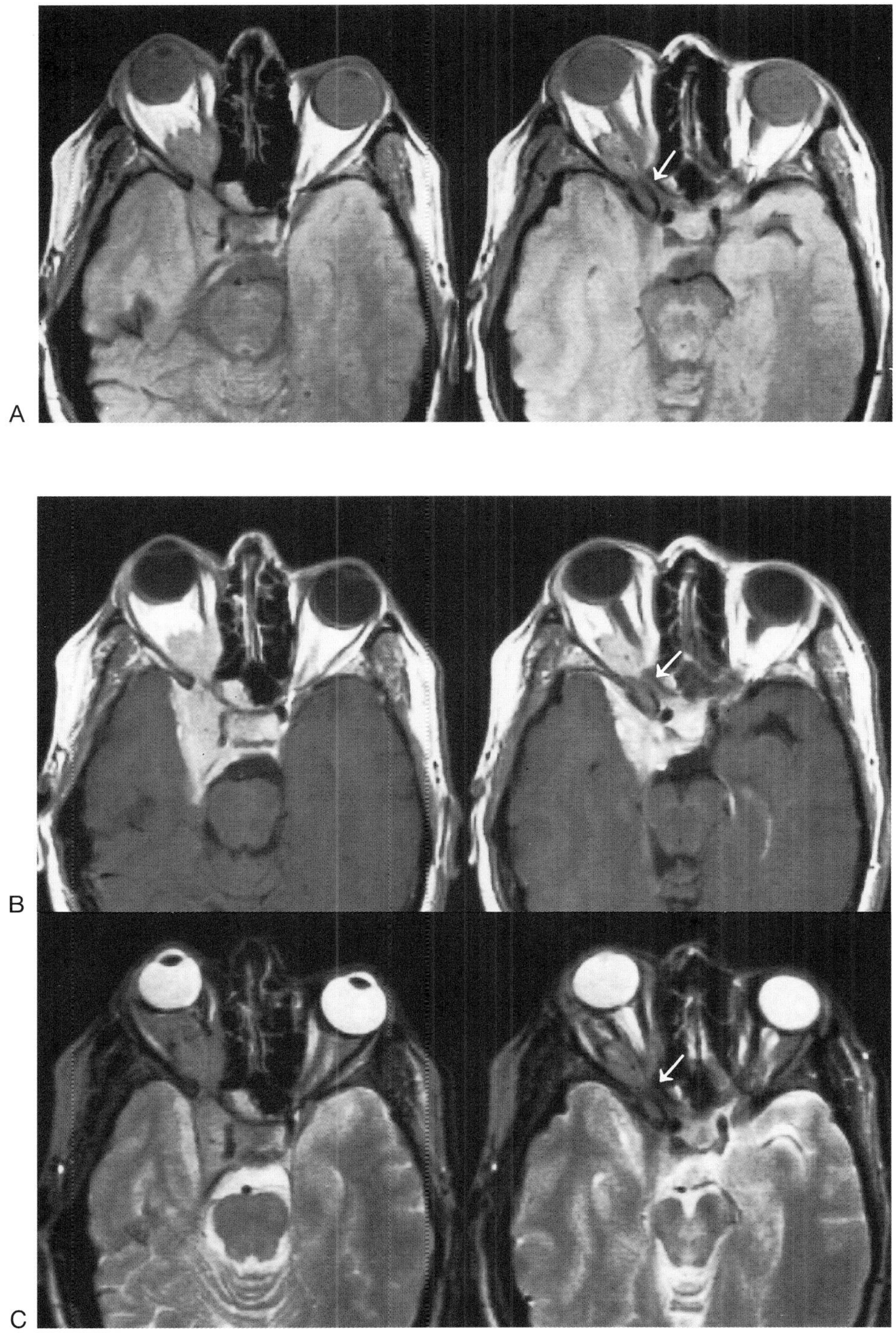

Fig. 18. *Right sphenocavernous meningioma.* 53-year-old woman with right oculomotor palsy and exophthalmos. Only after GD-DTPA enhancement (B) the real tumor spread and its anatomical relationships are well depicted. The meningioma occupies the right cavernous sinus, Meckel's cave, the sella, the posterior portion of the orbit and the clinopetrosal ligament. Note the relationships between the meningioma and the optic nerve and the integrity of the bone walls of the optic canal (↙). The right I.C.A. is surrounded by the tumor. Corresponding proton density- (A) and T_2- (C) weighted images.

A B

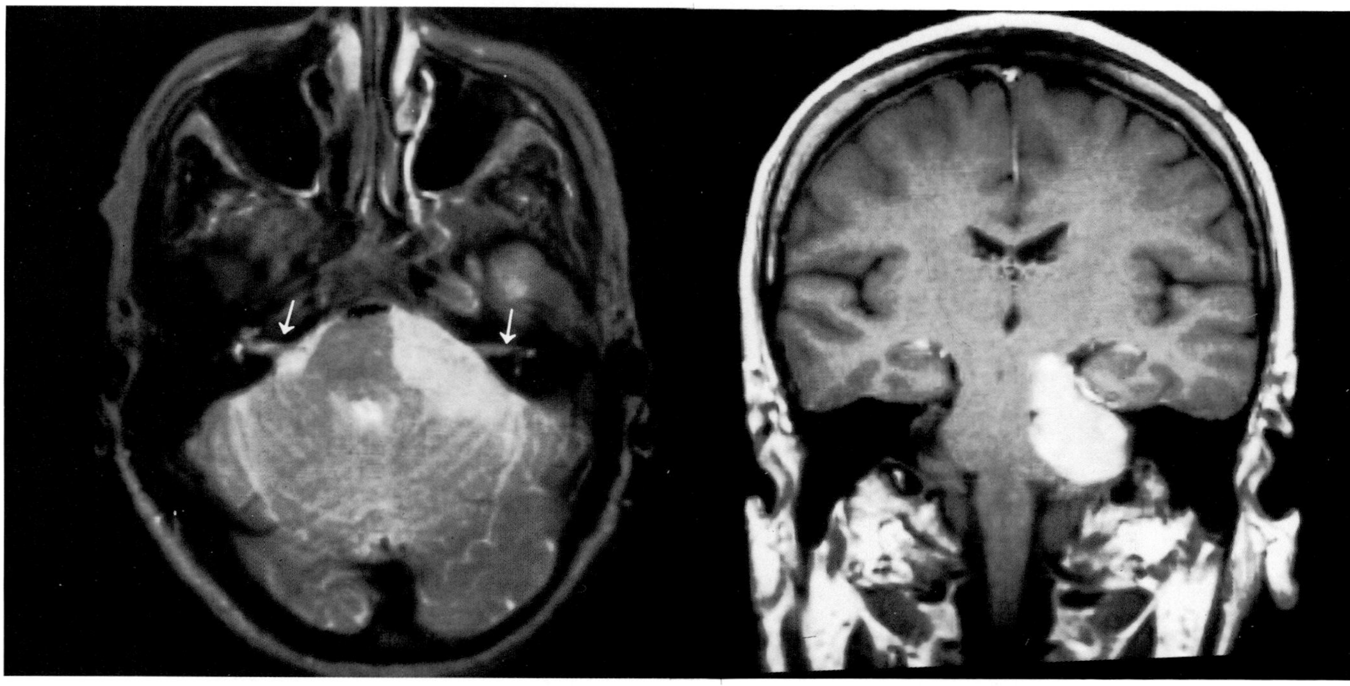

Fig. 19. *Left petrous apex meningioma.* 62-year-old woman with sensorimotor loss in the fifth cranial nerve. T_2-weighted axial view (A): note the unusual hyperintensity of the meningioma and a large base of the tumor with mass effect on the pons. Observe also the symmetry of the auditory canals, where the facial-acoustic nervous bundle can be identified (↓). The coronal scan after GD-DTPA portrays the craniocaudal spread of the neoplasm.

A B

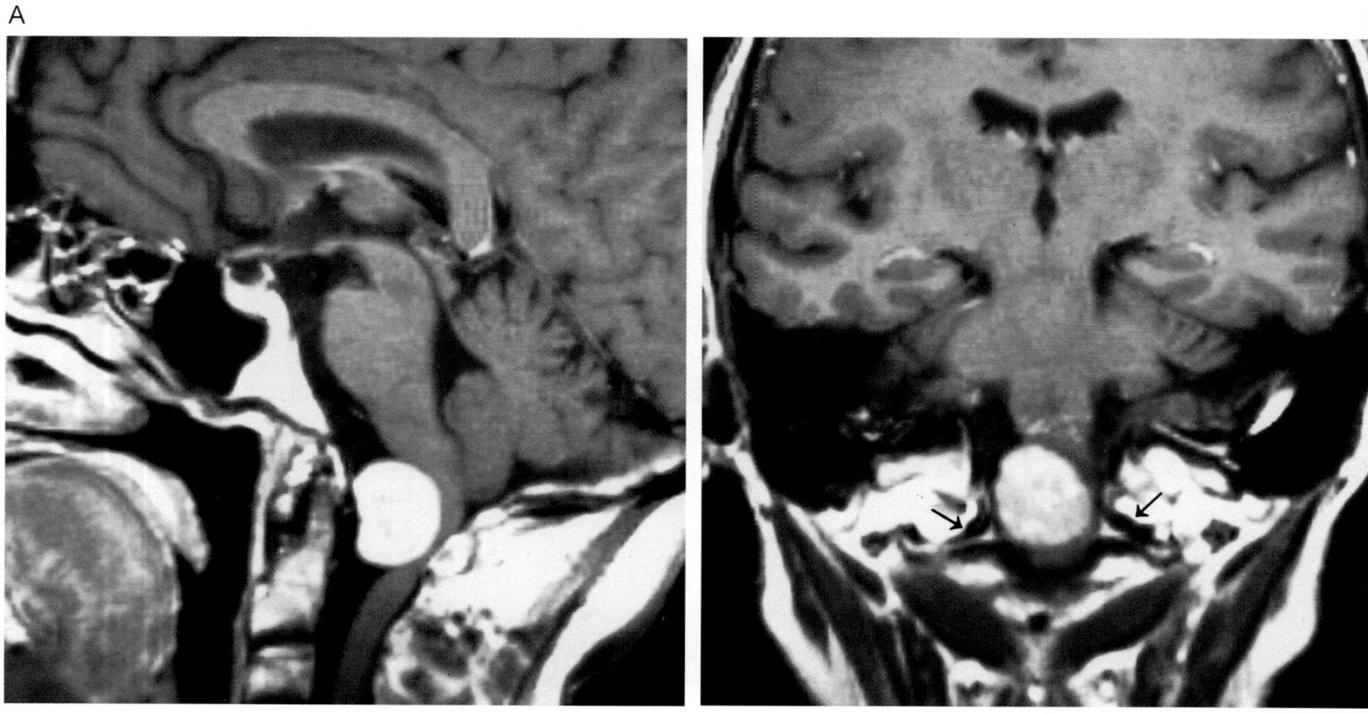

Fig. 20. *Meningioma of the anterior margin of the occipital foramen.* 67-year-old woman with severe spastic tetraparesis. A – T_1-weighted mid-sagittal section after i.v. GD-DTPA. The rounded mass markedly enhances, displaces the medulla oblongata backwards and compresses it against the posterior arch of the atlas. A hypointense CSF cleavage plane is evidenced between the tumor and the bulb. B – T_1-weighted coronal view after GD-DTPA. The tumor is slightly eccentric to the right. The arrows indicate the vertebral arteries at their inlet into the neurocranium.

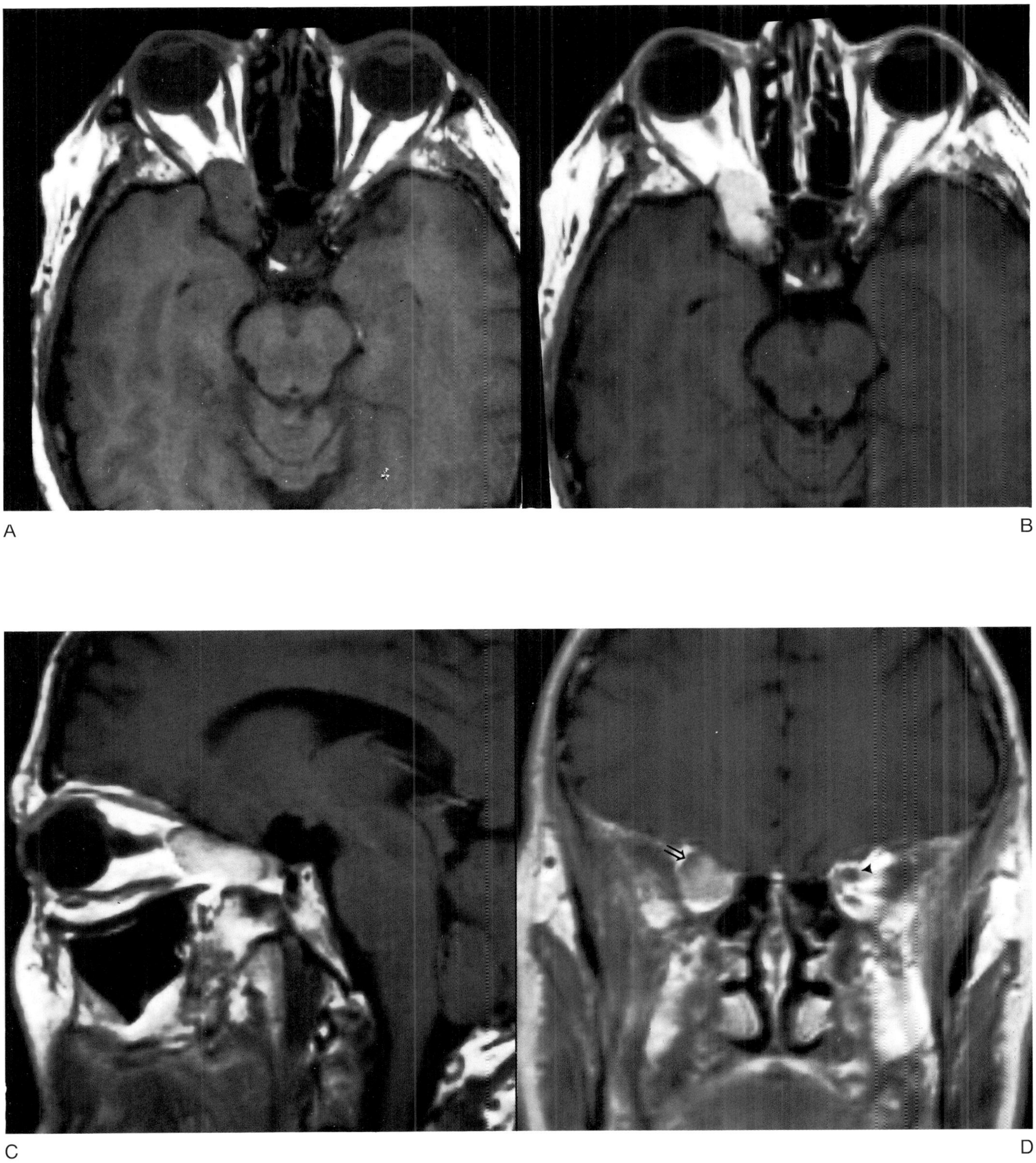

Fig. 21. *Right optic nerve sheath intracanalicular meningioma.* 54-year-old woman with several years of right blindness. T_1-weighted axial cuts before (A) and after (B) GD-DTPA. A – The mass is isodense and ovoid. It extends to the orbital and intracranial compartments, encasing the muscular attachments at the level of the anulus. B – Post-c.e. C – The meningioma fills the optic canal. D – Eccentric position of the optic nerve (⇓) with respect to the meningioma. The contralateral optic nerve is indicated (◀).

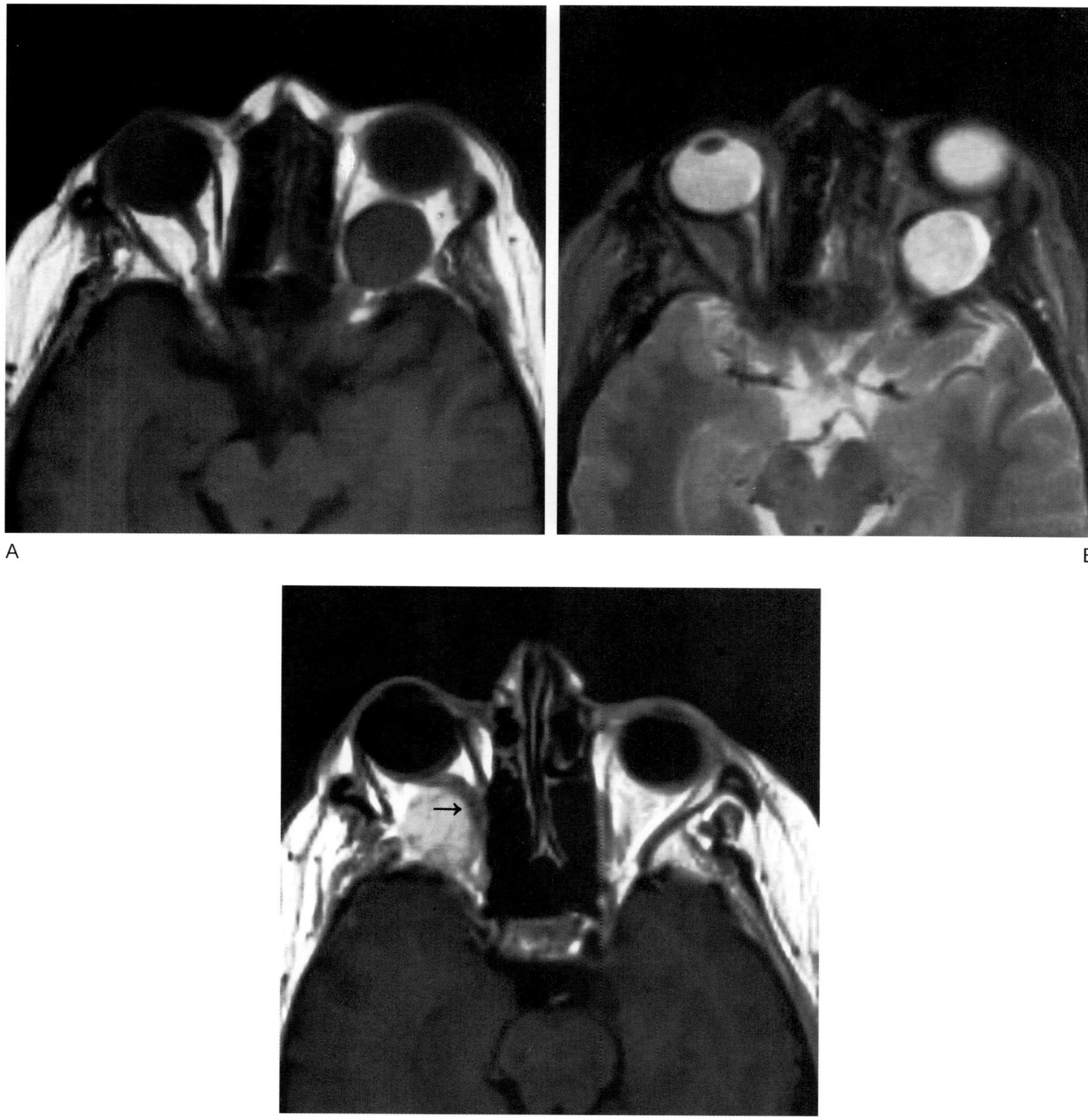

Fig. 22. *Left optic nerve meningioma.* 54-year-old woman with non-reducible exophthalmos and unaffected vision. The T_1- and T_2-weighted axial views (A, B) show the major diameter of the tumor. In A, the meningioma appears to be isointense and occupies the posterior part of the orbital compartment without entering into the optic canal. In B, the mass enhances with non-typical meningioma behavior. The chiasm is well visualized thanks to the cisternographic effect. C – More caudal scan after GD-DTPA: the neoplasm has an intense and homogeneous perfusion and is well demarcated from the medially displaced optic nerve (←). These signs are the most significant for diagnostic purposes.

References

1. Berry I, Brandt-Zawadzki M, Osaki L et al. (1986) Gd-DTPA in clinical MR of the brain. 2. Extraaxial lesions and normal structures. AJNR 7:789–793
2. Bird CR, Hasso AN, LeBeau DJ (1989) Meningiomas and skull base neoplasms. Top Magn Reson Imaging 1:52–68
3. Brant-Zawadzki M, Badami JP, Mills CM et al. (1984) Primary intracranial tumor imaging. A comparison of magnetic resonance and CT. Radiology 150:435–440
4. Breger RK, Paphe RA, Pojunas KW et al. (1987) Benign extraaxial tumors: contrast enhancement with Gd-DTPA. Radiology 163:427–429
5. Bronen RA, Sze G (1990) Magnetic resonance contrast agents: theory and application to the central nervous system. J Neurosurg 73:820–840
6. Cushing H, Eisenhardt L (1938) Meningiomas: Their Classification, Regional Behaviour, Life History, and Surgical End Results. Charles C. Thomas, Springfield, Illinois
7. Elster AD, Challa VR, Gilbert TH et al. (1989) Meningiomas: MR and histopathologic features. Radiology 170:857–862
8. Felix R, Shorner W, Laniado M et al. (1985) Brain tumors: MR imaging with gadolinium-DTPA. Radiology 156:681–688
9. Gadian DG, Payne JA, Bryant DJ et al. (1985) Gadolinium-DTPA as a contrast agent in MR imaging: theoretical projections and practical observations. J Comput Assist Tomogr 9:242–251
10. Gilbert JJ, Paulseth JE, Coates RK et al. (1983) Cerebral edema associated with meningiomas. Neurosurgery 12:599–605
11. Goldsher D, Litt AW, Pinto RS (1990) Dural "tail" associated with meningiomas on Gd-DTPA-enhanced MR images: Characteristics, differential diagnostic value, and possible implications for treatment. Radiology 176 447–450
12. Haughton VM, Rimm AA, Czervionke LF et al. (1988) Sensitivity of Gd-DTPA enhanced imaging of benign extraaxial tumors. Radiology 166:829–833
13. Harsh GR, IV, Wilson CB (1990) Peritorcular meningiomas. In: Wilkins RH, Rengachary SS (eds) Neurosurgery Update II. McGraw-Hill, New York, 428–433
14. Kepes JJ (1986) Presidential address: the histopathology of meningiomas. A reflection of origins and expected behaviour. J Neuropathol Exp Neurol 45:95–107
15. Mac Carthy CS, Boyd AS, Childs DS (1970) Tumors of the optic nerve. J Neurosurg 33:439–444
16. Malis LI (1990) Surgical approaches to tentorial meningiomas. In: Wilkins RH, Rengachary SS (eds) Neurosurgery Update II. McGraw-Hill, New York, 399–408
17. Mulder DW, Swenson WM (1974) Psychologic and psychiatric aspects of brain tumors. In: Vinken PJ, Bruyn GW (eds) Handbook of Clinical Neurology, Vol 16. Tumors of the Brain and Skull, Part I. North-Holland, Amsterdam, 727–740
18. Newman SA, Jane JA (1991) Meningiomas of the optic nerve, orbit, and anterior visual pathways. In: Al-Mefty O (ed) Meningiomas. Raven Press, New York, 461–494
19. Nakasu S, Nakasu Y, Matsumura K et al. (1990) Interface between meningioma and the brain on Magnetic Resonance Imaging. Surg Neurol 33:105–116
20. Parent AD (1991) Multiple meningiomas. In: Al-Mefty O (ed) Meningiomas. Raven Press, New York, 161–168
21. Parizel PM, Degryse HL, Gheuens J et al. (1989) Gadolinium-DTPA enhanced MR imaging of intracranial lesions. Comput Assist Tomogr 13:378–385
22. Phelps PD, Lloyd GA (1989) Magnetic Resonance with Gadolinium-DTPA for the investigation of temporal bone tumours. Clin Otolaryngol 14:251–262
23. Pomeranz SJ (1989) MR of supratentorial neoplasia. In: Pomeranz SJ (ed) Craniospinal Magnetic Resonance Imaging. W. B. Saunders Co, Philadelphia, 208–247
24. Pomeranz SJ (1989) Posterior fossa, skull base, craniocervical junction. In: Pomeranz SJ (ed) Craniospinal Magnetic Resonance Imaging. W. B. Saunders Co, Philadelphia, 248–274
25. Schorner W, Schibeus P, Henkes H et al. (1990) Intracranial meningiomas. Comparison of plain and contrast-enhanced examinations in CT and MRI. Neuroradiology 32:12–18
26. Strobos RJ (1974) Temporal lobe Tumors. In: Vinken PJ, Bruyn GW (eds) Handbook of Clinical Neurology, Vol 16. Tumors of the Brain and Skull, Part I. North-Holland, Amsterdam, 281–295
27. Tokomaru A, O'uchi T, Eguchi T et al. (1990) Prominent meningeal enhancement adjacent to meningioma on Gd-DTPA-enhanced MR images: Histopathologic correlation. Radiology 175:431–433
28. Watabe T, Azuma T (1989) T1 and T2 measurements of meningiomas and neuromas before and after Gd-DTPA. AJNR 10:463–470

29. Wilms G, Lammens M, Marchal G et al. (1989) Thickening of dura surrounding meningiomas: MR features. J Comput Assist Tomogr 13:763–768
30. Yoshida K, Furuse M, Kaneoke Y et al. (1989) Assessment of T1 time course changes and tissue-blood ratios after Gd-DTPA administration in brain tumors. Magn Reson Imaging 7:9–15
31. Zimmerman RD, Fleming CA, Saint-Louis LA et al. (1985) Magnetic resonance imaging of meningiomas. AJNR 6:149–157
32. Zimmerman CF, Schatz NJ, Glaser JS (1990) Magnetic resonance imaging of optic nerve meningiomas. Enhancement with Gadolinium-DTPA. Ophthalmology 97:585–591
33. Zimmerman RD (1991) MRI of intracranial meningiomas. In: Al-Mefty O (ed) Meningiomas. Raven Press, New York, 209–223

CHAPTER VII

Intracranial neurinomas

Intracranial neurinomas (n.) or schwannomas originate from the Schwann cells of the cranial nerves before emerging from the neurocranium.

More than 90% of such tumors derive from the vestibular component of the eighth nerve, inside the internal acoustic foramen, and are called n. of the acoustic nerve *(Fig. 1)*. They may be bilateral in Recklinghausen's disease; in this disease, they may be associated with other intracranial tumors: gliomas of the optic nerve and meningiomas *(Fig. 4)*.

The sizes of n. of the eighth nerve are very variable upon observation and depend on early diagnosis. Therefore, intracanalicular n. *(Fig. 3)* and giant n. with a diameter exceeding 5 cm *(Fig. 2)* may be found. In growing, they occupy the cistern of the cerebello-pontine angle, displacing the brainstem and the cerebellum contralaterally, the facial and the trigeminal nerves anterosuperiorly, the glossopharyngeal, vagal and accessory spinal nerves inferiorly.

Clinical onset is silent, with ipsilateral hypoacusis and tinnitus. In the late stages, obstruction of the Sylvian aqueduct causes hydrocephalus and an intracranial hypertension syndrome, which may be associated with cerebellar impairment due to compression of the ipsilateral hemisphere *(Fig. 2)*. At times, n. of the eighth nerve are associated with a posterior satellite cyst, which can be inferred from the fact that the cistern of the cerebello-pontine angle is full of sequestrated CSF.

Since these are benign lesions, radical surgery is curative. The difficulties of the surgical procedure, requiring the operating microscope, are directly proportional to the size of the mass. The surgical objective is to remove the lesion avoiding damage to the nearby tumor-compressed nerves, especially the facial nerve, and to the brainstem.

The most common approaches are: translabyrinthine (for intracanalicular and also extracanalicular tumors, performed by the otolaryngologist); suboccipital (generally for extracanalicular tumors, performed by the neurosurgeon); and combined translabyrinthine and suboccipital. The most critical stages of the surgical procedure are the dissections of the mass from the cranial nerves, from the A.I.C.A.s and P.I.C.A.s and from the lateral surface of the brainstem.

If the procedure is performed correctly, it does not involve the mortality and morbidity rates which were still being reported in the late 60s.

N. which stem from other cranial nerves are more rare: trigeminal, glossopharyngeal, spinal accessory, facial. After n. of the eighth nerve, the most frequent are the n. of the fifth cranial nerve, which originate from the Gasserian ganglion and reach enormous sizes owing to their paucisymptomatology. Their excision, however, is relatively simpler, since they are mostly extradural. The rare n. of the inferior cranial nerves *(Fig. 6)* are instead hard to remove radically without impairing the nerves. They originate from the posterior foramen lacerum and often grow in a dumbbell fashion, as occurs with intra-extradural tumors *(Fig. 5)*.

Morphologically, they may be divided into: n. of type A, with a more compact structure, predominant in spinal sites and in neurofibromatosis and n. of type B, predominant in cranial sites, with frequent processes of hyaline and mucoid degeneration.

On T_1-weighted MRI sequences, n. appear as formations with regular and well-defined boundaries and average-low signal intensity; they are hypointense with the cerebellar tissue but produce a more intense signal than the CSF, from which they can easily be discriminated *(Fig. 2A)*. On T_2-weighted sequences, they have variable behavior, since they may appear either as hyperintense formations, occasionally inhomogeneous due to areas of necrosis and hyaline degeneration *(Fig. 2B)*, corresponding to n. of type B, or as low-signal lesions which can be easily differentiated from the high-signal CSF ("cisternographic effect"). The latter appearance is more typical in n. of type A and in neurofibromas of Recklinghausen's disease *(Figs. 3, 4)*. Paramagnetic contrast media (GD-DTPA) further increase the diagnostic sensitivity of MRI, especially in identifying n. of small size or those located in sites of difficult detection (intracanalicular or Gasserian ganglion n.), and in evaluating recurrences after surgery.

Since GD-DTPA selectively binds to the n., it reduces the n. T_1 relaxation time; on T_1-weighted sequences, it causes a definite rise in intensity of the signal from the lesion which will thus be more easily detected *(Fig. 4)*.

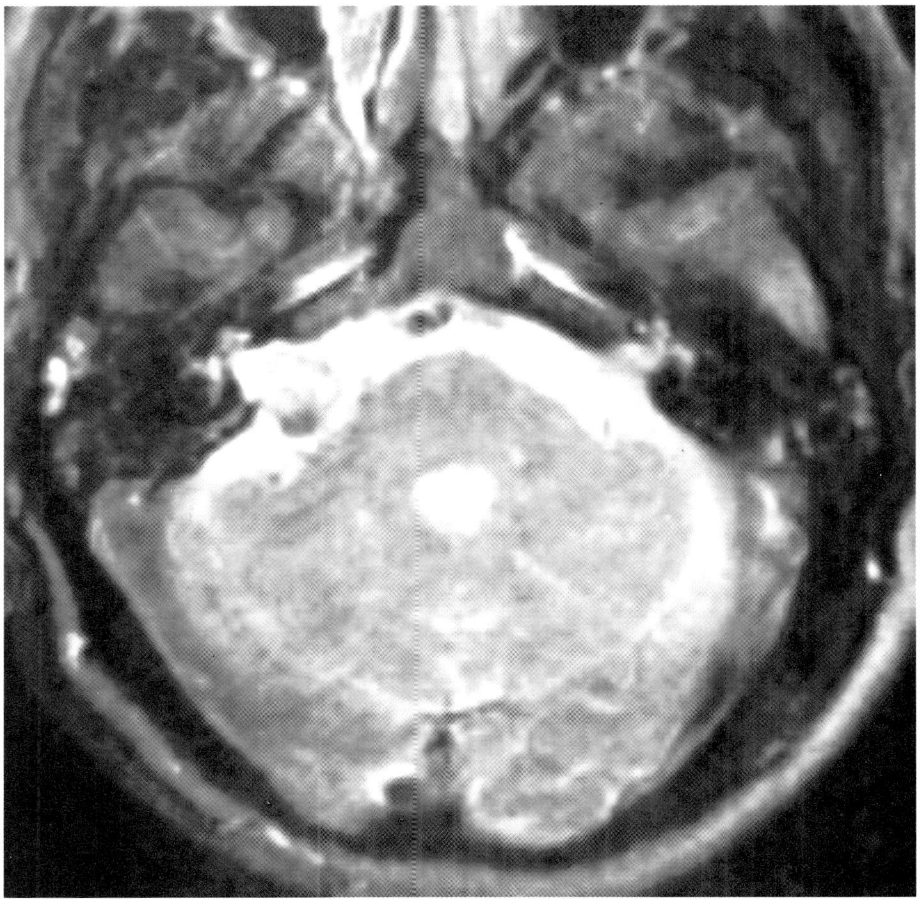

A

B

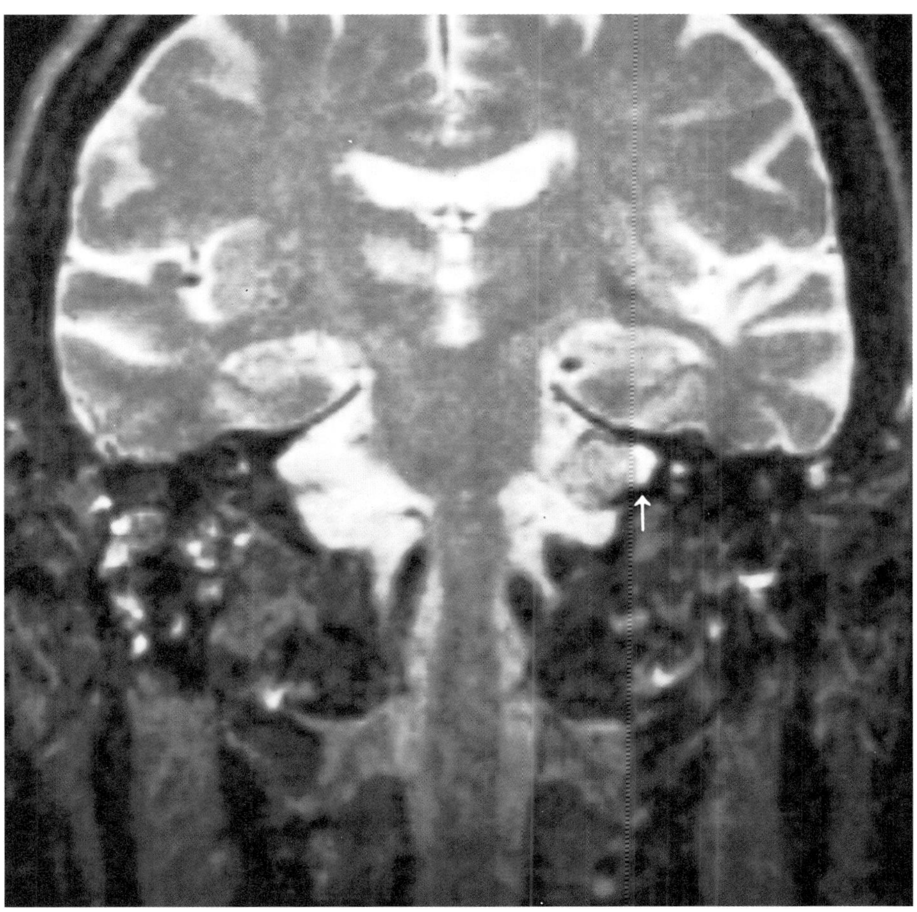

Fig. 1. *Left acoustic neurinoma* 80-year-old man with left deafness. For this symptom, he underwent CT scan, which showed a tumor of the cerebellopontine angle. A – T_2-weighted axial sequence. Given the width of the cisternal areas (atrophy), the neurinoma (1.5 cm diameter) does not cause brainstem compression. Its signal intensity is inhomogeneous. The coronal scan (B) better visualizes the considerable enlargement of the internal acoustic meatus and the spread of the neurinoma. The tumor does not involve the lateral portion of the acoustic canal, which is occupied by CSF (↑).

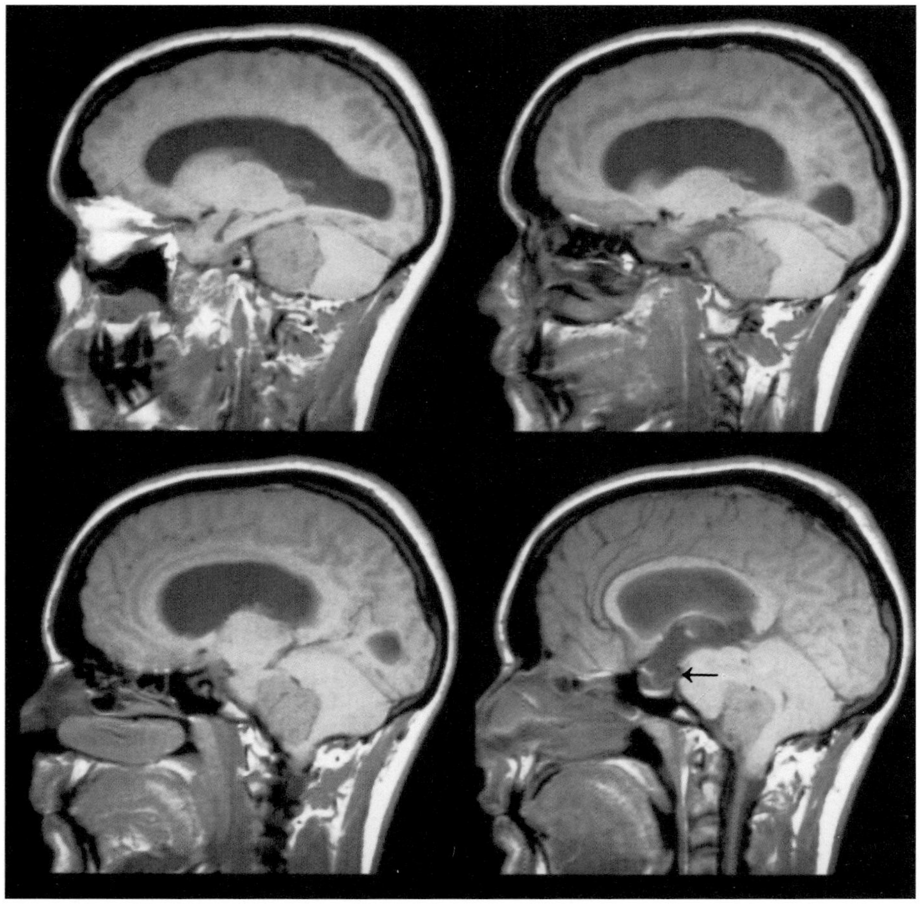

A

B

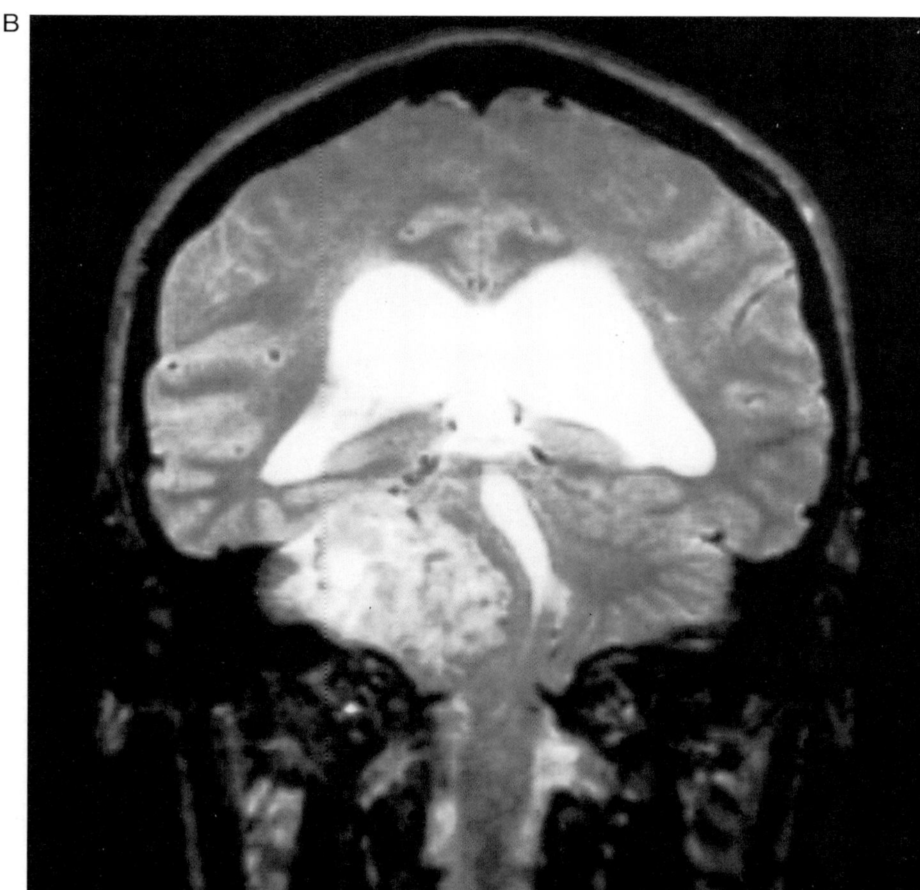

Fig. 2. *Right acoustic neurinoma*. 22-year-old woman with severe chronic intracranial hypertension. Plain films of the skull had shown all the signs of intracranial hypertension. A – TR 550 msec, TE 15 msec, sagittal scan. Observe the triventricular hydrocephalus secondary to the space-occupying lesion in the left cerebellopontine angle. The mass is hypointense with respect to the compressed and displaced cerebellar tissue. Note the third ventricle dilatation, causing secondary empty sella (←). B – TR 2,500 msec, TE 90 msec, coronal scan. The lesion has a high and inhomogeneous signal. Note the contralateral displacement of the fourth ventricle and of the aqueduct, dilated cranially to the obstruction.

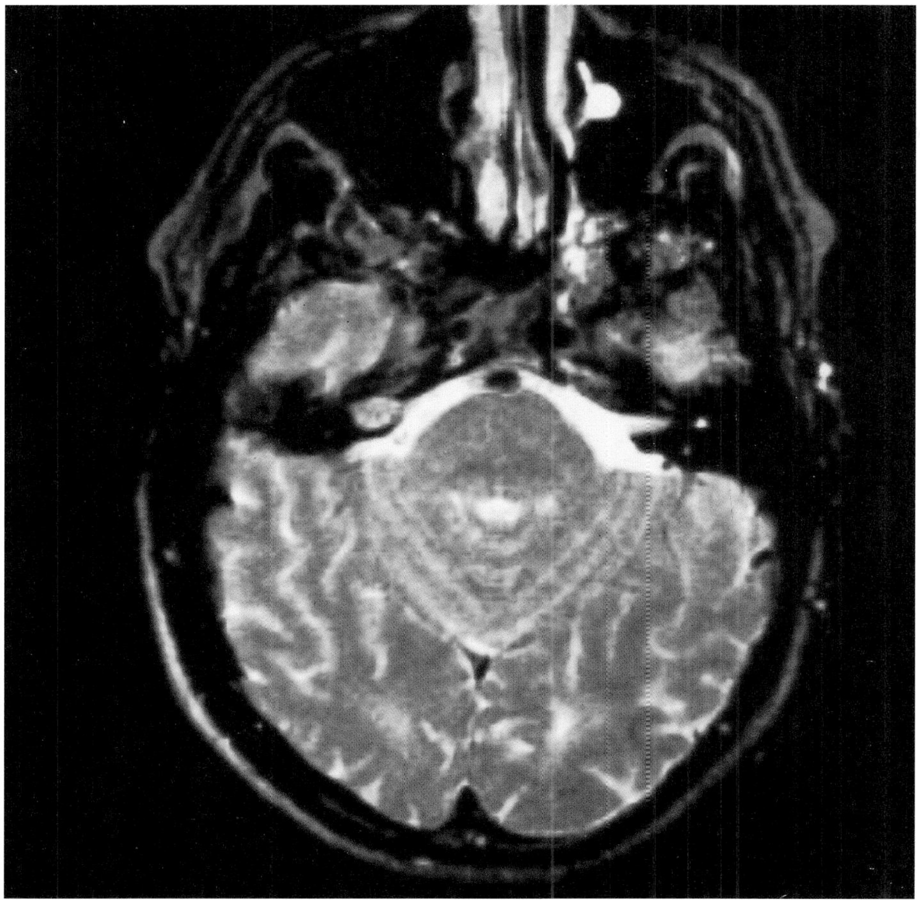

A

B

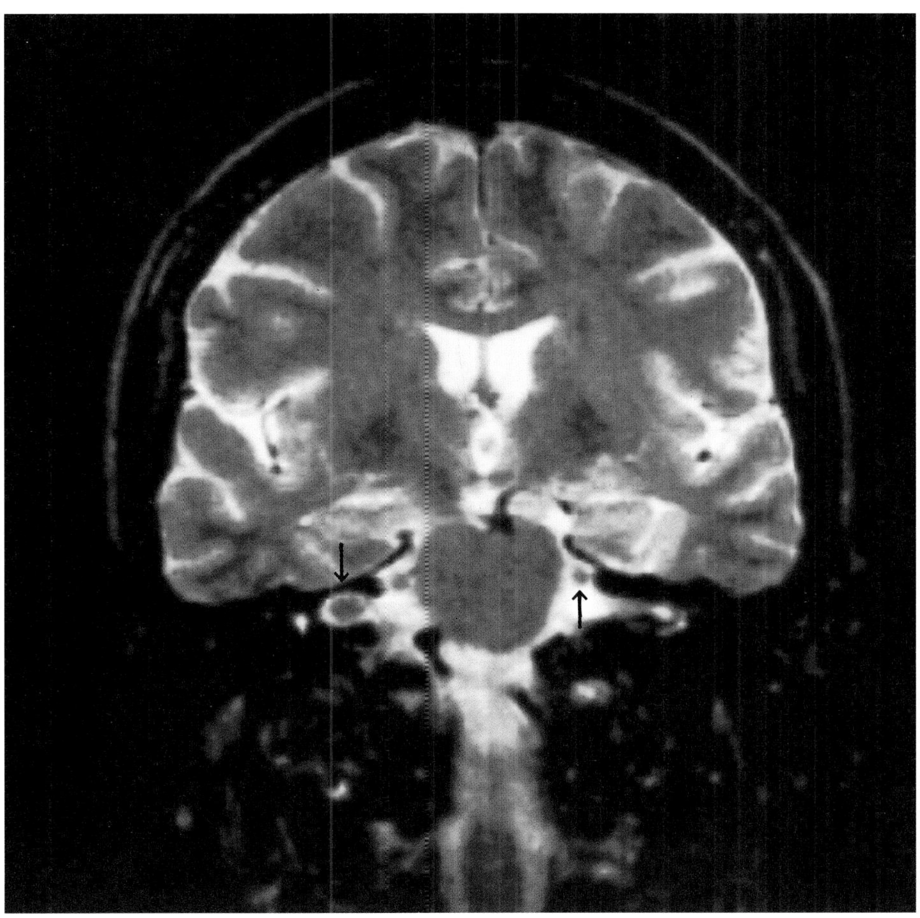

Fig. 3. *Right intracanalar neurinoma*. 45-year-old man with tinnitus and initial auditory loss. T_2-weighted sequence. A – axial scan, B – coronal scan. The intense "cisternographic effect" portrays an intracanalar neurinoma (↓), size 3 × 4 mm, and, bilaterally, the origin of the fifth cranial nerve (↑).

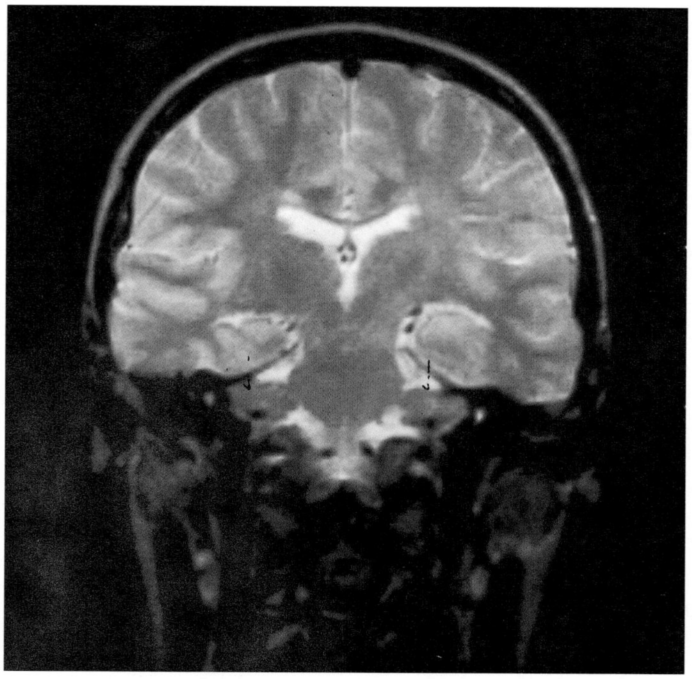

A

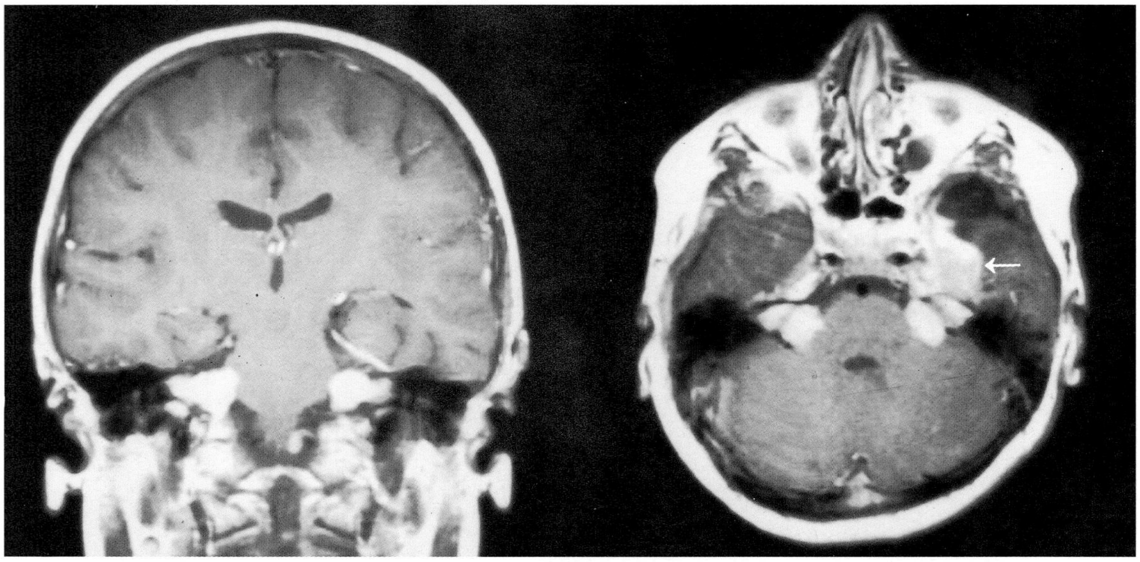

B

Fig. 4. *Recklinghausen's disease.* 12-year-old patient with neurofibromatosis, bilateral neurinomas of the eighth cranial nerve and partially resected meningioma of the internal third of the sphenoid wing (A). TR 2,500 msec, TE 90 msec, coronal view. The cerebellopontine cisterns are obliterated by the two neurinomas (max. diameter 2.5 cm). Note the typical dumbbell shape of the intracanalicular component of the tumor (↓). B – After i.v. GD-DTPA, TR 550 msec, TE 15 msec: high signal from the neurinomas with respect to standard MRI. The axial image shows the marked c.e. of the remnant meningioma (←). The tumor grows from the left anterior clinoid along the clinopetrosal ligament and the dura of the middle cranial fossa to the petrous bone. The low-signal focus of the temporal lobe is indicative of surgical sequelae.

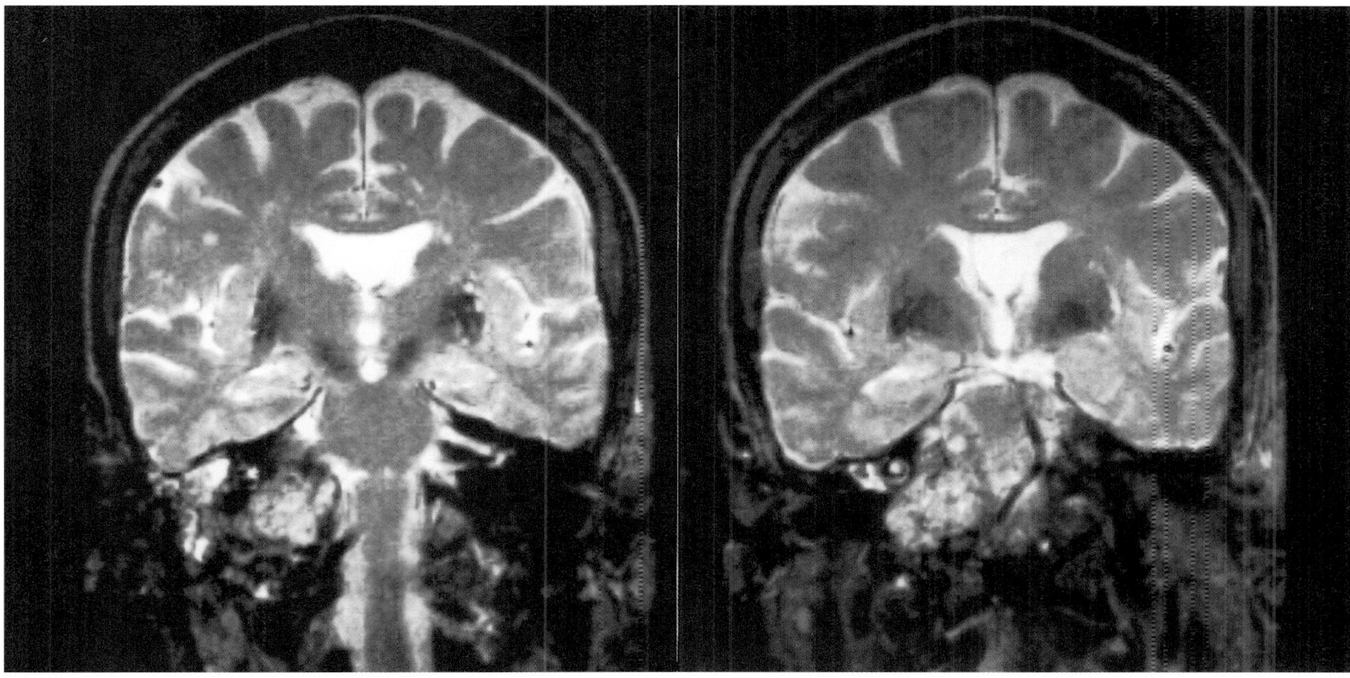

A

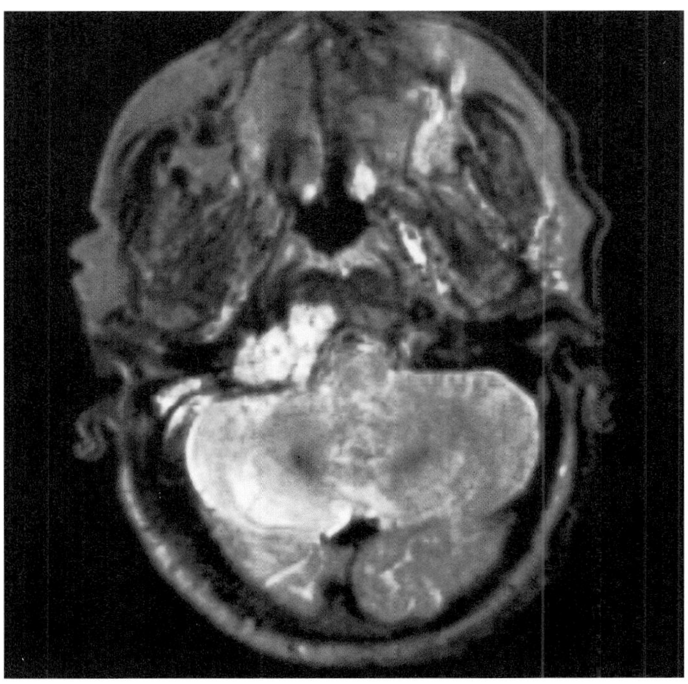

B

Fig. 5. *Right eleventh cranial nerve neurinoma.* 67-year-old woman with swallowing, phonation and gait disorders. The patient previously underwent diagnostic surgery via the suboccipital approach and a presumably eleventh cranial nerve neurinoma was partially removed. TR 2,500 msec, TE 90 msec, SE coronal (A) and axial (B) sequences. A huge, high-signal neoplasm occupies the posterior foramen lacerum, anteriorly to the brainstem, and extends caudally as far as the atlas and cranially as far as the petrous bone apex, mostly in an extradural location. The right cerebellar hemisphere shows the signs of the prior surgical procedure.

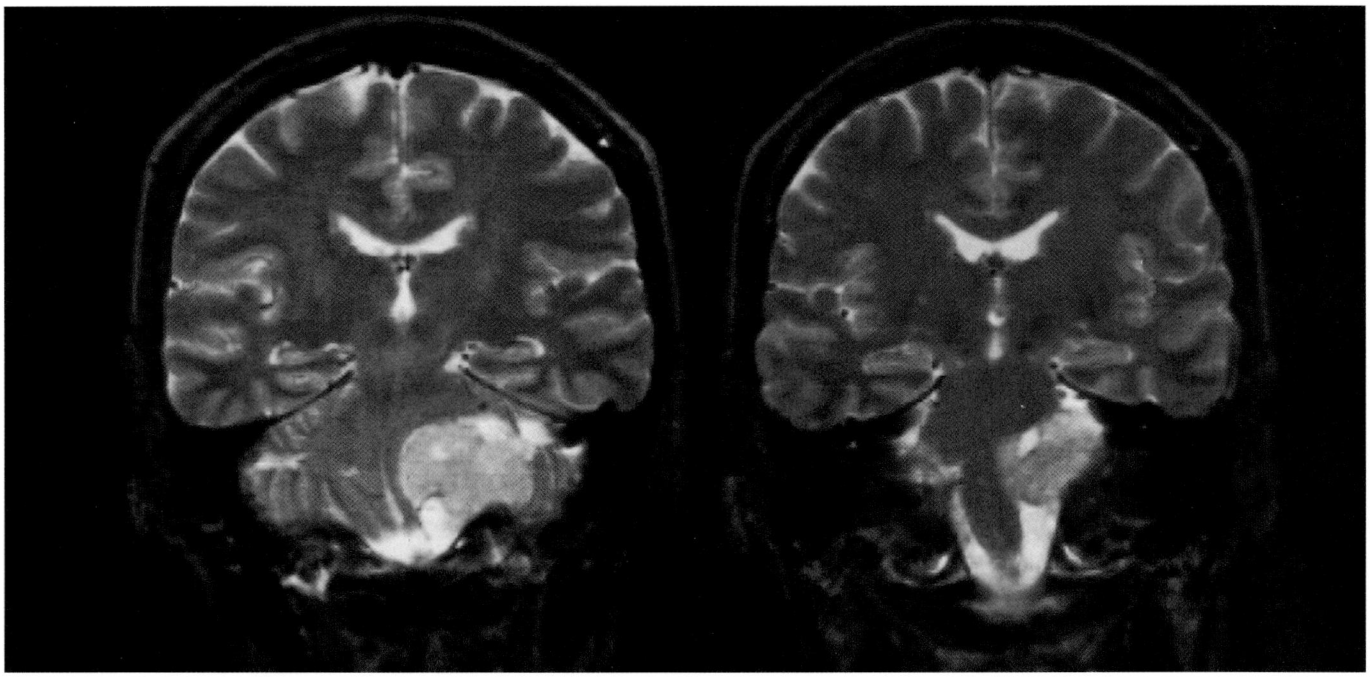

Fig. 6. *Left ninth cranial nerve neurinoma.* 61-year-old man with phonation and swallowing disturbances. The T_2-weighted coronal images show an extraaxial space occupying lesion in the left posterior cranial fossa. The tumor has intermediate-high intensity and cystic areas. It compresses the left cerebellar hemisphere and displaces the bulbopontine region contralaterally.

References

1. Bassi P, Piazza P, Cusmano F et al. (1990) MR cisternography of the cerebello-pontine angle and internal auditory canal in diagnosis of intracanalicular acoustic neuromas. Neuroradiology 31:486–491
2. Berry I, Brandt-Zawadzki M, Osaki L et al. (1986) Gd-DTPA in clinical MR of the brain. 2. Extraaxial lesions and normal structures. AJNR 7:789–793
3. Brant-Zawadski M, Badami JP, Mills CM et al. (1984) Primary intracranial tumor imaging A comparison of magnetic resonance and CT. Radiology 150:435–440
4. Breger RK, Paphe RA, Pojunas KW et al. (1987) Benign extraaxial tumors: contrast enhancement with Gd-DTPA. Radiology 163:427–429
5. Bronen RA, Sze G (1990) Magnetic resonance contrast agents: theory and application to the central nervous system. J Neurosurg 73:820–840
6. Curati WL, Graif M, Kingsley DPE et al. (1986) Acoustic neuromas: Gd-DTPA enhancement in MR imaging. Radiology 158:447–451
7. Felix R, Shorner W, Laniado M et al. (1985) Brain tumors: MR imaging with gadolinium-DTPA. Radiology 156:681–688
8. Flickinger JC, Lunsford LD, Coffey RJ et al. (1991) Radiosurgery of acoustic neuromas. Cancer 67:345–353
9. Gadian DG, Payne JA, Bryant DJ et al. (1985) Gadolinium-DTPA as a contrast agent in MR imaging: theoretical projections and practical observations. J Comput Assist Tomogr 9:242–251
10. Haughton VM, Rimm AA, Czervionke LF et al. (1988) Sensitivity of Gd-DTPA enhanced imaging of benign extraaxial tumors. Radiology 166:829–833
11. House JW, Waluch V, Jackler RK et al. (1986) Magnetic resonance imaging in acoustic neuroma diagnosis. Ann Otol Rhinol Laryngol 95:16–20
12. Jackler RK, Shapiro MS, Dillon WP et al. (1990) Gadolinium-DTPA enhanced magnetic resonance imaging in acoustic neuroma. Diagnosis and management. Otolaryngol Head Neck Surg 102:670–677
13. Litt AW, Kondo N, Bannon KR, Kricheff II (1990) Role of slice thickness in MR imaging of the internal auditory canal. J Comput Assist Tomogr 14:717–720
14. Loneragan R, Doust B, Fagan P et al. (1988) Magnetic Resonance Imaging evaluation of cerebellopontine angle tumours. Australas Radiol 33:47–55
15. Massengill R Jr, Johnstone W, Robbins J (1990) Diagnosis of acoustic neuroma by magnetic resonance imaging. J Tenn Med Assoc 83:124–126
16. Monsell EM, Rock JP (1990) Sensorineural hearing loss and the diagnosis of acoustic neuroma. Henry Ford Hosp Med J 38:9–12
17. Mulvinill JJ, Parry DM, Sherman JL et al. (1990) NIH Conference. Neurofibromatosis 1 (Recklinghausen disease) and Neurofibromatosis 2 (bilateral acoustic neurofibromatosis). An update. Ann Intern Med 113:39–52
18. Parizel PM, Degryse HL, Gheuens J et al. (1989) Gadolinium-DTPA enhanced MR imaging of intracranial lesions. Comput Assist Tomogr 13:378–385
19. Pomeranz SJ (1989) Posterior fossa, skull base, craniocervical junction. In: Pomeranz SJ (ed) Craniospinal Magnetic Resonance Imaging. W. B. Saunders Co, Philadelphia, 248–274
20. Sidman JD, Carrasco VN, Whaley RA, Pillsbury HC (1989) Gadolinium. The new gold standard for diagnosing cerebellopontine angle tumors. Arch Otolaryngol Head Neck Surg 115:1244–1247
21. Stack JP, Ramsden RT, Antoms NM et al. (1988) Magnetic resonance imaging of acoustic neuromas: The role of gadolium-DTPA. Br J Radiol 61:800–805
22. To SY, Lufkin RB, Rand R et al. (1990) Volume growth rate of acoustic neuromas on MRI post-stereotactic radiosurgery. Comput Med Imaging Graph 14:53–59
23. Waluch V, Dyck P (1990) Magnetic resonance imaging of posterior fossa masses. In: Wilkins RH, Rengachary SS (eds) Neurosurgery Update I. McGraw-Hill, New York, 30–46

CHAPTER VIII

Pituitary adenomas and craniopharyngiomas

Pituitary adenomas (p.a.) are benign epithelial tumors which originate from the cells of the adenohypophysis. They should be classified on the basis of the hormone that they release and of the clinical syndrome that they induce: prolactin (PRL)-secreting, growth hormone (GH)-secreting, adrenocorticotropin (ACTH)-secreting, which give rise to amenorrhea-galactorrhea, acromegaly and to Cushings's syndrome, respectively. Very rare pituitary tumors produce thyroid-stimulating hormone (TSH) and gonadotropins (FSH and LH). Furthermore, there are mixed adenomas, generally PRL- and GH-secreting, and nonfunctioning p.a.

Anatomically, their classification is based on size and growth direction: microadenoma (diameter <1 cm), intrasellar, suprasellar, supra-laterosellar and invasive p.a. The invasive types tend to disrupt the bone and to infiltrate the cavernous sinuses, even if they are histologically benign and different from the rare primary pituitary adenocarcinomas.

Microadenomas occupy a single part of the pituitary gland and their position reflects the normal topology of adenohypophyseal cells: PRL- and GH-secreting p.a. are generally lateral *(Figs. 1, 2, 3)*, whereas ACTH-releasing ones are anterior *(Fig. 5)*. Macroadenomas displace the cavernous sinuses and the I.C.A.s laterally *(Figs. 9, 10)*; when they occupy the suprasellar cistern, they displace the chiasm and the A.C.A.s upwards *(Fig. 8)*. Giant p.a. occupy the third ventricle and may cause obstructive hydrocephalus *(Fig. 12)*.

Frequently, p.a. undergo regressive and/or hemorrhagic events, taking the appearance of cystic lesions. Therefore, they should be differentiated from the "empty sella", which often simulates a nonfunctioning p.a. *(Fig. 6)* clinically and radiologically. The association of both these diseases is not an uncommon finding *(Fig. 7)*.

Women in fertile age almost exclusively have microadenomas: any event, which modifies the pituitary anatomy and which causes a disorder of the portal venous flow between the hypothalamus and the pituitary at the stalk level, also increases PRL release and impacts the menstrual cycle. This is the symptom which allows early diagnosis of these tumors. PRL release is under the inhibitory control of the hypothalamus which, by releasing dopaminergic amines, inhibits PRL synthesis. If the transport mechanism of inhibitors is altered, PRL secretion increases. Therefore, plasma assays show PRL increase even in non-PRL-secreting adenomas; in these cases, however, PRL levels generally remain below 100 ng/ml (normal values: 8–20). In PRL-secreting adenomas, instead, plasma PRL levels will exceed 100 ng/ml.

In males and in post-menopausal women, macroadenomas are more frequent, since their symptomatology is more silent *(Figs. 9, 10)*. They manifest themselves with a progressive panhypopituitary syndrome which is in part offset by the few functioning cells. Patients are thus diagnosed at a late stage and are generally referred to the specialist owing to visual disorders caused by chiasmatic compression.

In the study of p.a., MRI is currently the most sensitive modality to demonstrate small alterations. Additionally, it provides data on the anatomical relationship between the pituitary lesion and the surrounding structures: pituitary stalk, optic chiasm, carotid sinuses and parasellar cisterns. Diagnostic results are conditional upon an adequate technique for evaluating small-sized anatomical structures. As a consequence, use of high magnetic field (1–1.5 T) equipment is necessary. This equipment has a more favorable signal-to-noise ratio (SNR), affords maximum spatial and contrast resolution and allows contiguous thin sections (3 mm) to be obtained. The pituitary region is studied on coronal scans, which are more suitable for establishing morphological symmetry and size and for discriminating possible signal changes. Finally, sagittal scans provide an accurate and comprehensive anatomical picture of the sella, of the pituitary and of its stalk, of the optic chiasm, of carotid sinuses, of suprasellar cisterns and of the third ventricle. The axial projection is only occasionally used to derive further details on the relationship between the adenoma, the C.A.s and the cavernous sinuses *(Fig. 11)*.

The study is basically performed with T_1-weighted spin-echo sequences (short TRs and TEs), which offer the best anatomical details, highlighting microadenomas as foci of lower signal intensity vs. the normal glandular tissue *(Figs. 1, 4, 7)* and macroadenomas as iso- or hypointense formations vs. the cerebral tissue *(Figs. 8, 12)*. At times, microadenomas may be isointense with the pituitary gland and may be identified only through indirect signs, such as asymmetric protrusions on the gland profile, contralateral shift of the stalk or displacement of the carotid siphon *(Fig. 1)*. In these cases or on normal T_1-weighted images vs. a positive clinical picture for adenoma, the study should be supplemented with a coronal T_2-weighted scan, in order to evidence hyperintense areas which may point to a microadenoma *(Fig. 2)*. In macroadenomas, T_2-weighted SE sequences may be useful to demonstrate the presence of cystic or degenerating areas within them *(Figs. 9, 13)*, to better evaluate the extrasellar component or for a differential diagnosis with respect to other diseases of the region (meningiomas).

The use of GD-DTPA in p.a. diagnostics is quite recent and its diagnostic role was validated by multiple observations. In our experience, on images after perfusion with GD-DTPA, the contrast between the gland and the microadenoma may increase significantly. Microadenomas may appear as lower signal areas *(Fig. 4)* or as more perfused areas *(Fig. 3)*, depending on the extent of the vascular neoformation of the tumor. In macroadenomas, GD-DTPA may allow the identification of the residual pituitary tissue that enhances more than the adenoma *(Figs. 9, 10)*.

GD-DTPA is more indicated in the study of invasive macroadenomas before surgery, to better evaluate their relations with the cavernous sinuses and the C.A.s, and for follow-up after surgical and/or radiation therapy. For the sake of completeness, there are reports of p.a. which develop a hyperintense signal on T_1-weighted images, expressing a hemorrhagic event inside the neoplasm. Paramagnetic contrast media are an obvious option for the differential diagnosis between p.a. and meningiomas of the sellar region. The latter tumors have very intense perfusion, unlike p.a. whose signal enhancement is moderate.

The treatment of choice is surgery. The procedure may be very simple for intrasellar p.a., which are reached via the transrhinosphenoidal approach. Larger p.a., especially if they have a laterosellar extension, require the subfrontal or frontotemporal transcranial approach. This procedure is undoubtedly challenging but allows the entire neoplasm-affected region to be dominated. Occasionally, a partial resection of giant p.a. through the transrhinosphenoidal approach may be useful; the resection should be followed by a cycle of radiation therapy to which they are usually very sensitive. If the neoplasm is soft and diffluent, as is often the case, most of the tumor can be excised with a low-risk procedure. This fact can easily be predicted with an MRI examination.

PRL-secreting adenomas may also be successfully treated with bromocryptine. This dopaminergic agent inhibits prolactin overproduction by neoplastic cells and blocks their growth, at least during its administration. Very recently, also GH-producing tumors were treated with somatostatin, which selectively inhibits GH-producing cells. Many studies are ongoing to evaluate its definite clinical efficacy.

Craniopharyngiomas (c.) are epithelial tumors originating from the remnants of Rathke's pouch of the fetal pharynx, from which the adenohypophysis grows. These are nonfunctioning tumors which are located on the midline in sellar and/or suprasellar sites and which may reach considerable sizes. They are often cystic and their fluid is laden with products of epithelial exfoliation and with cholesterin crystals. In mixed-structure craniopharyngiomas, the cyst wall and the solid components, which are occasionally dominant, are laden with keratoid material which tends to calcify. This heterogeneity in tumoral components translates into evident signal inhomogeneities on MR images *(Fig. 16)*. The cystic formations with high cholesterin content have a pathognomonic behavior: they show high signal intensity *(Figs. 14, 16)* on T_1-weighted sequences, which is further enhanced on highly T_2-weighted sequences. However, cystic components can be observed in c. which have a more or less low signal intensity on T_1-weighted sequences, depending on the viscosity of the fluid, and a high signal only on T_2 sequences *(Fig. 19)*. Inside the solid components of the neoplasm imaged with T_2 sequences, inhomogeneities can be found which are due to calcifications (low signal intensity), keratoid material *(Fig. 18)* or degeneration areas *(Fig. 17)*. Calcifications are typical of this disease and can easily be demonstrated by conventional radiology and CT: however, especially when they are small-sized, they may be difficult to identify via MRI. This diagnostic limitation is widely offset by the greater detail which MRI provides on anatomical relations between the neoplasm and the neighboring structures.

GD-DTPA may enhance the walls in cystic c. *(Fig. 15)* as well as the fleshy solid components.

Clinically, c. present with visual impairment (e.g. bitemporal hemianopsia as in p.a.) and with signs of pituitary hypofunction. Diabetes insipidus is frequent, denoting important damage of the pituitary stalk and of the posterior lobe of the pituitary and/or of the hypothalamus. Unlike p.a., albeit large-sized, diabetes insipidus is a frequent finding in c.

During their growth, c. strongly adhere to the surrounding tissues, in particular to the chiasm, the hypothalamus and the cavernous sinuses. Therefore, their resection may be difficult and risky. Sometimes, they grow posteriorly until they obliterate the interpeduncular cistern and establish relations with the anterior aspect of the brainstem and the B.A., from which they are however separated by an arachnoid membrane.

The planning of their excision calls for a careful analysis of the relations between the tumor and the above-mentioned structures. The surgical approach will be subfrontal, frontotemporal or trans-callosal, depending on the location of the tumor with respect to the chiasm and to the third ventricle. As occurs with p.a., also the exclusively intrasellar c. can be removed via the transrhinosphenoidal approach *(Fig. 15)*.

Another therapeutical option for cystic c. is stereotactic puncture and drainage of the cystic component with an extrathecal "reservoir" *(Fig. 18)*. This is a low-risk procedure which may give good results, especially if it is combined with periodical intracavitary administration of bleomycin *(Fig. 19)* and should be considered for some adults and/or in very compromised patients. In adults, the solid component has a slow growth rate and the clinical syndrome is mostly ascribable to the presence of the cyst.

A rare lesion, similar to the c. but without proliferative potential, is the cyst of Ratkhe's pouch. It has a sellar *(Fig. 20)* or suprasellar location. It consists of a wall of monolayered cubic epithelium and has a whitish jelly-like content which justifies its high signal intensity on T_1-weighted images. Clinically, the lesion gives scarce symptoms and may be an occasional finding. However, it may cause diabetes insipidus. The surgical procedure is easy, because the cyst is well resectable and its marsupialization may be sufficient.

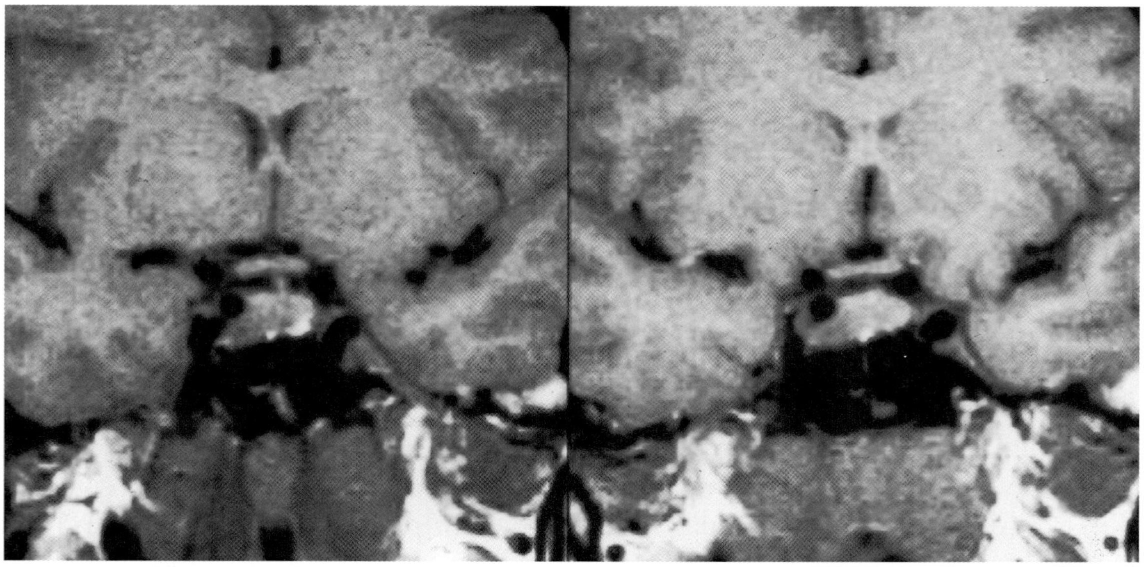

Fig. 1. *PRL-secreting microadenoma.* 23-year-old woman with secondary amenorrhea and hyperprolactinemia (190 ng/ml). SE (TR = 550 msec, TE = 15 msec) coronal scan with 3 mm-thick slices: hypointensity of the right half of the pituitary, extending below the cavernous sinus and elevating the intracavernous portion of the I.C.A. Observe the mass effect on the pituitary stalk, which is displaced contralaterally.

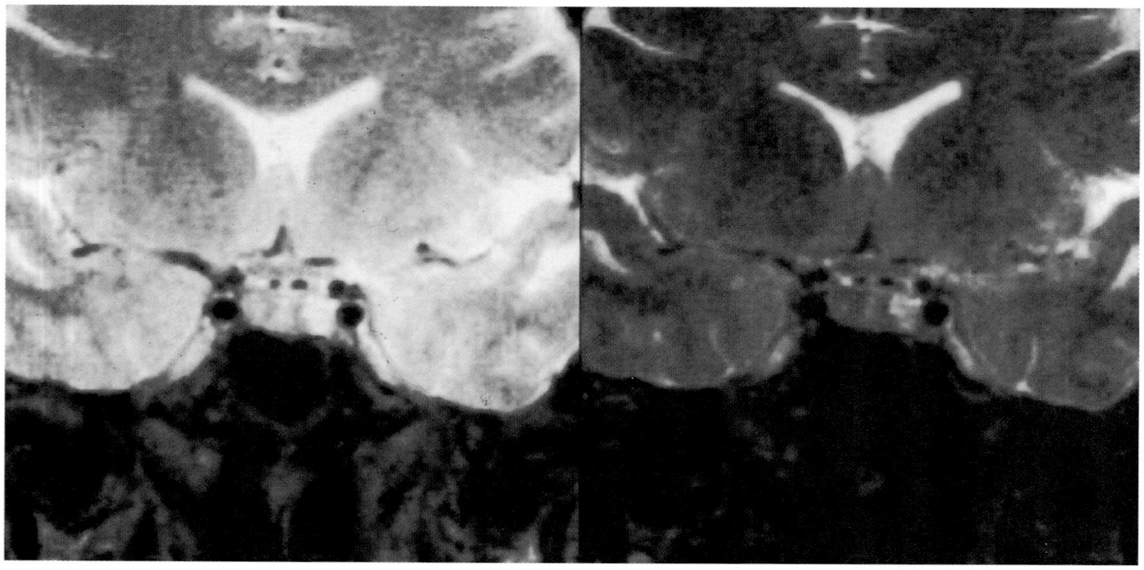

Fig. 2. *PRL-secreting microadenoma.* Multi-echo SE images (TR = 2,550 msec, TE = 30–60–120–160 msec). The late echoes enhance the signal from the microadenoma due to its high protein content.

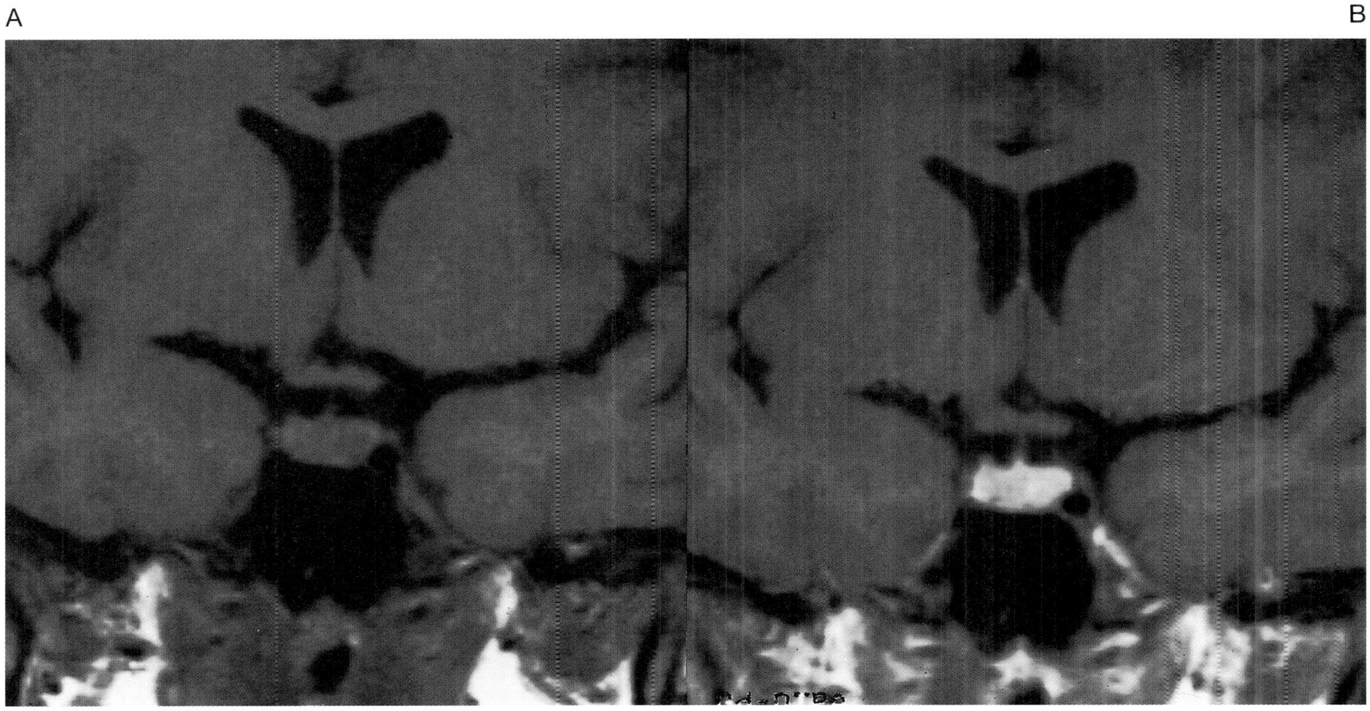

Fig. 3. *PRL-secreting microadenoma.* A – T_1-weighted SE sequences visualizing the adenoma in the left half of the pituitary as a focus of lower signal vs. the remaining part of the gland. B – Same section and sequence after i.v. GD-DTPA: the microadenoma enhances vs. the normal pituitary owing to hypervascularization.

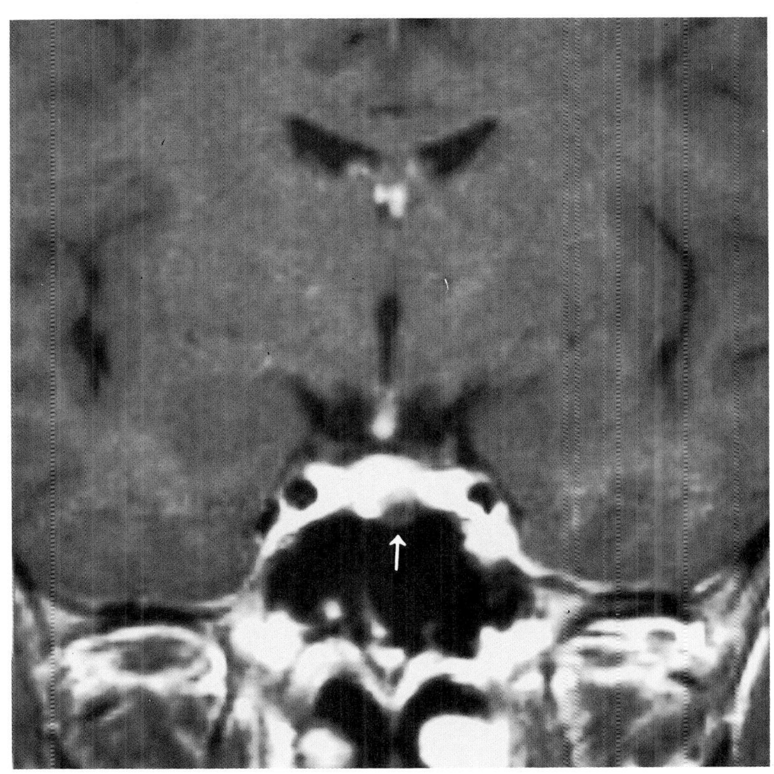

Fig. 4. *Non-secreting pituitary adenoma.* 27-year-old woman with prior amenorrhea. T_1-weighted image after GD-DTPA: coronal scan. Observe the signal enhancement of the pituitary, whereas the microadenoma (located on the left lower margin of the pituitary) remains markedly hypointense (↑).

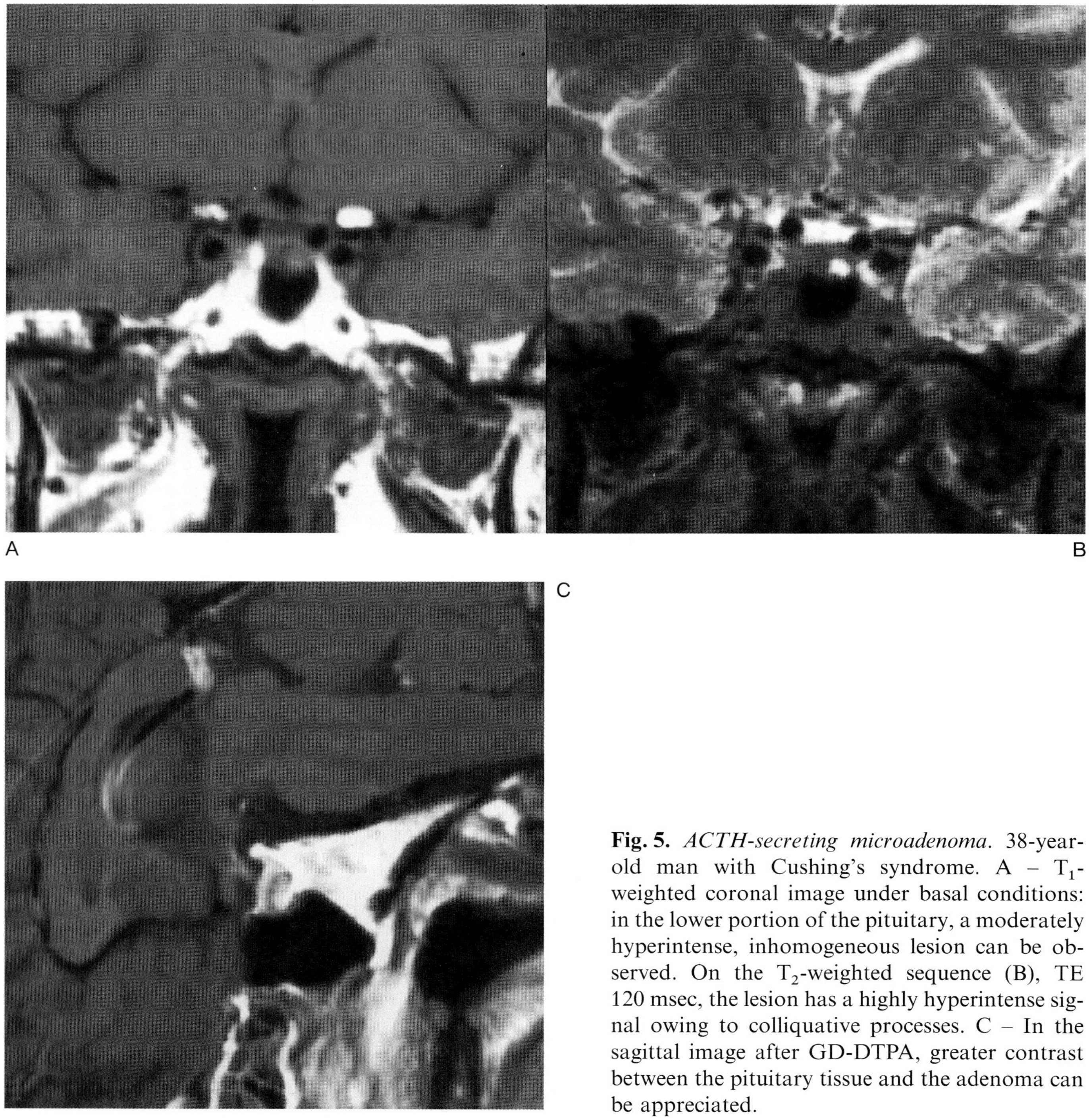

Fig. 5. *ACTH-secreting microadenoma.* 38-year-old man with Cushing's syndrome. A – T_1-weighted coronal image under basal conditions: in the lower portion of the pituitary, a moderately hyperintense, inhomogeneous lesion can be observed. On the T_2-weighted sequence (B), TE 120 msec, the lesion has a highly hyperintense signal owing to colliquative processes. C – In the sagittal image after GD-DTPA, greater contrast between the pituitary tissue and the adenoma can be appreciated.

Fig. 6. *Primary empty sella.* 42-year-old woman with amenorrhea, galactorrhea and moderate rise in prolactinemia. T_1-weighted images (A – sagittal; B – coronal): enlargement of the sellar cavity, whose content has a CSF-like signal in continuity with the suprasellar cistern. The pituitary stalk is displaced backwards, flattened downwards and the gland is deformed and compressed on the sellar floor. In B, note the chiasm and the optic nerves (↙), the intra- and supracavernous I.C.A.s, the A.C.A.s and the anterior clinoids, which are hyperintense owing to bone marrow (⇑).

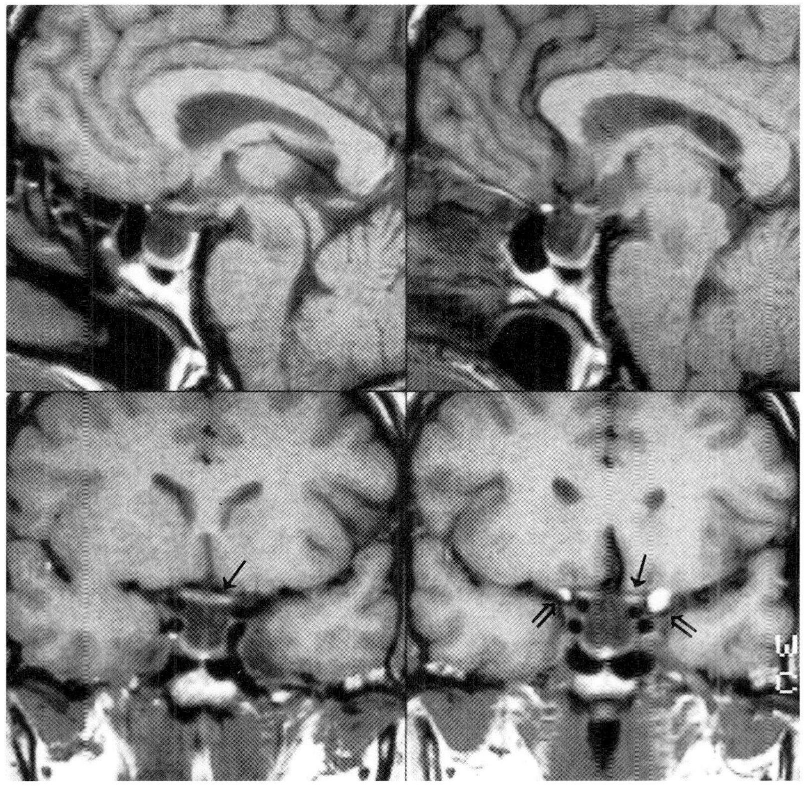

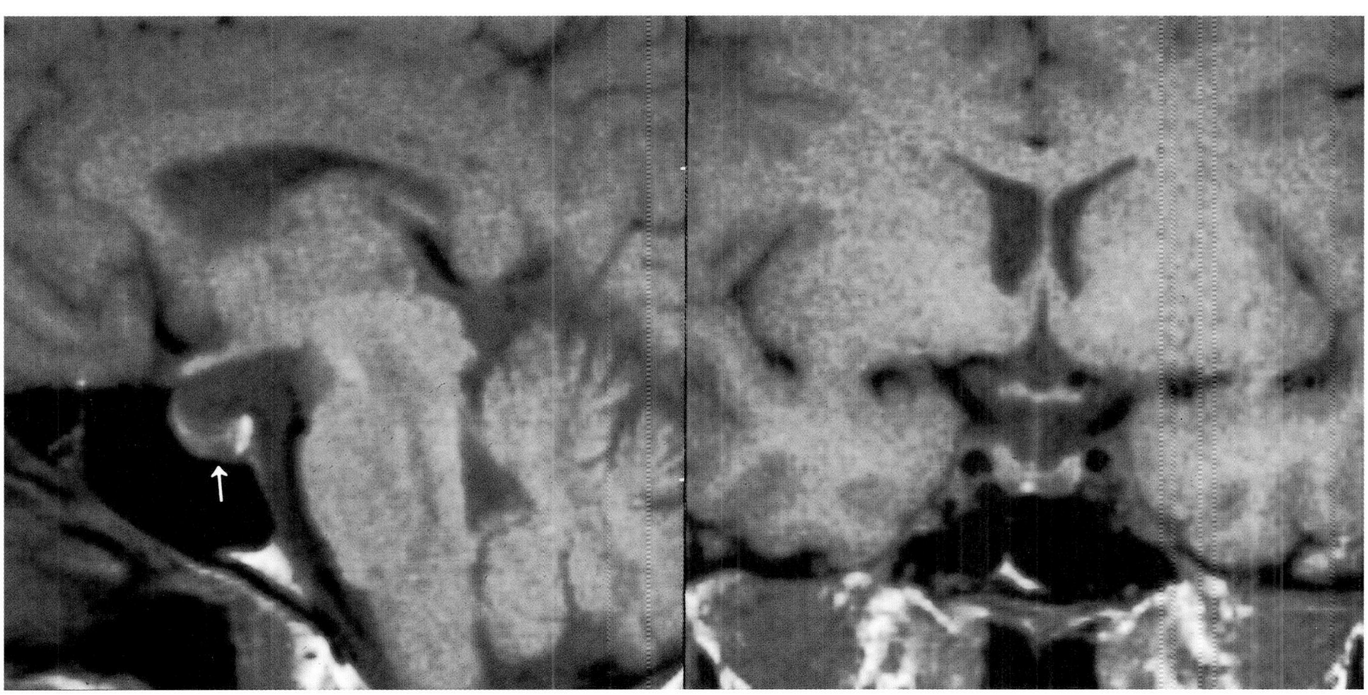

Fig. 7. *Non-secreting microadenoma and empty sella.* T_1-weighted sagittal and coronal scans. 4-mm diameter microadenoma (↑) in the left half of the pituitary. Note the mild empty sella.

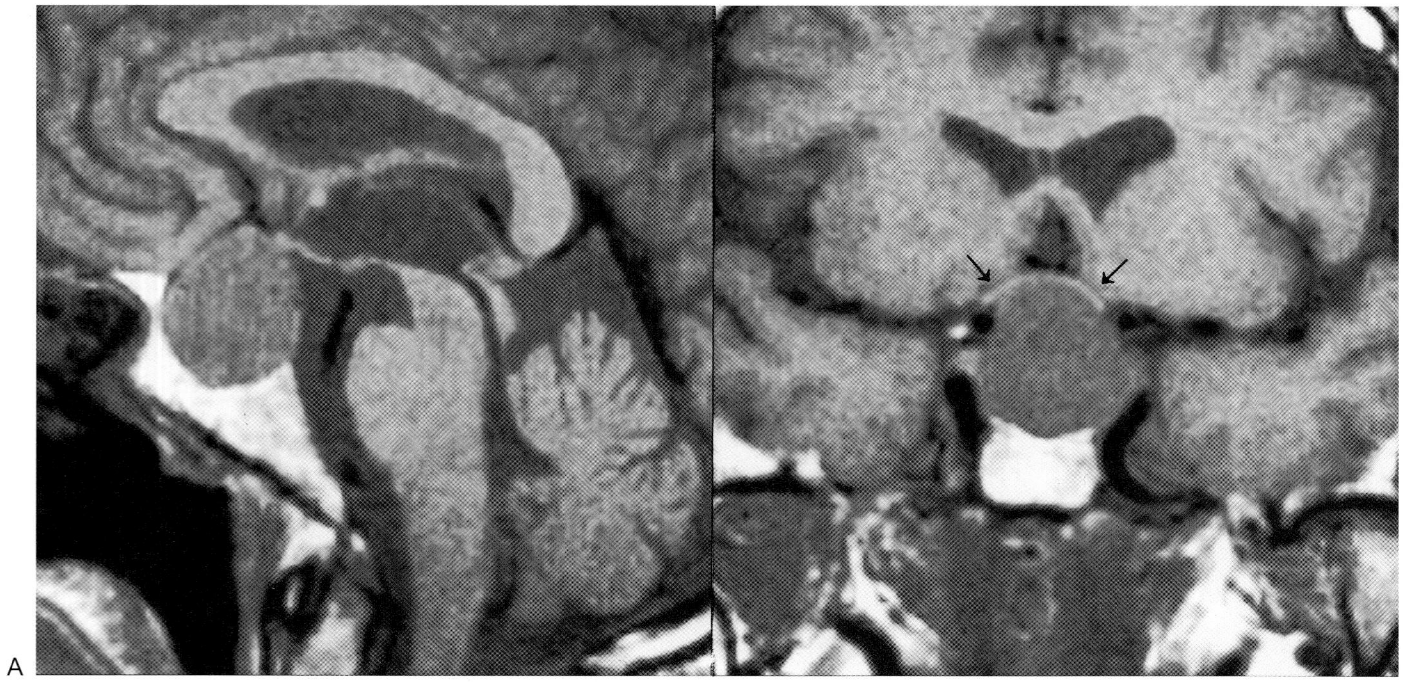

Fig. 8. *PRL-secreting macroadenoma.* 53-year-old man with bitemporal hemianopsia, impotence, loss of libido, asthenia and prolactinemia values of 500 ng/ml. T_1-weighted sagittal (A) and coronal (B) sections. The sella turcica is very wide and the neoplasm occupies the suprasellar cistern, amputating the anterior aspect of the third ventricle. The chiasm (↙) is uplifted and flattened with a lower concavity. The intracavernous and supraclinoid portions of the I.C.A. are lateralized. The neoplasm is homogeneous and isointense with the cerebral tissue.

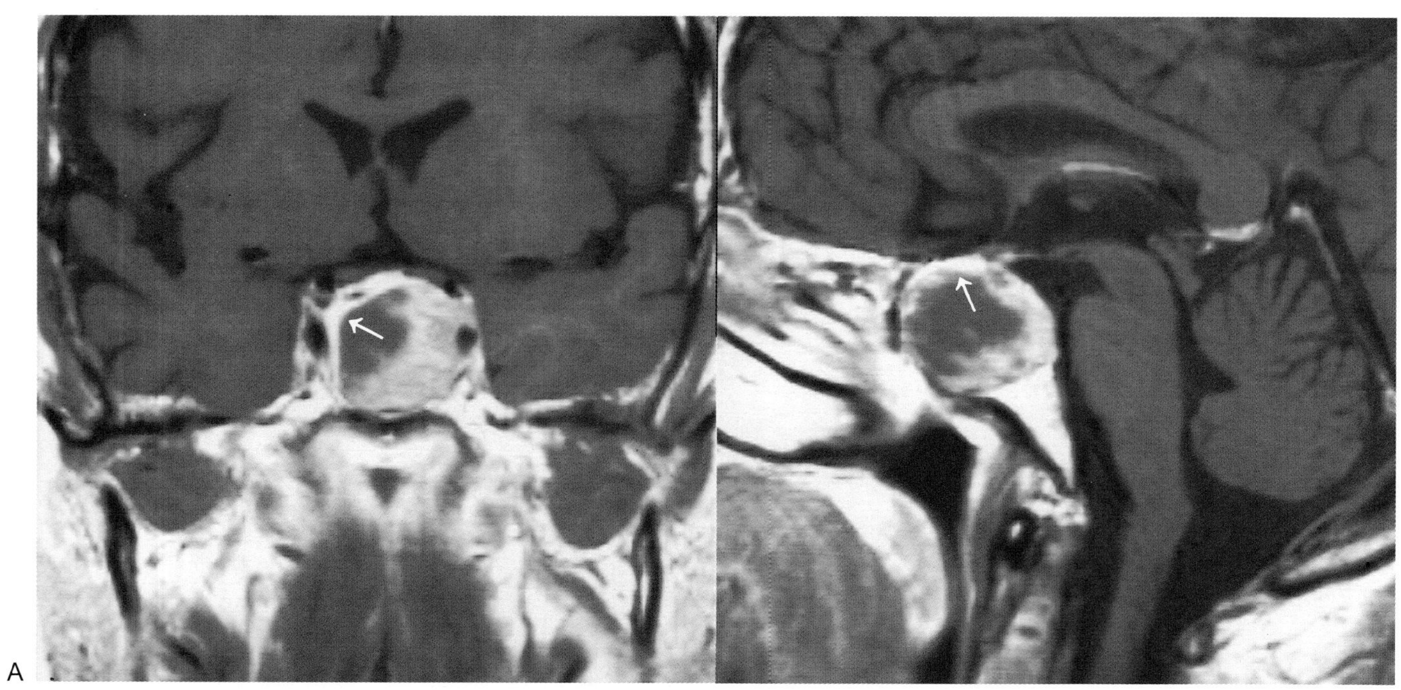

Fig. 9. *PRL-secreting macroadenoma.* 52-year-old man with predominantly left-sided bitemporal hemianopsia and impotence. T_1-weighted coronal (A) and sagittal (B) views after GD-DTPA. The GD-DTPA enhancement shows an inhomogeneous adenoma with a necrotic focus and a solid component which infiltrates the left cavernous sinus. On the right side, the adenoma is separated from the cavernous sinus by a highly hyperintense rim, representing the compressed and displaced pituitary tissue (↖).

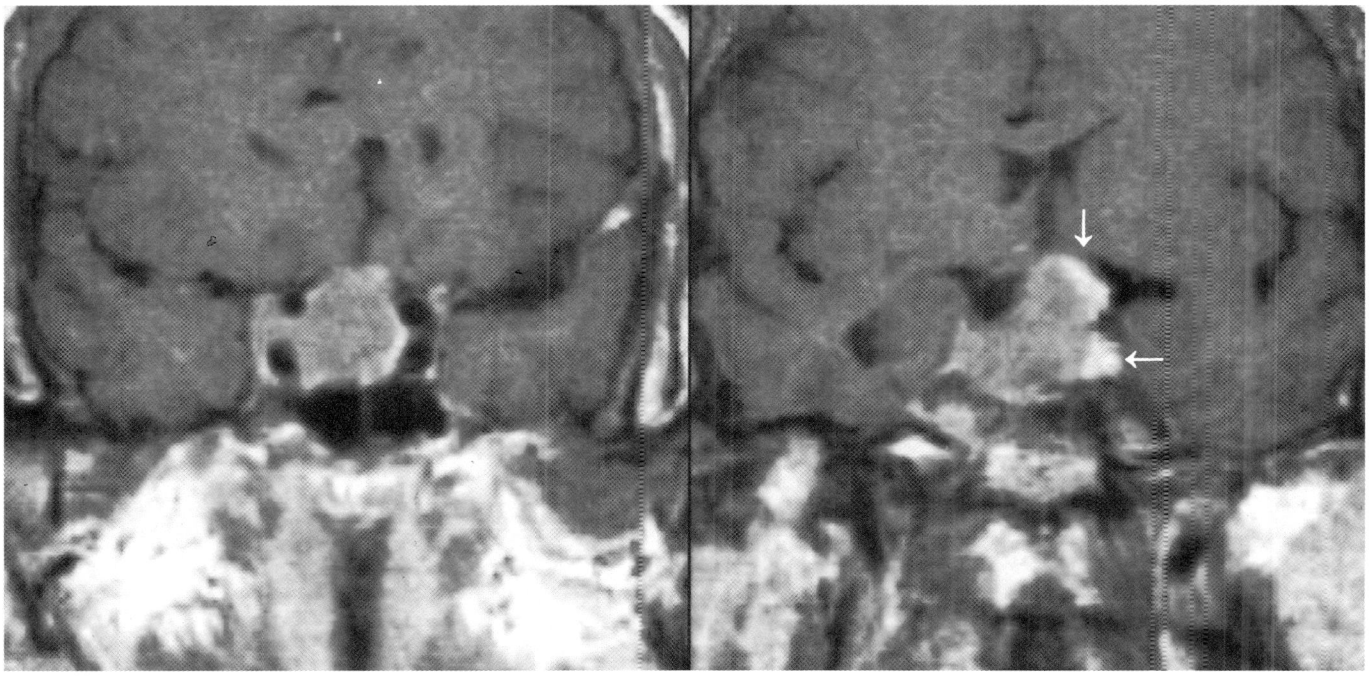

Fig. 10. *GH-secreting macroadenoma.* 52-year-old woman with acromegaly. T_1-weighted coronal views after GD-DTPA. The tumor predominantly occupies the supra- and laterosellar right side, encasing the C.A. in its intracavernous and supraclinoid portion. On the left side, it displaces the vessels without infiltrating them. The marked c.e. of the pituitary healthy tissue is shown (←).

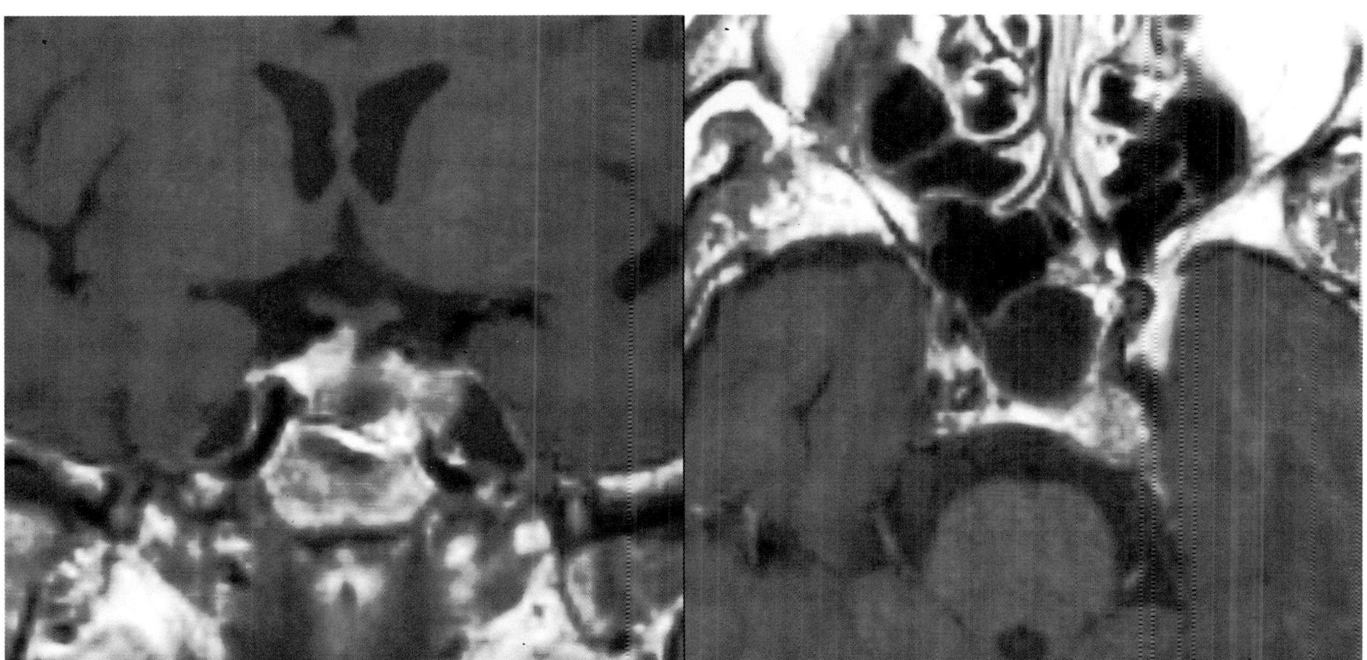

A B

Fig. 11. *Remnants of GH-secreting macroadenoma* 61-year-old man operated on and irradiated twenty years before these images. T_1-weighted coronal (A) and axial (B) scans after GD-DTPA: observe the post-surgical empty sella and the highly enhancing left parasellar tissue. The tumor grows along the clinopetrosal dural planes and partially involves Meckel's cave.

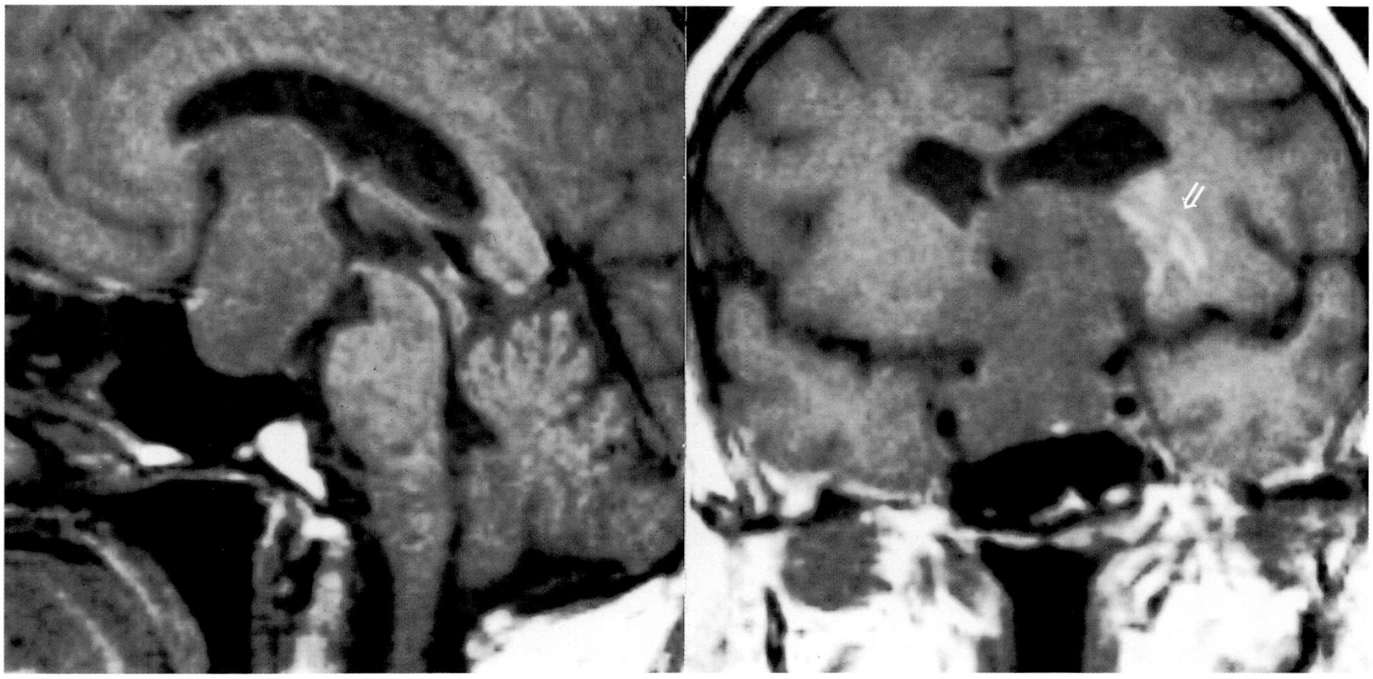

A B

C

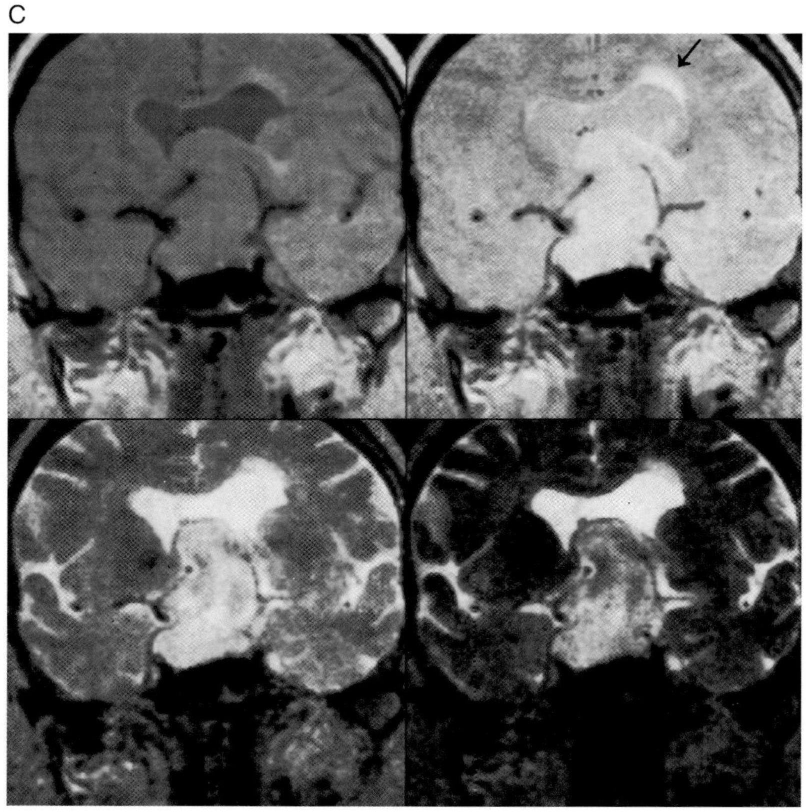

Fig. 12. *Non-secreting giant adenoma.* 62-year-old woman with severe ideomotor disorders, moderately severe mixed aphasia, severe visual impairment. T_1-weighted images. A – sagittal image: the tumor occupies the third ventricle completely and indents the lateral ventricles. B – coronal image: distension of the left lateral ventricle owing to obstruction of Monro's foramen with contralateral displacement of the septum pellucidum and damage of the left basal ganglia owing to direct compression (⇓). C – The multi-echo sequence depicts a fairly homogeneous neoplasm and the periventricular interstitial edema (↙) secondary to transependymal CSF reabsorption, typical of obstructive hydrocephalus. The relationships between the neoplasm and the vessels are well visualized.

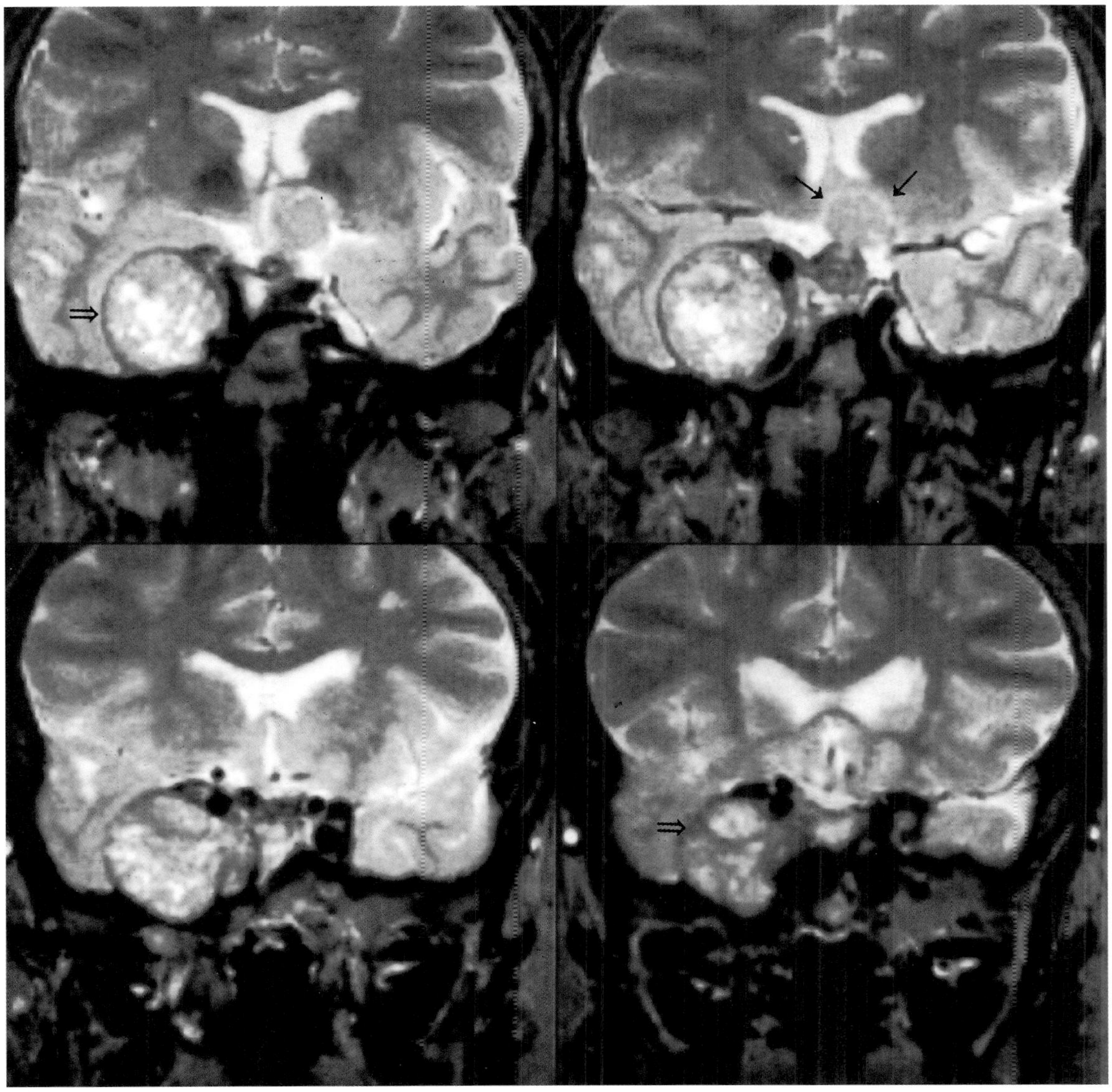

Fig. 13. *Dumbbell recurrence of intra- and extradural non-secreting macroadenoma.* 18-year-old young woman, operated on 3 years earlier owing to severe drop in visual acuity. 3 mm-thick, T_2-weighted coronal sections: iso-intense, homogeneous, small supra-retrosellar mass (↘) and larger, right temporal mass with inhomogeneous structure, necrotic and cystic high-signal foci (⇒). The latter lesion penetrates the right cavernous sinus, uplifts and medializes the I.C.A. and spreads extradurally. The temporobasal dura mater produces the low-signal rim (⇒) which surrounds the lesion.

A

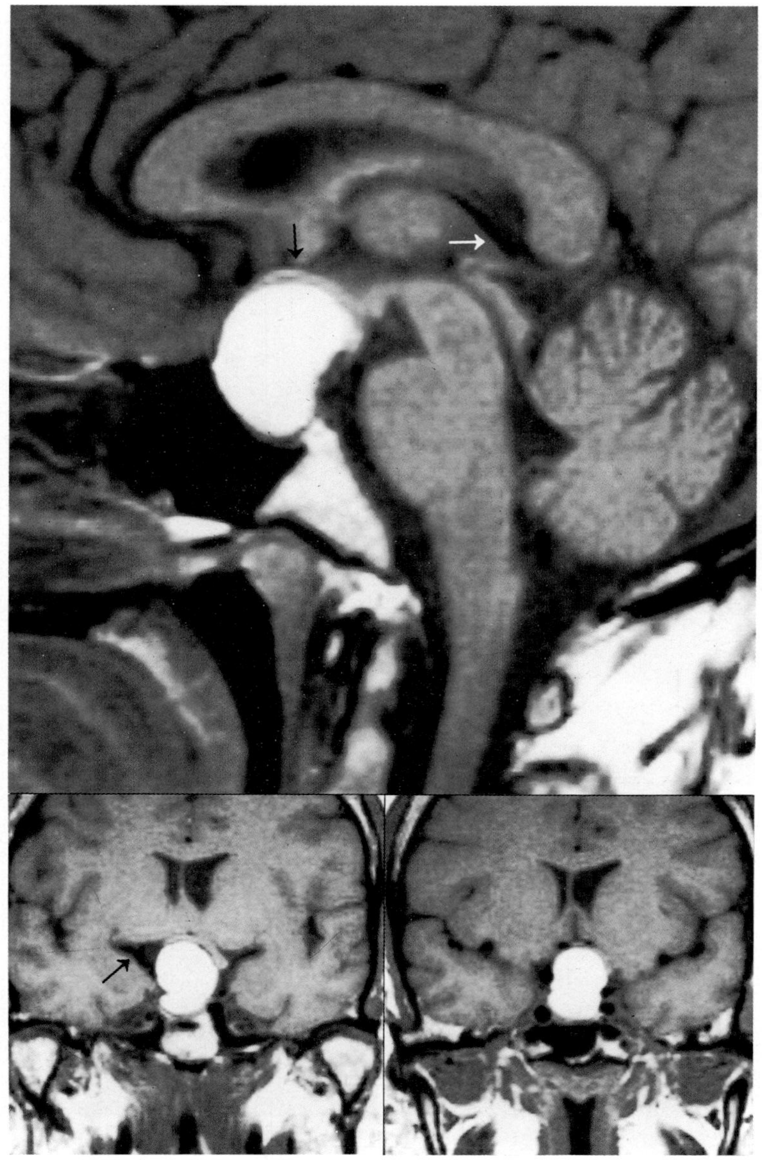

B

Fig. 14. *Intra- and suprasellar cystic craniopharyngioma.* 48-year-old woman with bitemporal hemianopsia. A – T_1-weighted sagittal scan: ovoid lesion with fat-like high signal; the lesion is due to a cholesterin-laden cyst. The anterior aspect of the third ventricle and the chiasm are uplifted (↓). The signal void (→) projecting along the roof of the third ventricle is the image of an internal cerebral vein. B – Same sequence but coronal section: observe the relationships of the cystic craniopharyngioma to the cavernous sinuses, the intracavernous carotid artery, the vessels of the circle of Willis, in particular to the right carotid artery branching (↗) and to the chiasm. The asymmetry of the frontal horns is independent of the lesion.

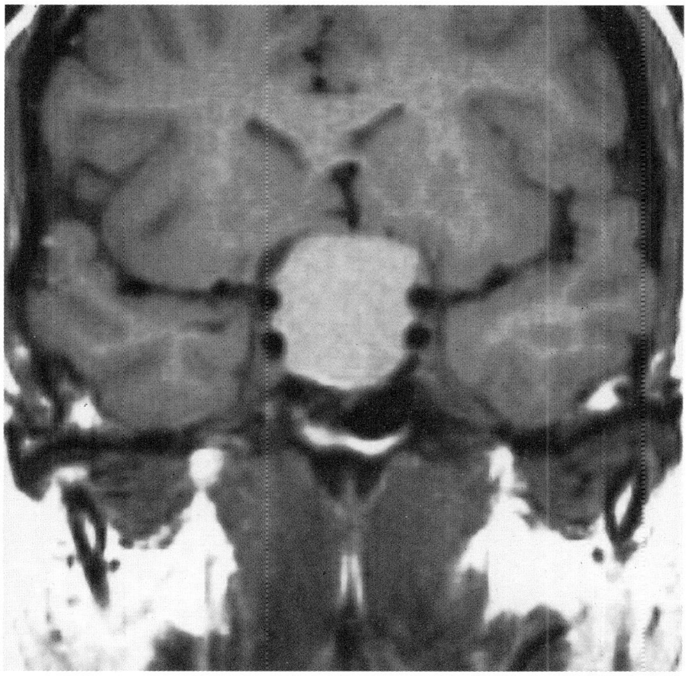

A

Fig. 15. *Intra- and suprasellar cystic craniopharyngioma.* 22-year-old woman with panhypopituitarism and bitemporal hemianopsia. T_1-weighted views pre- (A) and post- (B, C) i.v. GD-DTPA: intense peripheral enhancement of the cystic craniopharyngioma wall. The lesion totally occupies the sellar cavity, where the pituitary is no longer visible. It also divaricates the carotid siphons. Superiorly, it compresses the anterior aspect of the third ventricle and the chiasm.

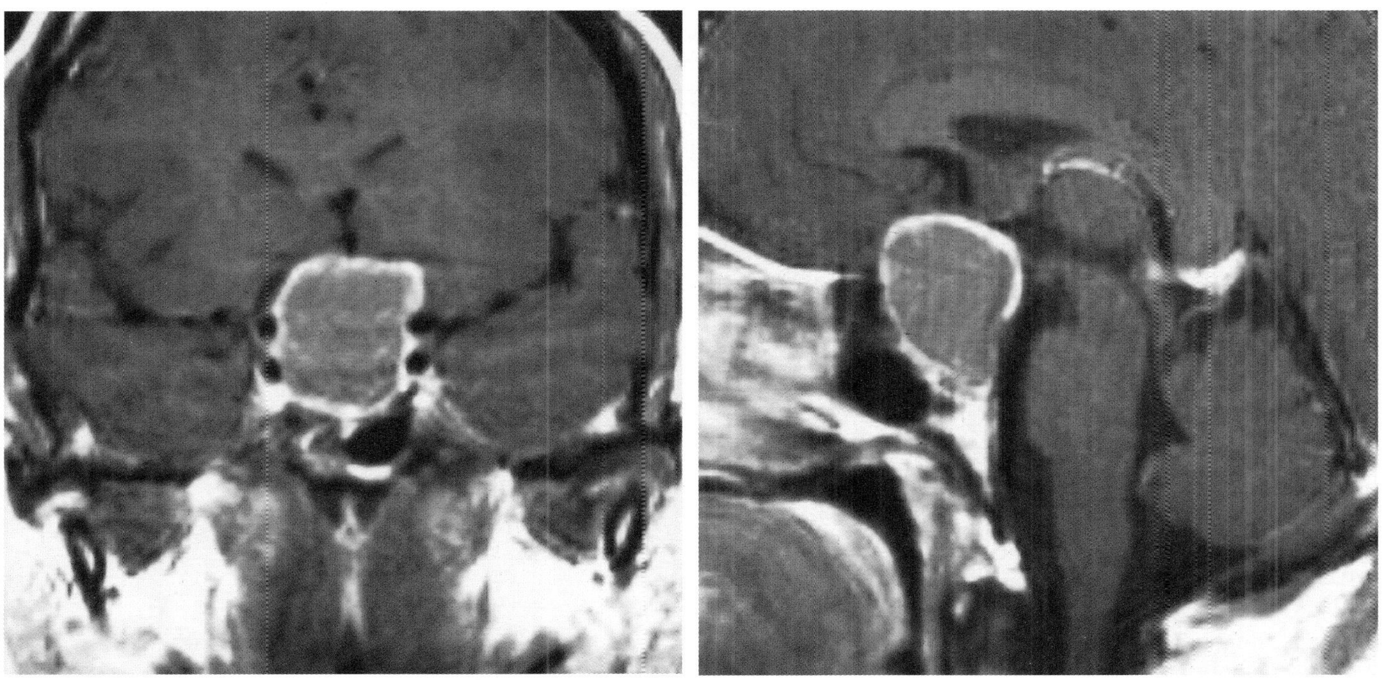

B

C

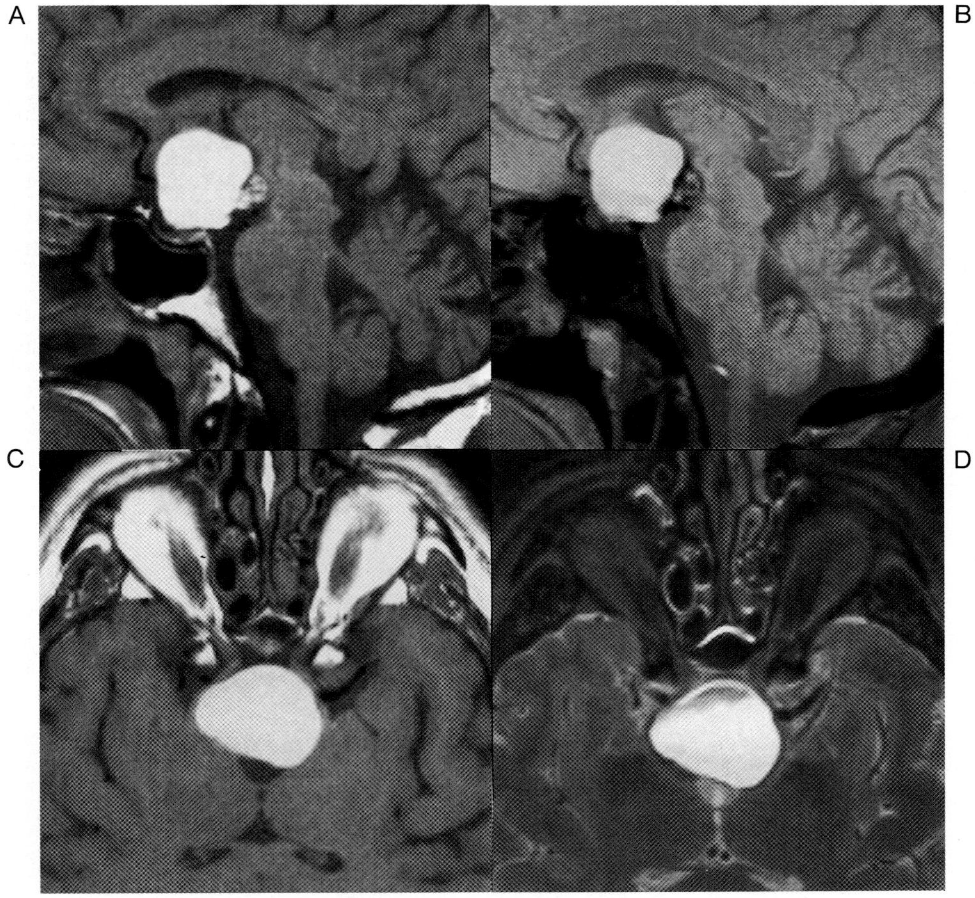

Fig. 16. *Suprasellar cystic craniopharyngioma.* 42-year-old man with right blindness and left temporal hemianopsia. Evidence of a space-occupying lesion above the sellar diaphragm with a predominantly cystic component. The signal is hyperintense on both the T_1-weighted sequence (A, C) and on the T_2-weighted one (D), which also shows nonuniformities of the tumor content. Posteriorly, observe a small solid component with calcifications, better visible on the gradient-echo image (B). The mass divaricates and compresses the optic tracts and the chiasm anteriorly and the cerebral peduncles posteriorly. The pituitary is compressed from above. Note the difference from the case of Fig. 15, where the tumor was operated on via a transsphenoidal approach because of its clear intrasellar growth. In this case, where the pituitary is clearly identifiable below the tumor, a transcranial approach is more suitable.

Fig. 17. *Invasive orbitoethmoidal recurrence of craniopharyngioma.* A – TR 2,500 msec, TE 15 msec; B – TR 2,500 msec, TE 90 msec: proton density-weighted images that show the anatomical details of the relationships between the tumoral mass and the orbital content. Right: mild compression of the posterior aspect of the orbital cone; left: invasion by the cystic formation (←). The solid tumor is inhomogeneous due to necrotic components; these are hypointense on early echoes and more intense on late echoes.

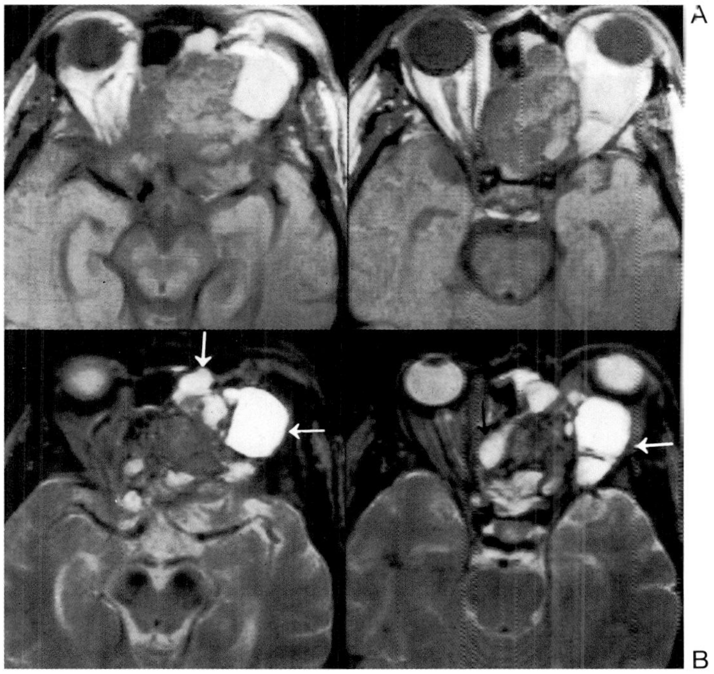

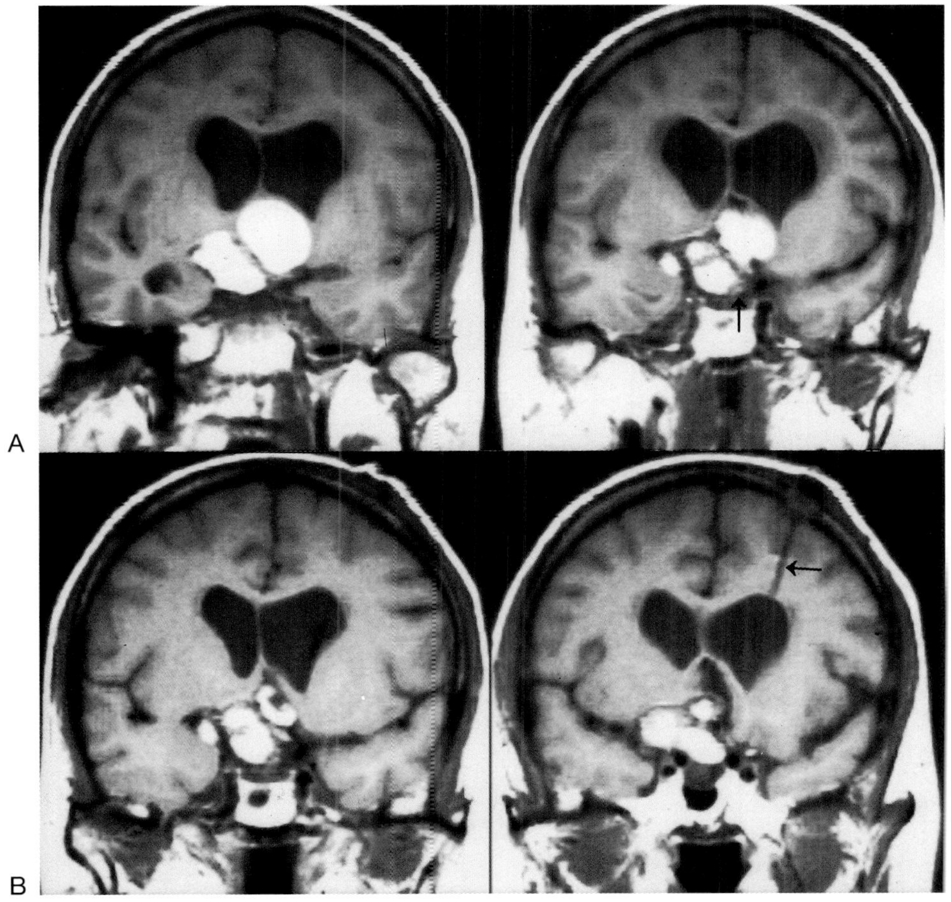

Fig. 18. *Partially cystic craniopharyngioma.* 50-year-old patient with diabetes insipidus and bitemporal hemianopsia. A – T_1-weighted sequence showing a solid component (↑) overlain by a markedly hyperintense cystic component. B – Same patient after drainage of the cyst and stereotactic placement of a subcutaneous reservoir. Note the catheter (←) and the cyst collapse which makes it possible to visualize the third ventricle.

A B

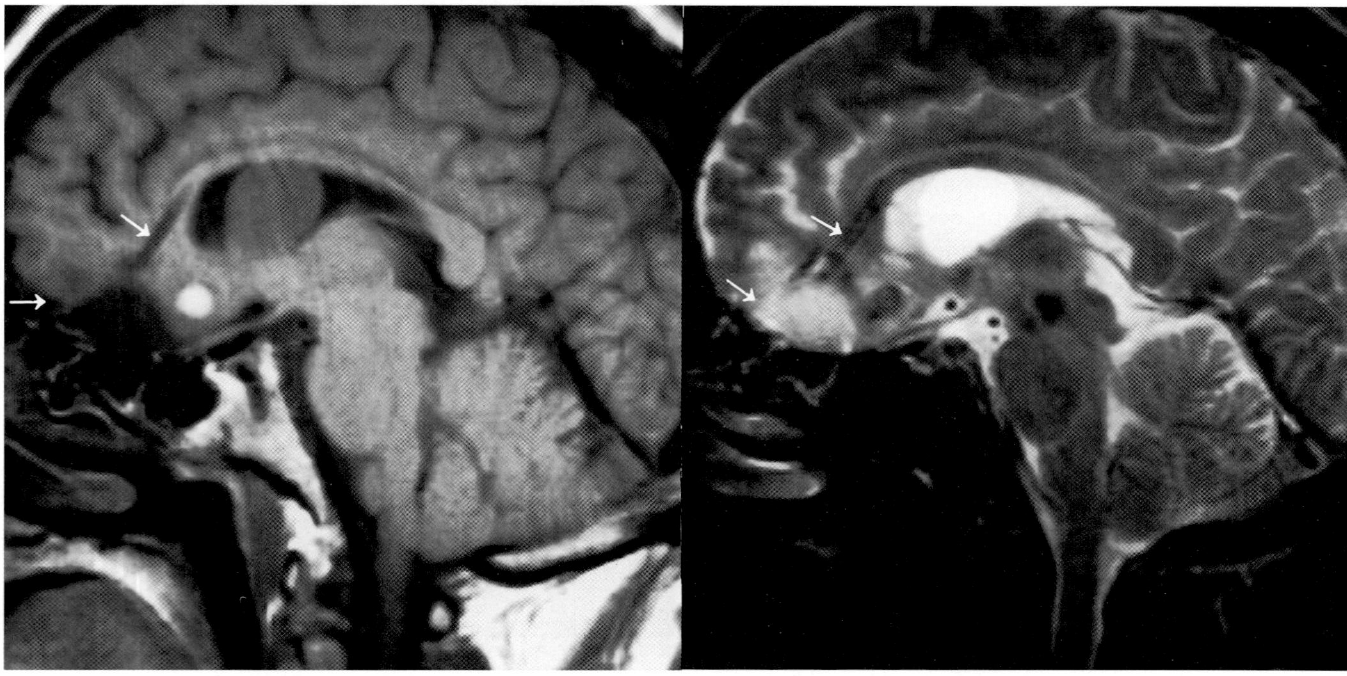

Fig. 19. *Partially cystic craniopharyngioma.* Follow-up examination of a 49-year-old patient with giant bifrontal cyst due to craniopharyngioma, treated with stereotactic drainage and repeated intracystic administration of bleomycine. Observe the remnants of the drained cystic cavity (→), containing a fluid producing a CSF-like signal; the catheter (↘); and a small focus, hyperintense on the T_1-weighted section (A) and hypointense on the T_2-weighted one (B); the focus reflects the solid, probably keratin-laden component. A third portion of the neoplasm occupies the right lateral ventricle; its signal is of the soft tissue type on T_1-weighted images and of the cystic type on T_2-weighted images, depending on its viscosity.

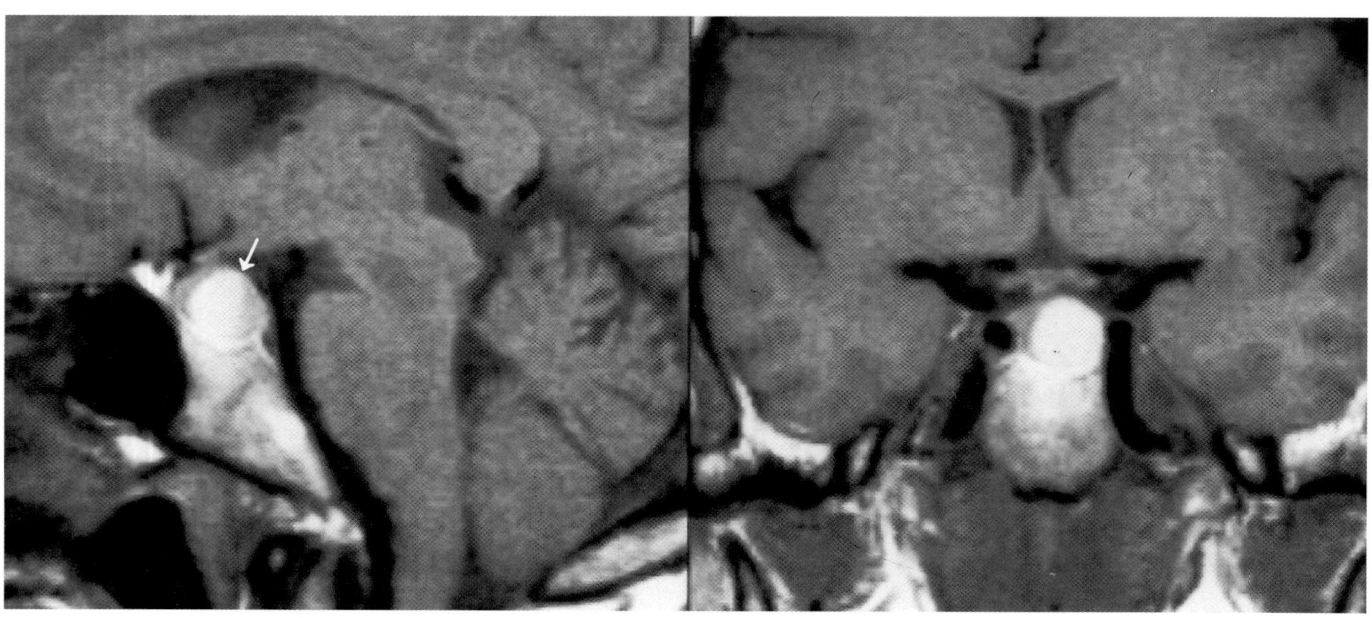

Fig. 20. *Rathke's pouch cyst.* 40-year-old woman with oligomenorrhea, moderate rise in prolactinemia and pulsating temporal headache. T_1-weighted sagittal and coronal views: intrasellar cyst uplifting the diaphragma. The pituitary is laminar and compressed upwards and to the right. Note the level images (↙), suggestive of inhomogeneity of the cystic content, with different signal intensity and different specific weight.

References

1. Akimura T, Kameda H, Abiko S et al. (1989) Infrasellar craniopharyngioma. Neuroradiology 31:180–183
2. Al-Mefty O, Hassounah M, Weaver P et al. (1985) Microsurgery of giant craniopharyngiomas in children. Neurosurgery 17:585–595
3. Apuzzo MLJ, Chihowani OK, Gott PS et al. (1982) Transcallosal interfornicial approaches for lesions affecting the third ventricle: Surgical considerations and consequences. Neurosurgery 10:547–554
4. Asari S, Ito T, Tsuchida S, Tsutsui T (1990) MR appearance and cyst content of Rathke's cleft cysts. J Comput Assist Tomogr 14:532–535
5. Ball WS Jr, Towbin RB (1989) MRI of pediatric central nervous system neoplasms. In: Pomeranz SJ (ed) Craniospinal Magnetic Resonance Imaging. W. B. Saunders Co., Philadelphia, 177–207
6. Barboriak PN, Neelon FA (1990) Medical treatment of pituitary neoplasms. In: Wilkins RH, Rengachary SS (eds) Neurosurgery. McGraw-Hill, New York, 14–18
7. Berry I, Brandt-Zawadzki M, Osaki L et al. (1986) Gd-DTPA in clinical MR of the brain. 2. Extraaxial lesions and normal structures. AJNR 7:789–793
8. Bronen RA, Sze G (1990) Magnetic resonance contrast agents: theory and application to the central nervous system. J Neurosurg 73:820–840
9. Chakeres DW, Curtin A, Ford G (1989) Magnetic resonance imaging of pituitary and parasellar abnormalities. Radiol Clin North Am 27:265–281
10. Chen JC, Kucharczyk W (1989) Hypothalamic pituitary region: Magnetic Resonance Imaging. Baillieres Clin Endocrinol Metab 3:73–87
11. Daniels DL, Pech P, Mark L et al. (1985) Magnetic resonance imaging of the cavernous sinus. AJNR 6:187–192
12. Davis PC, Hoffman JC, Spencer T et al. (1987) MR imaging of pituitary adenoma: CT, clinical, and surgical correlation. AJNR 8:107–112
13. Davis PC, Hoffman HC Jr, Malko JA et al. (1987) Gadolinium DTPA and MR imaging of pituitary adenoma: a preliminary report. AJNR 8:817–823
14. Doppmann JL, Frank KA, Dwyer AJ et al. (1987) Gadolinium DTPA enhanced MR imaging of ACTH secreting adenomas of the pituitary gland. J Comput Assist Tomogr 12:728–735
15. Dwyer AJ, Frank JA, Doppman JL et al. (1987) Pituitary adenomas in patients with Cushing disease: initial experience with Gd-DTPA-enhanced MR imaging. Radiology 163:421–426
16. Felix R, Shorner W, Laniado M et al. (1985) Brain tumors: MR imaging with gadolinium-DTPA. Radiology 156:681–688
17. Friedman HS, Oakes WJ (1987) Recurrent brain tumors in children. Pediatr Neurosci 13:233–241
18. Gadian DG, Payne JA, Bryant DJ et al. (1985) Gadolinium-DTPA as a contrast agent in MR imaging: theoretical projections and practical observations. J Comput Assist Tomogr 9:242–251
19. Guckel C, Benz-Bohm G, Wiedemann G, Thun F (1990) Resonance tomographic diagnosis of brain tumors in children and adolescents. A comparison with computed tomography. ROFO 153:313–320
20. Gudinchet F, Brunelle F, Barth MO et al. (1989) MR Imaging of the posterior hypophysis in children. Am J Roentgenol 153:351–354
21. Karande VC, Gole D, Kuhn JP, Crickard K (1990) Correlation between clinical, endocrinologic and Nuclear Magnetic Resonance findings in women with suspected pituitary adenomas. J Reprod Med 35:496–498
22. Komiyama M, Hakuba A, Yasui T et al. (1984) Magnetic Resonance Imaging of intracavernous pathology. Neurol Med Chir (Tokyo) 29:573–578
23. Konovalov AN (1987) Technique and strategies of direct surgical management of craniopharyngioma. In: Apuzzo MLJ (ed) Surgery of the Third Ventricle. Williams & Wilkins, Baltimore, 542–552
24. Koos WT, Miller MH (1971) Intracranial tumors of infants and children. Mosby, St Louis
25. Kucharczyk W, Peck WW, Kelly WM et al. (1987) Rathke cleft cysts: CT, MR imaging, and pathologic features. Radiology 165:491–495
26. Kucharczyk W, Smith RML (1990) Magnetic resonance imaging of sellar and parasellar lesions. In: Wilkins RH, Rengachary SS (eds) Neurosurgery Update I. McGraw-Hill, New York, 57–68
27. Kulkarni MV, Lee KF, McArdle CB et al. (1988) 1.5-T MR imaging of pituitary microadenomas: technical considerations and CT correlation. AJNR 9:5–11
28. Kwan E, Wolpert SM, Smith SP, Modic MT (1987) Radiology of third ventricular lesions. In: Apuzzo MLJ (ed) Surgery of the Third Ventricle. Williams & Wilkins, Baltimore, 262–300
29. Lambrecht L, Rubens R, Pevernagie D et al. (1989) MRI signal intensity profiles of sellar and perisellar lesions. Acta Clin Belg 44:303–310
30. Linden CN, Martinez CR, Gonzalvo AA, Cahill DW (1989) Intrinsic third ventricle craniopharyngioma: CT and MR findings. J Comput Assist Tomogr 13:362–363

31. Macpherson P, Hadley DM, Teasdale E, Teasdale G (1989) Pituitary microadenomas: Does Gadolinium enhance their demonstration? Neuroradiology 31:293–298
32. Newton DR, Dillon WP, Normal D et al. (1989) Gd-DTPA enhanced MR imaging of pituitary adenomas. AJNR 10:949–954
33. Packer RJ, Batzinski S, Cohen ME (1985) Magnetic Resonance imaging in the evaluation of intracranial tumors of childhood. Ann Neurol 18:217–277
34. Parizel PM, Degryse HL, Gheuens J et al. (1989) Gadolinium-DTPA enhanced MR imaging of intracranial lesions. Comput Assist Tomogr 13:378–385
35. Peck WW, Dillon WP, Norman D et al. (1989) High resolution MR Imaging of pituitary microadenomas at 1.5 T: Experience with Cushing disease. AJR 152:145–151
36. Pojunas KW, Daniels DL, Williams AL et al. (1986) MR imaging of prolactin-secreting microadenomas. AJNR 7:209–213
37. Pusey E, Kortman KE, Flannigan BD et al. (1987) MR of craniopharyngiomas: tumor delineation and characterization. AJNR 8:439–444
38. Sakamoto Y, Takahashi M, Korogi Y et al. (1991) Normal and abnormal pituitary glands: Gadopentetate Dimeglumine-enhanced MR Imaging. Radiology 178:441–445
39. Sheldon JJ (1989) MRI of the sella. In: Pomeranz SJ (ed) Craniospinal Magnetic Resonance Imaging. W. B. Saunders Co., Philadelphia, 275–314
40. Smith FW (1987) Magnetic Resonance Imaging of midline brain tumors using inversion recovery sequences at 0.08 T (3.4 MHz). Magn Reson Med 5:118–128
41. Snow RB, Johnson CE, Morgello S et al. (1990) Is Magnetic Resonance Imaging useful in guiding the operative approach to large pituitary tumors? Neurosurgery 26:801–803
42. Stadnik T, Stevenaert A, Beckers A et al. (1990) Pituitary microadenomas: diagnosis with two- and three-dimensional MR Imaging at 1.5 T before and after injection of gadolinium. Radiology 176:419–428
43. Stein AL, Levenick MN, Kletzky OA (1989) Computed Tomography versus Magnetic Resonance Imaging for the evaluation of suspected pituitary adenomas. Obstet Gynecol 73:996–999
44. Steiner E, Imhof H, Knosp E (1989) Gd-DTPA enhanced high resolution MR Imaging of pituitary adenomas. Radiographics 9:587–598
45. Vance ML, Lipper M, Klibanski A et al. (1990) Treatment of prolactin-secreting pituitary macroadenomas with the long-acting non-ergot dopamine agonist CV 205–502. Ann Intern Med 112:668–673
46. Yasargil MG, Curcic M, Kis M et al. (1990) Total removal of craniopharyngiomas. Approaches and long-term results in 144 patients. J Neurosurg 73:3–11
47. Youl BD, Plant GT, Stevens JM et al. (1988) Three cases of craniopharyngioma showing optic tract hypersignal on MRI. Neurology 40:1416–1419
48. Young SC, Zimmerman RA, Nowell MA et al. (1987) Giant cystic craniopharyngiomas. Neuroradiology 29:468–473
49. Yousem DM, Arrington JA, Kumar AJ, Bryan RN (1990) Bright lesions on sellar/parasellar T1-weighted scans. Clin Imaging 14:99–105
50. Zimmerman RA (1990) Imaging of intrasellar, suprasellar, and parasellar tumors. Semin Roentgenol 25:174–197

CHAPTER IX

Angiomas and tumor-like aneurysms

On the basis of their morphological and structural characteristics, angiomas (a.) are classified as:

- racemose a.
- cavernous a.

The group of racemose a. includes telangiectasias, varices, venous a. and arterovenous malformations (AVMs). Hemangioblastomas are real progressively-growing neoplastic lesions; hence, they are not dealt with in this chapter.

Telangiectasias, which are rather rare, are "capillary" angiomas, namely capillary dilatations and varicoses of the nerve tissue; small and isolated, they are generally located in the pons or in the roof of the fourth ventricle and only occasionally are they accompanied by hemorrhage.

Varices are small lesions characterized by dilated veins, often invisible to the naked eye.

The term venous a. defines a malformation that macroscopically looks like an AVM but that consists entirely of veins without arterovenous shunts *(Figs. 1, 2)*.

AVMs account for roughly 3–4% of the intracranial disorders that are of interest to the surgeon and for approximately 1/7 of intracranial aneurysms. Macroscopically, an AVM takes the form of a single dilated vessel or of an entanglement of vessels with one or more feeding arteries and one or more draining veins. The absence of arteriolar resistance brings about a progressive expansion in the volume of the a., caused by dilatation of the pathologic vessels.

The AVMs can be discovered by means of CT plus contrast media and MRI, as both methods clearly demonstrate the pathologic dilatation of the vessels. MRI depicts the tumoral vessels as serpiginous images with signal loss on both T_1- and T_2-weighted sequences *(Figs. 3, 6)*. Occasionally, owing to slow-flow-induced second-echo rephasing, draining vessels can be distinguished from the feeding artery as high-signal MR images.

The vessels most frequently involved are the M.C.A. and, in decreasing order, the A.C.A. *(Fig. 3)* and the P.C.A. *(Figs. 4, 5)*. Epilepsy and/or hemorrhage are the general mode of presentation of AVMs. Hemorrhages can be detected at a very early stage by CT or MRI scans. MRI is undoubtedly more sensitive in detecting hemorrhages in the subacute or chronic stages. Less frequent symptoms are headaches, paretic episodes or sensory disorders, bruit, visual disturbances, mental and gait disorders.

The possibility of successfully treating AVMs depends not only on usual factors, such as site, size, etc., but also on accurate hemodynamic evaluation of the lesion. This makes it imperative to carry out an accurate panangiographic study, even though MR angiography is an excellent method to show the feeding arteries and the nest of the AVM *(Fig. 4)*. Indeed, it is possible to recognize the arteries which, though supplying branches to the angioma, cross it in order to reach and feed the surrounding tissue. During surgery, it is advisable to spare the veins to the largest possible extent, so that venous drainage from the healthy brain tissue may occur normally. Finally, AVMs which are inoperable on account of site (critical areas) or size may be subjected to embolizing treatments via superselective catheterization or to stereotactic radiosurgery *(Fig. 6)*.

Cavernous a. are vascular abnormalities with sinusoidal dilatation, located mainly in the cerebral hemispheres *(Fig. 8)*. They may however occur in any district of the CNS *(Figs. 7, 8, 10, 11, 12)*. Upon observation, their diameter may range from a few millimeters to a few centimeters;

there is no brain tissue inside the sinusoidal spaces and typically they are not arterialized. Due to the lack of arterial flow inside the malformation, angiography does not generally show any vascular abnormality, but it can single out vessels displaced by the mass effect of the larger cavernous a. Also the CT scan is totally negative in the case of small cavernous a., whereas it is aspecific in the case of larger a., generally delineating a mildly hyperdense space-occupying lesion, occasionally with calcifications and without enhancement after contrast agents.

Conversely, MRI scans show cavernous a. as having typical and specific features: they take the form of images having a sharp outline, the signal being of mixed intensity on both sequences, since there are tissue elements characterized by both short T_1s and long T_2s. Weak signal areas are indicative of calcific and/or hemosiderin deposits, whereas intense signal areas are the equivalent of blood collections or clots. Moreover, they are typically surrounded by a thick low-signal rim, particularly evident on T_2-weighted images, which corresponds to the hemosiderin-laden ring *(Figs. 7, 8)*. Indeed, microhemorrhages are always present in cavernous a., even though they are clinically silent. In some cases, the hemorrhage may be of clinical importance but it is always restricted to the area underneath the tumor capsule *(Figs. 7, 10)*; by contrast, large hemorrhages *(Fig. 11)* are a rare occurrence. MRI is unquestionably the method of choice for this disease, because it can detect even small-sized tumors, which are often an occasional finding in asymptomatic patients or in patients with a history of seizures. Surgery is a successful option in cases where the lesion is symptomatic, also in critical areas.

The term giant aneurysm is used to refer to aneurysms having a diameter in excess of 2.5 cm. Of the various assumptions put forward to explain the formation of giant aneurysms, the most widely accepted invokes direct proportionality between width of the neck and diameter of the sac; a broad neck is supposed to favor greater blood turbulence and thus a progressive increase in sac volume; for this same reason, giant aneurysms often develop wall degeneration and internal thrombosis.

MRI portrays this variability in tissue components and flow dynamics via images having a rather inhomogeneous signal intensity on all the sequences. Calcium and hemosiderin deposits on the walls of the aneurysmal sac produce signals of increasingly lower intensity with echo time elongation, whereas the methemoglobin at the thrombus boundaries has high signal intensity on both short- and long-TR sequences. Finally, flow turbulence gives images with mixed signal intensity *(Fig. 14)*. In order to get a better view of the neck of the aneurysm or of the fast-flow part of the lumen, it is useful to resort to fast imaging with flow compensation, such as FISP or FLASH (TR 0.115 msec, TE 12 msec, FA 40°) *(Fig. 15)*.

Giant aneurysms are more common in women by a 3:1 ratio. They account for 5% of all intracranial aneurysms and at times they are associated with multiple aneurysms or AVMs. The symptomatology is that of a space-occupying lesion (tumor-like symptomatology) with headache, altered visual and oculomotor functions in carotid-ophthalmic and carotid-cavernous aneurysms, and deficits of other cranial nerves in vertebrobasilar aneurysms *(Fig. 15)*. The lesions originating from the A.C.A. produce slow-progressing mental and cognitive disorders, whereas those of the M.C.A. cause contralateral hemiparesis and seizures. Up to very recently it was commonly thought that giant aneurysms did not involve a high risk of rupture. Conversely, in examining the various series, a 30–80% frequency of subarachnoid hemorrhage is found. In effect, even the aneurysms that did not present with hemorrhage as a first symptom are likely to have had a history of sac rupture. Moreover, the finding of massive thrombosis inside the sac does not seem to be a protective factor against subarachnoid hemorrhage.

Surgery consists in closing the neck by means of a clip and in resecting the sac, where possible. Obviously, the decision to operate is influenced by such factors as age, general health of the patient, and above all by the anatomical position of the aneurysm. An alternative to surgery is superselective catheterization and embolization of the aneurysm. This technique is particularly indicated in giant C.A. aneurysms and in carotid-ophthalmic aneurysms.

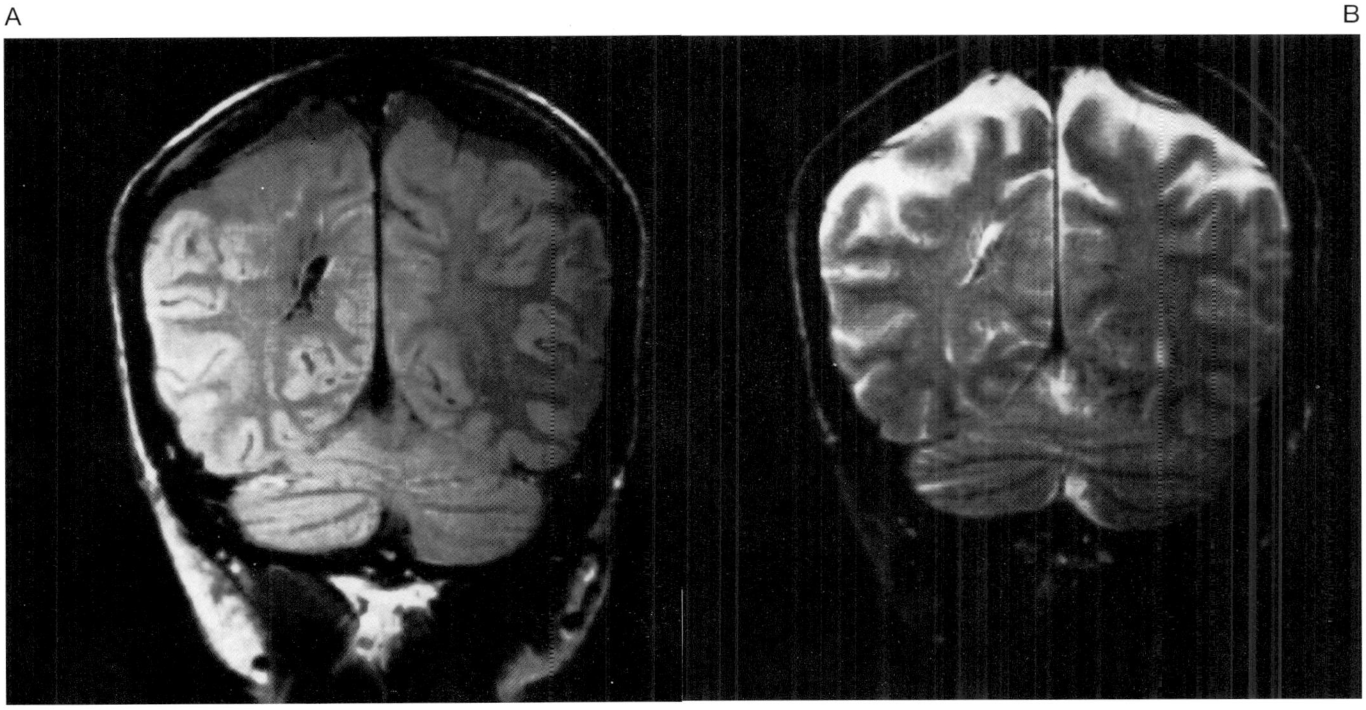

Fig. 1. *Right posterior parietal venous angioma.* The proton density- (A) and T_2-weighted (B) coronal scans show venous distension; slow flow causes the signal intensity to be different on early and late echoes owing to echo rephasing.

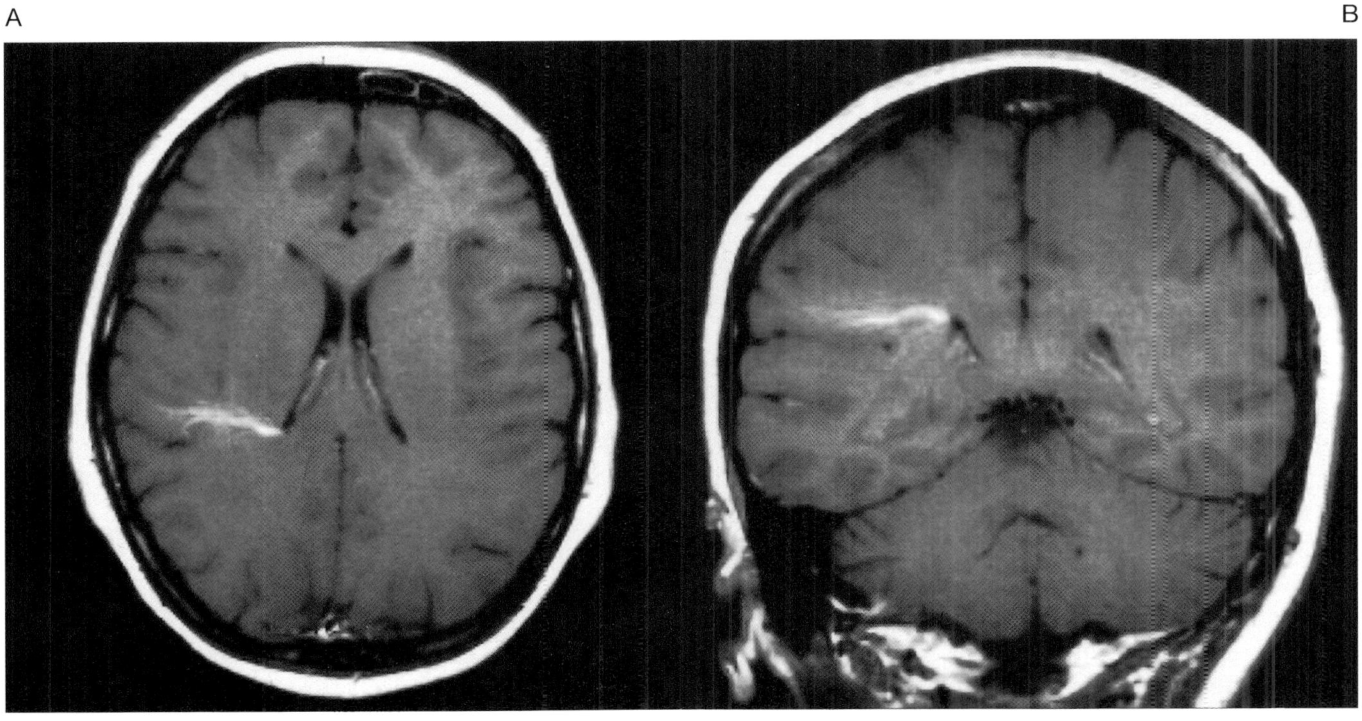

Fig. 2. *Right parietal venous angioma.* T_1-weighted axial (A) and coronal (B) views after i.v. GD-DTPA. The diagnosis of vascular malformation is facilitated by signal enhancement after contrast.

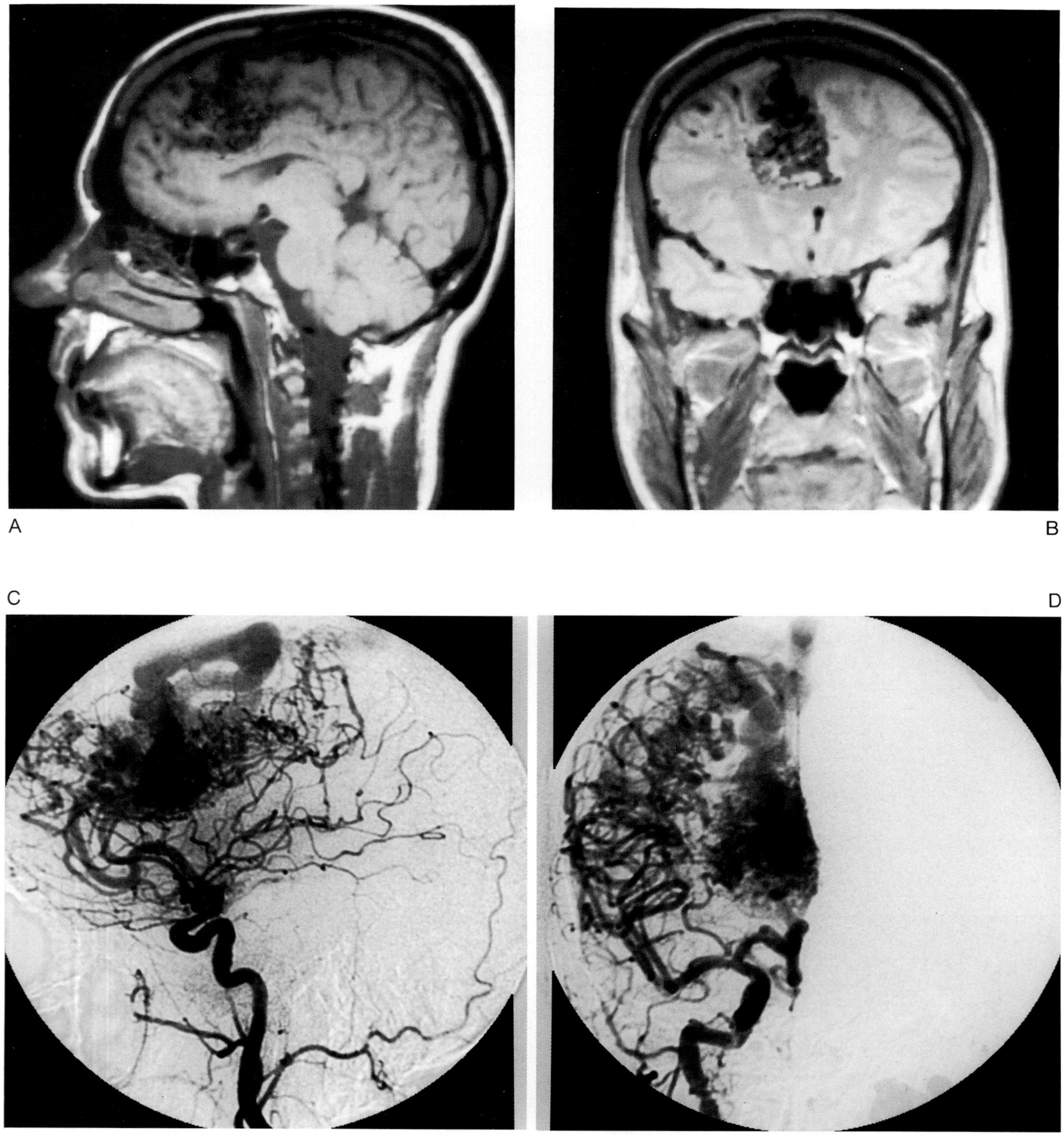

Fig. 3. *Right parasagittal frontal AVM.* 43-year-old woman with history of seizures and normal neurologic examination. Non-contrast CT evidenced a moderately hyperdense, space-occupying lesion with small calcifications and no perilesional edema. A – TR 550 msec, TE 15 msec, sagittal view: posterior frontal AVM with mass effect on the corpus callosum. The AVM vessels appear as a hypointense bundle. The hypertrophic draining vein has an even lower signal, indicative of fast flow. B – TR 2,500 msec, TE 15 msec, coronal view: the large veins draining into the S.L.S. and the contralateral transfalcal herniation are well outlined. Right carotid artery digital angiogram, lateral (C) and AP (D) views: marked hypertrophy of the right A.C.A. and of the posterior choroidal artery; AVM major feeding vessels; and evidence of large venous drainage into the S.L.S.

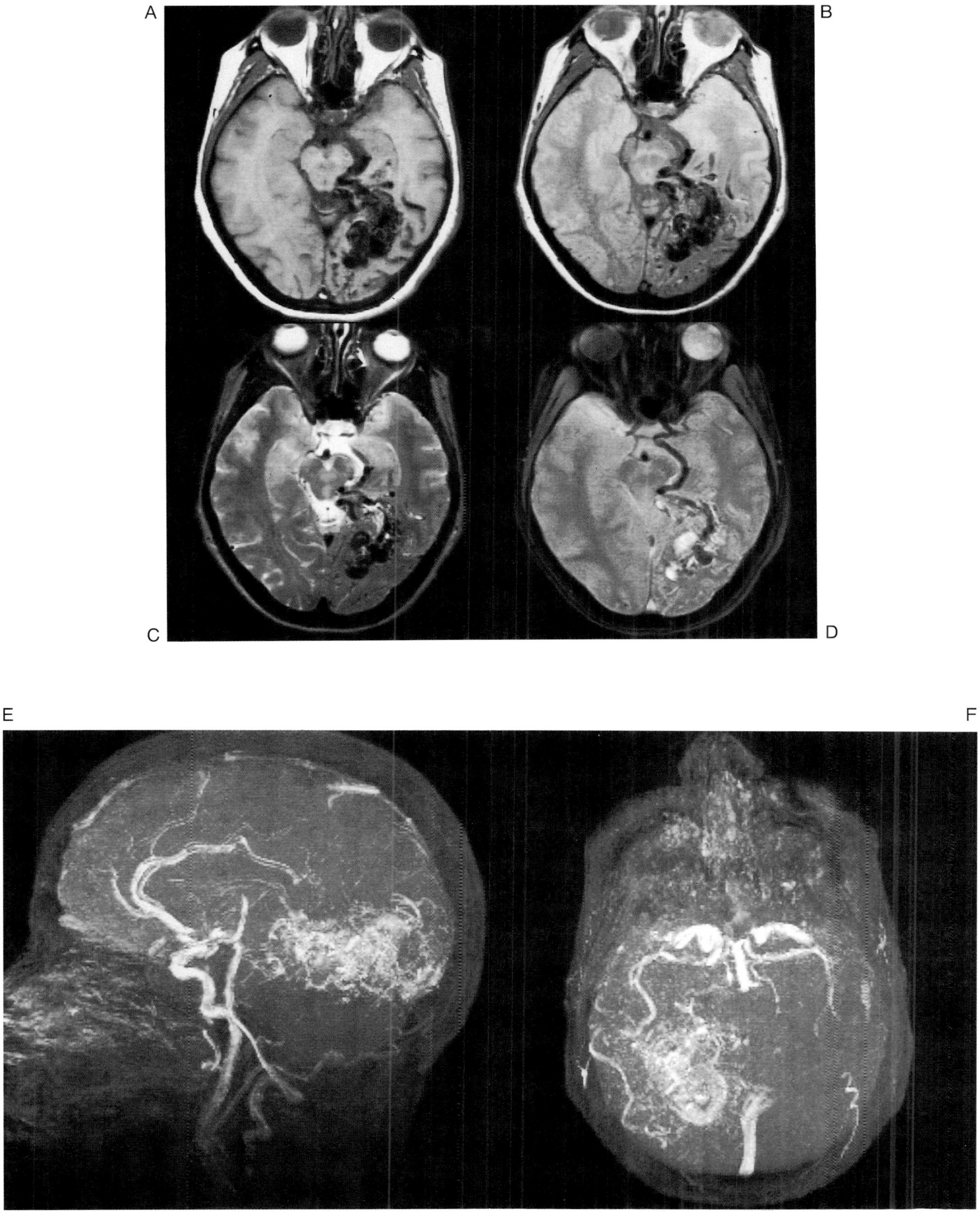

Fig. 4. *Left occipitotemporal AVM.* The T_1- (A), proton density- (B) and T_2- (C) weighted SE sequences well demonstrate the AVM and the relations of the hypertrophic feeding vessels to the deep structures. These vessels, which run on the medial surface of the temporal lobe, obliterate the cisterna ambiens and compress the left cerebral peduncle. D – The fast imaging sequence better visualizes the origin of the feeding vessel and differentiates the high- from the low-flow components of the AVM core. E, F – Vascular MRI (Flash 3D with flow compensation, TR 40 msec, TE 7 msec, FA 15°), sagittal and coronal views. They show both the AVM blush and its main feeding vessels.

A B

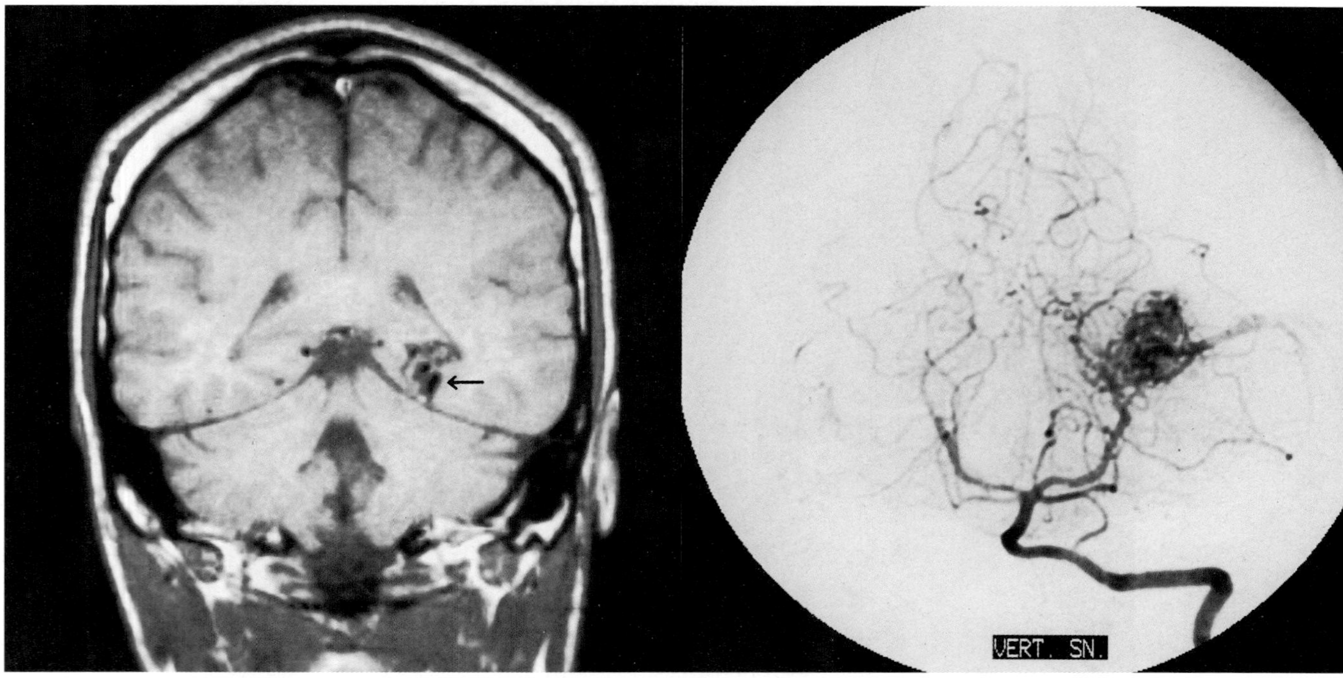

Fig. 5. *Deep left temporal AVM.* 18-year-old young man with seizures and normal neurologic examination. A – T_1-weighted coronal view: the lesion (←) is represented by a small, deep, temporal vessel entanglement, medial to the temporal horn. B – Left V.A. angiogram, axial view: small isolated malformation of the P.C.A. with evidence of early venous drainage.

A B

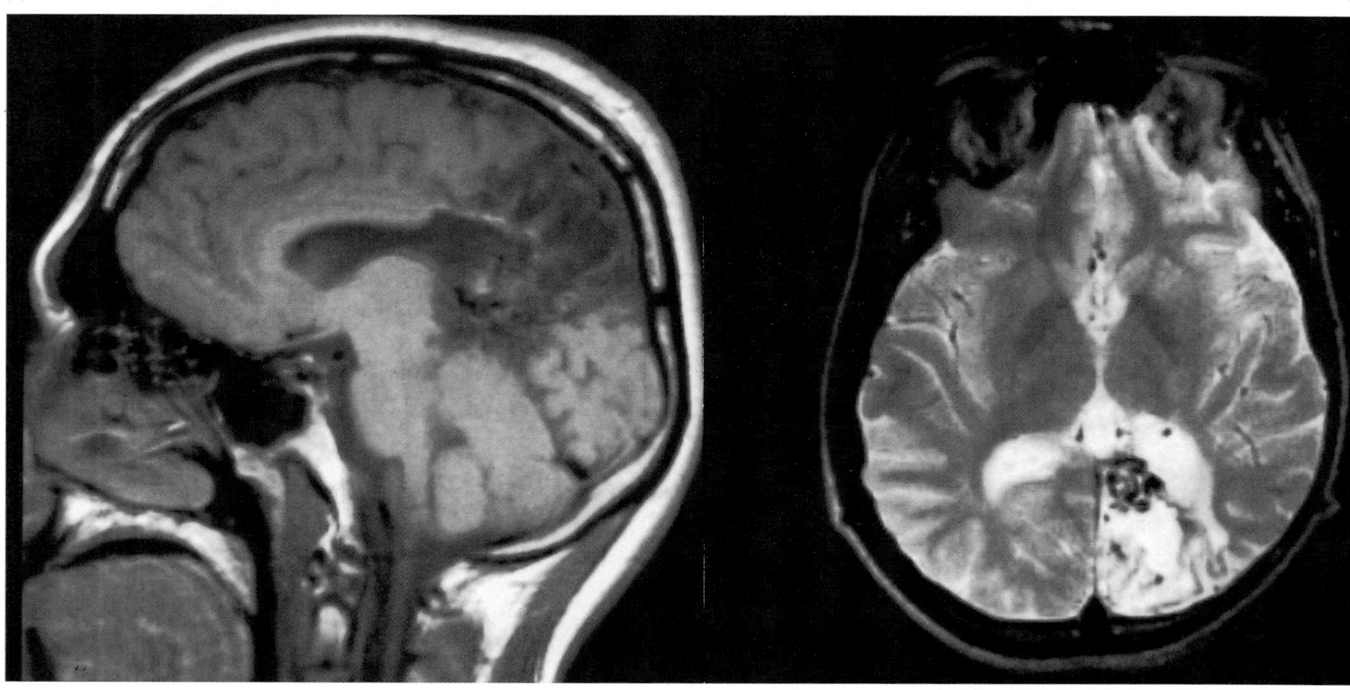

Fig. 6. *Parietooccipital AVM treated with embolization and radio-surgery.* 15-year-old boy with history of coma secondary to left parietooccipital intracerebral hematoma, demonstrated by CT and angiography. Embolization and radio-surgery of the malformation 2 years before MRI. A – The T_1-weighted sagittal scan evidences an extensive necrotic focus, hypointense with the healthy tissue. Inside the focus serpiginous images with signal void are visible. B – T_2-weighted axial scan: the residual vascular entanglement inside a post-radio-surgery high-signal focus is shown.

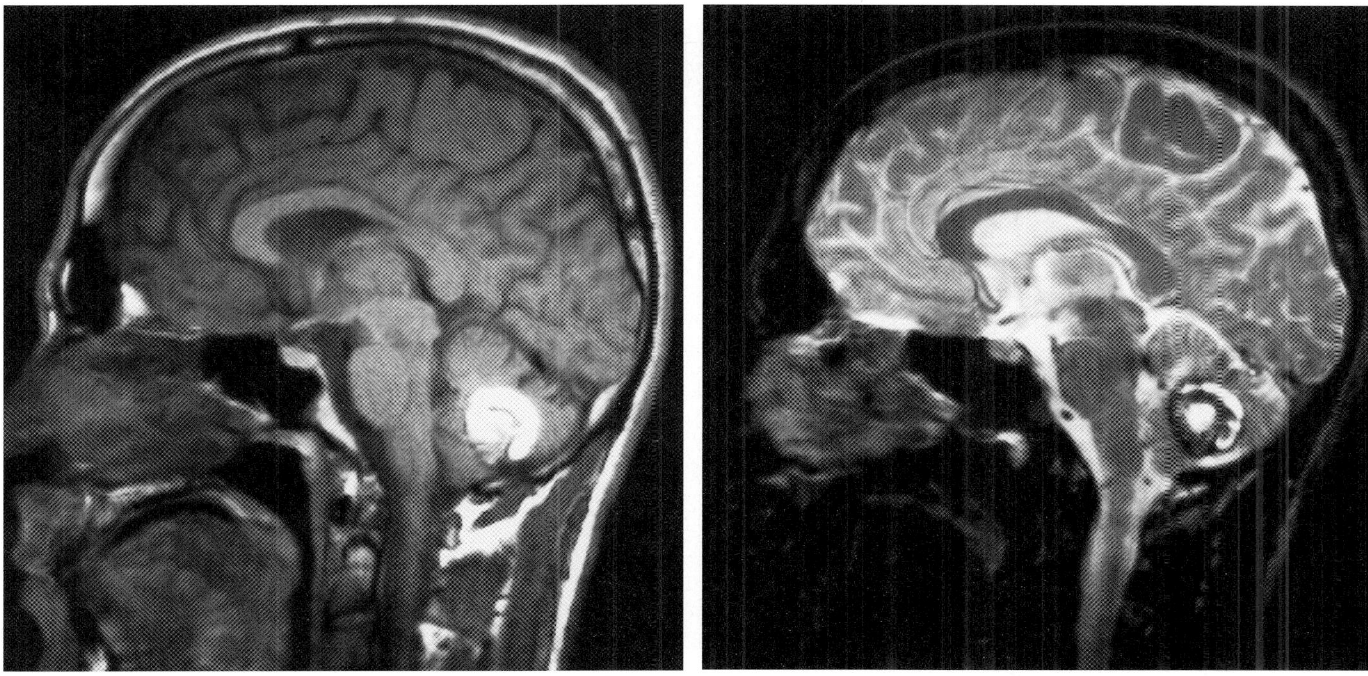

A B

Fig. 7. *Cavernous angioma of the vermis.* 20-year-old man with cerebro-meningeal bleed, severe headache, vomiting and ataxic disorders. On the T_1-weighted image (A), the lesion has a high signal due to: blood collections, typical for cavernous angioma; hemorrhagic-effusion methemoglobin in the neighbouring tissue. On the T_2-weighted image (B), the bloody areas and the recent hemorrhage maintain a high signal; conversely, the hemosiderin-laden fibrous pseudocapsule becomes markedly hypointense.

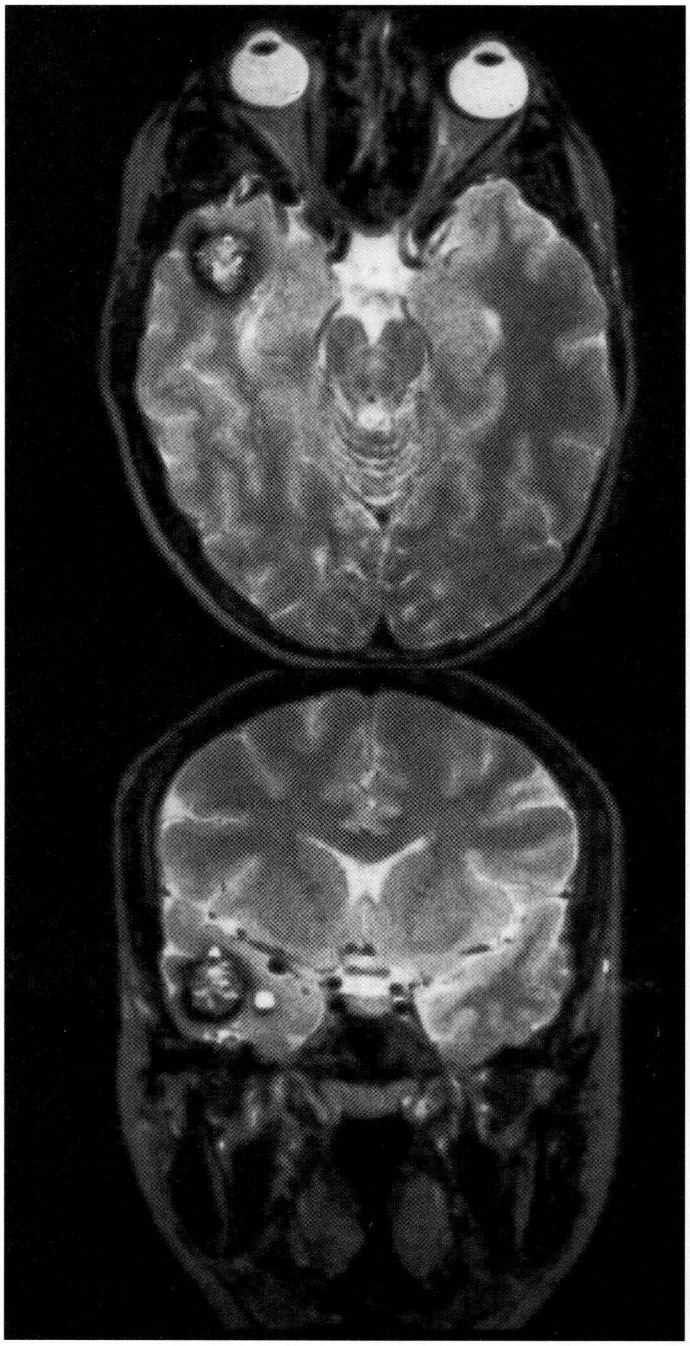

Fig. 8. *Right temporal cavernous angioma.* 19-year-old young woman with several years of seizures. T_2-weighted axial and coronal SE sequences: the cavernous angioma produces an inhomogeneous signal: intense in the central portion, markedly hypointense in the peripheral portion owing to hemosiderin. Note the large draining vein, medial to the mass; this was the only pathologic finding of the angiogram, that did not evidence any blush in the arterial phase.

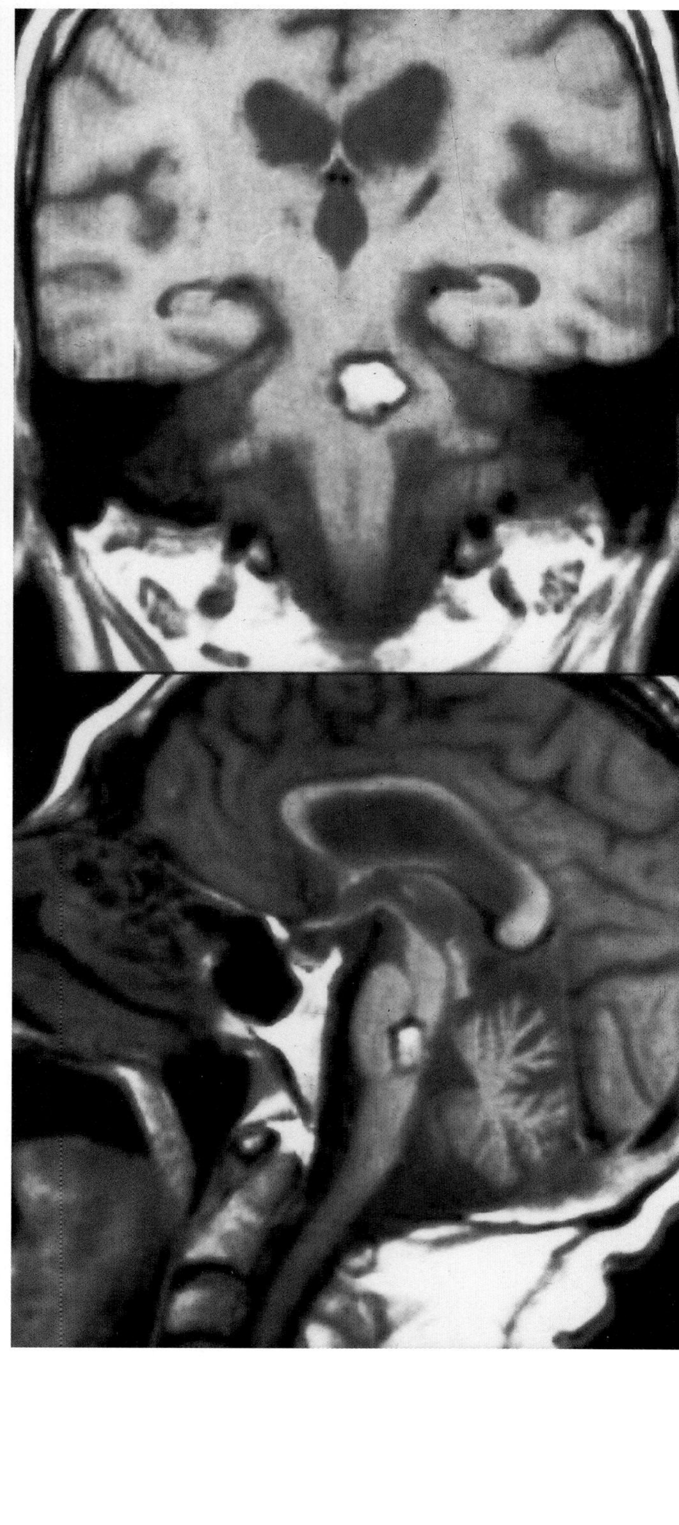

Fig. 9. *Brainstem cavernous angioma.* 45-year-old man with history of coma for unexplained reasons (normal brain CT). At present, consciousness disorders. T_1-weighted sagittal and coronal MRI characterizes the lesion which is located in the paramedian left middle cerebellar peduncle.

A B

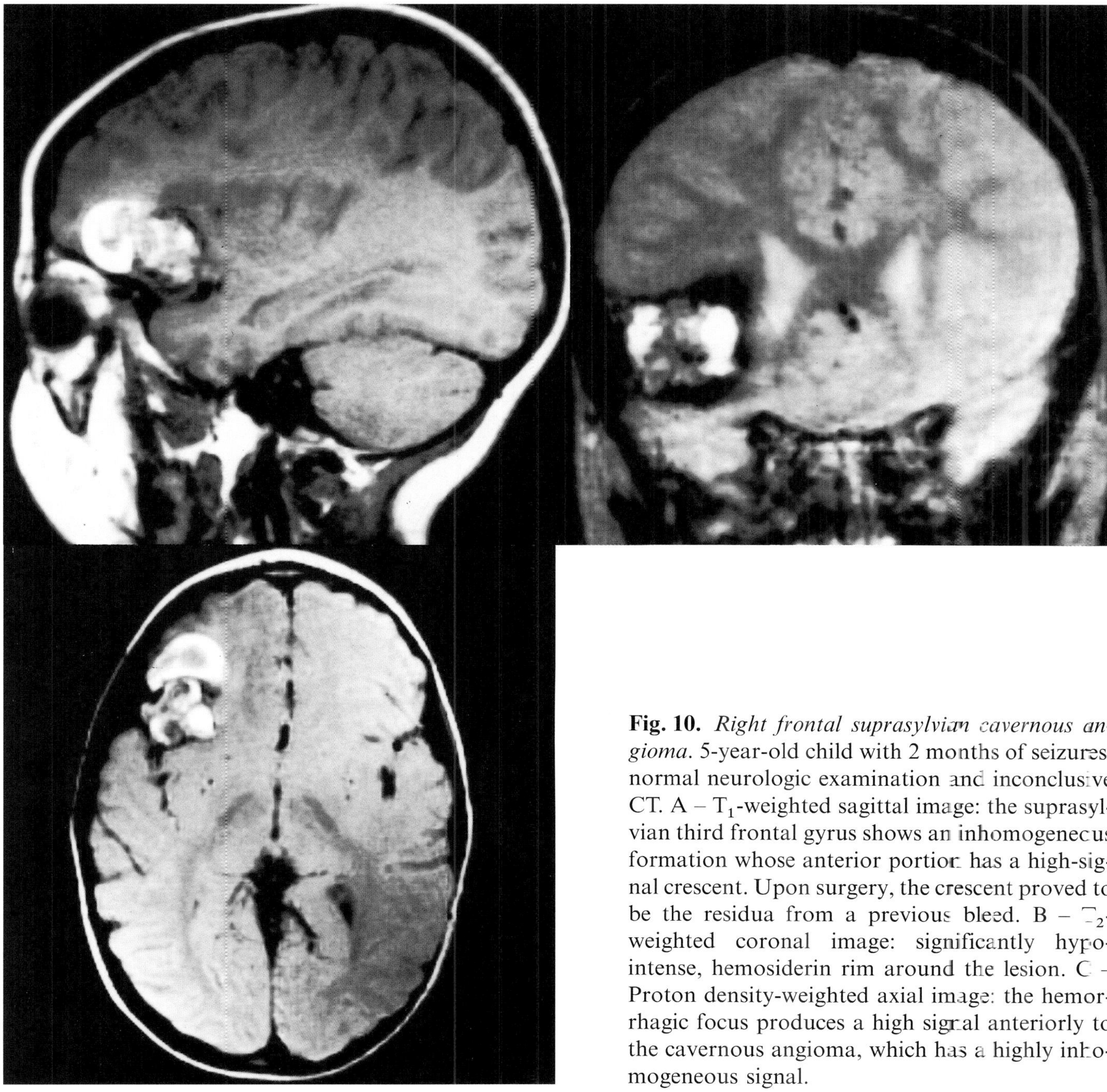

C

Fig. 10. *Right frontal suprasylvian cavernous angioma.* 5-year-old child with 2 months of seizures, normal neurologic examination and inconclusive CT. A – T_1-weighted sagittal image: the suprasylvian third frontal gyrus shows an inhomogeneous formation whose anterior portion has a high-signal crescent. Upon surgery, the crescent proved to be the residua from a previous bleed. B – T_2-weighted coronal image: significantly hypointense, hemosiderin rim around the lesion. C – Proton density-weighted axial image: the hemorrhagic focus produces a high signal anteriorly to the cavernous angioma, which has a highly inhomogeneous signal.

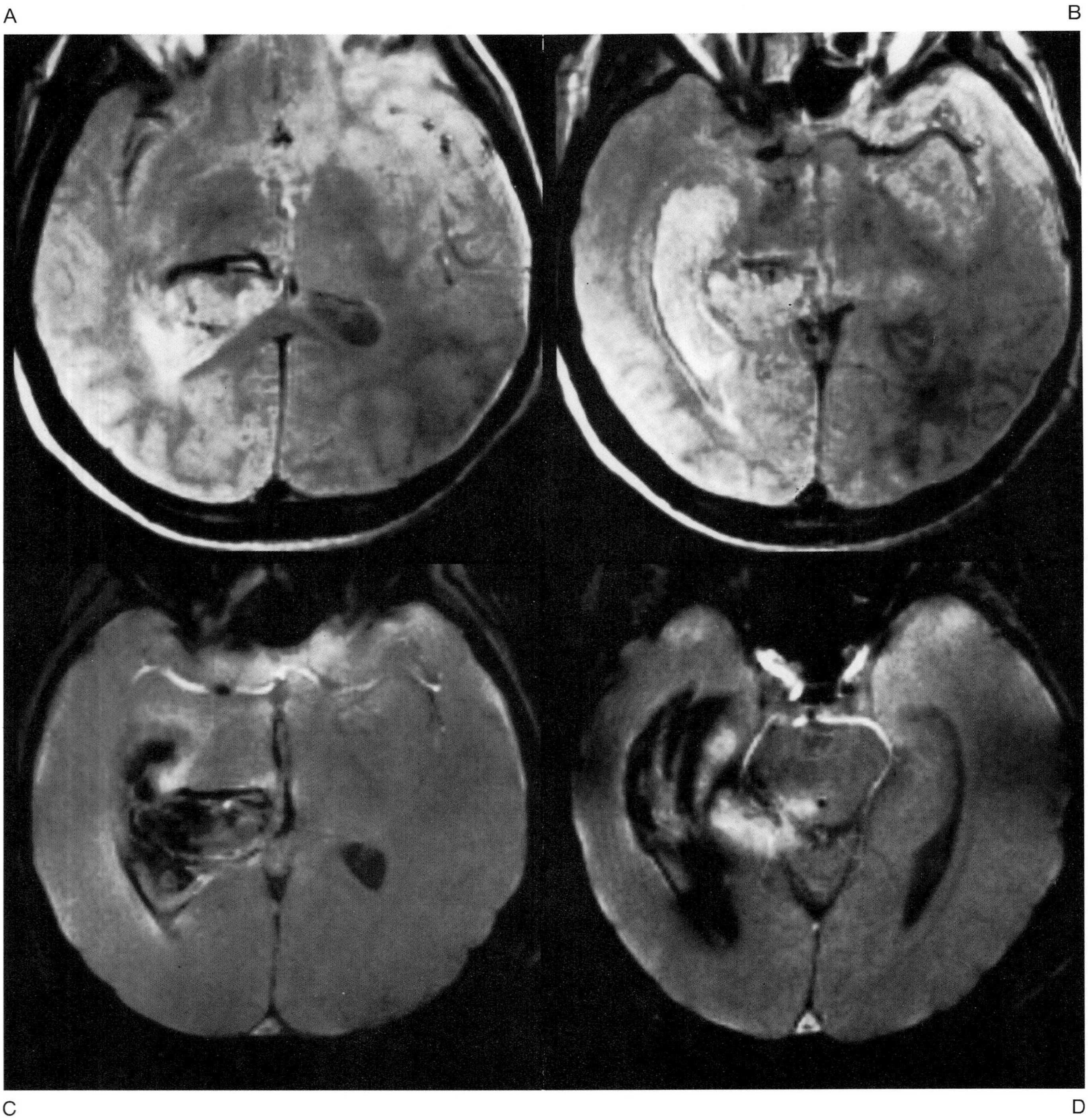

Fig. 11. *Right thalamus cavernous angioma.* A, B – The proton density-weighted axial images exhibit an angiomatous mass in the pulvinar; the mass is anteriorly delimited by hypointense hemosiderin deposits. The high signal inside the occipital and temporal horns indicates recent hemoventricle. The signal in the contralateral ventricle is different. C, D – The FISP sequence with flow compensation (TR 180 msec, TE 12 msec, FA 30°) evidences hyperintense vessels in the circle of Willis (M.C.A.s in C and P.C.A.s in D) with an angiogram-like effect.

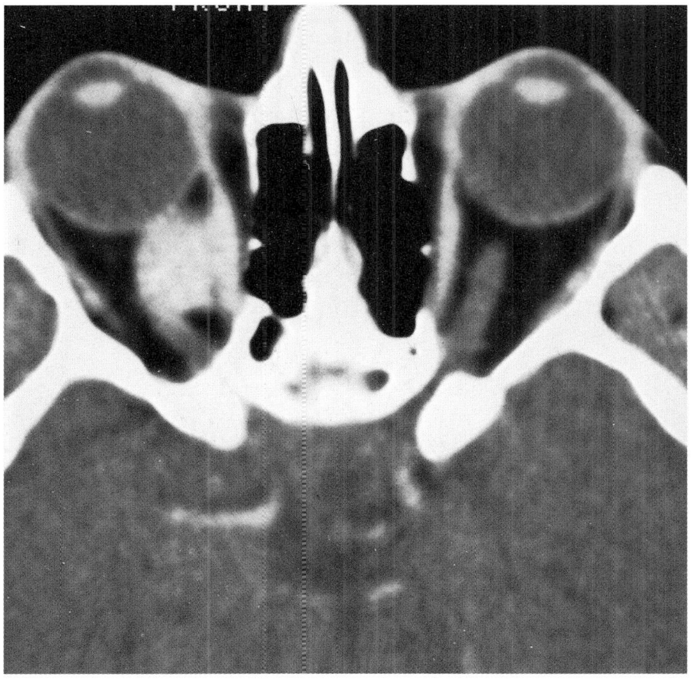

A

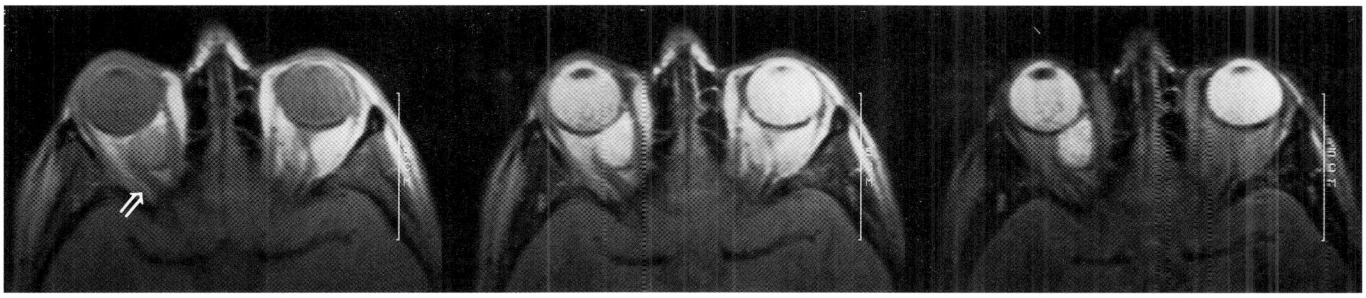

B

Fig. 12. *Right orbit cavernous angioma.* 38-year-old woman with decreased right-eye visual acuity and mild exophthalmos. A – Contrast CT: retrobulbar mass with intense c.e., apparently encasing and lateralizing the optic nerve; the mass suggests optic nerve sheath meningioma. B – The multi-echo sequence, instead, clearly shows that the neoplasm is separated from the optic nerve (⇑), questioning the diagnosis of meningioma. Histology proved the lesion to be a cavernous angioma.

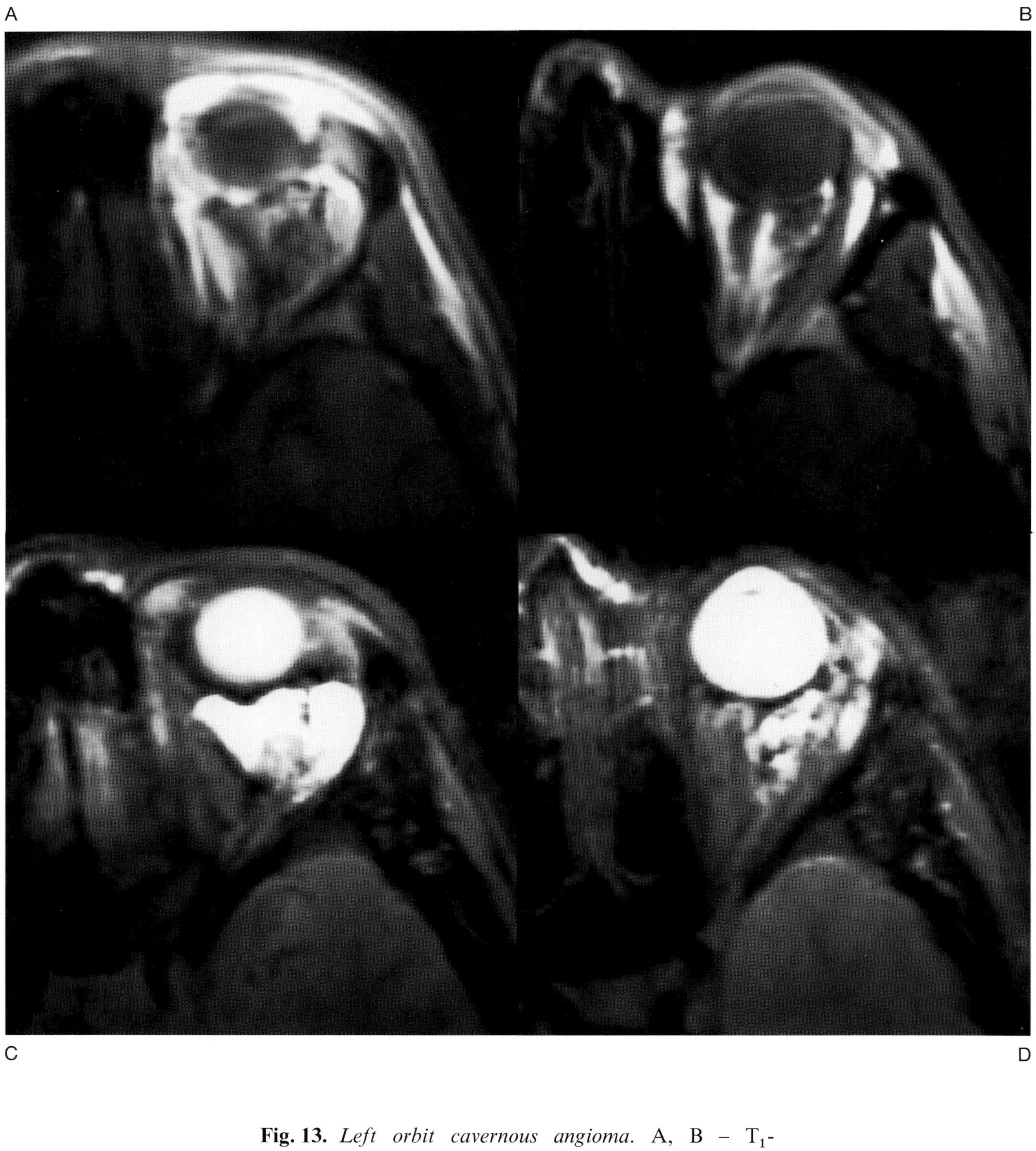

Fig. 13. *Left orbit cavernous angioma.* A, B – T_1-weighted images; C, D – T_2-weighted images. The T_1 images give a better view of the mass, that is intraconic between the optic nerve medially and the external rectus muscle laterally. The C and D images characterize the lesion, with typical, large bloody areas.

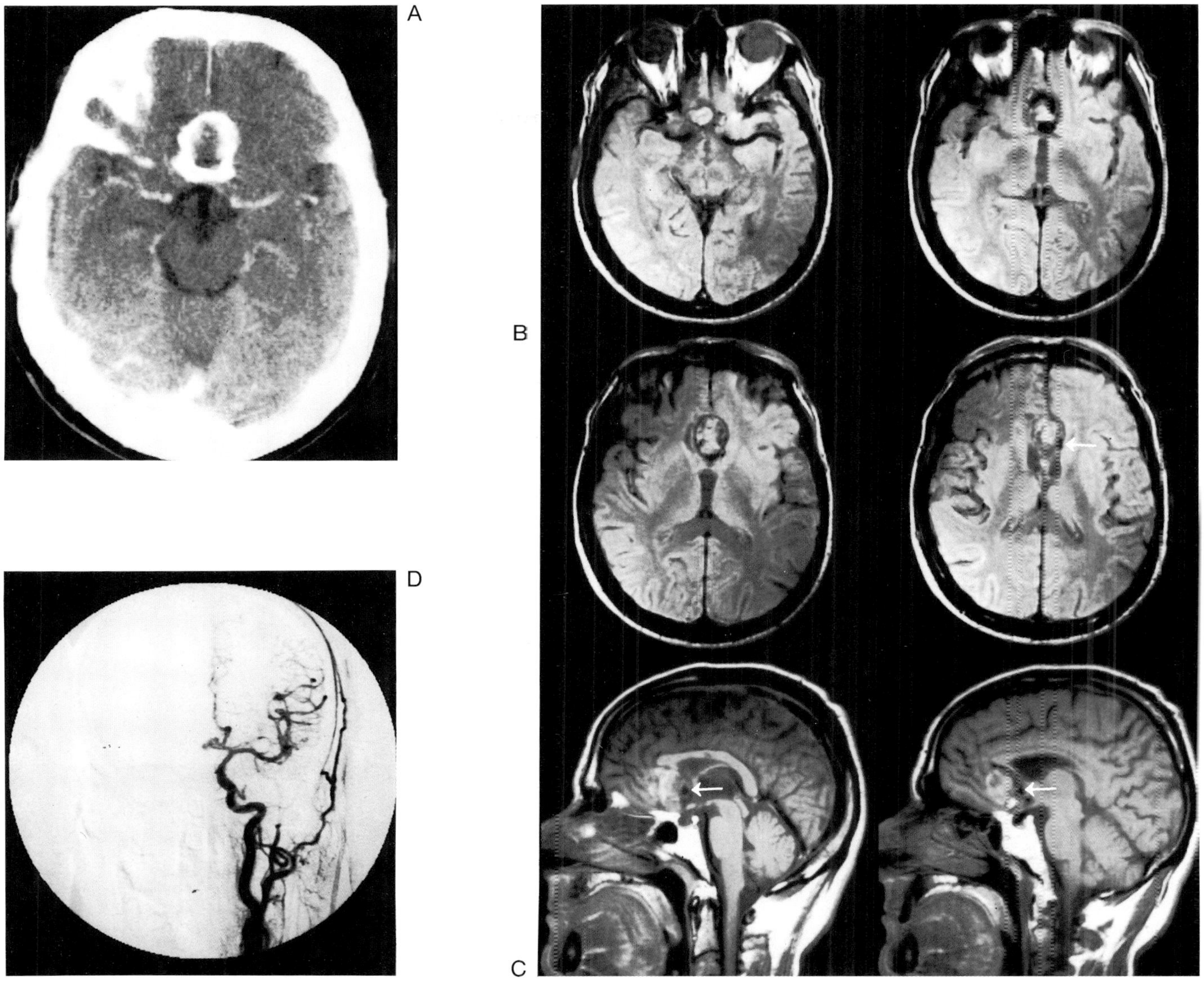

Fig. 14. *Giant aneurysm of the A.C.A.* 54-year-old man with slow-progressing psychic disorders and mental decay. A – Contrast CT: lesion with peripheral calcific rim and central isodense focus. No c.e. of this focus can be observed. Note the basal median frontal mass. B – Proton density-weighted SE sequence: inhomogeneous focus anterior to the circle of Willis; central area with high signal (clot) and peripheral area with low signal (parietal calcific component). The left A.C.A. (←) is displaced by the aneurysmal sac and the M.C.A.s are well delineated. C – T_1-weighted sagittal scan: validation of the inhomogeneity of the aneurysm and of the displacement of the A.C.A.s. The arrow (←) points to the signal void corresponding to the portion of the aneurysm with flow. D – Left carotid artery digital angiogram, axial view: note the small portion of the aneurysm with flow.

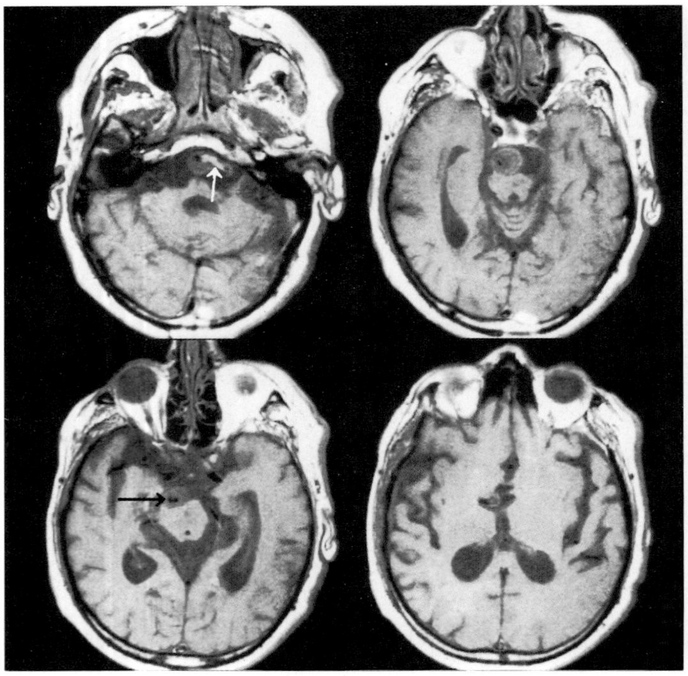

A

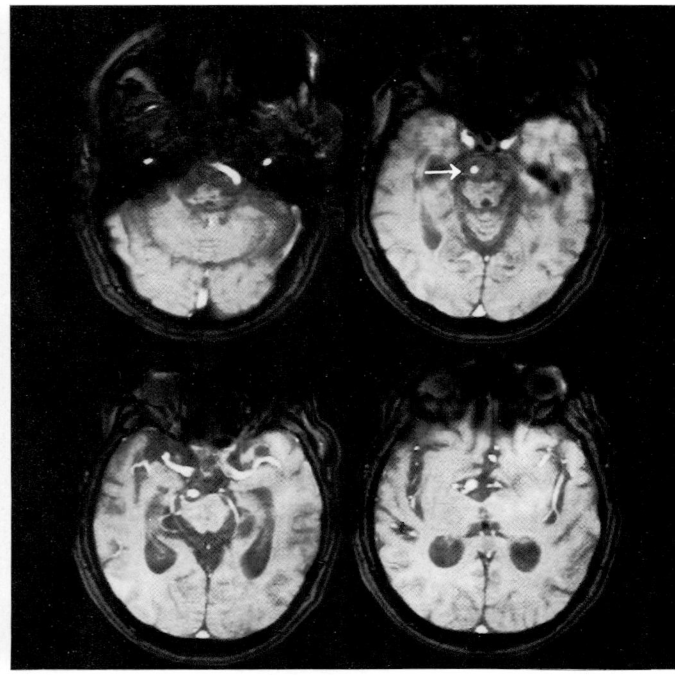

B

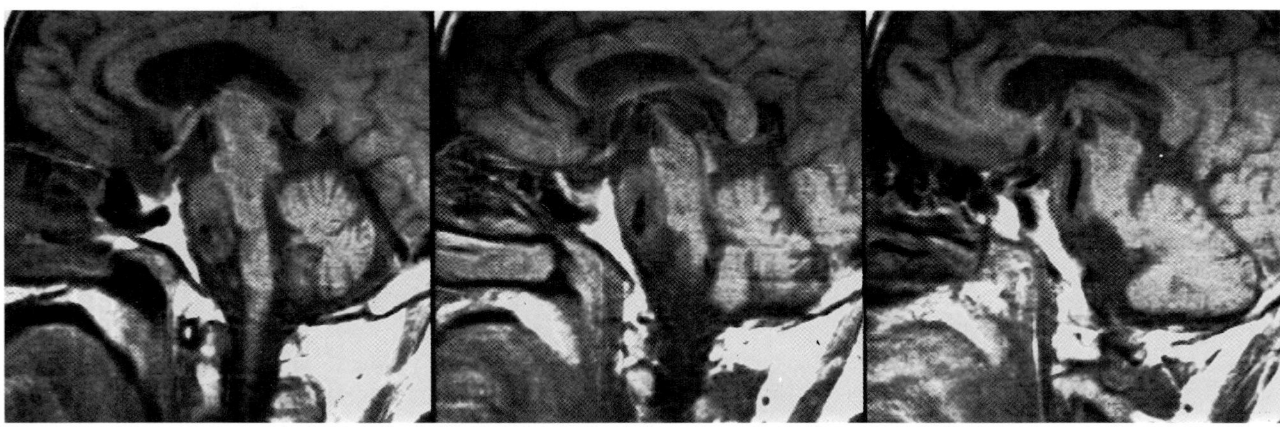

C

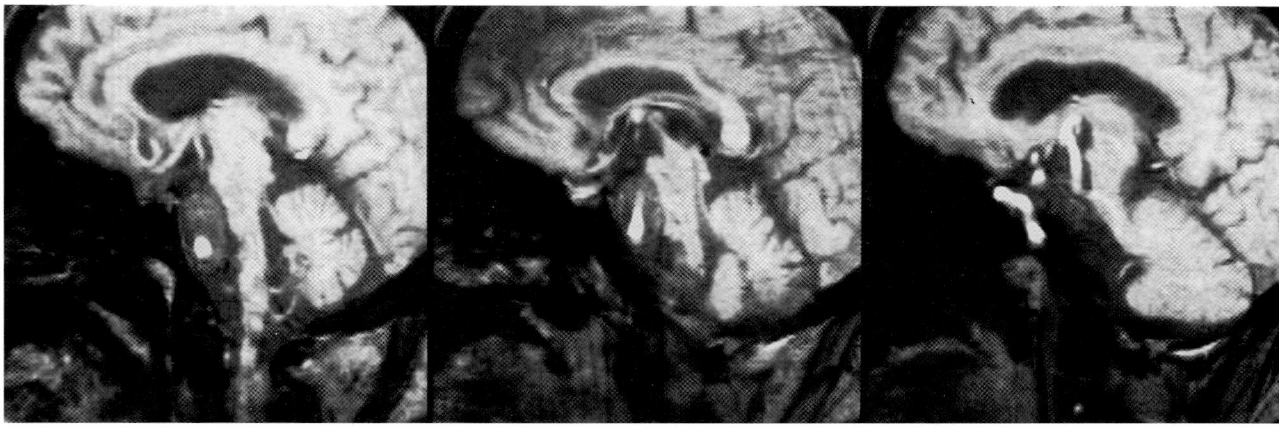

D

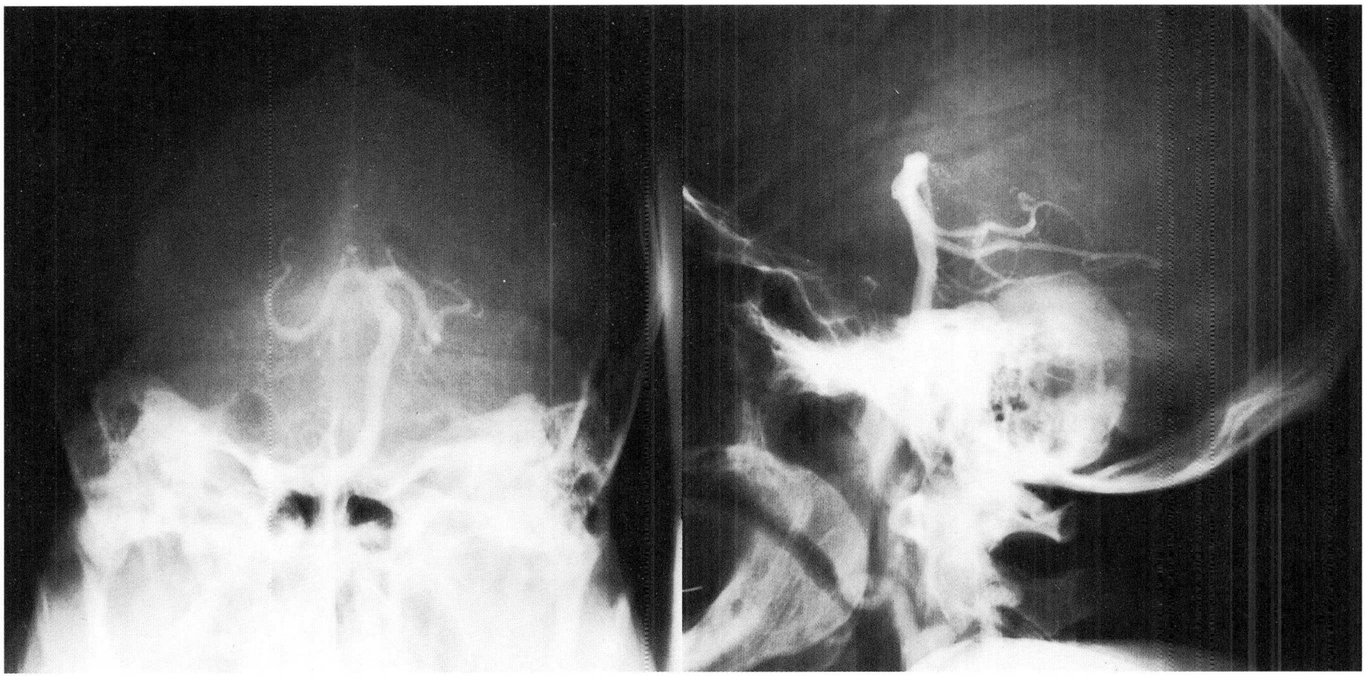

E F

Fig. 15. *Giant aneurysm in dolichomegabasilar artery*. 45-year-old man with spastic tetraparesis. The CT showed a hardly characterizable, space-occupying lesion anterior to the pons. A – T_1-weighted axial SE sequence: the aneurysm involves the B.A. completely from the confluence of the V.A.s (↑) to the origin of the P.C.A.s (→). The lumen of the artery is eccentric, occasionally shrunk but with flow. Observe the considerable thickness of the parietal thrombus. The aneurysm has a mass effect on the pons, which exhibits small tissue damage areas. B – Sections similar to the previous one but with fast imaging and flow compensation (TR 0.115; TE 12, FA 40°). These sections show the patency of the arterial lumen inside the aneurysm and of the vessels of the circle of Willis. The sagittal images, T_1-weighted (C) and with flow compensation (D), better demonstrate: verticalization of the B.A., whose distal end uplifts the lamina terminalis of the third ventricle in a "flap-like" fashion; and compression of the pons with posterior displacement of the brainstem. Anteroposterior (E) and lateral (F) conventional vertebral arteriogram: dolichomegabasilar artery without parietal changes or signs of aneurysmal alterations. In this case, MRI is conclusive for the characterization of the disease.

References

1. Atlas SW (1988) Intracranial vascular malformations and aneurysms. Current imaging applications. Radiol Clin North Am 26:821–837
2. Atlas SW, Grossman RI, Goldberg HI et al. (1987) Partially thrombosed giant intracranial aneurysms: correlation of MR and pathologic findings. Radiology 162:111–114
3. Atlas SW, Mark AS, Fram EK, Grossman RI (1988) Vascular intracranial lesions: Applications of gradient-echo MR imaging. Radiology 169:455–461
4. Augustyn GT, Scott JA, Olson E et al. (1985) Cerebral venous angiomas: MR imaging. Radiology 156:391–395
5. Barloon TJ, Yuth WT, Chiang FL et al. (1989) Lesions involving the fourth ventricle evaluated by CT and MR: A comparative study. Magn Reson Imaging 7:635–642
6. Belec L, Cesaro P, Brugieres P et al. (1988) Tumor-simulating giant serpentine aneurysm of the posterior cerebral artery. Surg Neurol 29:210–215
7. Biondi A, Scialfa G (1988) Morphological and blood flow MR findings in cerebral vascular malformations. J Neuroradiol 15:253–265
8. Biondi A, Scialfa G, Scotti G (1988) Intracranial aneurysms: MR Imaging. Neuroradiology 30:214–218
9. Bozzao L, Bastianello S, Fantozzi LM et al. (1988) Angiographic, CT and MRI study of cryptic brain stem vascular malformations. J Neuroradiol 15:148–159
10. Bradley WG Jr, Waluch V (1985) Blood flow: magnetic resonance imaging. Radiology 154:443–450
11. Bronen RA, Sze G (1990) Magnetic resonance contrast agents: theory and application to the central nervous system. J Neurosurg 73:820–840
12. Creasy JL, Price RR, Presbrey T et al. (1990) Gadolinium-enhanced MR angiography. Radiology 175:280–283
13. Destian S, Sze G, Krol G et al. (1988) MR imaging of hemorrhagic intracranial neoplasms. AJNR 9:1115–1122
14. Edelman RR, Mattle HP, Atkinson DJ (1990) Cerebral blood flow: assessment with dynamic contrast-enhanced T2-weighted MR imaging at 1.5 T. Radiology 176:211–220
15. Felix R, Shorner W, Laniado M et al. (1985) Brain tumors: MR imaging with gadolinium-DTPA. Radiology 156:681–688
16. Fontaine S, de la Sayette W, Gianfelice D et al. (1987) CT, MRI, and Angiography of venous angiomas: A comparative study. J Can Assoc Radiol 38:259–263
17. Fox JL (ed) (1983) Intracranial aneurysms. Springer, New York
18. Fortuna A, Ferrante L, Mastronardi L et al. (1989) Cerebral cavernous angioma in children. Childs Nerv Syst 5:201–207
19. Gadian DG, Payne JA, Bryant DJ et al. (1985) Gadolinium-DTPA as a contrast agent in MR imaging: theoretical projections and practical observations. J Comput Assist Tomogr 9:242–251
20. Gomori JM, Grossman RI, Goldberg HI et al. (1986) Occult cerebro-vascular malformations: high field MR imaging. Radiology 158:707–713
21. Gray L, Blinder RA, Djang WT (1990) Magnetic resonance imaging of cerebrovascular diseases. In: Wilkins RH, Rengachary SS (eds) Neurosurgery. McGraw-Hill, New York, 69–87
22. Griffin C, DeLaPaz R, Enzmann D (1987) Magnetic Resonance appearance of slow flow vascular malformations of the brainstem. Neuroradiology 29:506–511
23. Harder T, Dewes W, Solymosi L et al. (1989) MR tomography, CT and Angiography of vascular malformations of the central nervous system. ROFO 150:119–124
24. Hardy PA, Kucharczyk W, Henkelman RM (1990) Cause of signal loss in MR images of old hemorrhagic lesions. Radiology 174:549–555
25. Heffez DS, Zinreich SJ, Long DM (1990) Surgical resection of intrinsic brain stem lesions: an overview. Neurosurgery 27:789–797
26. Hendrix LE, Kneeland JB, Haughton VM (1990) MR Imaging of optic nerve lesions: Value of Gadopentetate Dimeglumine and fat-suppression technique. AJNR 11:749–754
27. Imakita S, Nishimura T, Yamada N et al. (1989) Cerebral vascular malformations: Applications of Magnetic Resonance Imaging to differential diagnosis. Neuroradiology 31:320–325
28. Koos WT, Miller MH (1971) Intracranial Tumors of Infants and Children. Mosby, St Louis
29. Kucharczyk W, Lemme-Pleghos L, Uske A et al. (1985) Intracranial vascular malformations: MR and CT imaging. Radiology 156:383–389
30. Leblanc R, Levesque M, Comair Y (1987) Magnetic resonance imaging of cerebral vascular malformations. Neurosurgery 21:15–20
31. Lee BCP, Herzberg L, Zimmerman RD et al. (1985) MR imaging of cerebral vascular malformations. AJNR 6:863–870

32. Levy RP, Fabrikant JI, Frankel KA et al. (1989) Stereotactic heavy-charged-particle bragg peak radiosurgery for the treatment of intracranial arteriovenous malformations in childhood and adolescence. Neurosurgery 24:841–852
33. Lo WW, Shelton C, Waluch V et al. (1989) Intratemporal vascular tumors: detection with CT and MR imaging. Radiology 171:445–448
34. Marchal G, Bosmans H, Van Fraeyenhoven L et al. (1990) Intracranial vascular lesions: optimization and clinical evaluation of three-dimensional time-of-flight MR angiography. Radiology 175:443–448
35. Matsumura K, Saito A, Nakasu Y et al. (1990) Magnetic Resonance Imaging of large and giant intracranial aneurysms. Neurol Med Chir 30:382–388
36. Needell WM, Maravilla KR (1988) MR flow imaging in vascular malformations using gradient recalled acquisition. AJNR 9:637–642
37. Olsen WL, Brant-Zawadzki M, Hodes J et al. (1987) Giant intracranial aneurysms: MR imaging. Radiology 163:431–435
38. Parizel PM, Degryse HJ, Gheuens J et al. (1989) Gadolinium-DTPA enhanced MR imaging of intracranial lesions. Comput Assist Tomogr 13:378–385
39. Rapacki TF, Brantley MJ, Furlow TM Jr et al. (1990) Heterogeneity of cerebral cavernous hemangiomas diagnosed by MR imaging. J Comput Assist Tomogr 14:18–25
40. Rigamonti D, Spetzler RF, Drayer BP et al. (1988) Appearance of venous malformations on Magnetic Resonance Imaging. J Neurosurg 69:535–539
41. Rigamonti D, Spetzler RF, Medina M et al. (1990) Cerebral venous malformations. J Neurosurg 73:560–564
42. Rigamonti D, Drayer BP, Johnson PC et al. (1987) The MRI appearance of cavernous malformations (angiomas). J Neurosurg 67:518–524
43. Sigal R, Krief O, Houtteville JP et al. (1990) Occult cerebrovascular malformations: Follow-up with MR imaging. Radiology 176:815–819
44. Sze G, Krol G, Olsen WL et al. (1987) Hemorrhagic neoplasms: MR mimics of occult vascular malformations. AJR 149(6):223–230
45. Tobias JA (1989) MRI of intracranial vascular disease with emphasis at low and intermediate field strengths (images at 0.35–1.0 T). In: Pomeranz SJ (ed) Craniospinal Magnetic Resonance Imaging. W. B. Saunders Co, Philadelphia, 315–350
46. Trussart V, Berry I, Manelfe C et al. (1989) Epileptogenic cerebral vascular malformations and MRI. J Neuroradiol 16:273–284
47. Waluch V, Dyck P (1990) Magnetic resonance imaging of posterior fossa masses. In: Wilkins RH, Rengachary SS (eds) Neurosurgery Update I. McGraw-Hill, New York, 30–46
48. Weil SM, Tew JM Jr (1990) Surgical management of brain stem vascular malformations. Acta Neurochir (Wien) 105:14–23
49. Worthington BS, Kean DM, Hawkes RC et al. (1983) NMR imaging in the recognition of giant intracranial aneurysms. AJNR 4:835–836
50. Yaşargil M (1988) Venous, cavernous and occult angiomas. In: Yaşargil M (ed) Microneurosurgery, Vol. IIIb. Thieme, Stuttgart, 405–438

CHAPTER X

Intracranial metastatic tumors

Intracranial metastases may be single *(Figs. 1, 3)*, multiple or diffuse *(Figs. 2, 9, 11, 13)*. The diffuse metastases have a meningeal location, whereas the others are commonly found in the tissue. They are believed to prefer the more richly vascularized districts (boundary between the cortex and the white matter), but this assumption is not unanimous, just as there are discordant views on their predilection for the left hemisphere.

Single metastases account for some 40–50% of all solid parenchymal metastases; they involve the brain in 80% of cases, the cerebellum in 16% and the brainstem in 4%.

Their incidence on tumor patients is 25–30%, but this percentage varies considerably depending on the organ affected by the primary tumor. Primary lung tumors and those that preferentially metastasize to the lung (breast carcinoma and melanoma) may reach a frequency of around 40%; they are followed by tumors of the urogenital tract, liver, pancreas and colon, and by sarcomas and systemic tumors, such as leukemias and lymphomas.

The time interval between diagnosis of the primary tumor and onset of metastases varies depending on oncotype and is shorter for lung tumors and longer for breast tumors.

Macroscopically, they appear as roundish and at times wedge-shaped nodules *(Fig. 16)*, with sharp contours, surrounded by edematous or gliotic brain tissue; inside such structures, vascular alterations may occur, that are typical of malignant glial tumors *(Fig. 15)*; this fact explains the fairly frequent intra- and perilesional hemorrhages and the necrotic and/or colliquative alterations of the abscess-type *(Fig. 14)* that accompany these metastases. In the absence of a positive tumor history, the neurological symptomatology is indistinguishable from that of other space-occupying intracerebral lesions and is therefore meaningless for diagnostic purposes. However, the presence of a fast-growing subcortical lesion surrounded by considerable cerebral edema (even when the lesion is small) may help make a correct diagnosis *(Fig. 12)*.

In the case of multiple metastases originated from the same primary tumor, various regressive events (necroses, hemorrhages or cysts), as well as various degrees of edema up to involvement of the whole hemisphere, may be observed. A differential diagnosis versus abscess-type, ischemic-hemorrhagic and parasitic lesions, or even multicentric gliomas, should be made, also by means of stereotactic biopsy.

The development of one or more metastases denotes *per se* the malignant nature of a neoplastic process, whose prognosis is therefore directly related to the oncotype and to its sensitivity to therapy. Nevertheless, sarcoma metastases seem to grow at a slower rate compared with malignant epithelial tumors. A similar behavior is noticed in breast and skin carcinomas, as well as in hypernephromas, in which the primary tumor grows rapidly and metastasizes at an early stage, whereas secondary lesions grow more slowly. While lung tumors have a rather slow local growth, their metastases develop rapidly and at an early stage.

On T_1 MR images, the metastases not complicated by regression phenomena produce an isointense or relatively hypointense signal with respect to the grey matter, while on T_2-weighted images their signal is relatively hyperintense.

The repetitive lesions of some oncotypes, such as melanomas and lung adenocarcinomas, may have special characteristics, owing to substances producing a paramagnetic effect: high signal on T_1-weighted images and/or very low signal on T_2-weighted sequences *(Figs. 5, 6, 7)*.

Metastases are often accompanied by hemorrhage which is due to their fast growth, abundant vascular neoformation or to predisposing factors such as coagulopathies or hypertension. The metastases that more frequently present hemorrhages are those of melanomas, hypernephromas, choriocarcinomas and at times of lung neoplasms. In such cases, the intensity of the signal will vary in relation to the acute, subacute or chronic stage of the bleeding.

The presence of intense edema is typical of metastatic lesions and at times it may be such as to partially mask the tumor focus, making it difficult to precisely evaluate size and number of foci. However, quite often there may be no edema at all. This is the case above all of the metastases from lung neoplasms, melanomas, and at times of the metastases from breast neoplasms. In such cases, especially if the lesion is small, MRI signal changes may not reflect repetitive lesions, since they are similar to those observed in gliosis caused by degenerative diseases and by chronic vascular insufficiency, alterations which may be concomitant with the metastases.

In order to make a differential diagnosis in such cases, it is necessary not only to establish whether they have a predominantly subcortical location *(Figs. 9, 10)* but also to use paramagnetic contrast agents to see whether there is a high degree of perfusion, typical of metastatic lesions *(Fig. 11)*.

I.v. administration of paramagnetic contrast agents is very useful in the diagnostic study of diffuse subependymal, choroidal and leptomeningeal metastases, which would otherwise be difficult to detect with a standard MRI examination *(Fig. 11)*.

Brain metastases can be treated with drugs, surgery, radiation therapy, chemotherapy and a combination of the foregoing methods. Medical therapy with corticosteroids alone is a palliative treatment, but in combination or in sequence with other treatments it contributes greatly to the reduction of brain edema.

In the case of a single metastasis, surgery is indicated when the primary tumor is not a fast-growing one and when it has not yet metastasized to other orgnas. Focal radiation therapy is to be preferred over radiation of the whole brain; the latter treatment is to be reserved for long-term survivors when new metastases appear. The type of chemotherapy varies depending on the primary tumor; its efficacy lies in the reduction of the volume of multiple brain metastases.

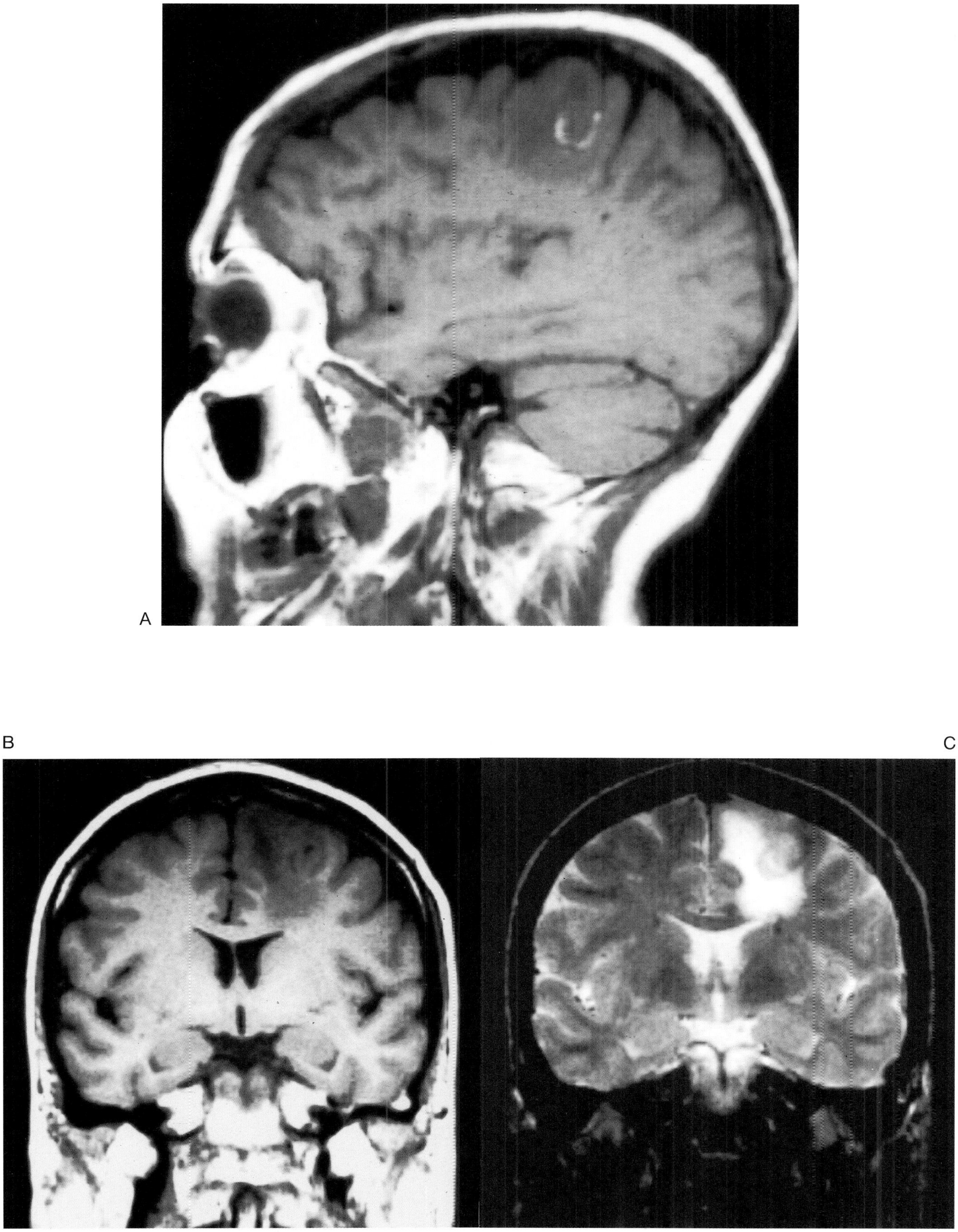

Fig. 1. *Single left parietal metastasis from lung neoplasm.* A – T_1-weighted sagittal section: the metastasis is demarcated from the surrounding edema by a hyperintense ring, ascribable to bleeding. B – Proton density-weighted coronal section: a rounded lesion with higher signal is evidenced inside the edema. C – T_2-weighted coronal image: the metastasis is better demarcated from the surrounding edema. The perilesional hemorrhage has low signal intensity owing to the presence of hemosiderin.

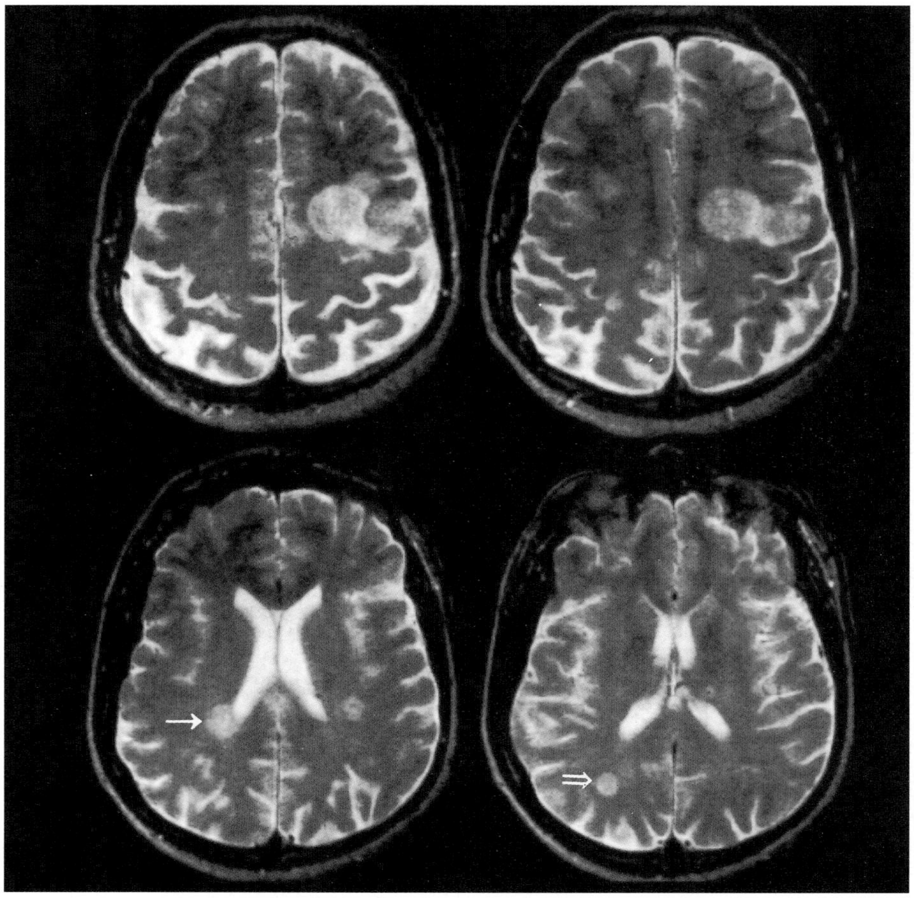

Fig. 2. *Multiple metastases from melanoma.* The T_2-weighted axial images visualize three conglomerate lesions in the left parietal region; their signal intensity is higher than that of the grey matter. Two other lesions can be noticed: in the periventricular area (→) and in the white matter of the occipital lobe (⇒).

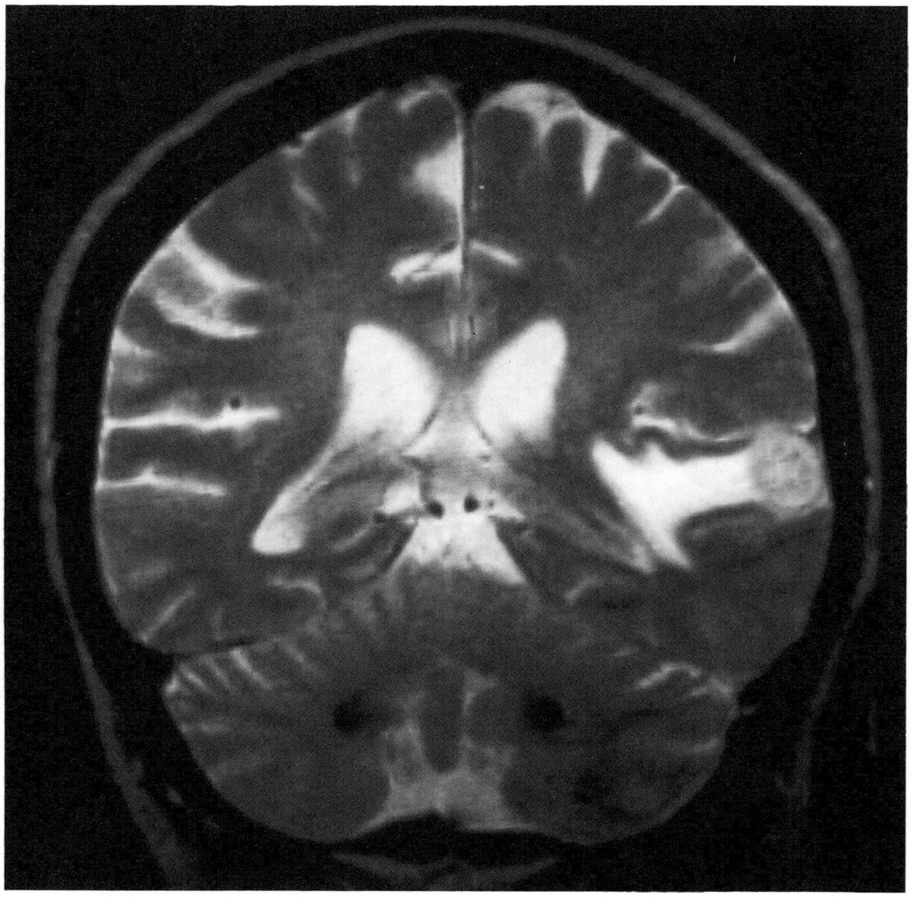

Fig. 3. *Single left subsylvian metastasis from breast neoplasm.* The T_2-weighted coronal image shows the cortical site of the metastasis with a medial edematous area.

A B

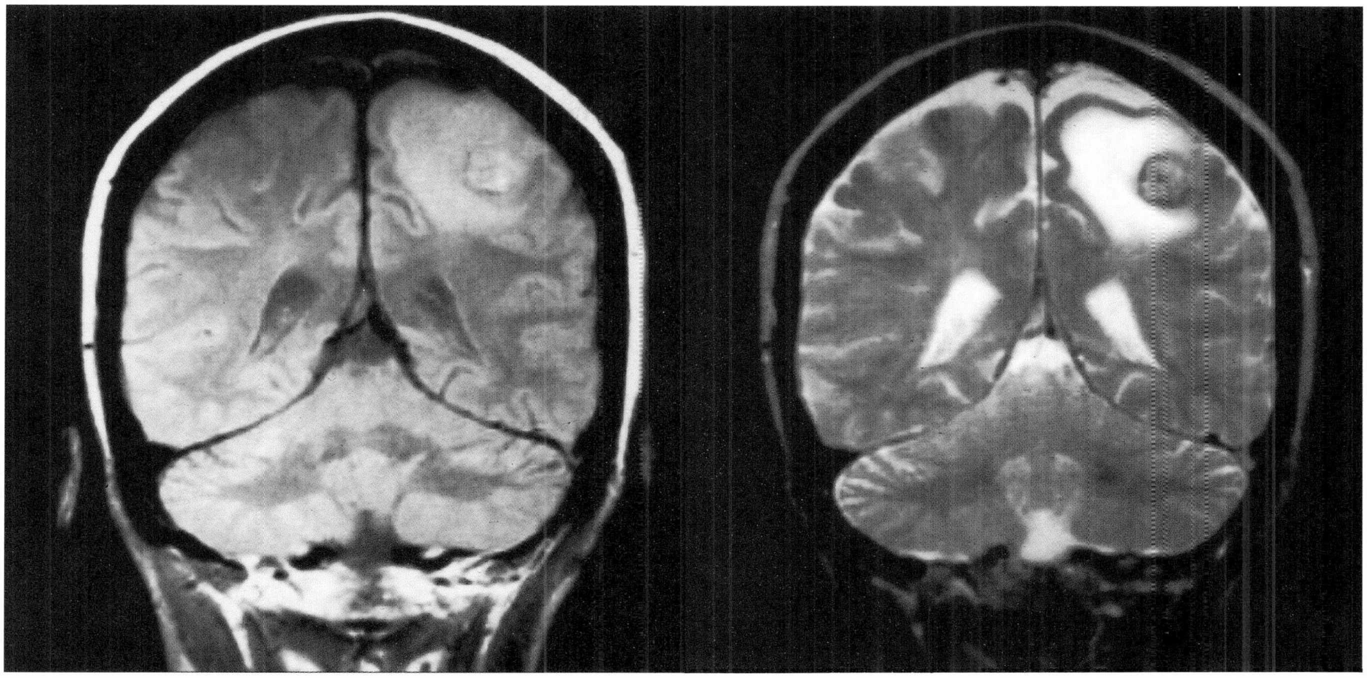

Fig. 4. *Left cortical parietal metastasis from breast tumor.* The CT was suggestive of a meningioma. Also on MRI examination, this metastasis presents some signal characteristics that are consistent with meningioma. However, the presence of edema and the subcortical site of the lesion on both T_1- (A) and T_2- (B) weighted images, together with patient history, suggest a metastasis. The lesion lies in a sulcus and the grey matter of the gyri is superficial with respect to the mass.

A B

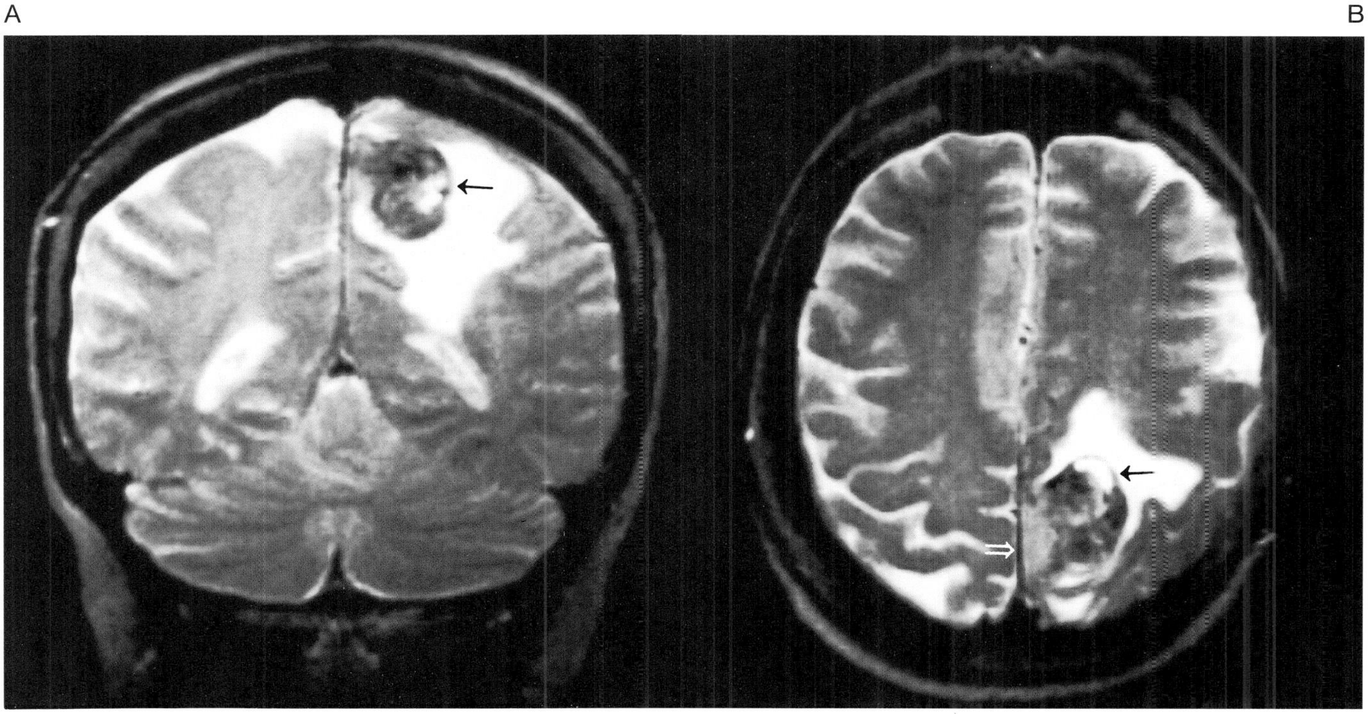

Fig. 5. *Left parasagittal parietal metastasis from melanoma.* T_2-weighted coronal (A) and axial (B) sections: as in the preceding case, the perilesional edema is clearly evident. The metastasis has a broad base (⇒) on the falx (meningiomatous appearance), an irregular signal with hemorrhagic foci (←), but above all low signal foci owing to the presence of material having paramagnetic effect (melanin).

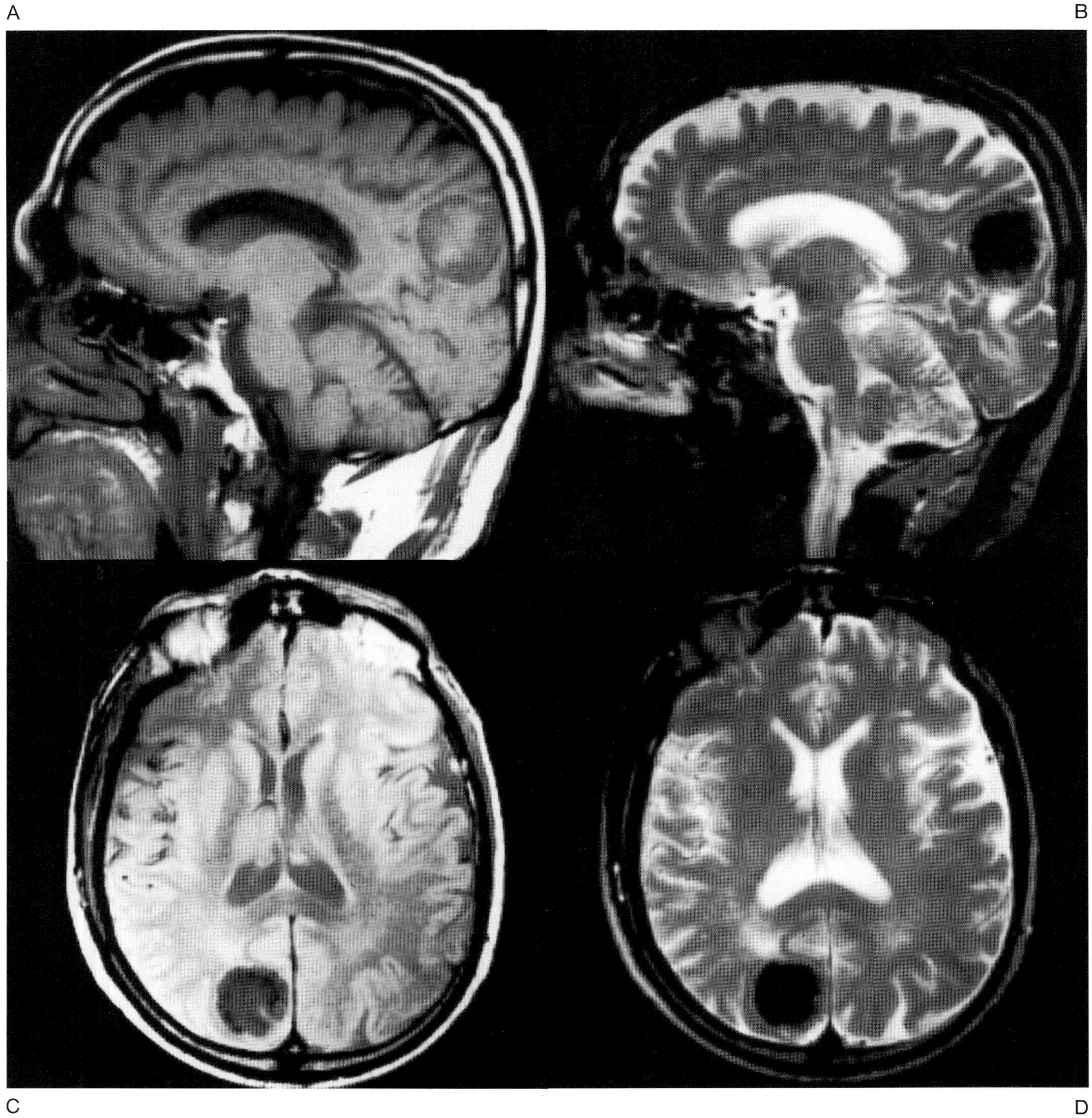

Fig. 6. *Right occipital metastasis from muciparous lung adenocarcinoma.* Huge, subcortical, non-edematogenic single metastasis producing an irregular signal with high intensity foci on the T_1-weighted view (A) and low intensity foci on both proton density- (C) and T_2- (B, D) weighted sequences owing to paramagnetic effect.

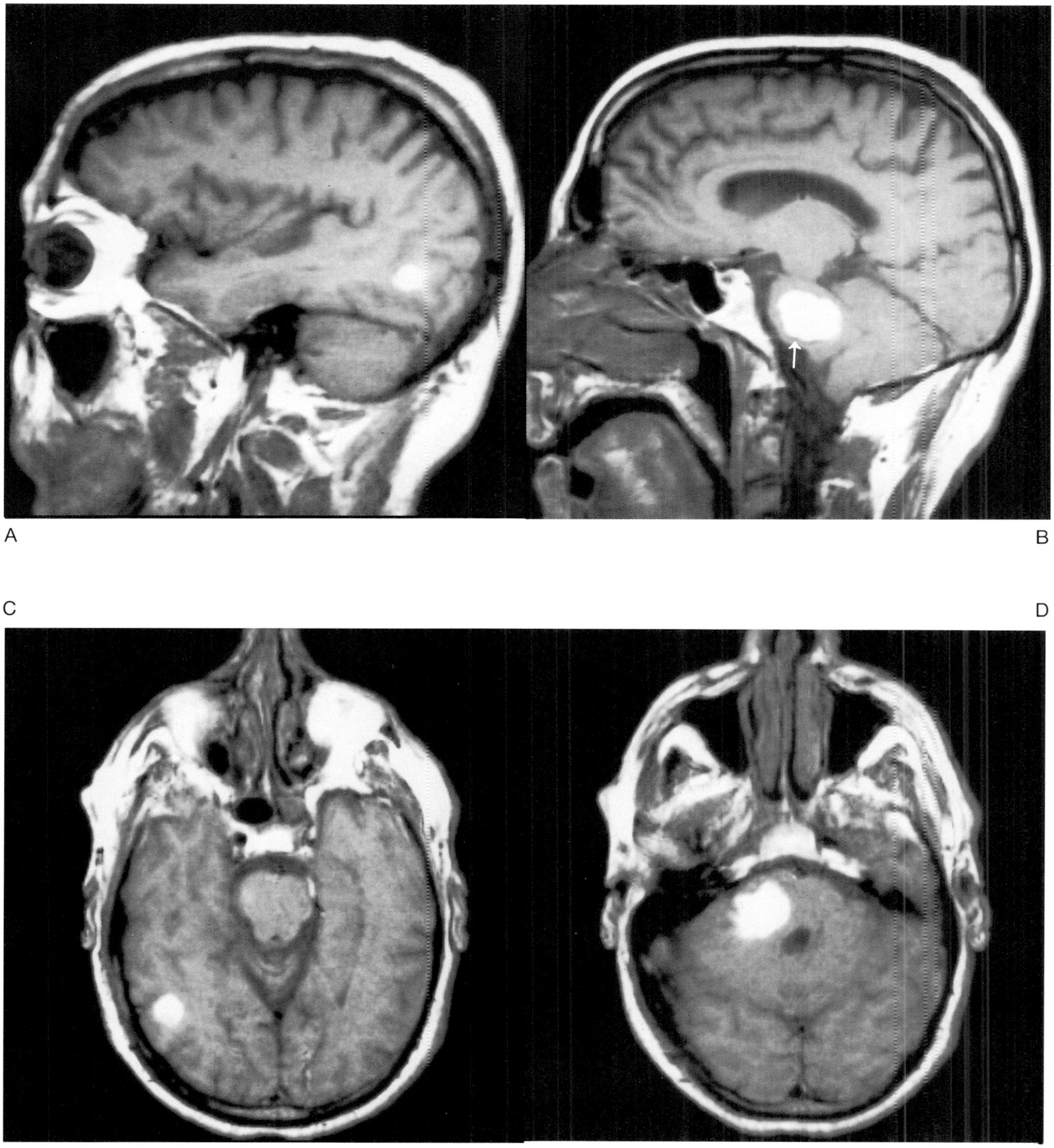

Fig. 7. *Multiple metastases from muciparous lung adenocarcinoma with cystic appearance*. The T_1-weighted sagittal (A, B) and axial (C, D) views demonstrate two lesions with a very high signal containing mucoid substances. Both lesions are not edematogenic. The CT scan had only visualized the metastases in the brainstem as a hypodense lesion surrounded by a thin perfusion ring (probably the wall of the cystic lesion). The arrow in B points to a thin hypointense wall (↑).

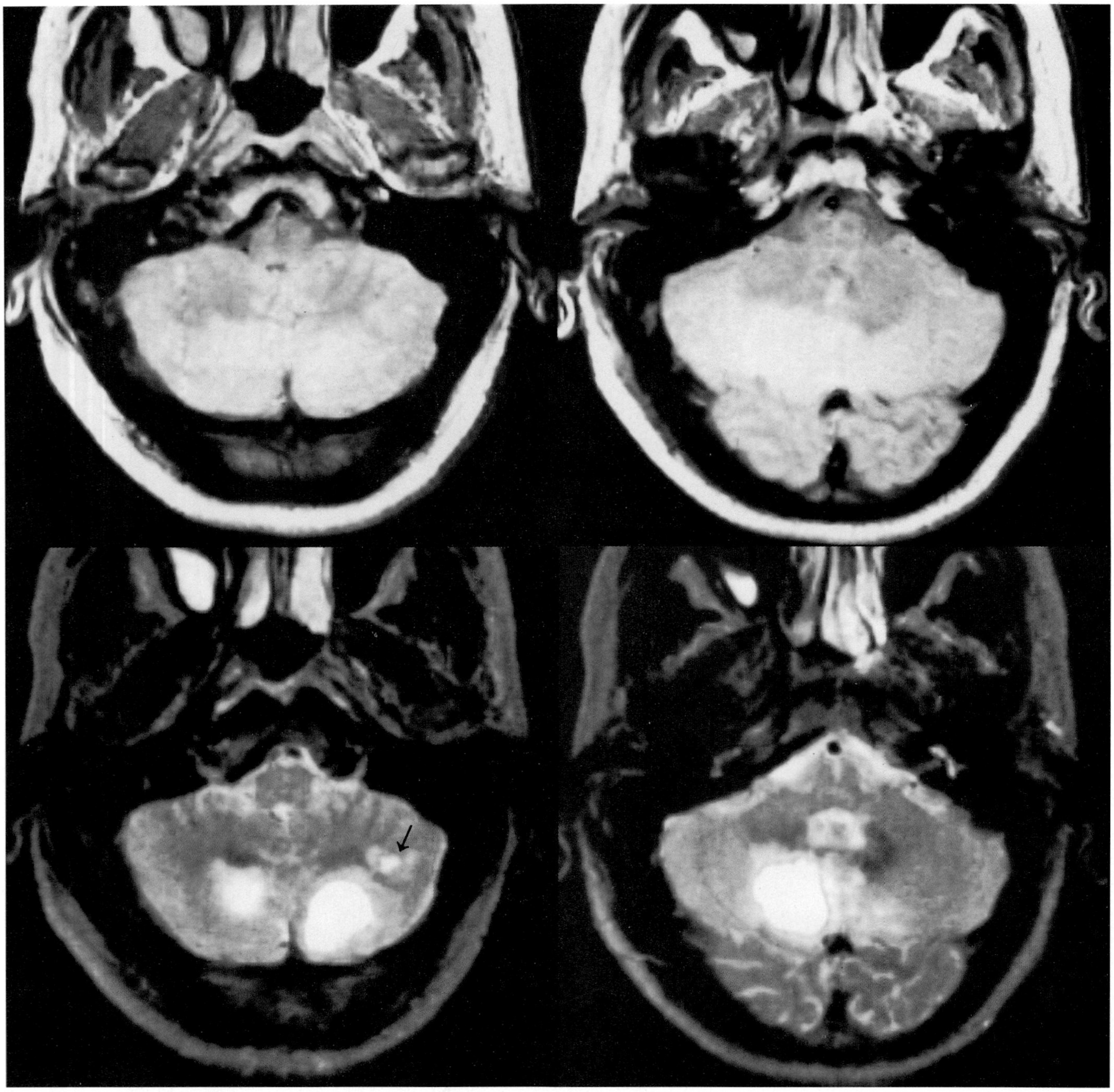

A B C D

Fig. 8. *Multiple metastases from lung neoplasm in the posterior cranial fossa.* Proton density- (A, B) and T_2- (C, D) weighted axial images: the metastases are well delineated in size and number and well differentiated from the surrounding edema only on the T_2-weighted images. Note the high sensitivity of MRI in evidencing even small-sized lesions (↙).

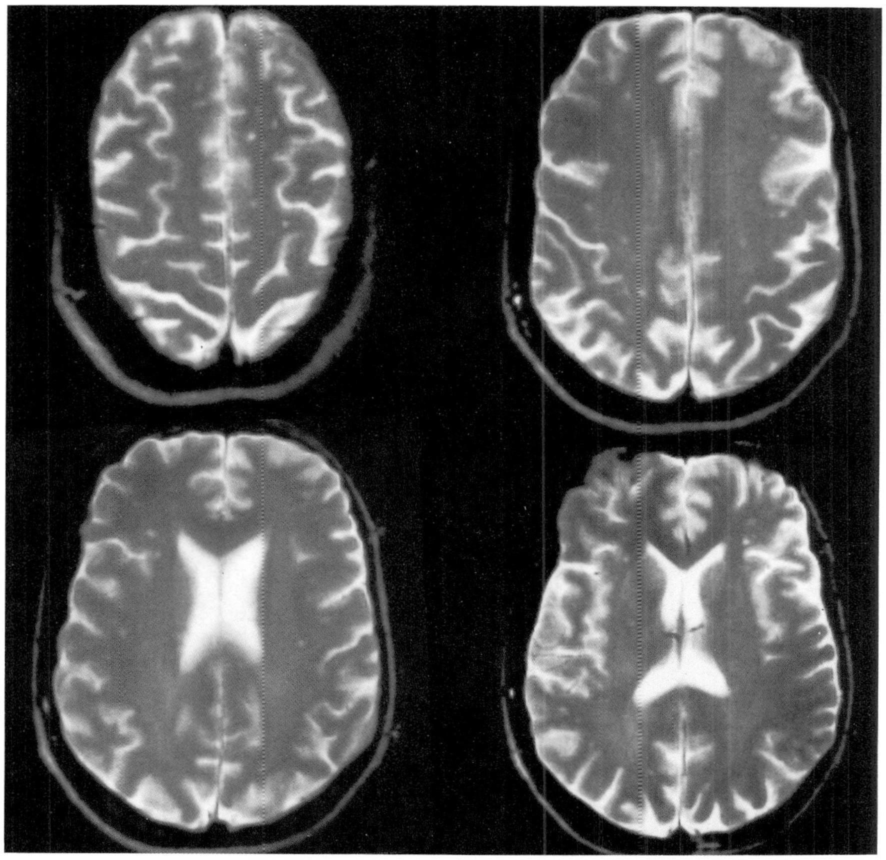

Fig. 9. *Multiple micrometastases from breast tumor.* The T_2-weighted axial views visualize minute, punctate, high-signal images which are consistent with metastases only on the basis of their subcortical location and of patient history.

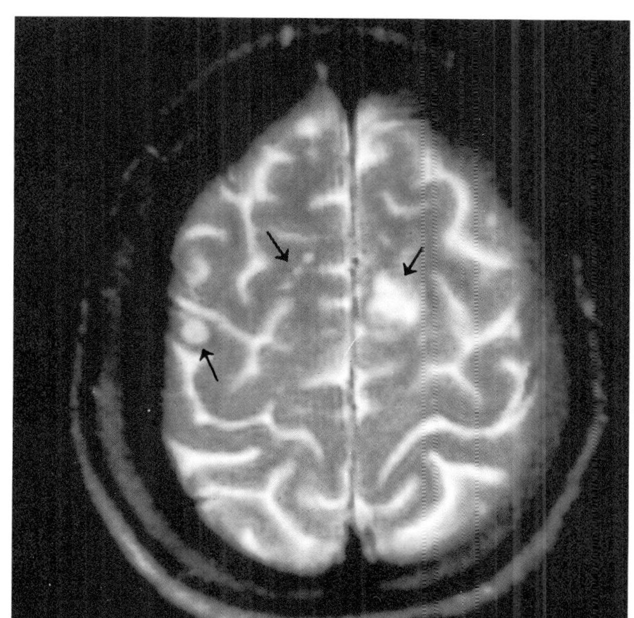

Fig. 10. *Frontal cortical metastases from lung neoplasm.* As in the previous case, the appearance of the lesion is not specific for repetitive lesions. In this case too, the clinical picture and site of the lesion are the basis for the diagnosis.

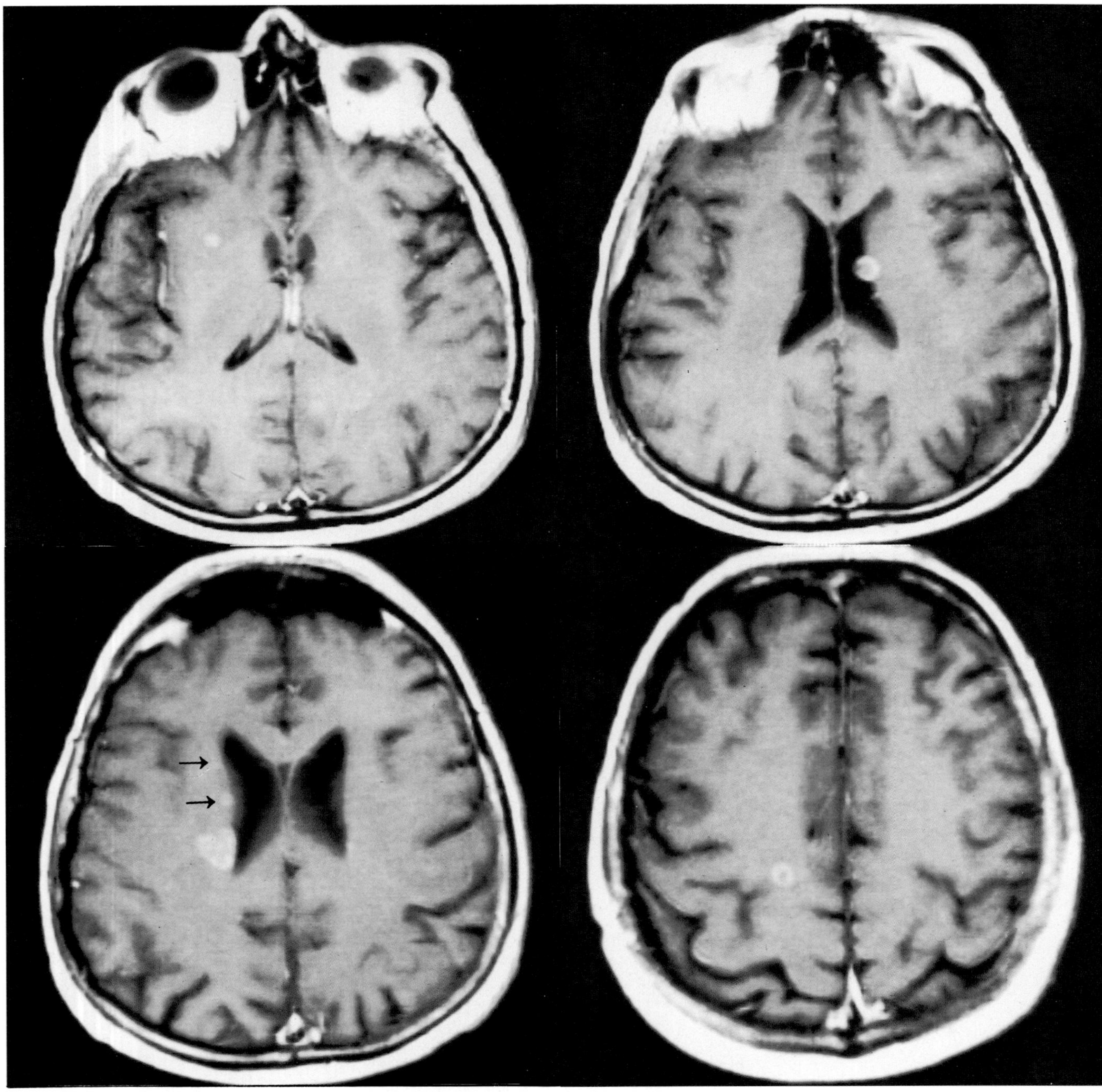

Fig. 11. *Multiple metastases from lung microcytoma.* T_2-weighted images after i.v. GD-DTPA. The paramagnetic contrast enhances the sensitivity of MRI in showing even very small lesions in the subependymal region (→). The larger lesions are necrotic at the center and do not present edema.

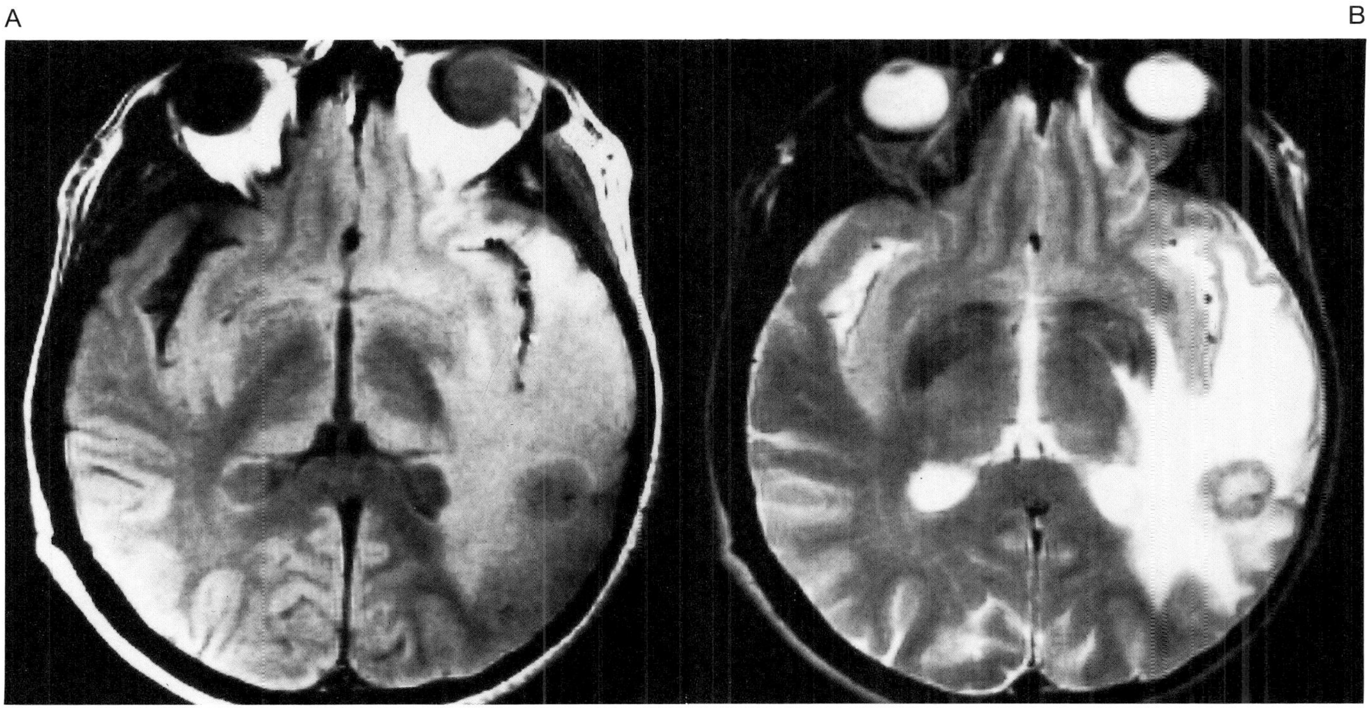

Fig. 12. *Subcortical left posterior temporal single metastasis from breast tumor.* Proton density- (A) and T_2- (B) weighted axial views: the neoplasm is sharply demarcated from the edema involving the whole of the temporal lobe. The T_2-weighted sequences visualize the central necrosis which presents high signal intensity.

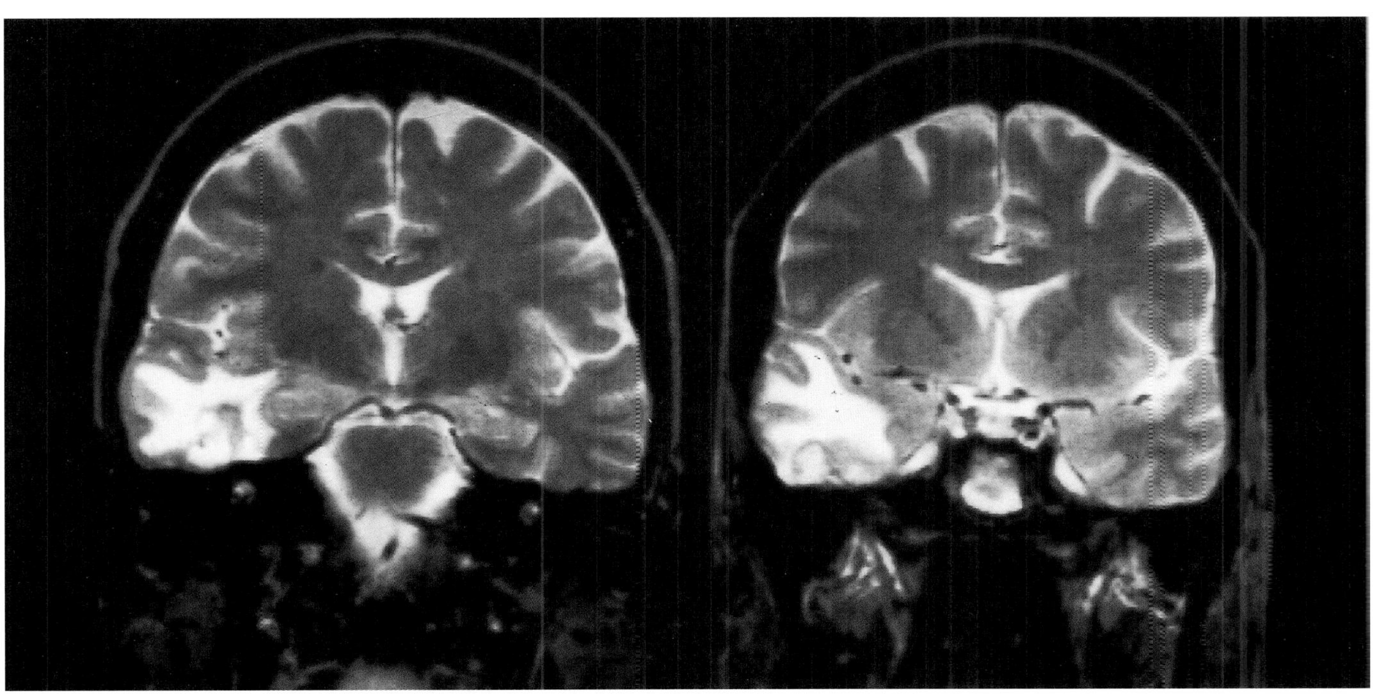

Fig. 13. *Right temporal basal leptomeningeal diffuse metastasis from breast carcinoma.* T_2-weighted coronal view: below an area of edema, a cluster of high-signal nodular lesions can be seen, which are in contact with the meningeal plane.

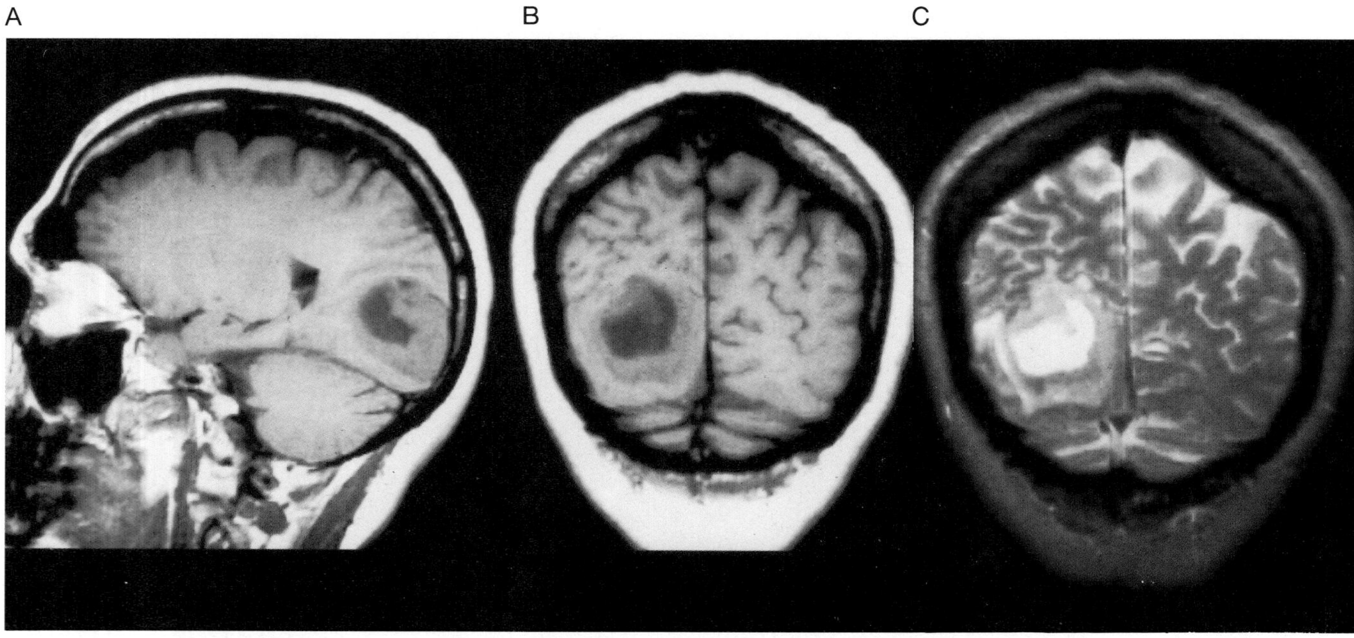

Fig. 14. *Right occipital single metastasis from breast neoplasm.* The lesion has a broad area of colliquative necrosis, whose signal intensity on the T_1- (A, B) and T_2- (C) weighted sequences is similar to that of the CSF. The internal morphology of the viable portion of the metastasis is irregular. Note the absence of edema.

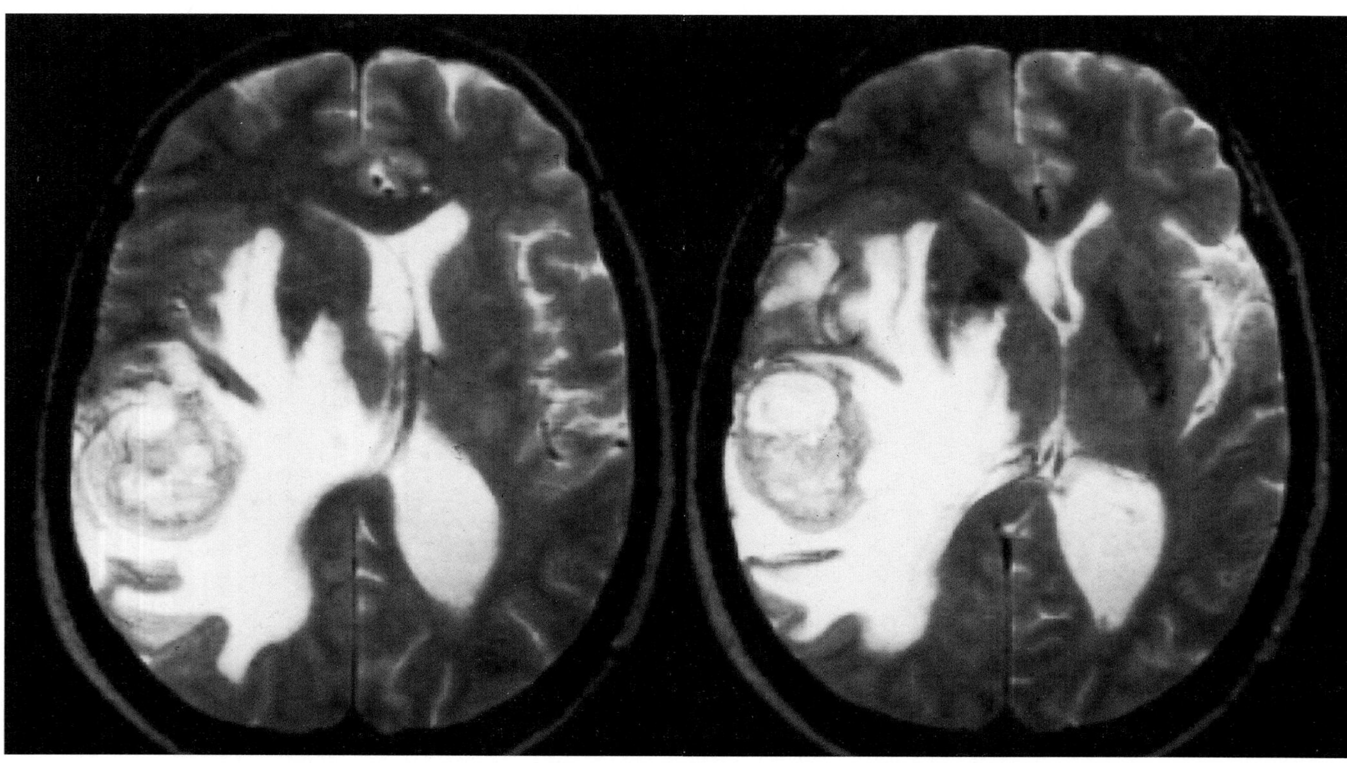

Fig. 15. *Right posterior temporal single metastasis from lung neoplasm.* Inside a vast edematous area, the T_2-weighted axial images show a lesion with highly irregular signal, simulating a malignant glial tumor. Note the considerable mass effect producing a contralateral displacement of the midline structures.

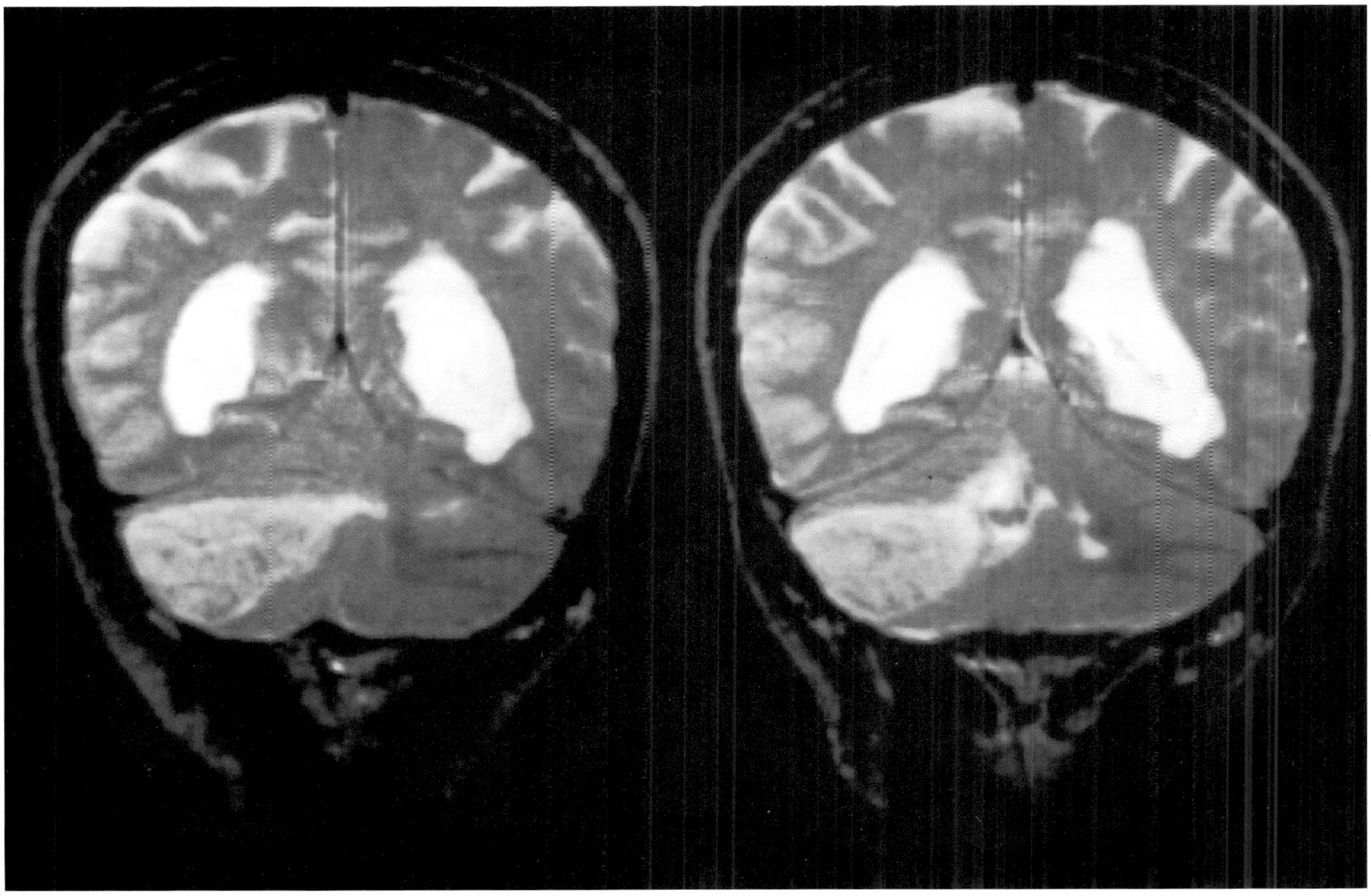

Fig. 16. *Right cerebellar metastasis from lung tumor*. The primary tumor was documented after cerebral MRI. The metastasis is wedge-like with the tip medially pointing to the right lateral recess of the fourth ventricle and with a homogeneous signal having an intensity slightly higher than that of the grey matter.

Fig. 17. *Metastasis of the pituitary gland and stalk from rectal carcinoma which presented with diabetes insipidus.* T_1-weighted sections before (A) and after (B, C) GD-DTPA. The dumbbell shape of the intra-suprasellar lesion is due to the sellar diaphragm (←). The intrasellar component grows especially on the right side and is eroding the floor and the ipsilateral anterior clinoid. The suprasellar portion occupies the chiasmal cistern, thus deforming the anterior aspect of the third ventricle. The metastasis is irregular owing to regressive events which are hypointense both before and after contrast.

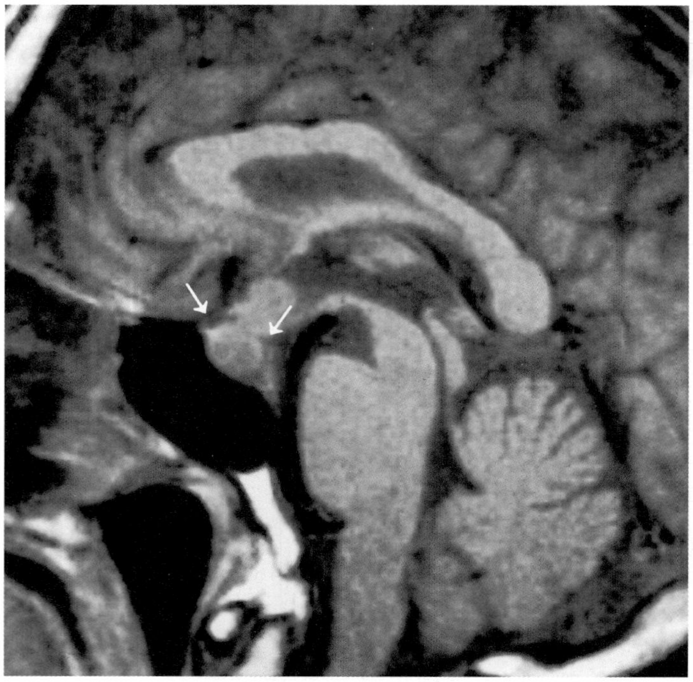

A

B

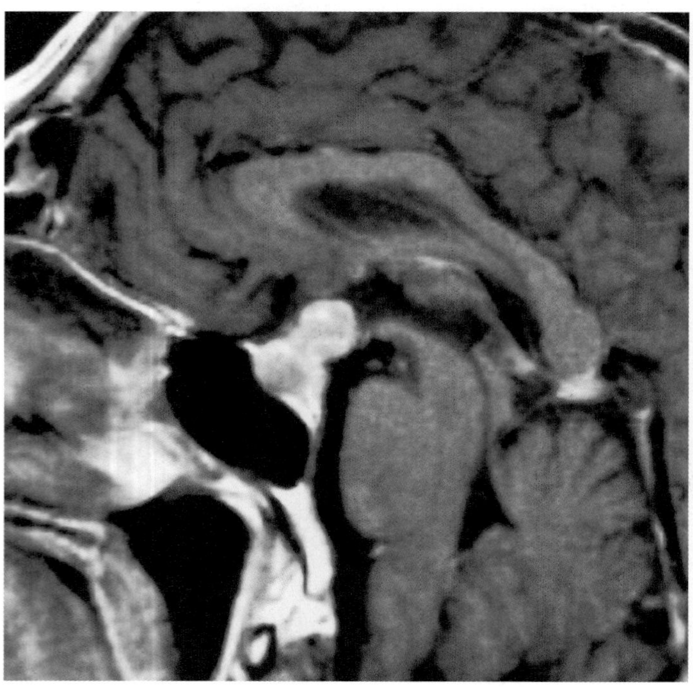

C

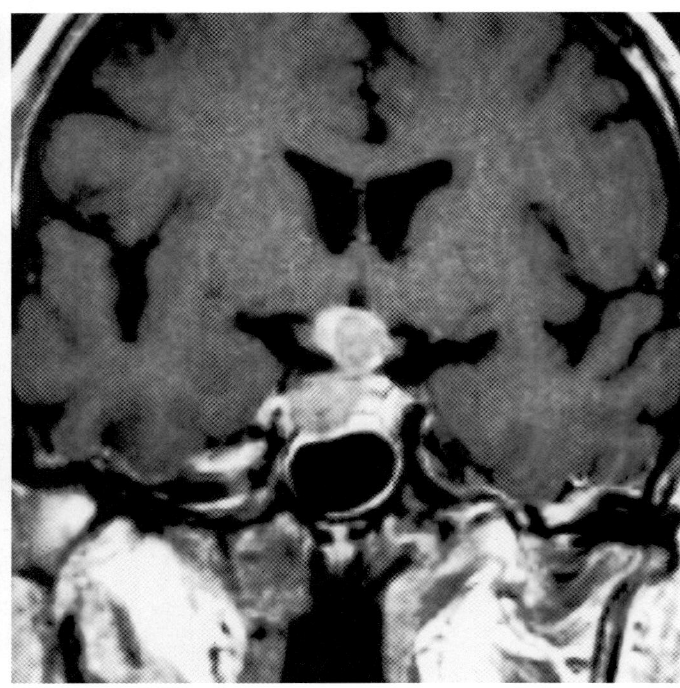

Fig. 18. *Intra-supra- and laterosellar metastasis.* 24-year-old patient with liposarcoma of the thigh. At the time of MRI examination, he complained of left opthalmoplegia and facial neuralgia, ascribable to an irritation of the first and second branch of the trigeminus. T_1-weighted images. On the sagittal view (A), the multilobular appearance of the neoplasm can be appreciated. It is isointense with the brainstem and part of its posterior portion protrudes into the interpeduncular cistern. The coronal view (B) visualizes the intrasellar invasion, the relationship to the optic chiasm and the involvement of the left cavernous sinus. On more posterior sections, note the extension of the neoplasm into the middle cranial fossa and the displacement of the medial gyri of the left temporal lobe (⇓).

A

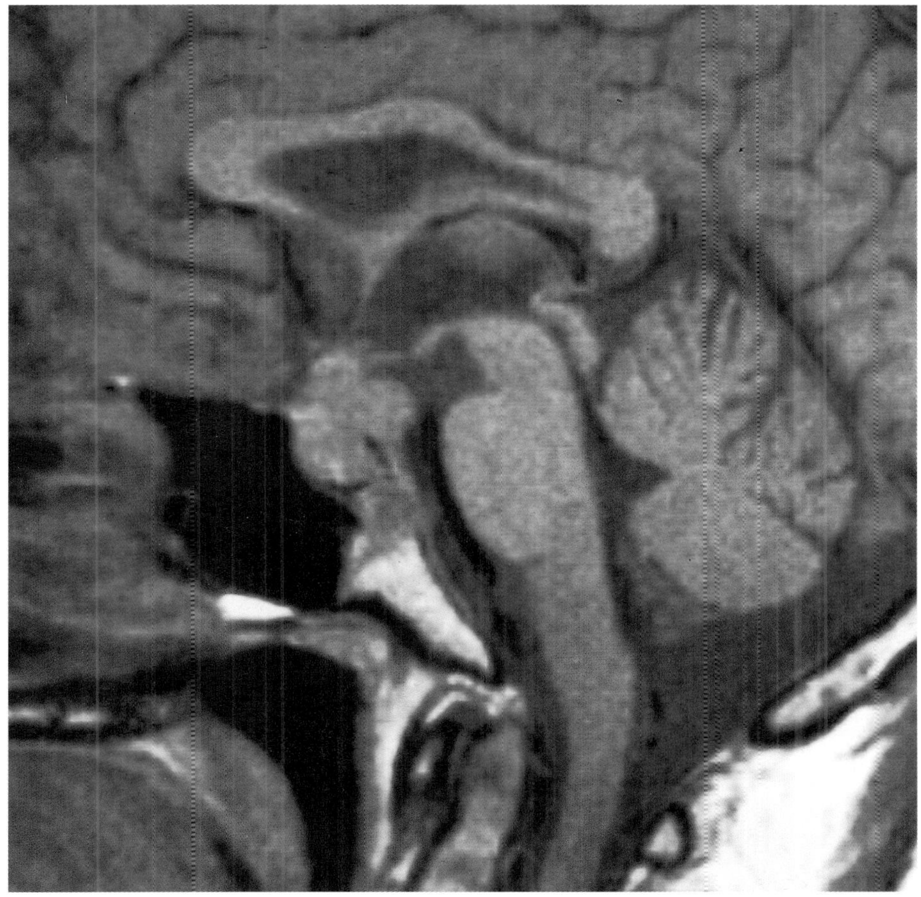

B

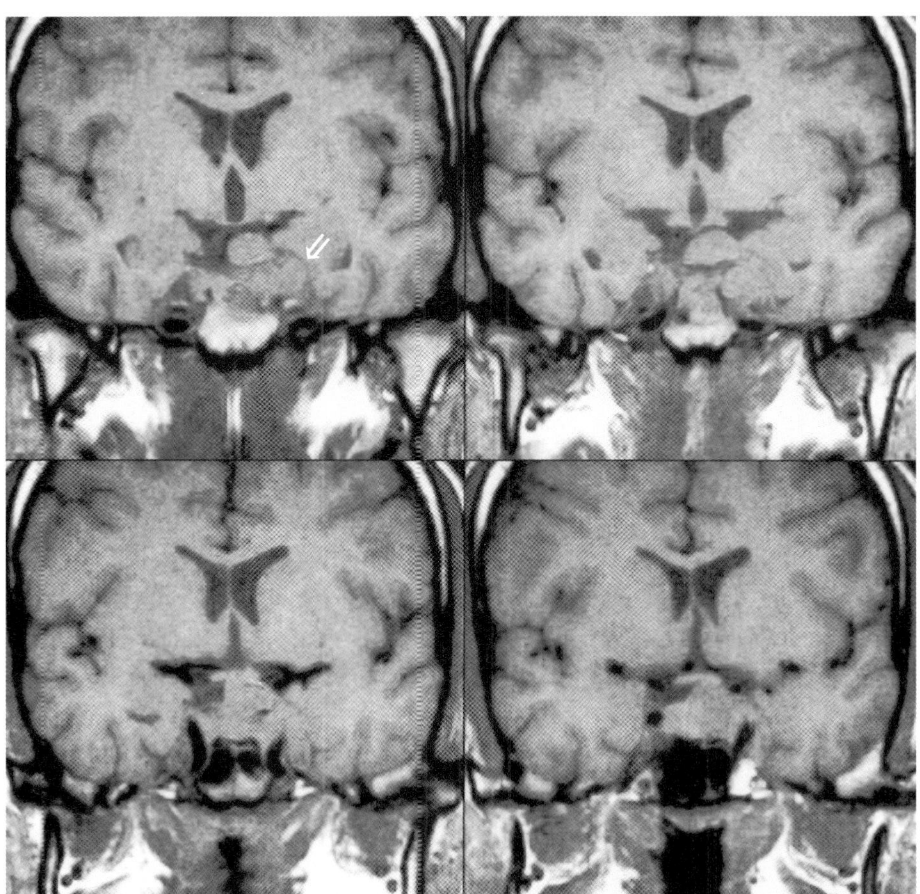

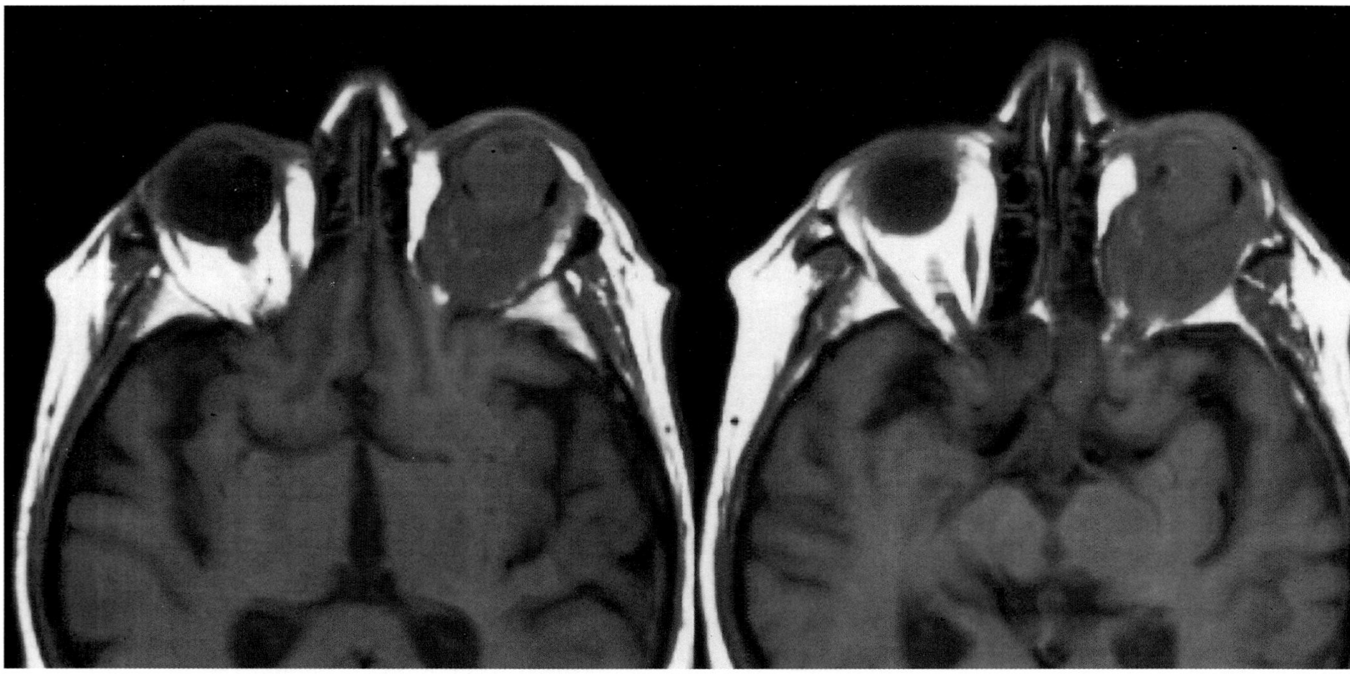

A

B

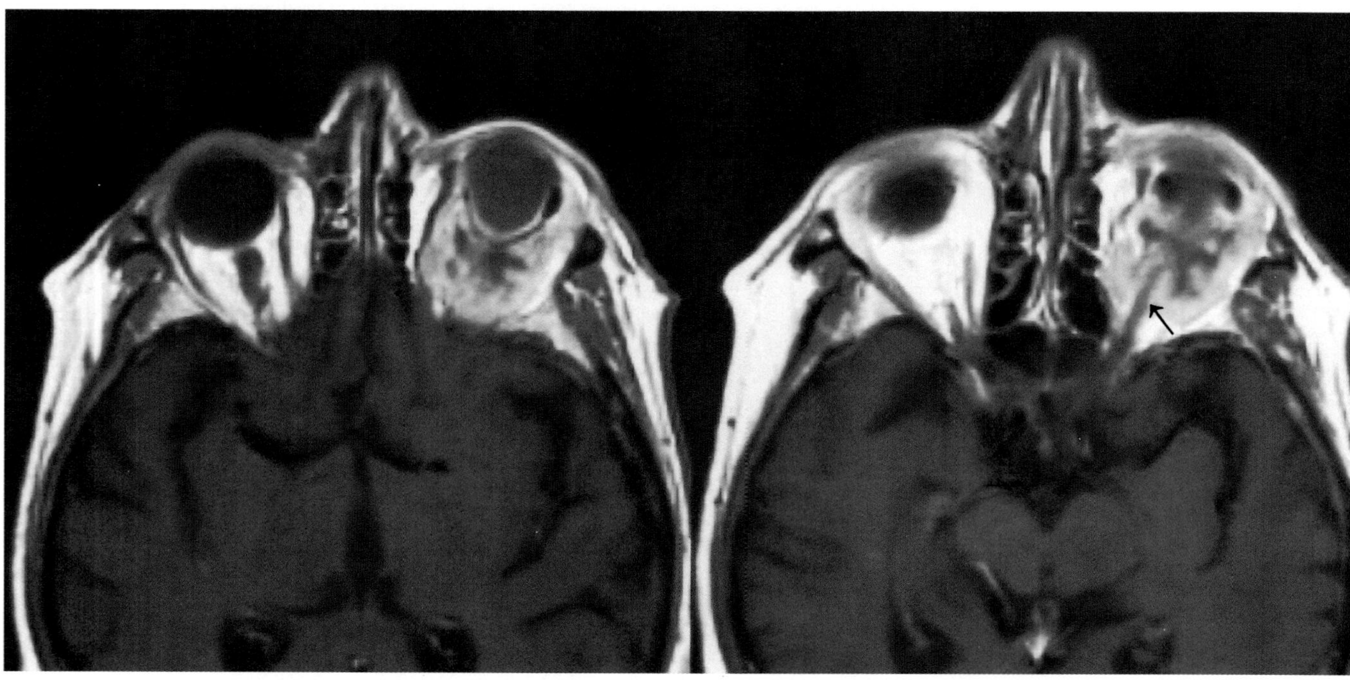

Fig. 19. *Left orbital metastasis from breast carcinoma.* T_1-weighted views pre- (A) and post- (B) GD-DTPA. The metastasis has infiltrated the muscular and fatty structures of the orbit, while the globe appears to be displaced anteriorly. The vitreous has a more intense signal than that of the contralateral one, probably due to disturbed circulation of the aqueous humor. The image after contrast shows the optic nerve (↖) and the inhomogeneous structure of the metastasis.

References

1. Bronen RA, Sze G (1990) Magnetic resonance contrast agents: theory and application to the central nervous system. J Neurosurg 73:820–840
2. Claussen C, Laniado M, Shorner W et al. (1985) Gadolinium-DTPA in MR imaging of glioblastomas and intracranial metastases. AJNR 6:669–674
3. Felix R,. Shorner W, Laniado M et al. (1985) Brain tumors: MR imaging with gadolinium-DTPA. Radiology 156:681–688
4. Gadian DG, Payne JA, Bryant DJ et al. (1985) Gadolinium-DTPA as a contrast agent in MR imaging: theoretical projections and practical observations. J Comput Assist Tomogr 9:242–251
5. Healy ME, Herselink JR, Press GA et al. (1987) Increased detection of intracranial metastasis with intravenous Gd-DTPA. Radiology 165:619–624
6. Parizel PM, Degryse HL, Gheuens J et al. (1989) Gadolinium-DTPA enhanced MR imaging of intracranial lesions. Comput Assist Tomogr 13:378–385
7. Pomeranz SJ (1989) MR of supratentorial neoplasia. In: Pomeranz SJ (ed) Craniospinal Magnetic Resonance Imaging. W. B. Saunders Co, Philadelphia, 208–247
8. Pomeranz SJ (1989) Posterior fossa, skull base, craniocervical junction. In: Pomeranz SJ (ed) Craniospinal Magnetic Resonance Imaging. W. B. Saunders Co, Philadelphia, 248–274
9. Sze G, Milano E, Johnson C et al. (1990) Detection of brain metastases: comparison of contrast-enhanced MR with unenhanced MR and enhanced CT. AJNR 11:785–791
10. Young B, Patchell RA (1990) Surgery for a single brain metastasis. In: Wilkins BH, Rengachary SS (eds) Neurosurgery Update II. McGraw-Hill, New York, 473–476

CHAPTER XI

Rare tumors and nontumoral space-occupying lesions

In this chapter we will focus on brain neoplasms that are not frequently reported and for which separate chapters would not be justified. We will also deal with mass-effect lesions due to malformations, parasitic and infectious diseases which have a tumor-like clinical behavior, together with some cases of lesions of the cranial vault. Given the differences among such lesions, their coverage in this chapter may appear as just another list of diseases, but the reader will soon realize that this is the corollary of previous chapters.

Epidermoids and dermoids

Epidermoids (e.) and dermoids (d.) arise from benign and slow-growing inclusions; the former account for 0.5%–1.5% and the latter for 0.3% of all intracranial tumors. The clinical onset of e. is reported to occur in the 20–40 age bracket, whereas d. are generally detected and treated in pediatric patients. The distinguishing feature between the two neoplasms lies in their histology: in e., the cyst capsule consists of stratified squamous epithelium, whereas in d. it consists of skin and derma elements, air and sebaceous glands. Both types develop as a result of the growth of the progressively-desquamating capsule components within the cyst. D. are more frequently sited on the midline *(Fig. 4)*, whereas e. are generally found in lateral positions *(Fig. 1)*, even though in some of the reported cases the tumor was located in the fourth ventricle *(Fig. 2)*.

Teratomas

Teratomas (t.) are dysembryogenic tumors and as such they may already be present at birth; they are more frequent in childhood and account for 0.3–0.5% of all intracranial tumors. The most common site of occurrence is the pineal gland (50%), followed, in order of frequency, by the pituitary (18%) *(Fig. 3)*, the spinal cord and the lateral ventricles. These tumors vary in size, but they can reach considerable dimensions owing to their very slow growth; macroscopically they are capsulated lesions, well delimited with respect to surrounding tissue and they generally have a distinct cleavage plane. Typical t. are to be distinguished from teratoid tumors where the structures belonging to the three embryonic layers are not so clearly distinct and the capsule is anchored to the surrounding tissues by adhesions. Like atypical t., teratoid tumors have malignant evolution.

T. have a smooth surface and are variegated in color owing to the presence of several hemorrhages and brown-colored cysts; they may contain mature tissues, premature forms of organs (for instance teeth) and material similar to that of dysembryogenic cysts (d., e.) and degradation products of prior hemorrhages.

The typical picture is a lesion which is well demarcated from the surrounding structures, large-sized and located on the midline in both pituitary and pineal sites; on both CT and MRI scans, the tumor is inhomogeneous and after administration of GD-DTPA, the signal produced by the tissue components is sharply enhanced; on T_2-weighted sequences, the capsule layers can be distinguished *(Fig. 3)*.

Symptomatology depends on the anatomical site of the lesion, which also conditions the possibility of total resection: where possible, total resection secures full recovery.

Lipomas

These are not real neoplasms and were more properly defined as "lipomatous hamartomas". The term lipoma might suggest that there is a neoplastic type of growth, whereas the term hamartoma implies a congenital origin with evident, small and often multiple masses *(Fig. 4)*, consisting of altered tissue but which is normally present in the CNS. Hamartomas are often associated with other midline lesions, such as colloid and dermoid cysts and angiomatosis.

Colloid cysts

These "tumors" are located at the roof of the third ventricle and adhere to the tela choroidea; they reach sizes of between 1 and 3 cm; they account for 0.6–1.5% of intracranial tumors and in most cases they cause biventricular hydrocephalus due to obstruction of Monro's foramina. They consist of a smooth capsule of varying thickness, greyish in color, housing a jelly-like substance. The most widely accepted pathogenetic assumption is that they originate from an abnormal exfoliation of the neuroepithelium that will form the roof of the third ventricle. These lesions are treated by biventricular-peritoneal CSF shunts, cyst drainage via stereotactic puncture *(Fig. 5)* and open neurosurgery via the transventricular frontal or transcallosal approach.

Papillomas of the choroid plexus

These are slow-growing, benign, ependymal tumors arising from the choroid plexus of the ventricles. They are usually associated with hydrocephalus, resulting from obstruction of the CSF flow, CSF overproduction and obliteration of the subarachnoid spaces caused by the frequent bleedings from the tumor surface. They are the most frequent oncotype in children under the age of three, in whom the papillomas are generally situated in the lateral ventricles *(Fig. 6)*; in adults, they are more usually found in the fourth ventricle *(Fig. 7)*.

Chordomas

These are rare lesions which account for some 0.15–0.2% of intracranial tumors and which arise from the embryonic remnants of the notochord. Nearly all cases are related to the clivus; when the body and the dorsal portion are involved, they present as sphenooccipital or petrosal chordomas; when the inferior segment of the clivus is involved, they are clival chordomas of the anterior aspect of the foramen magnum *(Figs. 8, 9)*. In other cases, they manifest themselves as sellar and parasellar tumors (the most rostral extension of the notochord) or as nasopharyngeal tumors (ventral portion of the clivus). Their clinical symptomatology is site-dependent. Chordomas are usually well demarcated from the surrounding tissue by the presence of a pseudo-capsule; on the contrary, inside the bone it is difficult to distinguish the boundary between healthy bone and tumor. For this reason, surgery may not always lead to total resection. It is advisable to have surgery followed by radiation therapy.

Primary lymphomas

The primary lymphomas (l.) of the CNS are malignant lymphocyte-derived tumors. Together with the secondary, they account for 0.5% of intracranial neoplasms. They may take the form of either single or multiple lesions without a favorite site *(Figs. 11, 12, 13)*. Their most frequent macroscopic appearance is a homogeneous, circumscribed lesion, denser than the neighboring cerebral tissue and surrounded by edema, occasionally with necrosis and/or hemorrhage. Given the massive size of the edema and the volume increase of the mass, they may cause a severe intracranial hypertension syndrome. For diagnostic accuracy, an examination of the CSF is of help in that it may show glycorrhachia below normal values in case of meningoencephalic involvement. A cytological test is also of help, because if it is positive (approximately 50% of cases), it may lead to a diagnosis of a malignant l. The CSF levels of beta-2-microglobulin, if higher than serum levels, are indicative of a primary CNS l. Stereotactic biopsies for histological evaluation as well as radio- and chemotherapy represent the diagnostic and therapeutic measures to be adopted for these tumors.

Suprasellar cerebral granulomatosis

This terminology is currently preferred to indicate the granulomatous degeneration of eosinophilic cells of the stalk and of the pars nervosa of the pituitary gland, which occurs in the pathologic conditions (eosinophilic granuloma and Hand-Schüller-Christian and Letterer-Siwe diseases) falling under the general term of "Histiocytosis X". They generally appear as small tumors of the sellar region having granular cells; they are asymptomatic and are thus usually incidental post-mortem findings. When they are symptomatic, they cause severe disorders in the visual function as a result of compression on the pregeniculate optic pathways, diabetes insipidus, panhypopituitarism and psychic disturbances.

From the diagnostic point of view, this granulomatosis can be differentiated from: craniopharyngioma by the absence of calcifications on plain films; chiasmatic gliomas and pituitary adenomas by the presence of blush in the suprasellar region on angiograms. In the absence of cerebral edema, the presence of a hyperdense, well-circumscribed mass on CT scan, combined with clinical and MRI findings can correctly guide the diagnosis *(Fig. 14)*.

If the conclusion is that the neoplasm is granulocytic, without an intrasellar component and large in size, if the symptomatology progresses and if the lesion grows symmetrically as often occurs, it would be preferable to excise it via the right subfrontal approach. Macroscopically, these lesions are compact and gummy, highly vascularized, more than the oncotypes that are typical of this region, without any connections with the dural plane; if the lesion can be easily resected from the structures that it involves, it can be totally removed, but this is not often the case. The role of radiotherapy has not been specified yet and the absence of a sufficient number of reports in the literature (only 30 cases of which 4 treated with radiotherapy) suggests to most centres that they should refrain from using such treatment.

For the diseases not dealt with in this chapter and described by the following MRI images, it was deemed unnecessary to go into the details pertaining to pathogenesis, clinical picture and treatment, leaving it up to the images to indicate the factors determining the differential diagnosis among malformations, parasitic, inflammatory lesions and tumoral lesions.

A B

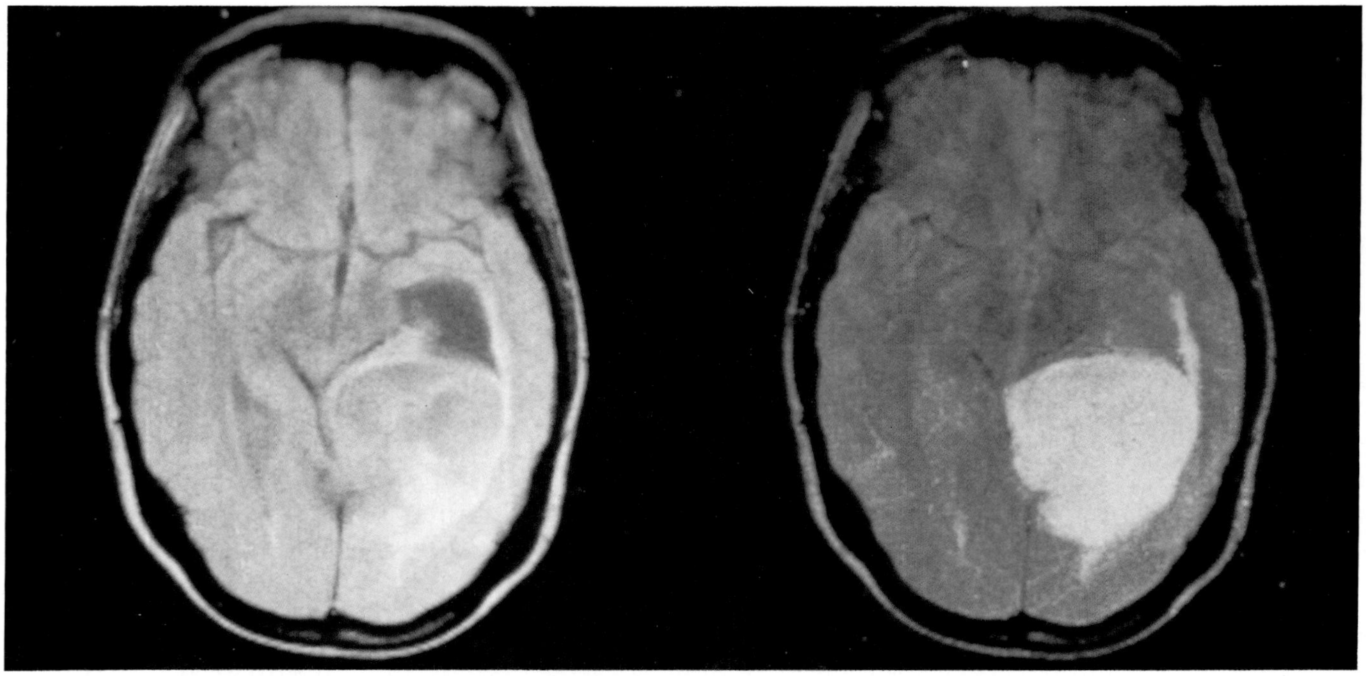

Fig. 1. *Epidermoid of the left lateral ventricle.* Proton density- (A) and T_2- (B) weighted axial sections. Observe a slightly inhomogeneous, large, rounded neoplasm starting from the trigonum and well separated from the surrounding tissue by a hyperintense rim on A. Anteriorly, the ipsilateral temporal horn is excluded and dilated. In B, the signal from the entire neoplasm is enhanced. Note the mild ependymal damage: crescentic hyperintensity lateral to the mass on (A) and (B) (by courtesy of L. Bozzao, M.D., Rome).

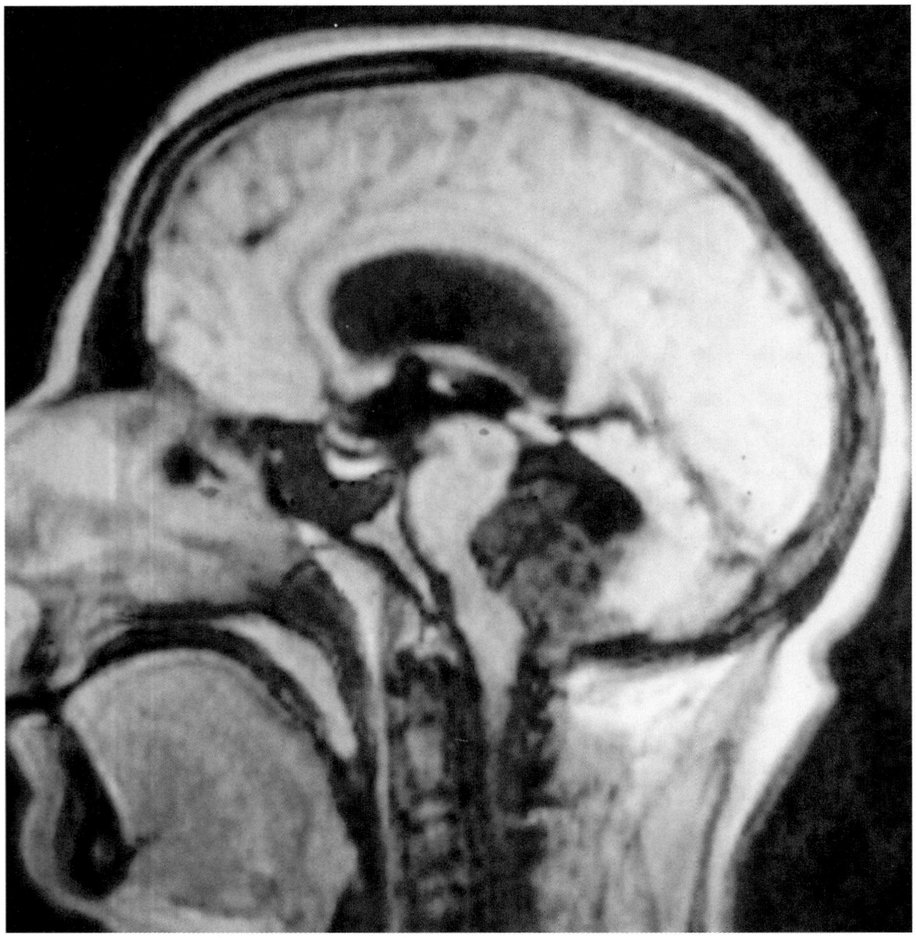

Fig. 2. *Epidermoid of the fourth ventricle.* T_1-weighted sagittal image; the mass is irregular and hyperintense with the brain tissue; it is larger in the fourth ventricle, hence dilating its upper portion (by courtesy of L. Bozzao, M.D., Rome).

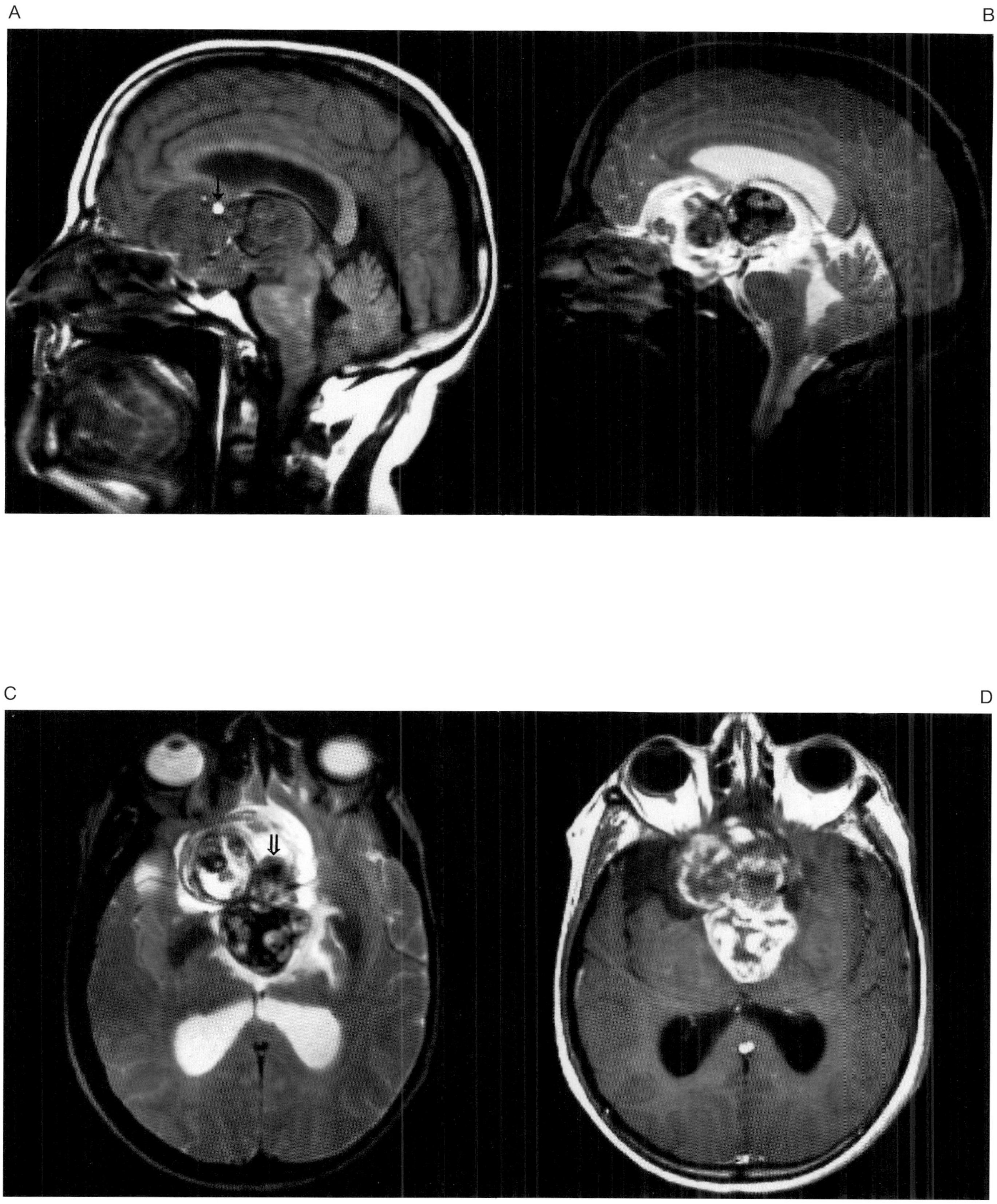

Fig. 3. *Suprasellar teratoma.* 60-year-old woman with somatic hypoevolutism, intracranial hypertension and psychoorganic syndrome. A, B – T_1- and T_2-weighted mid-sagittal images. C – T_2-weighted axial image. A huge tumor of the suprasellar and frontobasal region can be detected, whose upper portion occupies the third ventricle, inducing hydrocephalus of the lateral ventricles and displacing the midbrain backwards. The structure of the tumor is uneven due to different tissues: fat (↓), calcium (⇓), stratified keratin, solid parts of connective origin (relatively hyperintense on T_2-weighted images) and substances having paramagnetic effect (highly hypointense on T_2-weighted images). The picture in (C) highlights the damage to the surrounding brain: hyperintensity due to edema. GD-DTPA (D) delimits the parenchymatous components.

A B

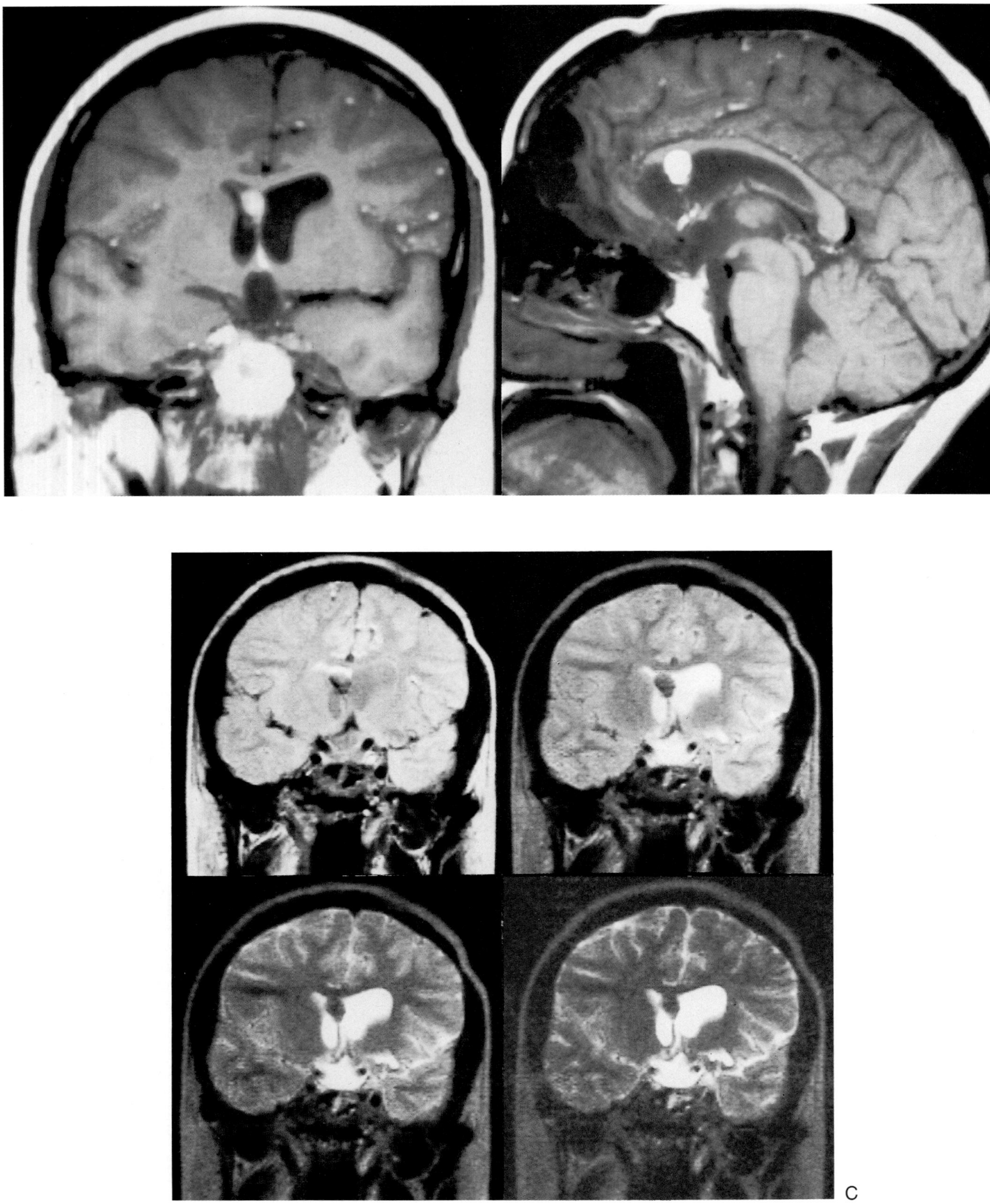

C

Fig. 4. *Lipoma of the septum pellucidum and diffuse lipomatosis.* 25-year-old woman operated on 5 years earlier to remove a dermoid in the sellar region. At surgery, small lipomas were found in the subarachnoid spaces of the cortex. T_1-weighted coronal (A) and sagittal (B) images. Observe: the sequelae of previous surgery; atrophy of the frontal pole and absence of the pituitary as well as a lipomatous lesion in the septum pellucidum, which had not been excised upon the first surgery; and numerous lipid "drops" in the CSF spaces. C – On the multi-echo sequence (TR 2,500 msec, TE 40, 90, 150, 210), the signal from the fat progressively decays as TE becomes longer. The early echoes exhibit a chemical shift artifact due to a fat/liquid interface.

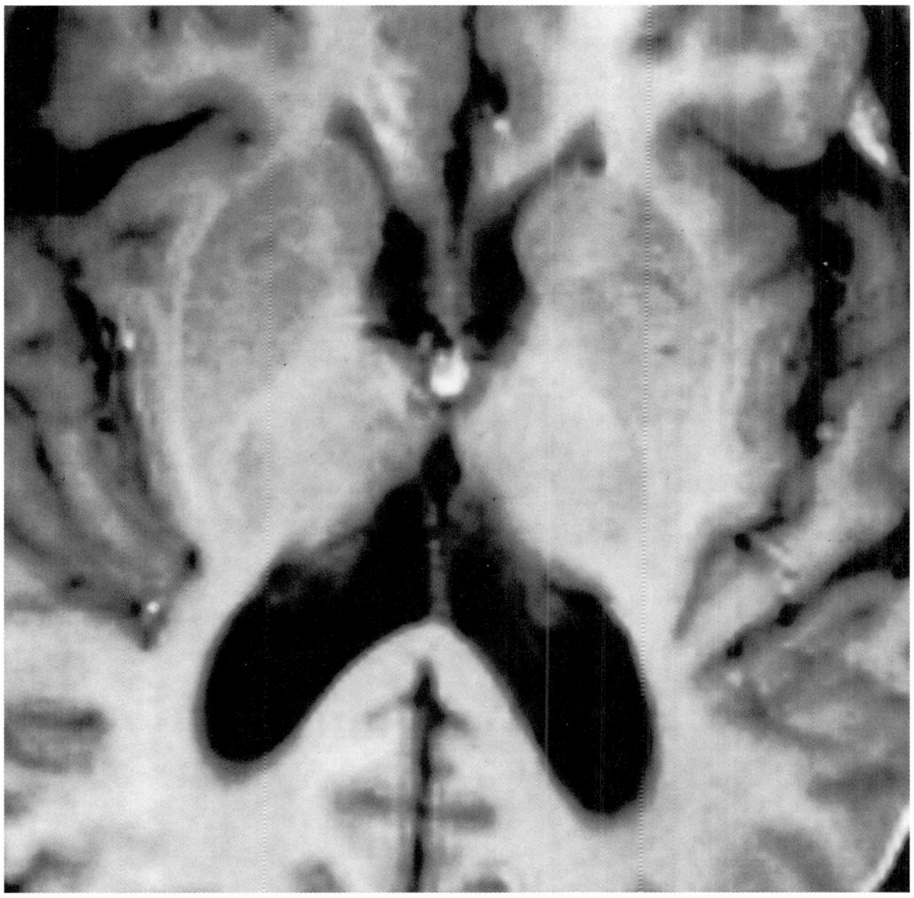

A

Fig. 5. *Colloid cyst of the third ventricle*. 60-year-old patient previously subjected to stereotactic drainage of the cyst. The T_1-weighted images show a small cyst remnant adhering to the tela choroidea of the third ventricle with typical high signal. In A, the basal ganglia are well outlined.

B

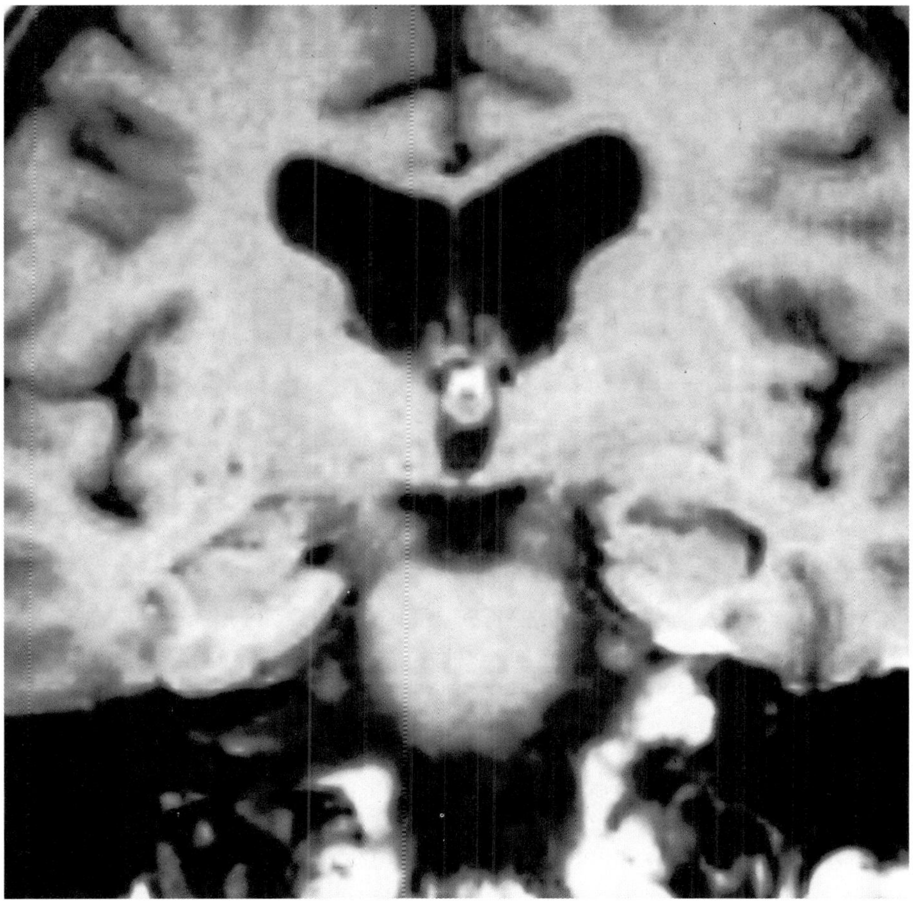

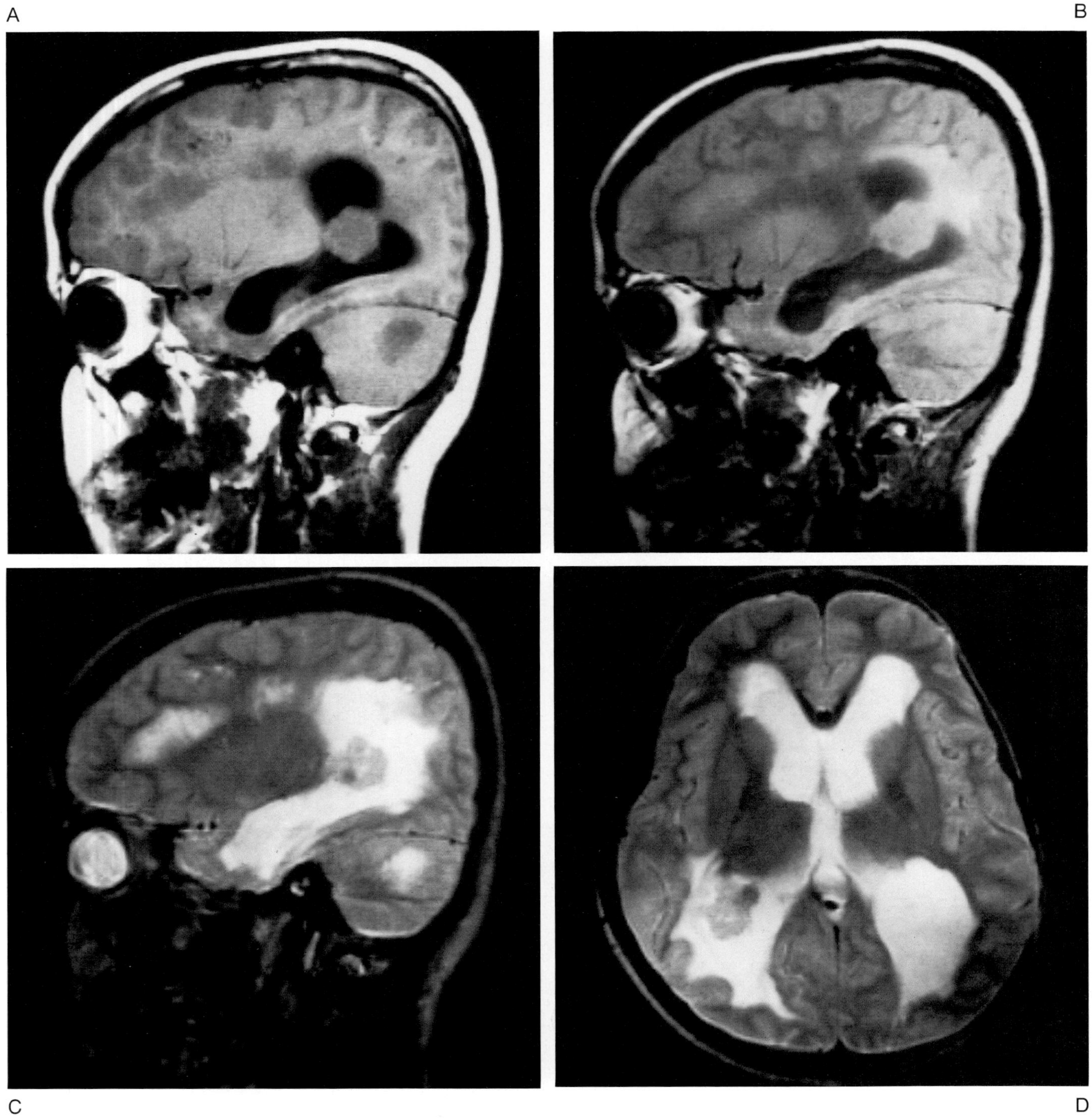

Fig. 6. *Papilloma of the choroid plexus of the right lateral ventricle.* 11-year-old girl with hydrocephalus due to concomitant space-occupying lesion of the posterior cranial fossa. A – The T_1-weighted sagittal view shows a small, berry-shaped mass in the trigonum of the right lateral ventricle whose density is identical to that of the cerebral tissue and which stands out against the markedly hypointense CSF. B, C, D – Long-TR sequence, first echo (B) and second echo (C, D). The lesion has a nonuniform signal due to calcifications (hypointense focus) and microcysts (hyperintensity); the latter microcysts are better visualized on T_2-weighted sequences. The lateral ventricles are dilated; on T_2-weighted sequences, they appear to be larger because of a transependymal reabsorption area. On proton density- (B) weighted images, the periventricular edema can be better discriminated and is evidenced by a crescentic hyperintensity above and behind the ventricular image.

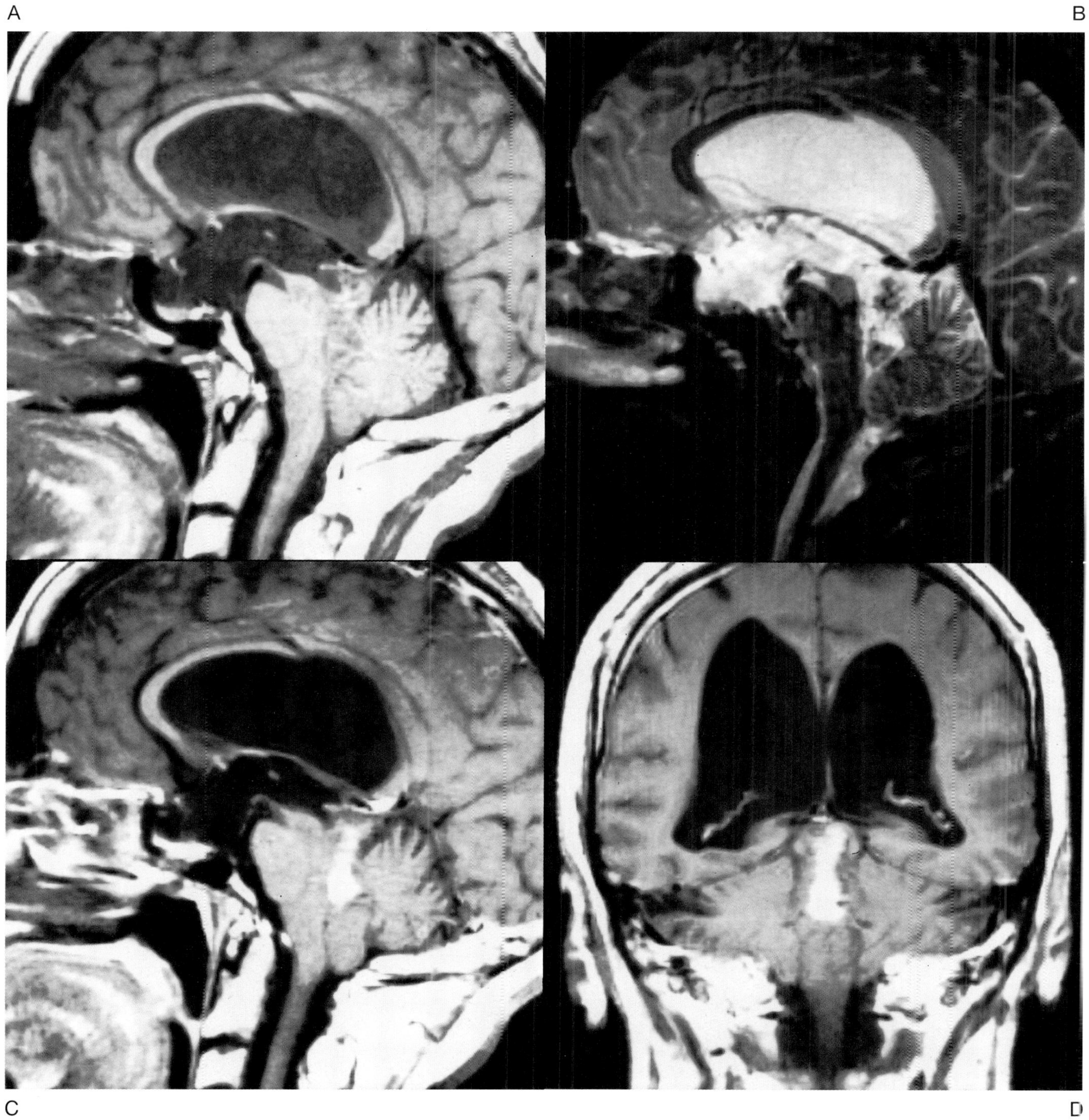

Fig. 7. *Papilloma of the fourth ventricle*. 63-year-old patient with intracranial hypertension due to triventricular hydrocephalus. The T_1- (A) and T_2- (B) weighted sagittal sections reveal a neoplasm which entirely occupies the fourth ventricle, the aqueduct and the posterior aspect of the third ventricle. The signal is inhomogeneous, especially on T_2-weighted images; on these images, the hypointense foci are likely to reflect prior intratumoral hemorrhages. GD-DTPA significantly enhances the signal (C, D).

Fig. 8. *Chordoma of the clivus.* 11-year-old girl with diplopia and occasional headaches. In the past, she had had an acute episode of forced rightward bending of the head. CT showed a partially calcific tumor of the clivus reaching C2–C3 and a mild supratentorial ventricular distension. There was palsy of the fifth, sixth, seventh and twelfth right cranial nerves with hemiatrophy of the tongue. A – T_1-weighted mid-sagittal section: alteration of the clivus morphology with posterior displacement of the whole brainstem (→). The isointense mass grows from the quadrigeminal plate to the C2–C3 interspace, anteriorly protruding into the retropharyngeal region. B – The T_2-weighted section, albeit disturbed by motion artifacts, better visualizes the mass which is hyperintense with the brainstem.

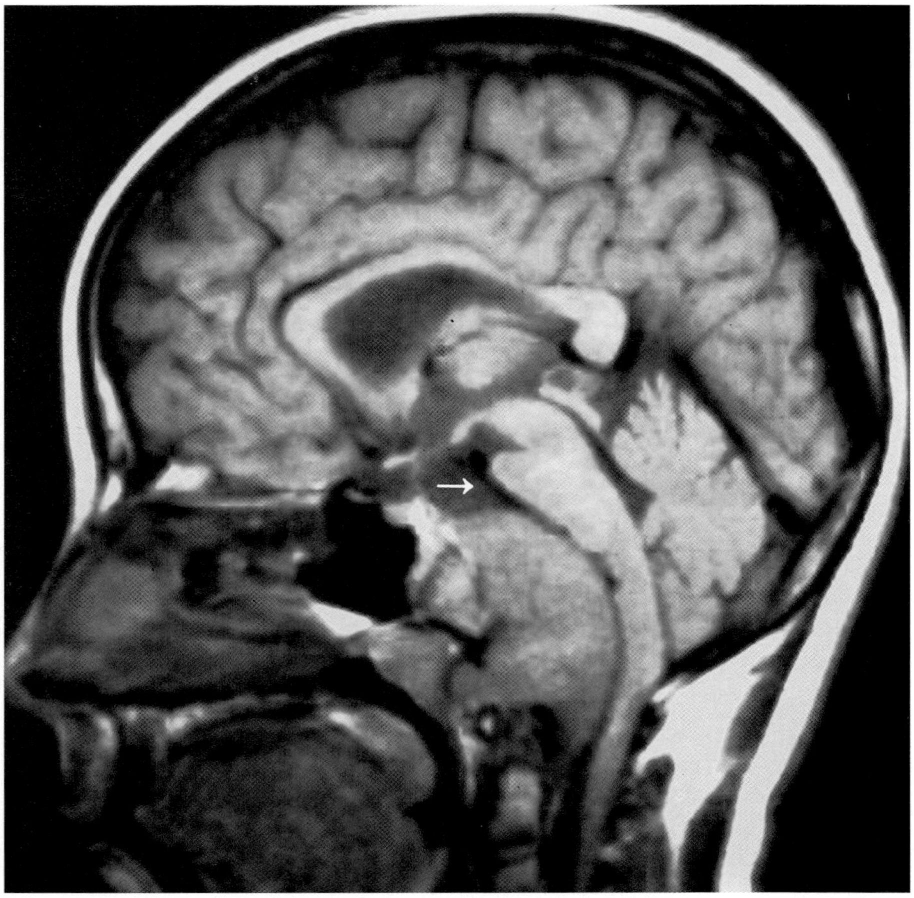

A

B

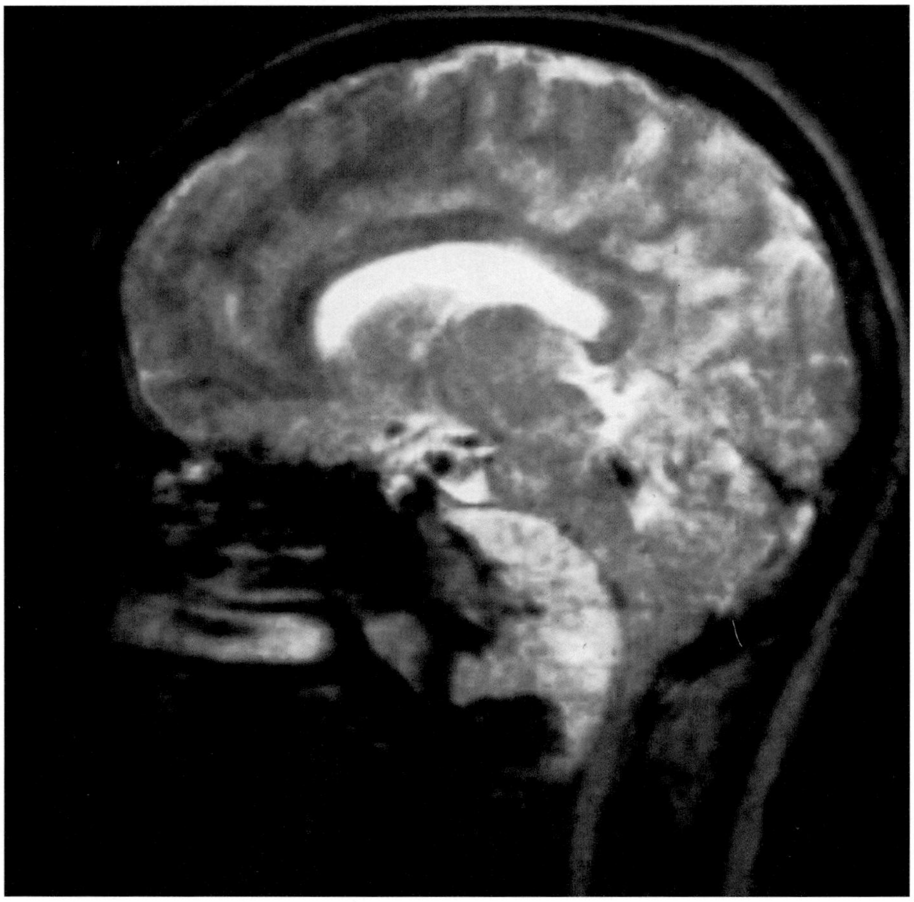

A B

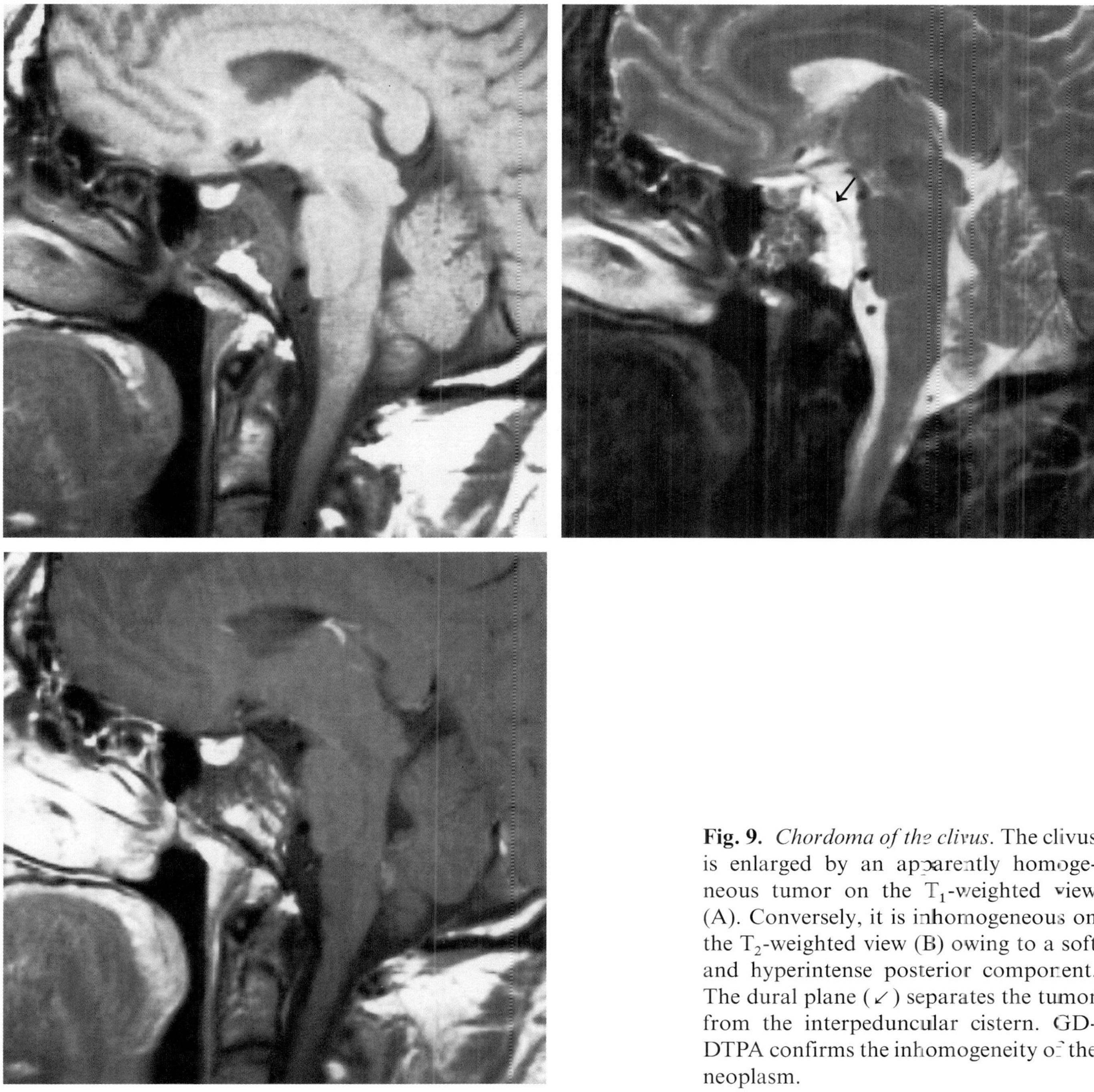

C

Fig. 9. *Chordoma of the clivus*. The clivus is enlarged by an apparently homogeneous tumor on the T_1-weighted view (A). Conversely, it is inhomogeneous on the T_2-weighted view (B) owing to a soft and hyperintense posterior component. The dural plane (↙) separates the tumor from the interpeduncular cistern. GD-DTPA confirms the inhomogeneity of the neoplasm.

Fig. 10. *Chondroma of the sella and of the upper clivus.* 27-year-old man with diplopia. The sella is distended and occupied by a mass, hyperintense after contrast (B, C), which anteriorly displaces the peduncle (↘) and the pituitary (⇗). The tumor grows into the upper clivus and is inhomogeneous; it seems to originate from the right posterior clinoid (→) on the axial view (C). Differential diagnosis with respect to a solid craniopharyngioma is difficult. A – T_1-weighted sequence.

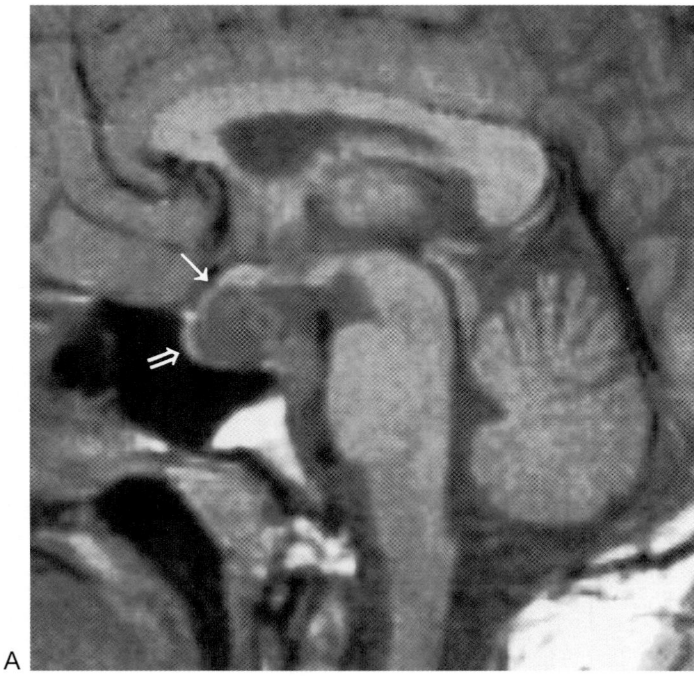

A

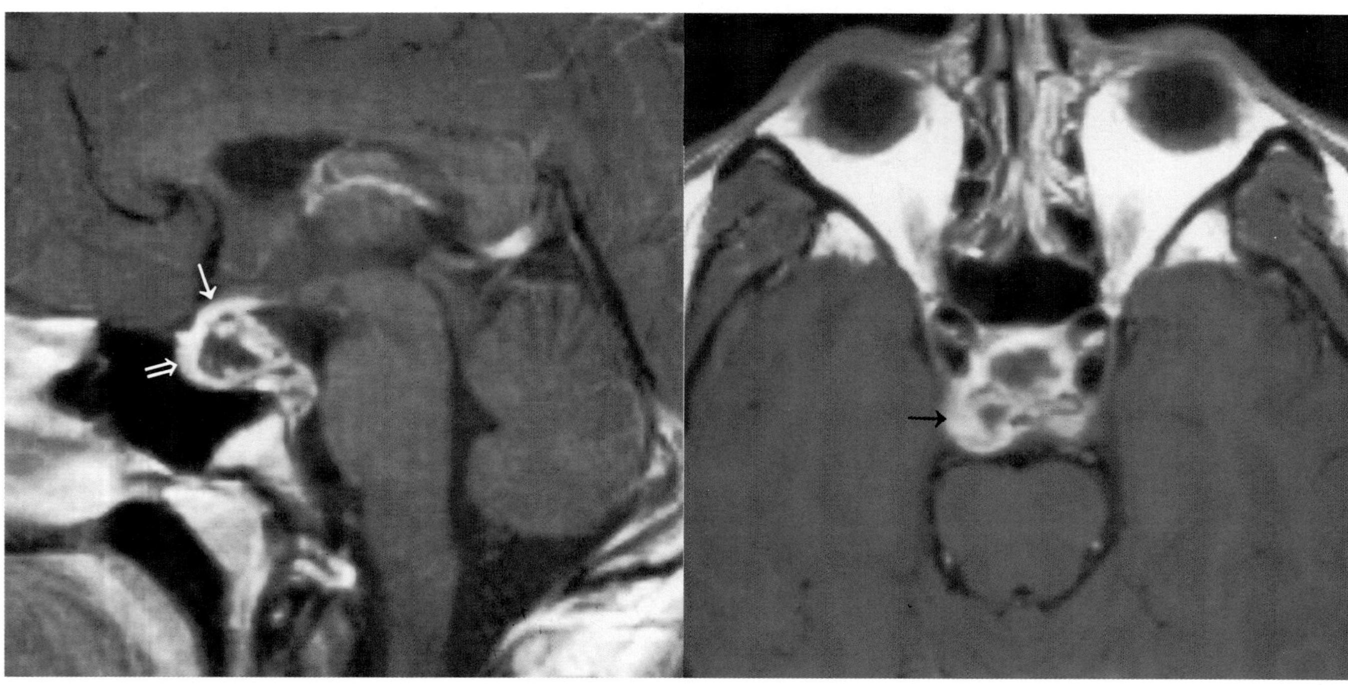

B C

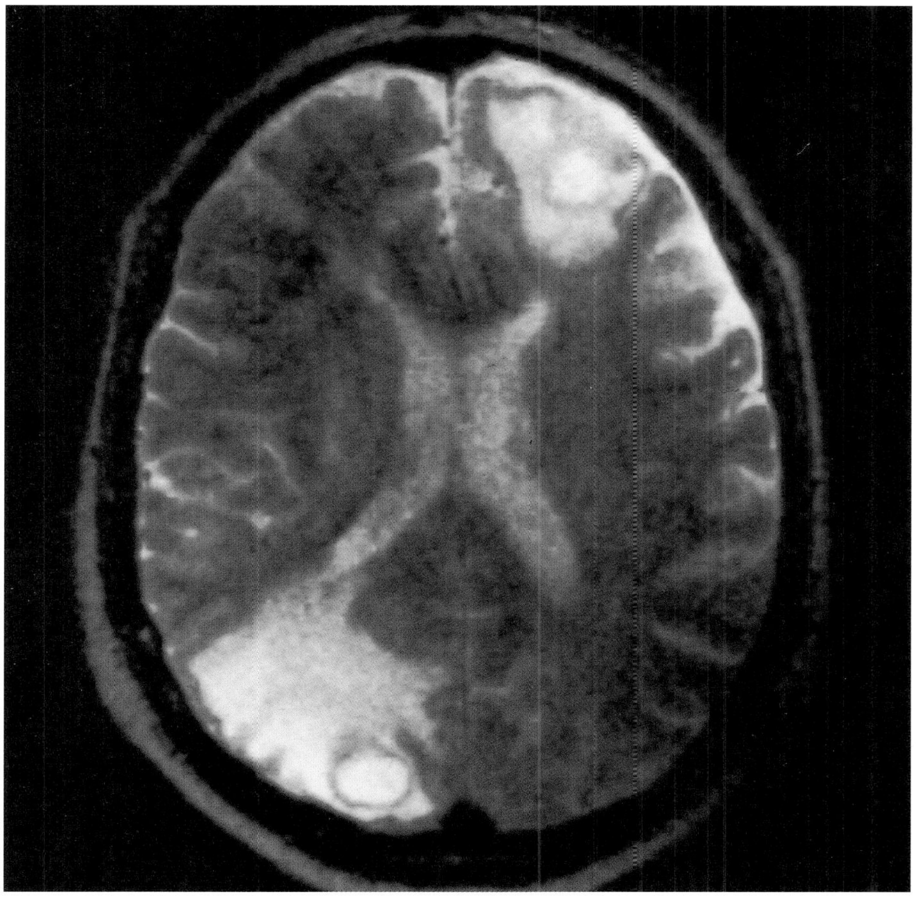

Fig. 11. *Non-Hodgkin lymphoma of the left frontal and right occipital regions.* 62-year-old man with 2-year history of nasopharyngeal lymphoma treated with combination chemotherapy. On admission to our department, he was found to have left hemiparesis mainly affecting the lower limb and bilateral papilledema. The T_2-weighted axial cut shows two significantly hyperintense foci with a hypointense rim. A concomitant white matter edema is visible.

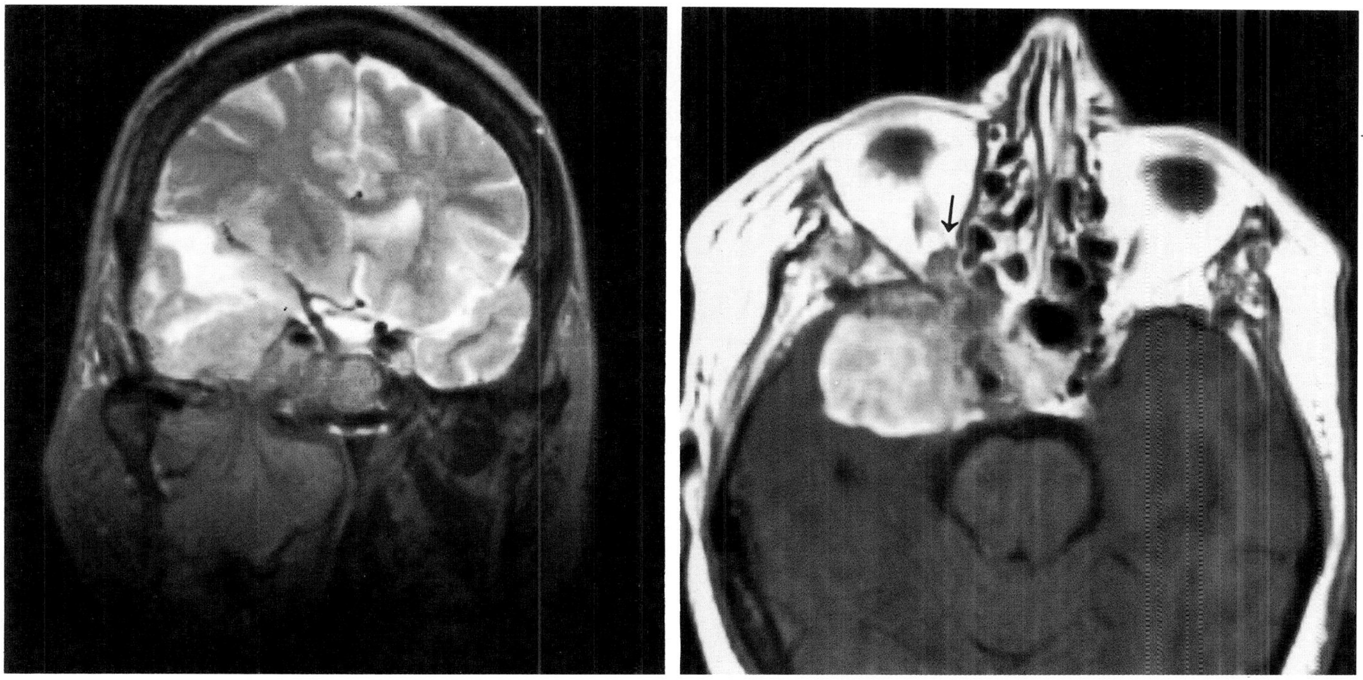

A B

Fig. 12. *Intra- and extracranial dumbbell lymphoma.* 60-year-old woman with right trigeminal neuralgia. A – T_2-weighted coronal view. B – T_1-weighted axial view after contrast. (A) demonstrates the intra-extracranial spread of the tumor which occupies the anterior aspect of the middle cranial fossa, Meckel's cave, and the sella. The tumor crosses the foramen ovale and grows into the infratemporal fossa. After enhancement (B), observe the infiltration of the right cavernous sinus, the tumor spread to the orbit (↓), and the integrity of the pontine cistern.

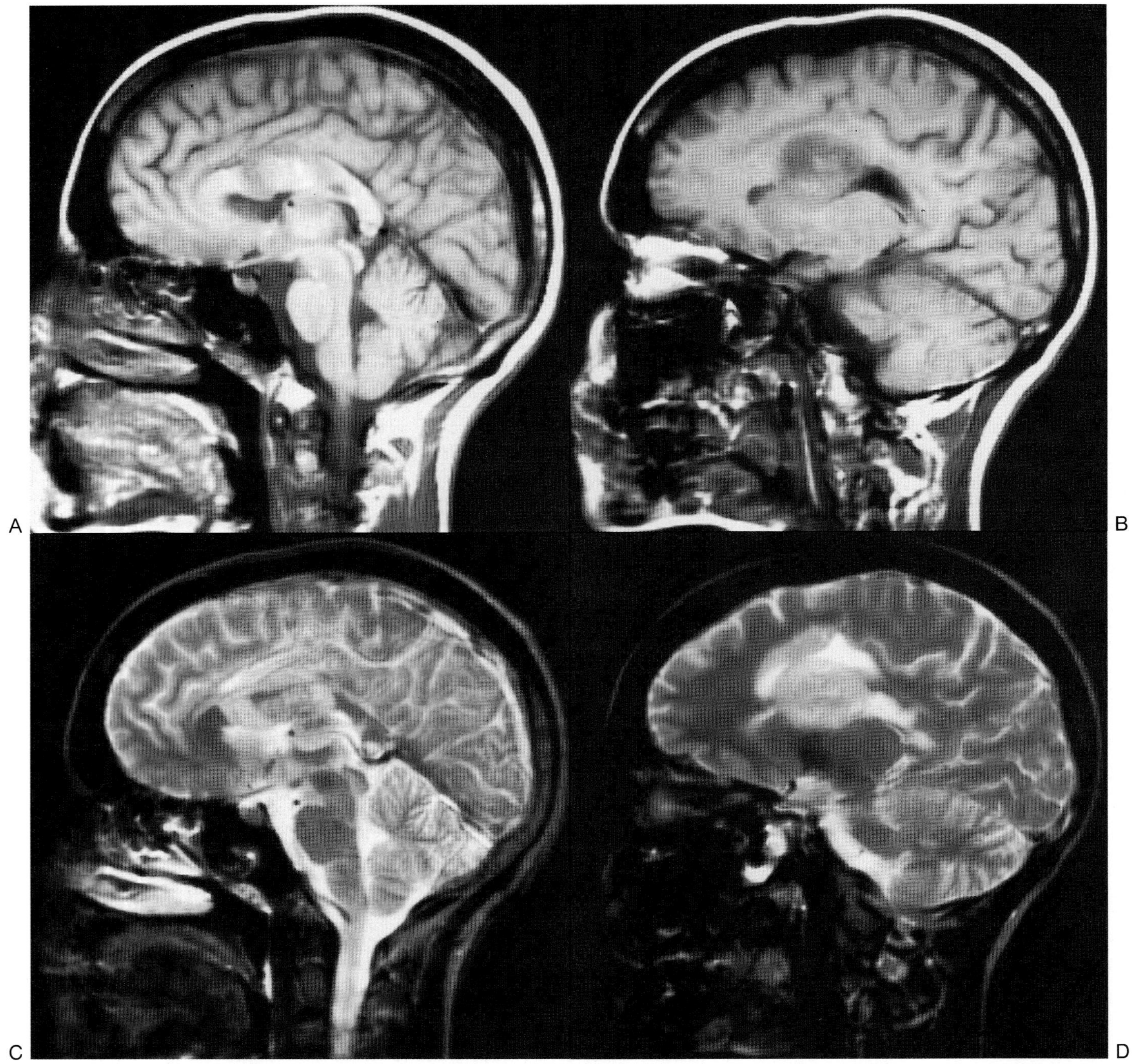

Fig. 13. *Lymphoma of the corpus callosum in an AIDS patient*. T_1- (A, B) and T_2- (C, D) weighted views. The nutform neoplasm of the corpus callosum is partially hemorrhagic and edematogenic, although well delimited from the surrounding tissue. The paramedian images (B, D) document the compression of the basal ganglia.

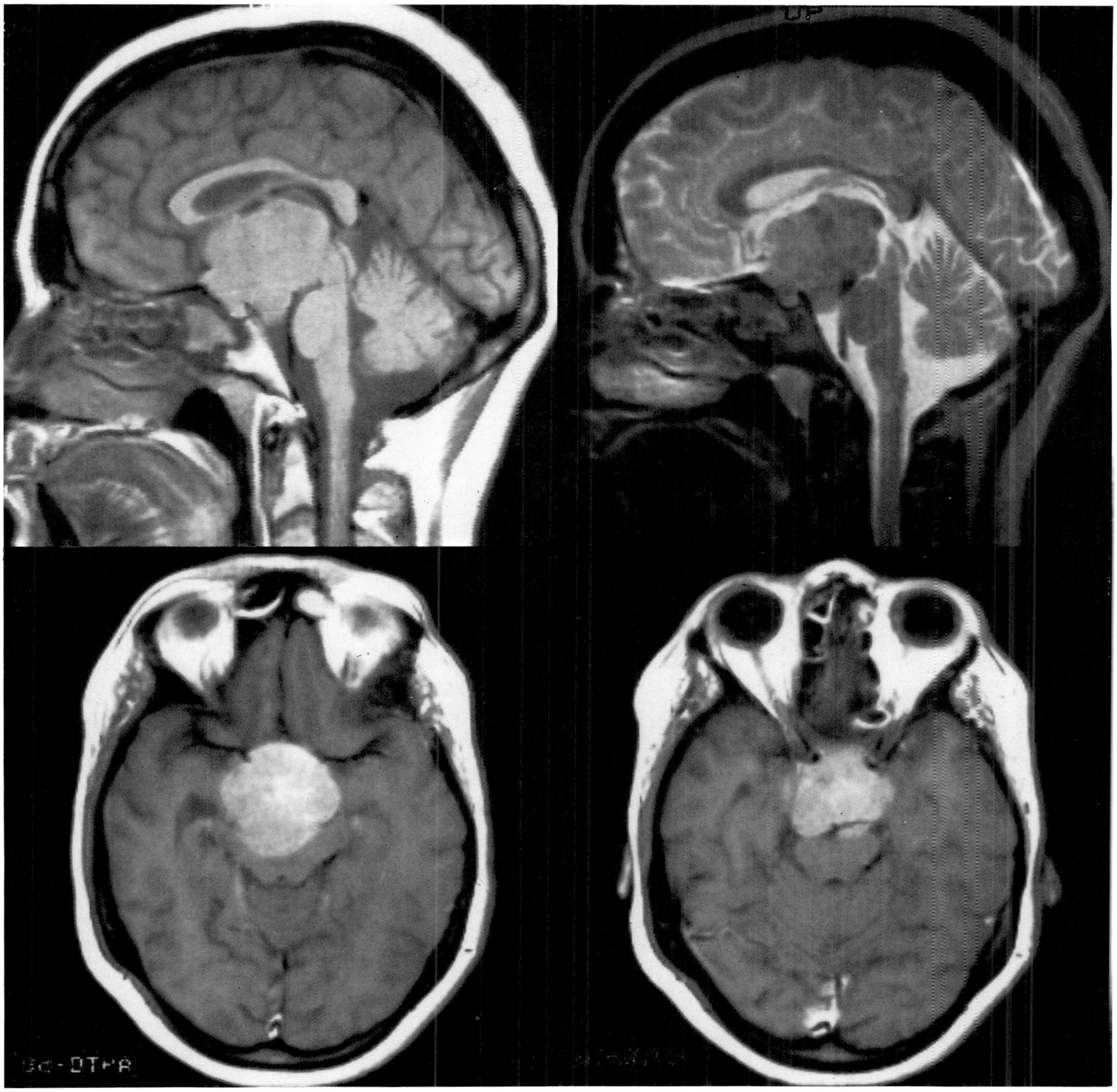

Fig. 14. *Granulomatosis of the hypothalamus.* 25-year-old woman with major visual deficit and obnubilation. A, B – T_1- and T_2-weighted sagittal sections. A huge, isointense mass occupies the entire hypothalamus and the third ventricle. The midbrain is compressed and displaced posteriorly. C, D – T_1-weighted sequences after GD-DTPA: the signal enhances and becomes slightly irregular. The axial images portray the compression of the midbrain and the widening of the cerebral peduncles (C). On D, the mass encases the left P.C.A. at its origin from the B.A. Note the optic nerves and the likely involvement of the chiasm.

A

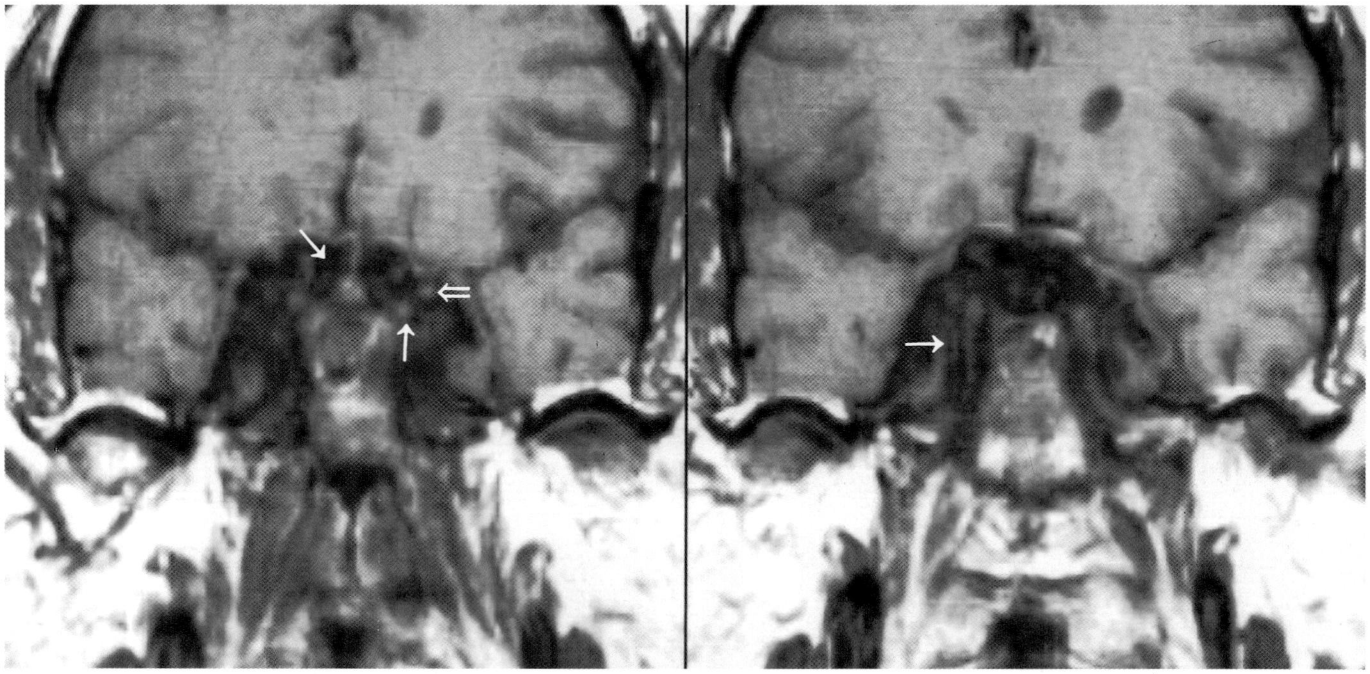

B

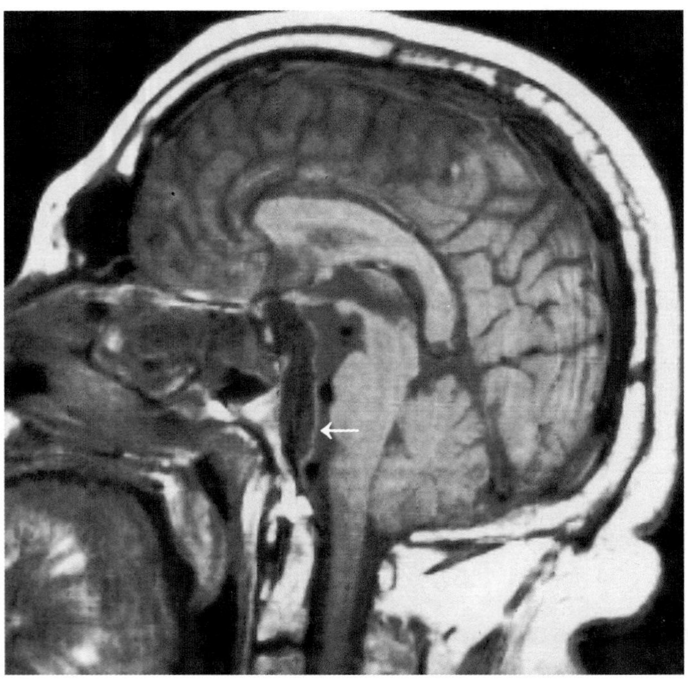

Fig. 15. *Sellar and parasellar chronic granulomatous aspecific meningitis.* 42-year-old man with diabetes inspidus, impotence and headache. A – T_1-weighted coronal views. Observe the thick plaque of hypointense tissue due to diffuse calcifications. The plaque extends bilaterally to the cavernous sinuses and to the sellar region and encases the pituitary (↘) and the cranial nerves, of which the third (⇐) and the sixth (↑) can be seen. The I.C.A.s (→) are obstructed owing to absence of flow in their intra- and supracavernous portions. This finding was confirmed by angiography. B – The sagittal view demonstrates the retroclival location of the lesion and its caudal spread. Note the separation from the CSF by a thick dural layer (←).

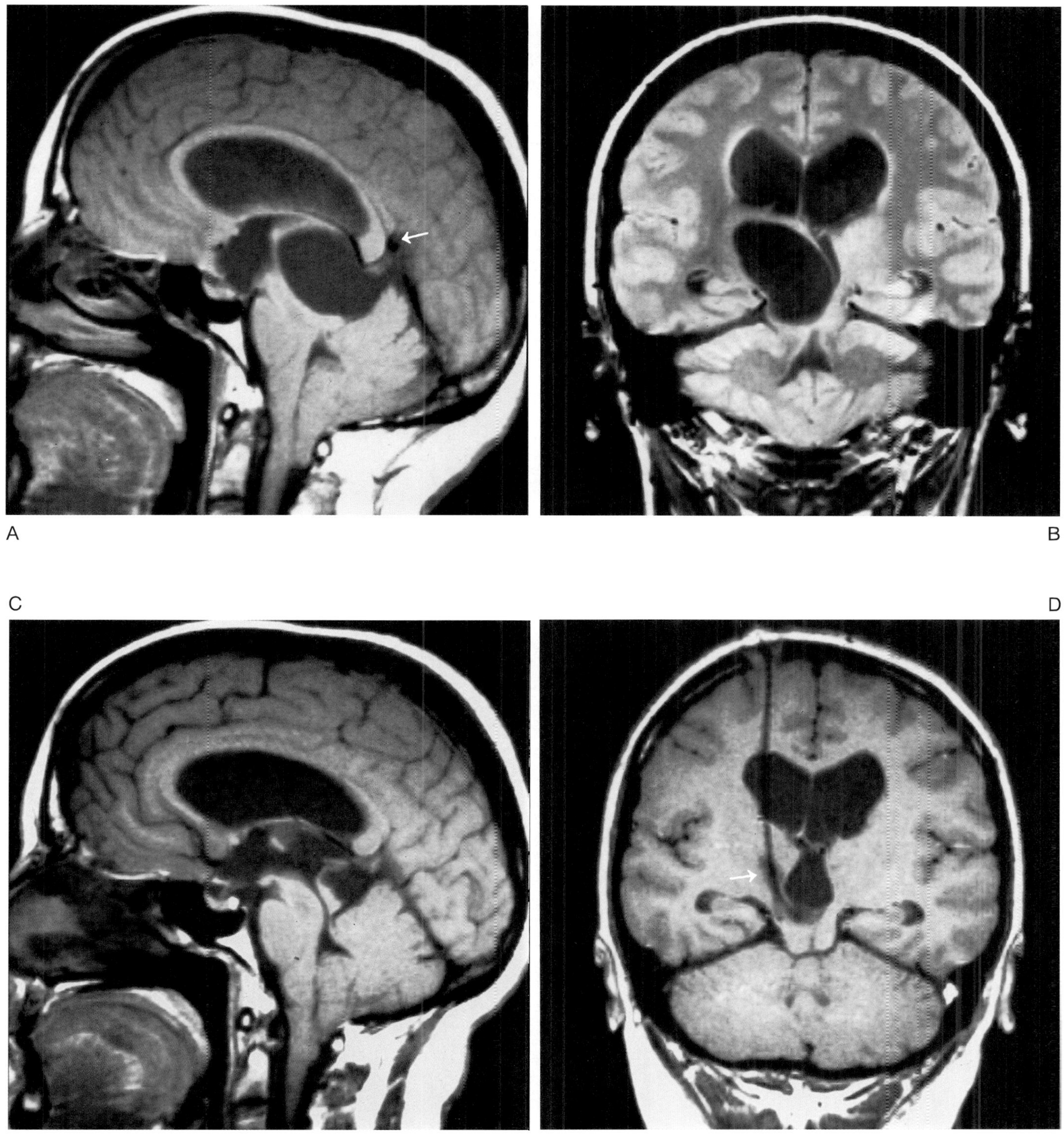

Fig. 16. *Arachnoid cyst of the right supracollicular pineal region.* 43-year-old woman with headache, paroxysmal arterial hypertension and tinnitus. For 2 years, she had had urinary incontinence and gait disturbances. CT showed a cyst in the third ventricle with hydrocephalus. A – The T_1-weighted mid-sagittal scan reveals a hypointense cystic lesion in the posterior aspect of the third ventricle, superiorly to the quadrigeminal plate. The lesion displaces the cerebellum and the fourth ventricle and occludes the Sylvian aqueduct. Note Galen's vein (←) and the herniation of the cerebellar tonsil in the occipital foramen. B – Proton density-weighted coronal scan. The supra- and sub-tentorial cystic lesion occupies the tentorial notch, displaces the third ventricle leftwards, compresses and obstructs the Sylvian aqueduct. With the CT-guided stereotactic technique, a shunt catheter was placed inside the cyst and a Rickam's reservoir was located under her scalp. Drainage punctures were performed until the cyst was completely emptied. C – T_1-weighted sagittal view. Observe the small remnant of the cyst and the patency of the Sylvian aqueduct. D – Coronal view. Reduction of hydrocephalus and visualization of the drainage catheter, whose tip is placed inside the remnant cystic cavity (→). The third ventricle is one the midline.

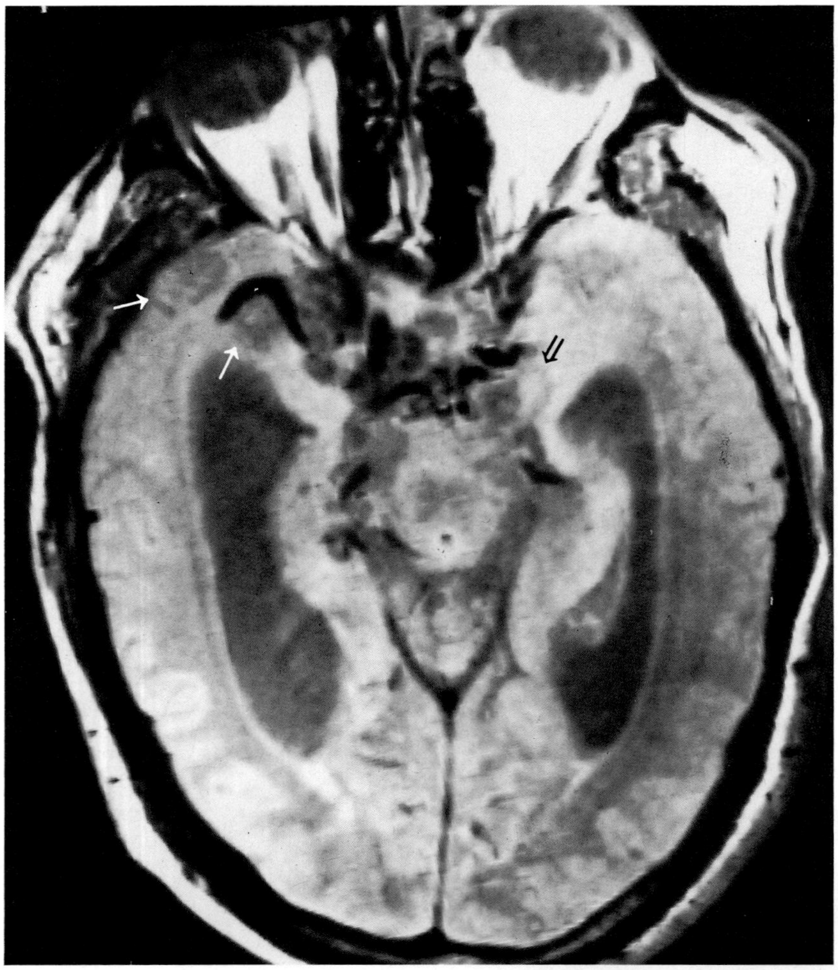

A

B

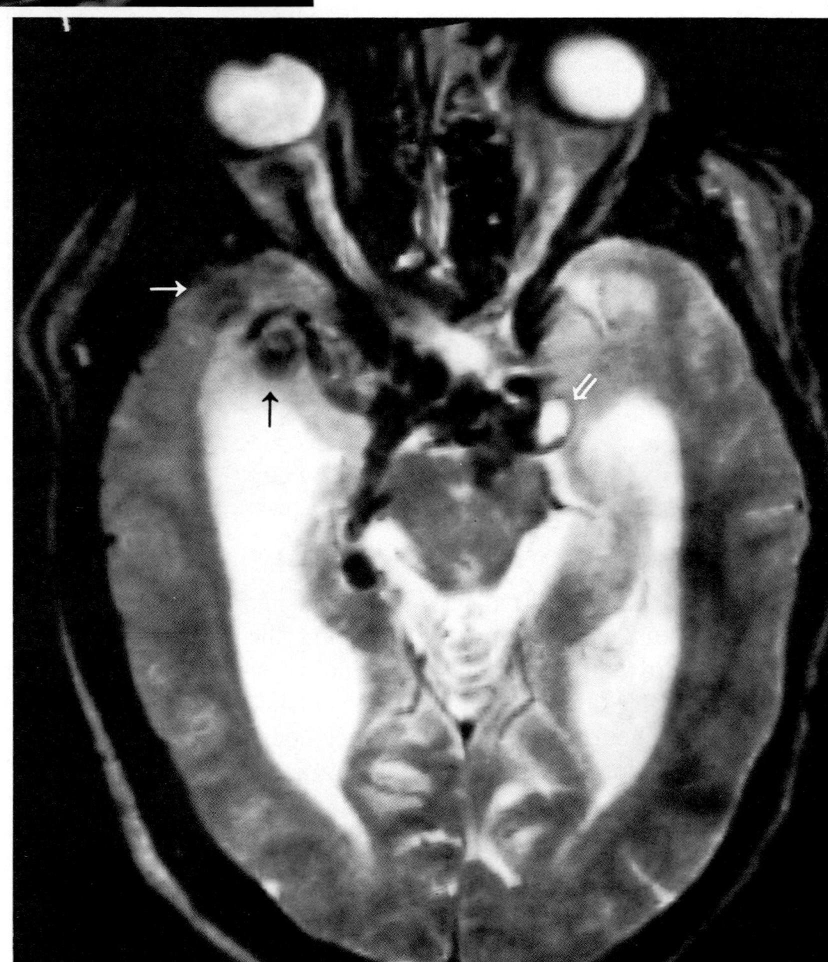

Fig. 17. *Encephalic cysticercosis.* 45-year-old patient with fixation amnesia and temporospatial disorientation. CT had shown numerous calcium deposits along the basal cisterns, consistent with craniopharyngioma. The proton density-(A) and T_2-weighted (B) axial cuts depict numerous calcium deposits which occupy the cisterns and encircle the vessels, the right optic nerve and the chiasm. The vessels can be easily distinguished from the calcifications on (A), where the former are markedly hyperintense. On T_2-weighted images (B), vessels and calcifications tend to elicit the same signal. Moreover, observe two hypointense, right temporo-polar nodular lesions (→↑), to be ascribed to the non-viable larva of the parasite. A third lesion (⇓) is suggestive of remnant adhesive arachnoiditis (sequestrated CSF), which also causes the concurrent hydrocephalus.

A B

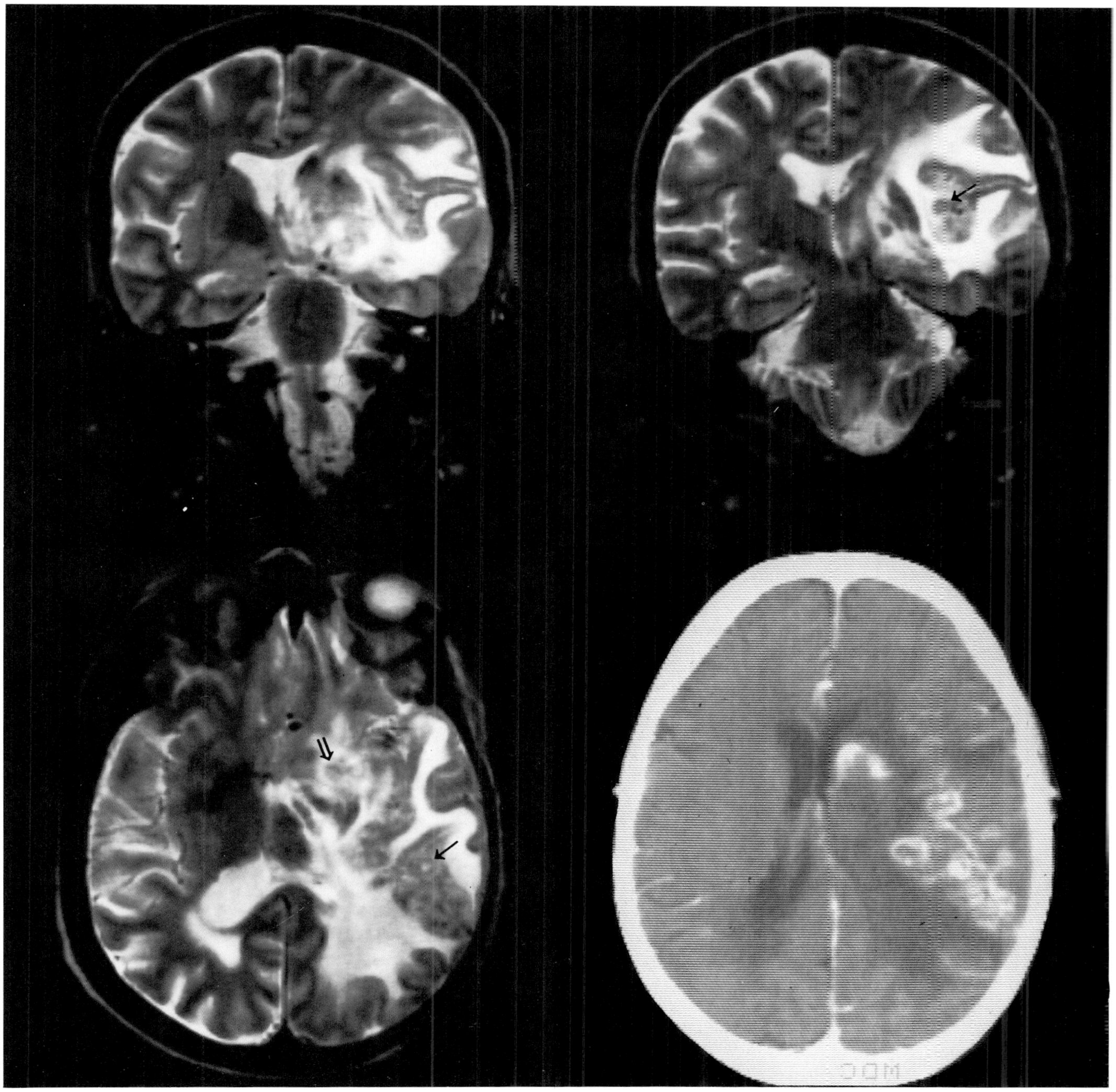

C D

Fig. 18. *Tuberculous meningoencephalitis.* 55-year-old woman with confusion and severe right hemiparesis. Based on an MRI performed one month earlier in another hospital, the patient was diagnosed as having a left frontotemporal glioma. In our MRI examination, the T_2-weighted images (A, B – coronal; C – axial) show a composite picture: intense edema of the white matter in the left hemisphere, nodular lesions with a "bull's eye" appearance (↙) in the grey matter. The deepest lesion (⇒), which had initially suggested a neoplasm, has the same nodular appearance. Contrast CT (D), carried out as a complementary study, confirms the nodular nature of the lesions. Stereotactic biopsy allowed us to make the diagnosis.

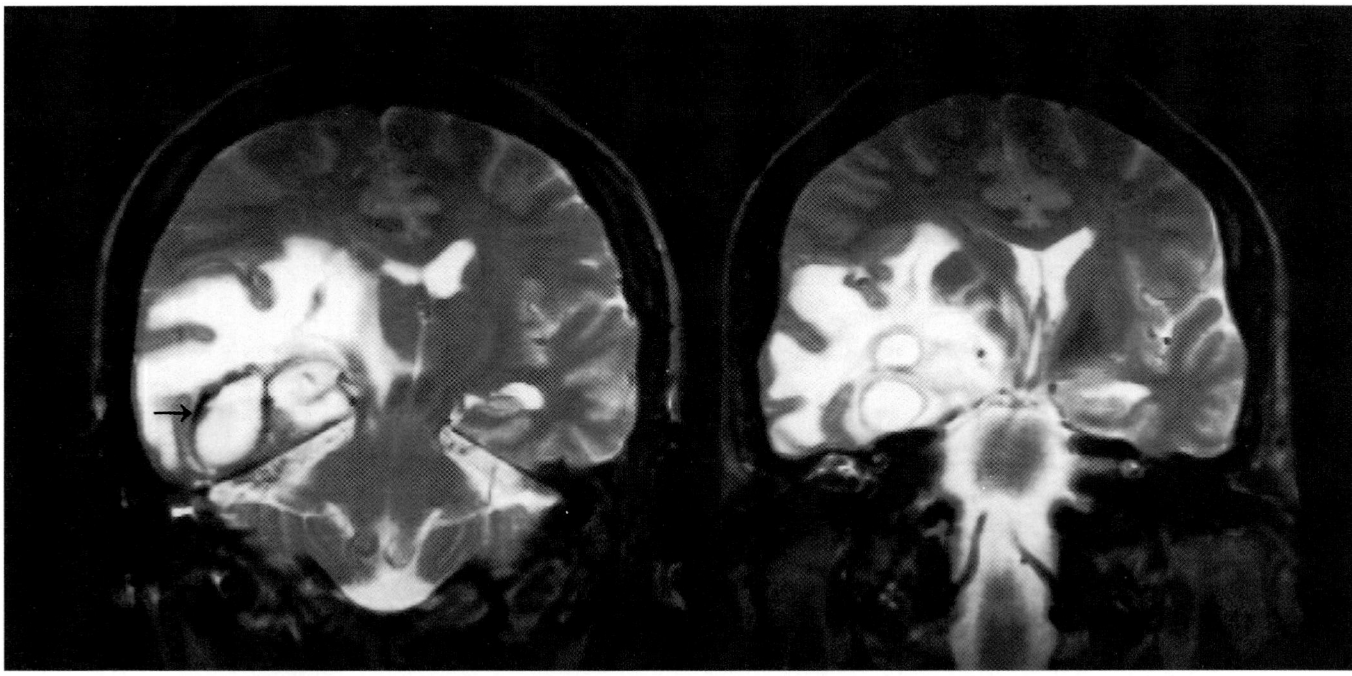

A

B

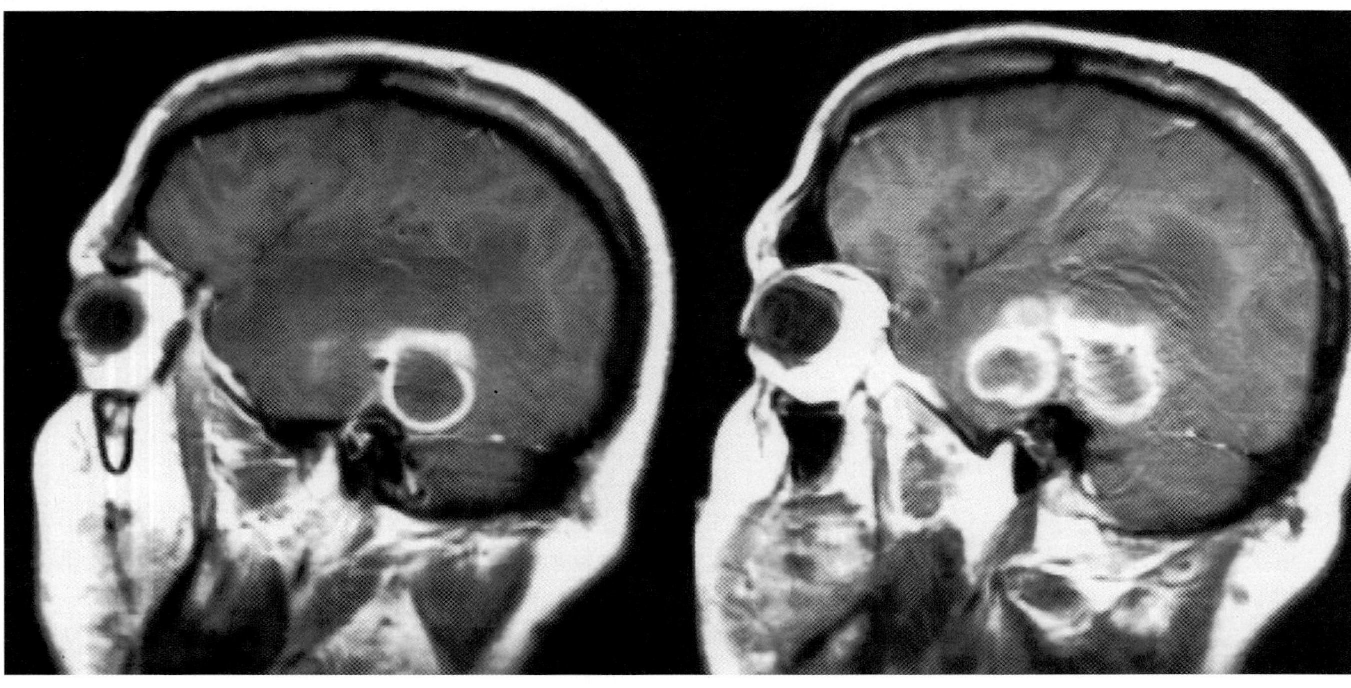

Fig. 19. *Multiple otogenic abscesses of the left temporal lobe.* 35-year-old man with progressive left hemiparesis and temporospatial disorientation. The T_2-weighted images (A) show the intensely edematogenic abscess components; their fibrotic walls are hypointense with the purulent fluid and with the edema. The outermost mass has a hemosiderin rim (→). In B, the contrast-enhanced rim of the abscess walls is well outlined after GD-DTPA administration.

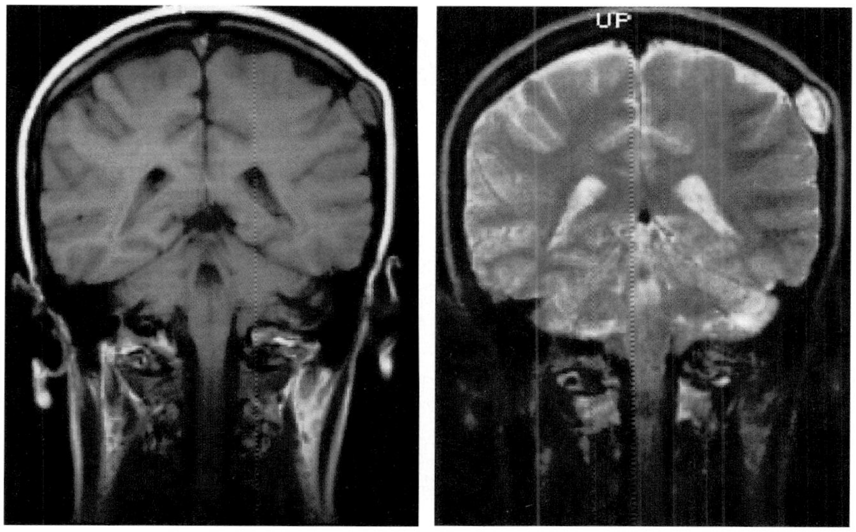

A B

Fig. 20. *Left parietal diploic angioma.* T_1- (A) and T_2- (B) weighted coronal cuts demonstrating an isointense (T_1) and hyperintense (T_2) intradiploic mass. Given the features of MRI, a more specific diagnosis is impossible. The T_2-weighted image demonstrates that the lesion has not completely eroded the inner diploe.

A B C

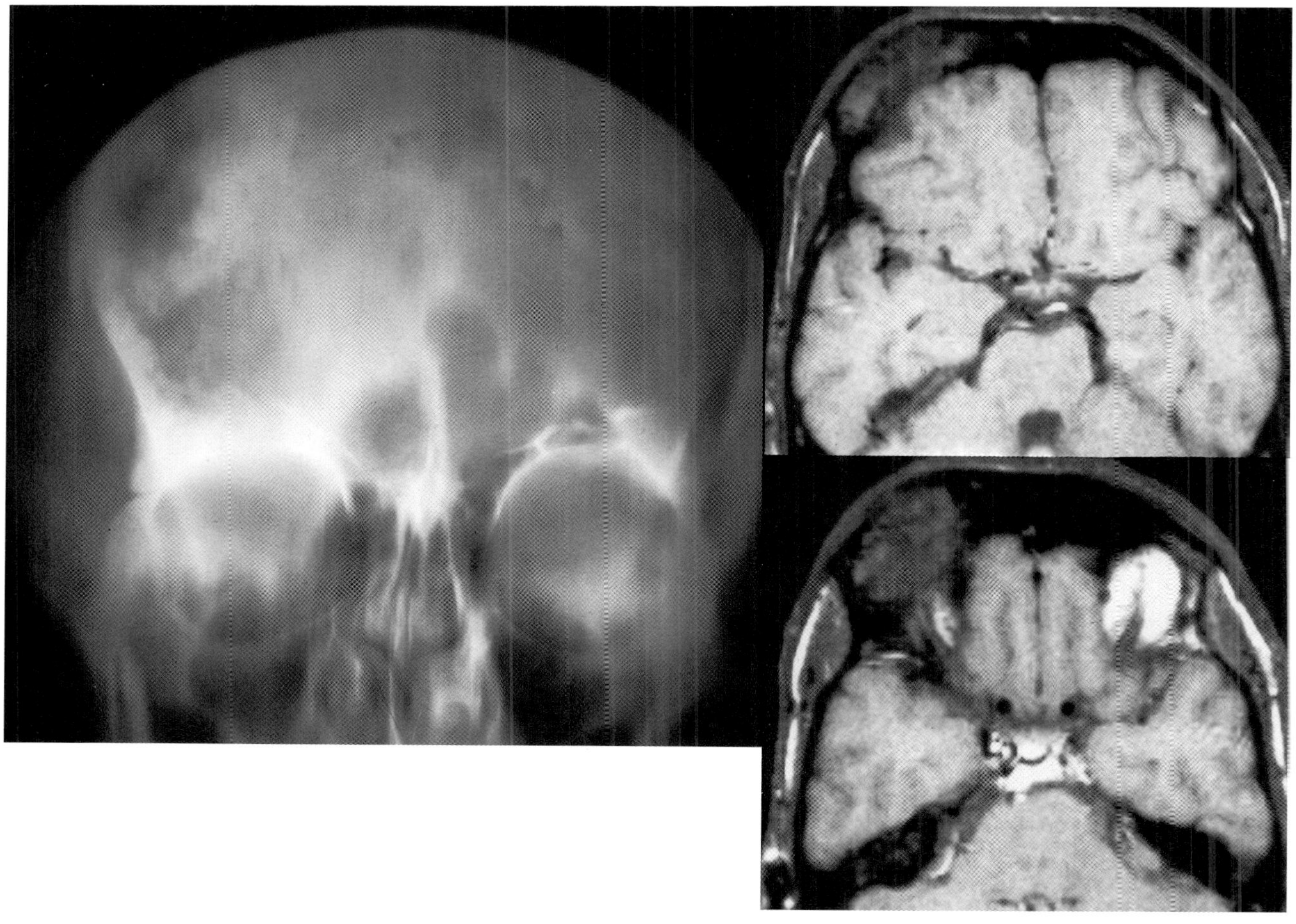

Fig. 21. *Right orbito-zygomatic fibrous dysplasia.* 33-year-old patient with pulsating headache and mildly tender, right supraorbital bone tumefaction. A – Conventional laminography of the fronto-orbital region: structural disruption of the frontal bone and hypertrophy of the zygomatic process. B, C – T_1-weighted axial cuts: they confirm the structural changes of the frontal bone, inhomogeneous hypointensity, integrity of the dural plane and no compression on the cerebral tissue. The upper margin of the orbital cavity is mildly deformed by the bone dysplasia.

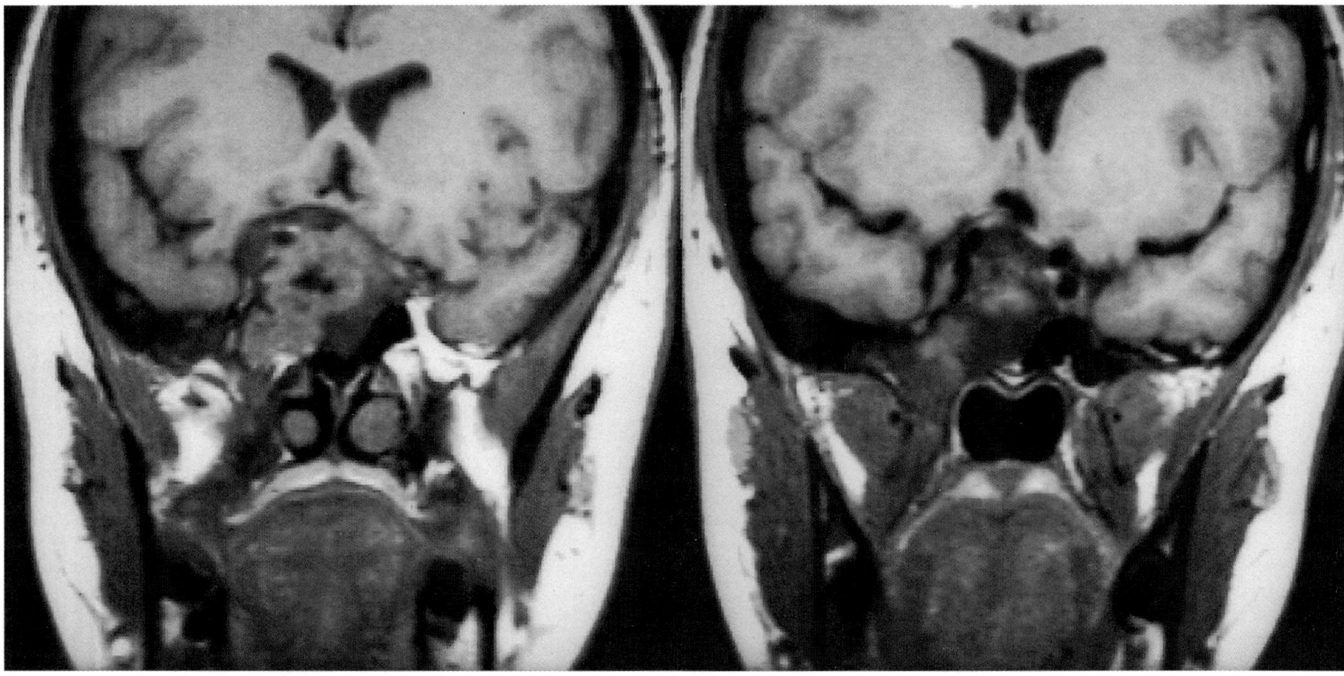

A

B

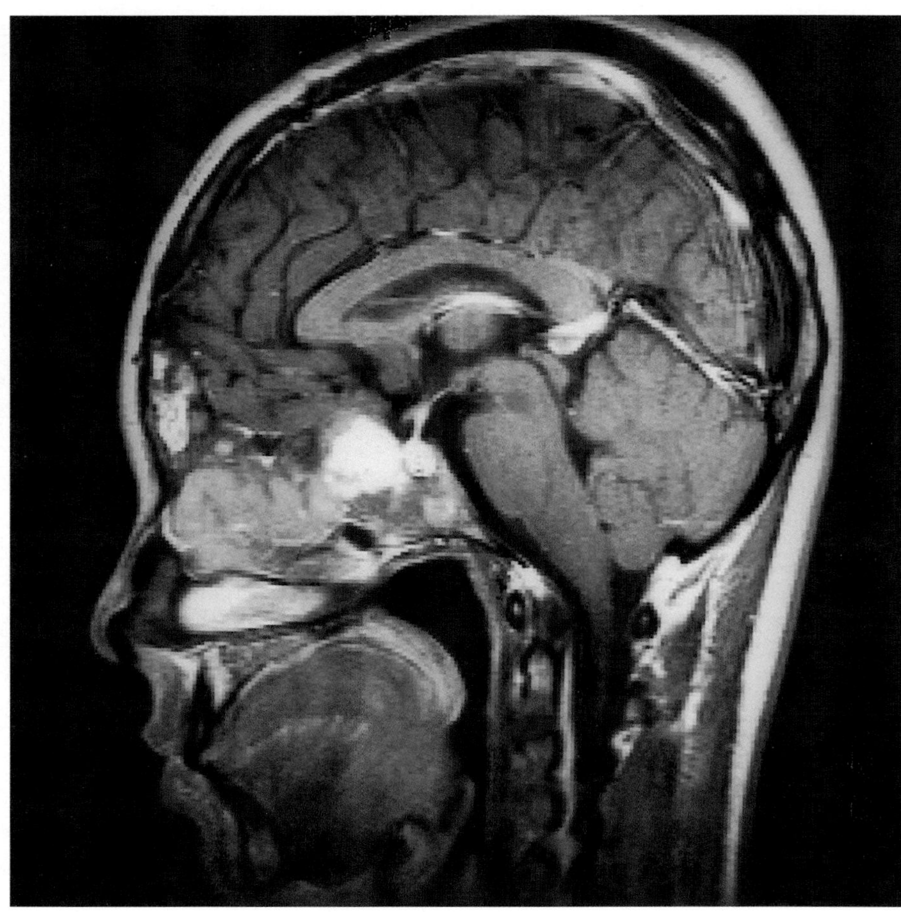

Fig. 22. *Orbitosphenoethmoidal fibrous dysplasia.* 22-year-old woman with prior surgery for decompression of the right optic nerve. Recently, she had had episodes of narcolepsy and oligomenorrhea. A – The T_1-weighted images show the altered and thickened bone which protrudes into the anterior cranial fossa, compresses the hypothalamus and elevates the optic tracts. On the sagittal view after GD-DTPA, note the significant enhancement of the fleshy components of the dysplastic process and of the pituitary, which is compressed into a small sella turcica.

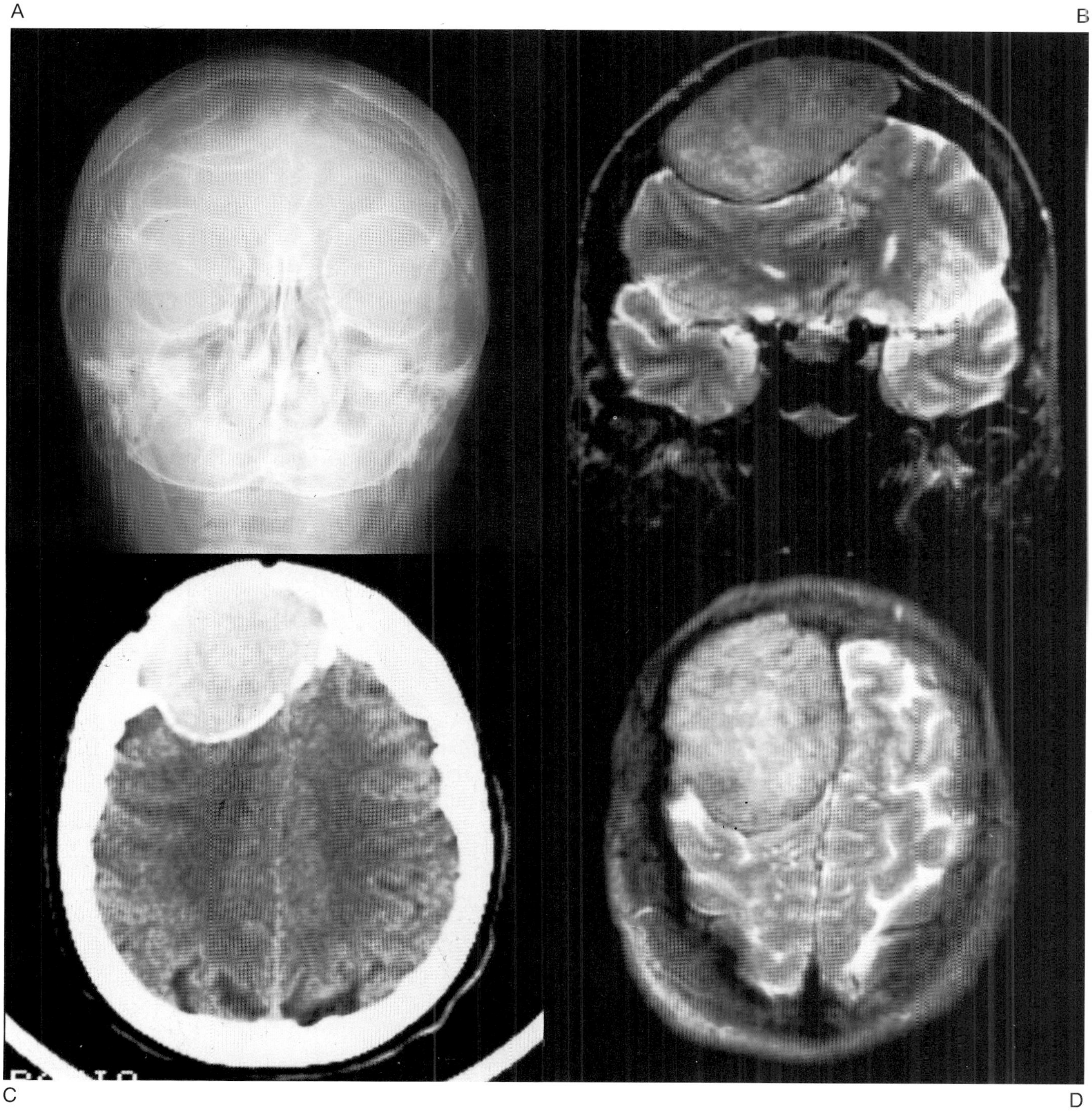

Fig. 23. *Right frontal plasmocytoma.* 66-year-old woman. Several years of progressive right frontal tumefaction. A – Plain film of the skull: osteolysis in the right frontal region with a sclerotic rim around the inner diploe. B – T_2-weighted coronal view: the lesion of diploic origin mainly grows outside the skull and leaves the inner and outer diploe unaffected; its structure is moderately inhomogeneous with average intensity signal. The internal theca appears as a sclerotic rim encircling the mass. C – Non-contrast CT: nutshell-shaped alteration of the right frontal bone which incorporates an approximately ovoid, slightly inhomogeneous, hyperdense core. D – T_2-weighted scan: the mass displaces the right frontal lobe and the cerebral falx; internally, it is inhomogeneous; posteriorly, it has a rim indicating the internal theca and intact dural plane.

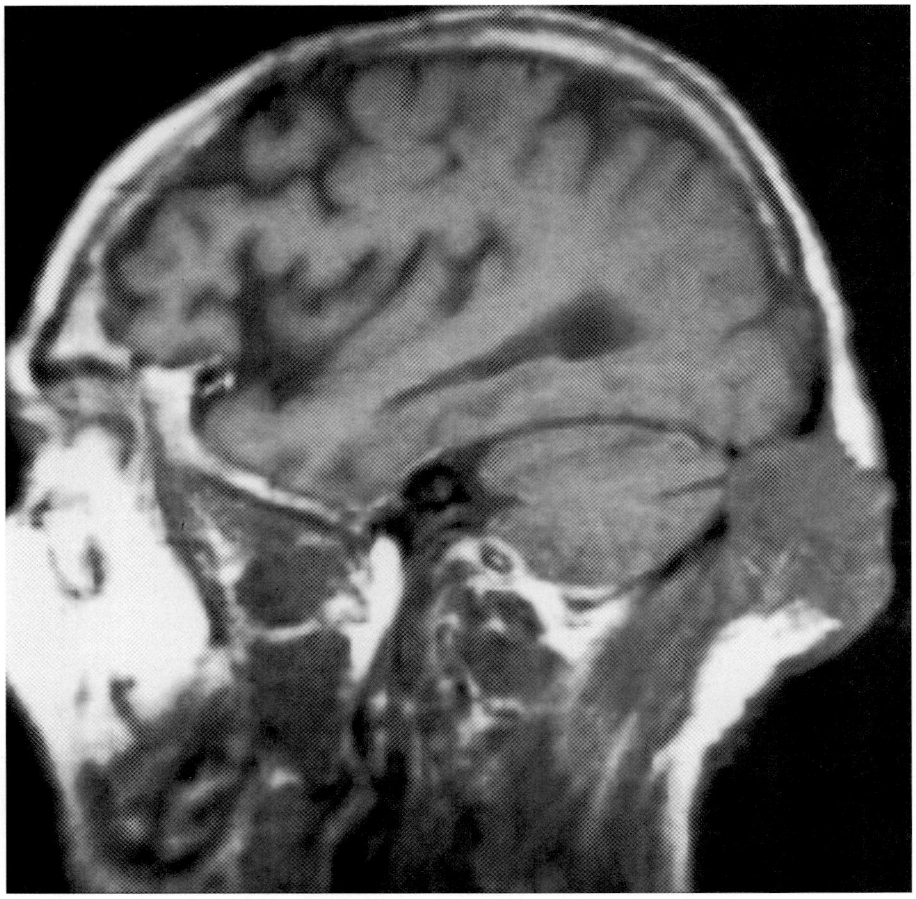

Fig. 24. *Basal cell epithelioma of the occipitonuchal region.* T_1-weighted paramedian sagittal scan. Extra- and intracranial lesion at the level of the torcular and of the left transverse sinus. Distally, the tumor infiltrates the nuchal muscles.

References

1. Anthony CD, Tucker JA (1990) Histiocytosis X affecting the nervous system. In: Wilkins RH, Rengachary SS (eds) Neurosurgery Update I. McGraw-Hill, New York, 36–41
2. Antunes JL, Louis KM, Ganti SR (1980) Colloid cyst of the third ventricle. Neurosurgery 7:450–455
3. Atlas SW (1990) Adult supratentorial tumors. Semin Roentgenol 25:130–154
4. Bosh DA, Rahn T, Backlund EO (1978) Treatment of colloid cysts of the third ventricle by stereotactic aspiration. Surg Neurol 9:15–18
5. Bronen RA, Sze G (1990) Magnetic resonance contrast agents: theory and application to the central nervous system. J Neurosurg 73:820–840
6. Byrd SE, Locke GE, Biggers S, Percy AK (1982) The computed tomographic appearance of cerebral cysticercosis in adults and children. Radiology 144:819–823
7. Carmel PW (1990) Brain tumors of disordered embryogenesis. In: Youmans JR (ed) Neurological Surgery, Vol. 5, 3rd edn. W. B. Saunders Co, Philadelphia, 3152–3170
8. Cobb CA III, Youmans JR (1990) Sarcomas and neoplasms of blood vessels. In: Youmans JR (ed) Neurological Surgery, Vol. 5, 3rd edn. W. B. Saunders Co, Philadelphia, 3152–3170
9. Dierckx IM, Appel B, Mortelmans LL (1990) Multifocal intracranial tumoral lesions: Neuroimaging and differential diagnosis with non-oncologic pathology. J Belge Radiol 73:7–14
10. Enzmann DR (1984) Imaging of Infections and Inflammations of the Central Nervous System: Computed Tomography, Ultrasound, and Nuclear Magnetic Resonance. Raven Press, New York
11. Favara BE, McCarthy RC, Mierau GW (1983) Histiocytosis X. Hum Pathol 14:663–676
12. Friedman RB, Segal R, Latchaw RE (1986) Computerized tomographic and magnetic resonance imaging of intracranial lipoma. J Neurosurg 65:407–410
13. Graif M, Pennock JM (1986) MR imaging of histiocytosis X in the central nervous system. AJNR 7:21–23
14. Guidetti B, Gagliardi FM (1977) Epidermoid and dermoid cysts: Clinical evaluation and late surgical results. J Neurosurg 43:12–18
15. Guidetti B, Spallone A (1981) The surgical treatment of choroid plexus papillomas; the results of 27 years experience. Neurosurg Rev 4:129–137
16. Helle TL, Britt RH, Colbi TV (1984) Primary lymphoma of the central nervous system. J Neurosurg 60:94–103
17. Higer HP, Pedrosa P, Schuth M (1989) MR Imaging of cerebral tumors: State of the art and work in progress. Neurosurg Rev 12:91–106
18. Ingraham FD, Bailey OT (1946) Cystic teratomas and teratoid tumors of central nervous system in infancy and childhood. J Neurosurg 3:511–532
19. Jack CR Jr, Reese DF, Scheithauer BW (1985) Radiographic findings in 32 cases of primary CNS lymphoma. AJNR 6:899–904
20. Jelinek J, Smirniotopoulos JG, Parisi JE, Kanzer M (1990) Lateral ventricular neoplasms of the brain: Differential diagnosis based on clinical, CT, and MR findings. Am J Roentgenol 155:365–372
21. Kjos BO, Brant-Zawadzki M, Kucharczyle W et al. (1985) Cystic intracranial lesions: Magnetic Resonance Imaging. Radiology 155:363–369
22. Koos WT, Miller MH (1971) Intracranial tumors of infants and children. Mosby, St Louis
23. Kortman KE, Van Dalsem W, Bradley WG (1985) MRI of intracranial epidermoid tumors. Radiology 157:71
24. Kwan E, Wolpert SM, Smith SP, Modic MT (1987) Radiology of third ventricular lesions. In: Apuzzo MLJ (ed) Surgery of the Third Ventricle. Williams & Wilkins, Baltimore, 262–300
25. Larson TC, Houser OW, Laws ER Jr (1987) Imaging of cranial chordomas. Mayo Clin Proc 62:886–893
26. Loftus CM, Biller J (1990) Management of multiple brain abscesses. In: Wilkins RH, Rengachary SS (eds) Neurosurgery. McGraw-Hill, New York, 282–285
27. Matsumoto J, Towbin RB, Ball WS Jr (1989) Cranial chordomas in infancy and childhood. A report of two cases and review of the literature. Pediatr Radiol 20:28–32
28. McGrath P (1971) Cysts of the sellar and pharyngeal hypophysis. Pathology 3:123–131
29. Neuwelt EA, Gumerbock MK, Dahlborg SA (1990) Lymphomas of the brain in adults. In: Youmans JR (eds) Neurological Surgery, Vol. 5, 3rd edn. W. B. Saunders Co, Philadelphia, 3137–3151
30. Oot RF, Melville GE, New PF et al. (1988) The role of MR and CT in evaluating clival chordomas and chondrosarcomas. AJR 151:567–575
31. Parizel PM, Degryse HL, Gheuens J et al. (1989) Gadolinium-DTPA enhanced MR imaging of intracranial lesions. Comput Assist Tomogr 13:378–385
32. Parker JC Jr, Dyer ML (1985) Neurologic infections due to bacteria, fungi, and parasites. In: Davis RL, Robertson DM (eds) Textbook of Neuropathology. Williams & Wilkins, Baltimore, 632–703

33. Pomeranz SJ (1988) MR of supratentorial neoplasia. In: Pomeranz SJ (ed) Craniospinal Magnetic Resonance Imaging. W. B. Saunders Co, Philadelphia, 208–247
34. Pomeranz SJ (1989) Posterior fossa, skull base, craniocervical junction. In: Pomeranz SJ (ed) Craniospinal Magnetic Resonance Imaging. W. B. Saunders Co, Philadelphia, 248–274
35. Rich TA, Shiller A, Suit HD et al. (1985) Clinical and pathologic review of 48 cases of chordoma. Cancer 56:182–187
36. Schorner W, Laniado M, Kornmesser W, Felix R (1989) Comparison of multi-echo and contrast-enhanced MR scans: Image contrast and delineation of intracranial tumors. Neuroradiology 31:140–147
37. Sekhar LN, Schramm VL Jr, Jones NF (1987) Subtemporal-preauricular infratemporal fossa approach to large lateral and posterior cranial base neoplasms. J Neurosurg 67:488–499
38. Sen CN, Sekhar LN, Schramm VL, Janecka IP (1989) Chordoma and chondrosarcoma of the cranial base: A 8-year experience. Neurosurgery 25:931–940
39. Simon JH, Szumowski J (1989) Chemical shift imaging with paramagnetic contrast material enhancement for improved lesion depiction. Radiology 171:539–543
40. Sze G, Zimmerman RD (1988) The Magnetic Resonance Imaging of infections and inflammatory diseases. Radiol Clin North Am 26:839–859
41. Tekenchi J, Mori K, Moritakes K et al. (1975) Teratomas in the suprasellar region: Report of five cases. Surg Neurol 2:247–255
42. terPenning B (1989) Inflammatory disease of the brain and spine. In: Pomeranz SJ (ed) Craniospinal Magnetic Resonance Imaging. W. B. Saunders Co, Philadelphia, 436–458
43. Waluch V, Dyck P (1990) Magnetic resonance imaging of posterior fossa masses. In: Wilkins RH, Rengachary SS (eds) Neurosurgery. McGraw-Hill, New York, 30–46
44. Yamada S, Kubota R, Yamada K (1990) T1 and T2 relaxation times on Gadolinium-Diethylenetriaminepentaacetic acid enhanced Magnetic Resonance images of brain tumors. Tohoku J Exp Med 160:145–148
45. Young SC, Grossman RI, Goldberg HI et al. (1989) MR of vascular encasement in parasellar masses: Comparison with Angiography and CT. AJNR 9:35–38
46. Yuh WT, Flickinger FW, Barloon TJ, Montgomery WJ (1988) MR Imaging of unusual chordomas. J Comput Assist Tomogr 12:30–35
47. Zimmerman RA (1990) Magnetic resonance imaging of intracranial infections. In: Wilkins RH, Rengachary SS (eds) Neurosurgery. McGraw-Hill, New York, 88–103
48. Zimmerman RA, Bilaniuk LT, Sze G (1987) Intracranial infection. In: Brant-Zawadzki M, Norman D (eds) Magnetic Resonance Imaging of the Central Nervous System. Raven Press, New York, 235–257

CHAPTER XII

Spinal Tumors

Spinal tumors are not classified according to the cell type they originate from, as was the case with intracranial tumors, but according to anatomical site, in particular in relation to the dura mater and to the SC. Hence, they may be extradural, intradural extramedullar, and intramedullar (Table I). Dysembryogenic tumors will be covered separately.

Amongst available diagnostic modalities, MRI is the method of choice for the study of spinal disorders because it provides a direct multilayered visualization of the content of the spine: cord, subarachnoid spaces and extradural structures.

Demonstrating the site of origin of the disease is thus easy, especially if a suitable technique is used, which will have to include T_1- and T_2-weighted sequences, sagittal and axial scans and often paramagnetic contrast media. T_2-weighted images are of paramount importance, given their greater sensitivity in direct visualization of the lesion and their "myelographic-like" intrathecal contrast effect. Such contrast, between the high signal of the CSF and the low signal of the cord and of the nerve roots, is absolutely necessary when evaluating whether there has been a complete or partial CSF pathway obstruction.

According to recent studies, also the i.v. administration of paramagnetic contrast medium proved to be of diagnostic importance in studying spinal tumors and absolutely necessary for identifying intramedullar neoplasms, leptomeningeal metastases and small neurinomas and meningiomas *(Fig. 15)*.

The extradural neoplasms located in the epidural space which compress the cord are mainly metastases and lymphomas. The epidural space may be subordinately compromised through the conjugation foramina and/or through extension of the tumor from its vertebral bone nidus *(Figs. 1, 2, 3)* or through the bloodstream.

Metastases in the extradural space are more frequently found because the life expectancy of cancer patients has become longer; they are predicted to occur in 5% of cases. The primary tumors that preferentially metastasize to the spine are lung, breast and gastrointestinal carcinomas, as well as melanomas. Lymphomas may first appear in the vertebrae or involve the spine in a systemic disease. The vertebra involved is very frequently the site of an osteolytic lesion with a possible somatic collapse, but at times, especially in Hodgkin's disease, there is an osteoblastic reaction evidenced by osteosclerosis. In the peridural lymphomatous locations, the tumor forms an infiltrating "sleeve", which stenoses the dural sac and which may grow considerably in length *(Fig. 7)*.

Clinical symptomatology is dominated by pain, often intractable by normal pain relievers and which responds only to surgical decompression or early radiation therapy. Sensorimotor deficits, secondary to cord compression and to radicular damage, may have an acute onset and evolve rapidly. To point out the importance of an early and correct diagnosis, it is worth recalling that a patient with complete paraplegia for more than 48 hours has very little prospect of recovery.

T_1-weighted MR images show the vertebral metastases as hypointense areas *(Fig. 1)* with respect to the bone marrow, that produces a relatively high signal owing to its fatty component; on the T_2-weighted images, the metastases are hyperintense *(Figs. 1, 2)* and may appear as inhomogeneous as a result of concurrent osteosclerosis. If sclerosis is prevalent, the metastatic focus will remain hypointense, even on T_2 images. In order not to make mistakes in the diagnosis, it is necessary to be aware of the way in which the bone signal varies as a function of age-related bone changes and/or of a degenerative disease.

Table 1. Guide to differential diagnosis of spinal tumors

Location Onchotype	Age (decades)	Favorite site	Symptoms
EXTRADURAL			
METASTASES			
lung carcinoma (c.) breast c.	4th–6th	Dorsal	Pain – sensorimotor deficiency
prostatic c.	6th–7th	Lumbar	Pain – radicular deficiency
LYMPHOMA MYELOMA	3rd–6th	Dorso-lumbar	Pain – sensorimotor deficiency
PRIMARY VERTEBRAL TUMORS			
chordoma	2nd–6th	Sacral	Pain – Cord and radicular deficiency
osteoblastoma		Dorsal	
INTRADURAL			
MENINGIOMA	4th–5th (fem.)	Cervico-dorsal	Slow-progressing cord deficiency
NEURINOMA	2nd–5th	Dorsal	Radicular pain – Slow-progressing deficiency
METASTASES (medulloblastoma, ependymoblastoma, germinoma)	1st–2nd	Ubiquitous	Radicular pain – Cord and radicular deficiencies
INTRAMEDULLAR			
ASTROCYTOMA	1st–5th	Cervico-dorsal	Slow-progressing cord deficiency
EPENDYMOMA	1st–5th	Cono-caudal	Slow-progressing cord deficiency
HEMANGIOBLASTOMA	3rd–4th	Ubiquitous	Slow-progressing cord deficiency
ANGIOMA	2nd–4th	Dorsal	Slow-progressing cord deficiency
METASTASES (lung c., breast c., melanoma)		Dorso-lumbar	Cord deficiency
INTRA-EXTRAMEDULLAR			
LIPOMA	1st–2nd	Cono-caudal	Lower limb distal deficiency Sphincteral deficiencies
EPIDERMOID	2nd–3rd	Dorso-lumbar	Recurrent aseptic meningites
DERMOID			Lower limb myelo-radicular deficiency
TERATOMA	1st	Ubiquitous	Cord deficiency

MRI signal characteristics T_1-weighted seq.	 T_2-weighted seq.	Signal changes after GD-DTPA–T_1-weighted seq.	Regressive processes	Other characteristics
Hypointensity	Hyperintensity			Osteolytic alterations (X-ray–CT) Vertebral collapse
Hypointensity	Hyper/hypointensity			Bone-densifying alterations (X-ray–CT)
Hypo/isointensity	Hyperintensity	Hyperintensity		Associated bone alterations Sleeve-shaped arrangement Multiple foci
Hypointensity	Hyperintensity	Hyperintensity	Calcifications	
Hypointensity	Hypointensity			
Hypointensity	Iso/hyperintensity	Hyperintensity	Calcifications	
Hypo/isointensity	Hyperintensity	Hyperintensity	Cysts Hyaline degeneration	Multiple neurinomas (Recklinghausen's disease) Intra-extradural neurinomas (dumbbell)
Hypo/isointensity	Hyperintensity	Hyperintensity		Neoplastic cells in the CSF
Hypo/isointensity	Hyperintensity	Inhomogeneous hyperintensity	Cysts Hemorrhage	Syringomyelia
Hypo/isointensity	Hyperintensity	Hyperintensity	Cysts Hemorrhage	Syringomyelia
Hypo/iso/hyperintensity vascular images	Hyper/isointensity Vascular images	High hyperintensity	Cysts Mural nodule	Syringomyelia Multiple hemangioblastomas (Hippel-Lindau's disease)
Serpiginous images with signal void	Hemosiderin deposits		Hemorrhage	
Isointensity	Hyperintensity	Hyperintensity		
Hyperintensity	Signal decrease			Associated dysrhafic state Dermal sinus
Inhomogeneous hypointensity	Inhomogeneous hyperintensity	None		Associated dysrhafic state
Hyperintensity	Hyperintensity			Dermal sinus
Inhomogeneity	Inhomogeneity		Calcifications	Possible malignant degeneration

Alterations such as intrasomatic Schmorl's nodules, degenerative sclerosis of the discosomatic limiting membranes and senile fibroses of the spine are not only site-specific but generate hypointense T_1 and T_2 images with a predominantly linear appearance. In active degenerative discopathy, however, low intensity foci may be observed on T_1 sequences, which become high intensity foci on T_2 images. Instead, the generally intrasomatic hyperintense focal areas, often displayed by T_1-weighted sequences, are to be ascribed to local build-up of bone marrow and, if larger, to bone lipomas proper. In these cases, signal intensity weakens on T_2 sequences, which is typical of fat tissue.

In terms of differential diagnosis, vertebral angiomas have variable intensities on T_1-weighted images, whereas on T_2 images they produce high signals and often show typical radial morphologies *(Fig. 11)*.

MRI is useful in primary bone neoplasms not so much for specificity as for a precise evaluation of the extent of the lesion and for establishing the involvement of the SC and of the nerve roots *(Fig. 10)*.

The surgical therapy of extradural neoplasms consists of decompressive laminectomy and removal of the tumor, which must be as extensive as possible. Surgery is indicated in the following cases: cord compression and spinal instability; neoplasm resistant to radiation therapy; relapse of cord compresison in long-term survivors. A pre-requisite is that the causal lesion should be a single one.

The primary tumors of the spine, which are mostly benign, are to be resected *en bloc,* using bone grafts and metal clamps to stabilize the spine.

Extramedullar intradural tumors are generally benign as in 90% of cases they are meningiomas and neurinomas.

Neurinomas arise from the roots of spinal nerves and may grow also outside the spine as occurs with dumbbell-shaped tumors *(Fig. 16)*. Multiple tumors can be found in patients with neurofibromatosis *(Fig. 15)*.

Neurinomas are characterized by an occasionally moderate increase in T_1 and T_2 relaxation times and are hypo-isointense on T_1 images *(Fig. 12)* and hyperintense on T_2-weighted ones *(Figs. 13, 14)*. They have sharp contours, are well encapsulated and may be round-shaped or oval; they model and displace the cord, which seldom shows signal changes. In order to evidence the growth of the lesion in the subarachnoid space and the contralateral displacement of the SC, thin slices should be obtained (4 mm) using the multi-echo technique along sagittal and axial planes. Moreover, axial scans are necessary for evaluating the extent of dumbbell neurinomas, because they show their intraforaminal component and their growth inside the paravertebral groove *(Fig. 16)*. On T_2-weighted images, large spinal neurinomas have a very inhomgeneous high intensity, due to regressive events of cystic type or of hyaline degeneration.

The incidence of spinal meningiomas is higher among females. Their favorite site is the dorsal spine both anteriorly and posteriorly to the SC *(Figs. 18, 20)*. They are typically sessile, the base by which they are attached to the dura mater being very large *(Fig. 19)*. They produce significant compression on the SC and as a result of their considerable density, they may deform contiguous bone structures. On T_1-weighted images, they are mostly hypo- or isointense with the SC and are moderately hyperintense on T_2-weighted images. However, these signal characteristics are not the rule. Both meningiomas and neurinomas can be more easily detected after i.v. administration of gadolinium (GD-DTPA), because they are both considerably enhanced *(Figs. 13, 14, 18, 20)*. Hence, the use of paramagnetic contrast proves to be particularly useful in identifying multiple or small-sized lesions *(Fig. 15)*.

Meningiomas and neurinomas are clinically characterized by a slow-growing neurological deficit, secondary to compression. Radicular pain is typical of neurinomas. Laterally-located tumors may cause the Brown-Séquard syndrome, characterized by ipsilateral paresis and sensory deficit of the epicritical sensitivity, combined with contralateral deficit of the protopathic sensitivity.

Therapy consists in radical resection of single tumors and of the symptomatic tumor/s in the case of multiple locations. In the cases of anterior meningiomas and of dumbbell-shaped neurinomas, surgery is very challenging and requires the cooperation of a general surgeon to remove the extraspinal component. A correct diagnosis, right from the beginning, evidencing the presence of a mediastinal or abdominal mass originating from within the spine, is of critical importance.

Finally, among intradural tumors, mention must be made of CSF-mediated metastases from cerebral neoplasms. The most common are those originating from medulloblastomas *(Figs. 21, 22, 23)*, ependymoblastomas and germinomas. Metastases from other neuroepithelial tumors are rare.

Intramedullar tumors may derive from neuroepithelial cells *(Figs. 24, 25, 26, 31)* or from vessels *(Figs. 27, 28, 29, 30)*. The former are fairly common also in childhood and may involve the SC in its entirety. In children, intramedullar tumors may cause local enlargement of the spinal canal, which is shown by plain radiograms. Intramedullar tumors may be distinguished in ependymomas, astrocytomas, spinal angiomas and hemangioblastomas, whose biological characteristics do not differ from the corresponding types arising in the brain (Table 1). Ependymomas may be cystic *(Fig. 31)* or papillary. The tumors of the filum terminale are peculiar since they grow to considerable sizes thanks to the availability of space.

Medullar astrocytomas may be cystic and well demarcated or infiltrating *(Figs. 25, 26)*; the highly dedifferentiated forms and the glioblastoma multiforme are rare. Other types of gliomas (e.g. oligodendrogliomas) are very rare. Intramedullar tumors become clinically manifest by slowly-ingravescent sensorimotor deficits. Angioblastomas may be multiple and associated with similar encephalic and retinal lesions (Von Hippel-Lindau disease). Onset may be acute with subarachnoid hemorrhage and/or hematomyelia, as with angiomas, that may also be responsible for a steal symptomatology (cord claudication). In intramedullar tumors, pain is neither constant nor typical. A unique feature is instead the "segmented anesthesia" produced by compression from inside, on the crossing of the fibers of the spinothalamic tract behind the ependymal canal.

Intramedullar neoplasms are responsible for enlargements of the SC that go well beyond the actual size of the tumor. MRI is not only capable of demonstrating the morphological changes of the SC, but also the neoplasm in its solid and/or cystic component, often differentiating it from edema or from reactive gliosis and almost always from rostral or caudal syringomyelic cavities *(Figs. 26, 31)*. This is done by accurately evaluating signal intensity changes on T_1-, proton density- and T_2-weighted sequences and the changes occurring after i.v. injection of paramagnetic contrast medium.

Of particular importance is the discrimination between neoplastic cysts and syringomyelic cavities because the surgical procedure is different: resection for the former and decompression for the latter.

Given their long T_1 and T_2, syringomyelic cavities have a typical, well-defined, CSF-like signal; in addition, they may have low intensity on T_2-weighted sequences as a result of transmission of CSF pulsatility. Instead, because of their greater protein content, neoplastic cysts have shorter T_1s and T_2s and hence a relatively enhanced signal on T_1 and proton density images. When differential diagnosis is difficult, i.v. gadolinium can be used, which will evidence peripheral perfusion and, in late imaging (1 h), it will show intracavitary concentration of the paramagnetic contrast agent *(Fig. 26)*. However, all intramedullar neoplasms may be associated with syringomyelic dilatations *(Figs. 27, 28, 31)*.

The MRI signal of ependymomas is hypointense on T_1 images, hyperintense on T_2 ones and is significantly enhanced following GD-DTPA at the level of the solid component of the neoplasm, especially at the poles of the tumor that are generally more vascularized. Perilesional hemosiderin deposits, markedly hypointense on long-TR sequences, are a frequent finding.

Astrocytomas are hypo-isointense on T_1-weighted sequences and hyperintense on T_2 ones. Infiltrating astrocytomas have blurred margins, produce slight deformations of the spinal cord and become unevenly perfused with contrast medium owing to different alterations of the BBB. The

MRI appearance of hemangioblastomas is that of an intra-extramedullar nodular neoformation with hypo-hyperintense areas on T_1 images and hyperisointense areas on T_2 ones, with no edema, occasionally associated with images of hypertrophic vessels. Hyperintensity is marked after GD-DTPA. Spinal AVMs are generally located in the subarachnoid space and at times also in the SC, and they can be detected as serpiginous or enlarged vessels. On spin-echo sequences, they produce a low signal owing to flow; on gradient echo (FA 5–10 degrees) images, their signal is instead high. Hemorrhagic complications can be detected on T_1 images as periradicular hematomas (high signal) or as sequelae (low signal caused by hemosiderin) on T_2-weighted images. Because of vascular disorders, angiomas may be associated with signal changes from the surrounding cord owing to edema and/or malacia. An angiographic study is however indispensable for deciding on the correct surgical treatment of angiomas and hemangioblastomas. MRI is best suited for the serial monitoring of this disease both during its natural course and during follow-up after surgery. Spinal cavernous angiomas have the same features as the cerebral ones *(Figs. 29, 30)*. Their diagnosis is crucial for the patient, as the small hemorrhages that are asymptomatic in the brain may cause disaster in the cord *(Fig. 30)*.

Ependymomas and astrocytomas, particularly if they are cystic, are well resectable; therefore, their total surgical removal is possible. At times, cyst drainage and marsupialization can give the patient long periods of relief. Conversely, infiltrating gliomas cannot be resected. Angiomas and angioblastomas are to be excised *en bloc* after closing the feeding and draining vessels. These lesions are always well demarcated from the SC even though cleavage from the surrounding healthy tissue may be difficult. It must however be emphasized that, from the surgical viewpoint, the SC is a much more vulnerable organ than the brain, because its vascular bed is not provided with sufficient anastomoses; consequently, any vascular lesion may entail enormous anatomical and functional damage.

Before MRI, intramedullar metastatic tumors were considered very rare. Nowadays, several cases have been reported in the literature. Breast carcinoma and melanomas are the most frequent tumors which give intramedullar metastases *(Figs. 32, 33)*.

Dysembryogenic tumors can be classified as either intramedullar or intra-extramedullar. They derive from embryonic residues trapped in the neural tube at the time of its closure. The most common forms are lipomas of the cauda which originate from the filum terminale *(Figs. 35, 36)*. Epidermoids, dermoids and teratomas are less frequent *(Fig. 34)*, and they too arise in the cauda. They are often associated with dysraphia. The disorders induced by these neoplasms are mostly related to the tethering of the SC; hence they become manifest in school children and during puberty when their growth is at its peak. They are characterized by distal deficits in the lower limbs with equinism and sphincteral disorders. The presence of epidermoids and dermoids may be suspected in the event of aseptic and relapsing meningites caused by debris shed by the tumor and also by the presence of a dermal sinus.

Lipomas are characterized by short T_1 and T_2 relaxation times; teratomas produce highly inhomogeneous signals on all sequences. In spite of cholesterin, epidermoids rarely elicit high intensity signals on T_1 sequences, unlike dermoids that are markedly hyperintense on these sequences. The resection of lipomas and epidermoids is extremely difficult because of the tough adhesions that they develop with the roots of the cauda. Given their low proliferation rate, it is often preferable to merely disengage the SC, partially resect the tumor and widen the spinal canal.

Mention must also be made of malformations which may be confused with neoplasms at a superficial examination. If densitometry is not performed correctly, thoracic meningoceles can be mistaken for dumbbell neurinomas on CT scans. In such cases, MRI is always capable of settling the dispute *(Figs. 37, 38)*.

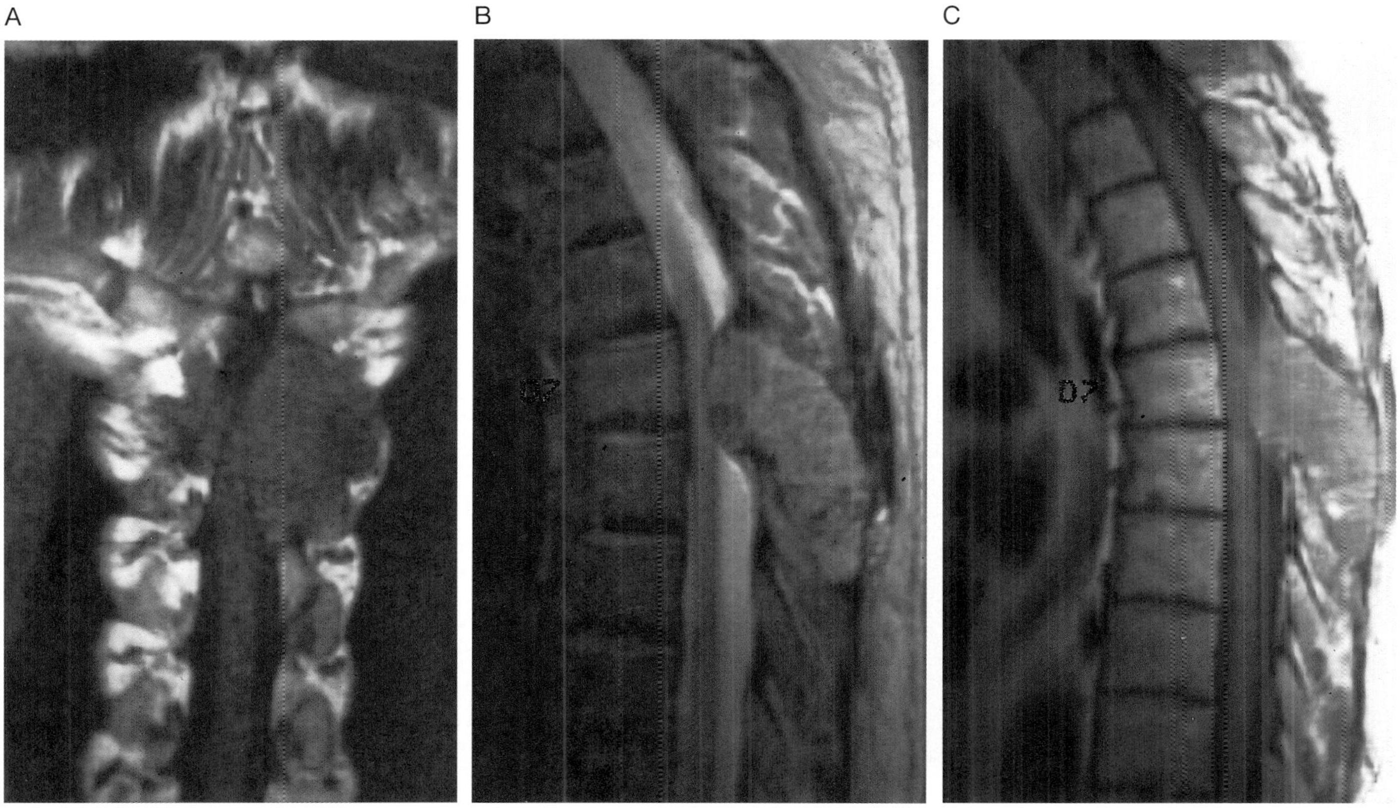

Fig. 1. *Metastasis from prostatic carcinoma.* The T_1-weighted coronal image (A) well demonstrates the spread of the neoplasm to the left laminae of D6, D7, D8 and to the right lamina of D7. The cord is displaced and sleeve-like compressed. The proton density- (B) and T_2-weighted (C) sagittal images show the obliteration of the posterior subarachnoid space and the cord compression. However, on these images, the compression appears less severe than on the coronal images.

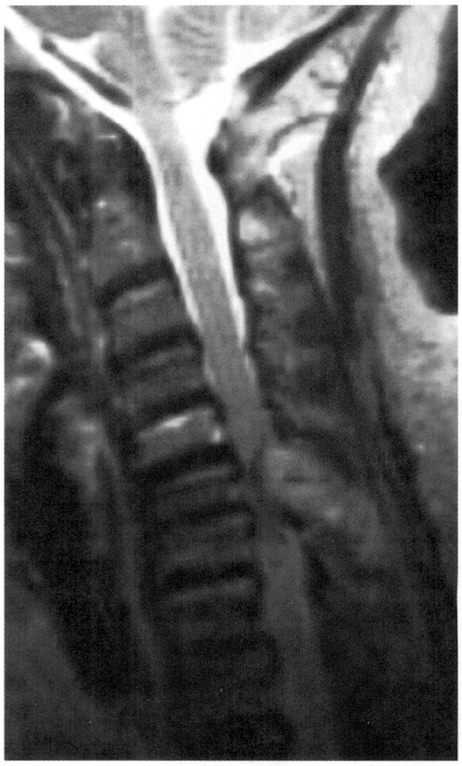

Fig. 2. *C5 bone metastasis from breast carcinoma.* T_2-weighted view: the lesion involves the spinous apophysis and the laminae. The spinal cord is markedly compressed.

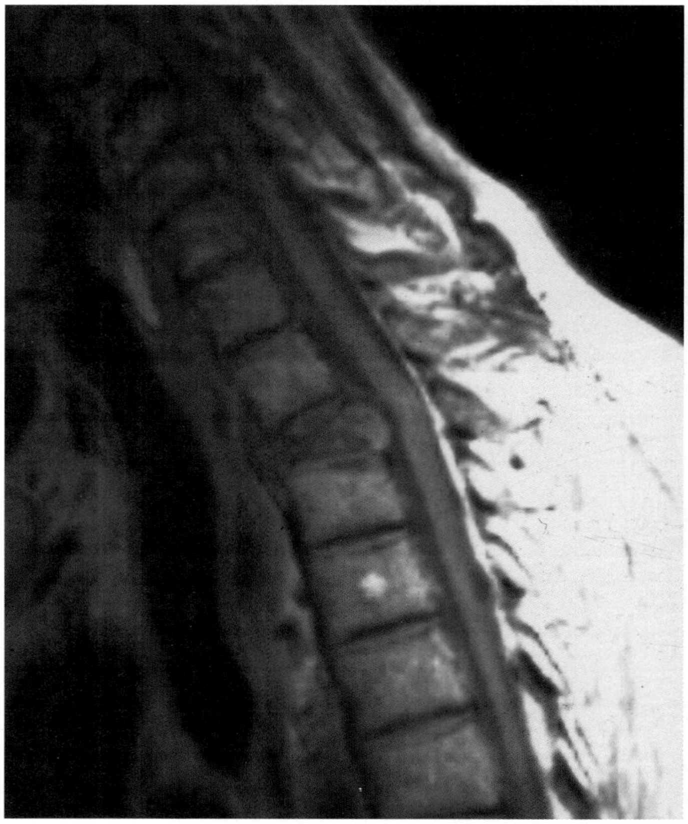

A

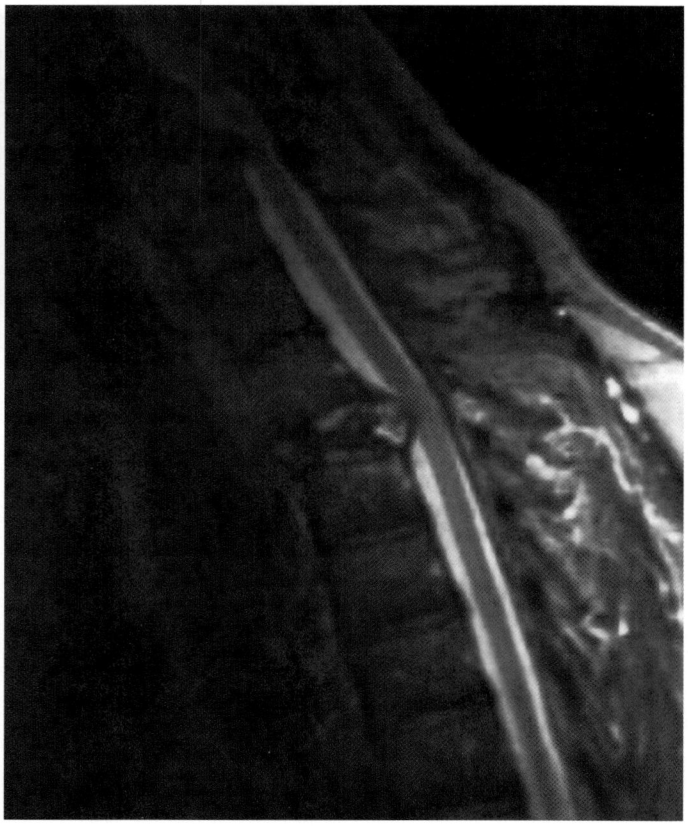

B

Fig. 3. *D2 bone-disrupting metastasis from gastric carcinoma.* A – TR 550 msec, TE 15 msec; B – TR 2,500 msec, TE 90 msec. Wedge-shaped deformation of the vertebral body with intact intervertebral disc spaces: the compression of the cord, displaced posteriorly against the laminae, is better seen on the T_2-weighted sequence (B), where the anterior subarachnoid space is totally obliterated by the neoplasm and crushed posteriorly against the laminae.

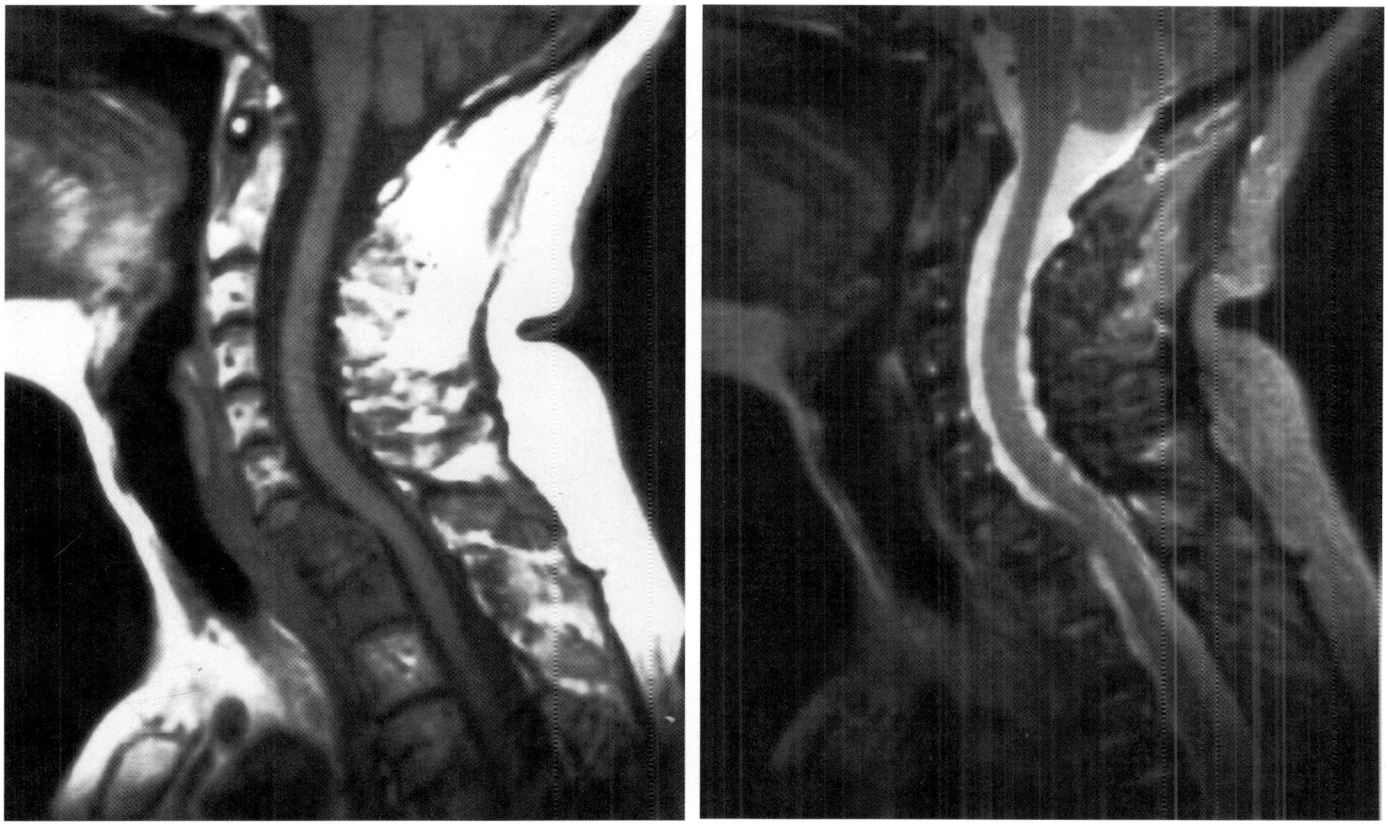

A B

Fig. 4. *C7–D1 somatic metastasis from lung carcinoma.* A – TR 550 msec, TE 15 msec; B – TR 2,500 msec, TE 90 msec. (A) shows a diffusely hypointense signal from the vertebral bodies whose posterior margin protrudes into the spinal canal. (B) depicts the effacement of the subarachnoid space and indentation of the spinal cord with unaltered signal. Note the integrity of the discs, which is an important finding in making a differential diagnosis with respect to inflammatory disorders (see Figs. 5 and 6).

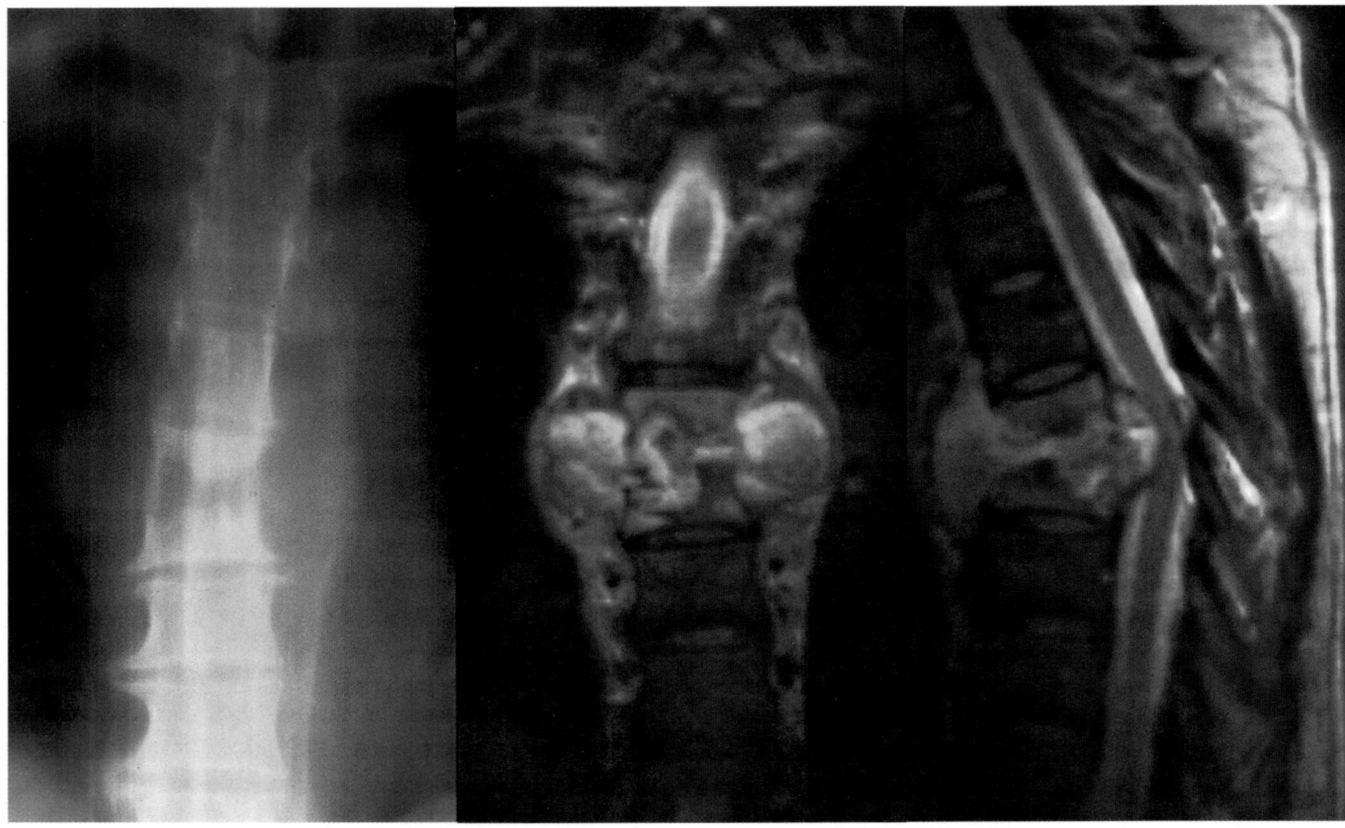

A B C

D

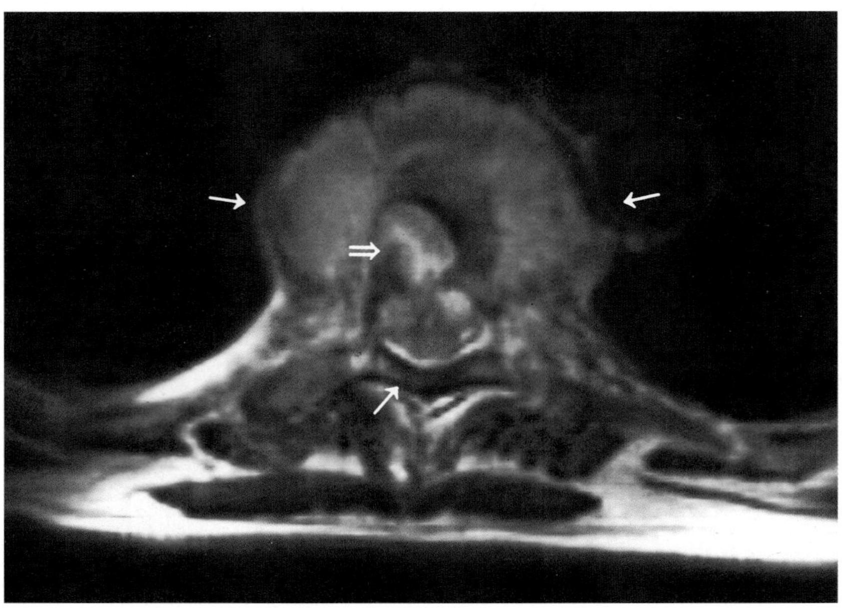

Fig. 5. *Tuberculous osteomyelitis.* 60-year-old woman with dorsal spinal pain and without previous specific diseases. The laminography of the spine shows a bone-disrupting process starting from the disc and spreading to the D6 and D7 bodies, associated with silent paravertebral abscess. The diagnosis is confirmed by MRI (T_2-weighted views) which clearly shows: bone cavitation with a sequestration (B); involvement of the disc and extent of the paravertebral abscess collections. On the sagittal view, the cord is deviated and compressed by the intraspinal component of the abscess. The axial view demonstrates that the ossifluent abscess tends to envelope the vertebral body (→←). Aortic involvement is also seen. The arrow (↗) indicates the posteriorly-displaced cord, the arrow (⇒) indicates the bone erosion.

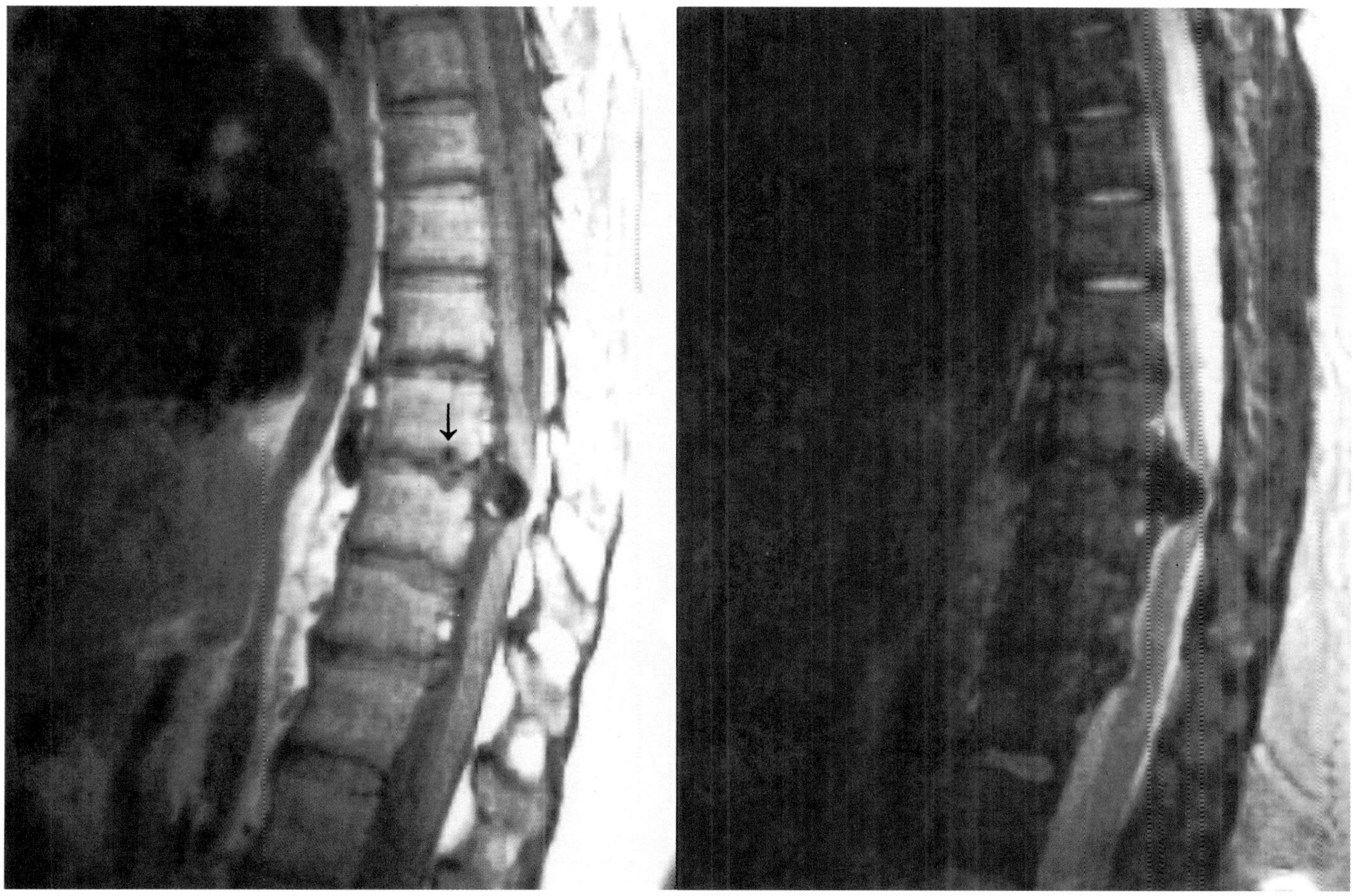

A

B

Fig. 6. *D9–D10 chronic discitis with calcific herniation.* 31-year-old woman with severe spastic paraparesis. A – T_1-weighted sequence. B – T_2-weighted sequence. Observe: the sequelae of the inflammatory process of the disc; the altered intervertebral disc limiting membranes but above all the coarse discal calcifications (↓) and the huge extruded herniation which occupies the entire canal, posteriorly displacing the cord, whose signal is altered.

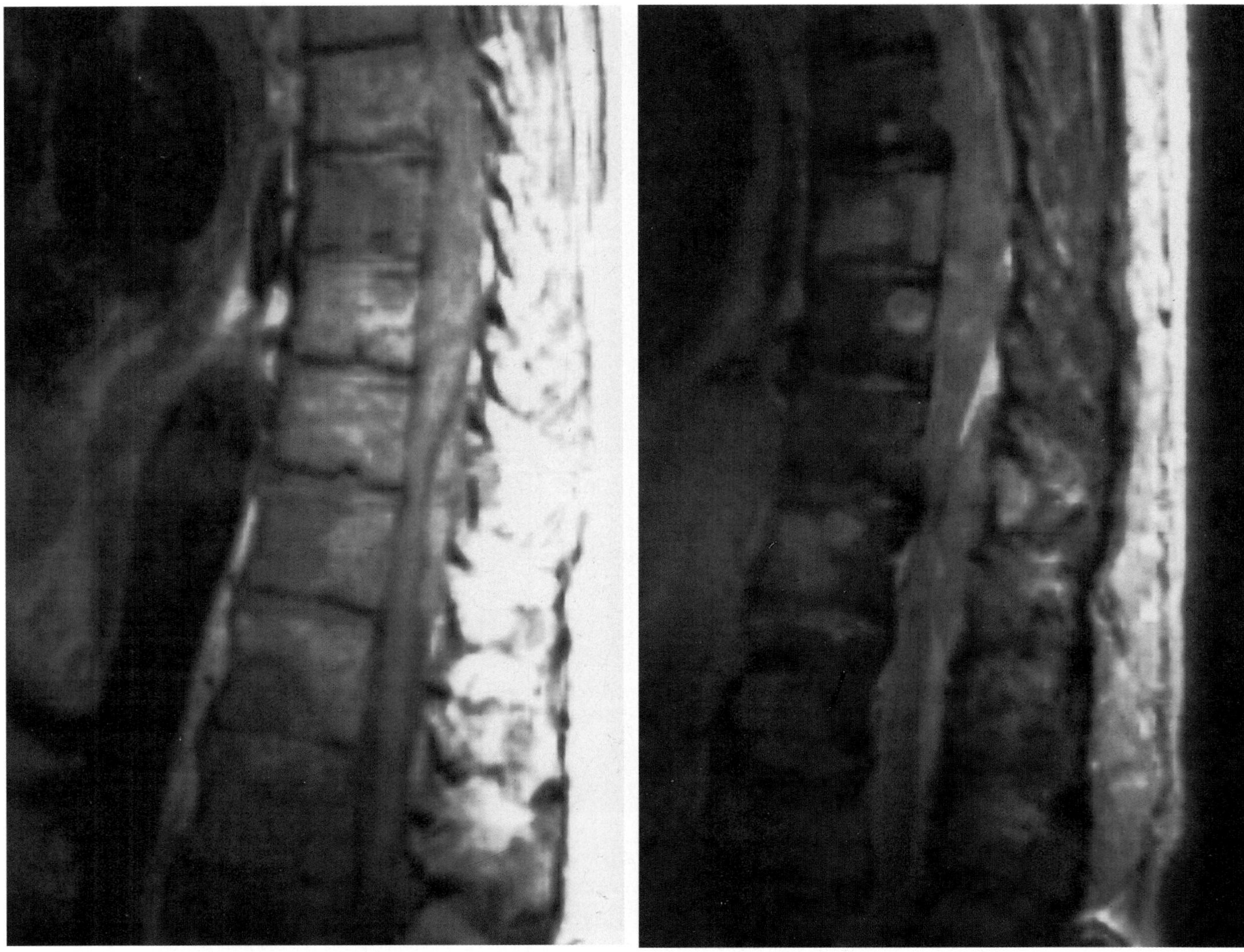

A B

Fig. 7. *Lymphoma with multiple vertebral involvement and sleeve-shaped extradural growth.* A – T_1-weighted mid-sagittal image showing the hypointense multiple vertebral loci of the tumor, especially at D8, D11, D12. The lymphomatous peridural mass extends over several metamers with maximum compression at D10–D11 and is slightly hypointense. B – T_2-weighted image of the lesions which are all hyperintense.

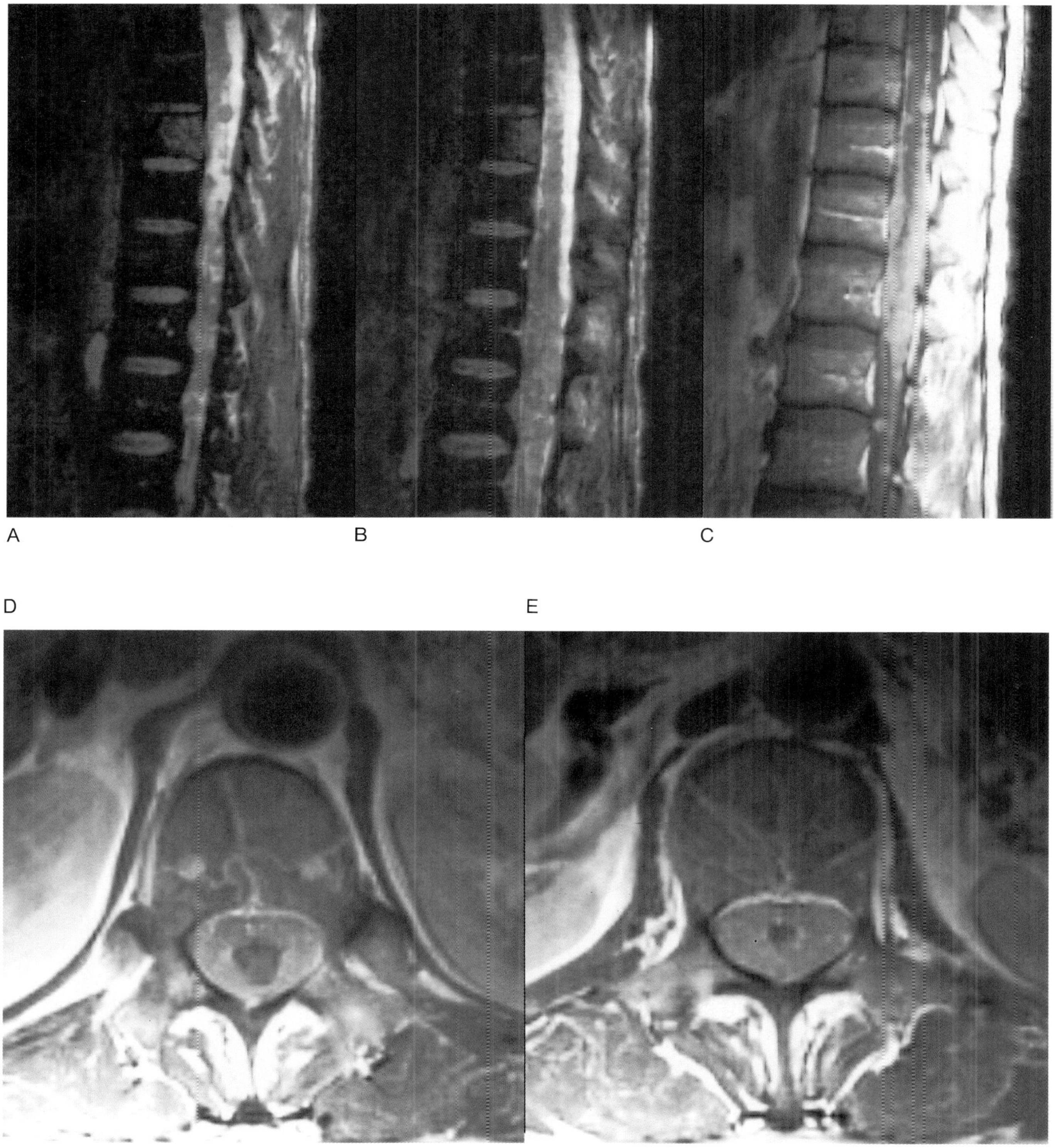

Fig. 8. *D9–D11 spinal intradural metastatic melanoma.* The myelographic effect of T_2-weighted images (A, B) shows numerous drop metastases in the lower dorsal region and a wide extramedullar plaque extending from D9 to D12. The tumoral areas enhance after contrast (C). The axial images after contrast (D, E) show the metastases which encircle the cord and the cone.

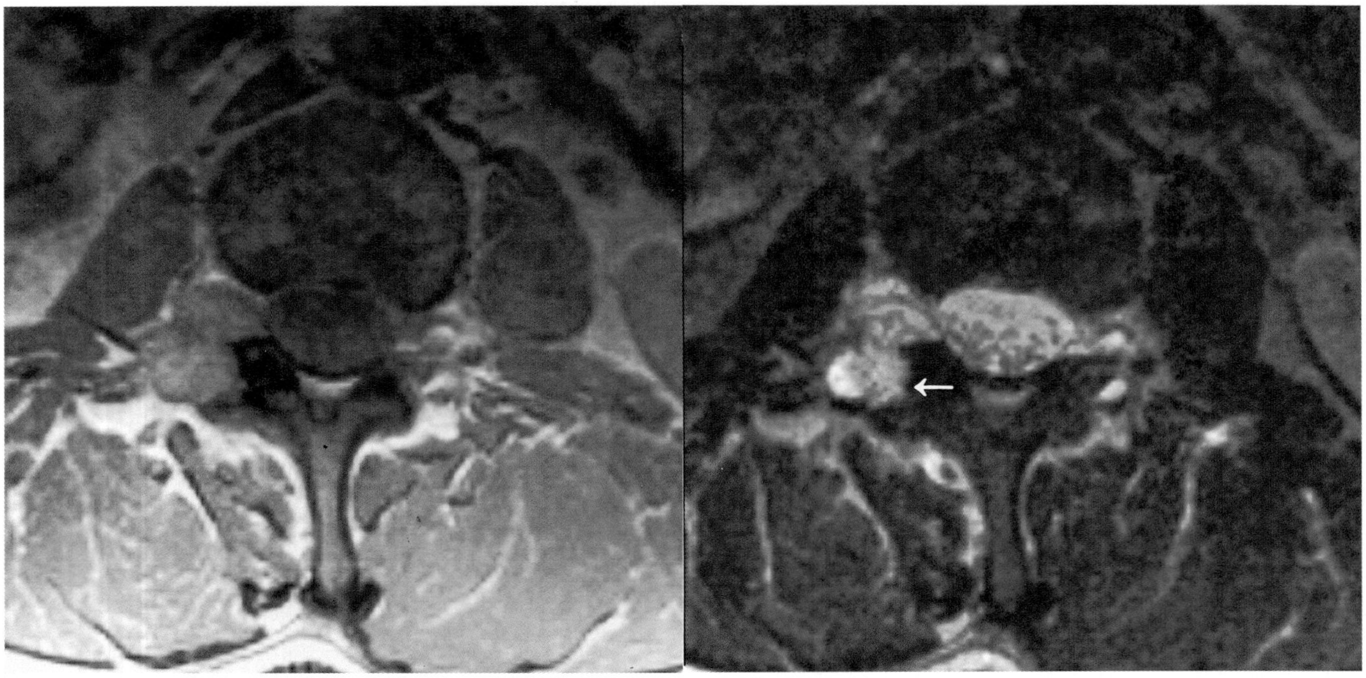

A B

Fig. 9. *L5 periradicular lymphangioma.* (A) T_1-weighted axial image after GD-DTPA. The right conjugation foramen is enlarged and occupied by a poorly enhancing dumbbell neoplasm that extends under the psoas from which it is well demarcated. (B) The corresponding T_2-weighted image shows the signal inhomogeneity of the lesion, having a more intense peripheral component, and the erosion of the articular facets (←). The caudal roots, hypointense with the CSF, are well outlined.

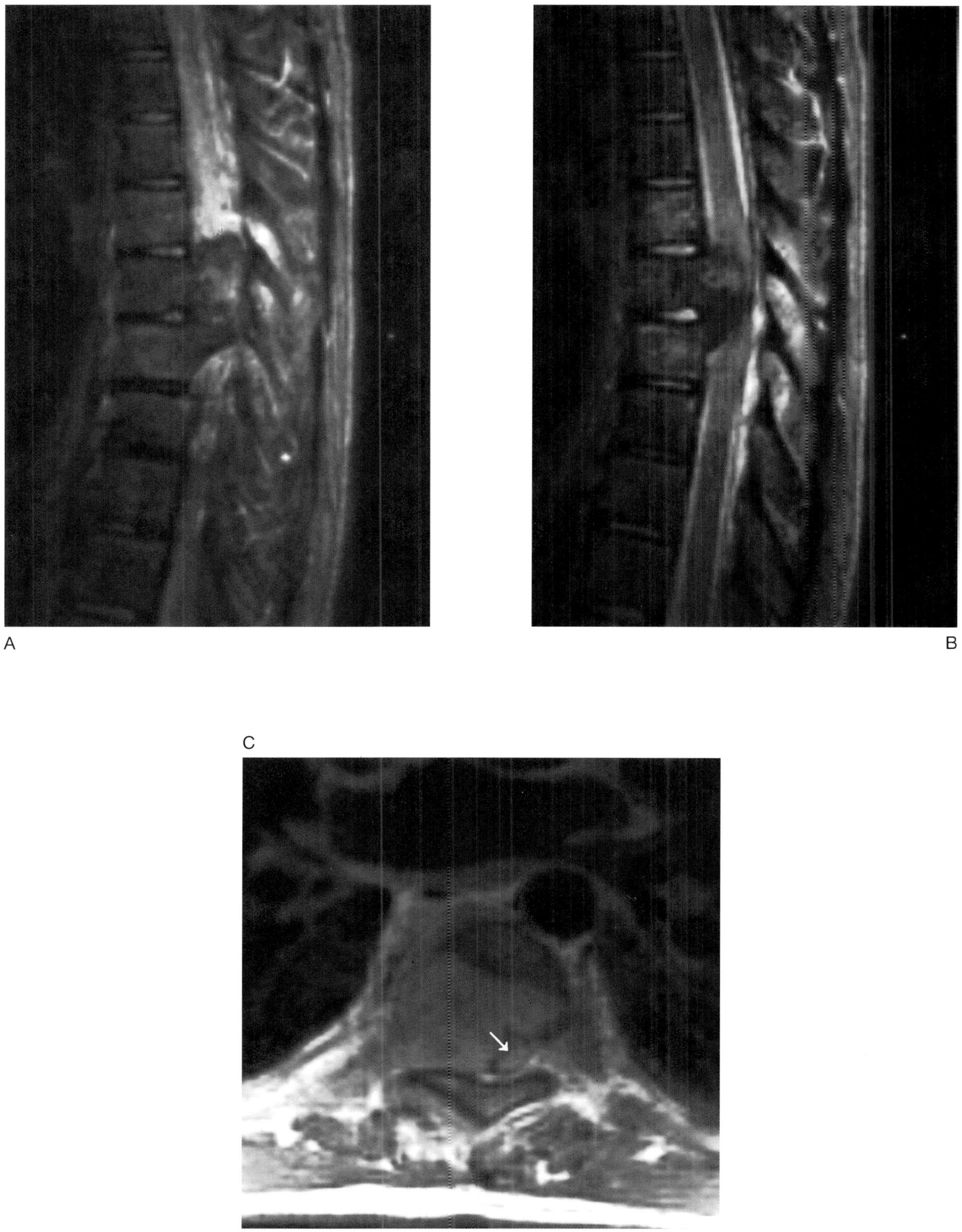

Fig. 10. *D6–D7 vertebral osteoblastoma.* 14-year-old girl with a slow-progressing spastic paraparesis. A, B – TR 2,500 msec, TE 90 msec, sagittal sections: the bone neoplasm originates from the right articular processes of D6–D7 and grows into the spinal canal, mainly occupying its right half (A). C – TR 550 msec, TE 15 msec; the axial section shows the cord compression (↘) and the transversal spread of the neoplasm, which is hyperintense with the healthy bone.

Fig. 11. *L3 vertebral angioma.* A – T_1-weighted coronal image. B – T_1-, proton density- and T_2-weighted images. Area of altered signal in the left half of the body; its boundaries are well delimited by a hypointense osteosclerotic rim. The signal decays with TE elongation. Note the radial area inside the lesion, seen to better advantage on (C).

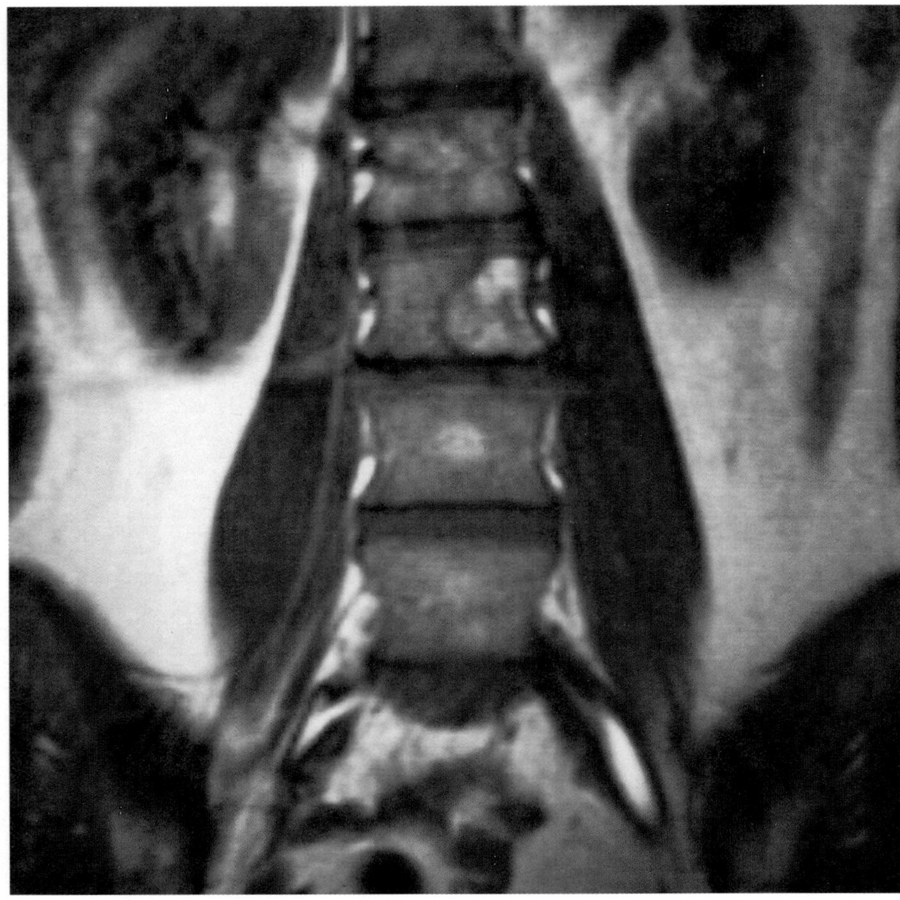

A

B C D

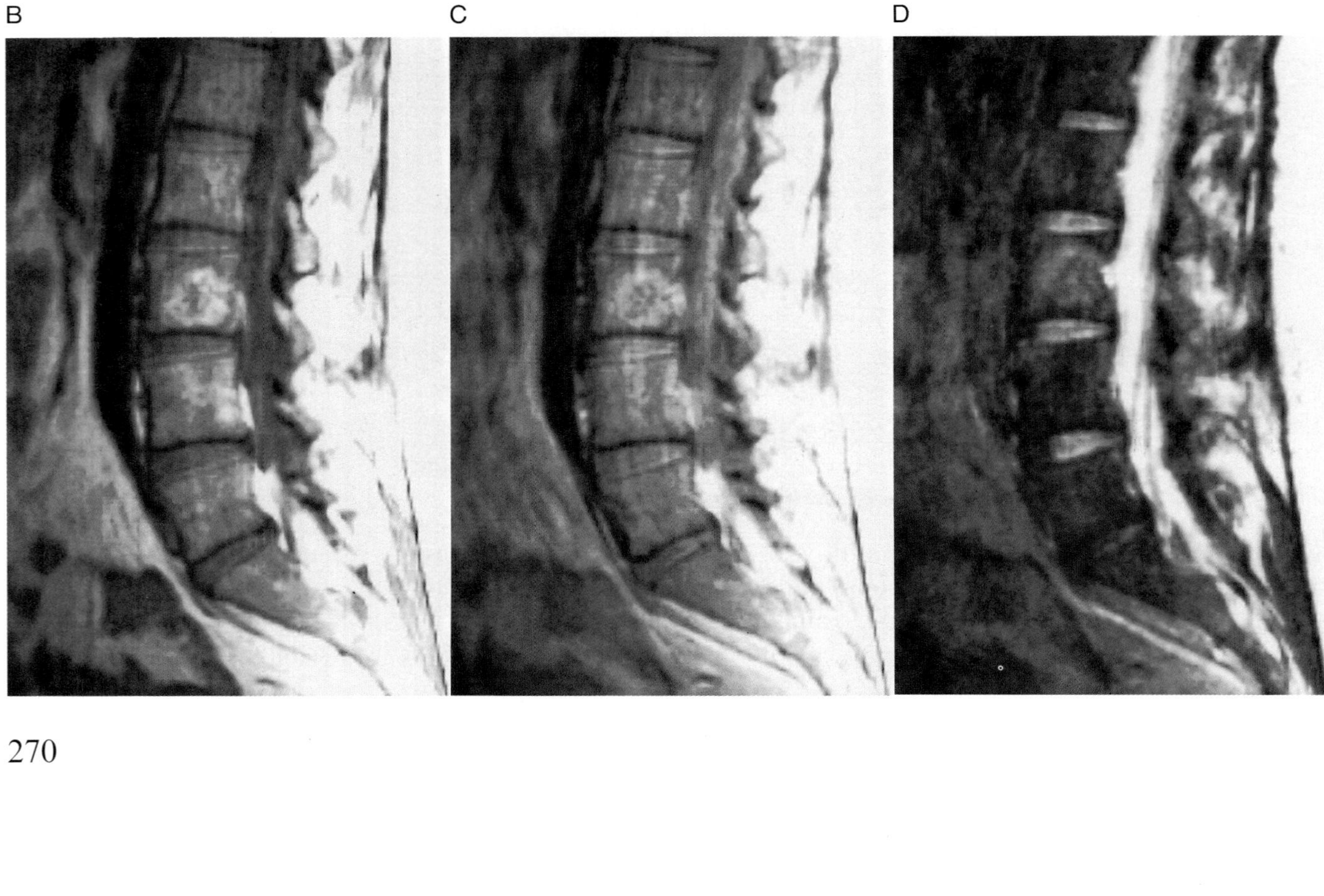

Fig. 12. *Neurinoma of the right D2 root.* The T_1-weighted section shows a small-sized extramedullar neoplasm, slightly hypointense with the cord, from which it is well demarcated. Note the cord compression and the central ependymal canal (→).

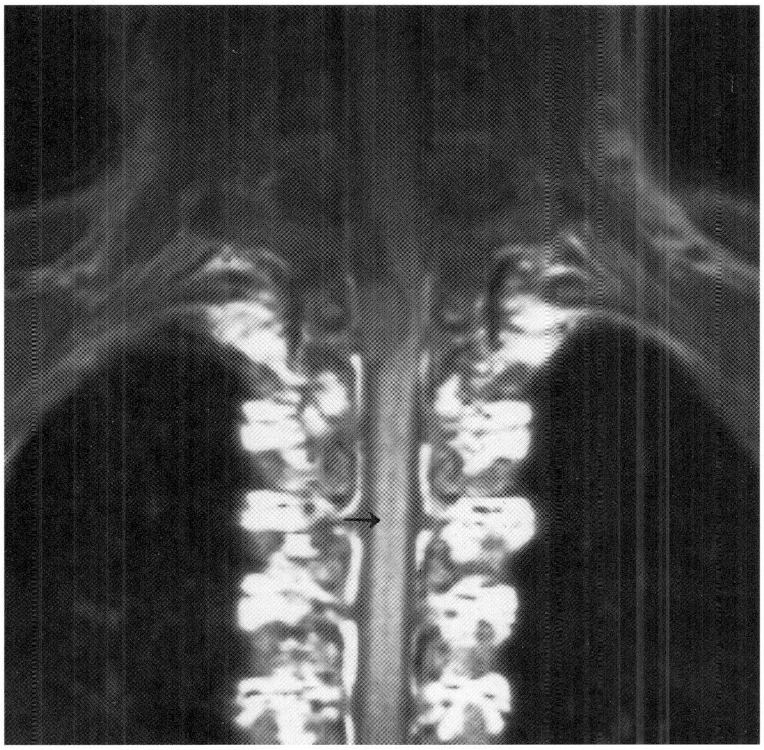

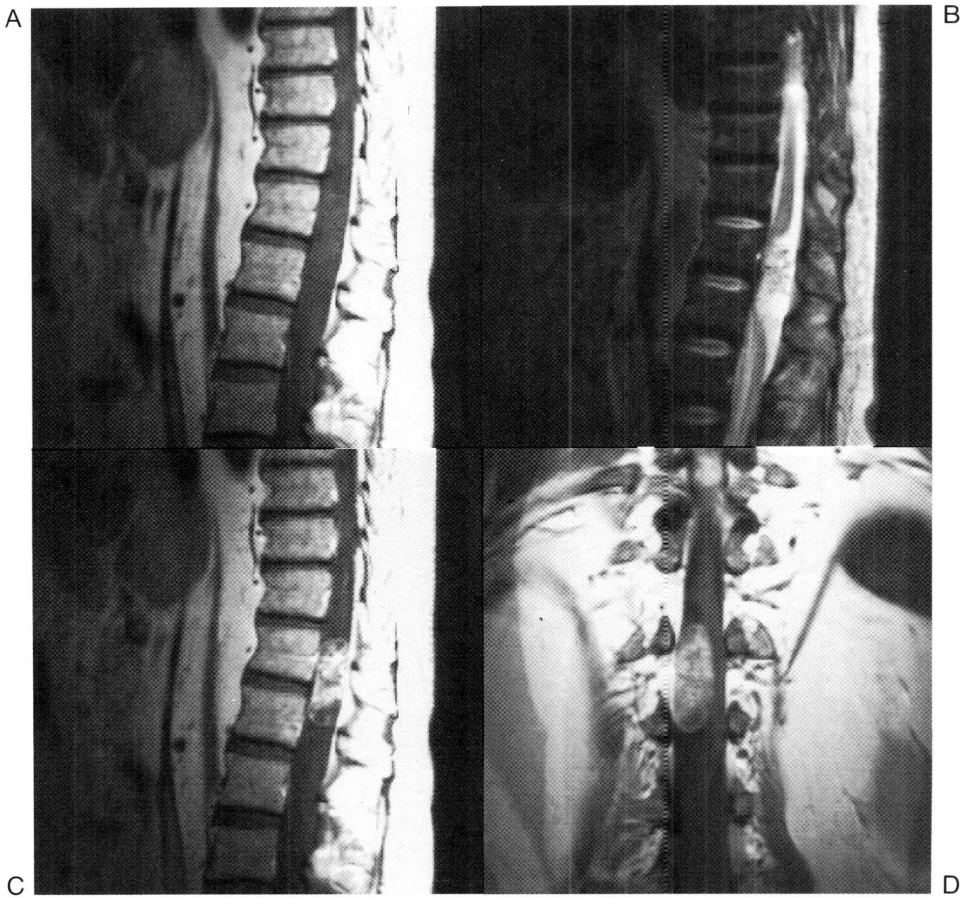

Fig. 13. *Right dorsal neurinoma (D9–D10).* 54-year-old man with severe long-standing paraparesis. The real morphology and structure of the neurinoma is well defined only on images after GD-DTPA (C, D). The T_2-weighted images well demonstrate the tumor relationships to the compressed spinal cord. The T_1-weighted image without GD-DTPA cannot demonstrate the neurinoma (A). Note the fatty degeneration of the skeletal muscles due to long-standing immobility.

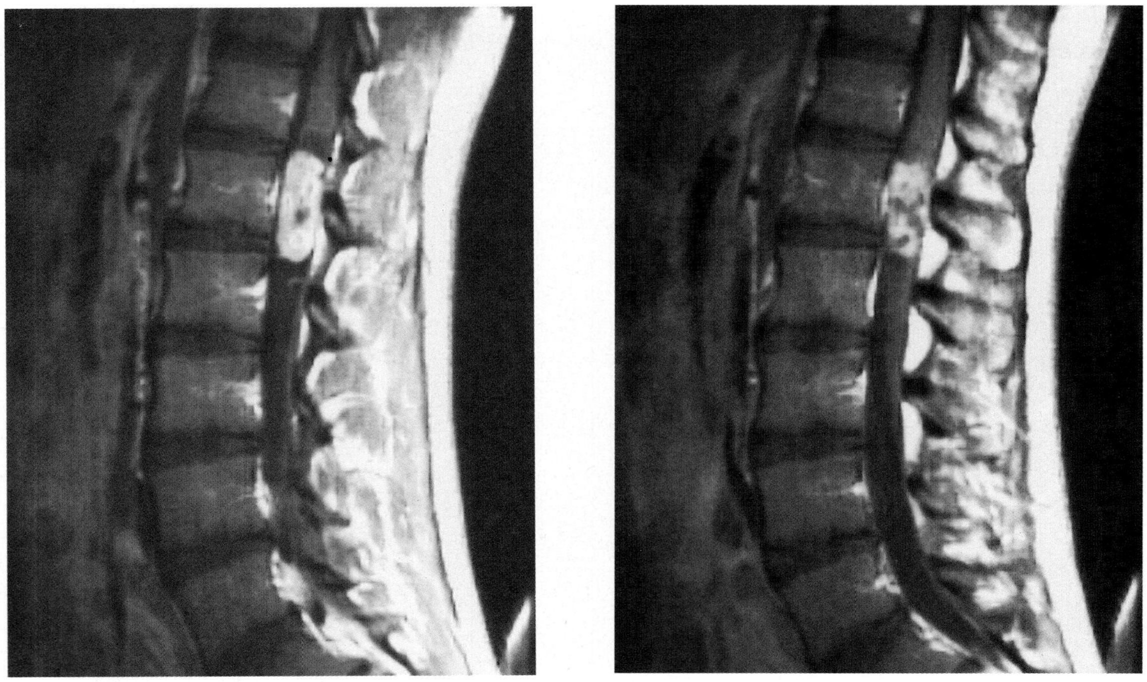

A B

Fig. 14. *D12 dorsal neurinoma.* The T_1-weighted views after GD-DTPA well demonstrate the neurinoma which compresses and displaces the cone. Within the tumor, non-enhancing necrotic areas are visible.

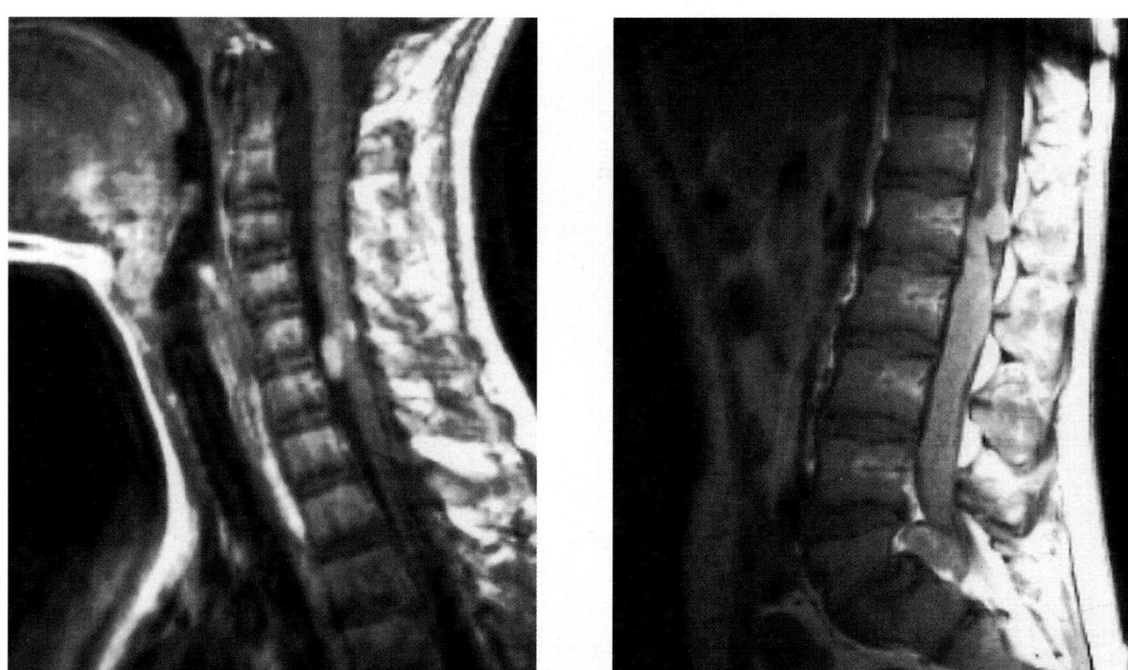

A B

Fig. 15. *Multiple neurinomas. Young man with neurofibromatosis (same case as in Fig. 4, Chap. VII).* The T_1-weighted images after GD-DTPA demonstrate small multiple neurinomas (→) and a huge pedunculated mass which occupies the dural sac below L1.

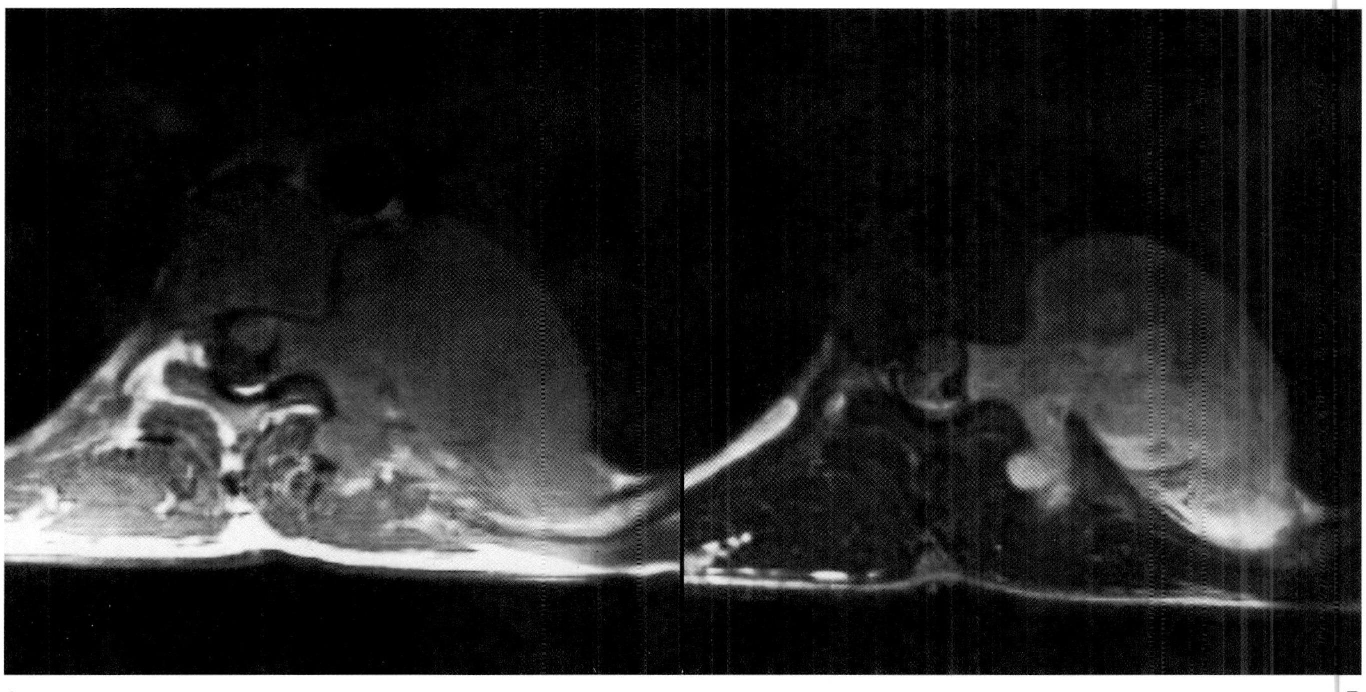

Fig. 16. *D8–D9 left dumbbell neurinoma.* Proton density- (A) and T_2- (B) weighted axial scan: the neoplasm originates from the conjugation foramen and grows mostly outside the spinal canal, forming a huge mass at the costovertebral junction. A tumoral tongue grows inside the paravertebral muscles. On late echoes, the signal is not uniform, as is often found with large-sized neurinomas, due to regressive events.

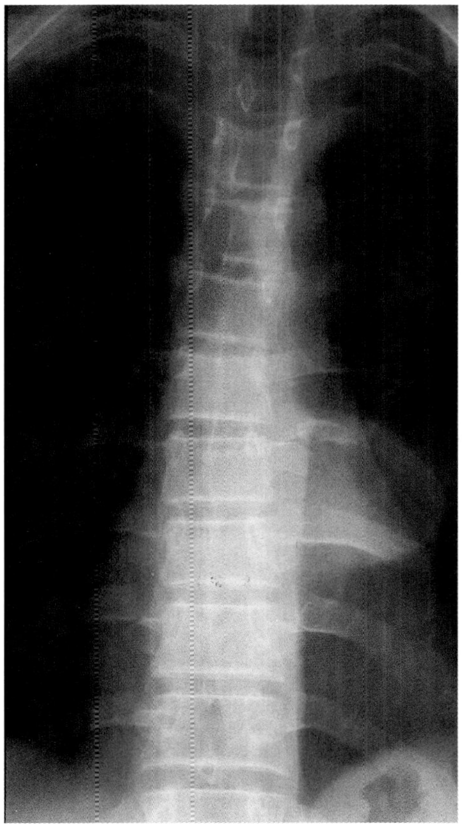

Fig. 17. *Same patient. Plain film of the spine.* Note the widening of the D8–D9 intercostal space with erosion of the 9th rib and a huge paravertebral mass.

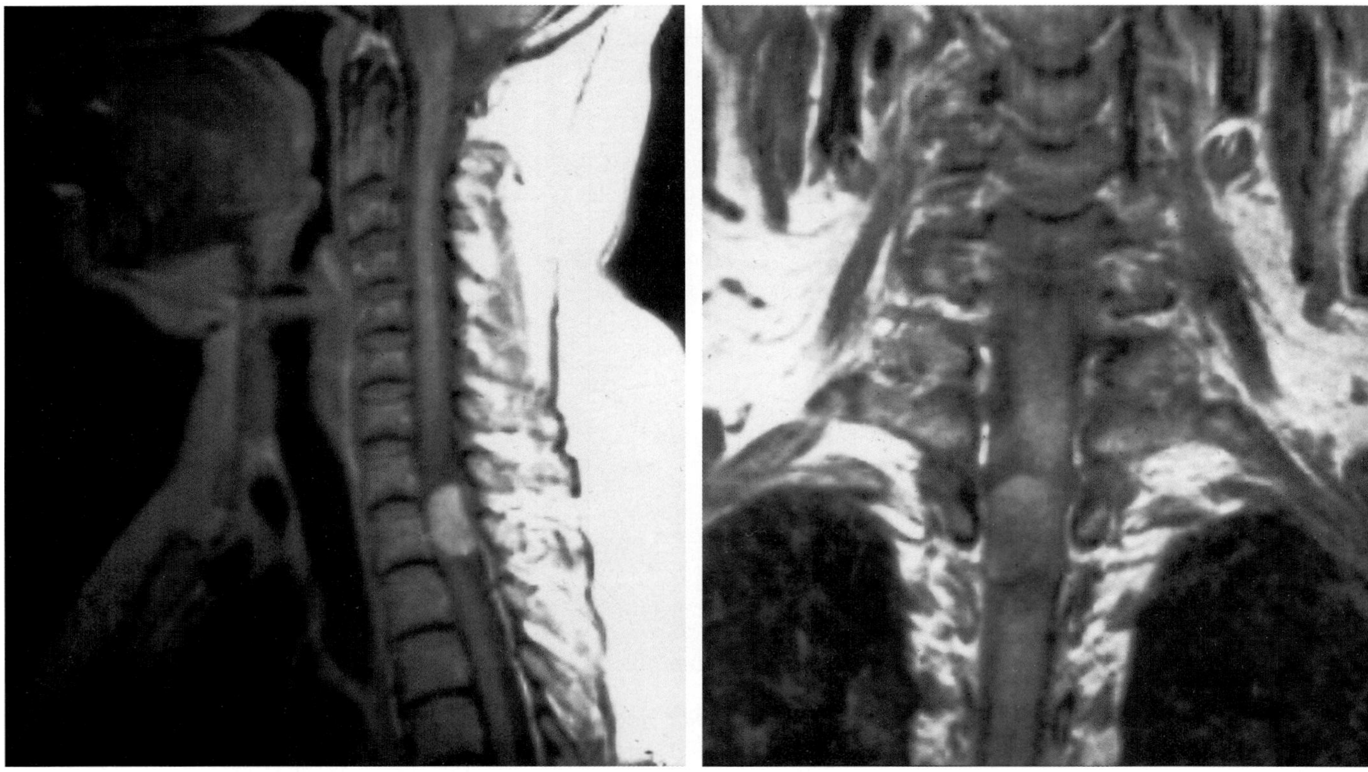

A B

Fig. 18. *D1–D2 right posterolateral meningioma.* T_1-weighted scan after GD-DTPA, sagittal (A) and coronal (B) views. The mass is located posteriorly to the spinal cord and has a large dural attachment.

A B

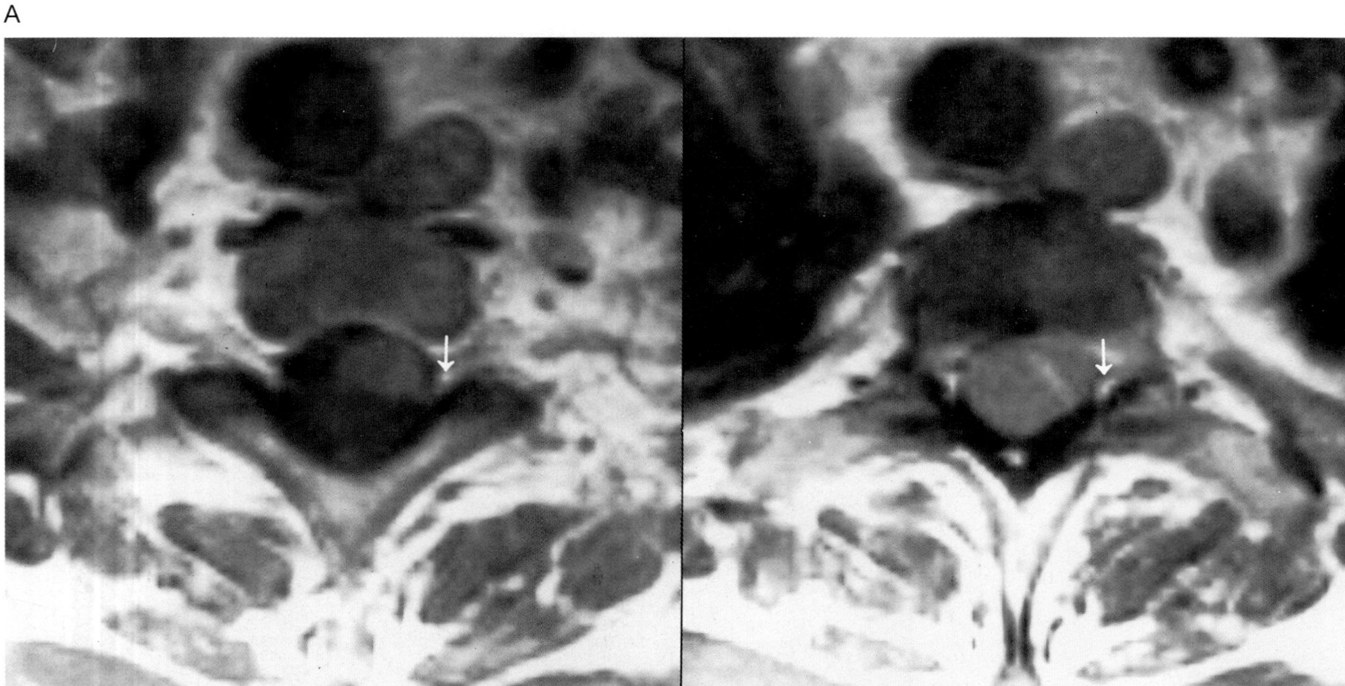

Fig. 19. Same case, axial scan. Late scans after GD-DTPA. The cord is displaced anteriorly to the left and is rotated clockwise. The arrows indicate its distorted roots. In B, the scan fully crosses the neoplasm and the cord can barely be recognized.

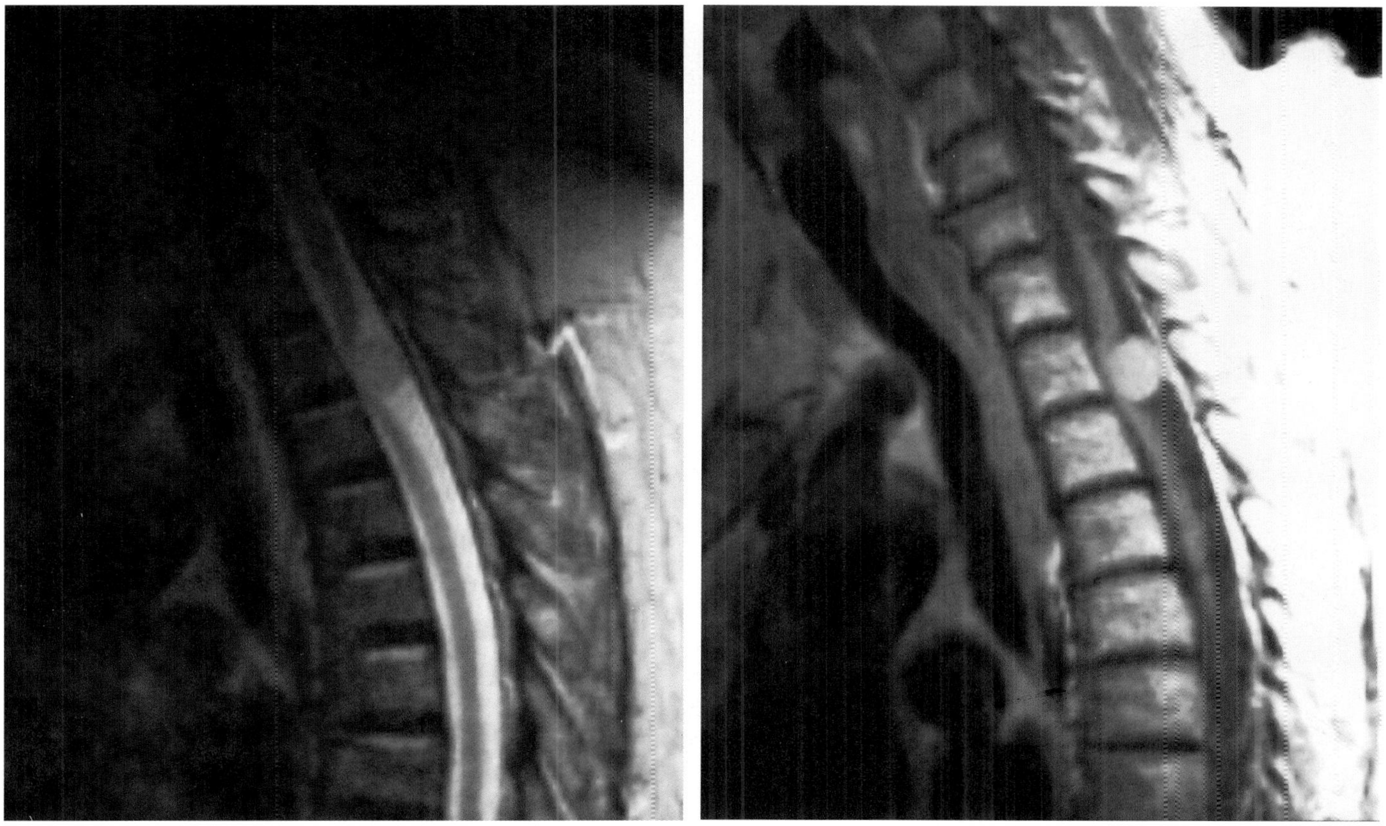

A

B

Fig. 20. *D2 posterolateral meningioma.* A – On the T_2-weighted sequence, the meningioma is seen as a hypointense focus in the CSF pathways (myelographic effect). B – T_1-weighted sequence: intense and homogenous perfusion of the neoplasm by GD-DTPA.

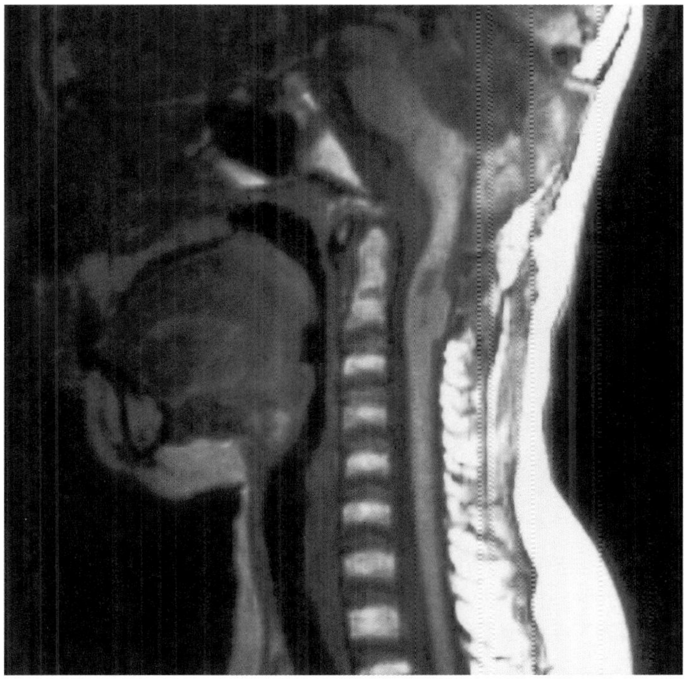

Fig. 21. *C2 subarachnoid spinal metastasis from cerebellar medulloblastoma.* 14-year-old boy operated on for a medulloblastoma of the vermis. T_1-weighted sagittal section: the cord is deformed by a hypointense posterior mass. Note the surgical sequelae on the cerebellum.

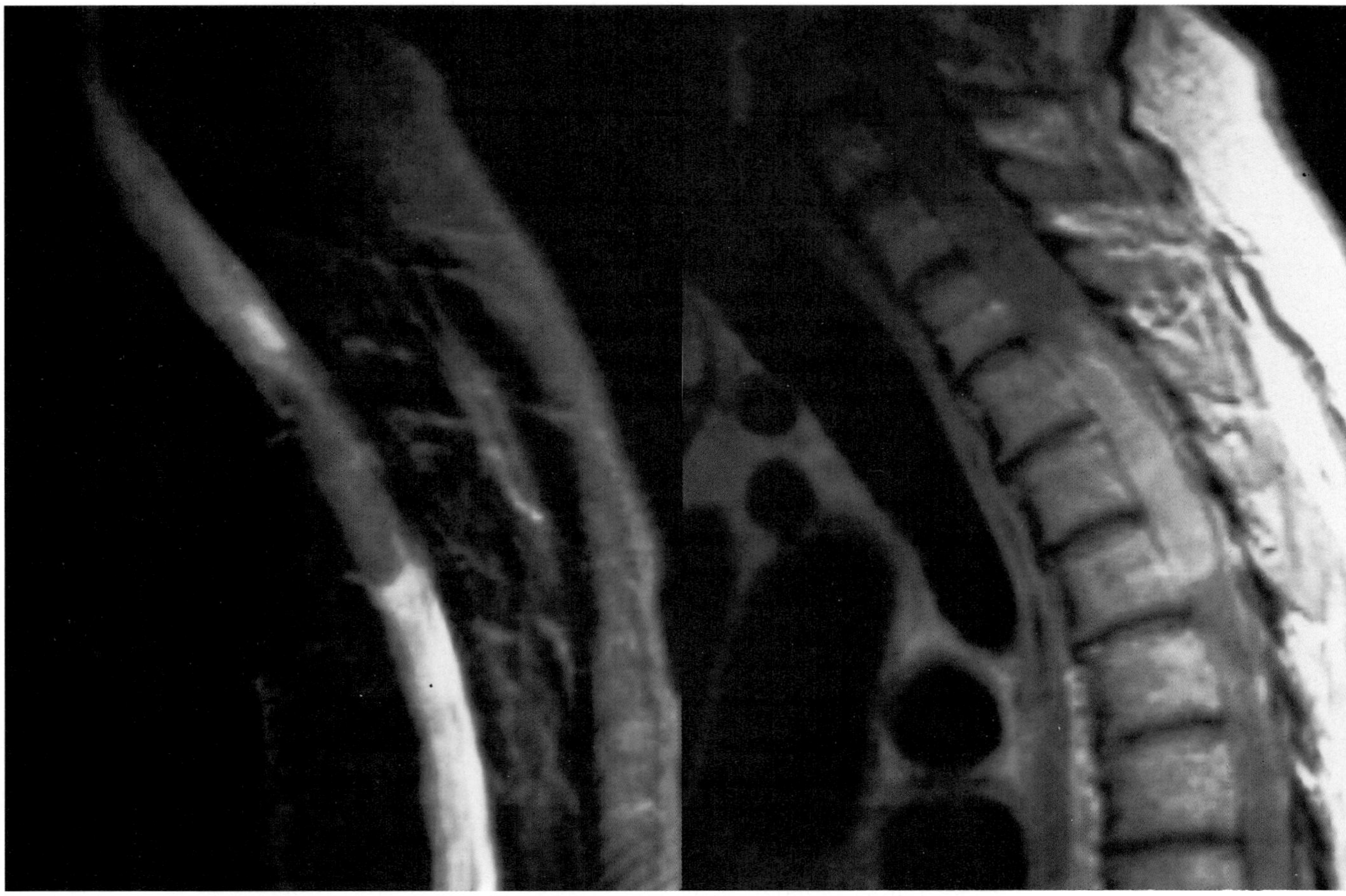

A B

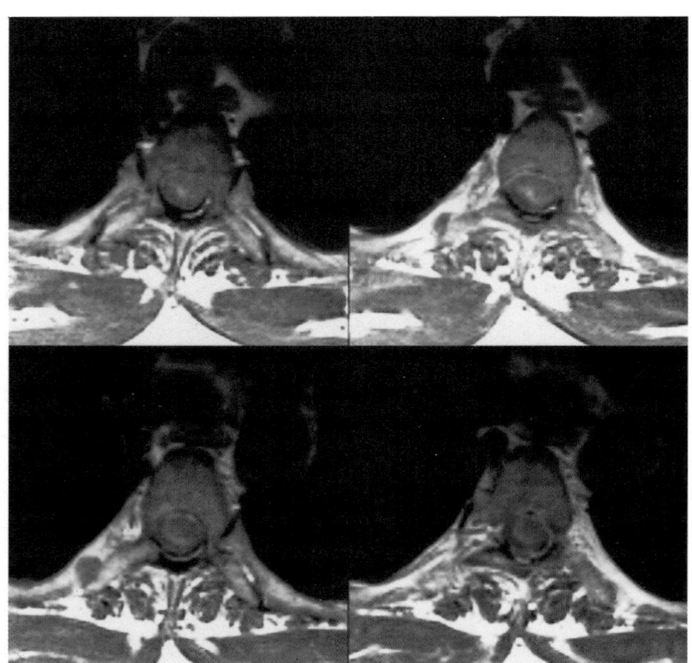

C

Fig. 22. *D3–D5 dorsal metastasis from cerebellar medulloblastoma.* The T_2-weighted sagittal view (A) depicts the longitudinal growth of the metastasis. The T_1-weighted view (B) shows hyperintensity of the lesion after i.v. GD-DTPA. On the axial views (C), the cord is displaced posteriorly to the right and compressed by the cylindrical lesion.

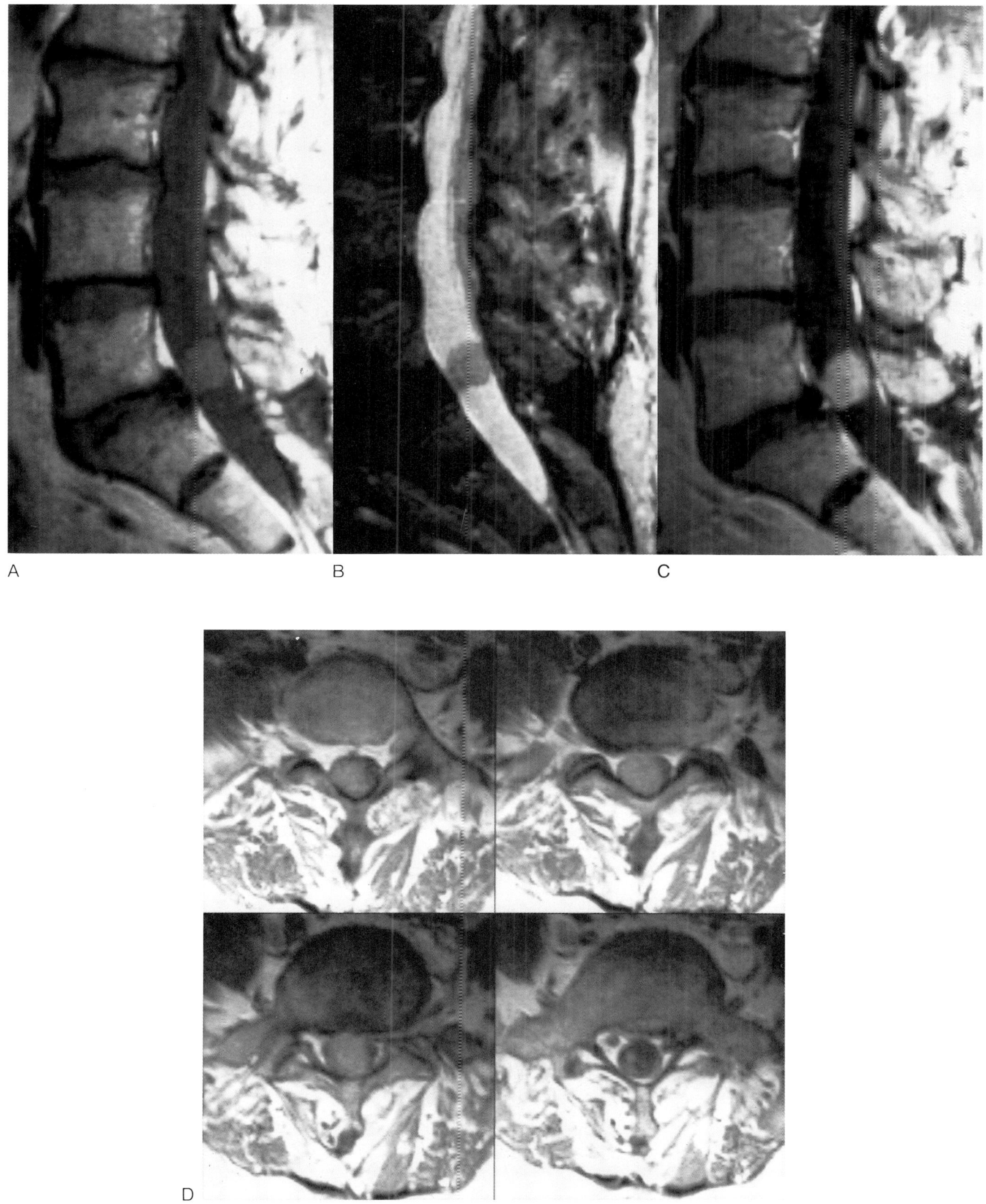

Fig. 23. Same patient as in the previous figure. Another metastasis in the dural sac at the level of the cauda is well documented on both the T_1-weighted views with (C) and without (A) GD-DTPA, and on the T_2-weighted views (B), where the lesion has a negative image. The axial T_1-weighted image after GD-DTPA (D) substantiates that the dural sac is totally occupied by the mass.

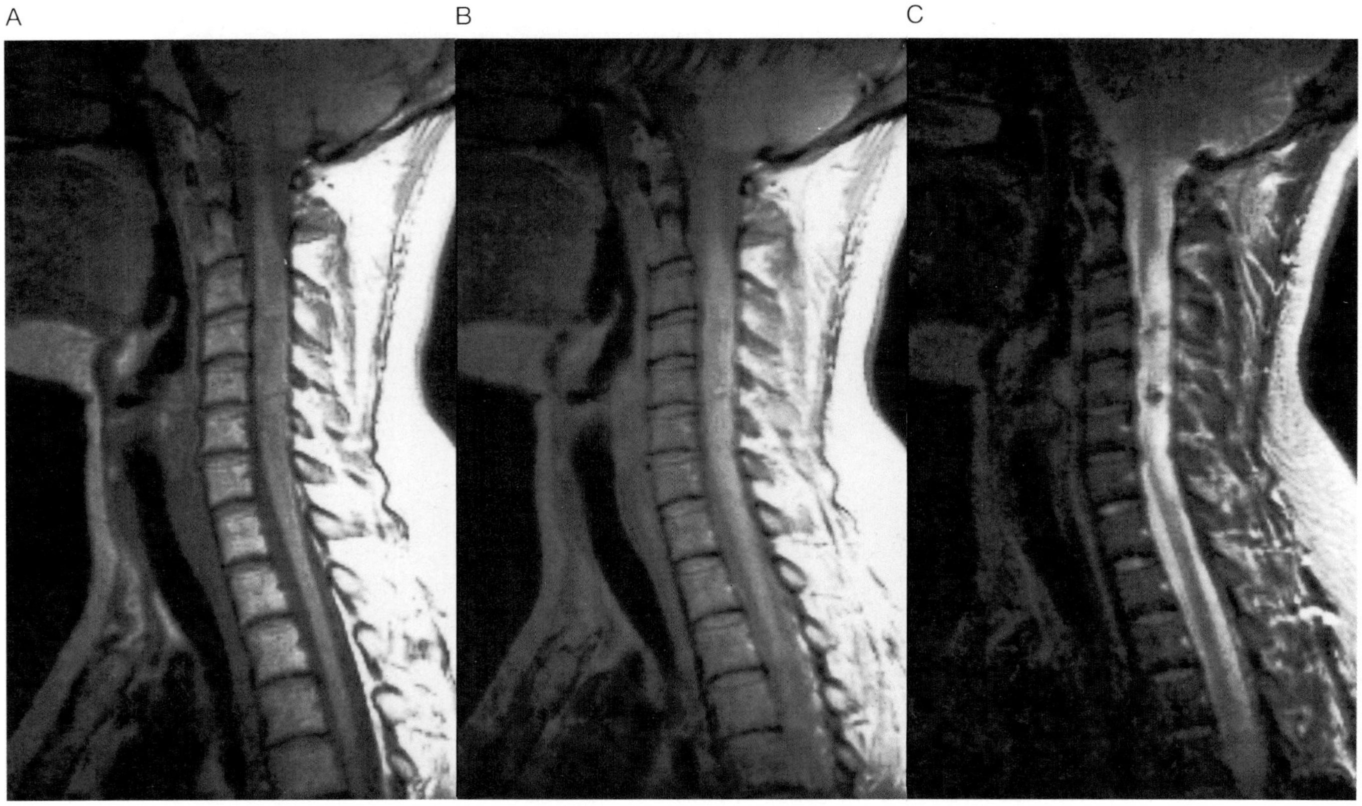

Fig. 24. *C3–C7 low-grade astrocytoma.* 39-year-old woman with progressive tetraparesis. Mid-sagittal sections: A – TR 550 msec, TE 15 msec; B, C – TR 2,500 msec, TE 20–90 msec. The cord is uniformly enlarged from C3 to C7, owing to a solid tumoral tissue which is homogeneous on (A) and (B) and inhomogeneous on (C) due to markedly hypointense foci, likely to be remnants of prior bleeds.

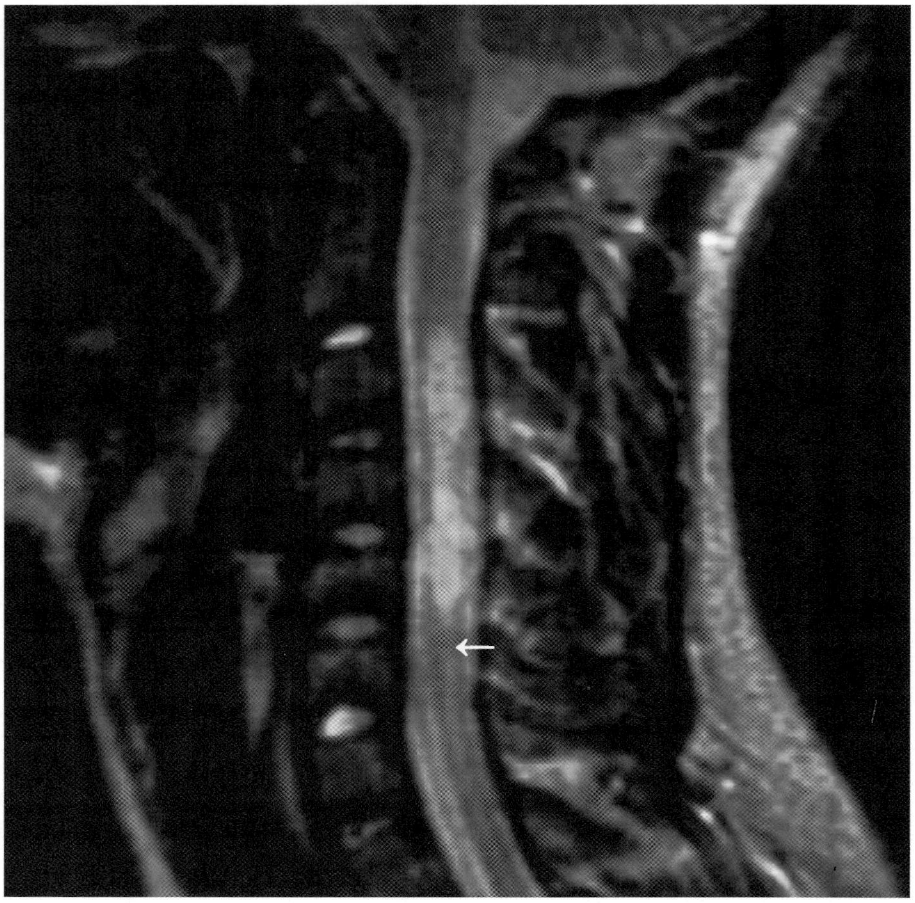

Fig. 25. *Cervical low-grade astrocytoma.* The T_2-weighted sagittal image delineates an altered signal focus from C3 to C6, in apparent continuity with the central ependymal canal (←). The neoplasm is of the infiltrating type, since the cord is scarcely enlarged.

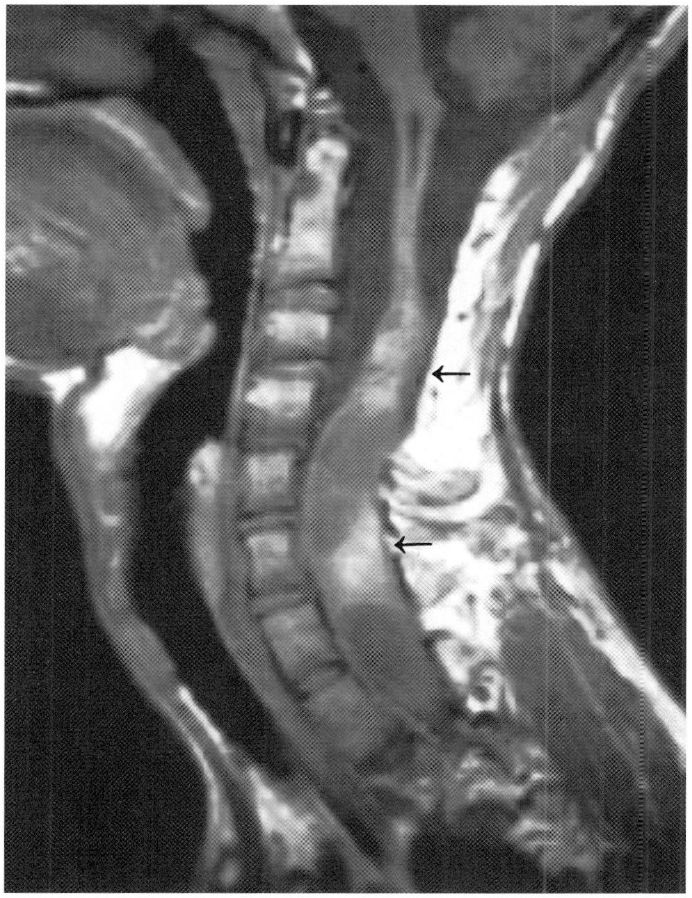

A

Fig. 26. *Bulbocervical low-grade astrocytoma.* 18-year-old man operated 10 years earlier for excision of a cerebellomedullar astrocytoma. At present, he is neurologically in good condition except for plegia of the right lower limb. A – T_1-weighted sagittal image after GD-DTPA. Note the flattening of the bulbomedullar tract with enlargement of the ependymal canal. Under the surgical site, the cord is enlarged by the neoplasm, which has important cystic components; the solid components enhance inhomogeneously. Early (B, C) and late (D, E) axial images after contrast: the solid components (←) of the neoplasm enhance on late scans. Also the largest neoplastic cyst enhances on late scans, since the contrast medium has accumulated inside the cavity (←).

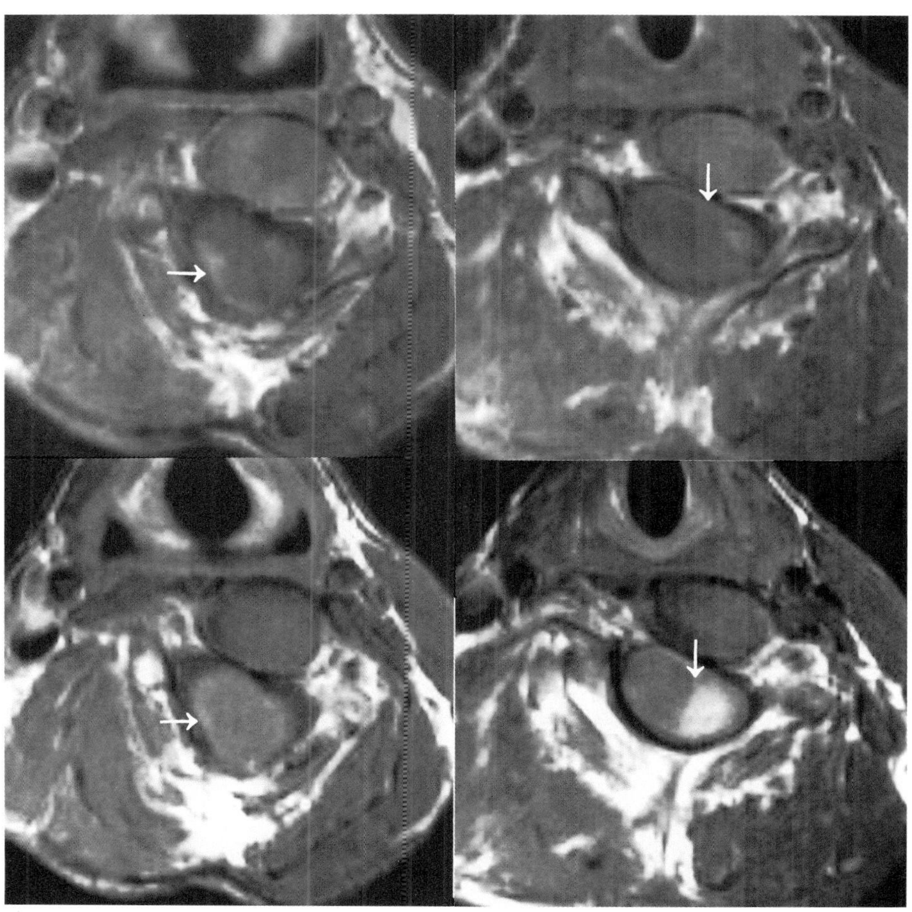

B C D E

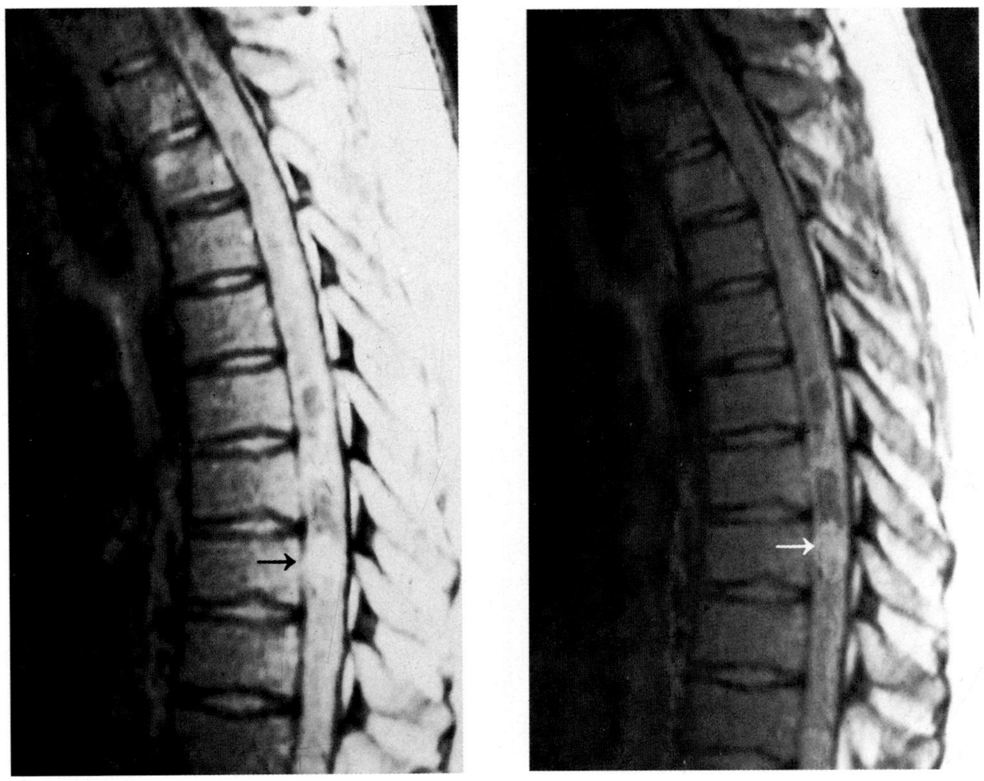

A B

Fig. 27. *D9 intramedullar angioblastoma.* 35-year-old man with spastic tetraparesis. A – T_1-weighted section showing a small hyperintense neoplasm (→) with proximal syringomyelic cavities, a frequent finding in this type of disease. B – On the proton density-weighted sections, the tumor enhances due to its high cellularity.

A

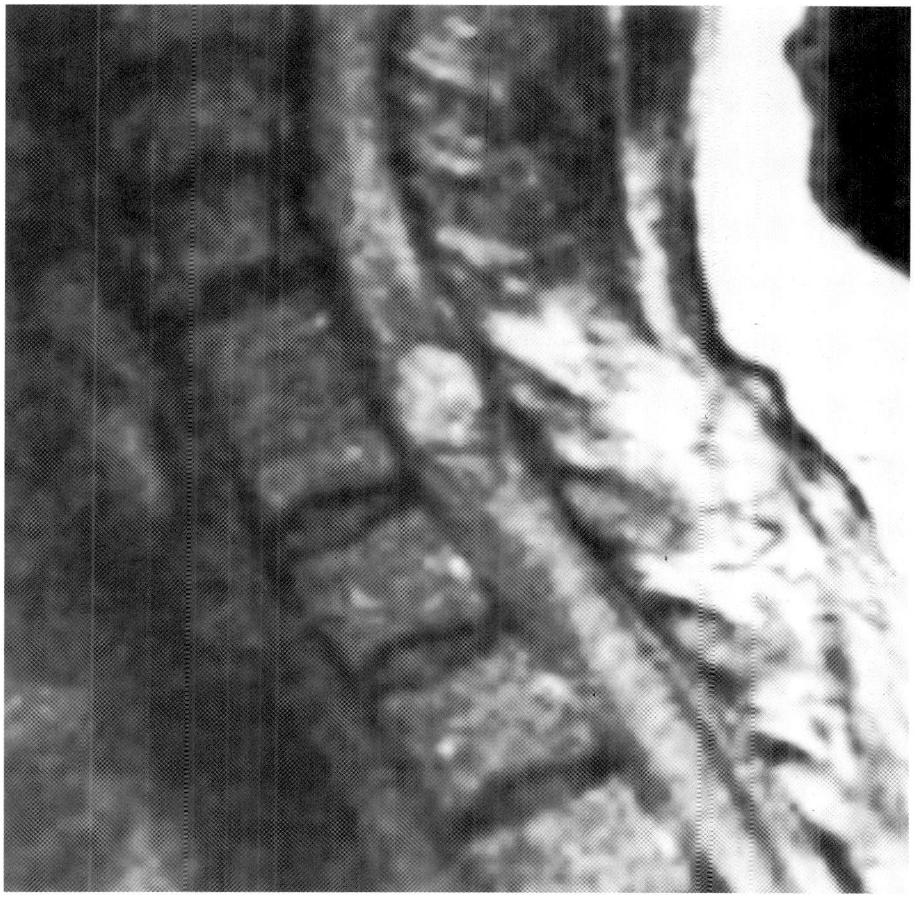

B

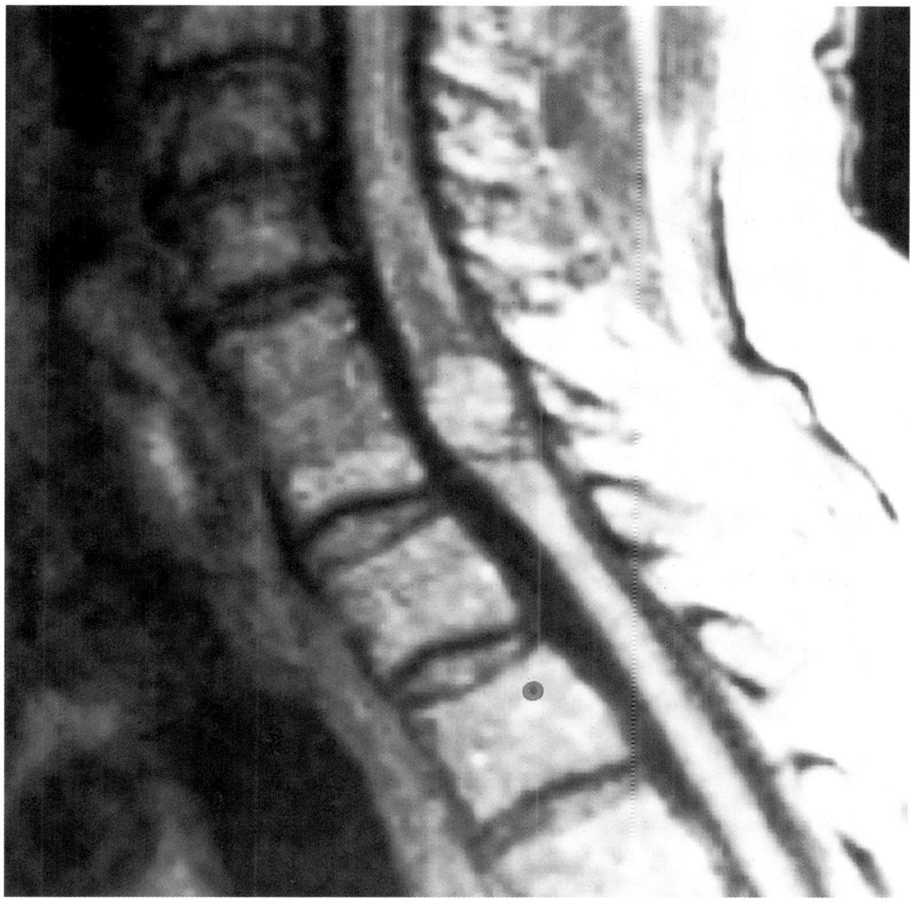

Fig. 28. *Cervical angioblastoma.* 59-year-old patient who underwent C5–C6 discectomy via the anterior approach with intervertebral arthrodesis. Both T_1- (A) and proton density- (B) weighted views show a high-signal, round-shaped, intramedullar neoplasm with proximal syringomyelia.

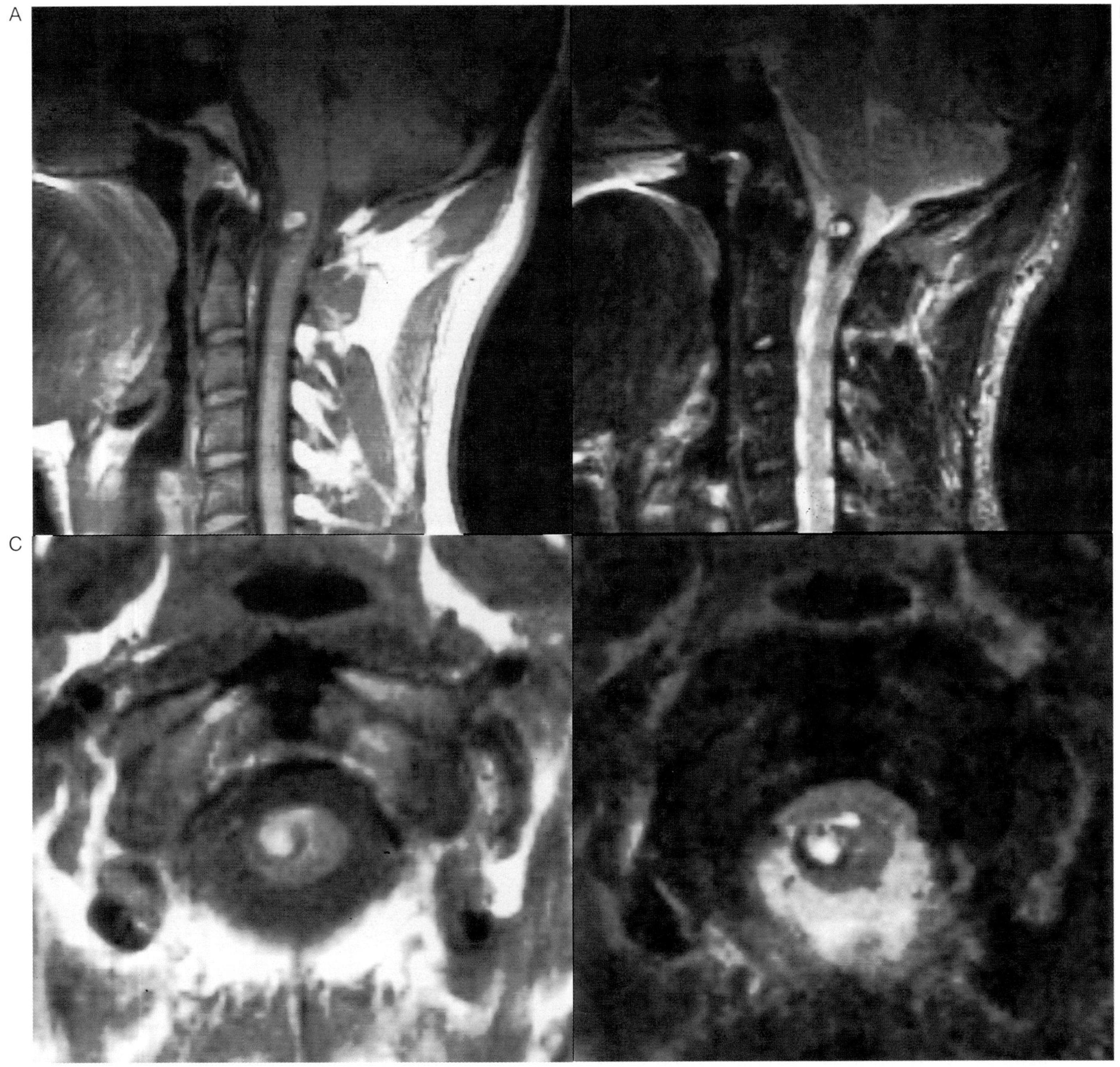

Fig. 29. *Intramedullar cavernous angioma (C1)*. 27-year-old man with left hemihypoesthesia. The T_1- (A) and T_2- (B) weighted images show a tumor with high-signal bloody areas. On both sequences, these areas are surrounded by a typical hypointense hemosiderin-laden rim, particularly visible on T_2. The axial images (C, D) document the eccentric position of the angioma, which outcrops at the surface of the cord.

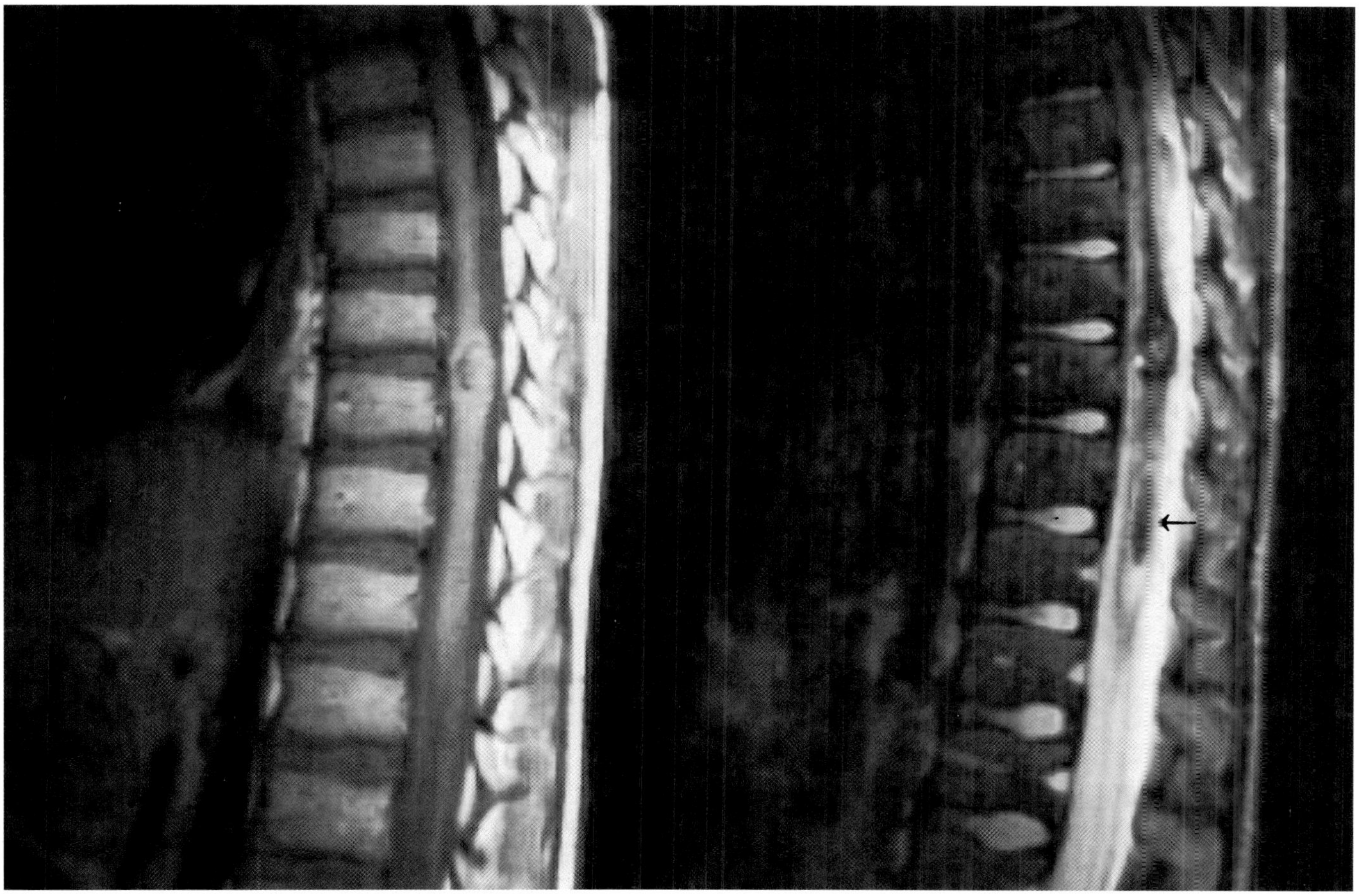

A B

Fig. 30. *D10–D11 intramedullar cavernous angioma.* 13-year-old boy with acute paraplegia. A – The T_1-weighted sagittal view shows a slightly hyperintense small lesion with a hypointense margin which deforms the cord profile. B – On the T_2-weighted view, the central part of the lesion keeps a high signal and the hemosiderin-laden rim is better visualized. The signal is still high for the central part of the lesion. More caudally, a syringomyelic distension with signs of recent hemorrhage can be observed. The arrow points to a hypointense focus due to desoxyhemoglobin. The latter finding is consistent with the acute onset of the clinical syndrome.

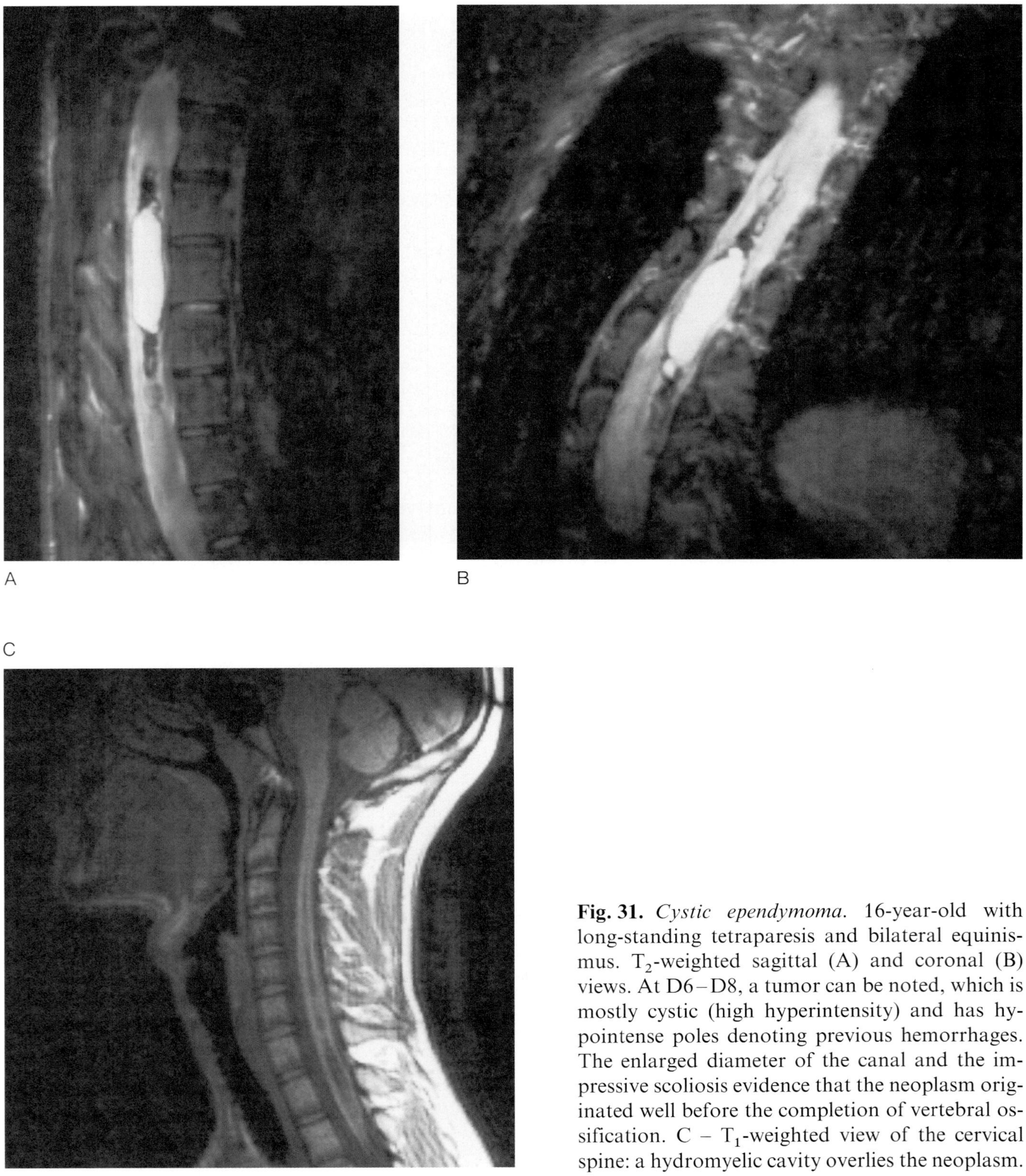

Fig. 31. *Cystic ependymoma.* 16-year-old with long-standing tetraparesis and bilateral equinismus. T_2-weighted sagittal (A) and coronal (B) views. At D6–D8, a tumor can be noted, which is mostly cystic (high hyperintensity) and has hypointense poles denoting previous hemorrhages. The enlarged diameter of the canal and the impressive scoliosis evidence that the neoplasm originated well before the completion of vertebral ossification. C – T_1-weighted view of the cervical spine: a hydromyelic cavity overlies the neoplasm.

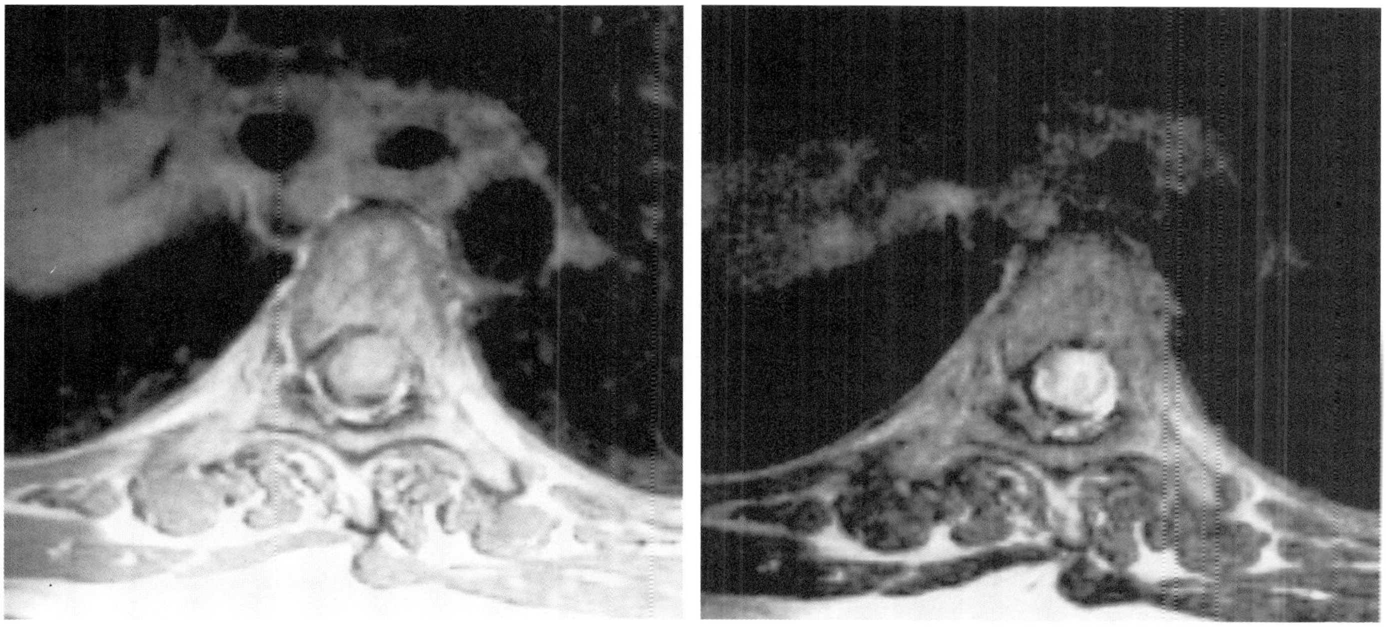

A B

Fig. 32. *D4–D5 intramedullar metastasis from breast carcinoma.* 34-year-old patient with progressive spastic paraparesis. A – Proton density-weighted axial cut: the intramedullar mass is slightly hyperintense with the tissue, which is compressed and displaced posteriorly and to the right. On the T_2-weighted sequence (B), the signal from the metastasis becomes typically more intense.

A B C

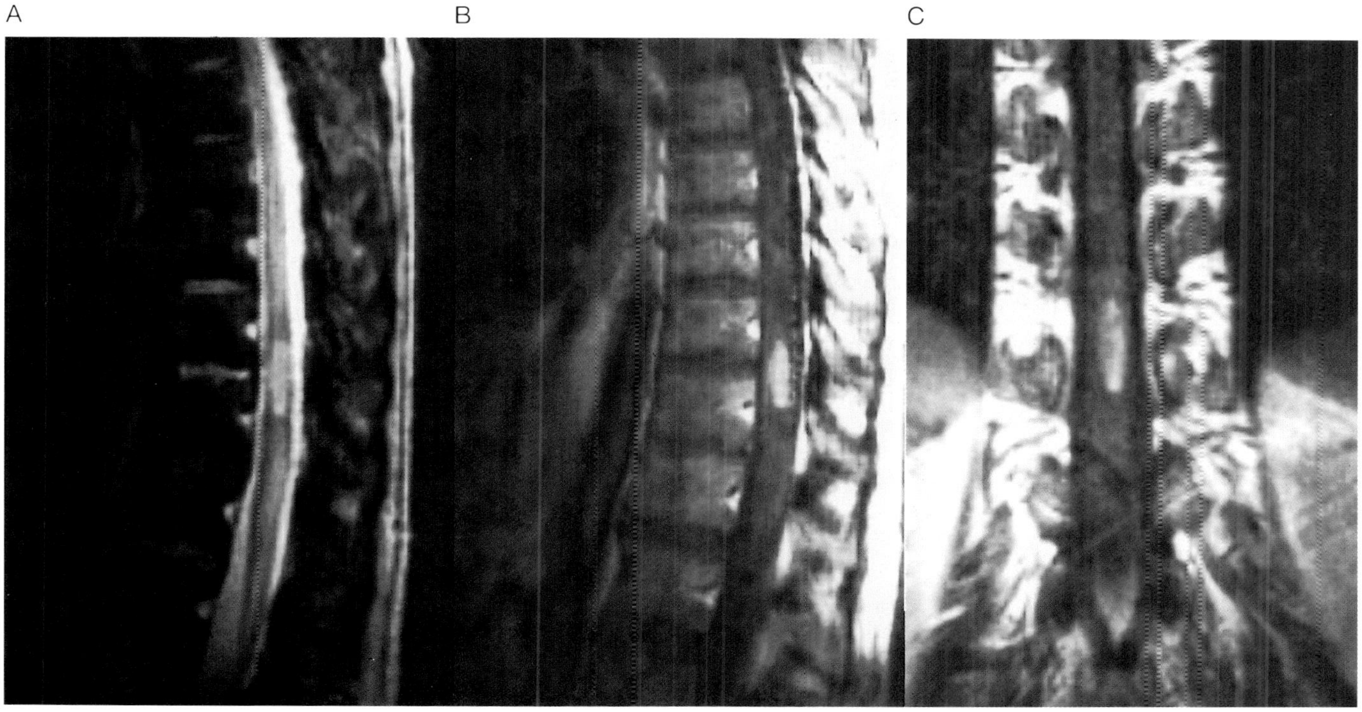

Fig. 33. *D11–D12 intramedullar metastatic melanoma.* A – The T_2-weighted sagittal scan shows an ovoid alteration of the signal from the cord without obliteration of the subarachnoid spaces. B and C – After GD-DTPA, the lesion enhances, suggesting the metastatic nature of the spinal alteration in a patient with diffuse metastatic melanoma.

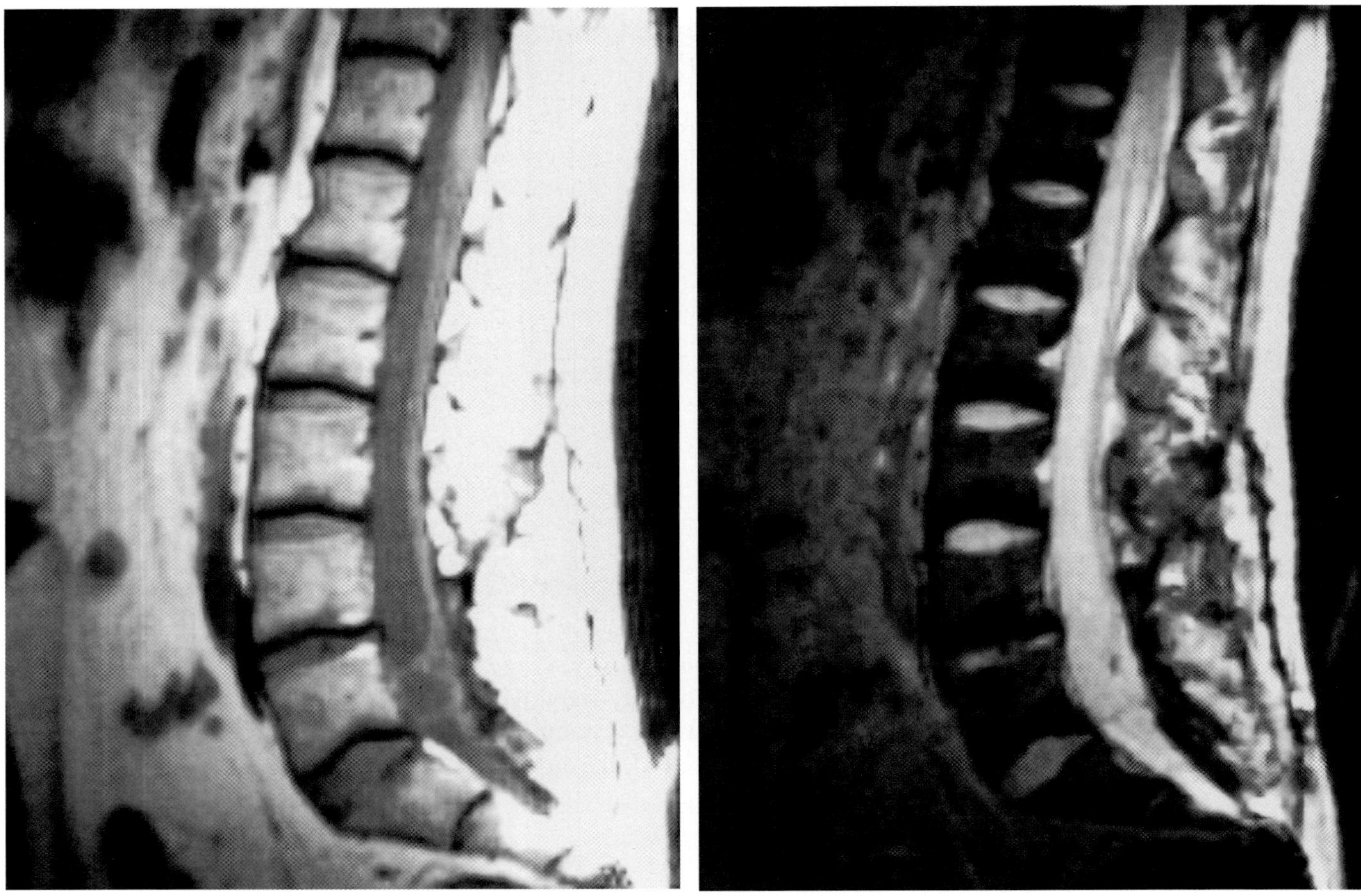

A B

Fig. 34. *Recurrent epidermoid of the cauda equina after partial resection.* 36-year-old man with sphincteral deficiency. A – T_1-weighted image showing a hypointense, round-shaped mass, whose rim is isointense with the filum terminale. B – T_2-weighted image: the intensity of the neoplasm is CSF-like. The MRI section is difficult to interpret. At surgery, an epidermoid growing between the sacral roots and the filum terminale was found. The mass was excised and the filum terminale sectioned.

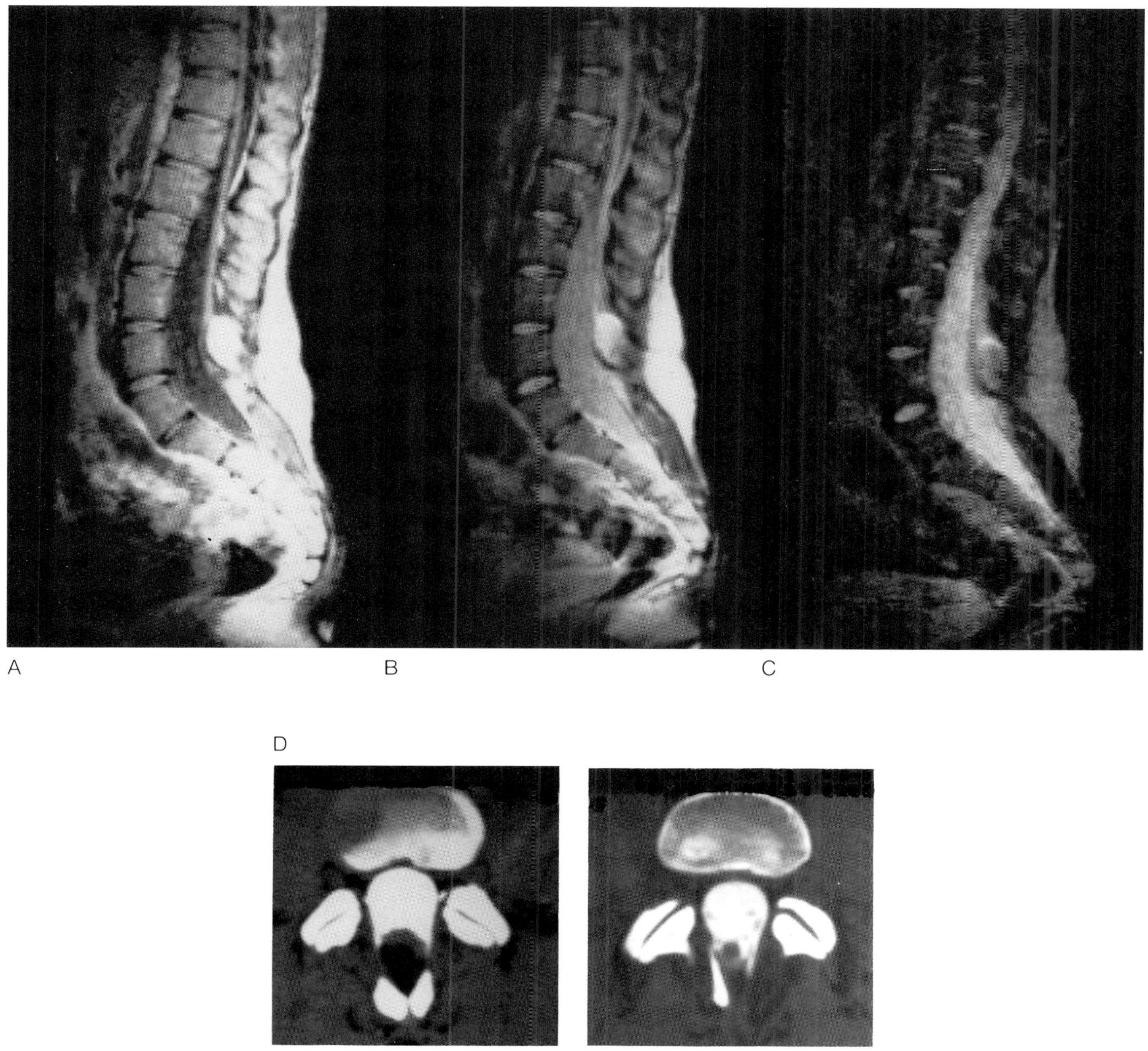

Fig. 35. *Lipoma of the cauda.* 22-year-old man with severe motor loss of the feet and occasional sphincteral deficiency. Typical signal from the lesion: hyperintensity on the T_1-weighted scan (A); progressive decrease with lengthening of the echo time on the T_2-weighted scans (B, C). Subcutaneous lipoma, lumbar schisis and dural megasac are also present. CT with intraspinal contrast medium (D) evidences the lipoma as a lesion with negative density values and the megasac anterior to the mass.

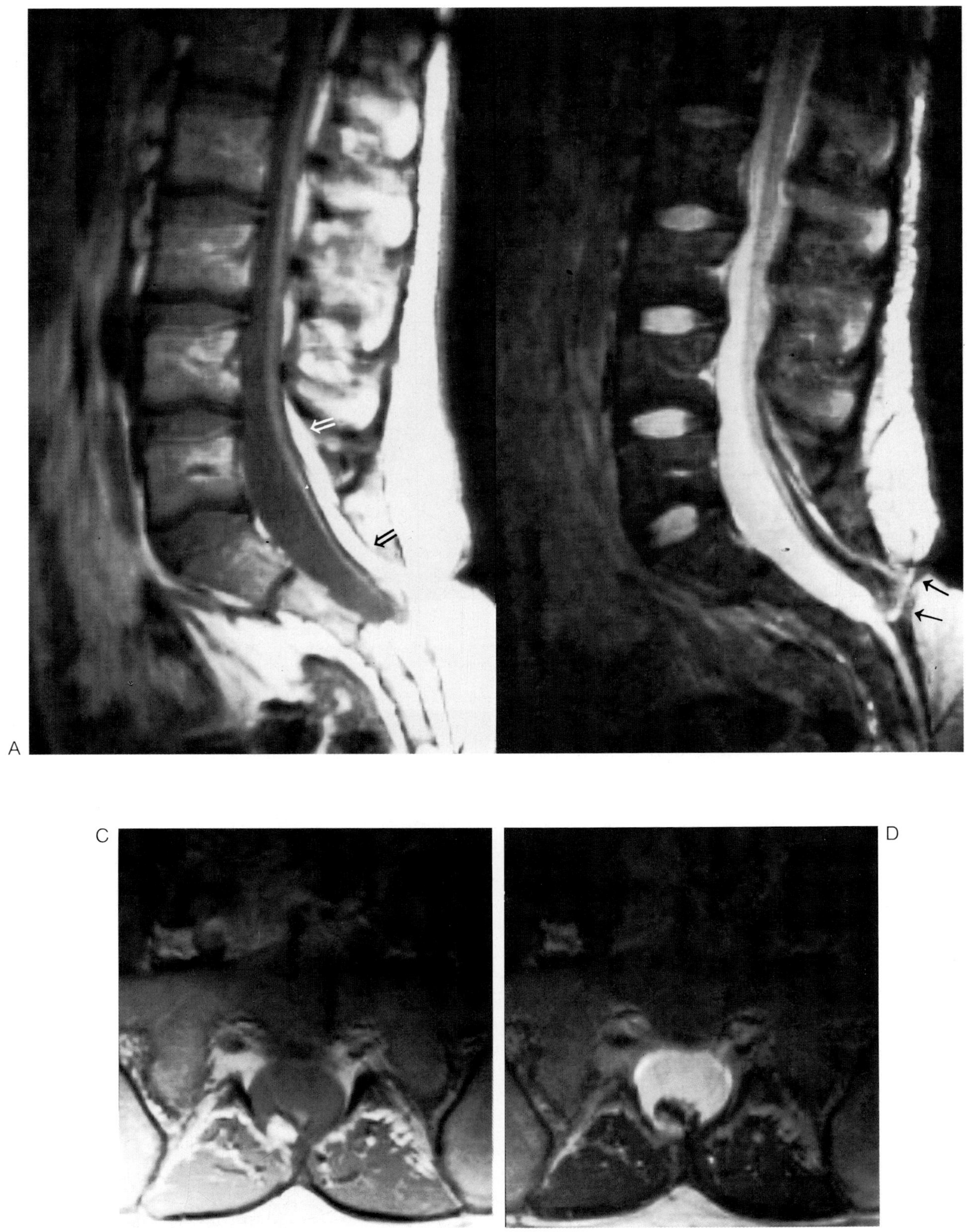

Fig. 36. *Dysrhafism of the lumbosacral region with intra-extradural lipoma and tethered cord.* 19-year-old young man with sphincteral incontinence since birth, which had recently turned into retention and perineal aneasthesia. These disturbances were underestimated in spite of the X-ray finding of a widespread lumbosacral schisis. The MRI study (A – TR 550 msec, TE 15 msec; B – TR 2,500 msec, TE 90 msec) demonstrates the introflexion of the cutaneous planes owing to dermal sinus (↗), the lipoma which extends posteriorly to L4 and the tethering of the lower part of the cord. C – TR 2500 msec, TE 25 msec; D – TR 2500 msec, TE 90 msec. The axial planes give a better view of the extra- and intradural site of the lipomatous mass and the posterior tethering of the filum terminale. The roots are visualized in their entirety thanks to their almost horizontal course. Typical signal from the lipoma: high on the T_1- (A) and proton density- (C) weighted sequences, low on the T_2- (B, D) weighted sequences.

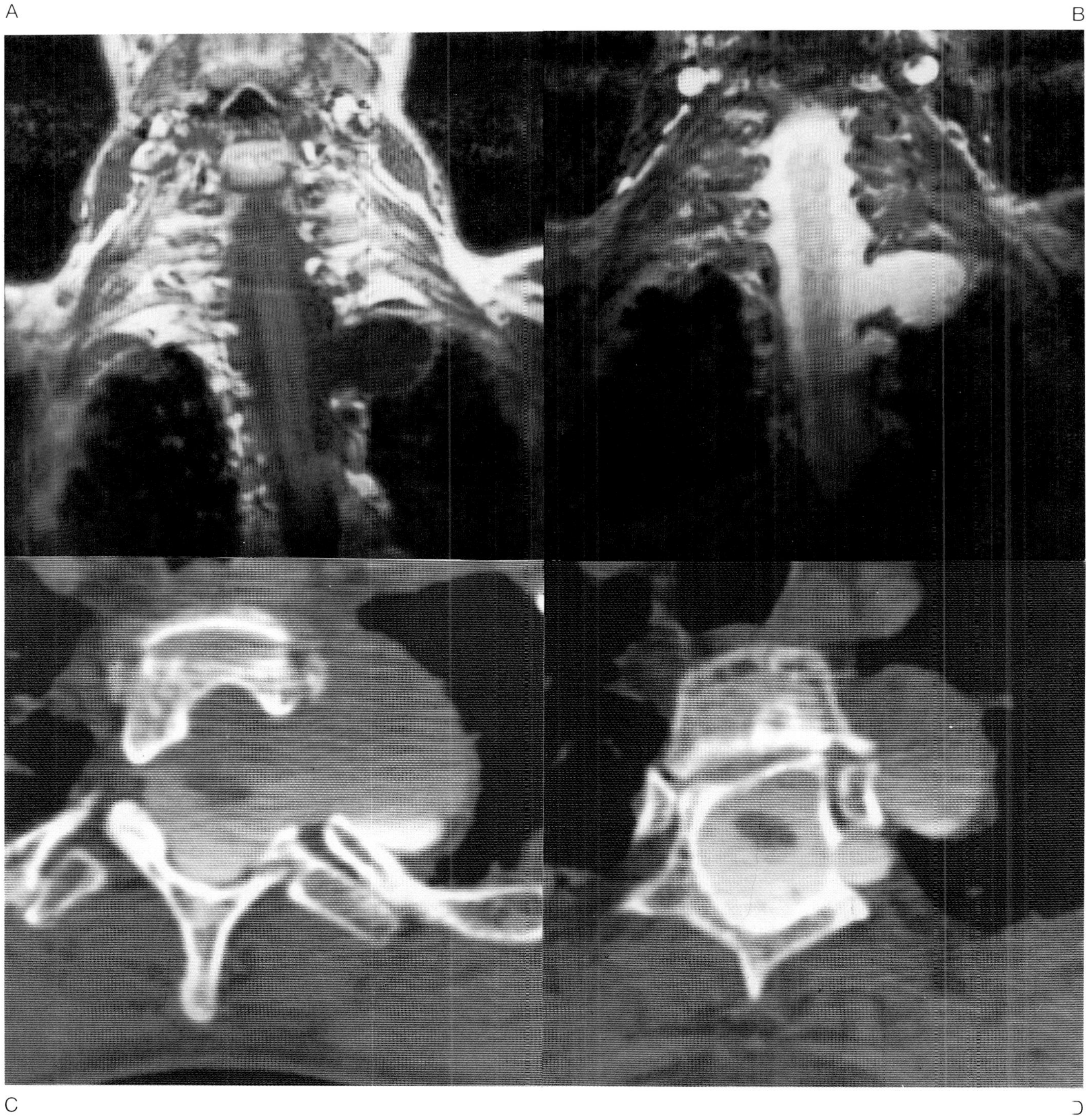

Fig. 37. *D2–D3 left lateral meningocele*. MRI investigation on clinically suspected dumbbell neurinoma. The T_1-(A) and T_2- (B) weighted coronal images visualize, at D2, the meningocele, the schisis, the correct position of the cord and its ependymal canal, as well as another small underlying pocket. The above features are also visible on CT after intrathecal iopamidol (C, D).

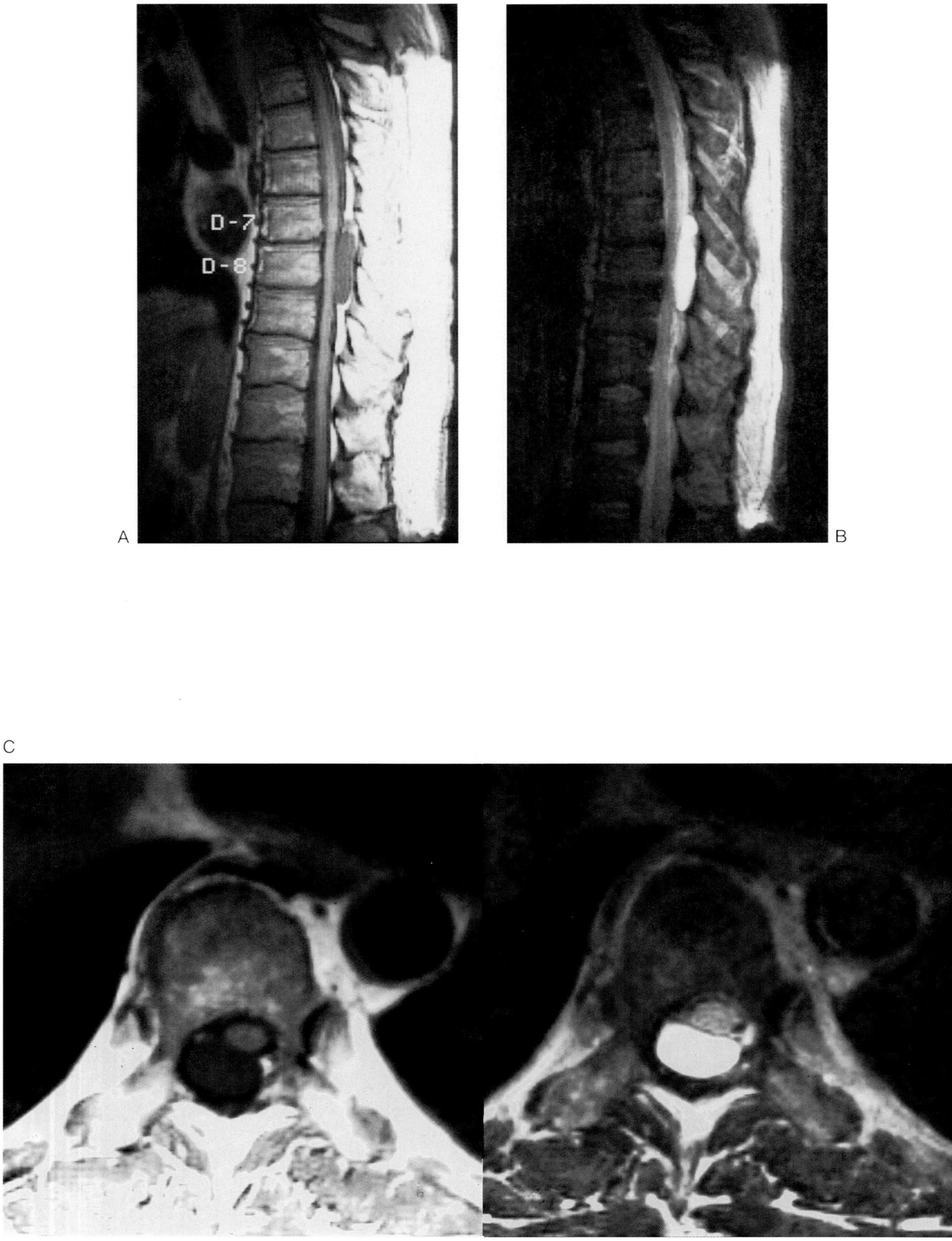

Fig. 38. *Dorsal arachnoid cyst.* The T_1- (A) and T_2- (B) weighted midsagittal images show, at D7–D8, an ovoid formation with its major axis in the longitudinal direction; the formation contains a fluid with CSF-like signal intensity. The T_1- (C) and T_2- (D) weighted axial images give a better view of the intradural site of the cyst and of its relations with the cord, displaced anteriorly to the left.

References

1. Asleson RJ, Haughton VM (1990) Magnetic resonance imaging of craniovertebral junction lesions. In: Wilkins RH, Rengachary SS (eds) Neurosurgery Update I. McGraw-Hill, New York, 47–56
2. Augenstein HM, Sze G, Becker R (1991) Imaging of spinal meningiomas. In: Al-Mefty O (ed) Meningiomas. Raven Press, New York, 603–613
3. Bronen RA, Sze G (1990) Magnetic resonance contrast agents: theory and application to the central nervous system. J Neurosurg 73:820–840
4. Czervionke LF, Daniels DL (1988) Cervical spine anatomy and pathologic processes: applications of new MR imaging techniques. Radiol Clin North Am 26:921–947
5. Czervionke LF, Daniels DL, Ho PSP et al. (1988) The MR appearance of gray and white matter in the cervical spinal cord. AJNR 9:557–562
6. Di Chiro G, Doppman JL, Dwyer AJ et al. (1985) Tumors and arteriovenous malformations of the spinal cord: assessment using MR. Radiology 156:689–697
7. Dillon WP, Norman D, Newton TH et al. (1989) Intradural spinal cord lesions: Gd-DTPA-enhanced MR imaging. Radiology 170:229–237
8. Fontaine S, Melanson D, Cosgrove R et al. (1988) Cavernous hemangiomas of the spinal cord: MR imaging. Radiology 166:839–841
9. Harkey HL, Crockard HA (1991) Spinal meningiomas: Clinical features. In: Al-Mefty O (ed) Meningiomas. Raven Press, New York, 593–601
10. Kent DL, Larson EB (1988) Magnetic resonance imaging of the brain and spine: is clinical efficacy established after the first decade? Ann Intern Med 107:402–424
11. Lee KS, Spetzler RF (1990) Spinal cord cavernous malformation in a patient with familial intracranial cavernous malformations. Neurosurgery 26:877–880
12. Mallon WJ, Harrelson JM (1990) Primary neoplasms of the spine. In: Wilkins RH, Rengachary SS (eds) Neurosurgery. McGraw-Hill, New York, 19–28
13. Miller KD Jr (1990) Magnetic resonance imaging of the vertebral column and spinal cord. In: Wilkins RH, Rengachary SS (eds) Neurosurgery. McGraw-Hill, New York, 104–118
14. Parizel PM, Baleriaux D, Rodesch G et al. (1989) Gadolinium-DTPA-enhanced MR imaging of spinal tumors. AJNR 10:249–258
15. Pomeranz SJ (1989) Posterior fossa, skull base, craniocervical junction: In: Pomeranz SJ (ed) Craniospinal Magnetic Resonance Imaging. W. B. Saunders Co, Philadelphia, 248–274
16. Pomeranz SJ (1989) Neoplasms of the spine. In: Pomeranz SJ (ed) Craniospinal Magnetic Resonance Imaging. W. B. Saunders Co, Philadelphia, 513–540
17. Sisti MB, Stein BM (1991) Surgery of spinal meningiomas. In: Al-Mefty O (ed) Meningiomas. Raven Press, New York, 615–620
18. Slasky BS, Bydder GM, Niendorf HP et al. (1987) MR imaging with gadolinium-DTPA in the differentiation of tumor, syrinx, and cyst of the spinal cord. J Comput Assist Tomogr 11:845–850
19. Smoker WRK, Goderski JC, Knutzon RK et al. (1987) The role of MR imaging in evaluating metastatic spinal disease. AJR 149:1241–1248
20. Solero CL, Fornari M, Giombini S et al. (1989) Spinal meningiomas: Review of 174 operated cases. Neurosurgery 25:153–160
21. Sze G, Krol G, Zimmerman RD et al. (1988) Gadolinium DTPA: malignant extradural spinal tumors. Radiology 167:217–233
22. Sze G, Abramson A, Krol G et al. (1988) Gadolinium-DTPA in the evaluation of intradural extramedullary spinal disease. AJR 150:911–921
23. terPenning B (1989) Inflammatory disease of the brain and spine. In: Pomeranz SJ (ed) Craniospinal Magnetic Resonance Imaging. W. B. Saunders Co, Philadelphia, 436–458
24. Wetzel LH, Levine E (1990) Pictorial essay. MR imaging of sacral and presacral lesions. Am J Roentgenol 154:771–775
25. Williams AL, Haughton VM, Pojuntas KW et al. (1987) Differentiation of intramedullary neoplasms and cysts by MR. AJR 149:159–164

Henri Duvernoy

The Human Brain

Surface, Three-dimensional Sectional Anatomy and MRI

In collaboration with
E. A. Cabanis,
M. T. Iba-Zizen,
J. Tamraz, and
J. Guyot

Illustrations by
J. L. Vannson

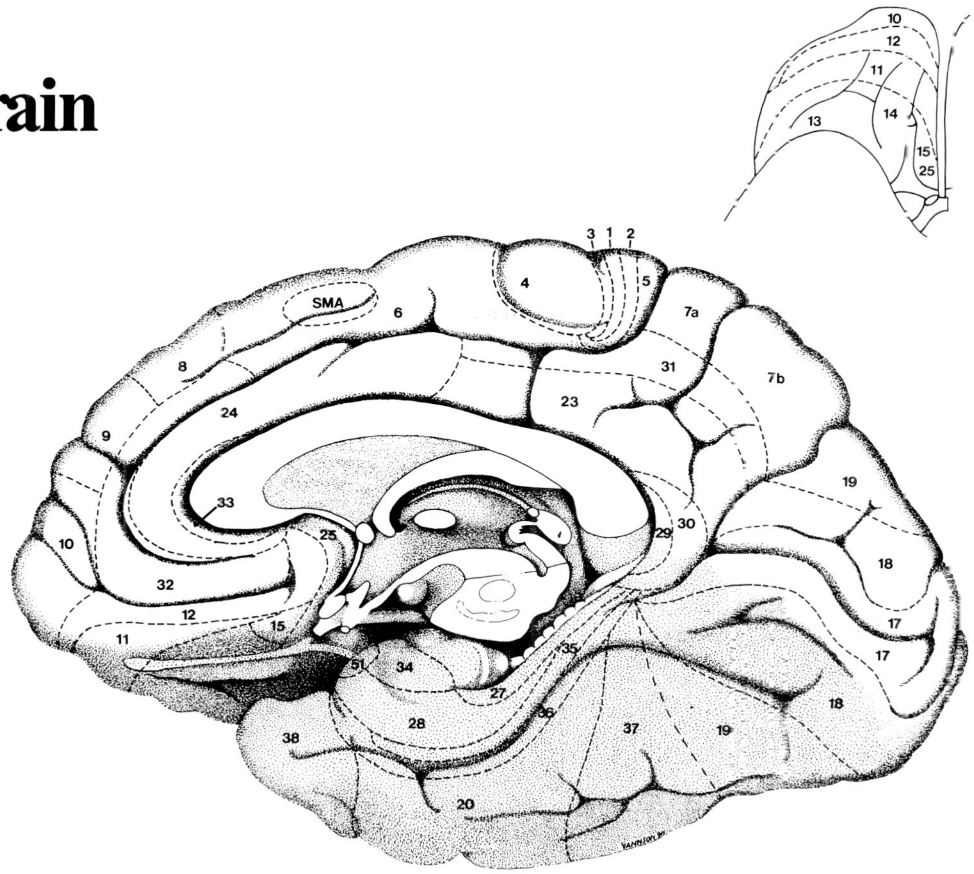

Fig. 25 and 25'. Cytoarchitectonic areas according to Brodmann. Inferomedial surface of the right hemisphere (Fig. 25). Orbital surface of the right hemisphere (Fig. 25').

1991. 191 figures.
VII, 354 pages.
Cloth DM 268,–, öS 1876,–
ISBN 3-211-82260-7

The recent progress of medical imaging due to CT, MRI, and the three-dimensional reconstruction of cerebral structures, calls for a better understanding of the anatomy of the brain. Therefore, this book comprises serial sections – 2 to 4 mm thick – of the cerebral hemispheres and diencephalon in the coronal, sagittal, and horizontal planes.

So as to point out the level of the sections more accurately, each of the sections are shown from different angles emphasizing the surrounding hemisphere surfaces. This three-dimensional approach has proved extremely useful to apprehend the difficult anatomy of the gyri and sulci of the brain. Certain complex cerebral structures such as the occipital lobe, the deep grey matter (basal ganglia and thalamus) and the hippocampus have been studied in greater detail. Wherever possible, MRI images of the same plane have been added so that they can be compared with the anatomical section.

Prices are subject to change without notice

Springer-Verlag Wien New York

Sachsenplatz 4–6, P.O. Box 89, A-1201 Wien · Heidelberger Platz 3, D-1000 Berlin 33
175 Fifth Avenue, New York, NY 10010 USA · 37-3, Hongo 3-chome, Bunkyo-ku, Tokyo 113, Japan

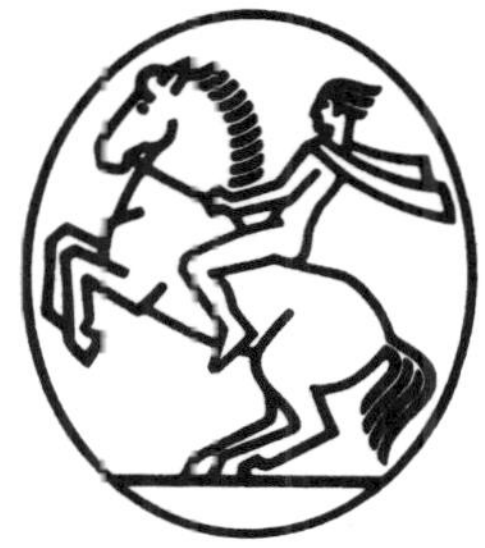

Wolfgang Seeger

Differential Approaches in Microsurgery of the Brain

In Collaboration with W. Mann

Springer-Verlag Wien New York

Prof. Dr. med. WOLFGANG SEEGER
Medical Director of the Department of General Neurosurgery
and Chairman of Neurosurgery of the Neurosurgical Clinic

Prof. Dr. med. WOLF MANN
Ear, Nose and Throat Clinic

University of Freiburg i. Br., Federal Republic of Germany

With 201 Figures

Printed in Austria

Library of Congress Cataloging in Publication Data. Seeger, Wolfgang, 1929– . Differential approaches in microsurgery of the brain. 1. Brain-Surgery. 2. Microsurgery. I. Mann, W. (Wolf) II. Title. RD594.S425 1985. 617'.481. 85-12724.

ISBN 3-211-81857-X Springer-Verlag Wien–New York
ISBN 0-387-81857-X Springer-Verlag New York–Wien

Preface

In the present volume various approaches to the same target area in the deep regions of the brain are described. In the previous volumes this aspect was taken little into account. The author endeavored to describe particularly the typical operative approaches and their principles to make it easier for the beginner to learn the microsurgical techniques in interventions in the central nervous system.

Now problematical processes in the immediate vicinity of the brainstem area have been exclusively selected. They have been separated into dorsal, lateral and ventral processes with locations mainly in the dorsal, lateral or ventral cisternal areas. Each of these three groups has been separated again into rostral, middle and posterior approaches to the rostrally lying, middle and posterior portions of the cisterns.

A particular example of the problems of operations in the depth of the cisternal area was shown to be the approach to the so-called "quadrigeminal" region. Only recently is information accumulating on successful operations in this region of the brain. In the literature so far too little has been mentioned that there are five different approaches to the so-called "quadrigeminal" region, all of which can be indicated. No single approach is exclusively to be recommended. Two factors influence the selection of the correct approach:

1. The individual anatomical conditions of the brain, which – as is well known – are subject to variations. Here the venous variations play a major role, therefore operative problems of the cerebral veins in particular have been discussed in the previous volume.
2. The type and size of the process, symmetrical or asymmetrical localization and its particular situation in relation to the surrounding brain structures and cerebral vessels. Here it is to be noted that the so-called "quadrigeminal" region consists not only of the Cisterna tecti, but the nearby fissures (Fissura transversa cerebri and Fissura horizontalis cerebelli) should also be included. The pathological processes do not generally confine themselves to the Cisterna tecti, but extend over the neighboring fissures. The Cisterna tecti extends without limits into the neighboring fissures and into the Cisterna ambiens.

As previously, besides personal operational experiences (which are not marked as such) also interventions are presented which have been carried out by co-workers. For further suggestions the author acknowledges the daily discussions with the co-workers, of whom Prof. Dr. J. Gilsbach, PD. Dr. H. R. Eggert, Dr. W. Hassler and Dr. A. Harders should be specially mentioned. The author also thanks Prof. Dr. M. G. Yaşargil, Zürich, Prof. Dr. K. Sugita, Nagoya, Prof. Dr. G. Baumgartner, Colmar, and Prof. Dr. J. Staubesand, Freiburg, for their suggestions. The otorhinological operations were all carried out by Prof. Dr. W. Mann, Ear, Nose and Throat Clinic, Freiburg (Director: Prof. Dr. Chl. Beck), together with Prof. Dr. J. Gilsbach, who was responsible for the neurosurgical parts of the operations.

The manuscript was typed by Mrs. Ermy Hilsenbek-Hottek, Mrs. V. Kullmann and Mr. Hans G. Förster (Neurosurgical Clinic, Freiburg). For the translation I thank Mrs. Dr. L. D. Ladurner, Salzburg. I would especially like to thank Springer-Verlag Wien–New York for the continually good cooperation, helpfulness and excellent makeup of the book.

Freiburg, July 1985 Wolfgang Seeger

Contents

Part I

General Remarks

(Figs. 1 to 5)

Chapter 1
General Remarks
(Figs. 1 to 5)

Fig. 1

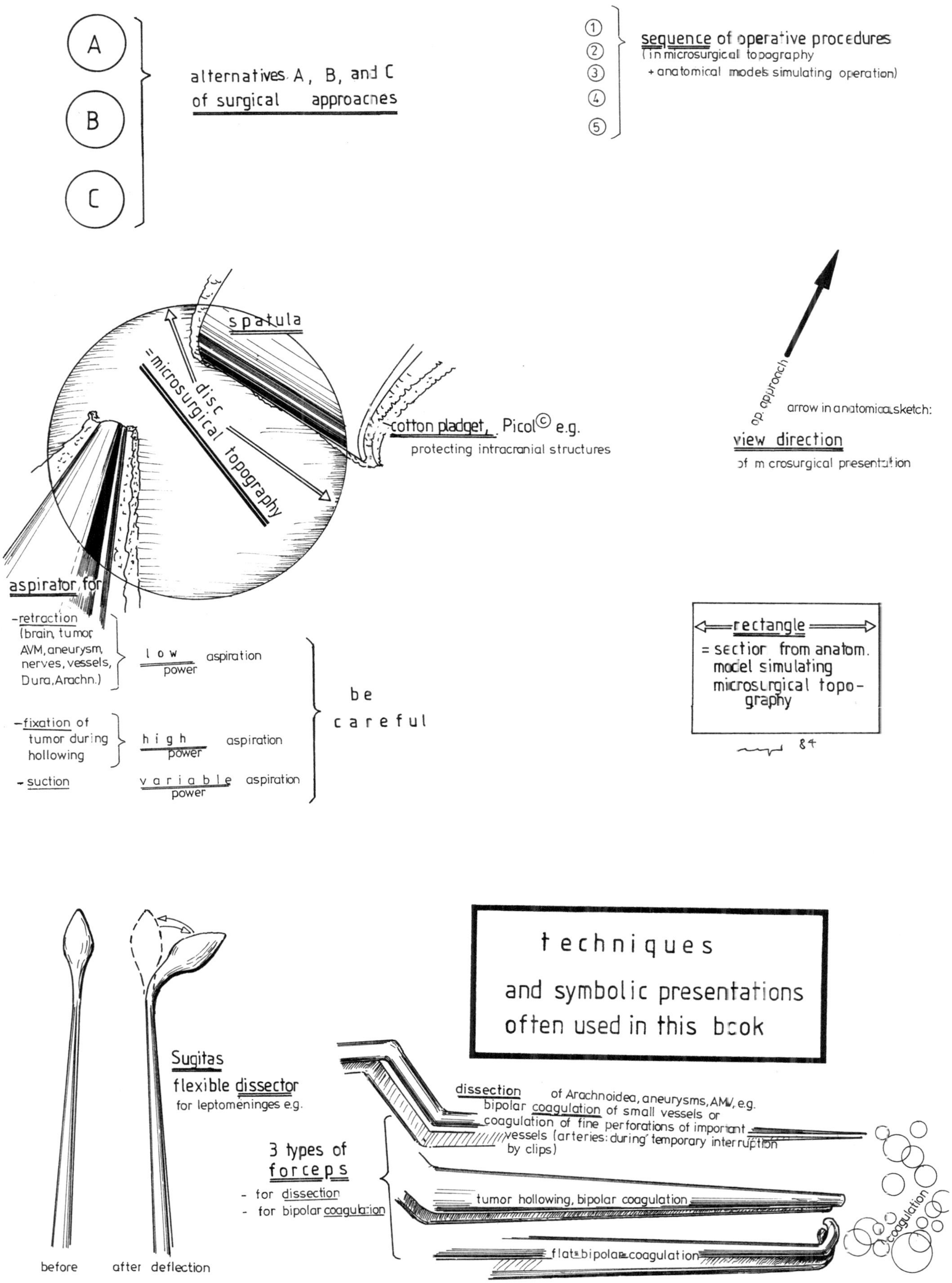

A
B
C
alternatives A, B, and C of surgical approaches
① ② ③ ④ ⑤
sequence of operative procedures (in microsurgical topography + anatomical models simulating operation)
spatula
disc = microsurgical topography
cotton pladget, Picol© e.g.
protecting intracranial structures
op. approach
arrow in anatomical sketch:
view direction
of microsurgical presentation
aspirator for
- retraction (brain, tumor, AVM, aneurysm, nerves, vessels, Dura, Arachn.)
low power aspiration
- fixation of tumor during hollowing
high power aspiration
- suction
variable power aspiration
be careful
rectangle
= section from anatom. model simulating microsurgical topography
84
techniques
and symbolic presentations
often used in this book
Sugitas
flexible dissector
for leptomeninges e.g.
before
after deflection
3 types of forceps
- for dissection
- for bipolar coagulation
dissection of Arachnoidea, aneurysms, AMV, e.g.
bipolar coagulation of small vessels or coagulation of fine perforations of important vessels (arteries: during temporary interruption by clips)
tumor hollowing, bipolar coagulation
flat bipolar coagulation
coagulation

Fig. 2

dorsal CSF - spaces close to the brainstem

anterior segment: Cisterna corporis callosi (rostral area) ·ccc·
- Chapter 2 -

middle segment: Fiss. transversa (medial area) ·ftm·
Cisterna tecti ·ct·
Fiss. horizontalis (medial area) ·fhm·
- Chapter 3 -

posterior segment : Cisterna cerebellomedull. ·ccm·
- Chapter 4 -

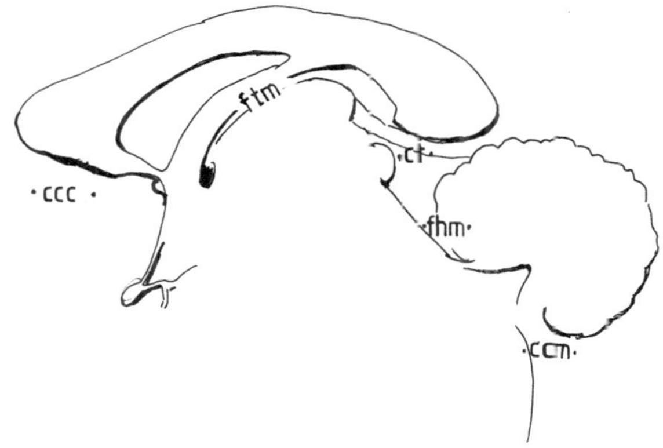

lateral CSF-spaces

(anterior segment: Sylvian fissure)
- -

middle segment: Fiss. transversa (lateral area) ·ftl·
Cisterna ambiens ·cam·
Fiss. horizontalis lateral area ·fhl·
- Chapter 5 -

posterior segment: Cisterna cerebellopontina ·ccp·
neurosurgical + o t o l o g i a l aspects (petrosectomy) ·pte·
Cisterna cerebellomecullaris lat. ·ccl·
- Chapter 6 -

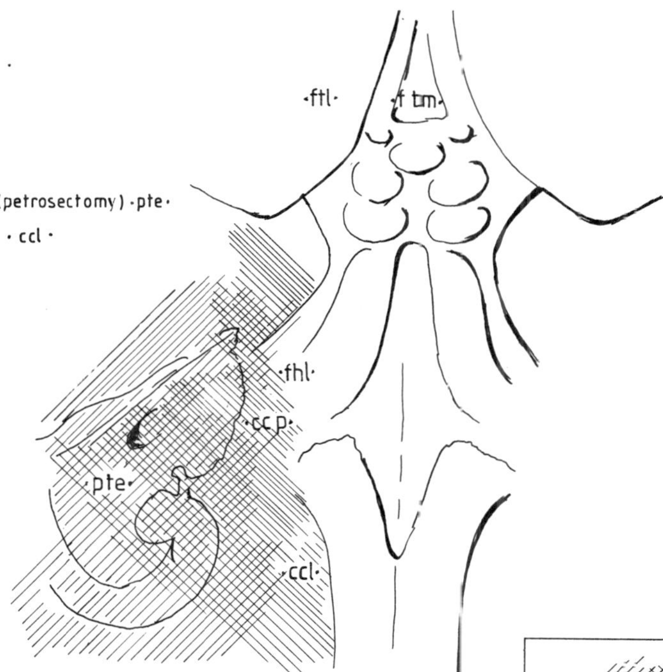

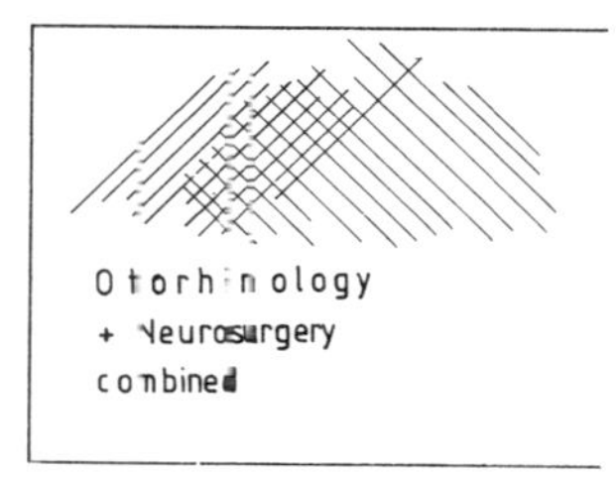

basal CSF-spaces

anterior segment : Cisterna opt. + frontal base/Cavum nasi ·cof· /·can·
neurosurgical + o t o r h i n o l o g i c a l aspects
- Chapter 7 -

middle segment: Cisterna interpeduncularis ·cip·
Cisterna pontis (rostral area) ·cpr·
neurosurgical + o t o r h i n o l o g i c a l aspects ·fca·
(faciocranial approach)
- Chapter 8 -

posterior segment : Cisterna pontis (caudal area) ·cpc·
Cisterna praemedullaris ·cpm·

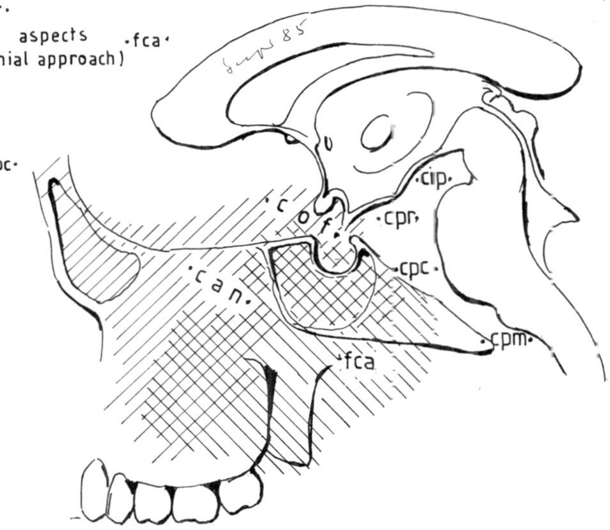

preformed CSF-spaces for approaches described in this book

Fig. 3. Dorsal CSF spaces of brainstem. The basal portions of the **cisterns of the Corpus callosum** are also considered dorsal, since they are situated dorsal from the Chiasma and Lamina terminalis and thus dorsal from the 3rd ventricle

The anterior and middle cistern regions merge into one another. The middle region (Fissura horizontalis cerebelli, rostral area) and the **posterior region** (Cisterna cerebello-medullaris) are separated by the 4th ventricle. The 4th ventricle connects with the Cisterna cerebello-medullaris over the Apertura mediana (Magendi). The 4th ventricle is **separated** from the Fissura horizontalis cerebelli and the Cisterna tecti only by the very thin Velum medullare ant., which pathological processes can destroy. In such cases, contact is produced during surgery between the Cisterna tecti, the Fissura horizontalis cerebelli (rostral area), the 4th ventricle, and the Cisterna cerebello-medullaris

Tumors and vascular deformations can spread from one CSF area into the other and frequently do not respect the boundaries between the anterior, middle, and posterior cranial fossa

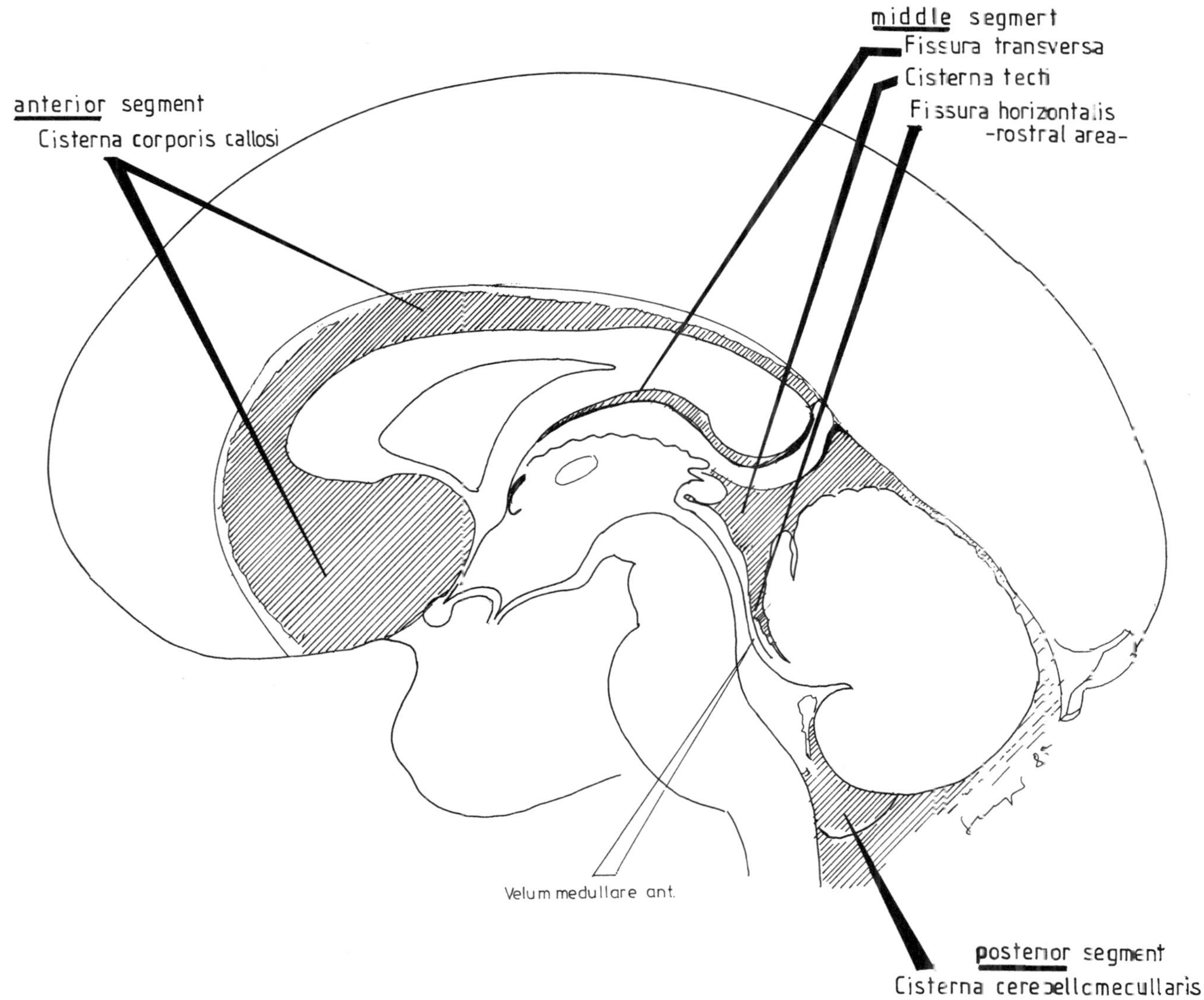

dorsal CSF-spaces close to the brainstem
- cisterns and fissures -

Fig. 4. Comparison of the lateral and dorsal CSF spaces
Anterior segment: Only the dorsal (and basal) CSF spaces are present
Middle segment: Fissura transversa in the area of the Trigonum is very wide
The Cisterna ambiens extends from the Cisterna tecti to the basal cistern area
The Fissura horizontalis cerebelli extends from the N. trigeminus to the midline and surrounds the middle and superior cerebellar peduncle (Brachium pontis and Brachium conjunctivum), as well as the Velum medullare ant. Because of the various operative approaches possible, a medial and lateral region had to be differentiated*
Posterior segment: The lateral cistern region is formed dorsolateral from the Cisterna cerebellopontina and basolateral from the Cisterna ponto-medullaris lateralis. A double-layered arachnoid membrane between the two cisterns covers the cranial nerves IX to XI. This arachnoid membrane has to be preserved in cases of acoustic neurinomas. The membrane adheres to the Plexus chor. of the Recessus lateralis with the so-called Foramen Luschkae (which may be closed)
The exact knowledge of the construction of the Arachnoidea of the brain is an essential condition for operating in the vicinity of the brainstem

* For some authors, only the Fissura horizontalis in its posterior portion, which lies between the Lobulus semilunaris sup. and the Lobulus biventer and which laterally extends to the Flocculus. The Fissura, however, continues on up in front and becomes deepest between the Velum medullare ant. and the Lobulus centralis cerebelli.

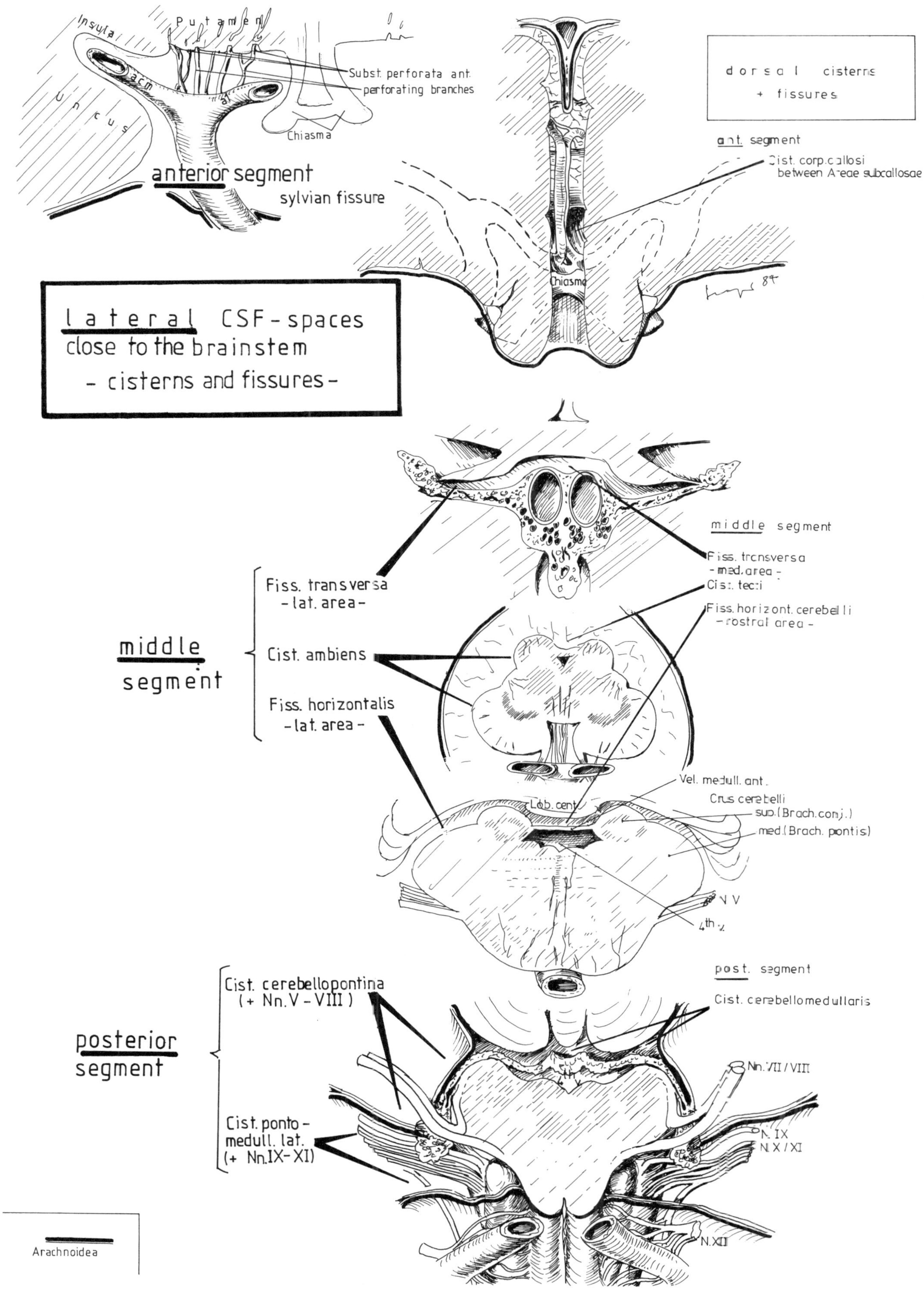
Insula
Putamen
Uncus
acm
aci
Subst. perforata ant.
perforating branches
Chiasma
anterior segment
sylvian fissure
dorsal cisterns
+ fissures
ant. segment
Cist. corp. callosi
between Areae subcallosae
Chiasma
lateral CSF-spaces
close to the brainstem
- cisterns and fissures -
middle segment
Fiss. transversa
- med. area -
Cist. tecti
Fiss. horizont. cerebelli
- rostral area -
Fiss. transversa
- lat. area -
middle
segment
Cist. ambiens
Fiss. horizontalis
- lat. area -
Vel. medull. ant.
Crus cerebelli
sup. (Brach. conj.)
med. (Brach. pontis)
Lob. cent.
N. V
4th v.
post. segment
Cist. cerebellomedullaris
Cist. cerebellopontina
(+ Nn. V - VIII)
posterior
segment
Nn. VII / VIII
Cist. ponto-
medull. lat.
(+ Nn. IX-XI)
N. IX
N. X / XI
N. XII
Arachnoidea

Fig. 5. Comparison of dorsal and basal cisterns
Dorsal CSF spaces:
Anterior segment = Cisterna corporis callosi. Adhesions may severely restrict the CSF fissure up to as far as the margin of the Falx
Middle segment: The Fissura transversa is usually narrow. Whenever this CSF space is opened, the Fornix and the Tela chorioidea are pushed away from each other, as is shown in the illustration (see double-pointed arrow). The Tela chorioidea of the 3rd ventricle is covered by a thin arachnoid layer, which guards the hypervascularized surroundings of the inner cerebral veins from surgical manipulation. There are no or only few vessels between the Tela chorioidea and the Fornix. On both sides of the V. magna Galeni there are small connections between the Fissura transversa and the Cisterna tecti
Posterior segment = Cisterna cerebello-medullaris
Basal cisterns: This cistern region is the most familiar, since most operations are performed there. All of the cisterns are separated from one another by gappy arachnoid membranes. For this reason, the arachnoid membranes between the various cisterns always have to be covered with cotton wool during surgery (if the operation is not extended to a neighboring cistern) to minimize the blood admixtures of the cisternal CSF

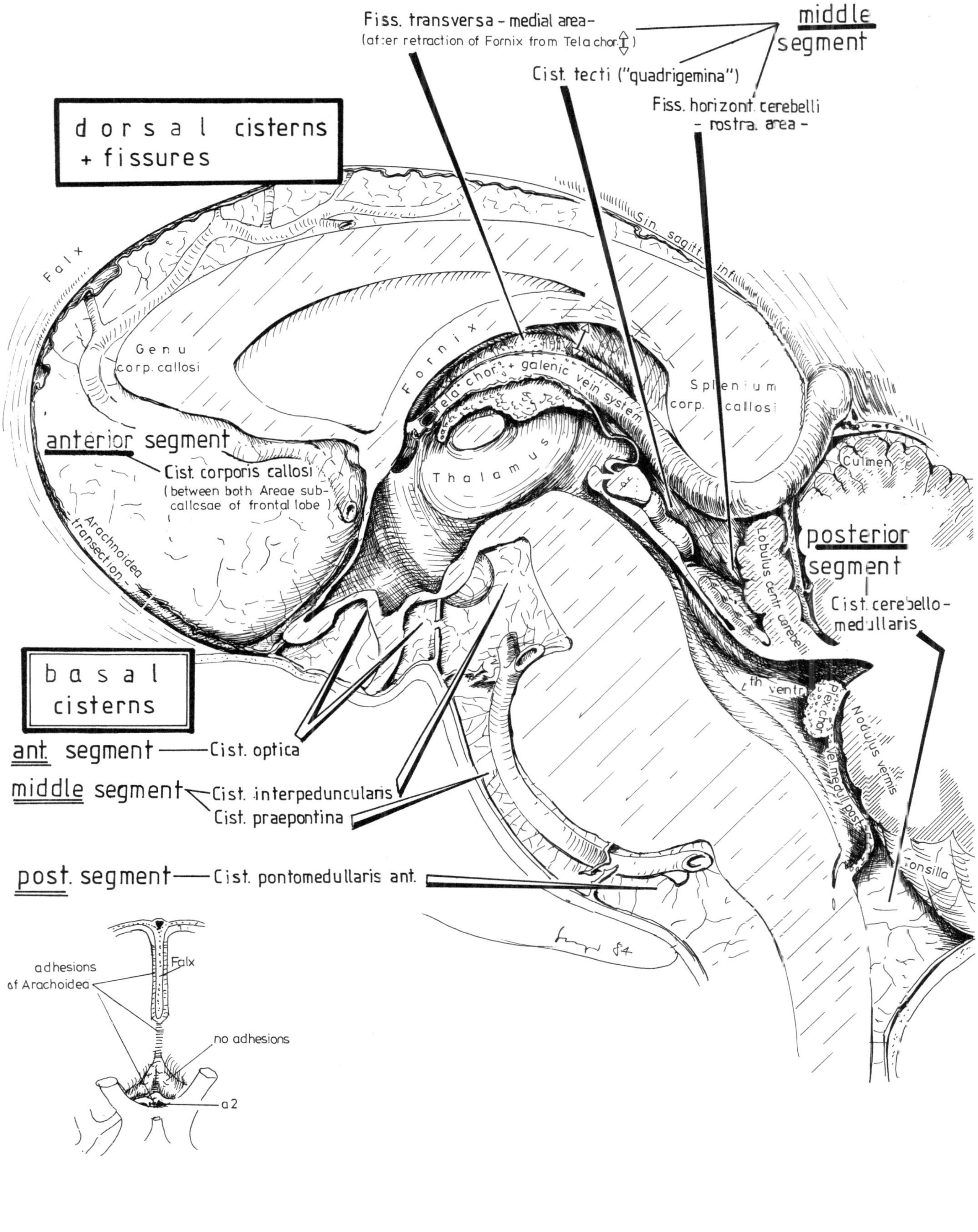
Fiss. transversa - medial area-
(after retraction of Fornix from Tela chor.)
middle
segment
Cist. tecti ("quadrigemina")
Fiss. horizont. cerebelli
- rostral area -
dorsal cisterns
+ fissures
Falx
Sin. sagitt. inf.
Genu
corp. callosi
Fornix
Tela chor. + galenic vein system
Splenium
corp. callosi
Thalamus
Culmen
anterior segment
Cist. corporis callosi
(between both Areae subcallosae of frontal lobe)
Arachnoidea transection
Lobulus centr. cerebelli
posterior
segment
Cist. cerebello-
medullaris
basal
cisterns
4th ventr.
plex. chor.
Nodulus vermis
vel. medull. post.
ant. segment
Cist. optica
middle segment
Cist. interpeduncularis
Cist. praepontina
post. segment
Cist. pontomedullaris ant.
Tonsilla
adhesions
of Arachoidea
Falx
no adhesions
a2

Part II

Special Microsurgical Aspects

(Figs. 6 to 201)

Chapter 2

Dorsal Cisterns and Fissures, Anterior Segment (Figs. 6 to 45)

Fig. 6. Relationships of the **Arachnoidea** to the Falx and the cranial base
In the front diagonal illustration, the arachnoidea is lifted from the basal dura, as can be done during operations without having to open the CSF spaces

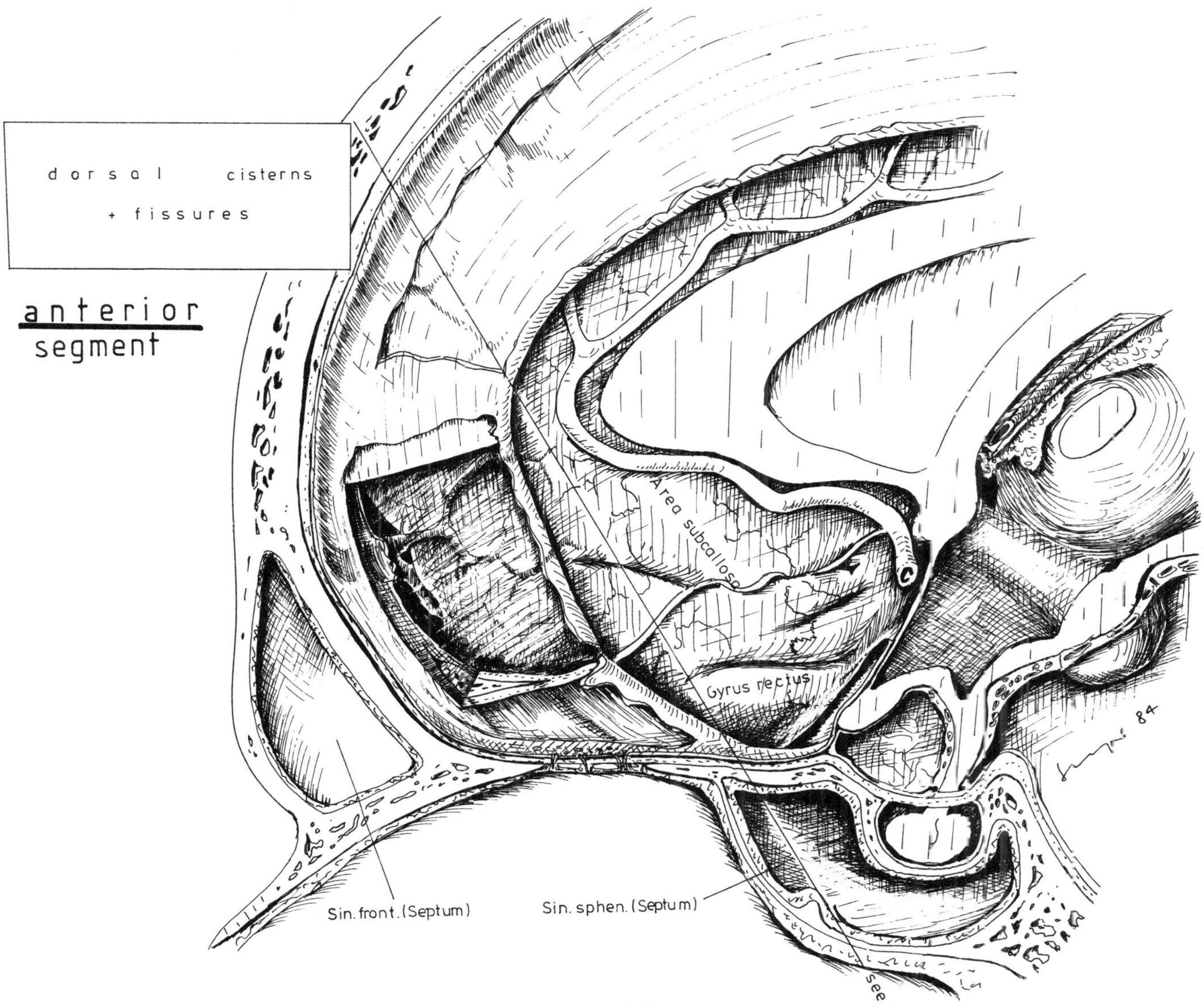

dorsal cisterns
+ fissures
anterior
segment
Area subcallosa
Gyrus rectus
Sin. front. (Septum)
Sin. sphen. (Septum)
see frontal oblique transection

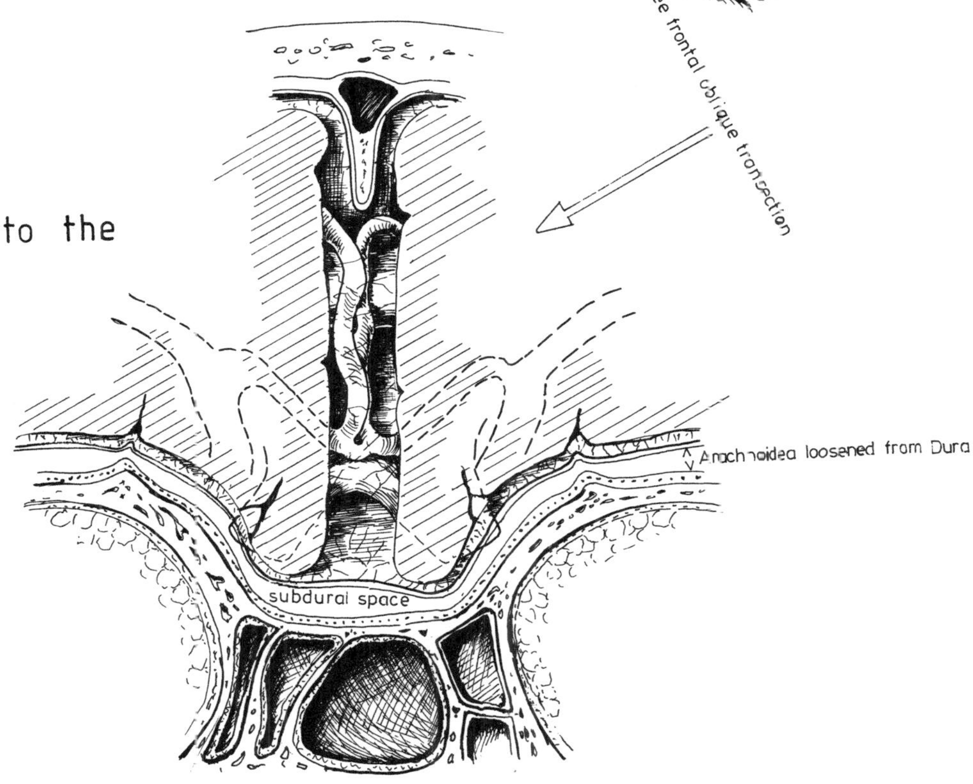

relationship to the
cranial base
Arachnoidea loosened from Dura
subdural space

Fig. 7. Surgical examples of frontomedial angiomas with connections to A1, A. communicans ant., A2, to the Corpus callosum and Gyri orbitales, basal ganglia and ventricular system.

A and **B** Two operative approaches

Main argument for **A:** A. cerebri ant. is deeply situated and all of the angioma portions are located near the midline

Main argument against **A:** large draining veins in the frontopolar area hinder the midline approach

Main argument for **B:** the laterobasal portions of the angioma are wide. Because vision is poor, there is danger of causing damage in the anterior part of this area

(A) midline - approach

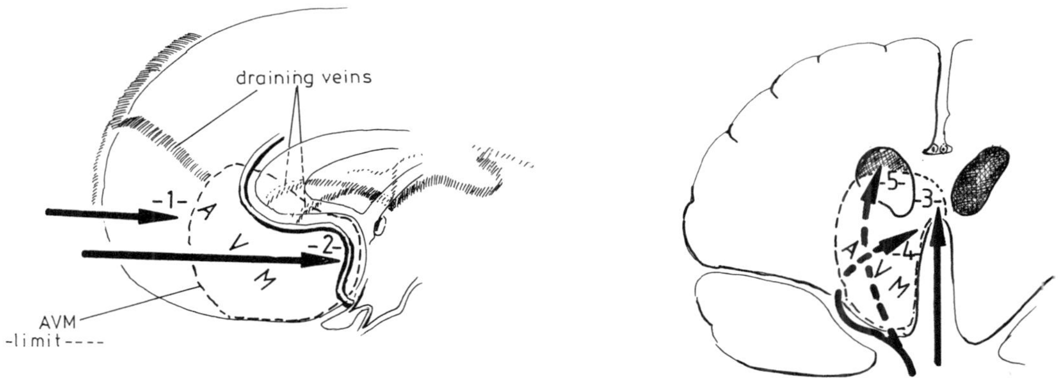

favorable	- if no blockage of midline-approach by thick-calibrated bridging and draining veins -1- - deep localized A2 less problematic -2- - portions of AVM in Corpus callosum less problematic -3-
unfavorable	- lateral and deeply localized (close to basal ganglia) portions of AVM -4- - portions of AVM in Cornu ant.- 5-

---

(B) pterional approach

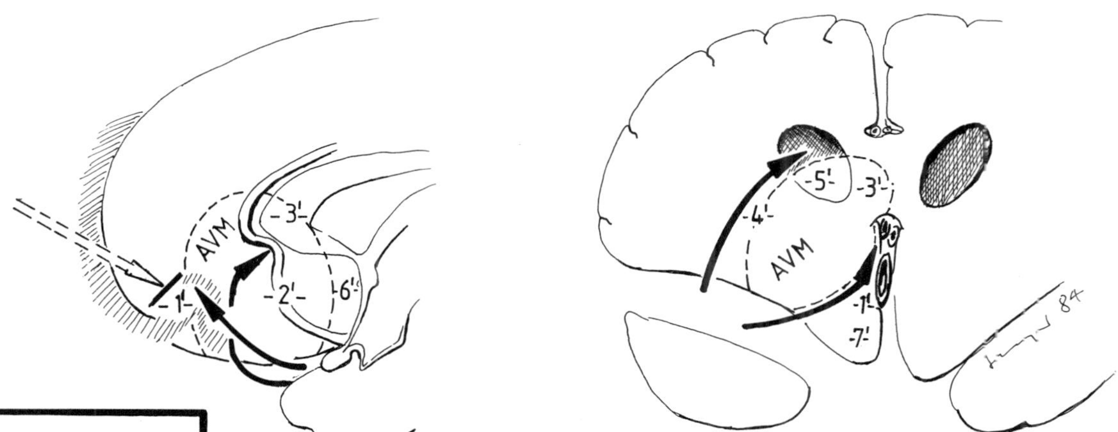

favorable	- localization lateral and close to basal ganglia -4'- and Cornu ant.-5'- less problematic - if Area subcallosa - 6' - and Gyrus rectus - 7'-are not involved - Allocortex may be preserved - - if midline-approach is blocked by veins -1'-
unfavorable	- A2, all variations - 2'- - Corpus callosum infiltrated by AVM - 3'-

Fig. 8. Surgery in two sessions **C** is to be considered when all of the adverse factors of **A** and **B** are given. Main argument for beginning the pterional operation: draining veins of the frontopolar area are avoided. The larger portion of the AVM can be isolated from here. The second operation is performed using the midline approach. It can be carried out immediately after the first operation or few weeks later *
None of the counterarguments is applicable for the second operation

---

* Presently, some authors recommend removing large AVM's in two separate operations so that the hemodynamics of the cerebral circulation can be gradually normalized.

FIG. 8

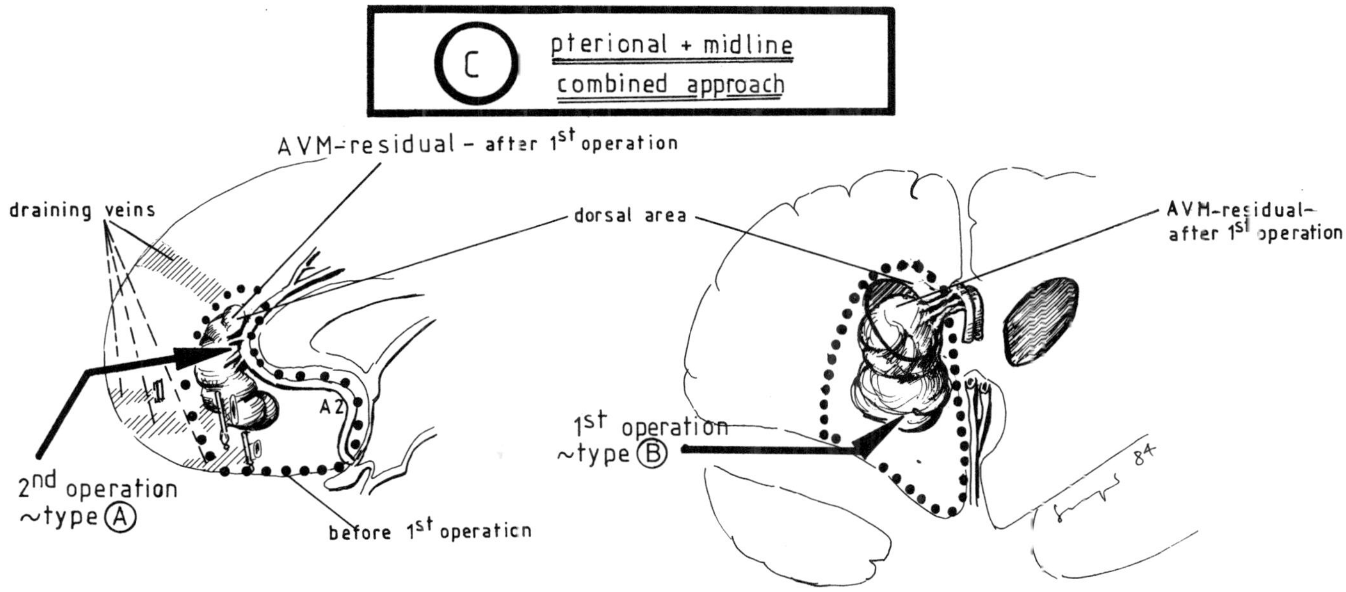

1st op. ~Ⓑ

favorable:	- lateral location - approach not hindered by frontomedial draining veins
unfavorable:	- A2 in dorsal area

2nd op. ~Ⓐ

favorable:	- A2, all variations - medial draining veins eliminated after 1st operation
unfavorable:	—

Fig. 9. Clinical examples* of the operative approaches **A** (midline) and **B** (pterional)

Differences:

A situated more medially in the basal area. Basal draining veins in the middle fissure are fewer (than in **B**).
Approach to N. opticus and to Aa. cerebri antt. is thus favorable

B base of the angioma is broader in the area of the orbital gyri. Area of the Gyrus rectus is left out

* Both patients without neurological or psychological deficits, both pre- and postoperatively.

FIG. 9

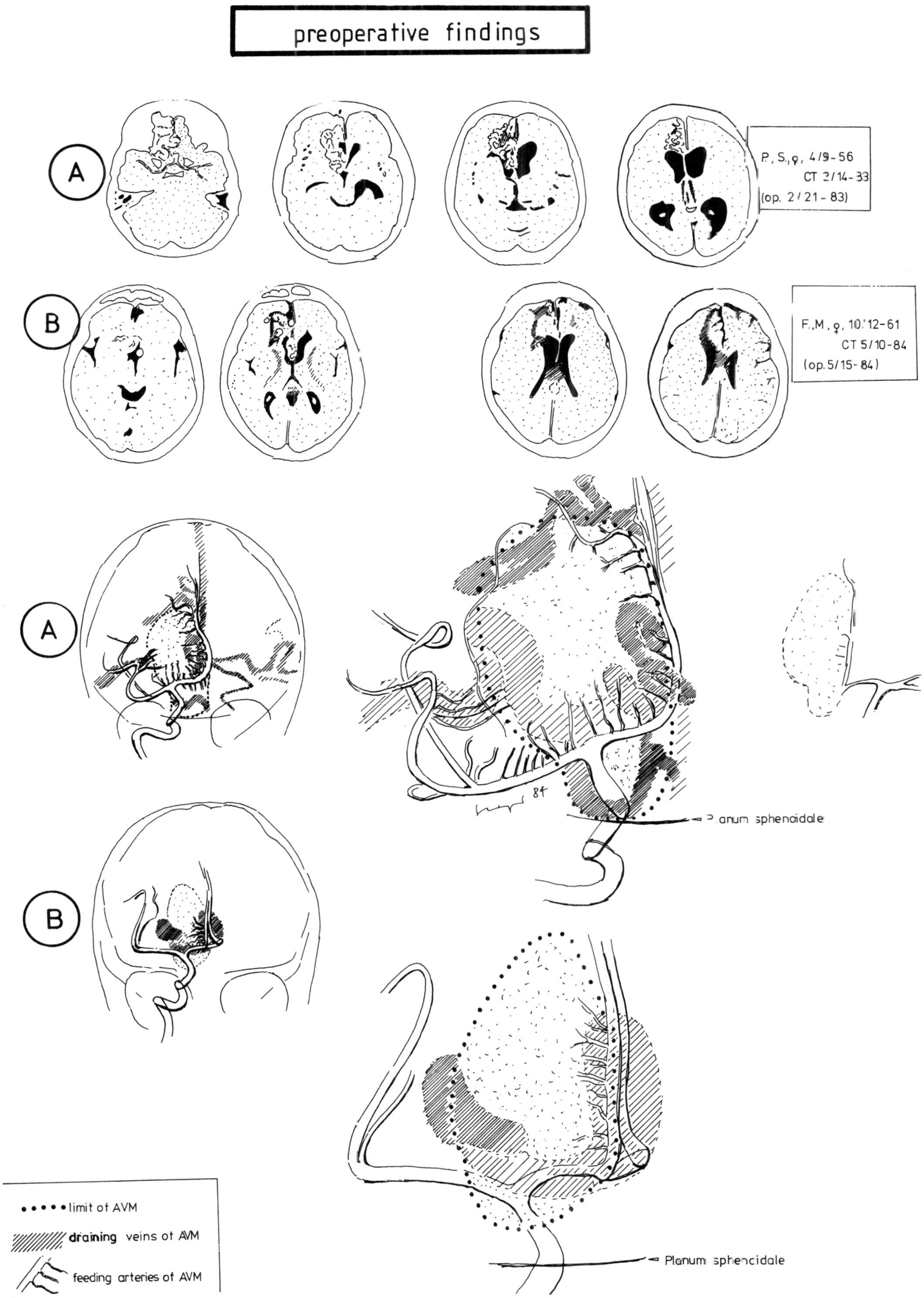
preoperative findings
A
P., S., ♀, 4/9-56
CT 2/14-33
(op. 2/21-83)
B
F.,M., ♀, 10/12-61
CT 5/10-84
(op.5/15-84)
A
B
84
Planum sphenoidale
Planum sphenoidale
limit of AVM
draining veins of AVM
feeding arteries of AVM

Fig. 10
A Complete extirpation of the angioma in one operation
B Residual AVM in dorsal A2 region, which was not detected when the pterional approach was used

FIG. 10

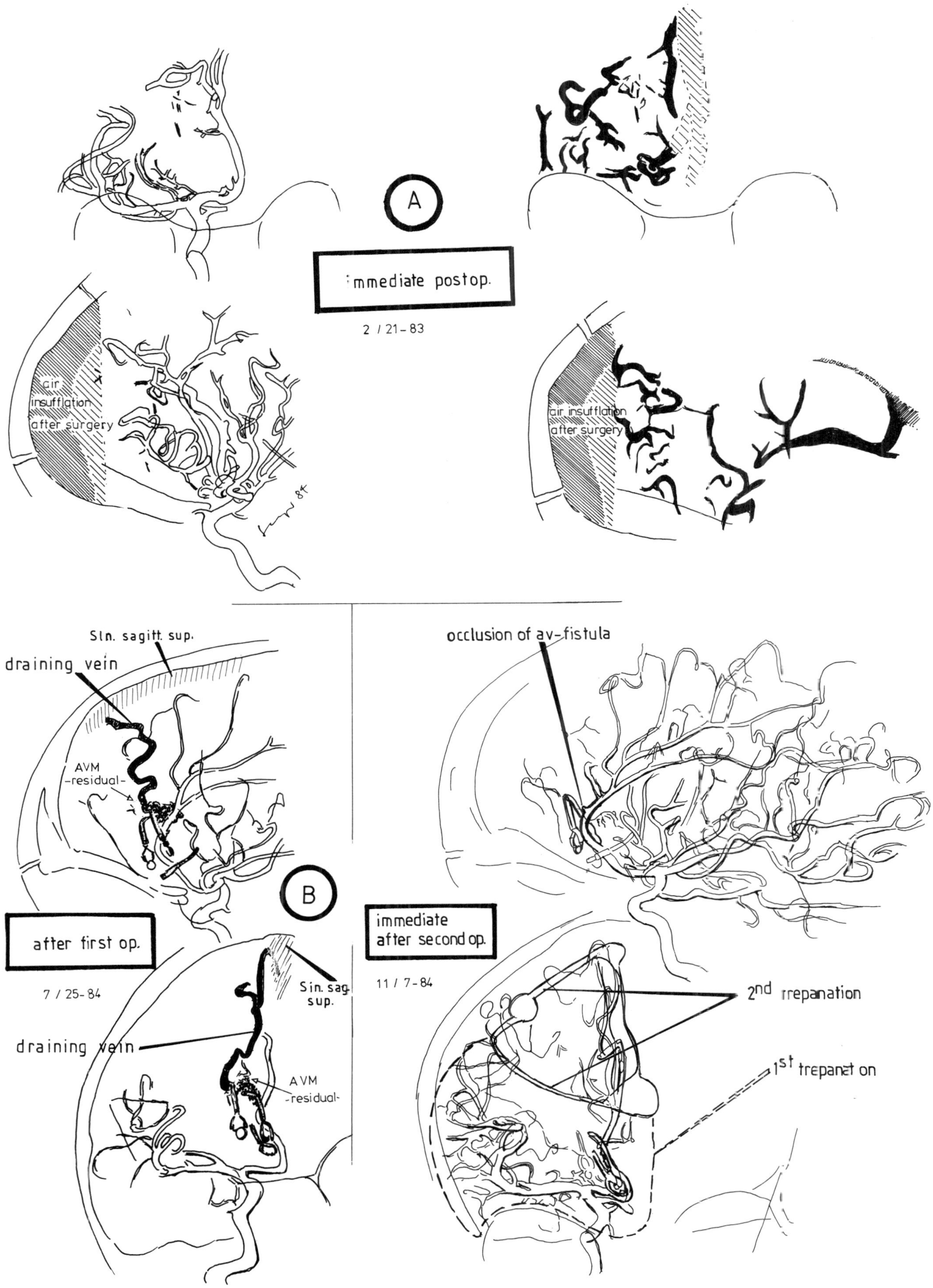
A
immediate postop.
2 / 21- 83
air insufflation after surgery
air insufflation after surgery
Sin. sagitt. sup.
draining vein
AVM -residual-
occlusion of av-fistula
B
after first op.
7 / 25- 84
immediate after second op.
11 / 7- 84
Sin. sag. sup.
draining vein
AVM -residual-
2nd trepanation
1st trepanation

Fig. 11. Position of both AVM's (**A**′ + **B**′) in the brain, as could be assumed from angiography and CT

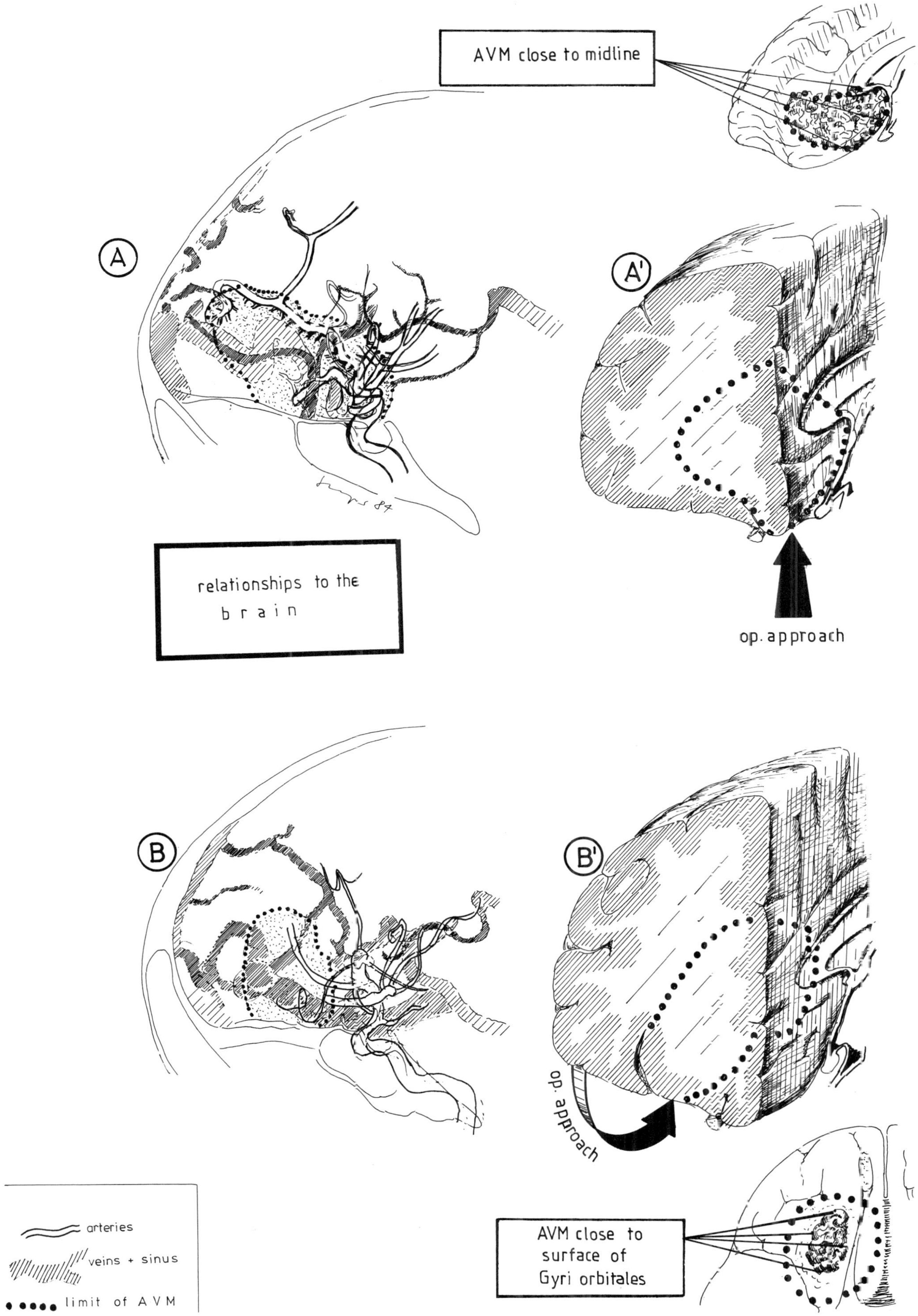
AVM close to midline
A
A'
relationships to the brain
op. approach
B
B'
op. approach
AVM close to surface of Gyri orbitales
arteries
veins + sinus
limit of AVM

Fig. 12. The assumed connections between the **arteries and brain structures** based on the angiogram

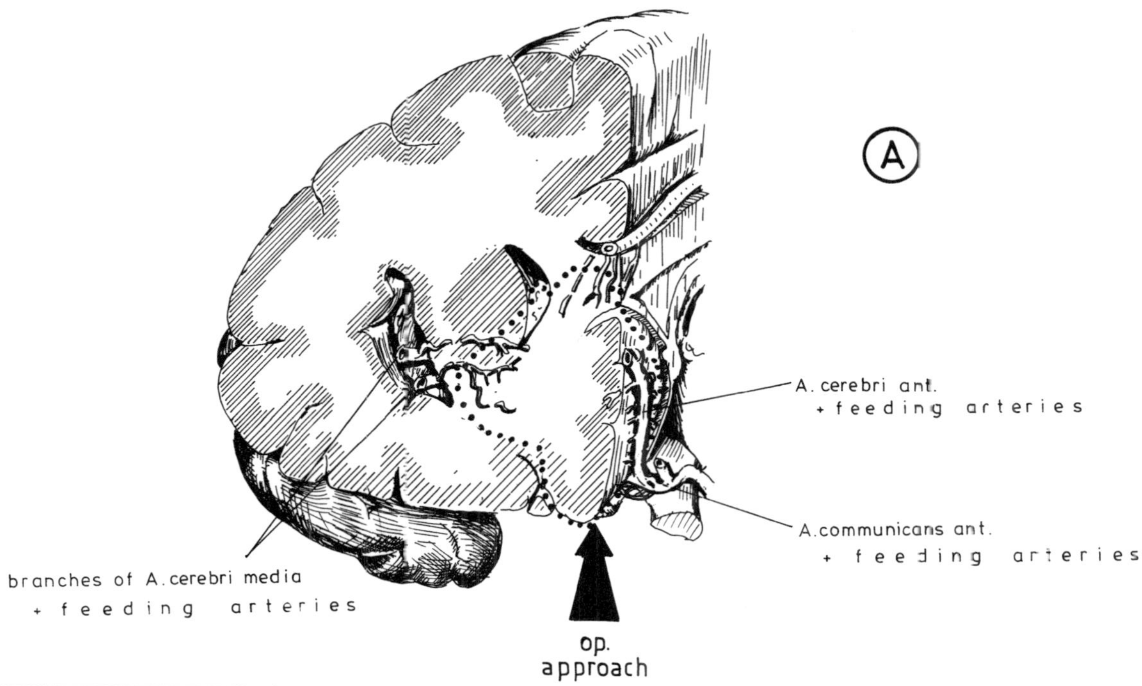

relationships to
arteries

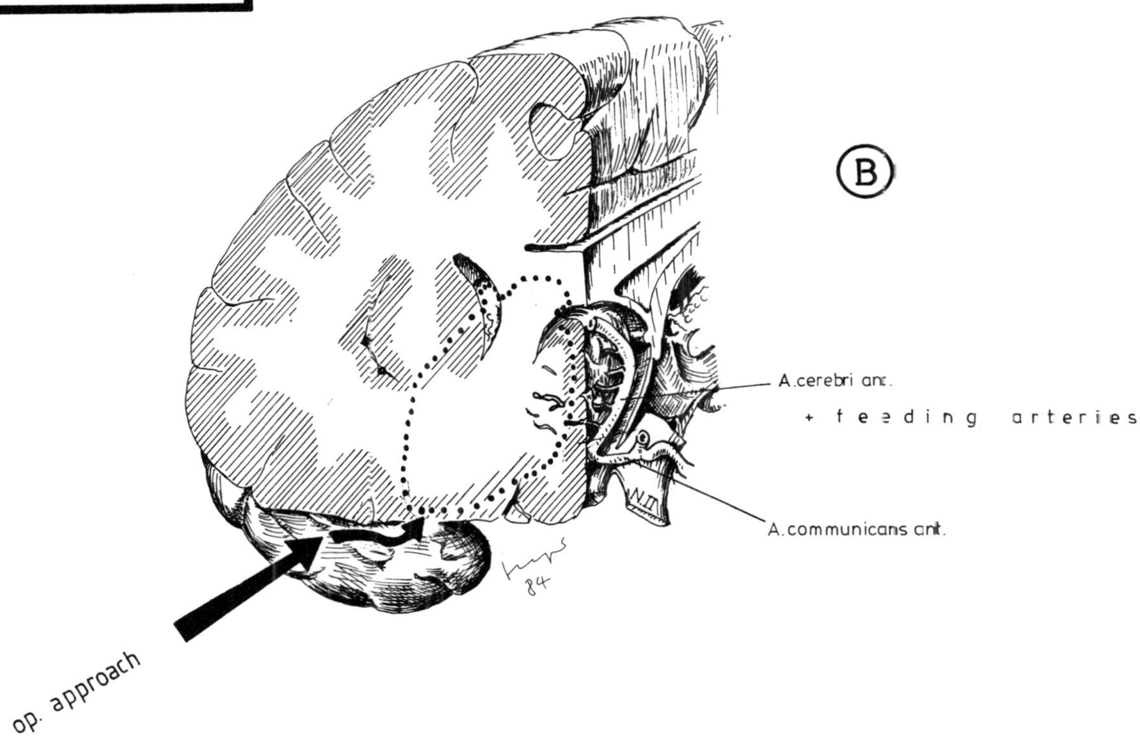

Fig. 13. On the basis of the angiogram of the two types of AVM **A** + **B** the possible anatomical location of the veins in the model is indicated. In **B** it seems questionable in which direction the basal draining vein should be positioned. This vein is always present also in healthy people, but here it has an exceptionally small calibre

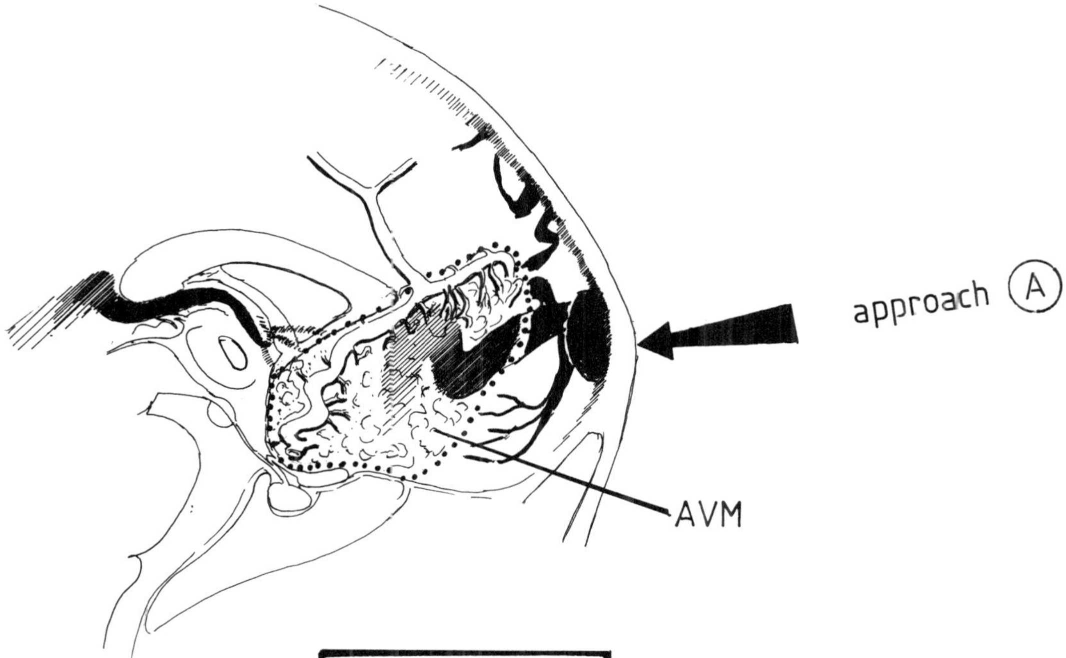

relationships to veins

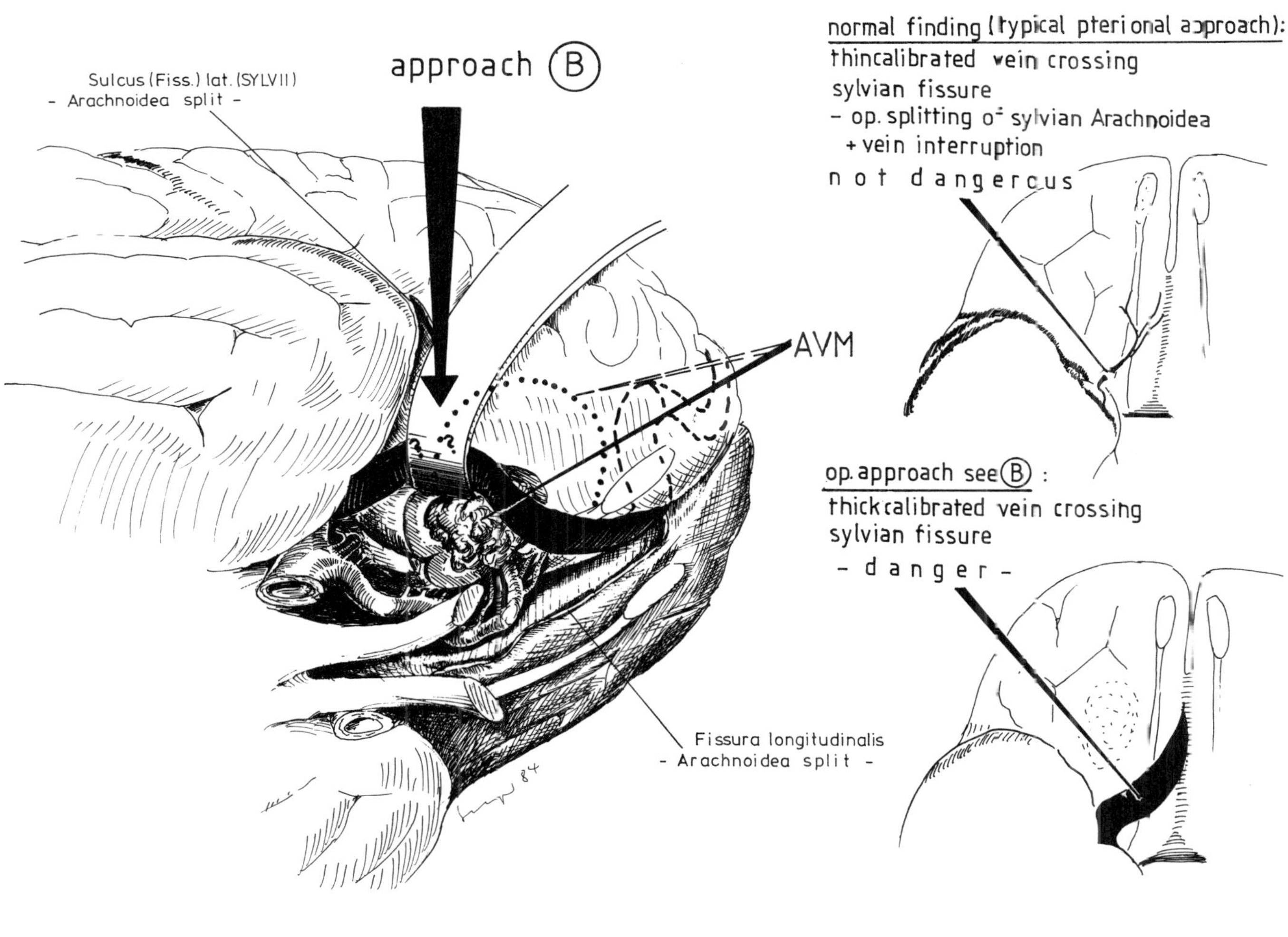

Fig. 14. Construction of the arachnoidea in its operative opening in the anatomical model

FIG. 14

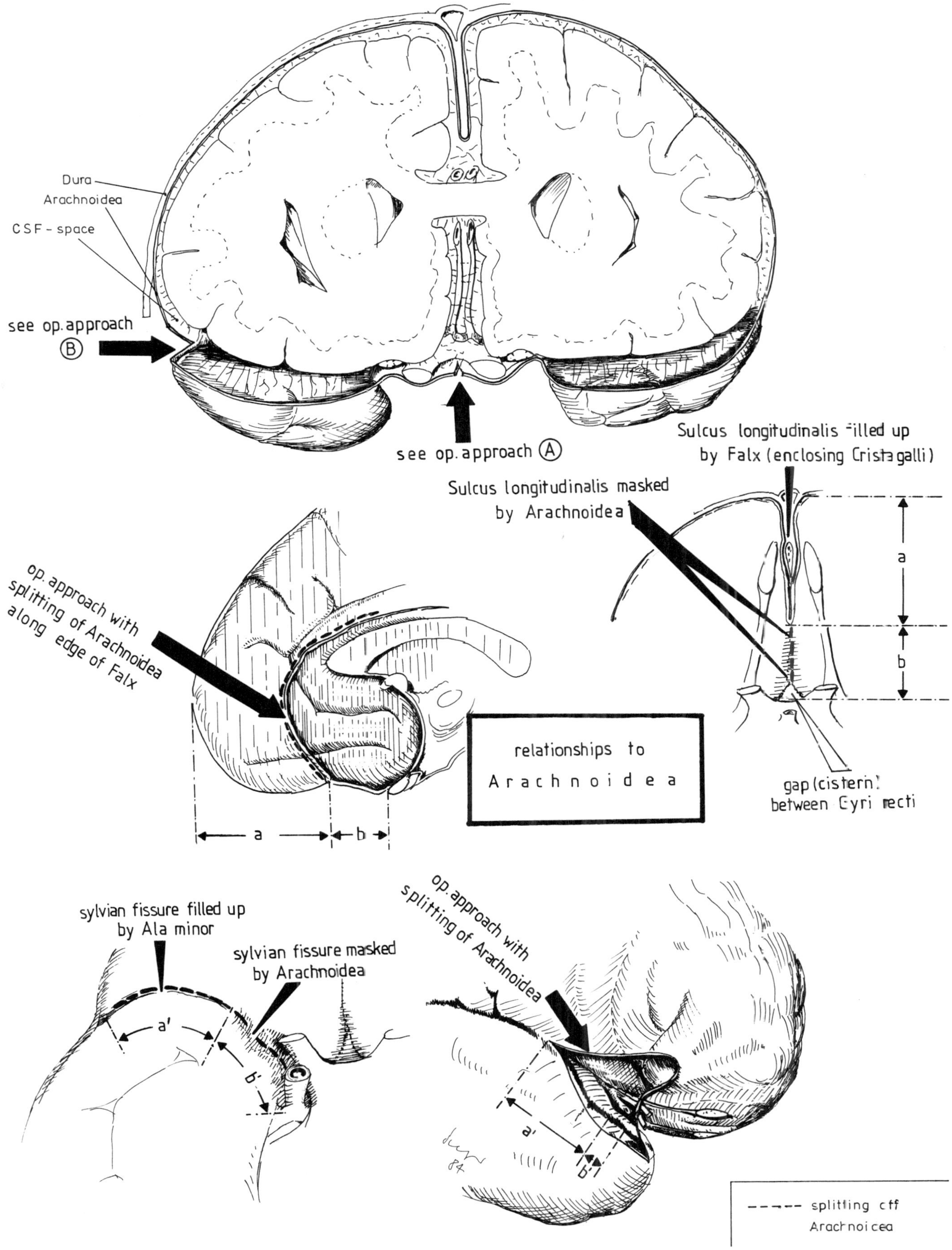

Dura
Arachnoidea
CSF - space
see op. approach
Ⓑ
see op. approach Ⓐ
Sulcus longitudinalis filled up
by Falx (enclosing Crista galli)
Sulcus longitudinalis masked
by Arachnoidea
a
b
op. approach with
splitting of Arachnoidea
along edge of Falx
relationships to
Arachnoidea
a
b
gap (cistern)
between Gyri recti
sylvian fissure filled up
by Ala minor
sylvian fissure masked
by Arachnoidea
a'
b'
op. approach with
splitting of Arachnoidea
a'
b'
splitting off
Arachnoidea

Fig. 15. In **A** and **B** are similar areas (**a** to **d** and **a′** to **c′**) reached by different routes (black arrow). Pale arrow: possible blocking of the operative approaches **A** and **B** due to draining veins. The angiogram allows no certain statement, because it is not known preoperatively how far the veins may be freed of arachnoidea and pulled to one side during the operation. Large veins should only at the end of the operation be interrupted. If interruption of the larger veins is necessary, then it must be certain that sufficient large veins remain preserved until the end of the operation. Otherwise an increase in pressure in the angioma is possible with danger of rupture and a generalized increase in intracerebral vascular pressure following sudden interruption of larger AV-shunts

FIG. 15

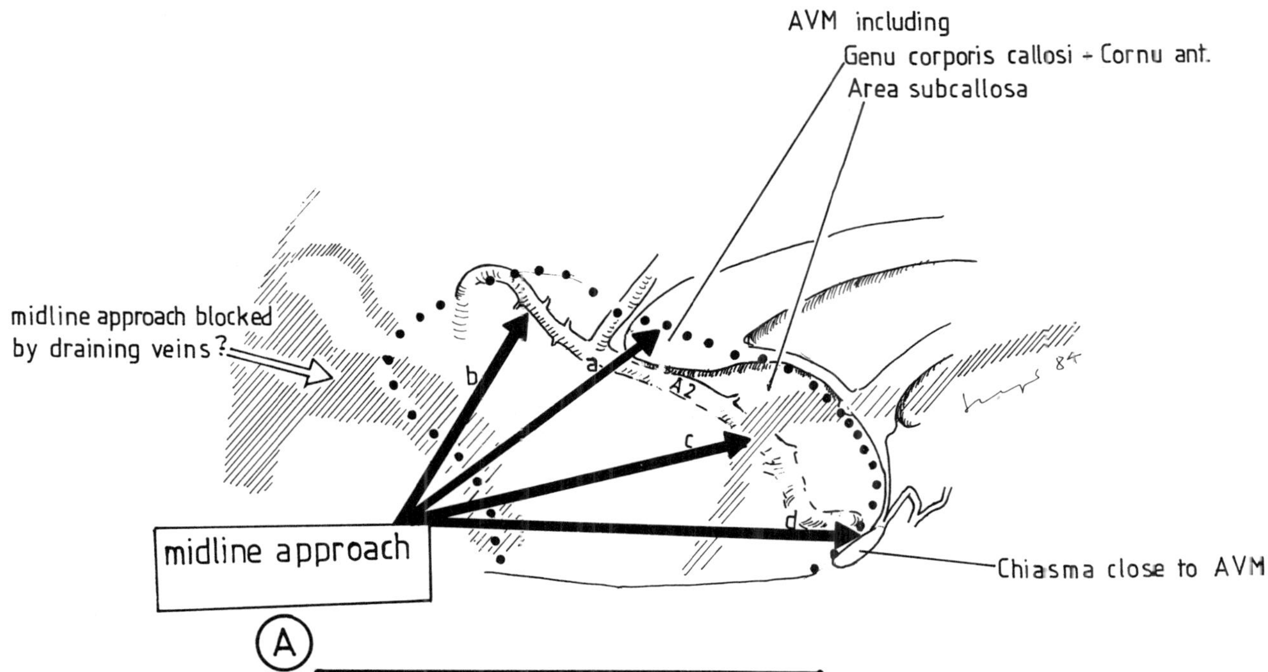

preop. problems and principles of operation

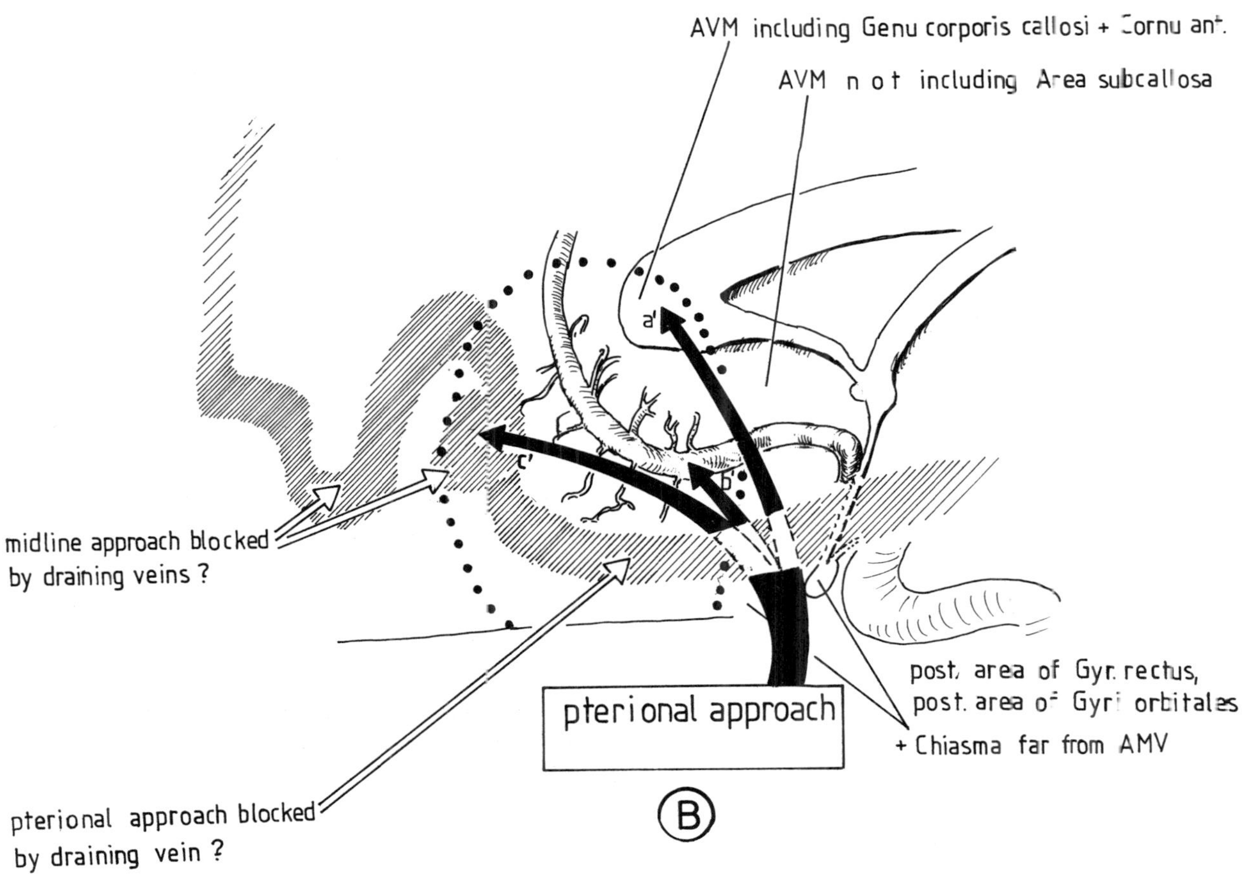

a to d op. approach Ⓐ
a' to c' „ „ Ⓑ similar a to d

Fig. 16. Preoperative planning of operation via the midline approach **A**

Preoperative problems:
1. Presupposition for the operation: no blocking of the approach by fronto-polar draining veins
2. Determination of the landmarks for orientation during the operation
3. Determination of the situation of the angioma in the brain tissue (Corpus callosum and frontal horn structures) and in relation to the anterior cerebral artery. The relations to the anterior cerebral artery allows the assessment of how far the AVM infiltrates essential structures (Lamina terminalis, 3rd ventricle) located behind the anterior cerebral artery.

Operational strategy:
1. Begin in the middle fissure. There is the approach easiest.
1st step: exposure of the anterior cerebral artery from distal to proximal. Via the pterional approach **B** this step is the most difficult and possibly not feasible, so that reoperation may be required
2nd step: exposure of both A1, the A. communicans ant., and the proximal part of A2. The 1st and 2nd steps can be reversed according to individual circumstances
3rd step: preparation of the anterior cerebral artery from distal to proximal. Depending on individual circumstances the preparation can also be carried out from proximal to distal. Even when the angiogram shows the AVM only in front of the anterior cerebral artery, it is still to be considered that angiographically not visualized parts of the angioma may also lie behind the anterior cerebral artery. **The chiasma and the entire Lamina terminalis including the rostral fibers of the Corpus callosum should always be also visualized**
4th step: isolation of the angioma in the longitudinal fissure on the frontal border. One draining vein possibly located here must if possible remain intact (if at least two deep lying veins of similar large calibre could be preserved until the end of the operation)

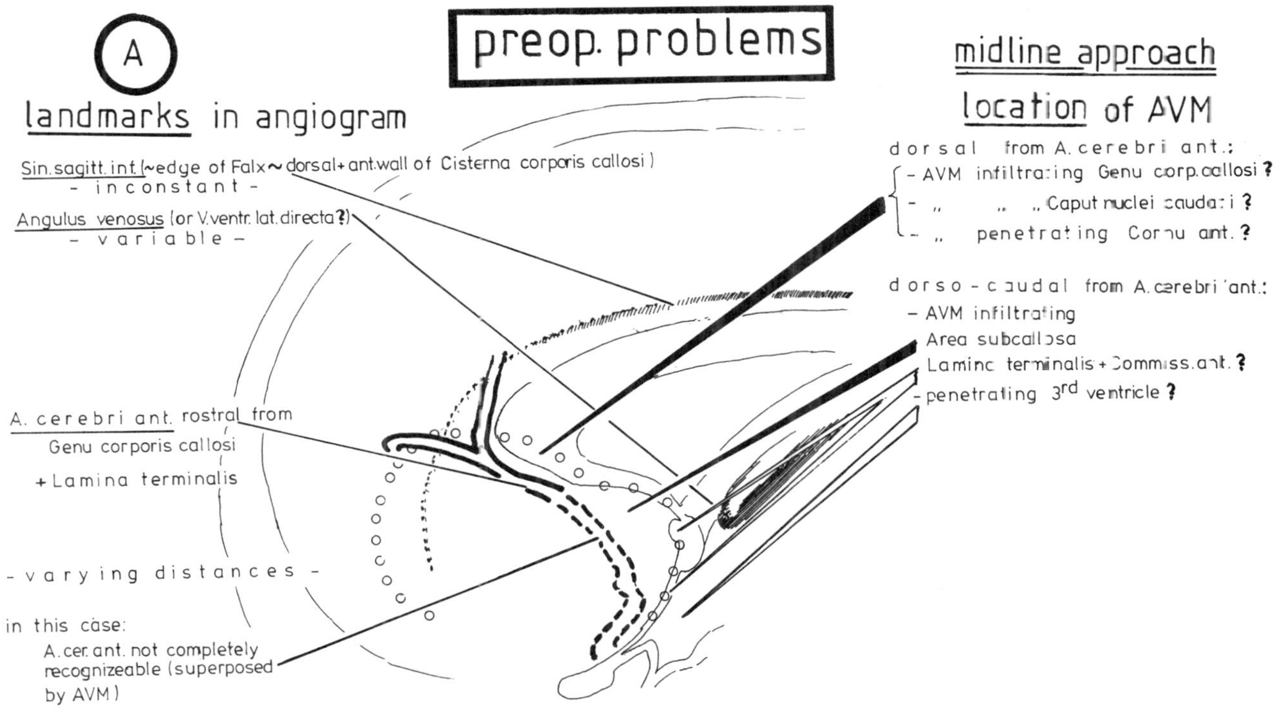

A
preop. problems
landmarks in angiogram
Sin.sagitt.int.(~edge of Falx ~ dorsal+ant.wall of Cisterna corporis callosi)
- inconstant -
Angulus venosus (or V.ventr. lat. directa?)
- variable -
A. cerebri ant. rostral from
Genu corporis callosi
+ Lamina terminalis
- varying distances -
in this case:
A.cer.ant. not completely recognizeable (superposed by AVM)
midline approach
location of AVM
dorsal from A.cerebri ant.:
- AVM infiltrating Genu corp.callosi ?
- " " " Caput nuclei caudati ?
- " penetrating Cornu ant. ?
dorso-caudal from A.cerebri ant.:
- AVM infiltrating
Area subcallosa
Lamina terminalis + Commiss.ant. ?
- penetrating 3rd ventricle ?

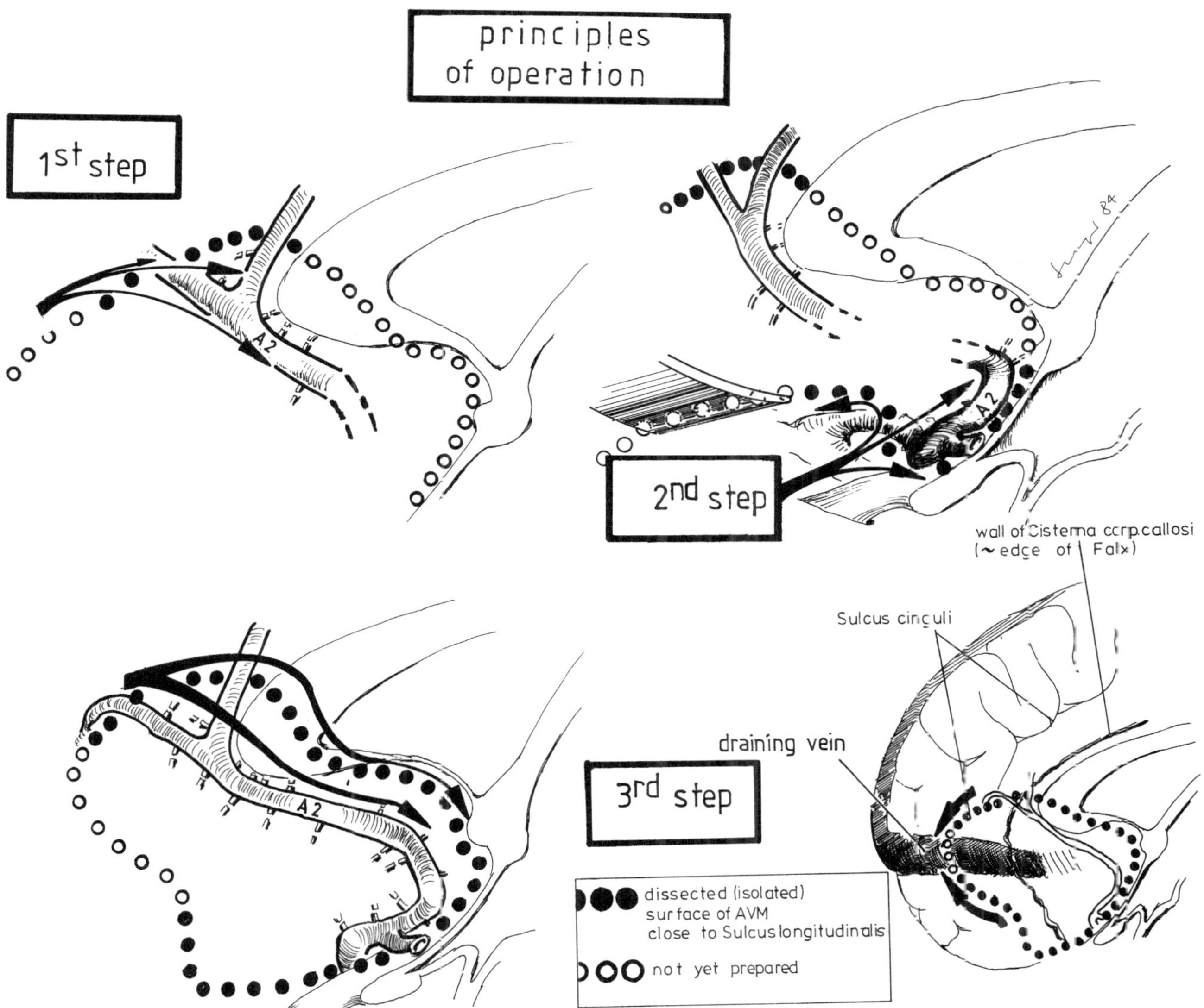

principles of operation
1st step
A2
2nd step
A2
wall of Cisterna corp.callosi
(~ edge of Falx)
Sulcus cinguli
draining vein
3rd step
A2
dissected (isolated) surface of AVM close to Sulcus longitudinalis
not yet prepared

Fig. 17. Preoperative surgical planning
Dissection of lateral part of angioma
This part of the midline approach is the most difficult when compared with the pterional approach. Following the **4th step** from medially the angioma is now isolated laterally and frontally. The lateral draining vein visualized in the angiogram should be preserved. During the operation it was clipped too early by mistake **(5th step)**
6th step: the numerous feeding vessels from branches of the middle cerebral artery visualized in the angiogram were interrupted, including those from the island and basal ganglia area
In the planning of the operation the importance of the lateral draining veins was underestimated. **Compression of other veins, for example in the middle fissure, can lead to increase in pressure in the angioma and to rupture of vessels when additional interruption of a large vein occurs**

FIG. 17

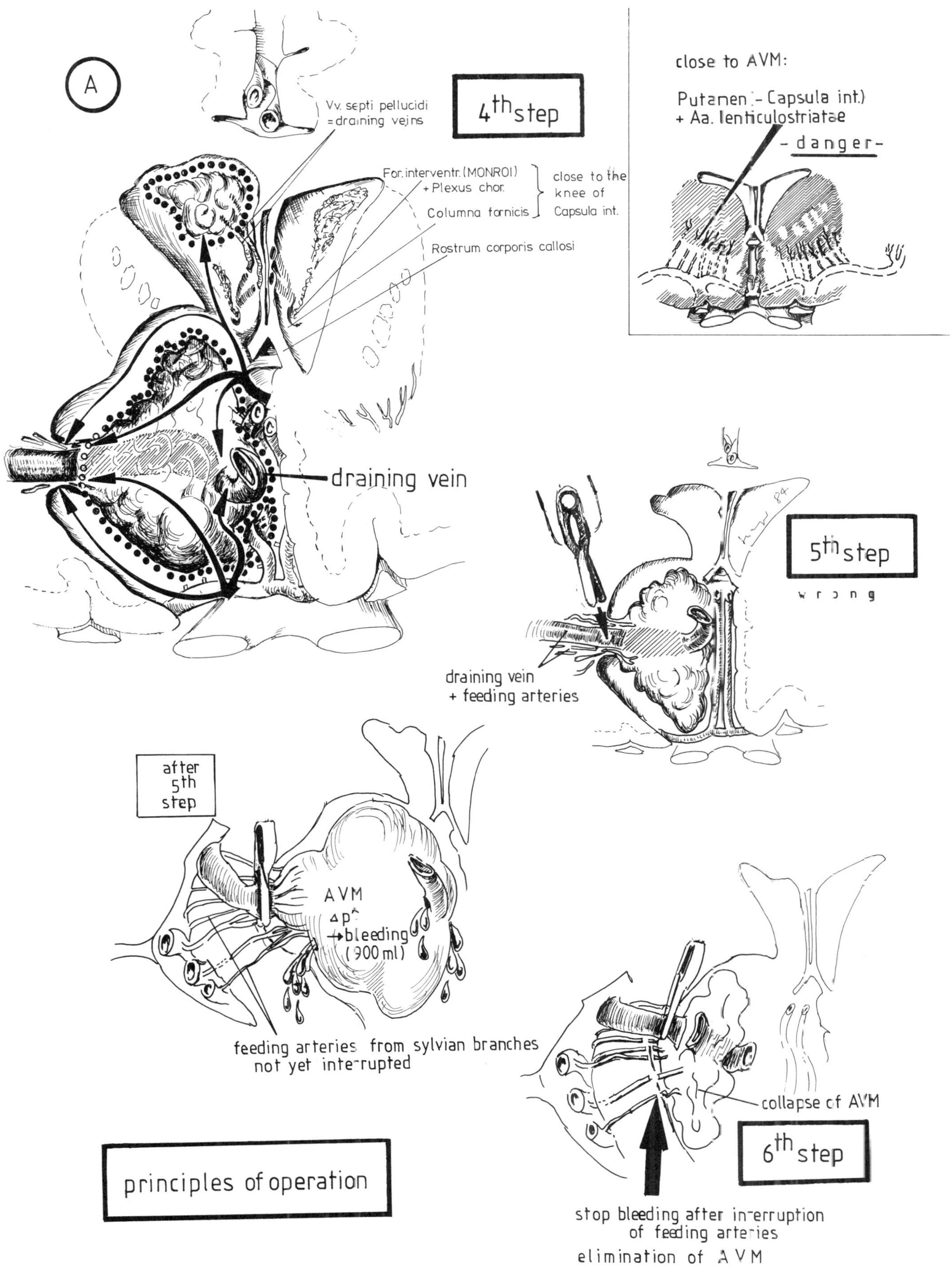
A
4th step
Vv. septi pellucidi
=draining veins
For. interventr. (MONROI)
+ Plexus chor.
Columna fornicis
close to the
knee of
Capsula int.
Rostrum corporis callosi
draining vein
close to AVM:
Putamen (- Capsula int.)
+ Aa. lenticulostriatae
- danger -
5th step
wrong
draining vein
+ feeding arteries
after
5th
step
AVM
Δp↑
→bleeding
(900 ml)
feeding arteries from sylvian branches
not yet interrupted
collapse of AVM
6th step
stop bleeding after interruption
of feeding arteries
elimination of AVM
principles of operation

Fig. 18. Start of the operation
Postoperative x-ray pictures to demonstrate the location of the trepanation (**A** + **B**)
Anatomical positioning sketches of the trepanation (**A′** + **B′**). **Not only with the midline approach but also the pterional approach one must leave both the operational possibilities open, since it is never foreseeable whether the commenced approach can be continued or whether it has to be combined with a second approach**

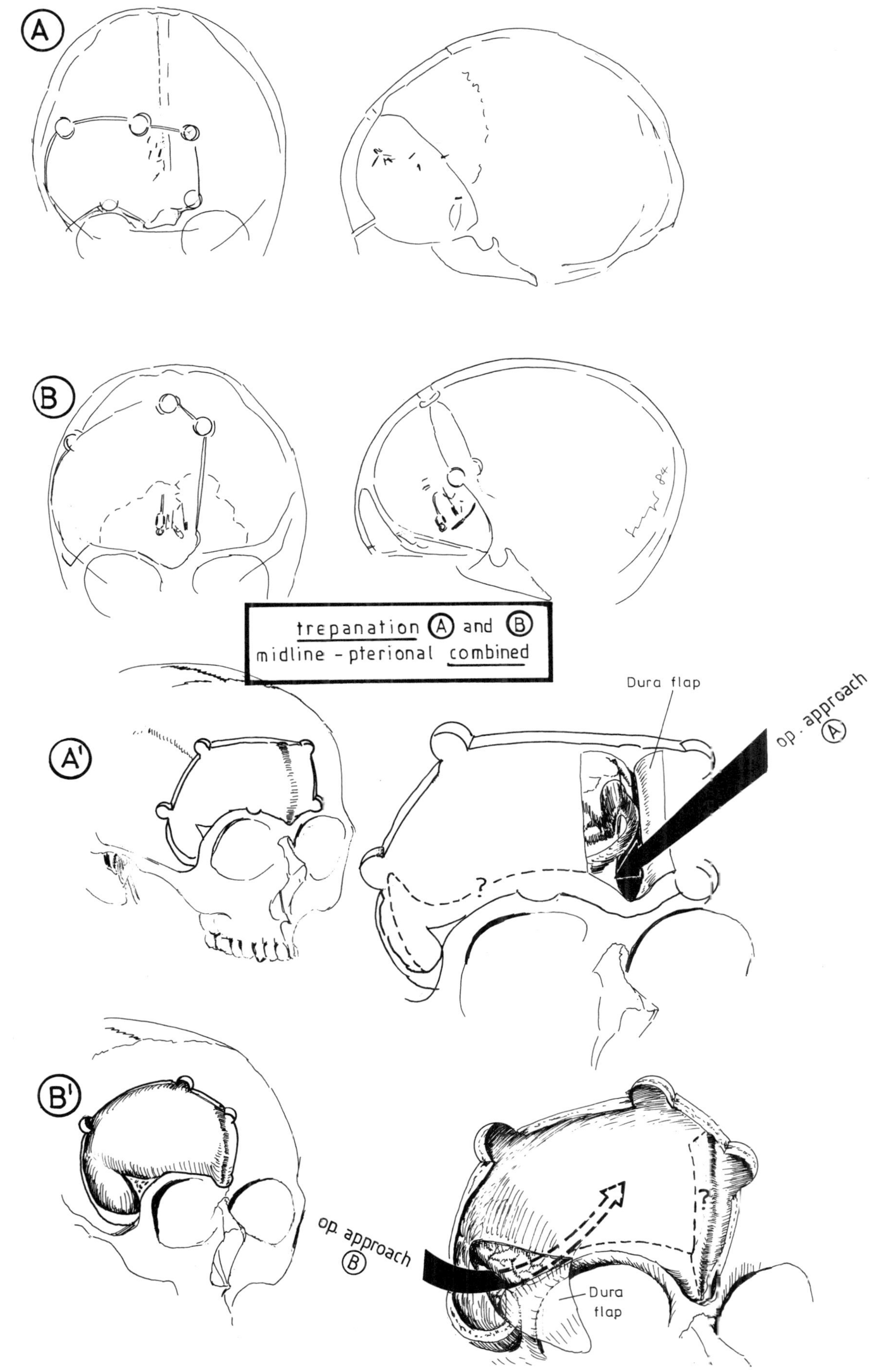
A
B
trepanation A and B
midline - pterional combined
A'
Dura flap
op. approach A
?
B'
op. approach B
Dura
flap
?

Figs. 19–23. Carrying out of the midline operation **A**

Fig. 19. Anatomical positioning sketches of the micro-surgical site of the subsequent pictures

FIG. 19

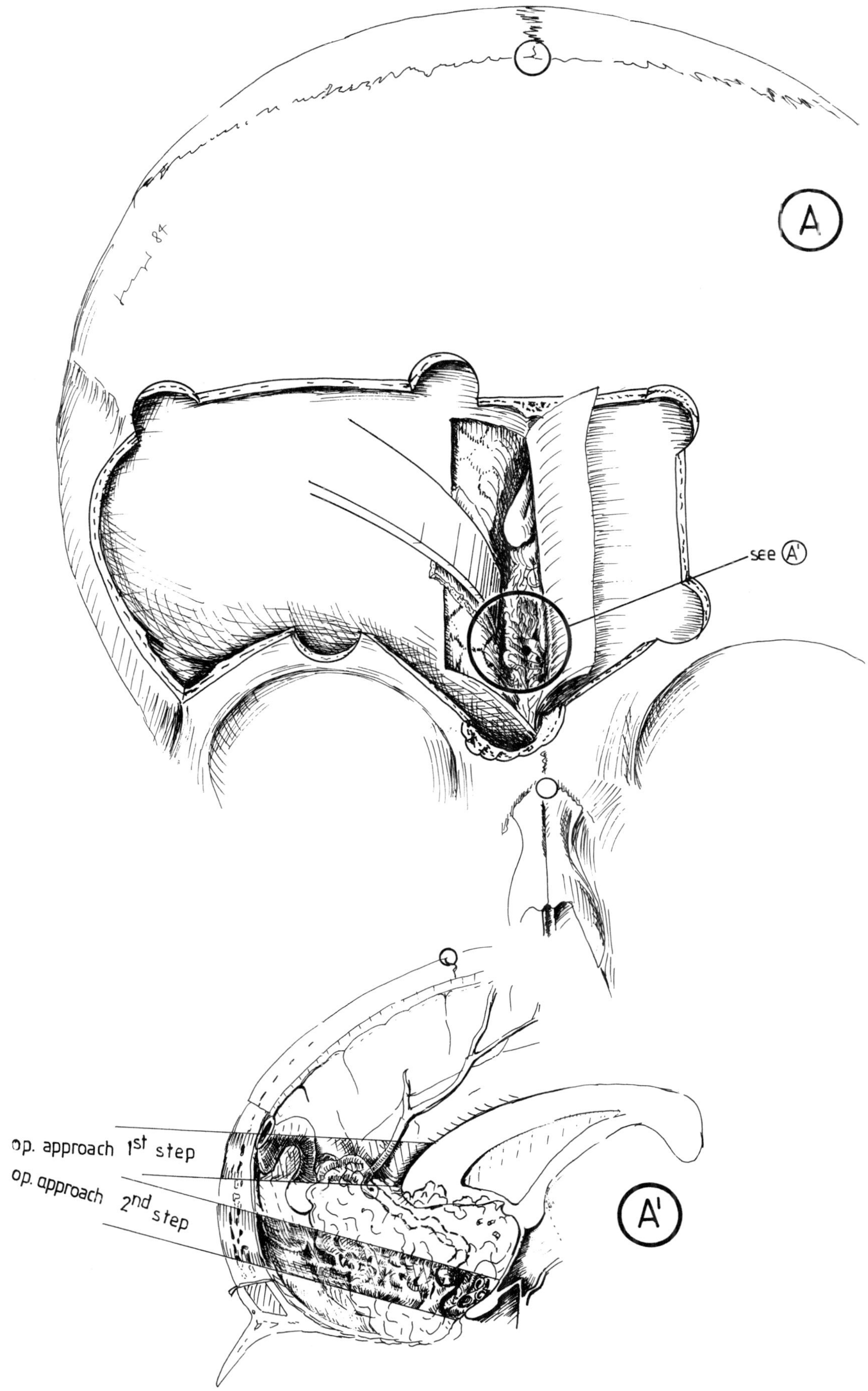

Fig. 20. **1st step:** search for the pericallosal artery and its exit from the angioma. Microsurgical site – **A** – with anatomical positioning sketch – **A′**

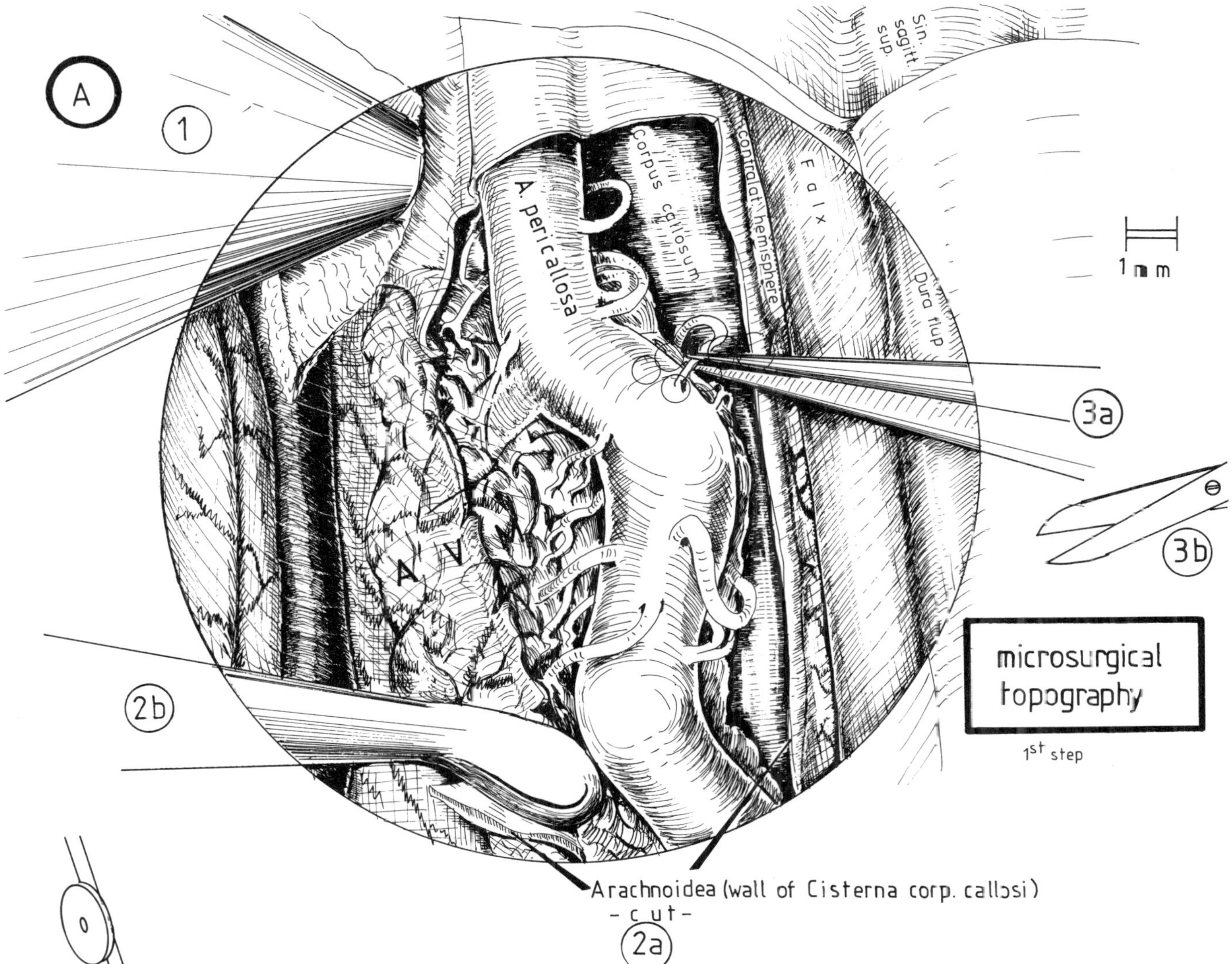
A
1
Sin. sagitt. sup.
Corpus callosum
contralat. hemisphere
F a l x
Dura flap
A. pericallosa
1 mm
3a
3b
A V
2b
microsurgical topography
1st step
Arachnoidea (wall of Cisterna corp. callosi)
- c u t -
2a

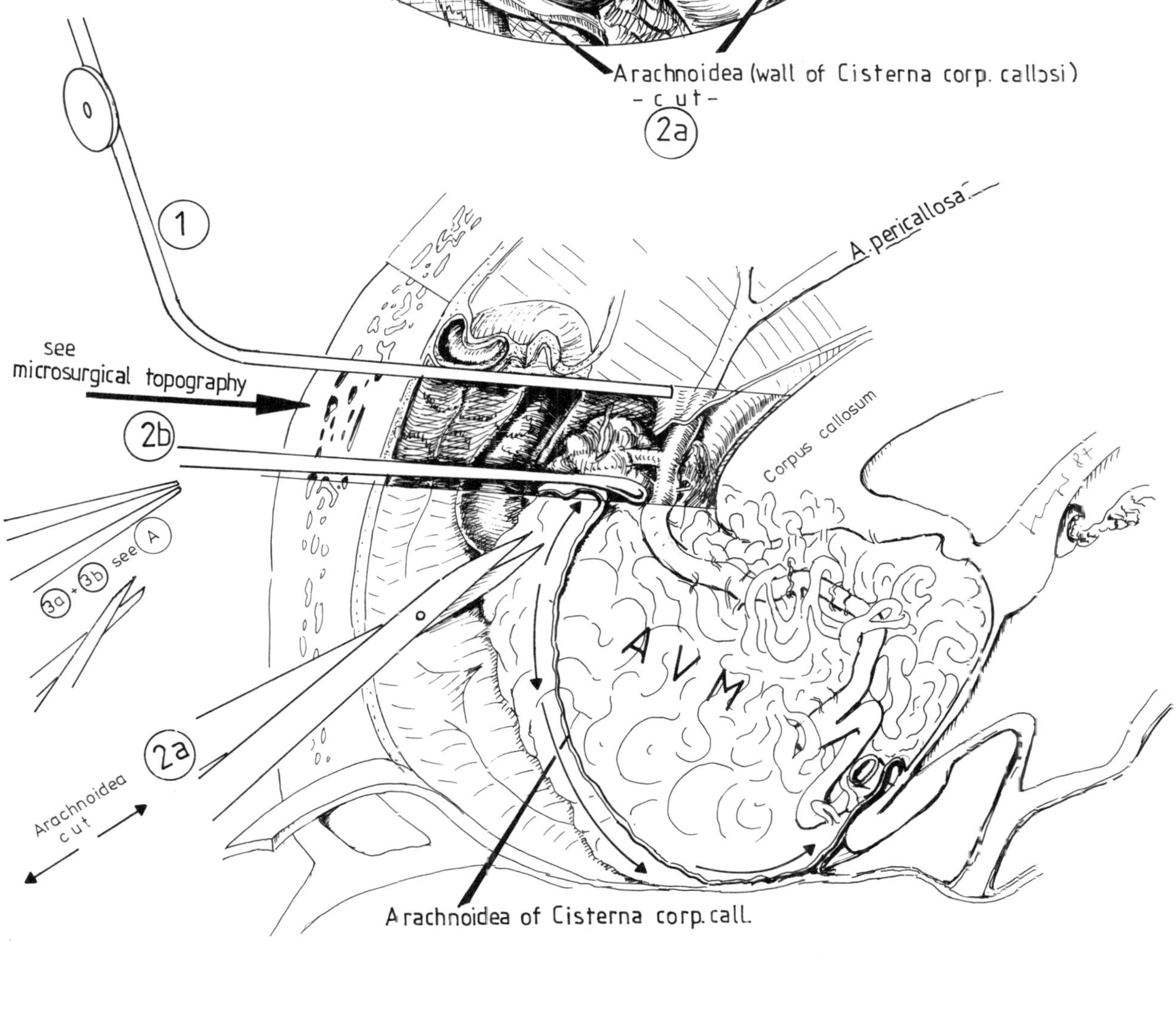
1
A. pericallosa
see
microsurgical topography
2b
Corpus callosum
3a + 3b see A
2a
AVM
Arachnoidea cut
Arachnoidea of Cisterna corp. call.

Fig. 21. **2nd step:** exposure of the anterior cerebral artery, A1 and A2 sections both sides and the anterior communicating artery from proximal to distal. The anatomical normal variations – prefixed chiasma – make the orientation easier. Microsurgical site – **A** – with anatomical positioning sketch

 FIG. 21

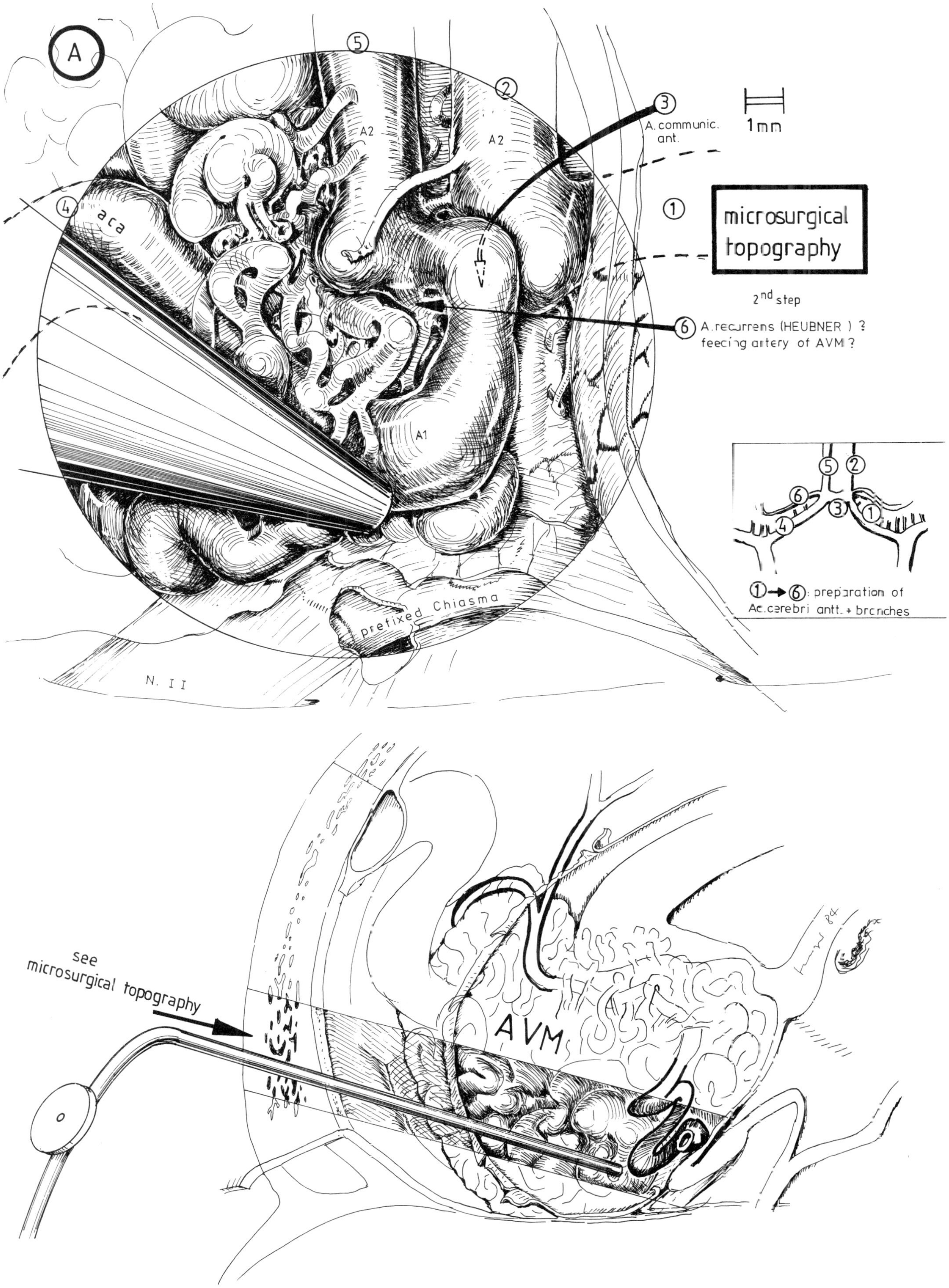
A
⑤
②
③
A. communic. ant.
1mm
A2
A2
④ aca
①
microsurgical topography
2nd step
⑥ A. recurrens (HEUBNER) ?
feeding artery of AVM ?
A1
prefixed Chiasma
N. II
⑤ ②
⑥ ③ ①
④
①→⑥: preparation of Ac. cerebri antt. + branches
see microsurgical topography
AVM

Fig. 22. **3rd** and **4th steps:** the medial limits of the angioma are meanwhile exposed, the arachnoidea surrounding the angioma is cut and the angioma isolated laterally, dorsally and basally
During freeing of the basal ganglia area adjacent to part of the angioma and from the forceps radiation of the Corpus callosum the Cornu anterius is opened. Removal of intraventricular part of the angioma. Microsurgical site – **A** with anatomical positioning sketch

FIG. 22

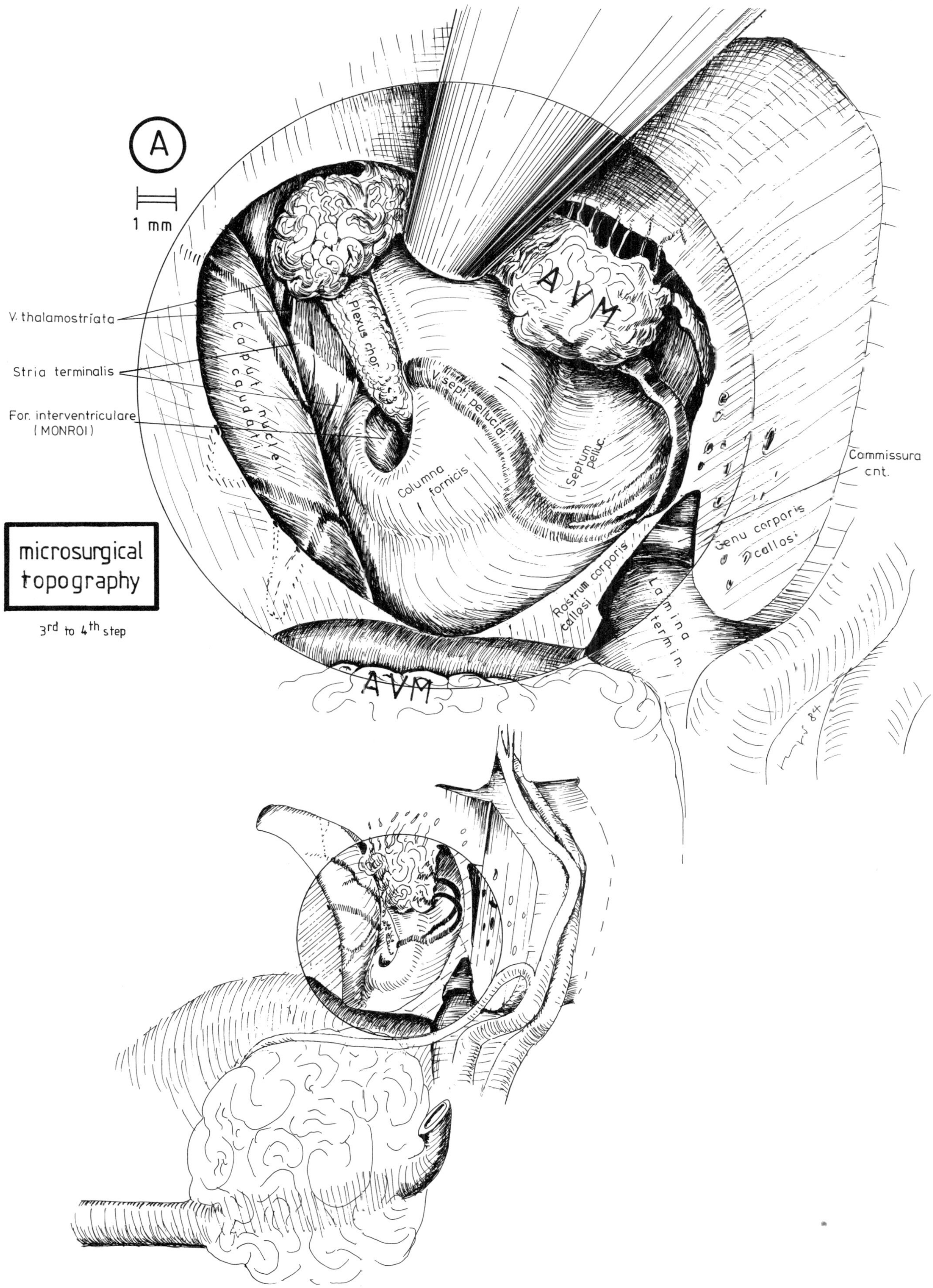

A
1 mm
V. thalamostriata
Stria terminalis
For. interventriculare
(MONROI)
Caput nuclei caudati
Plexus chor.
V. septi pellucidi
AVM
Columna fornicis
Septum pelluc.
Commissura ant.
Genu corporis callosi
Rostrum corporis callosi
Lamina termin.
AVM
microsurgical topography
3rd to 4th step

Fig. 23. **5th step:** after clipping of the lateral draining vein inflation of the AVM and rupture of several AVM vessels. Correction of mistake:
1. Use of a temporary clip which can be removed immediately.
2. Reduction of the pressure of the spatula on the angioma in order to minimize the compression of large veins far away.
3. Interruption of the last of the angioma's feeding arteries
The mistaken early closure of the large draining vein occurred because the author thought that all feeding arteries had already been interrupted. Hidden behind the vein even more feeding arteries were found, after whose interruption the bleeding stopped and it was possible to remove the angioma **(6th step).**
If the AVM inflates during the operation and begins to bleed diffusely, an extensive coagulation of the angioma surface is dangerous because the bleeding increases and cannot be stopped by coagulation. Applying and pressing on cotton and waiting for several minutes prevents loss of blood and usually leads to spontaneous cessation of bleeding
Dangers: occult bleeding from the posterior surface of the angioma with severe bleeding, recognizable by the general increase in intracranial pressure
Microsurgical site – **A** – with anatomical sketch

FIG. 23

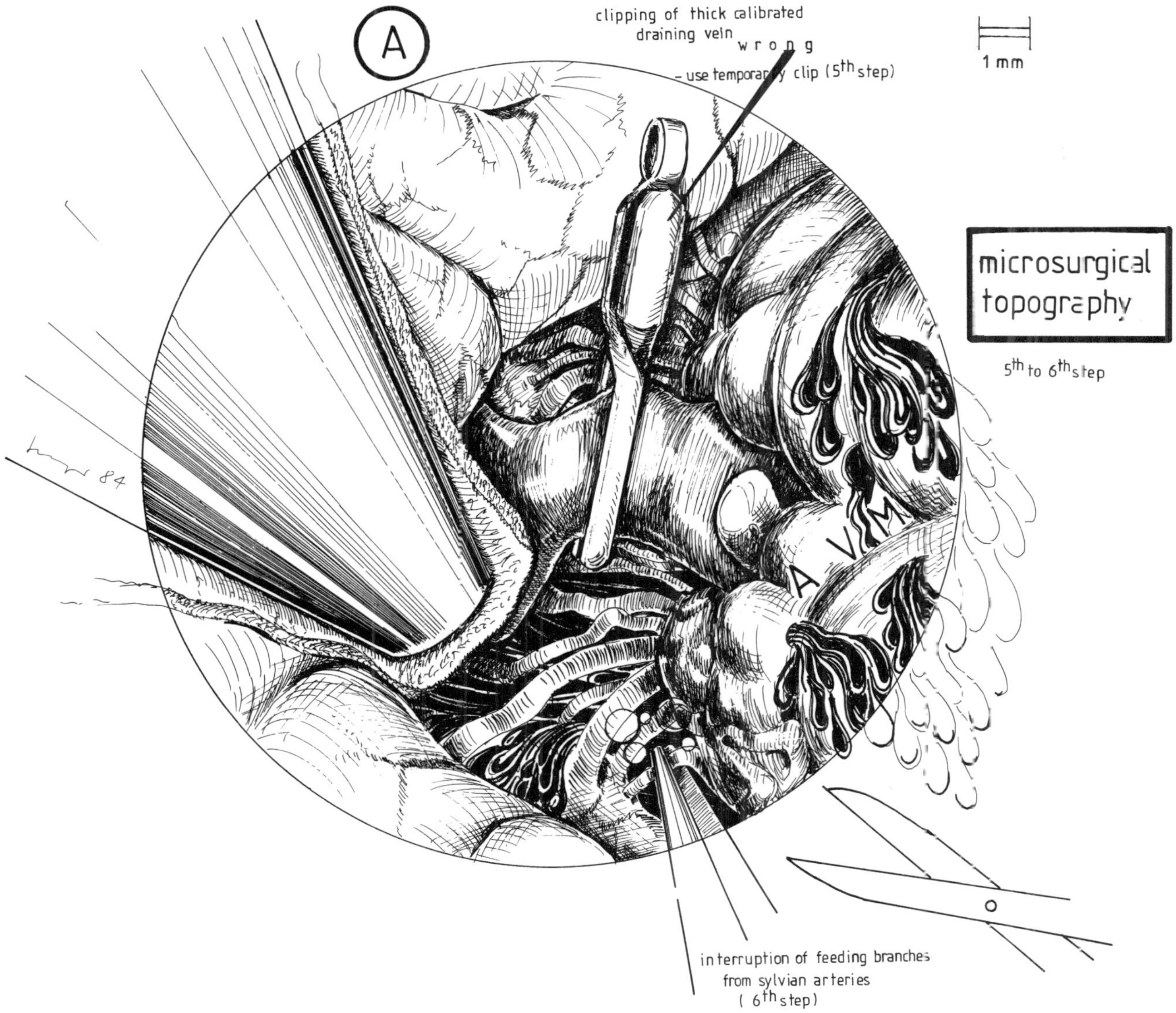
A
clipping of thick calibrated draining vein wrong
– use temporary clip (5th step)
1 mm
microsurgical topography
5th to 6th step
AVM
interruption of feeding branches from sylvian arteries (6th step)

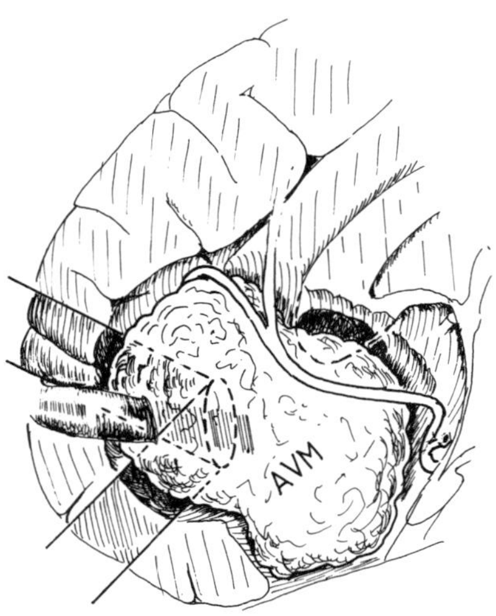
AVM

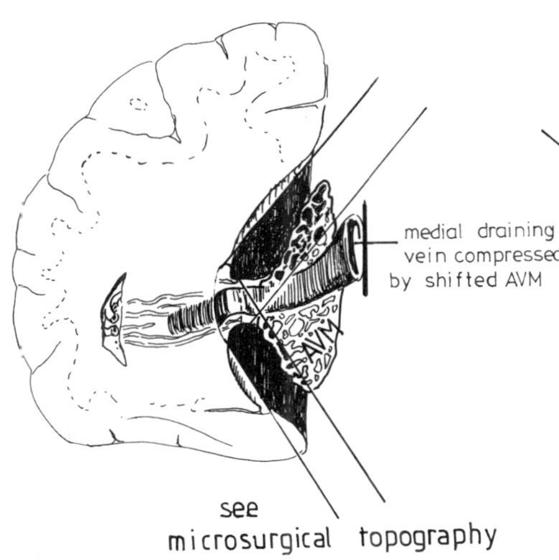
medial draining vein compressed by shifted AVM
AVM
see microsurgical topography

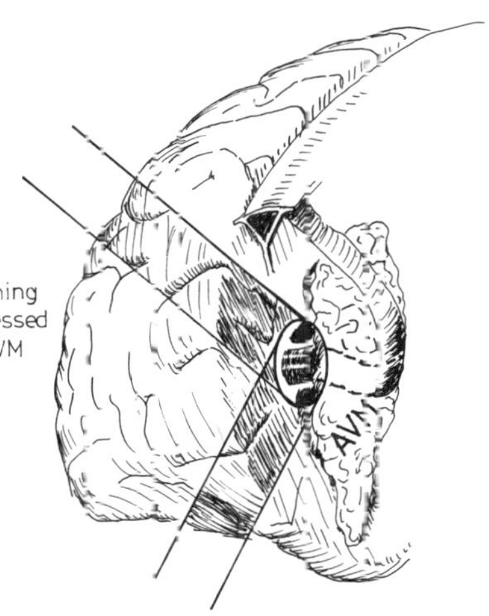
AVM

Fig. 24. From the pterional approach the most difficult parts of the AVM to reach are those in the area dorsal to the Genu corporis callosi and their feeding arteries from the anterior cerebral artery. The landmarks are particularly important here. AVM parts posterior to the anterior cerebral artery allow the assumption that the Genu corporis callosi, the anterior horn and the anterior part of the basal ganglia are penetrated by the angioma. Probably the angioma has not penetrated the Lamina terminalis because the anterior cerebral artery (A1) penetrates the AVM from underneath and behind the Genu corporis callosi

(B) **pre op. problems** pterional approach

landmarks in angiogram — location of AVM

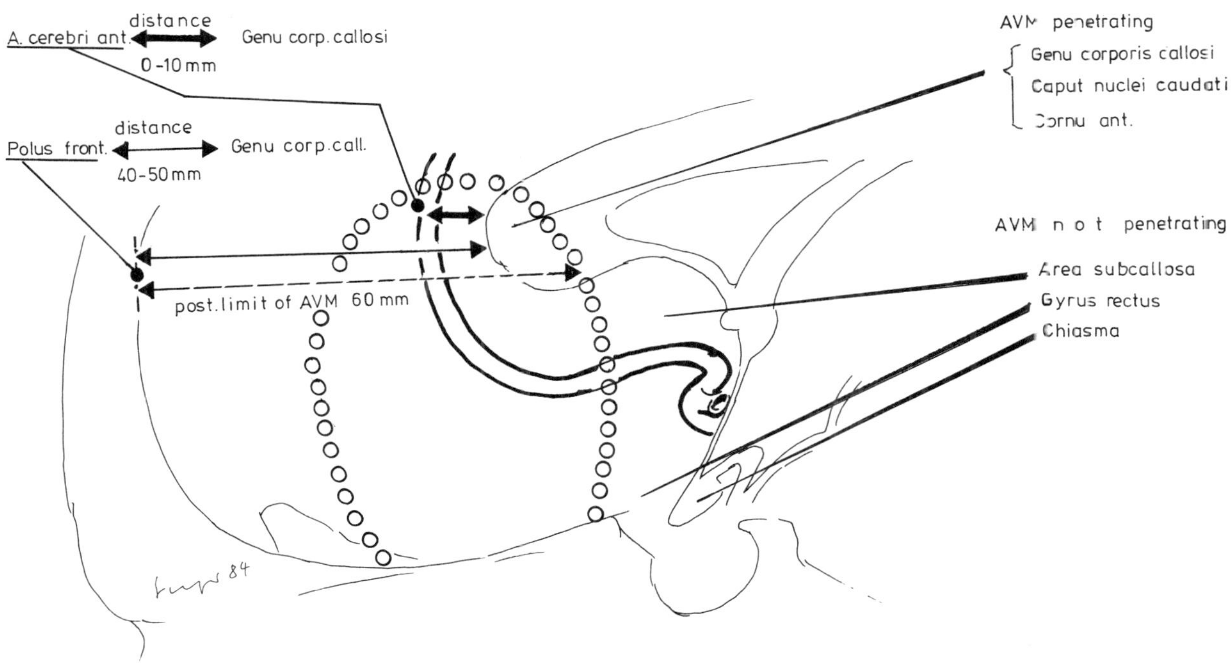

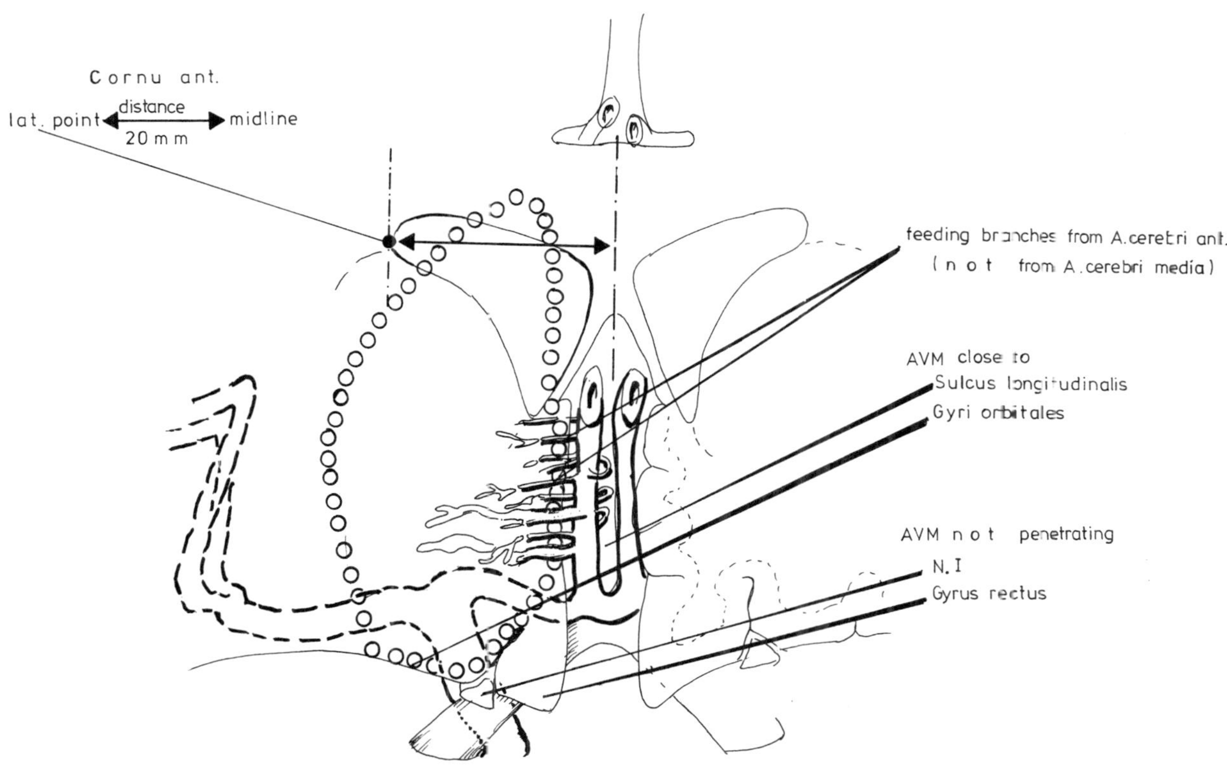

Fig. 25. The most important advantage of the pterional approach as compared to the midline approach: a large part of the lateral surface of the angioma with its feeding arteries from the cerebral artery may be clearly exposed. The Gyrus rectus belonging to the limbic system remains intact

FIG. 25

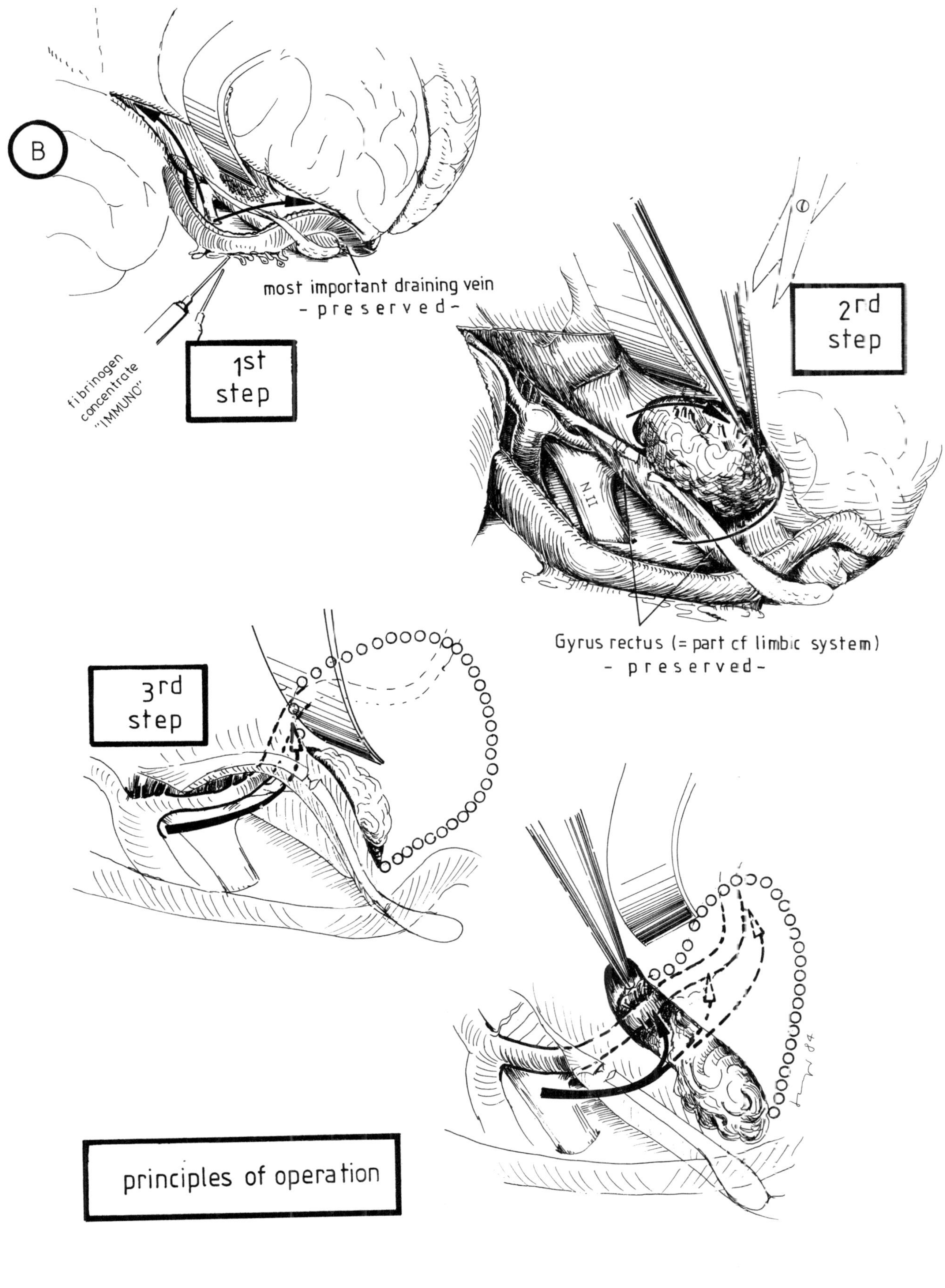

principles of operation

Fig. 26. The medial portions of the AVM in the area of the longitudinal fissure are easily isolated next. Even parts of the AVM which have infringed on the Cornu anterius are still visible – 3rd + 4th step
Problematical are the parts dorsal to the area of the Genu corporis callosi. Due to the restricted vision a small residual of the AVM was left unnoticed, which was removed some months later – 5th step

FIG. 26

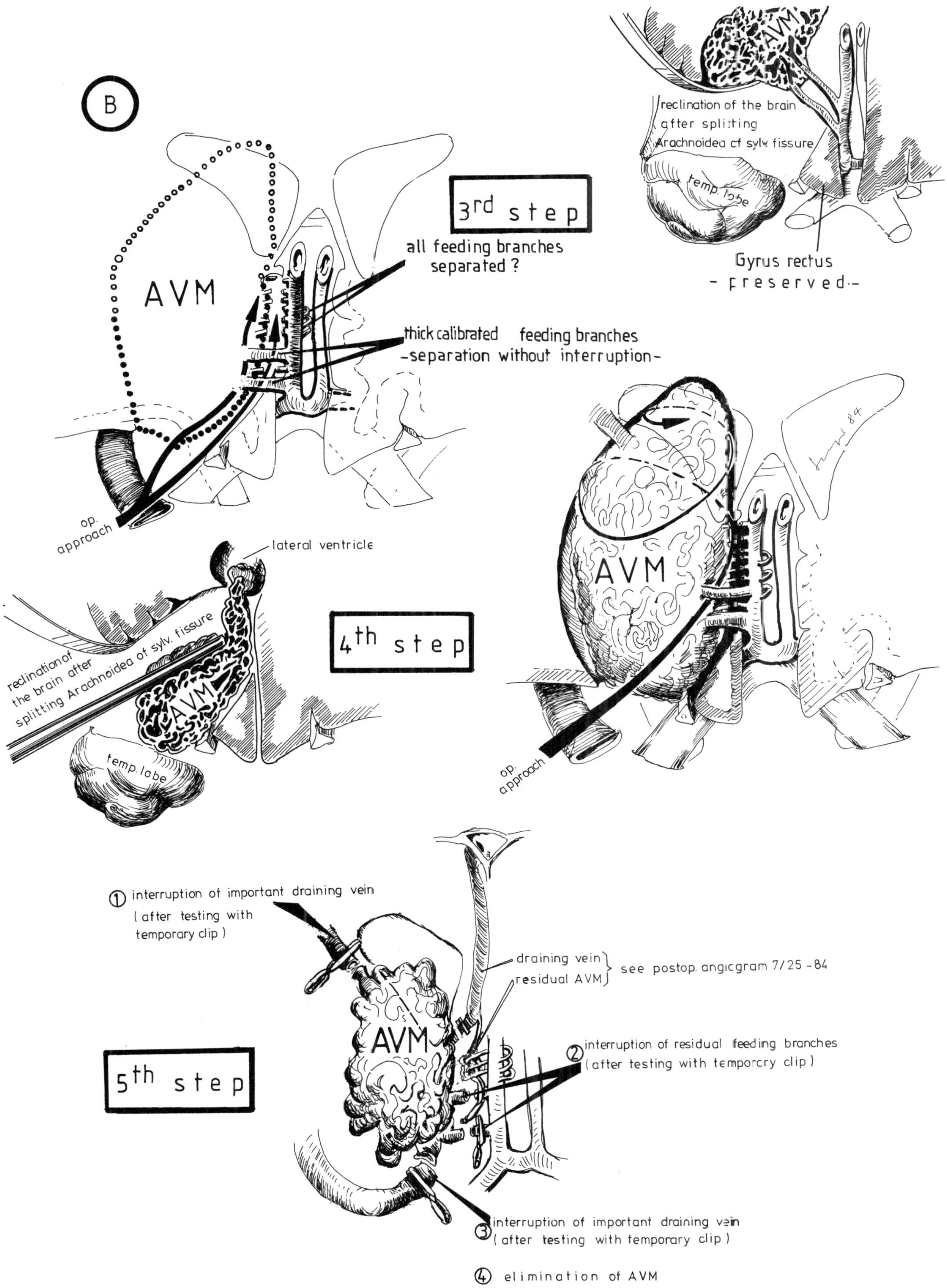

B
reclination of the brain
after splitting
Arachnoidea of sylv. fissure
temp. lobe
Gyrus rectus
- preserved -
AVM
3rd step
all feeding branches
separated ?
thick calibrated feeding branches
-separation without interruption-
op. approach
lateral ventricle
reclination of the brain after splitting Arachnoidea of sylv. fissure
4th step
AVM
op. approach
① interruption of important draining vein
(after testing with
temporary clip)
draining vein
residual AVM
see postop. angiogram 7/25 -84
5th step
② interruption of residual feeding branches
(after testing with temporary clip)
③ interruption of important draining vein
(after testing with temporary clip)
④ elimination of AVM

Fig. 27. Operation
1st and **2nd steps:** opening of the Sylvian fissure with exposure of the penetration point of the carotid artery and second nerve. Preparation of a basal draining vein and exposure of the Olfactorius. After separation of the Olfactorius one knows that the AVM has not reached to the Gyrus. **This part of the limbic system stays intact, also later in the operation**

FIG. 27

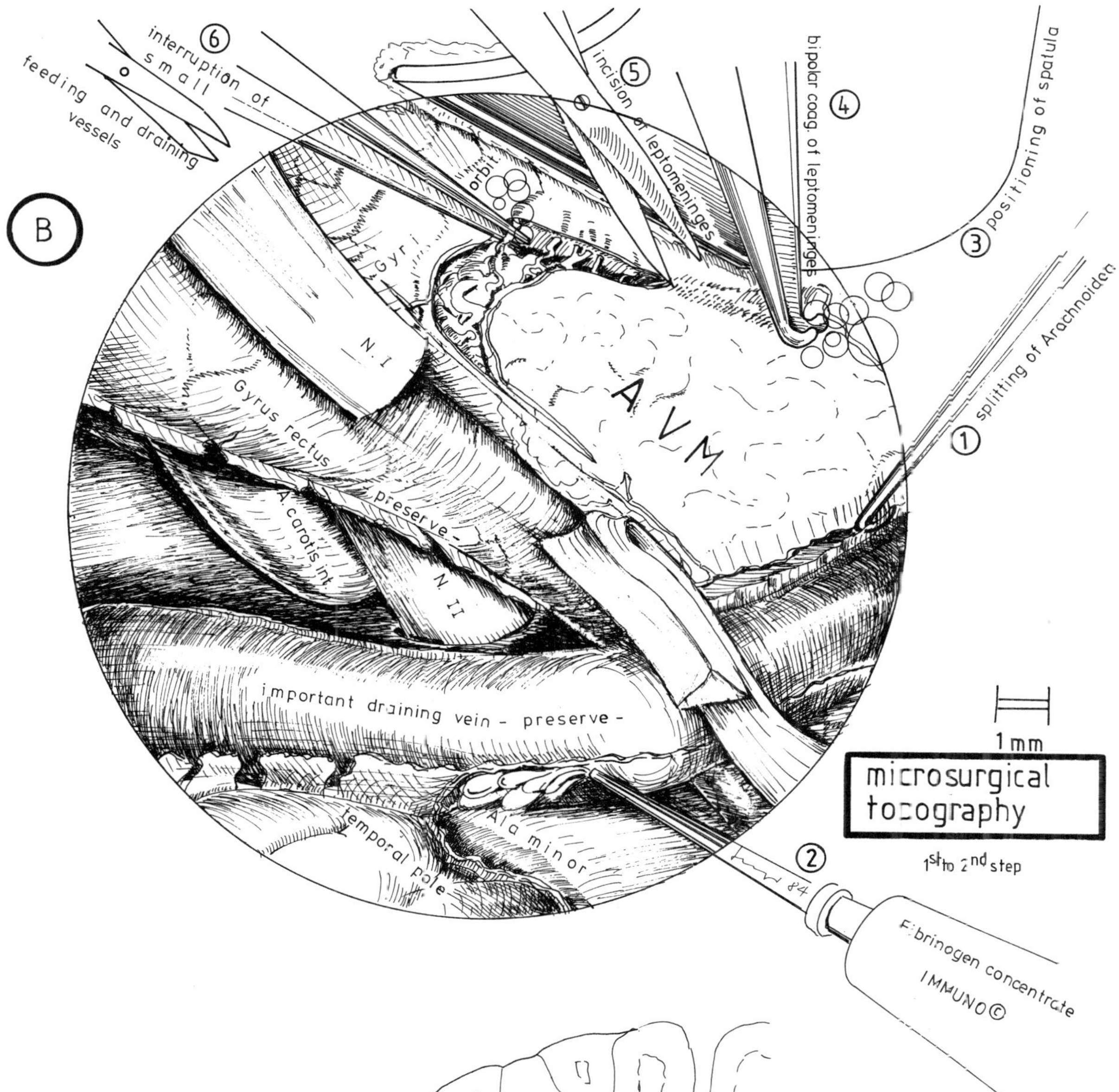

B
interruption of small feeding and draining vessels
⑥
⑤ incision of leptomeninges
④ bipolar coag. of leptomeninges
③ positioning of spatula
① splitting of Arachnoidea
②
orbit
Gyri
N. I
AVM
Gyrus rectus
preserve
A. carotis int.
N. II
important draining vein - preserve -
temporal pole
Ala minor
Fibrinogen concentrate
IMMUNO©
1 mm
microsurgical topography
1st to 2nd step

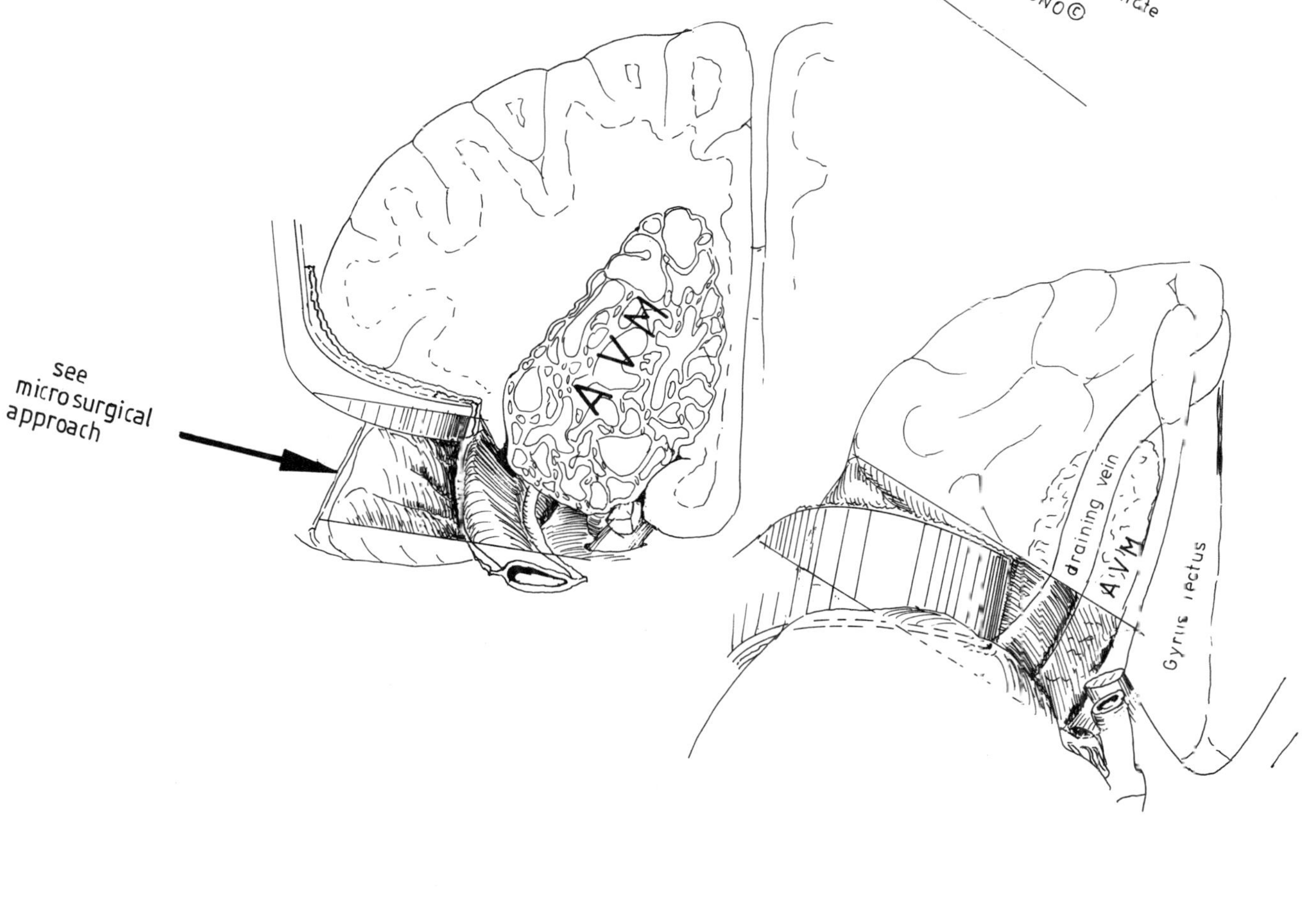

see microsurgical approach
AVM
draining vein
AVM
Gyrus rectus

Fig. 28. **3rd step:** further opening of the Sylvian fissure, exposing the Chiasma and over it the Sulcus longitudinalis with both anterior cerebral arteries (A1 and A2 both sides)

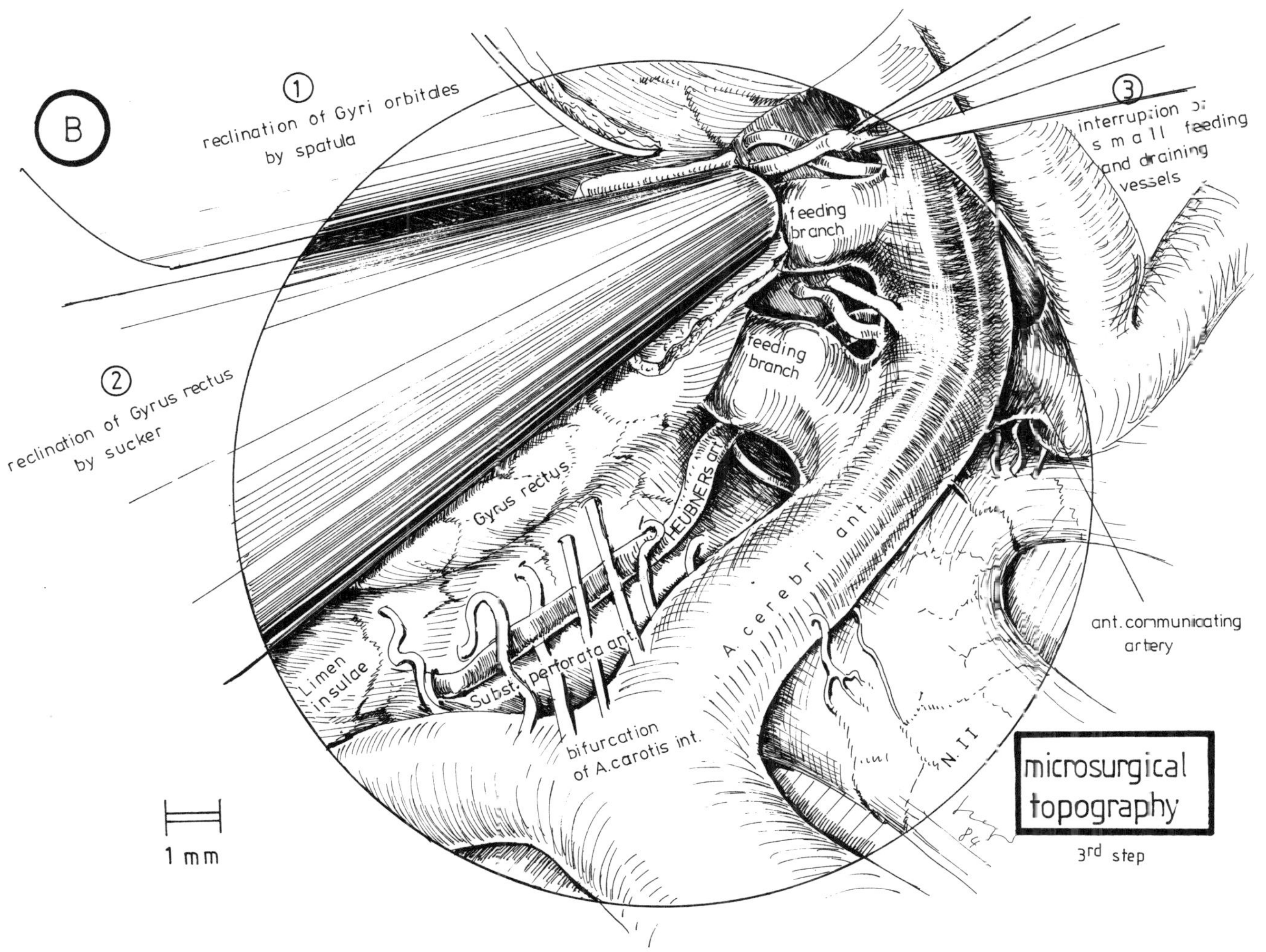
B
① reclination of Gyri orbitales by spatula
② reclination of Gyrus rectus by sucker
③ interruption of small feeding and draining vessels
feeding branch
feeding branch
Gyrus rectus
HEUBNERs art.
Limen insulae
Subst. perforata ant.
A. cerebri ant.
bifurcation of A. carotis int.
N. II
ant. communicating artery
1 mm
microsurgical topography
3rd step

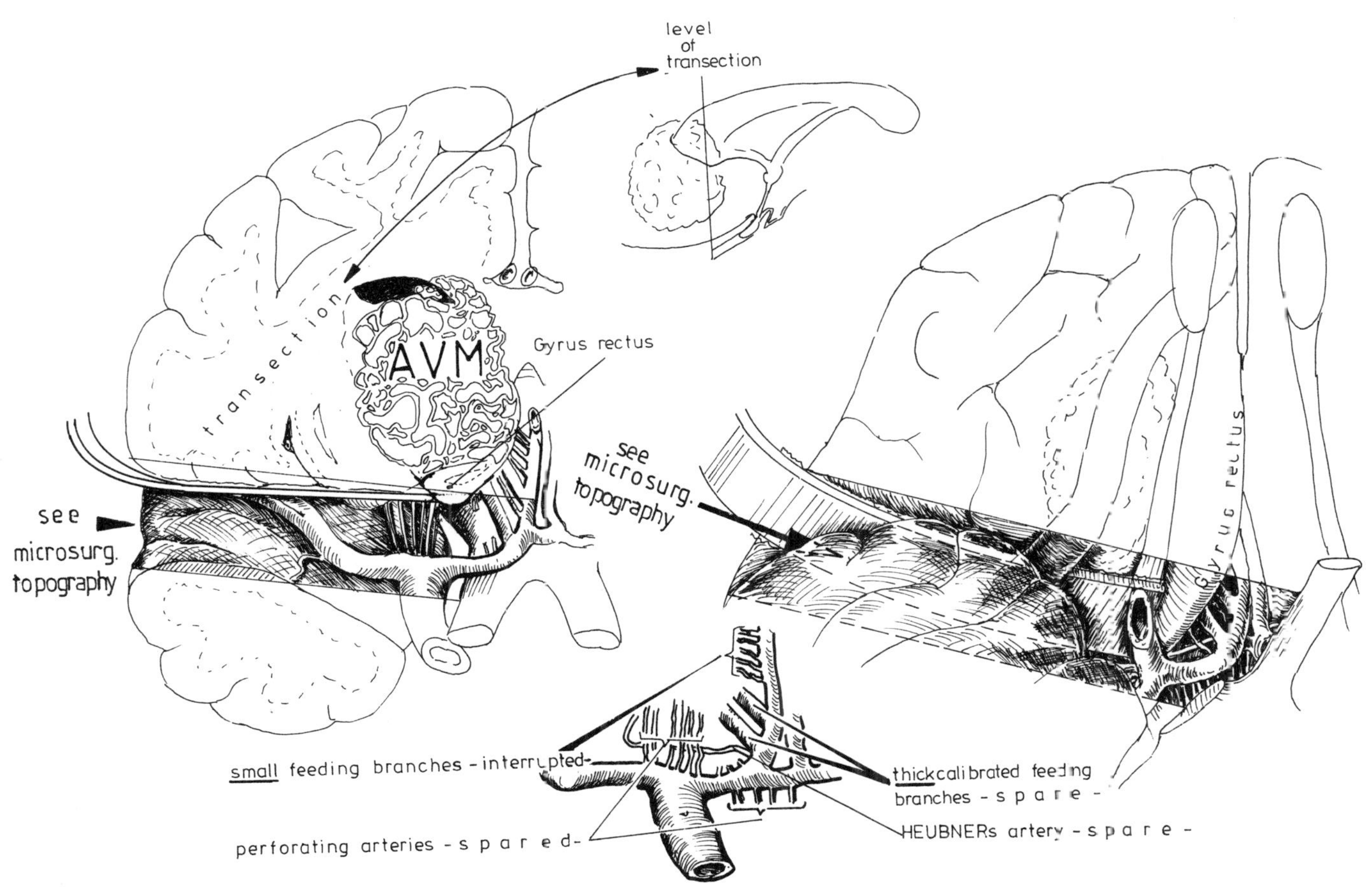
level of transection
transection
AVM
Gyrus rectus
see microsurg. topography
see microsurg. topography
Gyrus rectus
small feeding branches - interrupted-
perforating arteries - s p a r e d-
thickcalibrated feeding branches - s p a r e -
HEUBNERs artery - s p a r e -

Fig. 29. **3rd step.** Continuation: preparation in the Fissura longitudinalis along the anterior cerebral artery (A2)

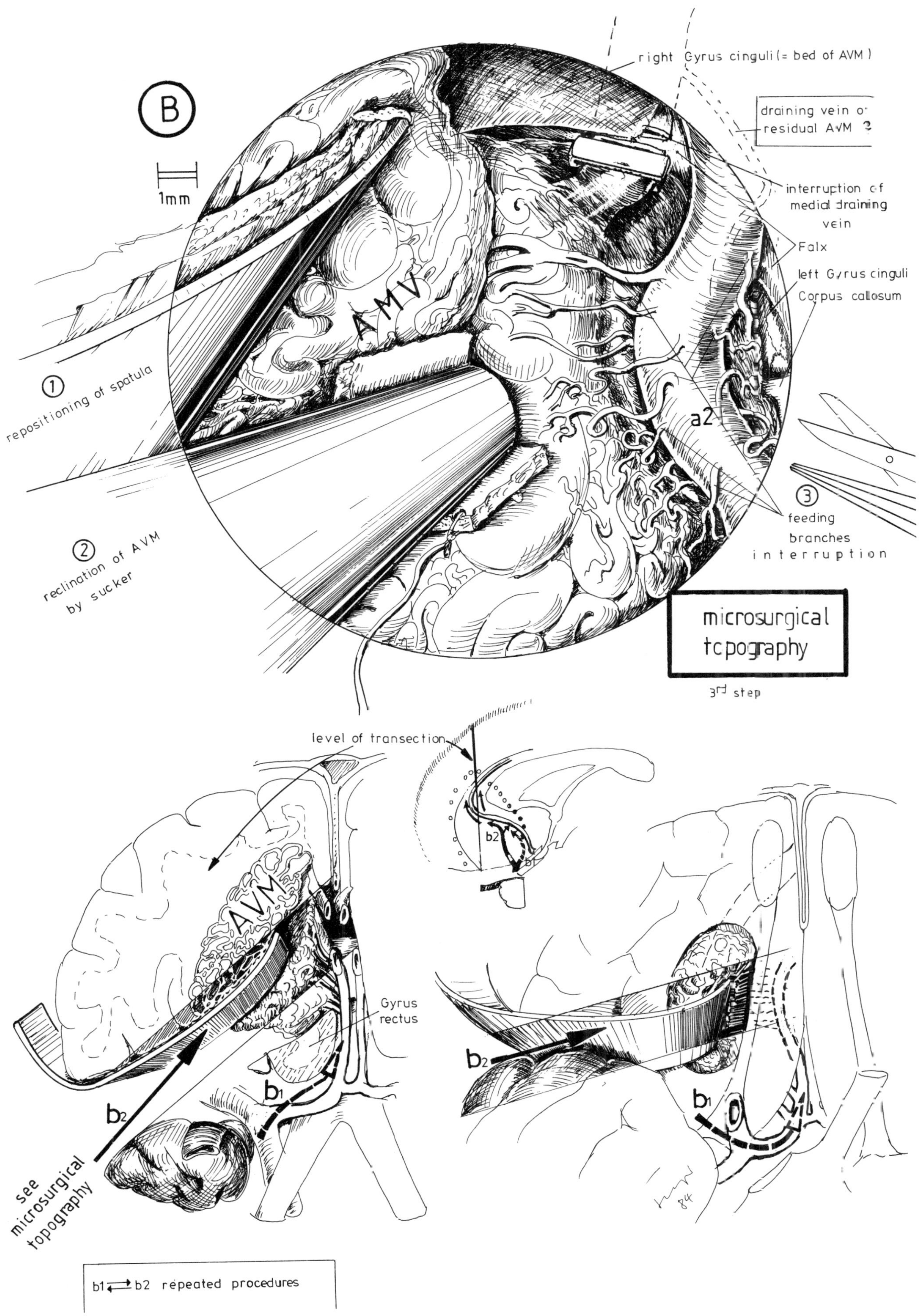
B
1mm
right Gyrus cinguli (= bed of AVM)
draining vein of residual AVM ?
interruption of medial draining vein
Falx
left Gyrus cinguli
Corpus callosum
AMV
a2
① repositioning of spatula
② reclination of AVM by sucker
③ feeding branches interruption
microsurgical topography
3rd step
level of transection
b2
b1
AVM
Gyrus rectus
see microsurgical topography
b1 ⇄ b2 repeated procedures

Fig. 30. **4th step:** preparation of the Genu corporis callosi. Separation of the AVM portions from the right Cornu anterius. Separation on all sides of the isolated AVM. **By the Genu corporis callosi the preparation was particularly difficult to visualize, so that an AVM fistula dorsal on the Corpus callosum was not reached.** This is typical for the pterional operation of this type of AVM

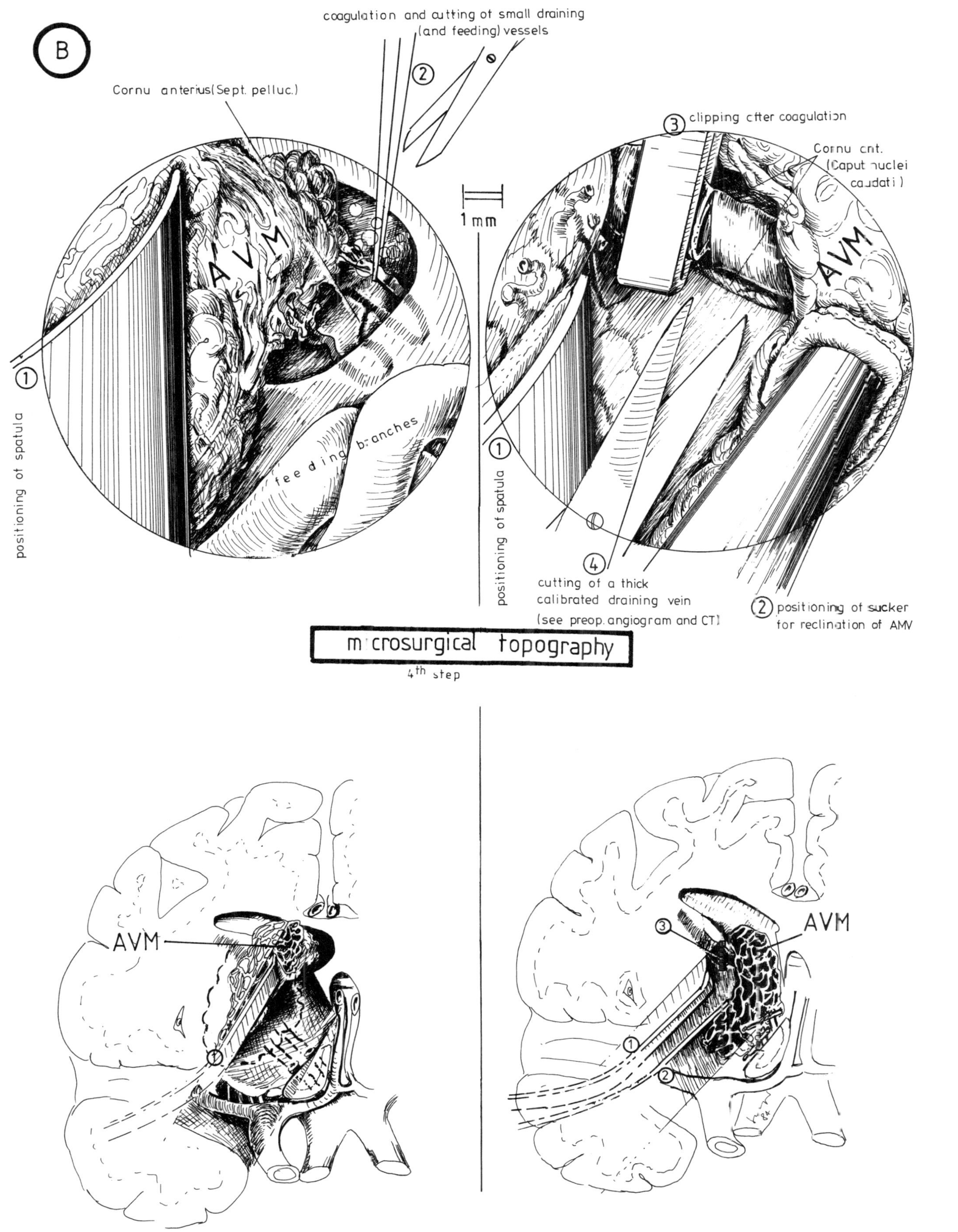
B
coagulation and cutting of small draining (and feeding) vessels
②
Cornu anterius (Sept. pelluc.)
AVM
① positioning of spatula
feeding branches
1 mm
③ clipping after coagulation
Cornu ant. (Caput nuclei caudati)
AVM
① positioning of spatula
④ cutting of a thick calibrated draining vein (see preop. angiogram and CT)
② positioning of sucker for reclination of AMV
microsurgical topography
4th step
AVM
①
AVM
③
①
②

Fig. 31. Some months later: removal of the residual AVM from high frontally avoiding the old operational area.
Principle of the operative approach
1st step: look for the pale red blood carrying draining vein on the Fissura longitudinalis. Both clips and the characteristic branching areas of the vessels allowed a more certain orientation of the small residual AVM
2nd step: the preparation was performed from the Sulcus corporis callosi between the Gyrus cinguli and Genu corporis callosi. The residual AVM was caused by the insufficient placement of the clip *a*. After testing – *2* – interruption of the fistula.
3rd step: Control: several veins containing dark blood. Closure of the open anterior horn – *2*

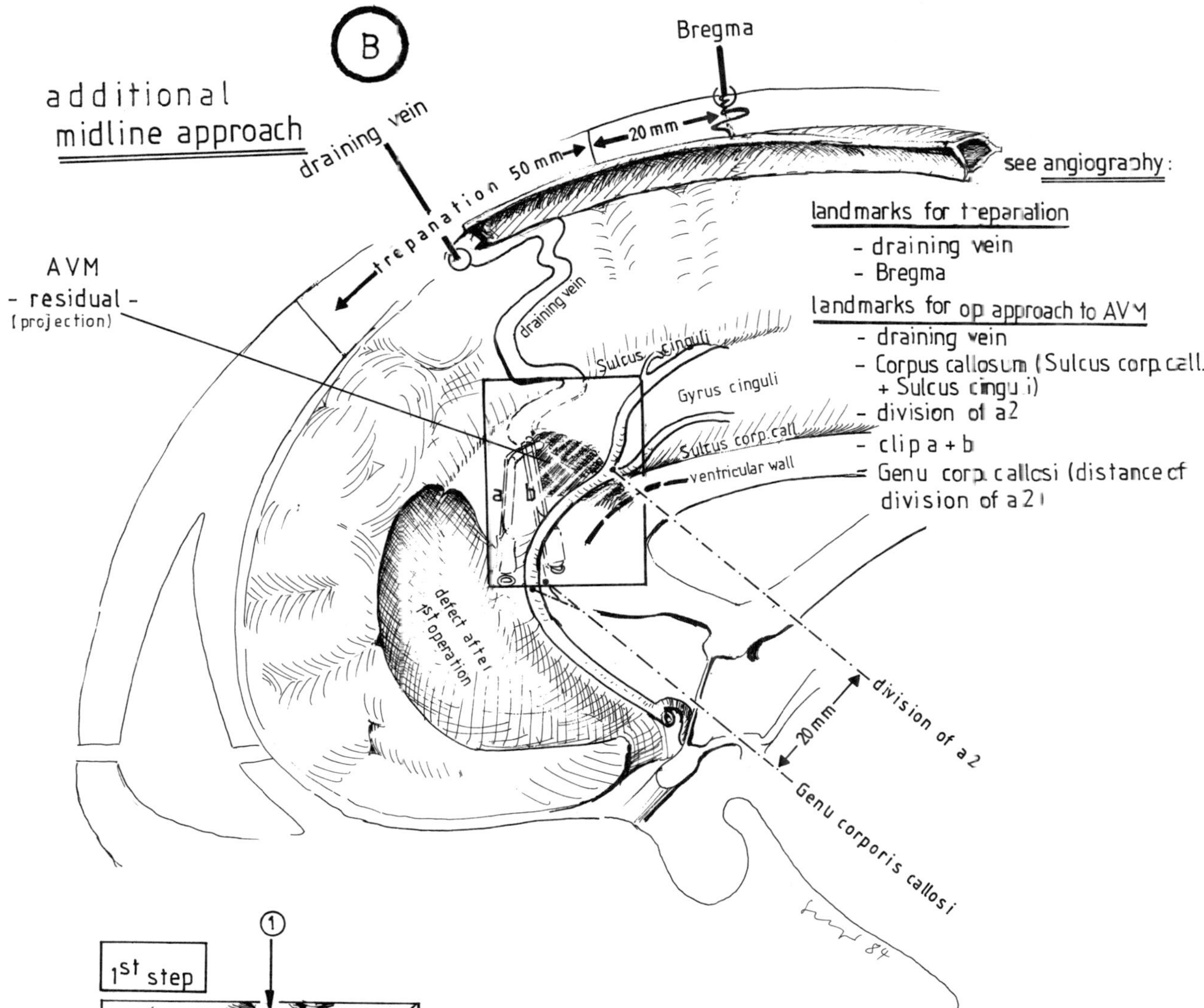

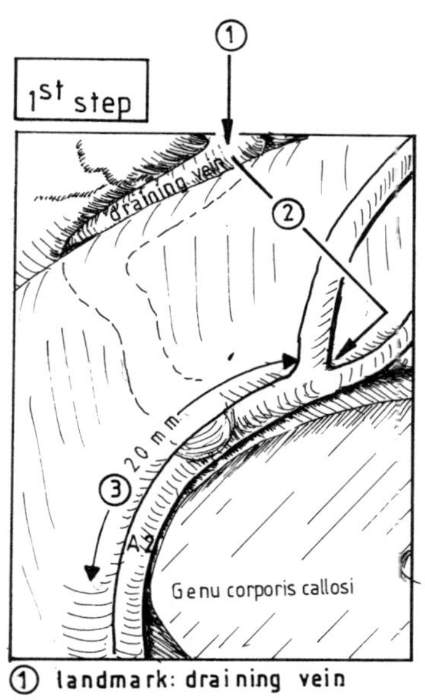

1. landmark: draining vein
2. landmark: division of A2
3. landmark: distance between division of a2 and Corpus callosum

principles of operation

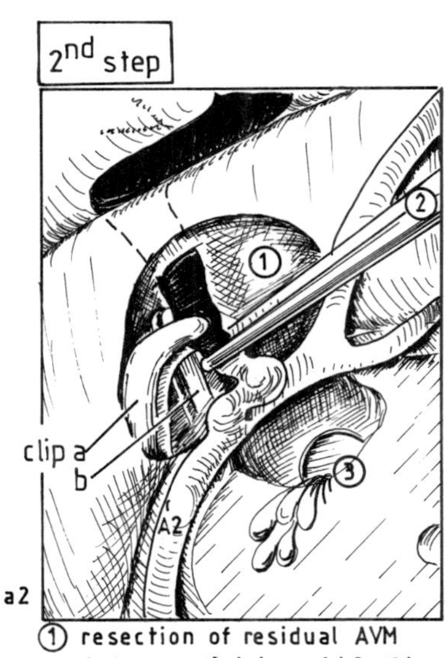

1. resection of residual AVM between division of A2 and clips a+b
2. during compression of av-fistula draining vein carries dark blood
3. Cornu ant. open

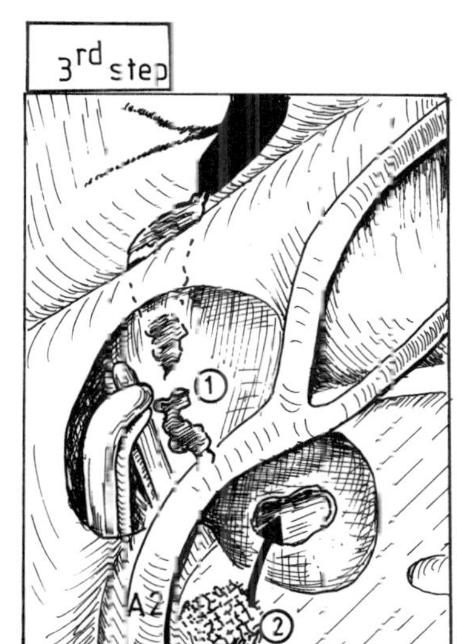

1. interruption of av-fistula
2. gap covered by tabotamp® e.g.

Fig. 32. Microsurgical site. The topographical anatomical landmarks are recognizable: on the surface the pale red blood-containing vein; deeper the branch of A2 and the two clips. The cause of the AV fistula is recognizable: the crooked clip had only closed a part of the anterior cerebral artery – A2 – arteriovenous fistula. Through the remaining lumen arterial blood can flow into the vein

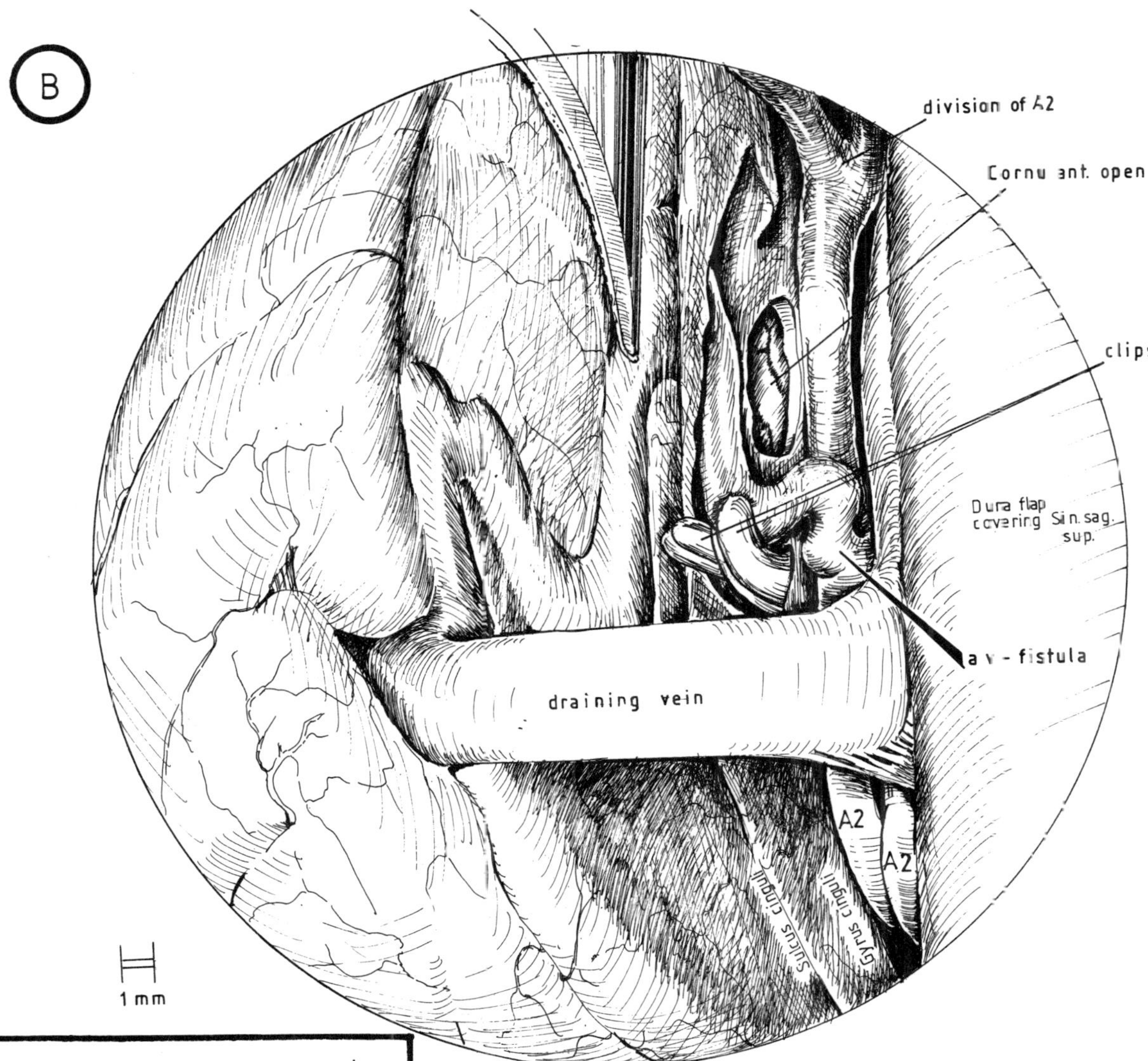

microsurgical topography

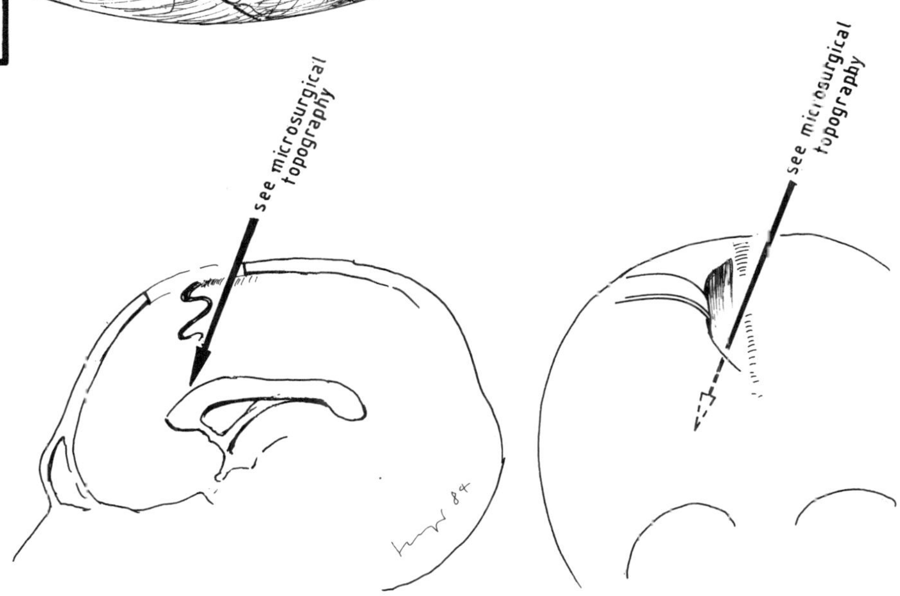

Fig. 33. Pterional and midline combined approach, operative approach type **C**
40-year-old patient, normal preoperatively, postoperatively 24 hours comatose, with passing right oculomotor paresis, reduction of visus, temporary psychosyndrome
Combined approach necessary, since the disadvantages of the pterional and midline approaches are present. **Disadvantage of the midline approach:** – midline approach hindered by draining veins. – AVM extends extensively laterally

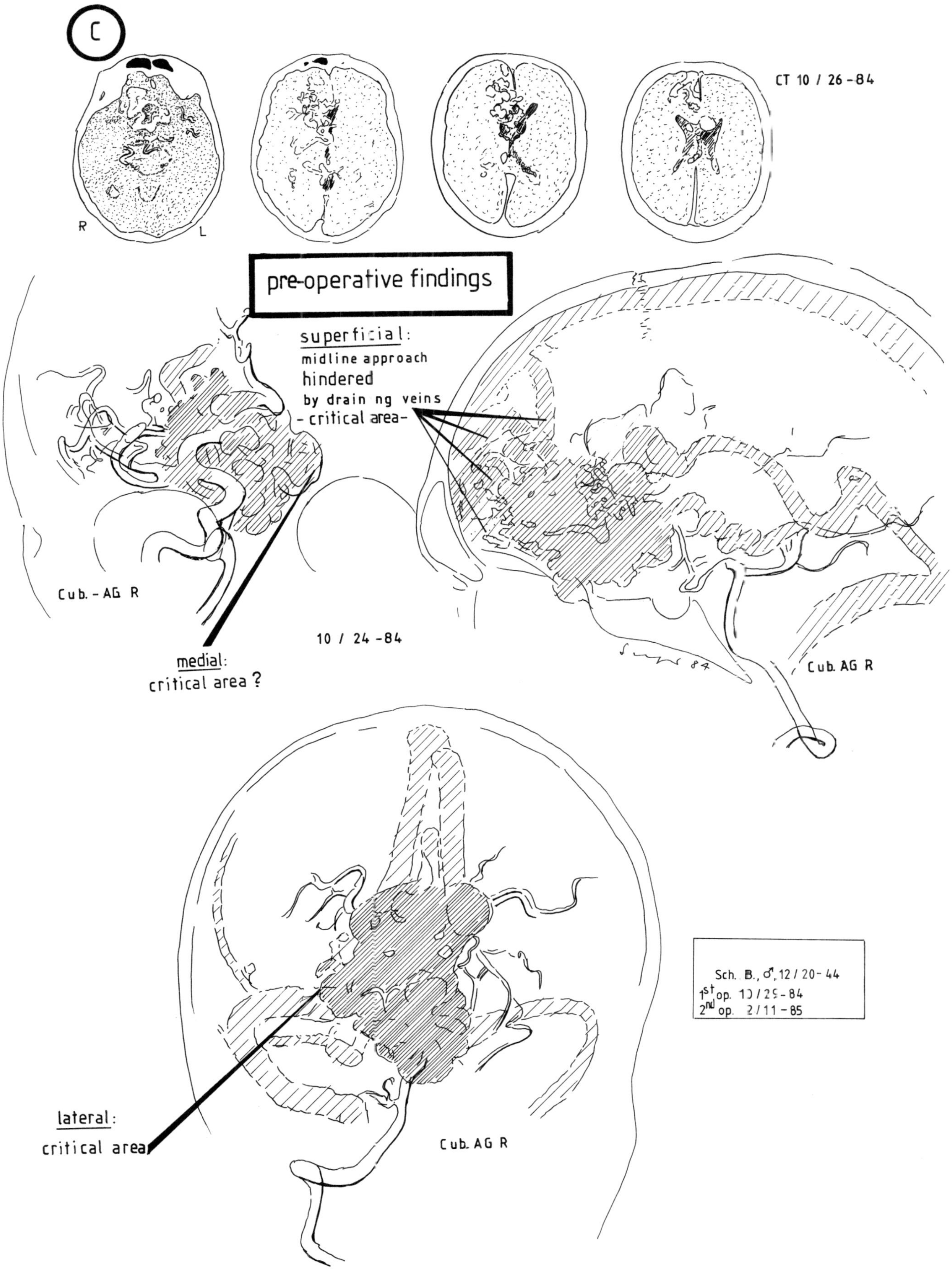
C
CT 10 / 26 - 84
R
L
pre-operative findings
superficial:
midline approach
hindered
by draining veins
- critical area -
Cub. - AG R
10 / 24 - 84
medial:
critical area ?
Cub. AG R
Sch. B., ♂, 12 / 20 - 44
1st op. 10 / 29 - 84
2nd op. 2 / 11 - 85
lateral:
critical area
Cub. AG R

Fig. 34. Disadvantage of the pterional approach: extensive bulging of the AVM dorsally

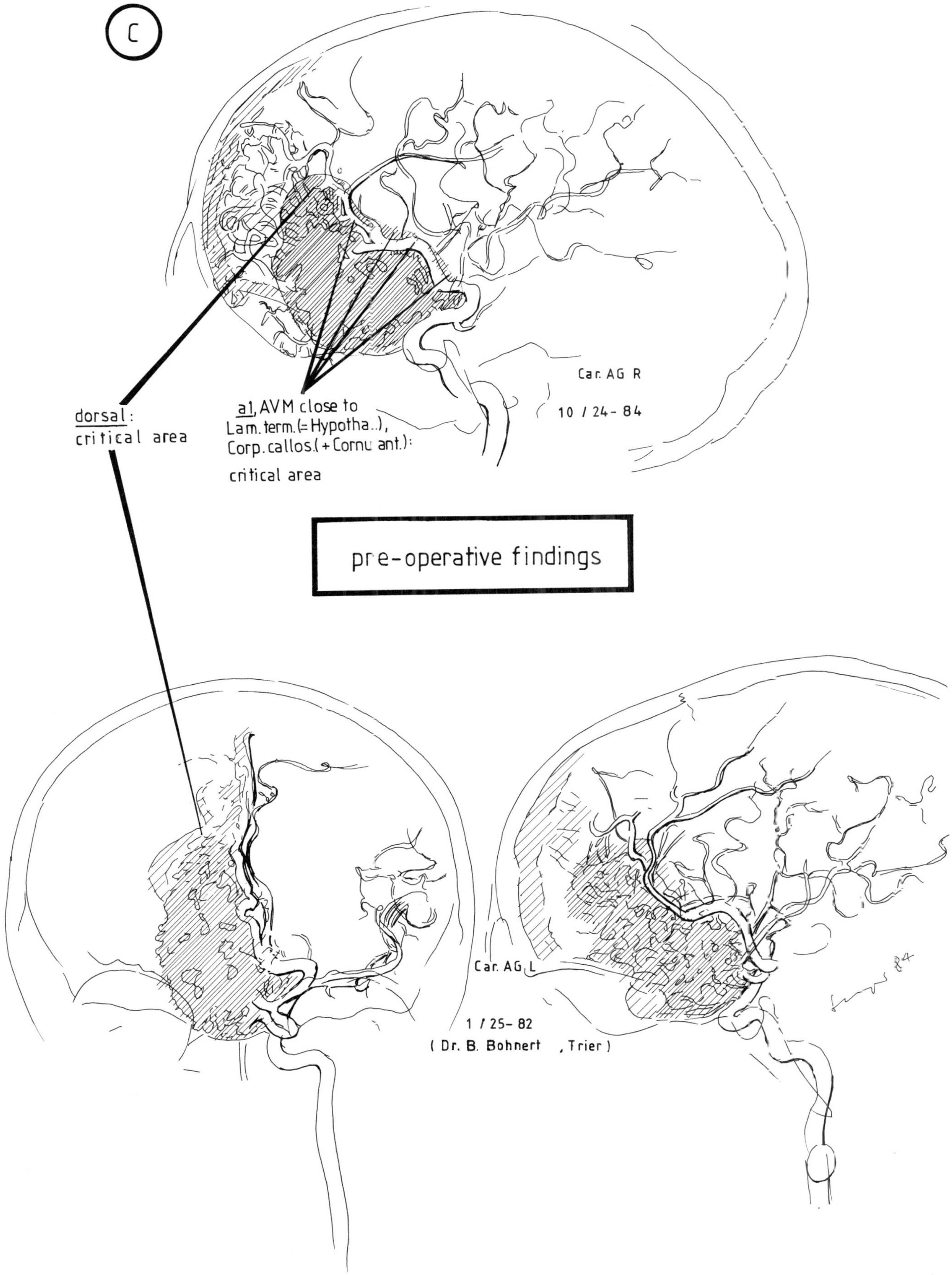
C
dorsal:
critical area
a1, AVM close to
Lam. term. (= Hypotha..),
Corp. callos. (+ Cornu ant.):
critical area
Car. AG R
10 / 24- 84
pre-operative findings
Car. AG L
1 / 25- 82
(Dr. B. Bohnert , Trier)

Fig. 35. Postoperative residual angioma. Feeding vessels and draining veins only dorsally. This region was difficult or impossible to reach using the pterional approach. The provided sketch shows the operative topography

FIG. 35

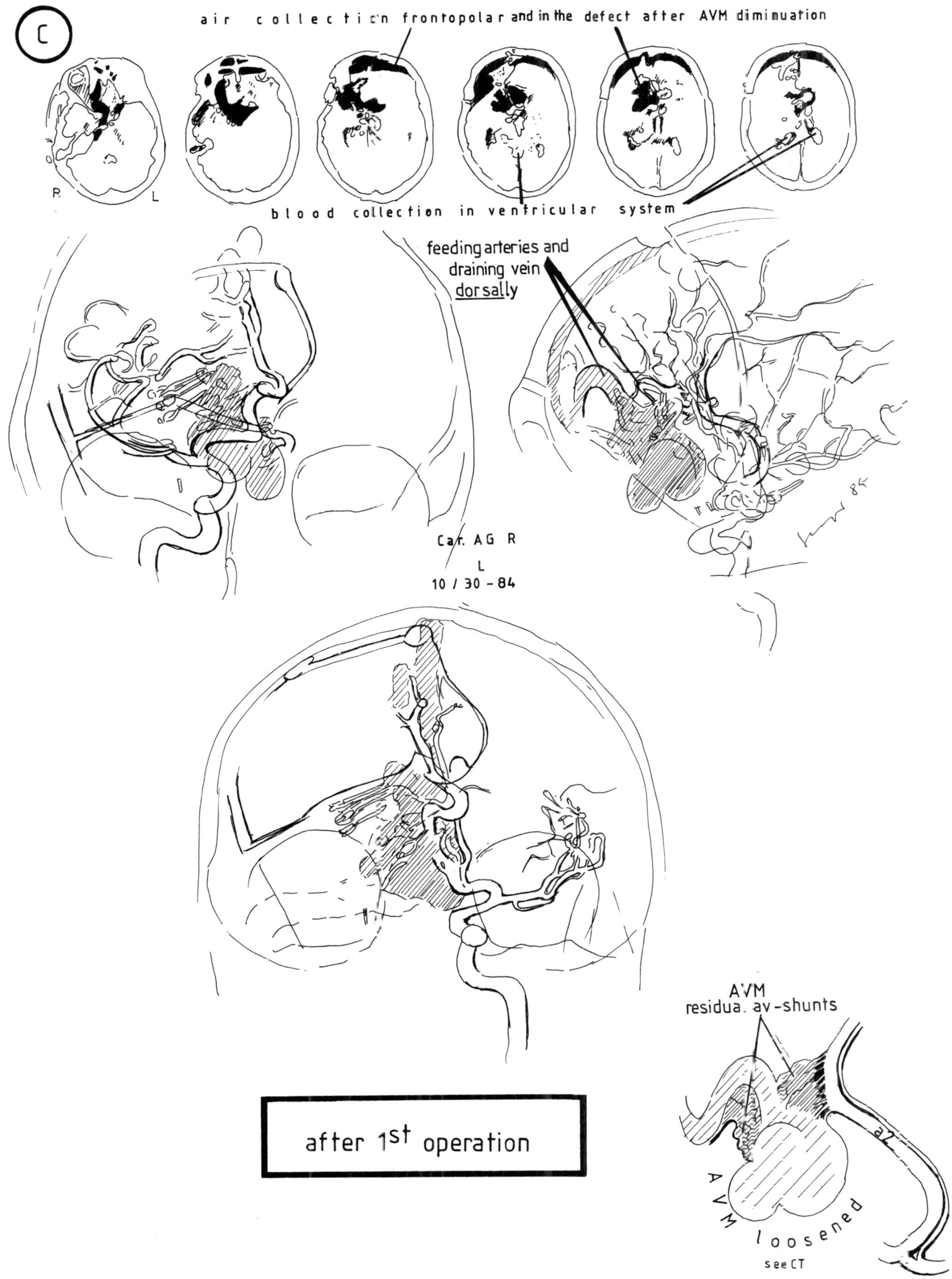
C
air collection frontopolar and in the defect after AVM diminuation
R
L
blood collection in ventricular system
feeding arteries and draining vein dorsally
Car. AG R
L
10 / 30 - 84
after 1st operation
AVM
residual av-shunts
a2
AVM loosened
see CT

Fig. 36. Angiogram before and after total removal of the residual angioma

FIG. 36

before 2nd operation

C

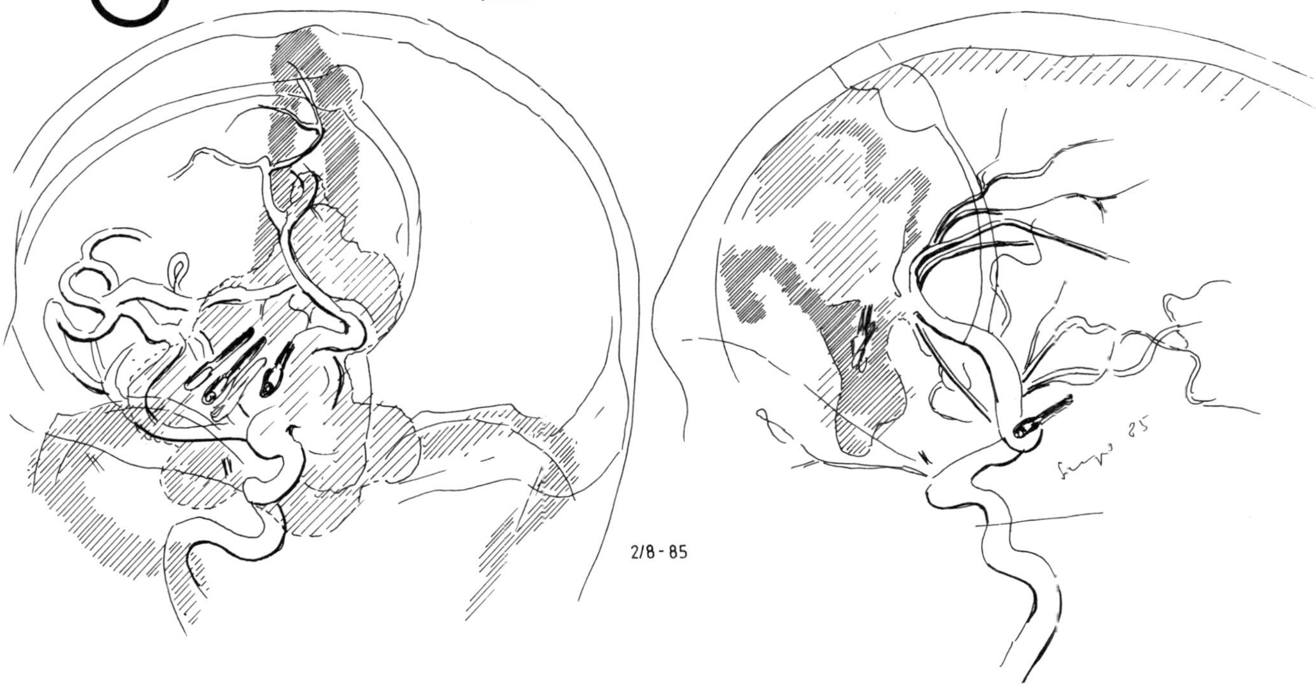

after 2nd operation

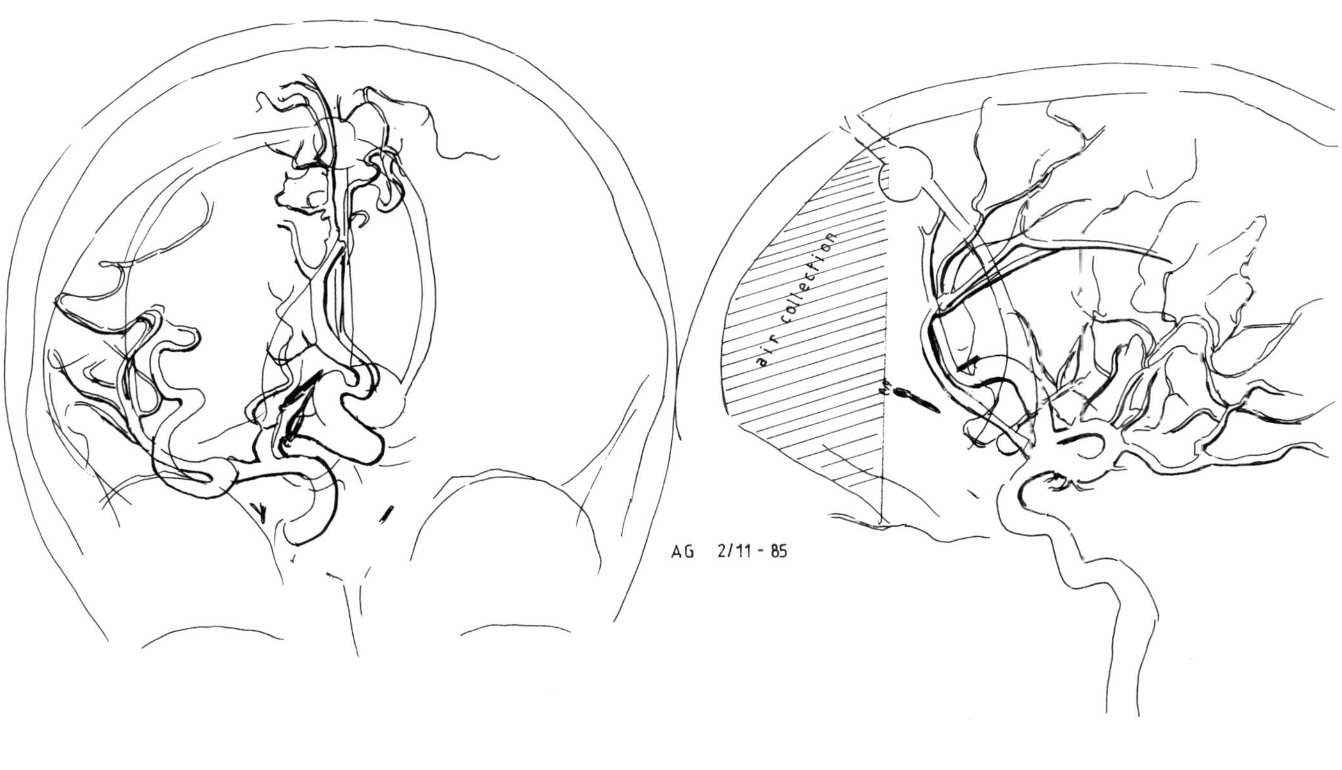

Fig. 37. The combined operation **C** starts pterional
1st step: opening of the Sylvian fissure and exposure of the anterior circle of Willis both sides. The Lamina terminalis – *3* – only requires opening if extensive adhesions of the basal cisterns (from previous bleeding) hinder the suction of CSF
2nd step: next is the cortex cut further medially, where one can reach the angioma the least deep. Only secondarily, after pushing away the brain tissue in a lateral direction, one looks for the limits sideways – *1* –. The midline is opened basally from behind, not in front, in order to prepare the anterior cerebral artery from proximal to distal
3rd step: the operation is interrupted because the anterior cerebral artery is not anymore clearly visible dorsally. By the Genu corporis callosi a residual part of the angioma remains, which will later be operated using a midline approach

FIG. 37

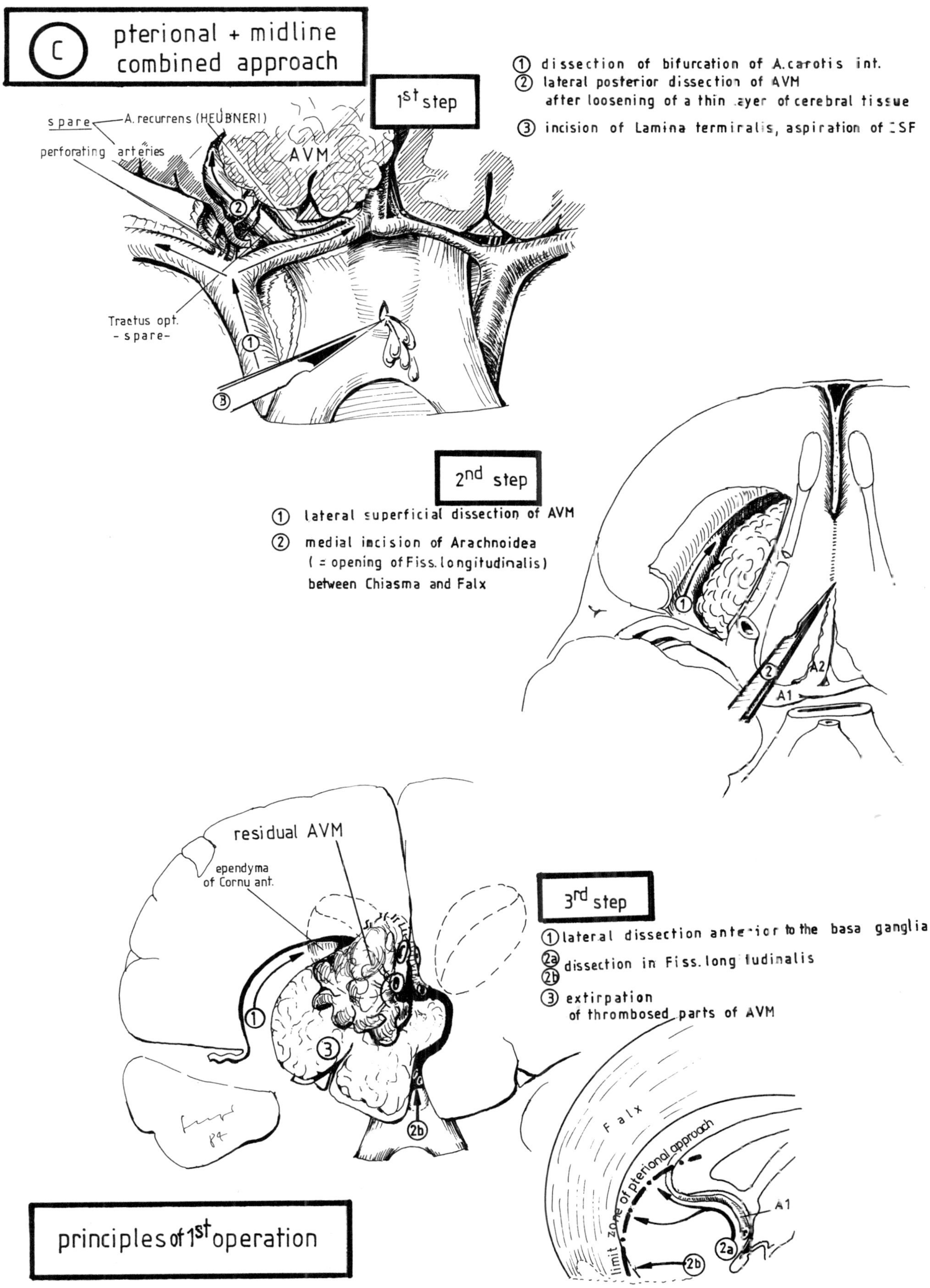
C pterional + midline combined approach
1st step
① dissection of bifurcation of A. carotis int.
② lateral posterior dissection of AVM after loosening of a thin layer of cerebral tissue
③ incision of Lamina terminalis, aspiration of CSF
spare
A. recurrens (HEUBNERI)
perforating arteries
AVM
Tractus opt. - spare -
2nd step
① lateral superficial dissection of AVM
② medial incision of Arachnoidea (= opening of Fiss. longitudinalis) between Chiasma and Falx
A2
A1
residual AVM
ependyma of Cornu ant.
3rd step
① lateral dissection anterior to the basal ganglia
2a dissection in Fiss. longitudinalis
2b
③ extirpation of thrombosed parts of AVM
Falx
limit zone of pterional approach
A1
2a
2b
principles of 1st operation

Fig. 38. **1st step:** start of the microsurgical topographical isolation of the angioma with exposure of the circle of Willis. Identification of the perforating arteries and the A. recurrens Heubneri

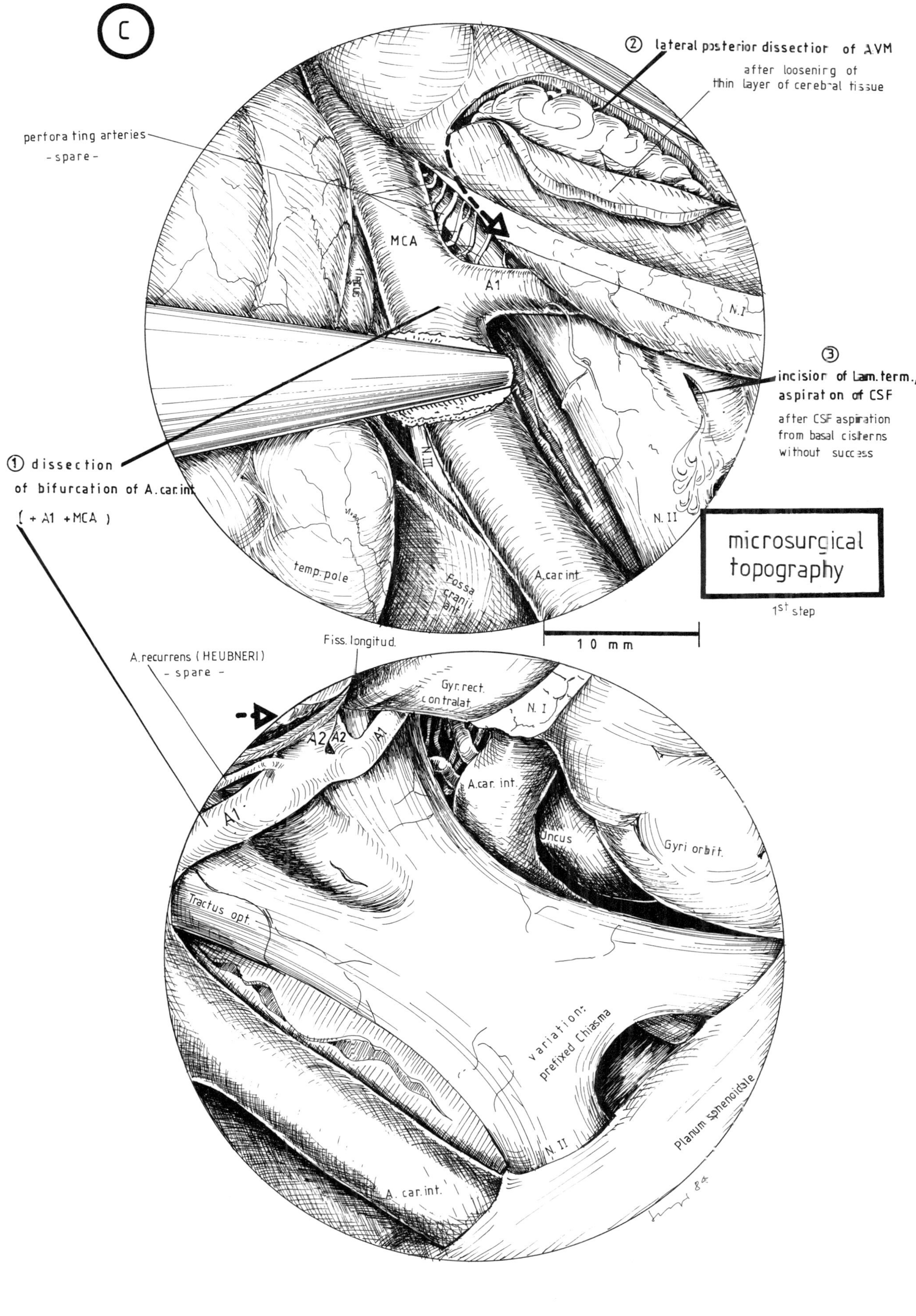
C
② lateral posterior dissection of AVM
after loosening of
thin layer of cerebral tissue
perforating arteries
- spare -
MCA
A1
N. I
③
incision of Lam. term.,
aspiration of CSF
after CSF aspiration
from basal cisterns
without success
① dissection
of bifurcation of A. car. int
(+ A1 + MCA)
N. III
N. II
microsurgical
topography
1st step
temp. pole
Fossa cranii ant.
A. car. int
10 mm
Fiss. longitud.
A. recurrens (HEUBNERI)
- spare -
Gyr. rect.
contralat.
N. I
A2
A2
A1
A1
A. car. int.
Uncus
Gyri orbit.
Tractus opt.
variation:
prefixed Chiasma
Planum sphenoidale
N. II
A. car. int.

Fig. 39. **2nd step:** superficial circular isolation of the border of the angioma

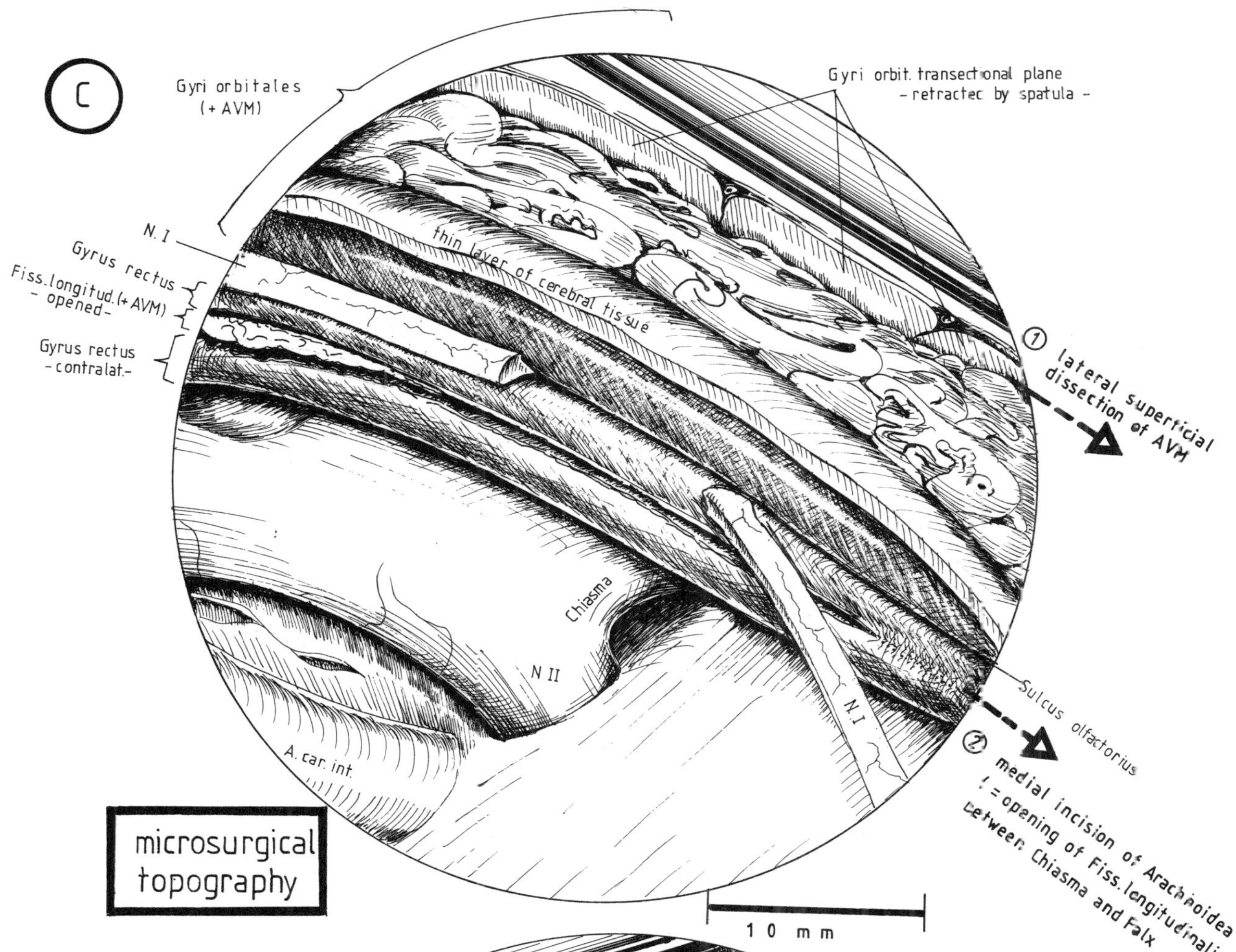

microsurgical topography

2nd step

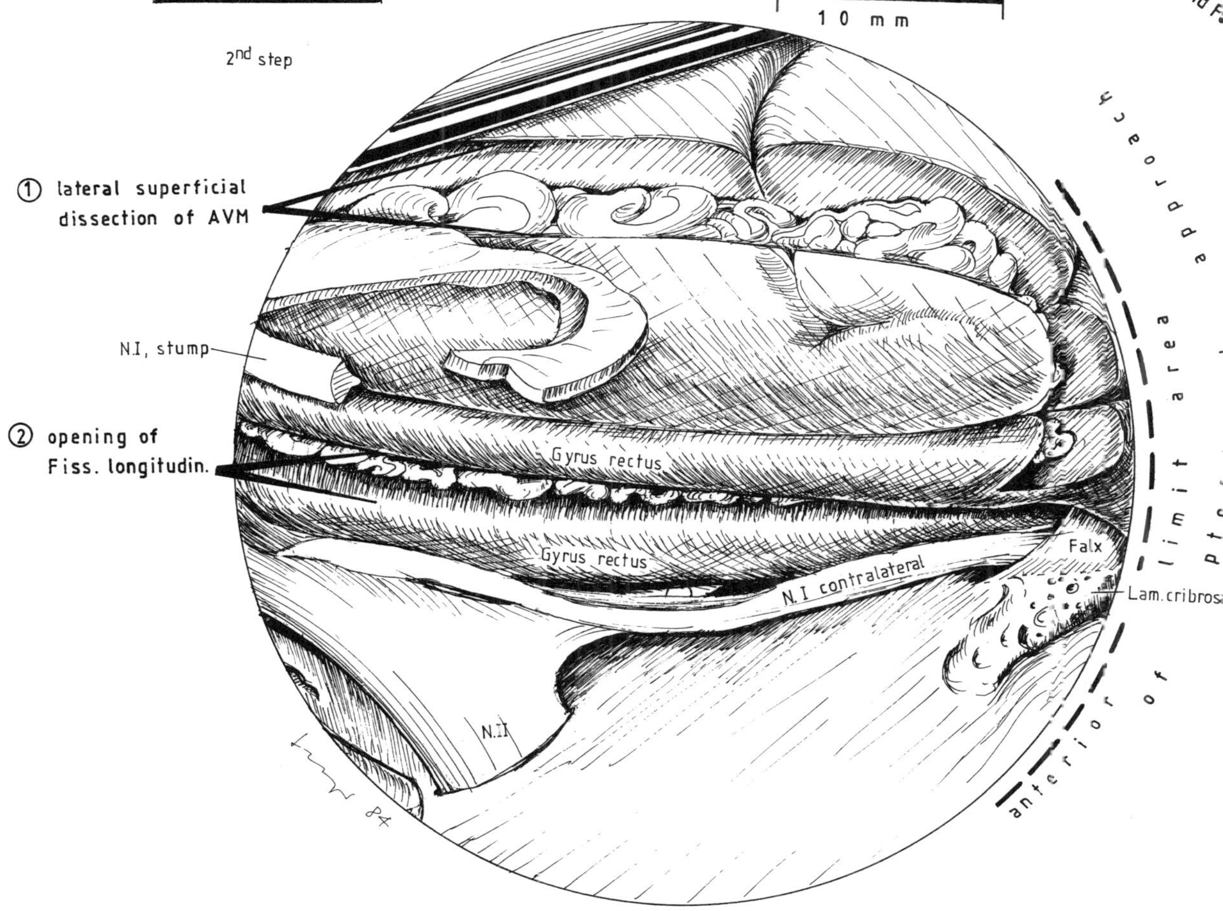

Fig. 40. **3rd step:** isolation of the part of the angioma in the midline and dorsally in the region of the Genu corporis callosi

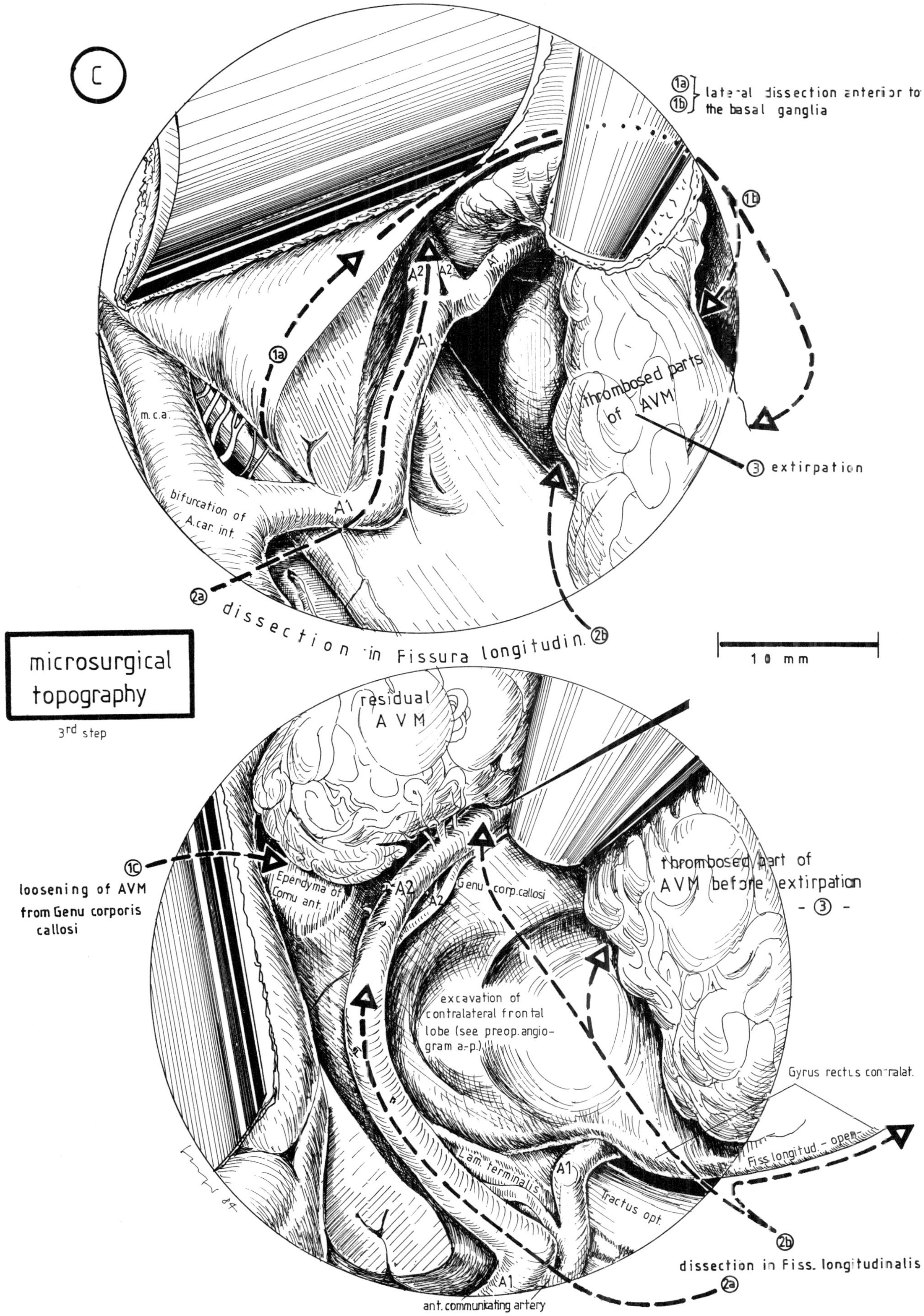
C
1a } lateral dissection anterior to
1b } the basal ganglia
1a
1b
A2
A2
A1
A1
m.c.a.
thrombosed parts of AVM
3 extirpation
bifurcation of A.car. int.
A1
2a
dissection in Fissura longitudin. 2b
10 mm
microsurgical topography
3rd step
residual AVM
1c
loosening of AVM from Genu corporis callosi
Ependyma of Cornu ant.
A2
A2
Genu corp.callosi
thrombosed part of AVM before extirpation
- 3 -
excavation of contralateral frontal lobe (see preop. angiogram a.-p.)
Gyrus rectus contralat.
Fiss.longitud. - open-
Lam. terminalis
A1
Tractus opt.
2b
dissection in Fiss. longitudinalis
2a
A1
ant. communicating artery

Fig. 41. At the start of the intervention acute appearance of brain prolapse. It was assumed that the temporary clipping of a draining vein had led to intracerebral haemorrhage. Since the haemorrhage could not be localized, a CT had to be carried out before the intervention could be continued

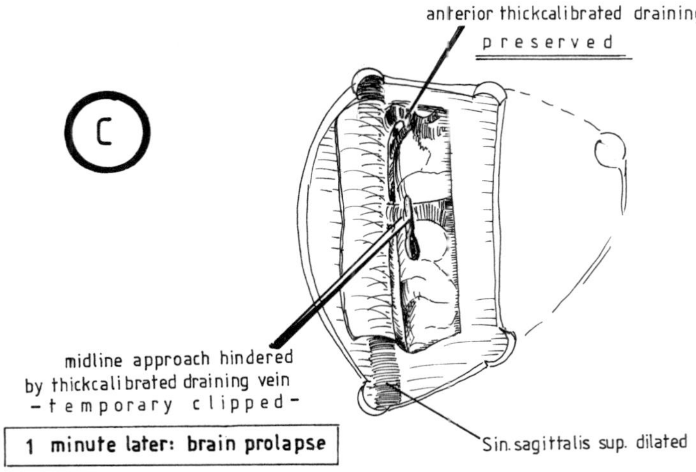

complication at begin of 2nd operation

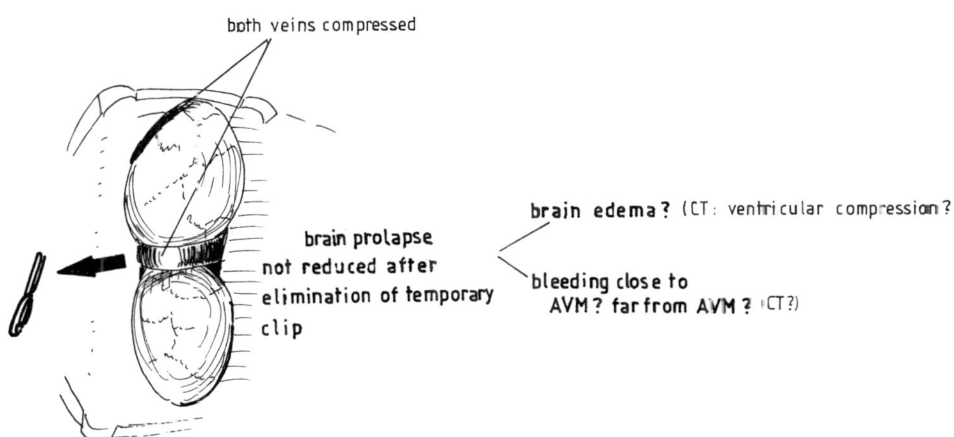

- PEEP reduced, position of the head elevated: brain prolapse idem
- suture of Dura mater stops brain prolapse, wound closure, CT

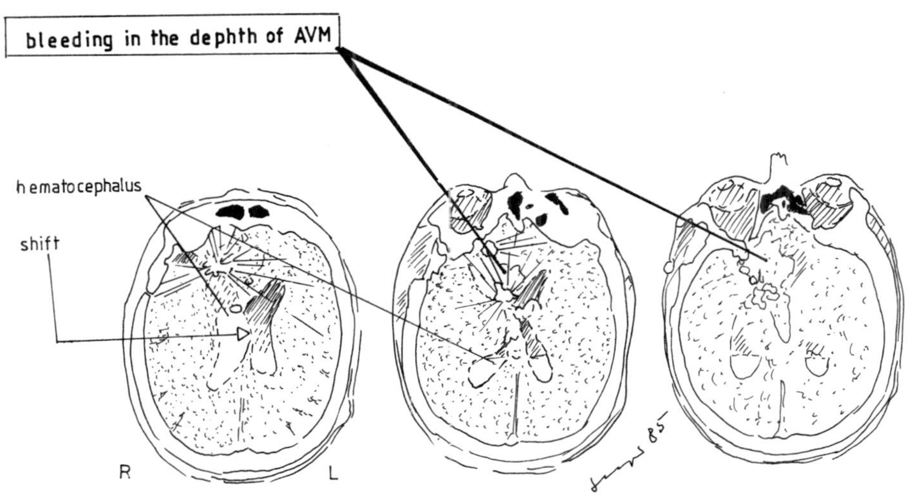

- wound reopened -

Fig. 42. The resection of the brain prolapse proved to be unproblematical since the angioma lay closely under the brain surface. The preoperative angiogram had suggested a deeper location of the angioma

FIG. 42

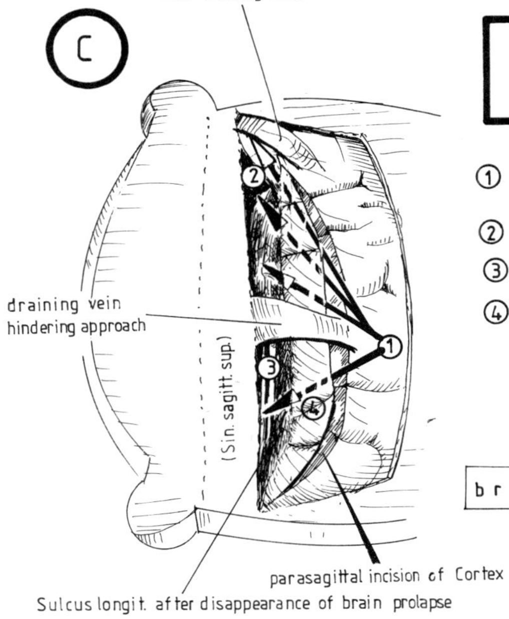

1st step

1. dissection of AVM in Sulcus longitud.
2. partial evacuation of hematoma
3. dissection of Aa. pericallosae
4. small rim of brain tissue resected

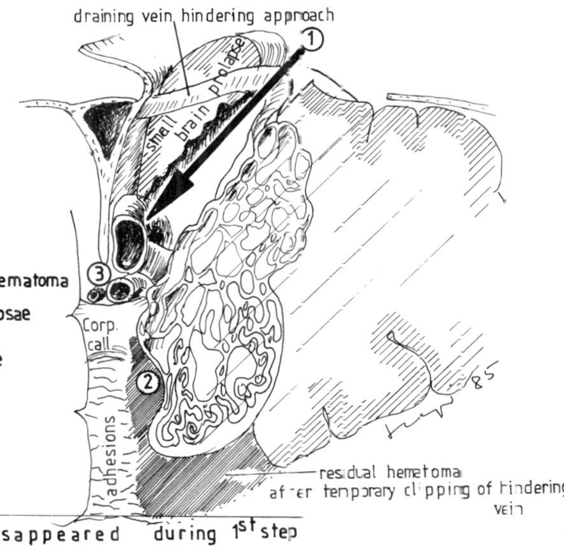

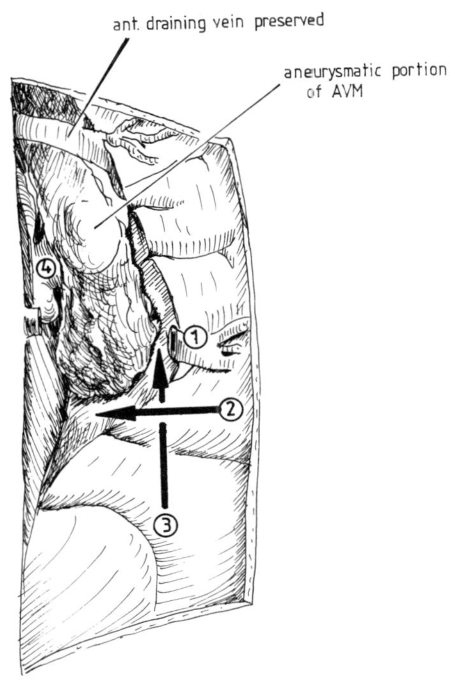

2nd step

1. hindering vein cut (after 1st step thrombosed)
2. dissection of post. portion of AVM
3. " " lat. " " "
4. " " short thick calibrated feeding artery

at this step relationships between A2 and short feeding arteries are unclear

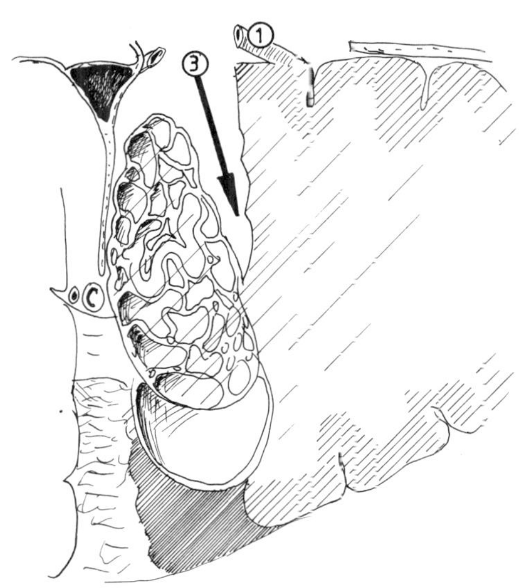

principles of 2nd operation

Fig. 43. Right up to the end of the intervention were the large feeding arteries and main draining veins preserved. Only at the end were the main feeding artery from the A2 and the main draining vein interrupted, resulting in haemorrhaging

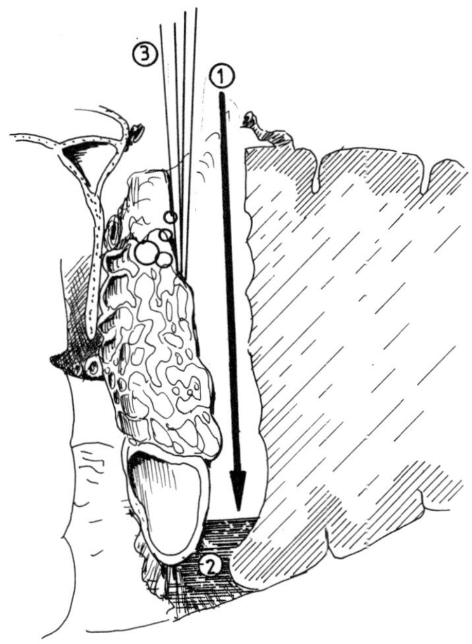

① lateral dissection of AVM

② evacuation of residual hematoma

③ shrinking of AVM by bipolar coagulation

3rd step

④ medial dissection of AVM

during ④ rupture of aneurysmatic portion of AVM

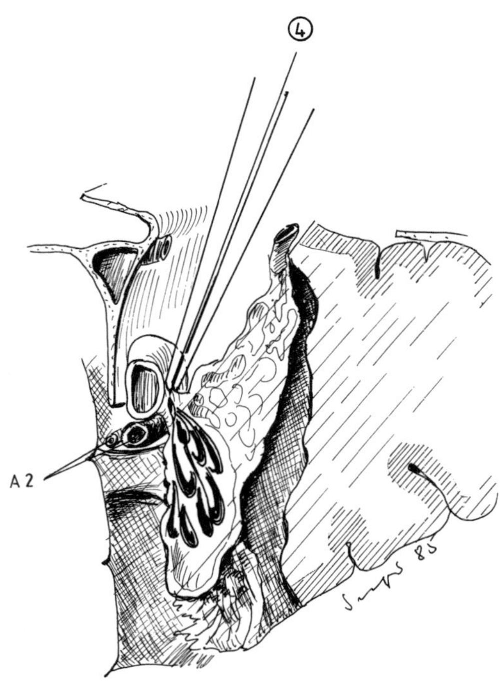

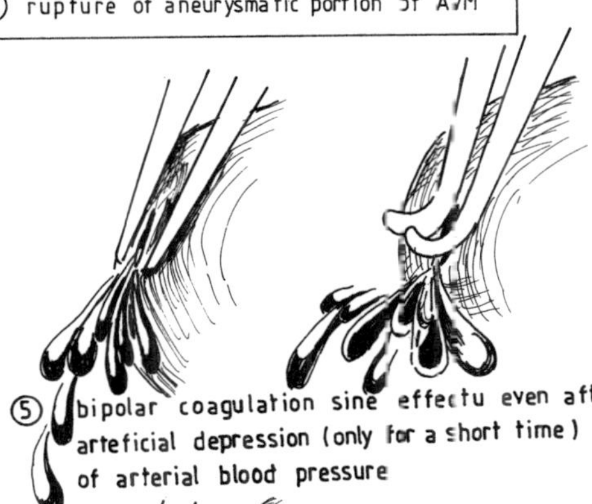

⑤ bipolar coagulation sine effectu even after arteficial depression (only for a short time) of arterial blood pressure

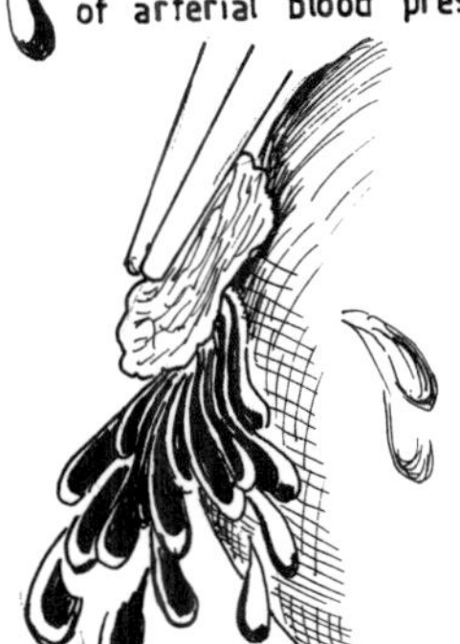

⑥ compression of bleeding vessel by cotton pledget even during hypotension sine effectu

temporary pilot clip see 4th step

Fig. 44. Principle of interruption of the main shunts of the AVM with control of the haemorrhaging

FIG. 44

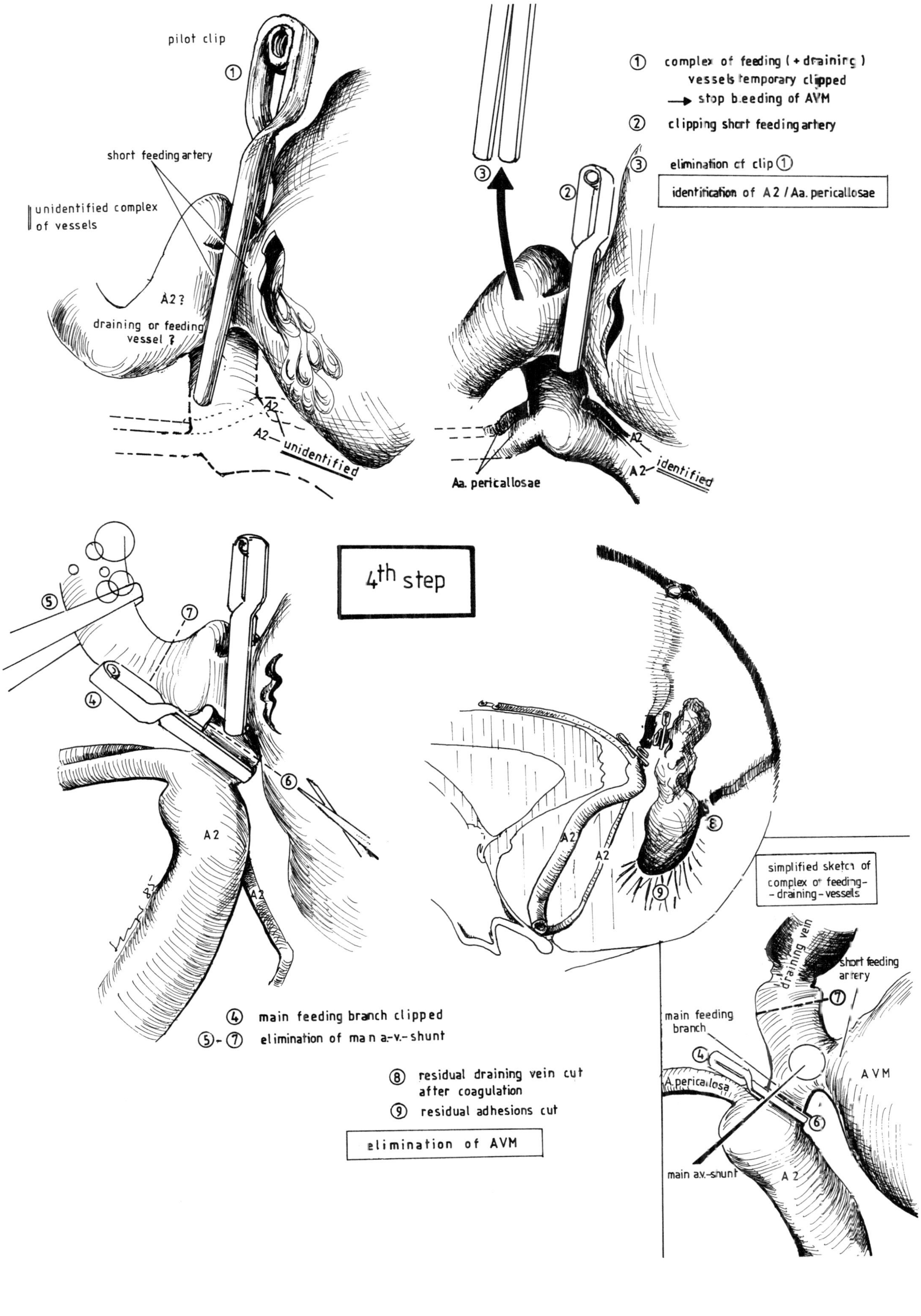

pilot clip
①
short feeding artery
unidentified complex of vessels
A2 ?
draining or feeding vessel ?
A2
A2
unidentified
① complex of feeding (+ draining) vessels temporary clipped → stop bleeding of AVM
② clipping short feeding artery
③ elimination of clip ①
identification of A2 / Aa. pericallosae
③
②
Aa. pericallosae
A2
A2
identified
4th step
⑤
⑦
④
⑥
A2
A2
A2
A2
⑧
⑨
simplified sketch of complex of feeding- - draining - vessels
draining vein
short feeding artery
⑦
main feeding branch
④
A. pericallosa
AVM
⑥
main a.v.-shunt
A 2
④ main feeding branch clipped
⑤ - ⑦ elimination of main a.-v.-shunt
⑧ residual draining vein cut after coagulation
⑨ residual adhesions cut
elimination of AVM

Fig. 45. The same situation as in Fig. 44 but at the microsurgical site

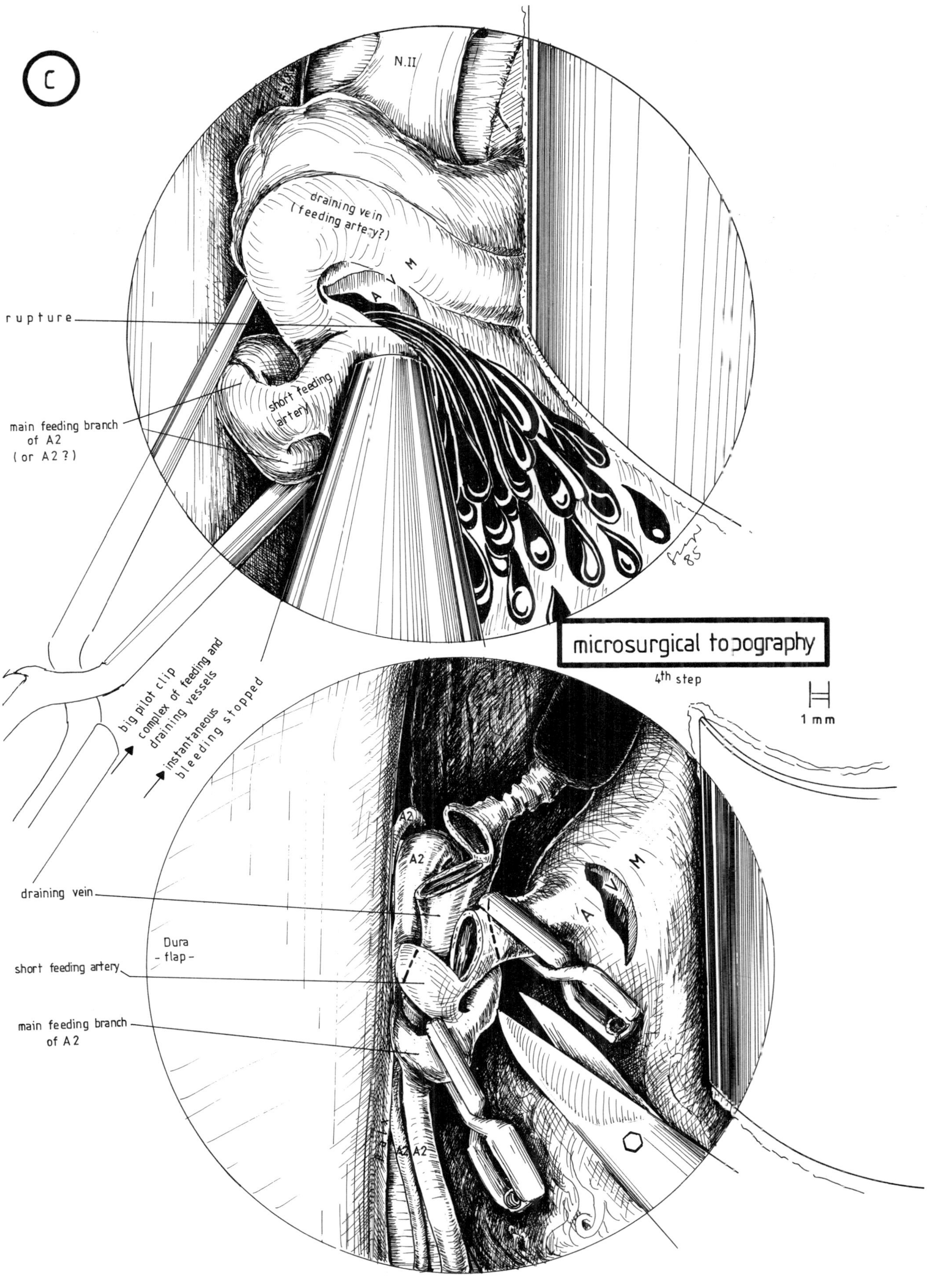
C
N.II
draining vein
(feeding artery?)
AVM
rupture
short feeding artery
main feeding branch of A2 (or A2?)
85
microsurgical topography
4th step
1 mm
big pilot clip complex of feeding and draining vessels
instantaneous bleeding stopped
A2
A2
AVM
draining vein
Dura - flap -
short feeding artery
main feeding branch of A2
A2 A2

Chapter 3
Dorsal Cisterns and Fissures, Middle Segment
(Figs. 46 to 99)

Fig. 46

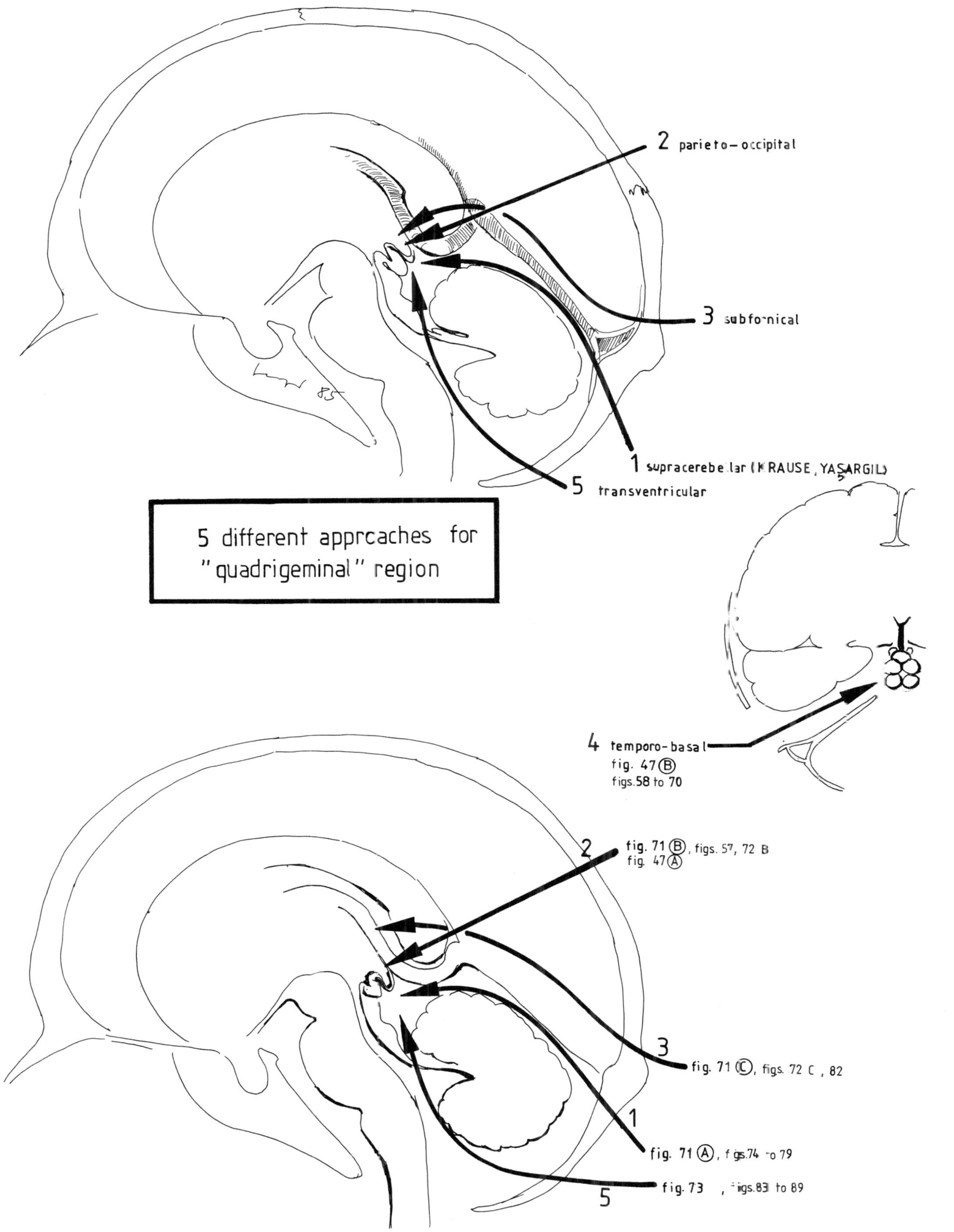

5 different apprcaches for "quadrigeminal" region

Fig. 47. Galenic AVM with typical location in the Fissura transversa cerebri
Usual approach parieto-occipital **A**
Here a variation was chosen as an example, which allowed a different angle of vision on the angioma. Via approaches **A** and **B** the operative steps are the same. This example shown here is didactically better, because in this case due to widening of the subdural space, the vision from the atypical approach **B** was better

variation : combination
galenic AMV + subdural hygroma

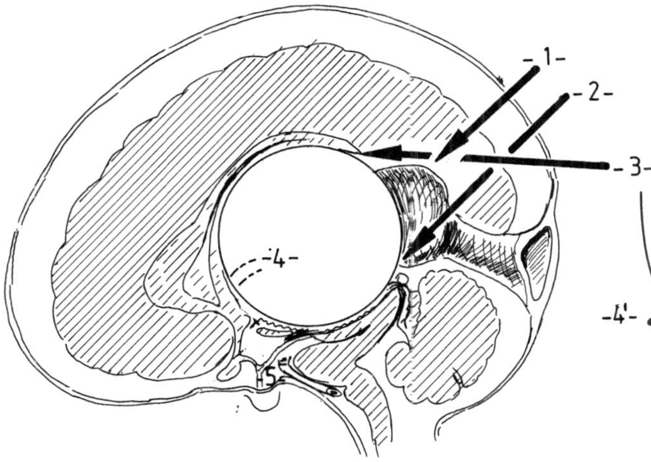

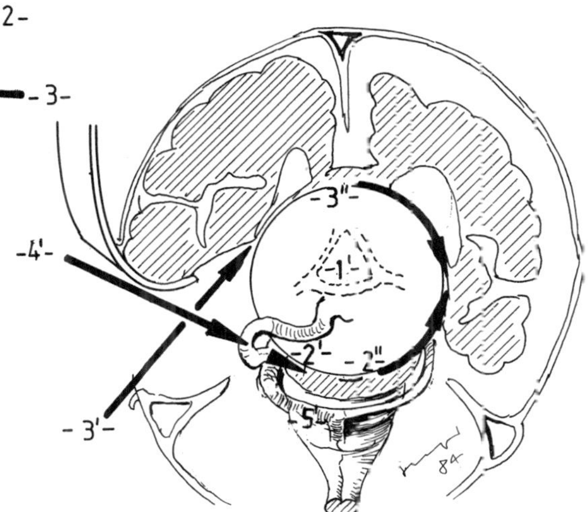

Ⓐ parieto-occipital approach

temporo-basal approach Ⓑ

favorable:

- draining veins less problematic -1-
- bilateral approach to floor -2- and roof -3- of Fissura transversa

- location of feeding artery -4'- and bifurcation of A.basil. -5'-
- right side approach to floor -2'- and roof -3'- of Fissura transversa

unfavorable:

- location of feeding artery -4-
- location of bifurcation of A.basilaris -5-

- left side approach to floor -2" - and roof -3"- of Fissura transversa
- location of draining veins -1'-

Fig. 48. Anatomical position of the Fissura transversa cerebri. There is a smooth limited capillary narrow CSF space. **The Fissura transversa cerebri is the part of the outer CSF space whose deep situation between the dorsal brainstem (Tela chorioidea of the 3rd ventricle) and the cerebrum (floor structures of the lateral ventricles = Fornices) is difficult to localize.** The anatomically inexperienced would mistake this structure for a part of the ventricular system. Hence the detailed exposure of the morphology of this region

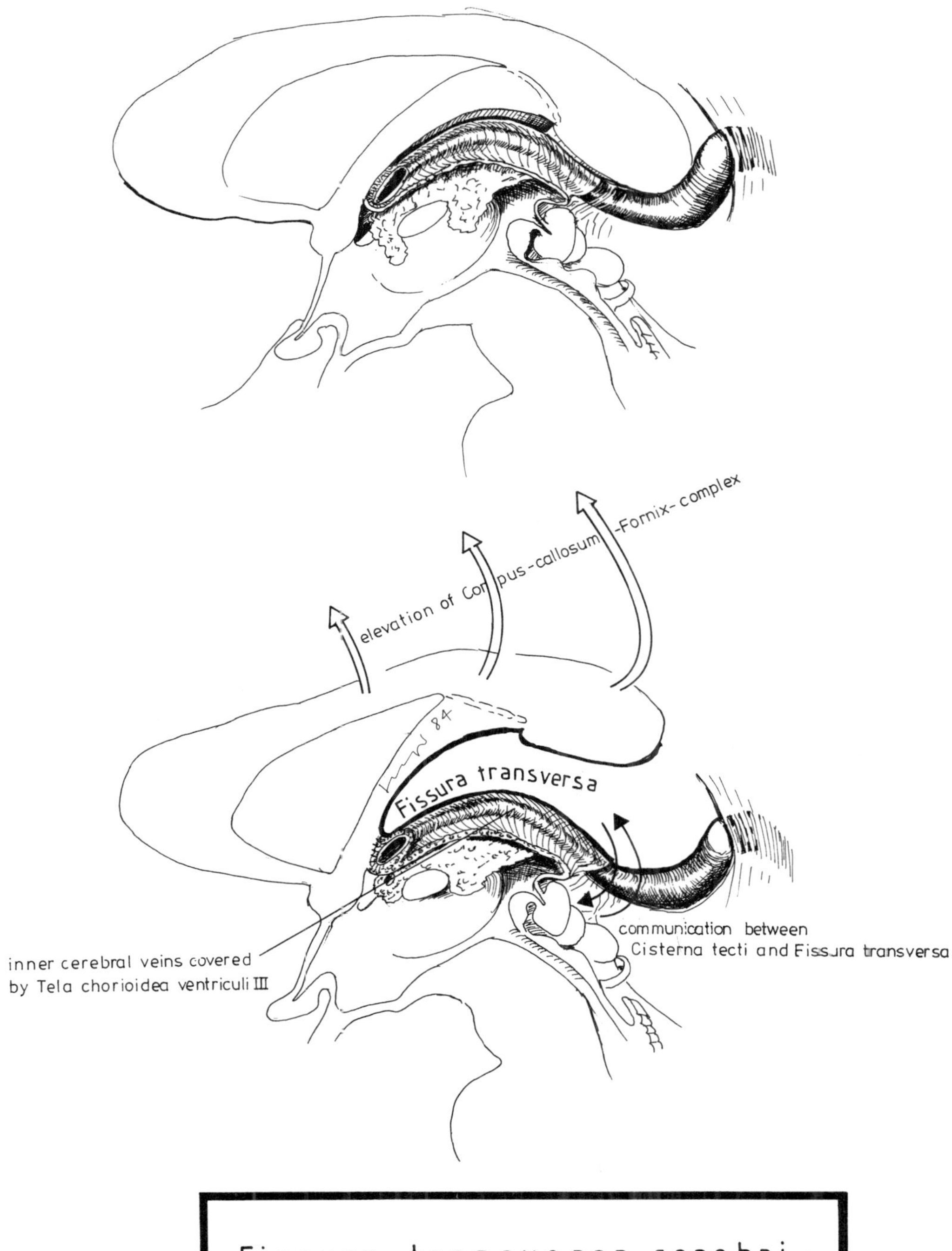

Fissura transversa cerebri :
location of galenic AVM

Fig. 49. The av-angioma is fed by a large feeding artery, usually with some additional small arteries. All feeding arteries derive from choroid group. The draining vein is the V. magna Galeni which dilates. At the early stage the Vv. cerebri intt. are still there. The dilatation of the V. Galeni is first limited to the region below the Splenium corporis callosi. **The aneurysmatic expansion of the Galenic AV-angioma starts in the posterior part of the Fissura transversa**

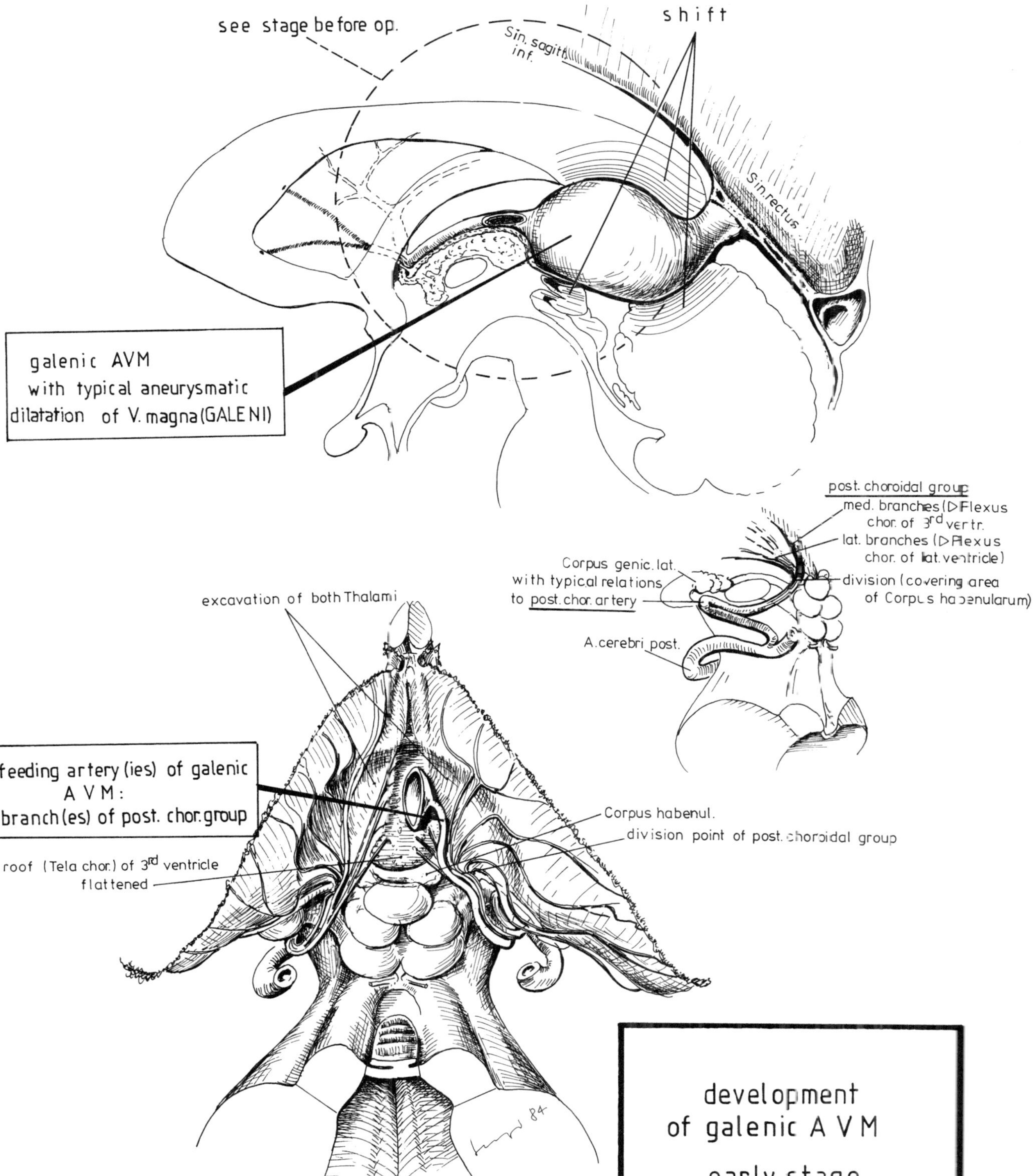

development
of galenic A V M
- early stage -

Fig. 50. Late stage: the galenic AVM fills the entire Fissura transversa and the Cisterna tecti resulting in compression of the brainstem and rostral part of the cerebellum
Without displacement only the **Galenic point** remains in the same place
(Galenic point: entry point of the V. magna Galeni on the frontal border of the Falx/Tentorium). **Site of** the most important **feeding artery**

FIG. 50

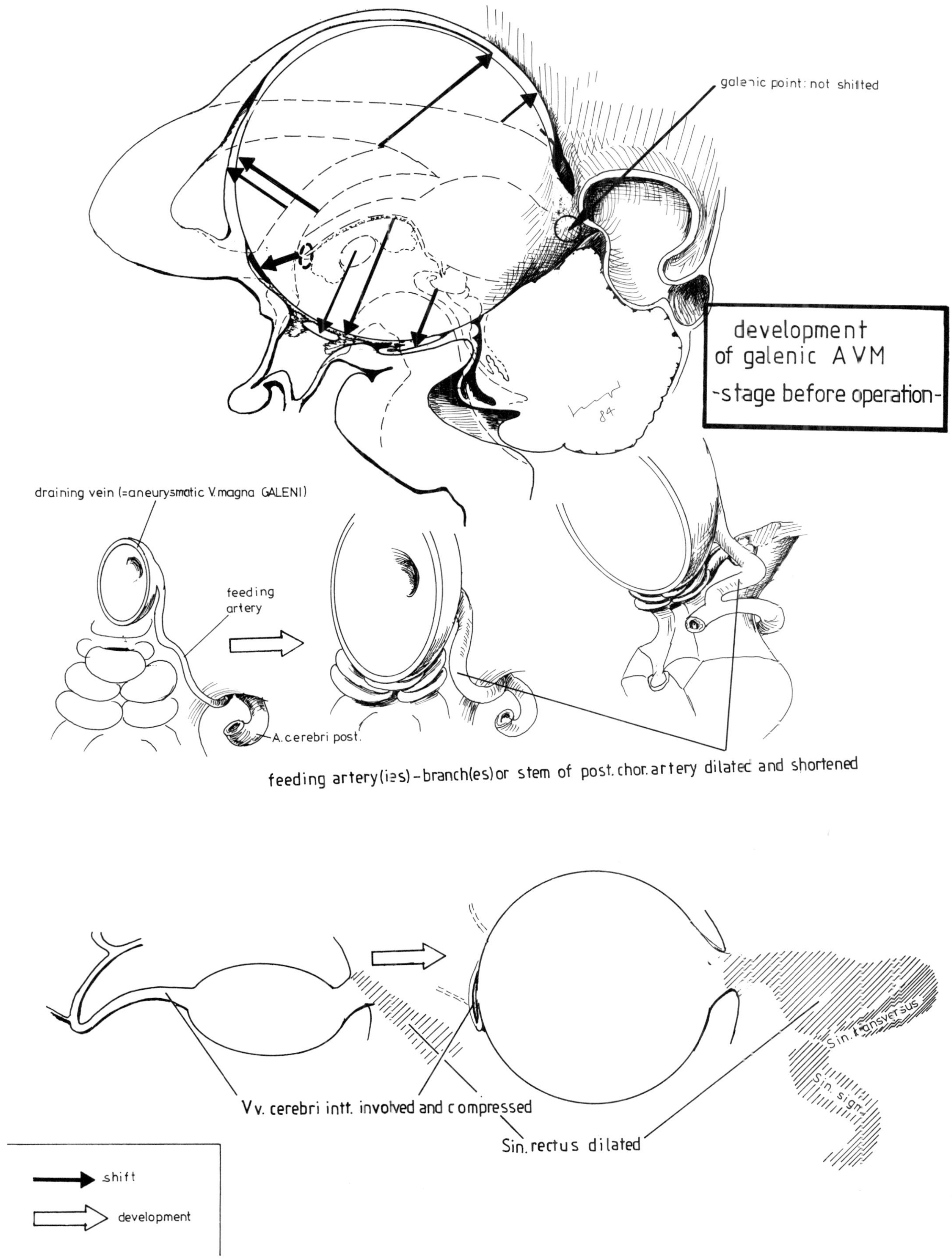

galenic point: not shifted
development of galenic AVM -stage before operation-
draining vein (=aneurysmatic V. magna GALENI)
feeding artery
A. cerebri post.
feeding artery(ies) - branch(es) or stem of post. chor. artery dilated and shortened
Sin. transversus
Sin. sign.
Vv. cerebri intt. involved and compressed
Sin. rectus dilated
shift
development

Fig. 51. AVM and ventricle system: Because the AVM lies basal from the lateral ventricles, a dorsal raising and lateral displacement of both lateral ventricles occurs. The basal and lateral displacement of the brainstem is understandable, when the relationship between the inferior horn and Tractus opticus is observed

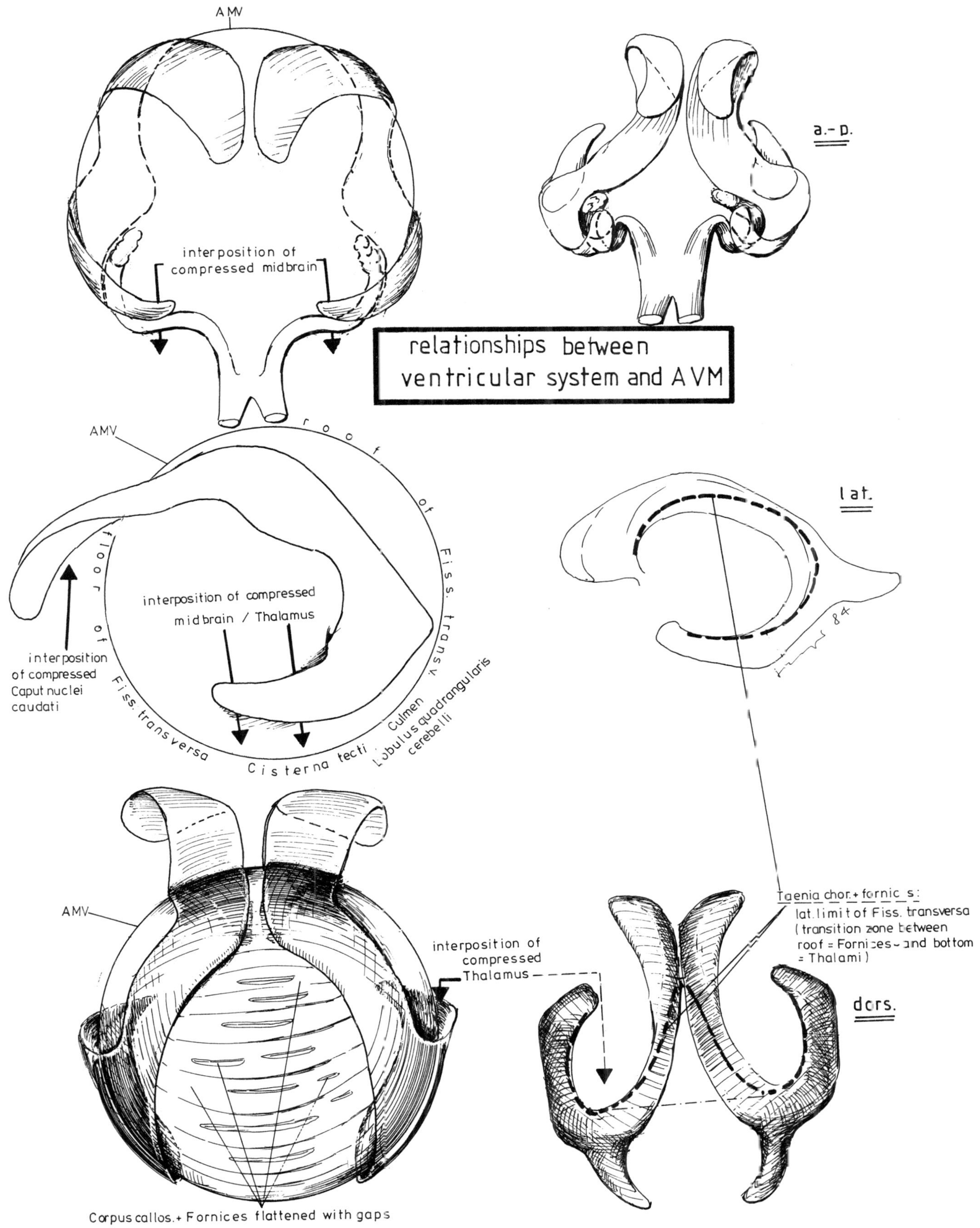
AMV
a.- p.
interposition of
compressed midbrain
relationships between
ventricular system and AVM
AMV
roof of Fiss. transv.
floor of Fiss. transversa
interposition of compressed
midbrain / Thalamus
interposition
of compressed
Caput nuclei
caudati
Cisterna tecti
Culmen
Lobulus quadrangularis
cerebelli
lat.
AMV
interposition of
compressed
Thalamus
Taenia chor.+ fornic s:
lat. limit of Fiss. transversa
(transition zone between
roof = Fornices - and bottom
= Thalami)
dors.
Corpus callos.+ Fornices flattened with gaps

Fig. 52. **Shift of the brainstem** (dashed lines) before and after compression of the brainstem due to the AVM

FIG. 52

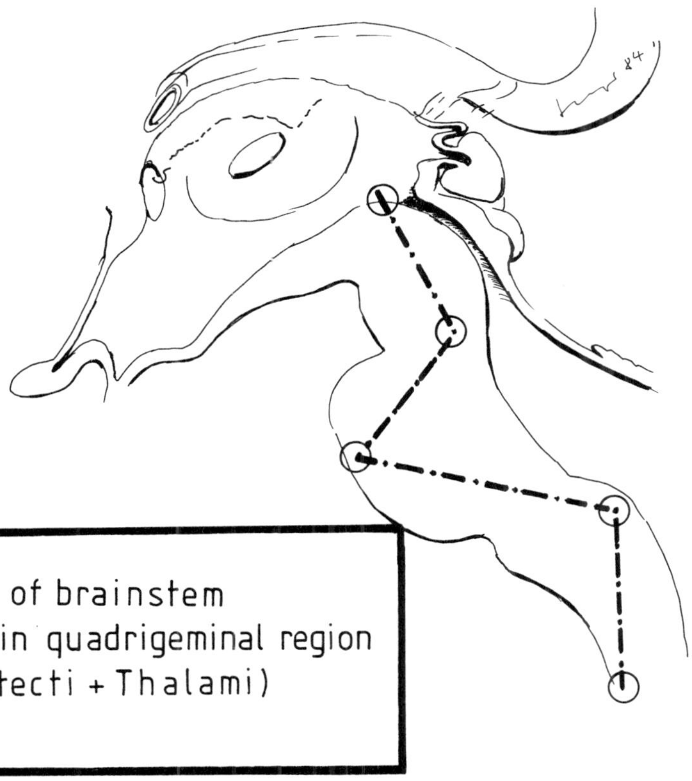
shift of brainstem
maximal in quadrigeminal region
(Lamina tecti + Thalami)

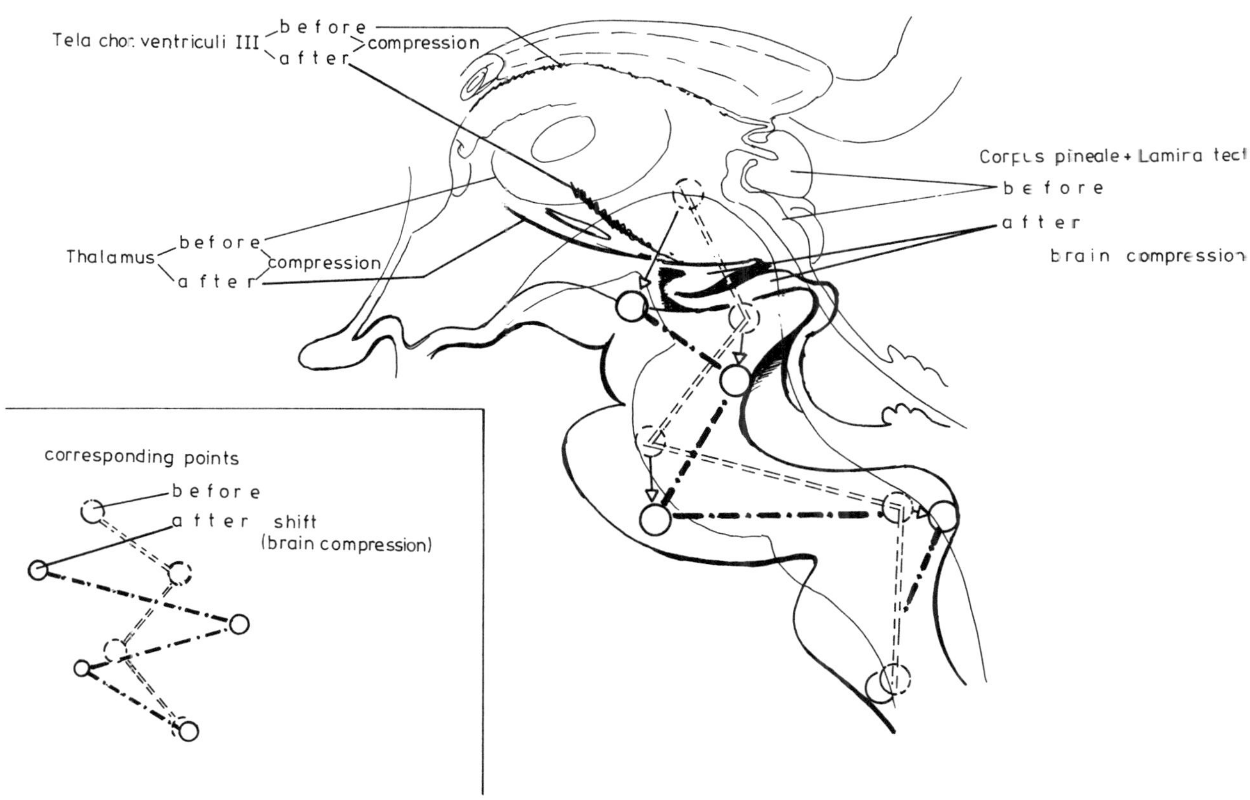
Tela cho: ventriculi III
before
after
compression
Corpus pineale + Lamina tecti
before
after
brain compression
Thalamus
before
after
compression
corresponding points
before
after shift
(brain compression)

Fig. 53. With the shift of the brainstem an accompanying **shift of the basal artery occurs**
The basal artery can normally extend deep into the operatively hardly accessible Fossa interpeduncularis. After an axial shift of the brainstem it moves deeper and is more easily accessible for operation

FIG. 53

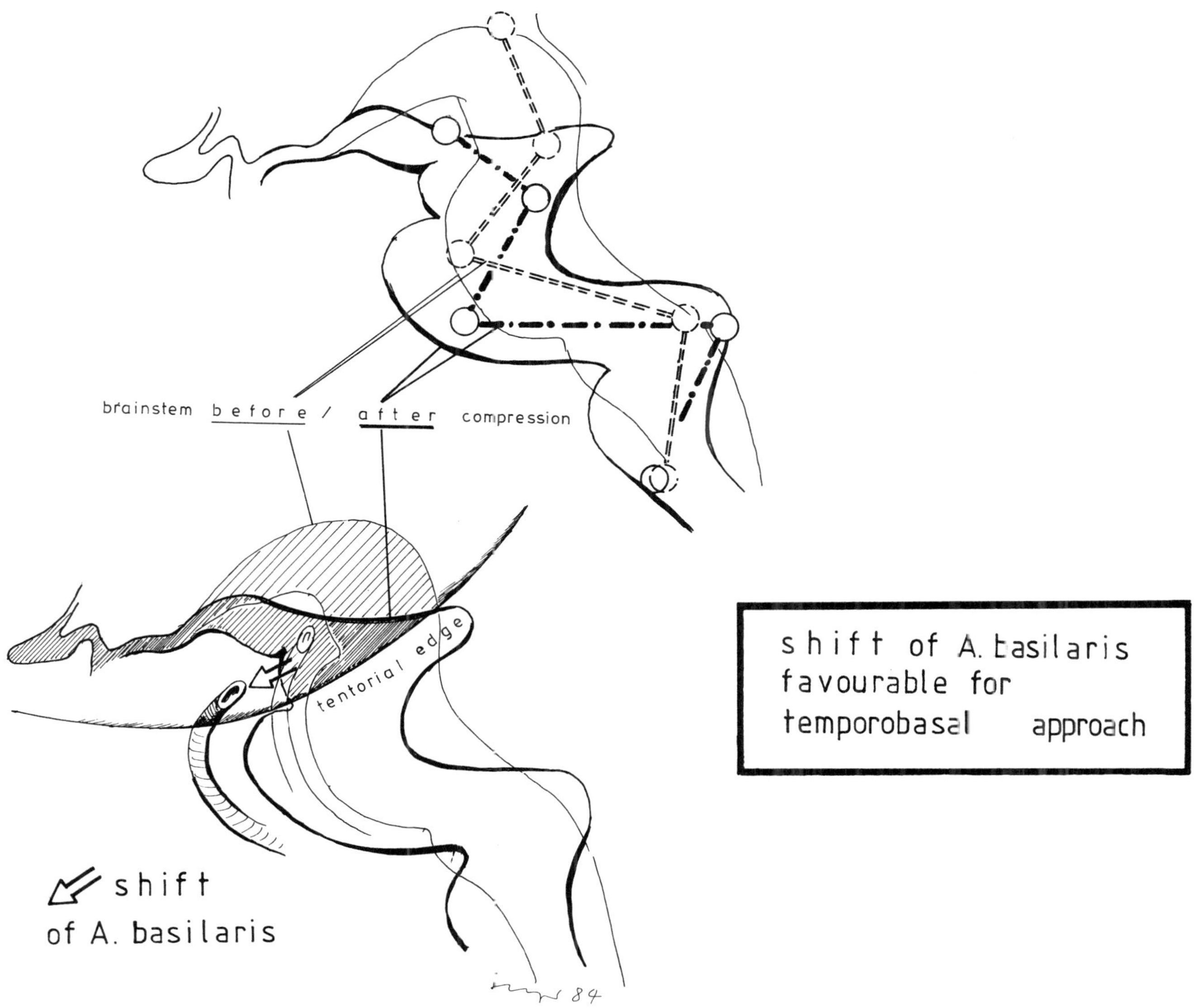
brainstem before / after compression
shift of A. basilaris favourable for temporobasal approach
tentorial edge
shift
of A. basilaris

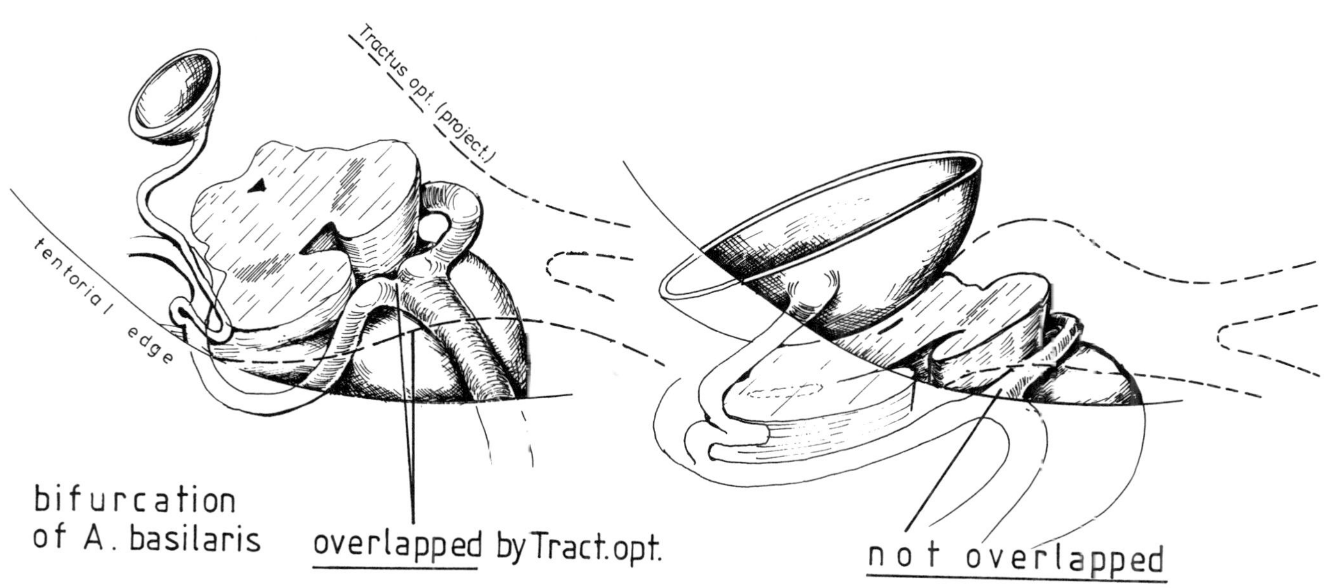
Tractus opt. (project.)
tentorial edge
bifurcation
of A. basilaris
overlapped by Tract.opt.
not overlapped

Fig. 54. AVM + Cisterna ambiens and Cornu inf.: With further enlargement of the AVM the Thalamus is not only compressed laterally but also in a rostral direction. Thereby the inferior horn and the Cisterna ambiens are shortened and the feeding artery is accessible both laterally and dorsally. As a landmark the Corpus geniculatum mediale – *gm* – is suitable. Normally it is only accessible for operation via the infratentorial approach, since it is overlapped laterally by the Tractus opticus and Pulvinar thalami. With a Galenic angioma it is squeezed out laterally and visible via the temporal approach. The Corpus geniculatum laterale, the end of the Tractus opticus, is even in the normal anatomical brain preparation difficult to distinguish, during the operation in the normal brain and in the presence of a Galenic AVM it is difficult to identify

For abbreviations – see upper part of picture.

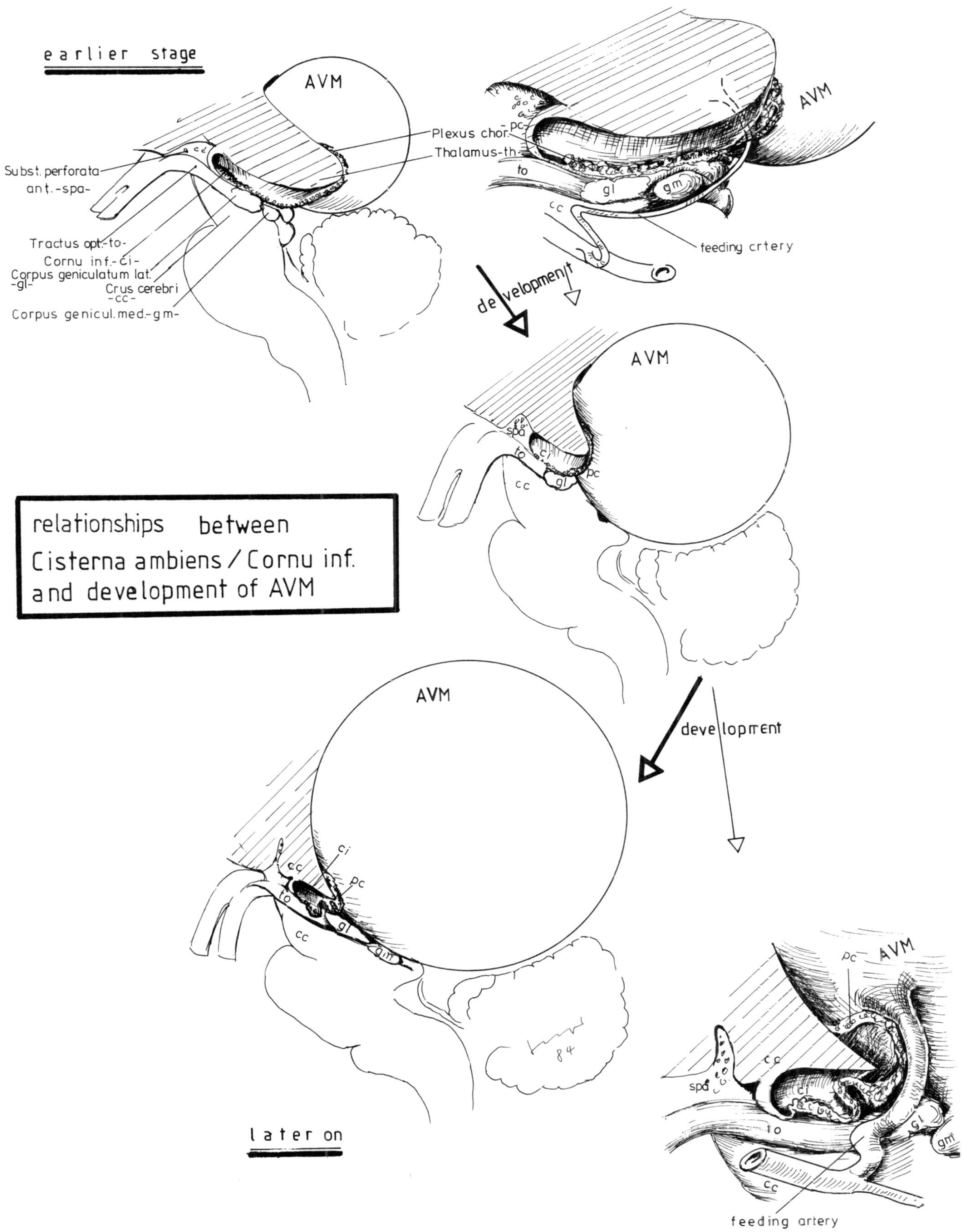
earlier stage
AVM
Subst. perforata ant.-spa-
Tractus opt.-to-
Cornu inf.-ci-
Corpus geniculatum lat. -gl-
Crus cerebri -cc-
Corpus genicul. med.-gm-
Plexus chor. pc
Thalamus-th
to
gl
gm
cc
feeding artery
development
AVM
spa
to
ci
cc
gl
pc
relationships between
Cisterna ambiens / Cornu inf.
and development of AVM
AVM
development
ci
cc
pc
to
gl
cc
gm
later on
pc
AVM
cc
spa
ci
to
gl
gm
cc
feeding artery

Fig. 55

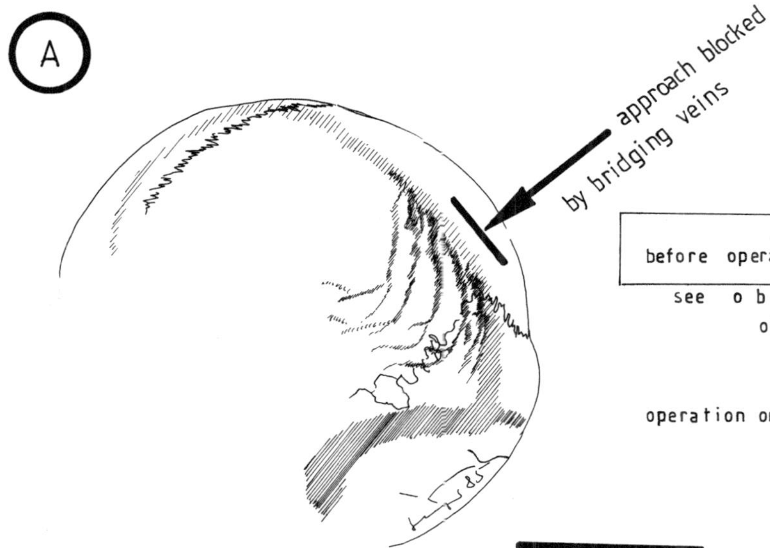

before operation :

see o b l i q u e presentation of angiogram

operation on the side without blocking veins

1st step

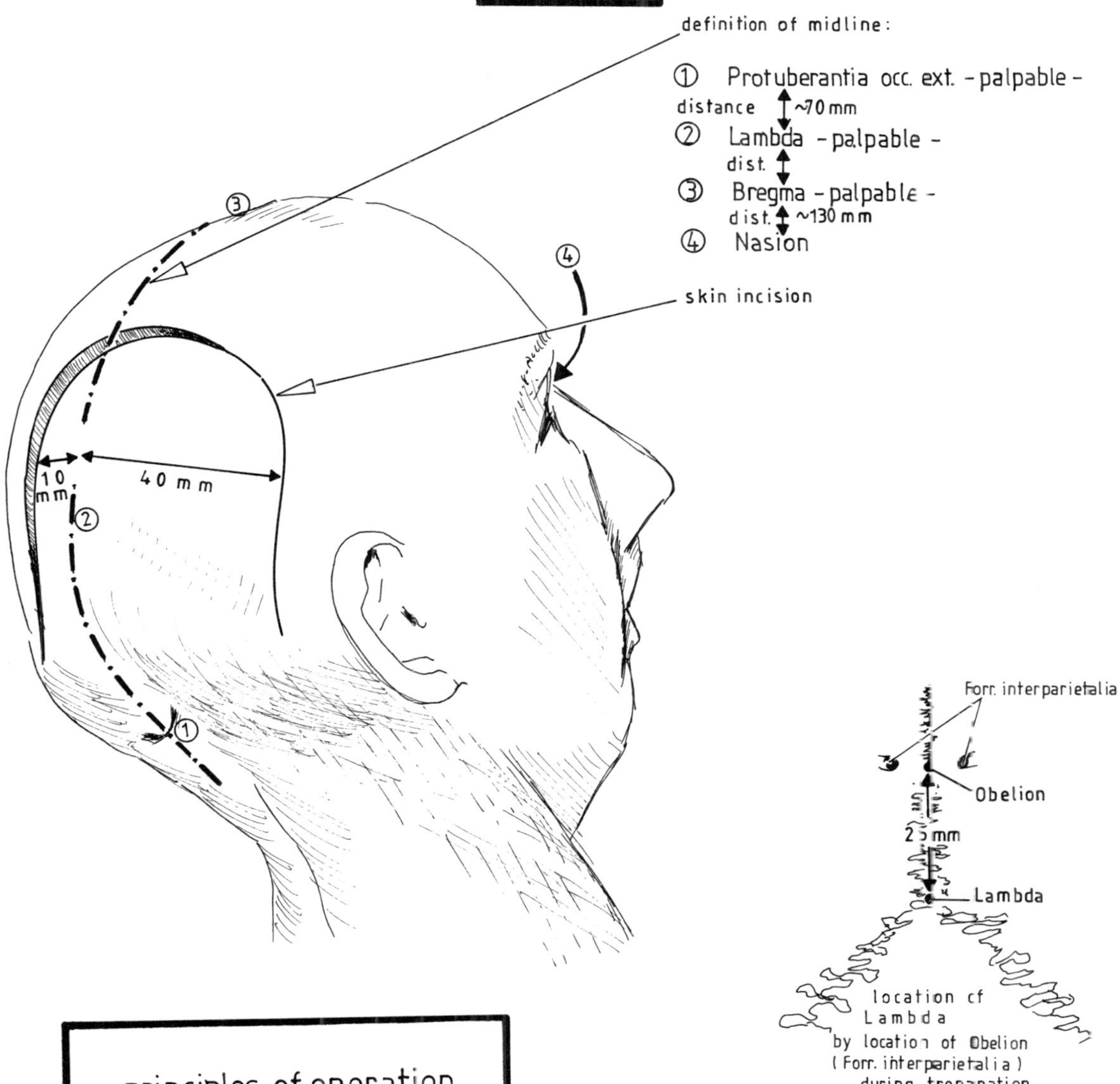

principles of operation

Fig. 56

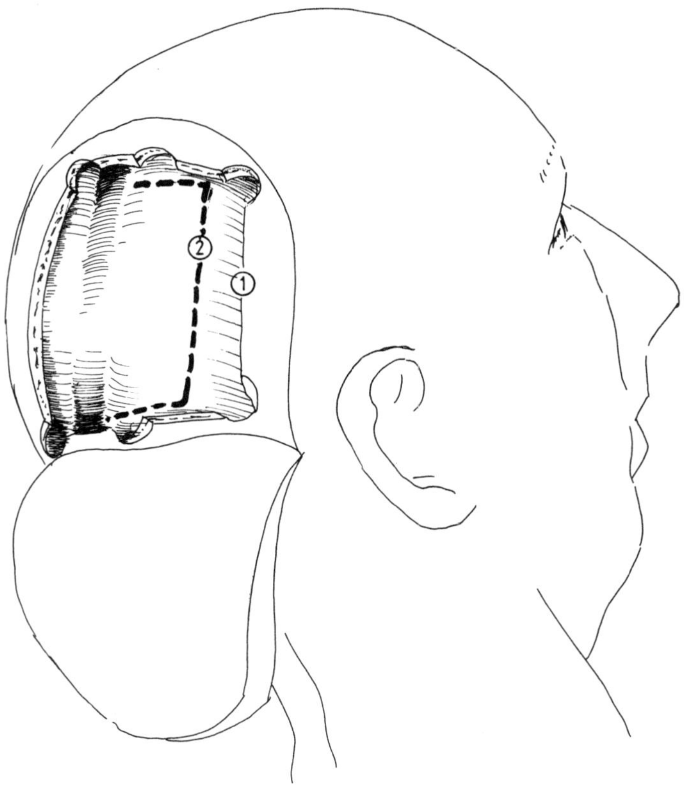

2nd step

① trepanation

② Dura incision

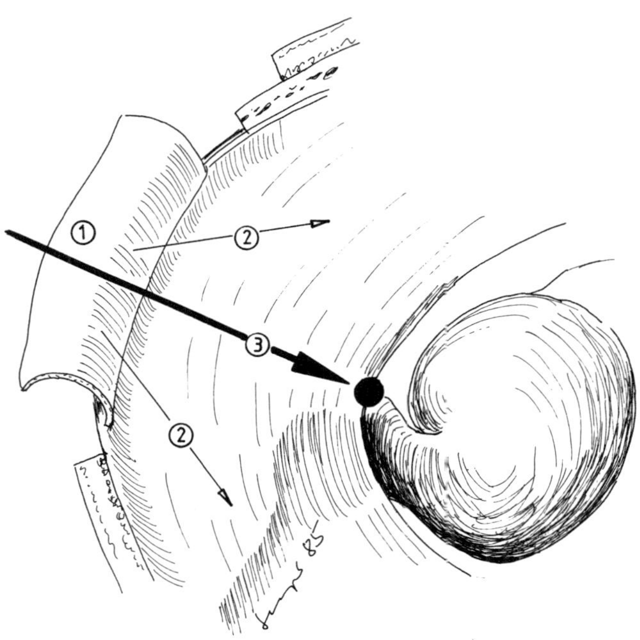

3rd step

① eversion of Dura flap

② dissecting Arachnoidea in Sulcus (Fiss.) long i.

③ location of galenic point (~ post. part of AVM)

following steps see approach (B)
1st to last step

Fig. 57. Clinical example of a Galenic AVM. Six years ago two operations in another hospital, with interruption of three feeding arteries originating from the right posterior cerebral artery. A postoperatively right-sided oculomotor paresis which later disappeared. Following some increase in size another operation was indicated (and performed by Prof. Dr. J. Gilsbach, coworker of the author). Straight after the operation paresis of ocular movement upwards and right oculomotor paresis. Deficits later improved. The microsurgical topography shows the situation after clipping of the main feeding artery, just before sectioning of the feeding artery and extirpation of the completely isolated AVM

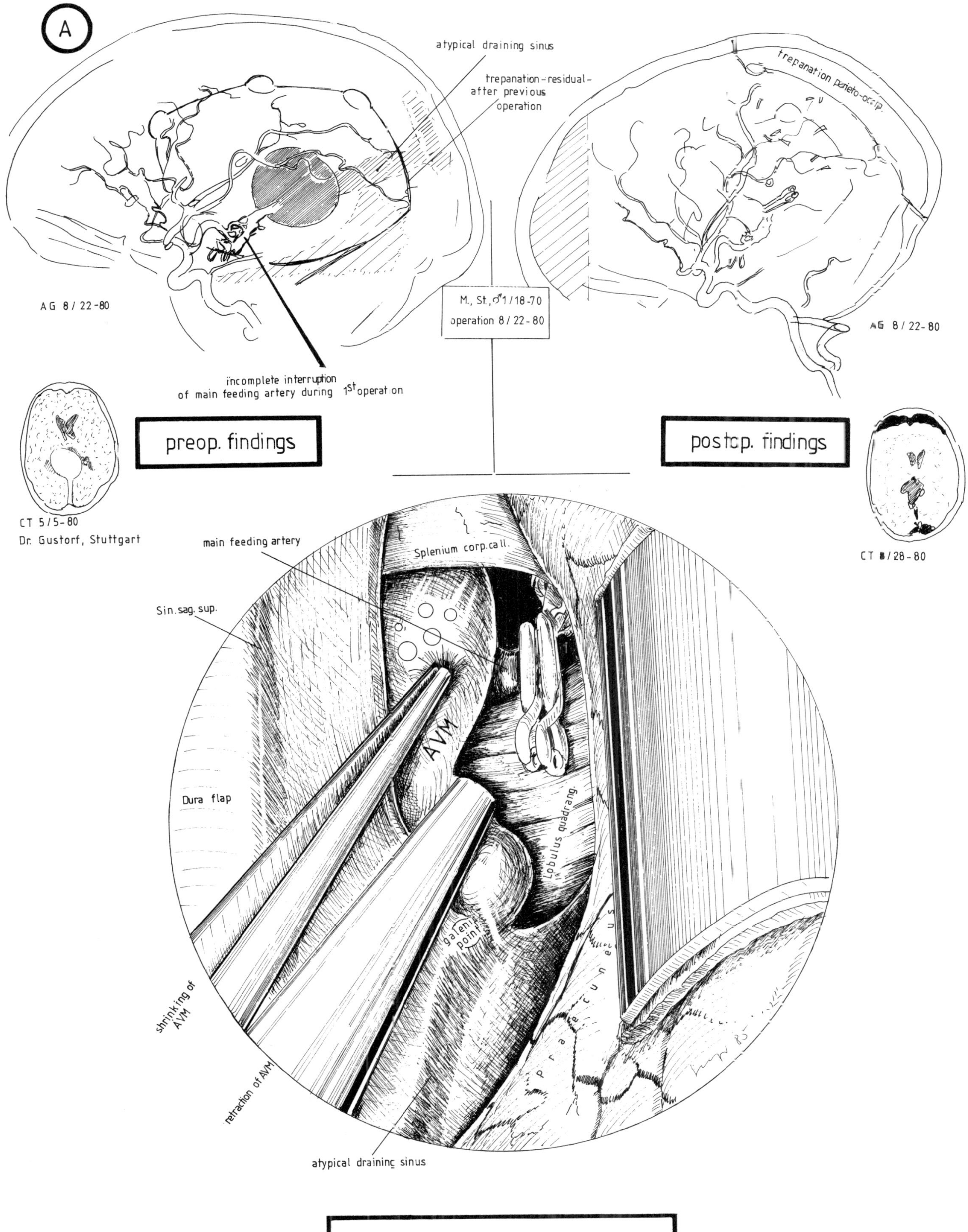

microsurgical topography

Fig. 58. Up until surgery a 10-month-old child had a considerably retarded psychic and motor functional development with a head cirumference of 52 cm and a right hemiparesis. In the prone position the head was only briefly lifted. Immediately postoperatively the child was awake with no further deficits. Recovery was rapid after the operation. During a follow-up period of 4 years no seizures and recovered psychic development. He seems still retarded with unsteady fine motor function, somewhat atactic gait, standing on one foot, hopping and walking on heels not possible, and a slight convergent strabismus. Sometimes shunt problems

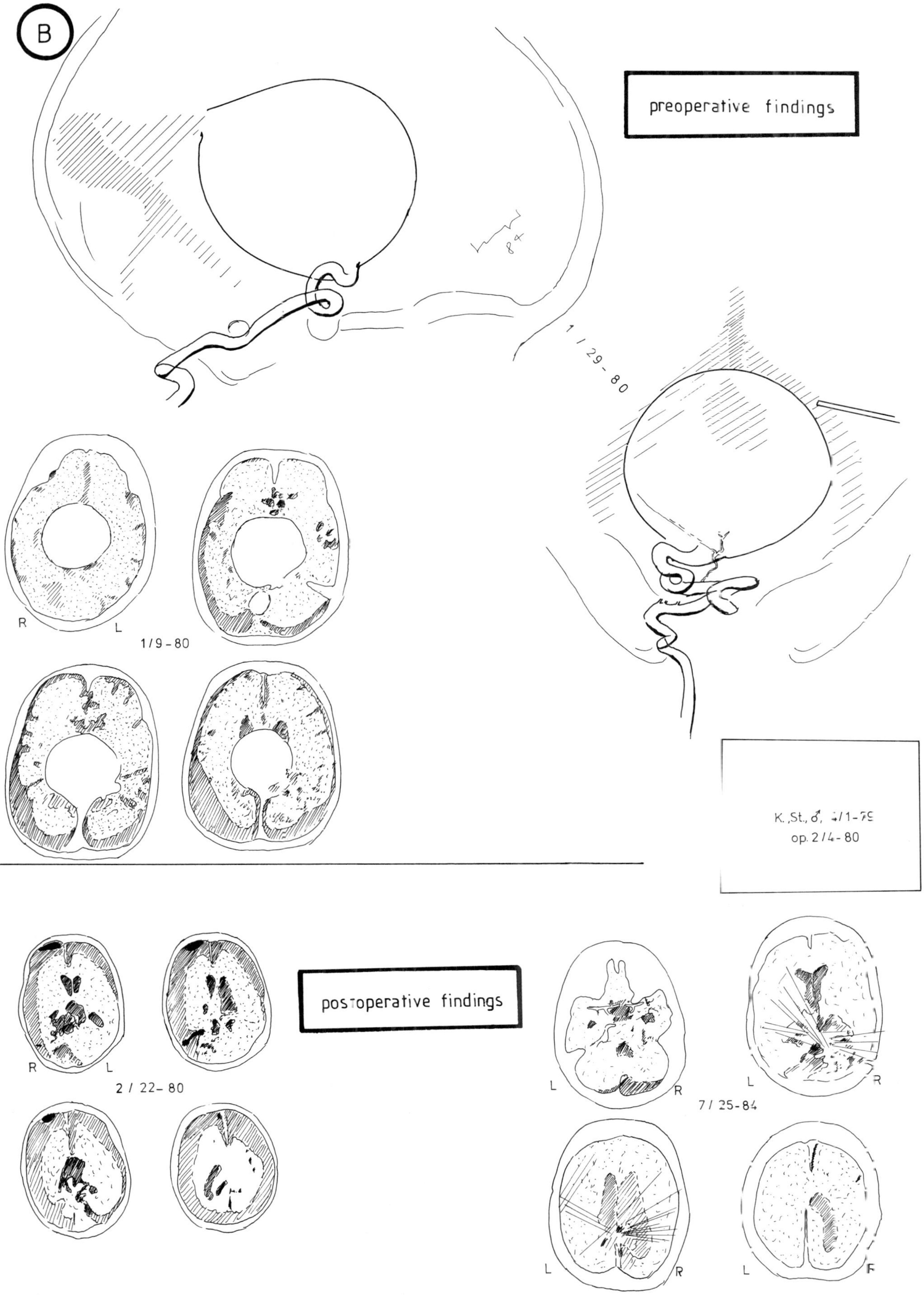
B
preoperative findings
1 / 29 - 80
R
L
1/9 - 80
K.,St.,♂, 4/1-79
op. 2/4 - 80
postoperative findings
R
L
2 / 22 - 80
L
R
7/ 25 - 84
L
R
L
R

Fig. 59. Principles of operation:
1st and 2nd steps: in contrast to tumor operations the arachnoidal layer, which covers the pathologic process, is removed. Thus, when operating a Galenic AVM, brain tissue is protected by two arachnoidal layers:
– the arachnoid of the AVM and the arachnoidal wall of the cistern
3rd step: after temporary clipping of the feeding artery the angioma is considerably shrunk by electrocoagulation because the pressure in the angioma is greatly reduced. However, opening of the angioma is not indicated as it would further bleed from small vessels nearby

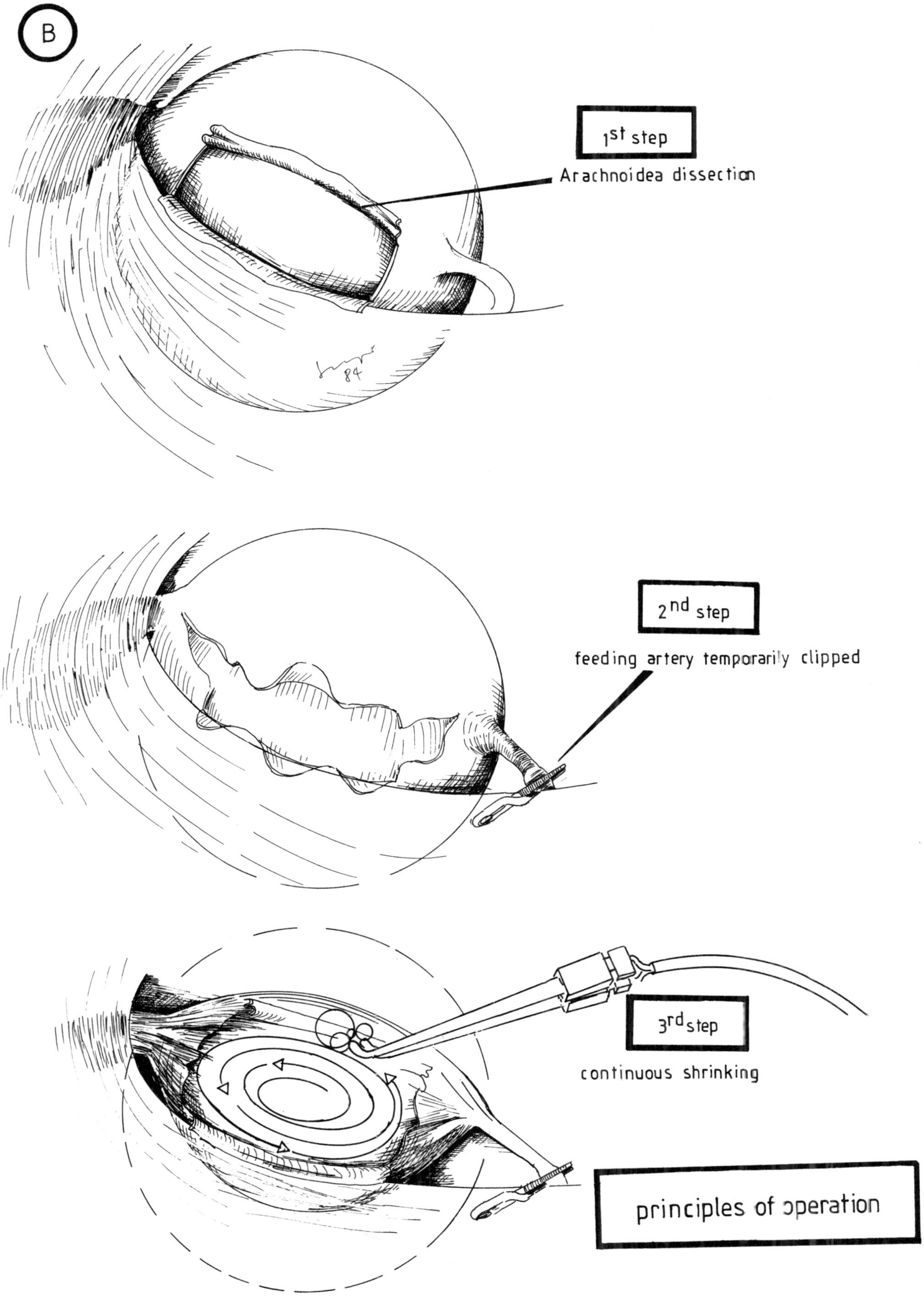
B
1st step
Arachnoidea dissection
2nd step
feeding artery temporarily clipped
3rd step
continuous shrinking
principles of operation

Fig. 60. **4th–8th steps:**
after clipping and cutting of the feeding artery the angioma is shrunk from rostral to occipital. Only then the circular preparation of the AVM is possible at the Galenic point.
By the parieto-occipital midline approach the Galenic point is nearer, but just as difficult to prepare. Some authors recommend a fenestration of the Falx. This can only be done close to the region of the V. magna Galeni, and not via the Fornix (further rostrally), so as to preserve the limbic system and prevent serious psychic damage. The interruption of small feeding vessels is easy, in constrast to other typical angiomas in other locations
Preserving the arachnoidea freed from the AV-angioma: the CSF spaces remain as intact as possible

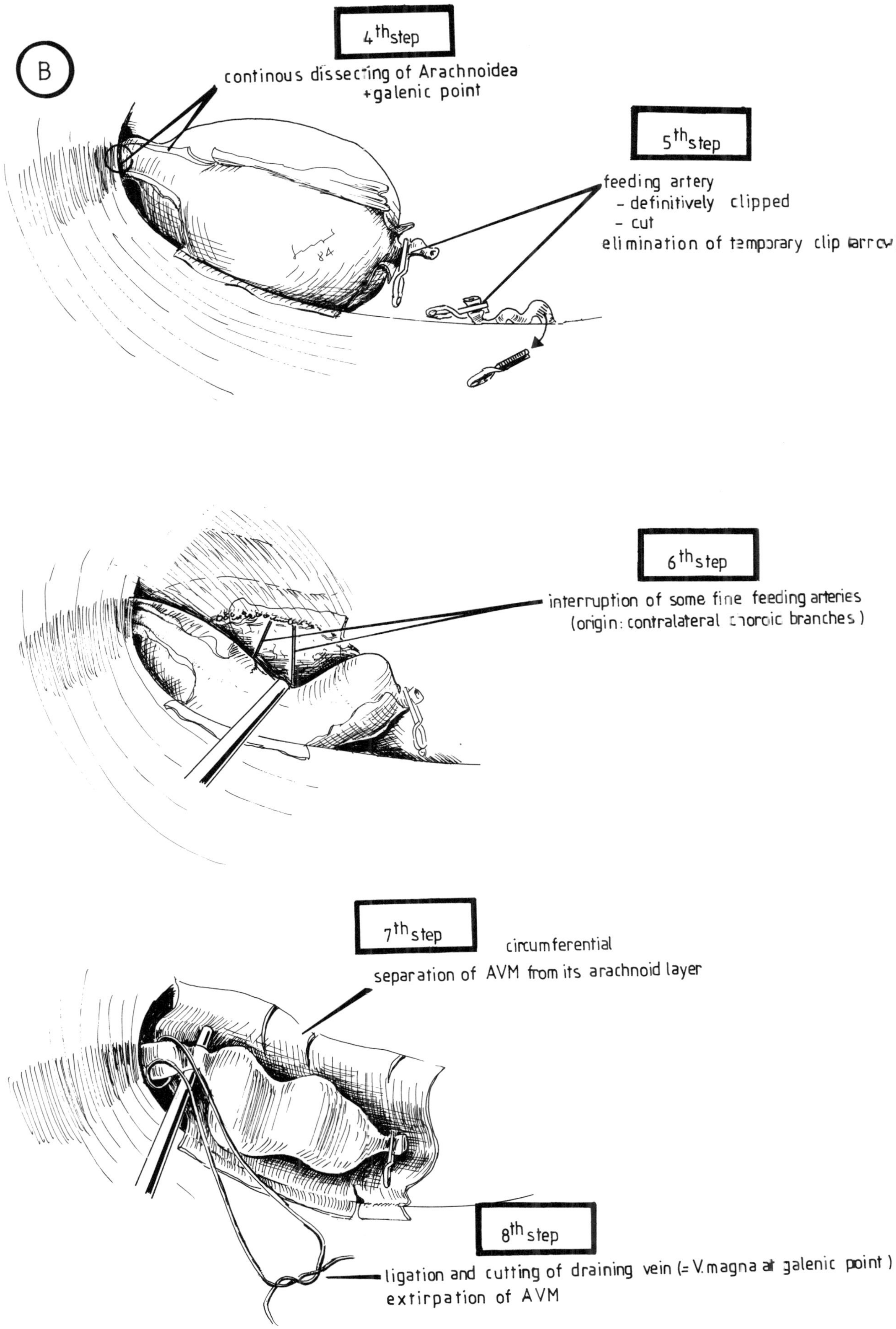
B
4th step
continous dissecting of Arachnoidea +galenic point
5th step
feeding artery
- definitively clipped
- cut
elimination of temporary clip (arrow)
6th step
interruption of some fine feeding arteries (origin: contralateral choroic branches)
7th step
circumferential separation of AVM from its arachnoid layer
8th step
ligation and cutting of draining vein (= V.magna at galenic point)
extirpation of AVM

Fig. 61. Operation: essential is the approach over the tentorium as far basal as possible. Described is the atypical approach **B.** For comparison the typical approach **A** is shown below. With **A** there are problems with the sinus and bridging veins, which have been already exposed in detail *

* See Seeger, W., Microsurgery of Cerebral Veins. Wien–New York: Springer. 1984.

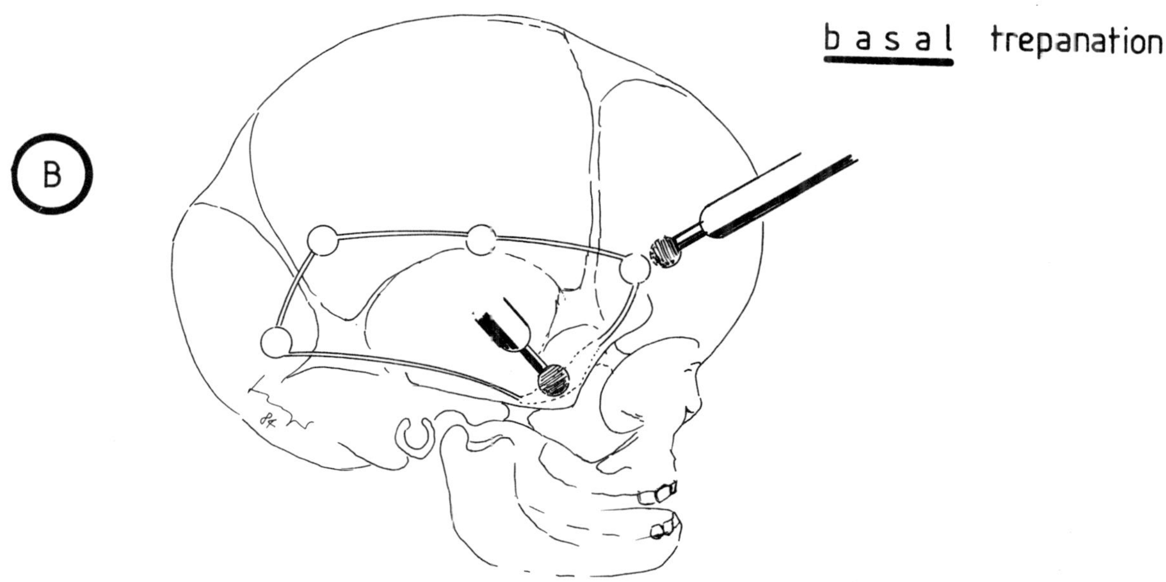
b a s a l trepanation
B

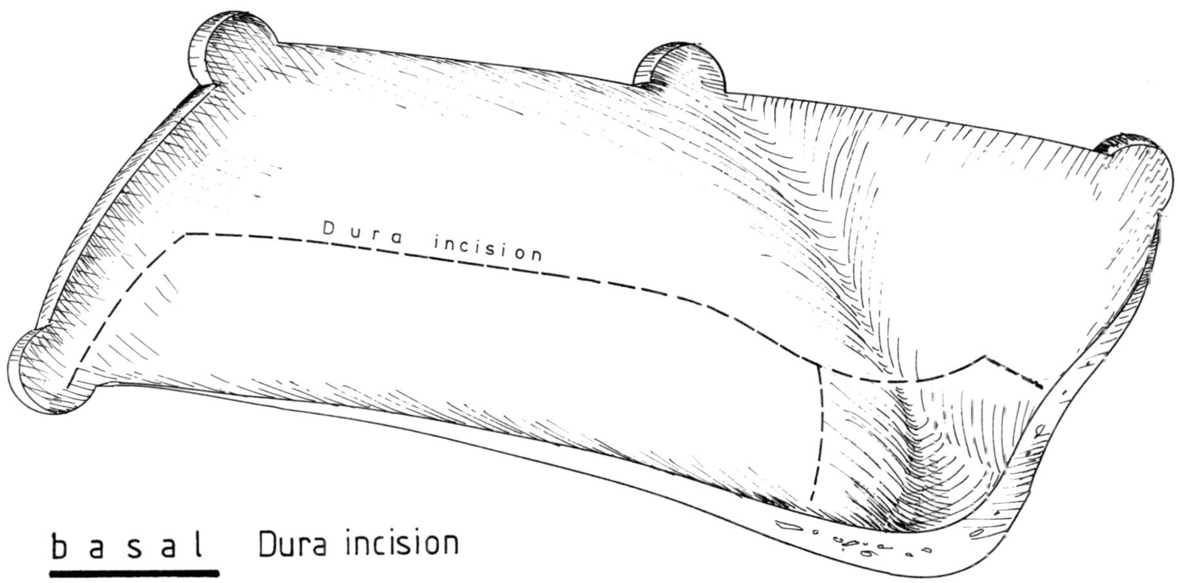
Dura incision
b a s a l Dura incision

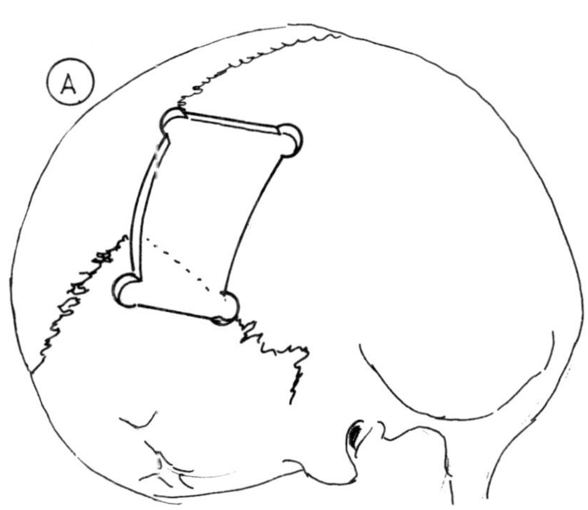
A

Fig. 62. Preservation of the temporo-basal veins as far as possible. The more extensive the trepanation towards the base, the better the basal cerebral veins can be preserved which are stretched from the base to the tentorium

FIG. 62

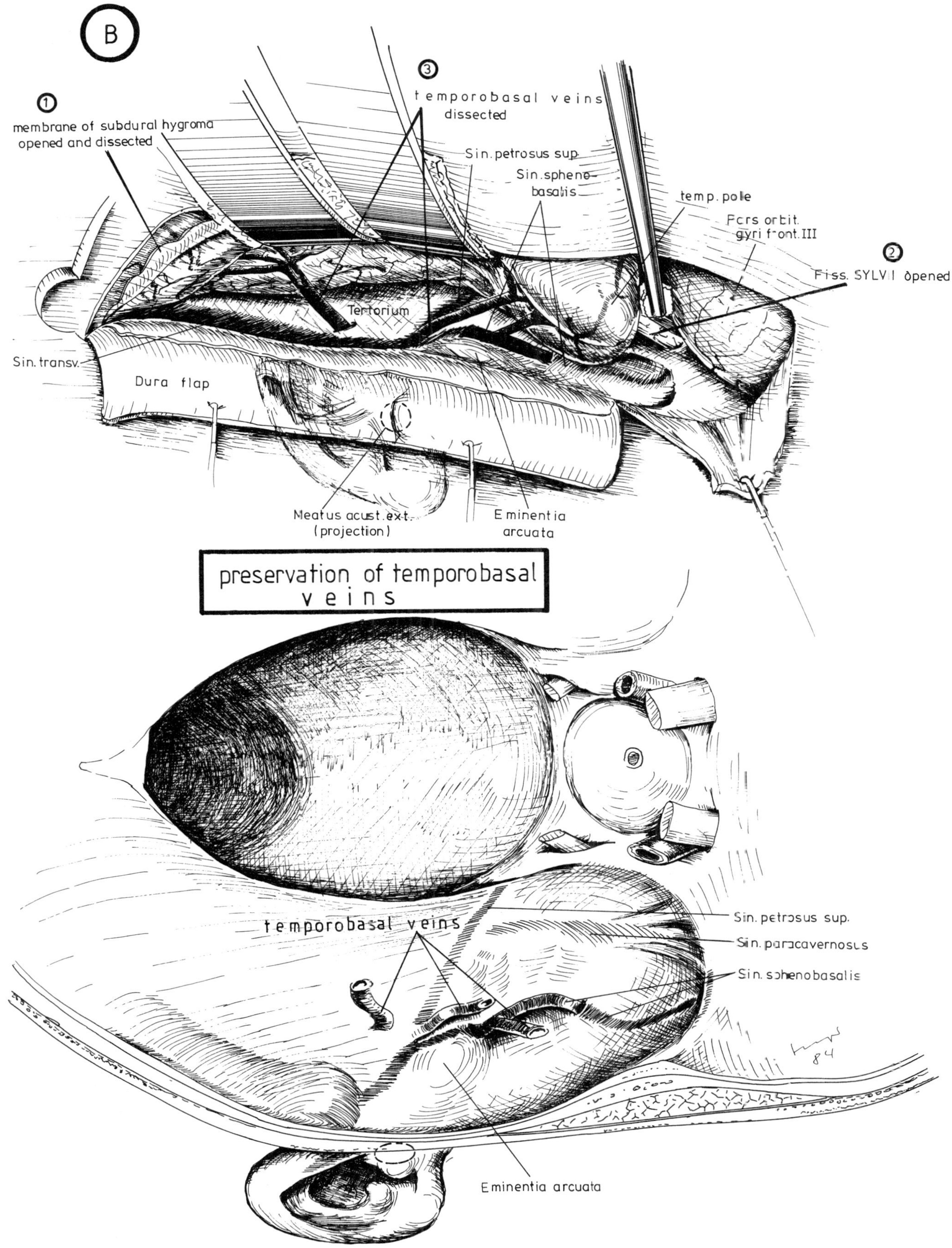
B
① membrane of subdural hygroma opened and dissected
③ temporobasal veins dissected
Sin. petrosus sup.
Sin. sphenobasalis
temp. pole
Pars orbit. gyri front. III
② Fiss. SYLVII opened
Tentorium
Sin. transv.
Dura flap
Meatus acust. ext. (projection)
Eminentia arcuata
preservation of temporobasal veins
temporobasal veins
Sin. petrosus sup.
Sin. paracavernosus
Sin. sphenobasalis
Eminentia arcuata

Fig. 63. **1st step:** the wall of the AVM is smoothly limited. The deepest arachnoidal layer covering the AVM is easily removed (which distinguishes it from tumorous arachnoidea). The fornix and thalamus are well protected when one succeeds in freeing the AVM from its arachnoidal capsule and pushing the capsule against the neighbouring structures. This is the result of the anatomical situation (see the accompanying sketches)

FIG. 63

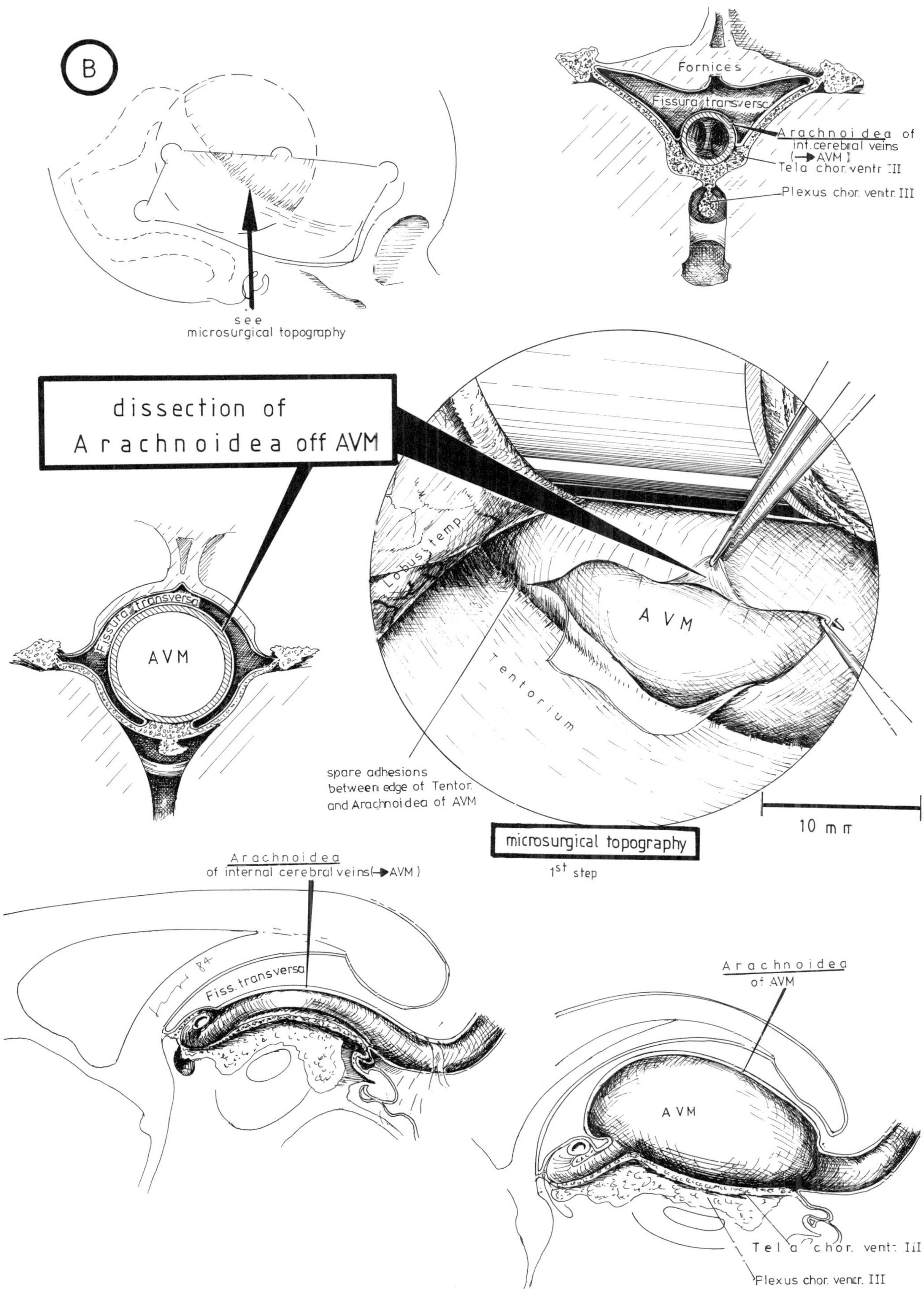

B
see
microsurgical topography
Fornices
Fissura transversa
Arachnoidea of
int. cerebral veins
(→AVM)
Tela chor. ventr. III
Plexus chor. ventr. III
dissection of
Arachnoidea off AVM
Fissura transversa
AVM
Lobus temp.
AVM
Tentorium
spare adhesions
between edge of Tentor.
and Arachnoidea of AVM
10 mm
microsurgical topography
1st step
Arachnoidea
of internal cerebral veins (→AVM)
Fiss. transversa
Arachnoidea
of AVM
AVM
Tela chor. ventr. III
Plexus chor. ventr. III

Fig. 64. **2nd step:** due to its dorsolateral location to the thalamus the feeding artery is better accessible via the temporo-basal approach than the parieto-occipital **A**

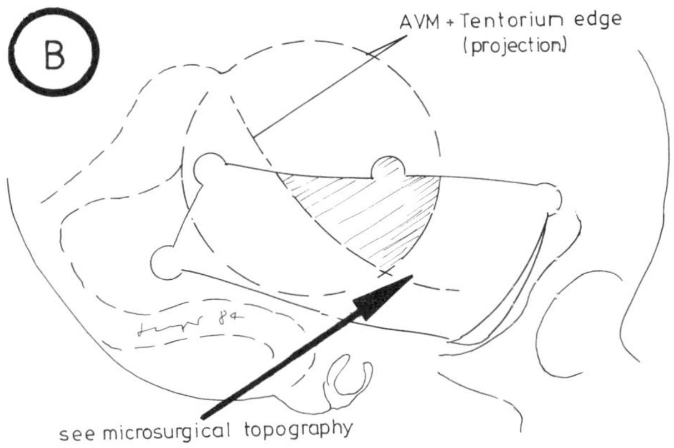

temporary clipping of feeding artery

10 mm

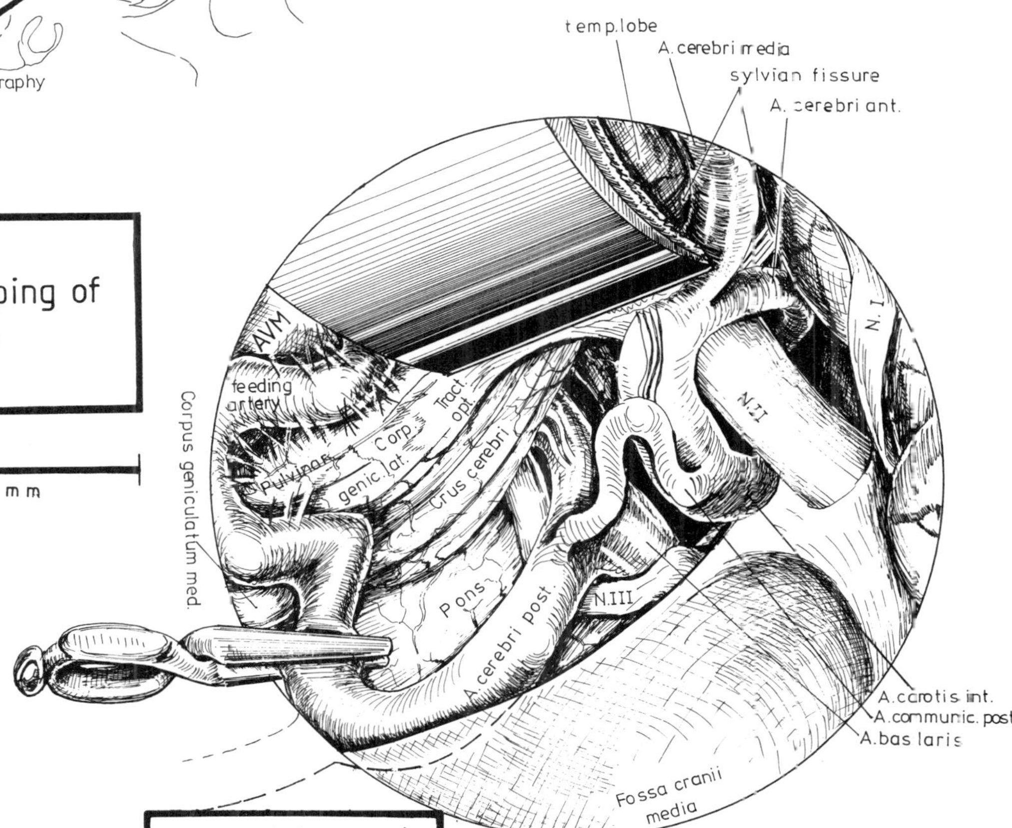

microsurgical topography

2nd step

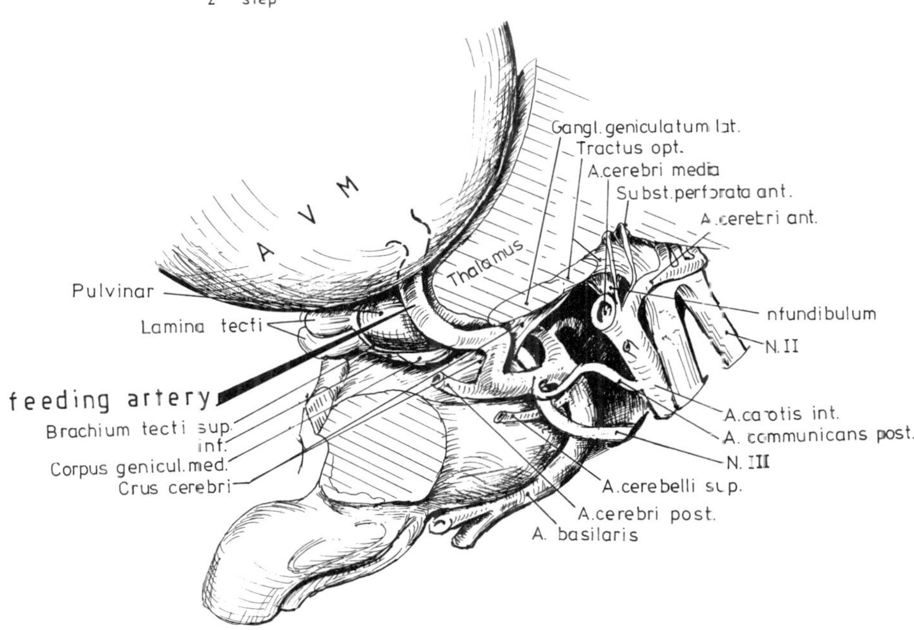

Fig. 65. **3rd and 4th steps:** as soon as the feeding artery is clipped the continuation of the operation is easier: after clipping of the artery the pressure in the angioma sinks. With electrocoagulation the angioma shrinks considerably

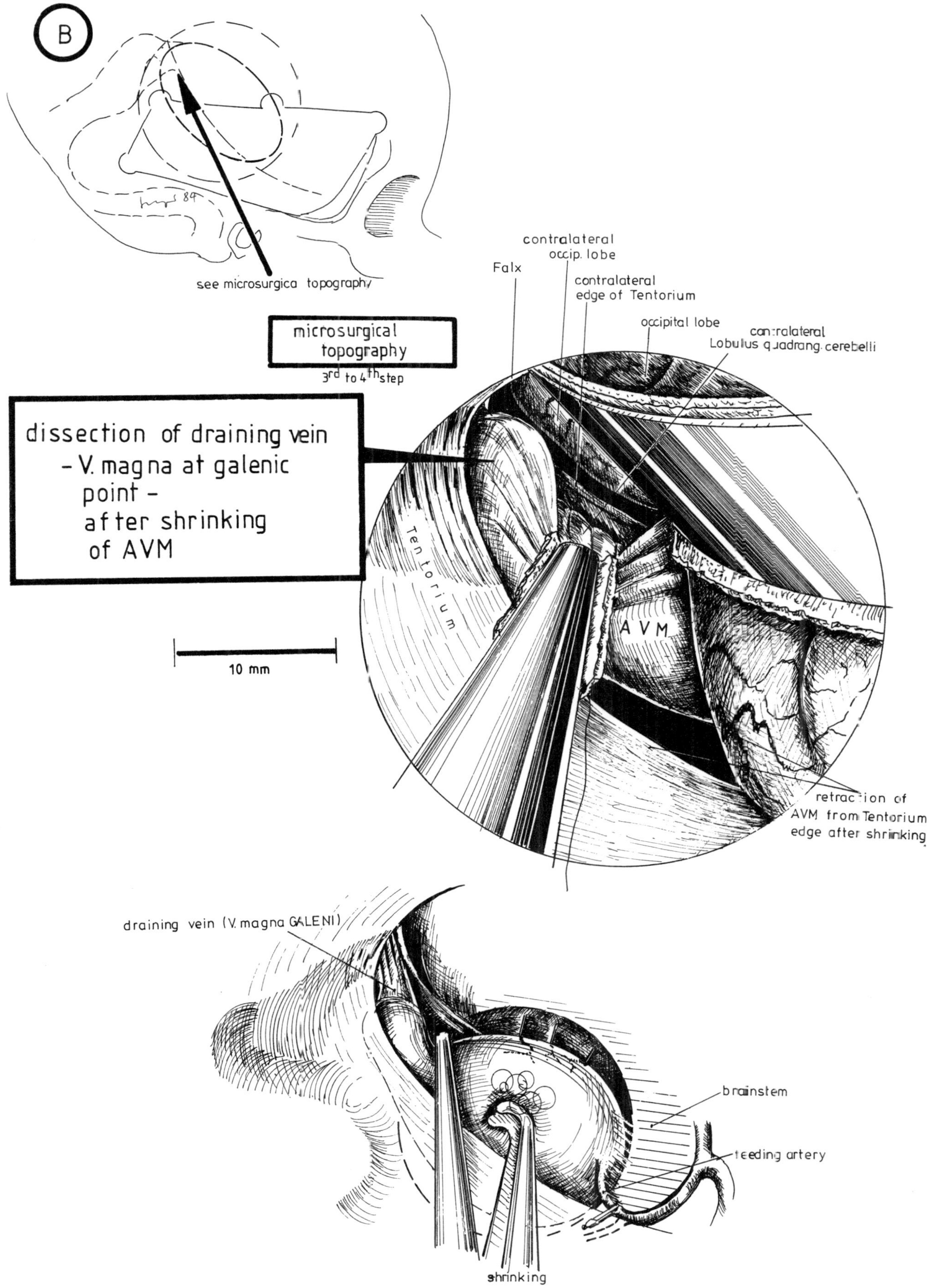
B
see microsurgica topography
microsurgical topography
3rd to 4th step
dissection of draining vein - V. magna at galenic point - after shrinking of AVM
10 mm
contralateral occip. lobe
Falx
contralateral edge of Tentorium
occipital lobe
contralateral Lobulus quadrang. cerebelli
Tentorium
AVM
retraction of AVM from Tentorium edge after shrinking
draining vein (V. magna GALENI)
brainstem
feeding artery
shrinking

Fig. 66. After decrease of pressure in the AVM more CSF can be lost. Sucking away of CSF leads to a sinking back of the brain and blood flow disturbances, which after refilling of the CSF space with Ringer solution quickly improves

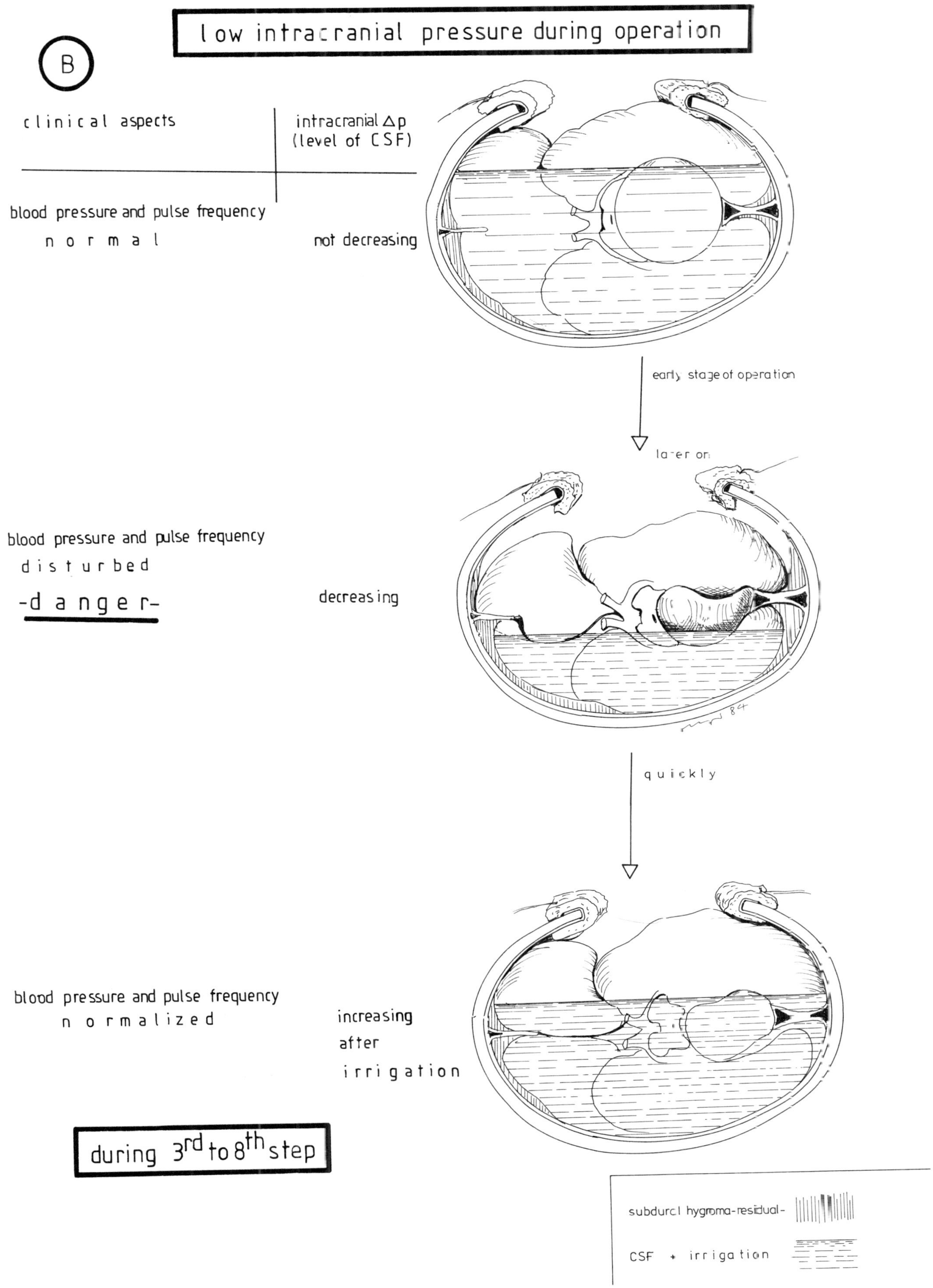
low intracranial pressure during operation
B
clinical aspects
intracranial Δp
(level of CSF)
blood pressure and pulse frequency
normal
not decreasing
early stage of operation
later on
blood pressure and pulse frequency
disturbed
-danger-
decreasing
quickly
blood pressure and pulse frequency
normalized
increasing
after
irrigation
during 3rd to 8th step
subdurcl hygroma-residual-
CSF + irrigation

Fig. 67. **5th step:** only after shrinkage of the AVM can the feeding artery be well prepared and definitively clipped far proximally

B

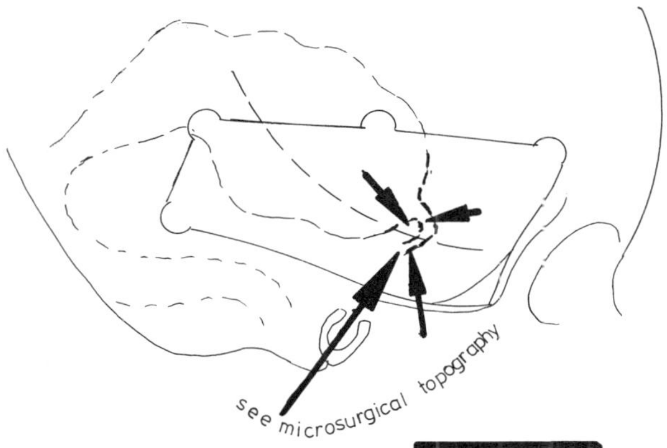

microsurgical topography
5th step

interruption of feeding artery

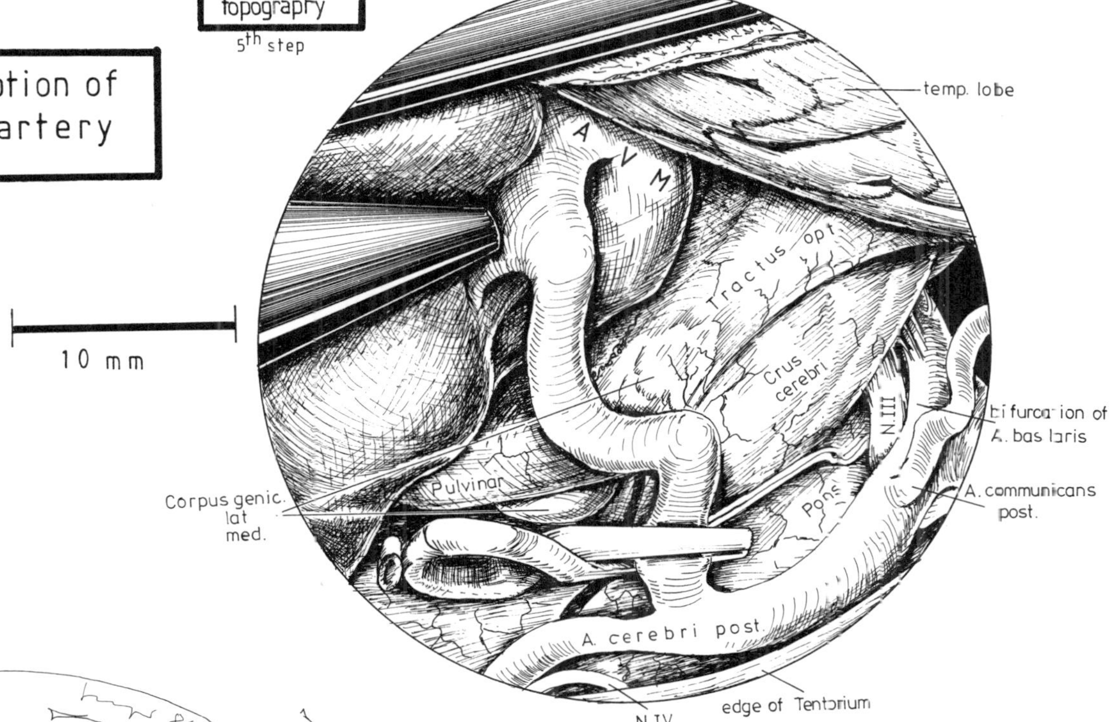

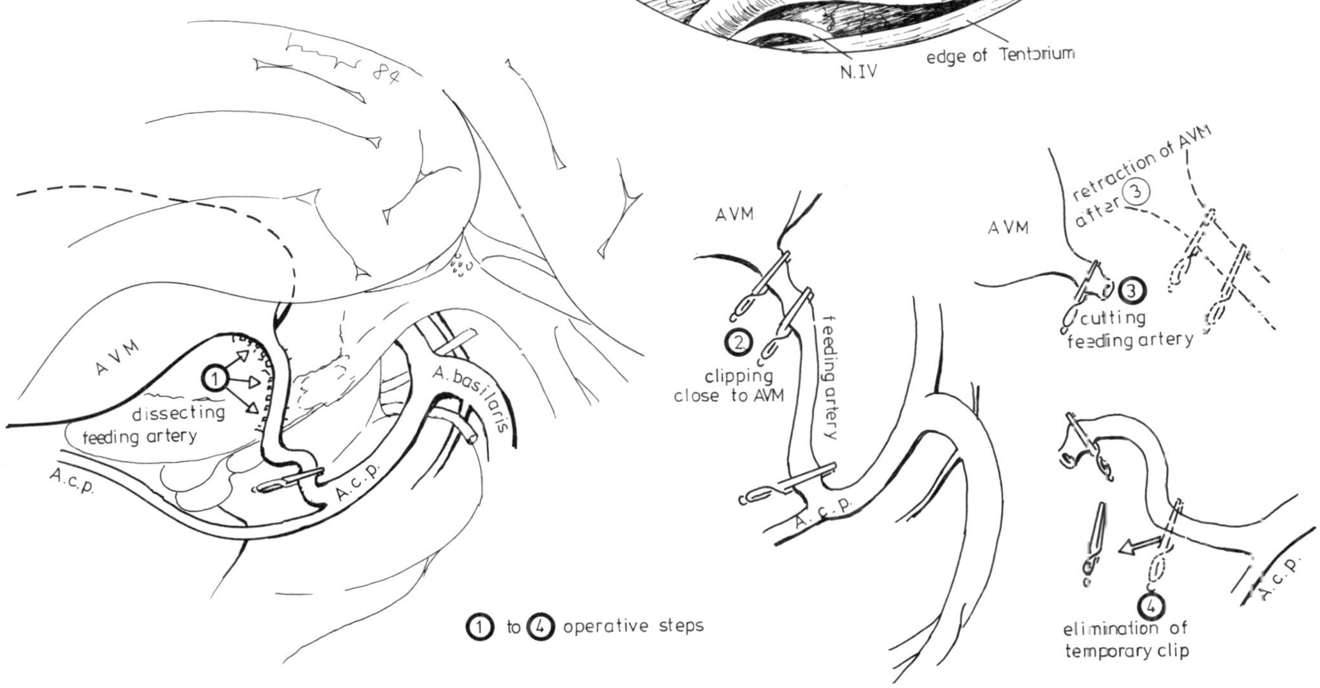

Fig. 68. **5th and 6th steps:** shrinkage and freeing of the AV-angioma from the floor and roof of the Fissura transversa are carried out. Since the Tela chorioidea, Taenia chorioidea and the Taenia fornicis are very much thinner due to the angioma, flow of CSF from the lateral ventricle can occur. At the microsurgical site the Corpus geniculatum mediale is indicated as landmark and the positions of Corpus geniculatum laterale and Tractus opticus are also indicated, but both difficult to identify during the operation. On the other hand, the Brachium colliculi inferioris is well identifiable when the angioma is considerably shrunk and the flattened brain has again achieved its relief

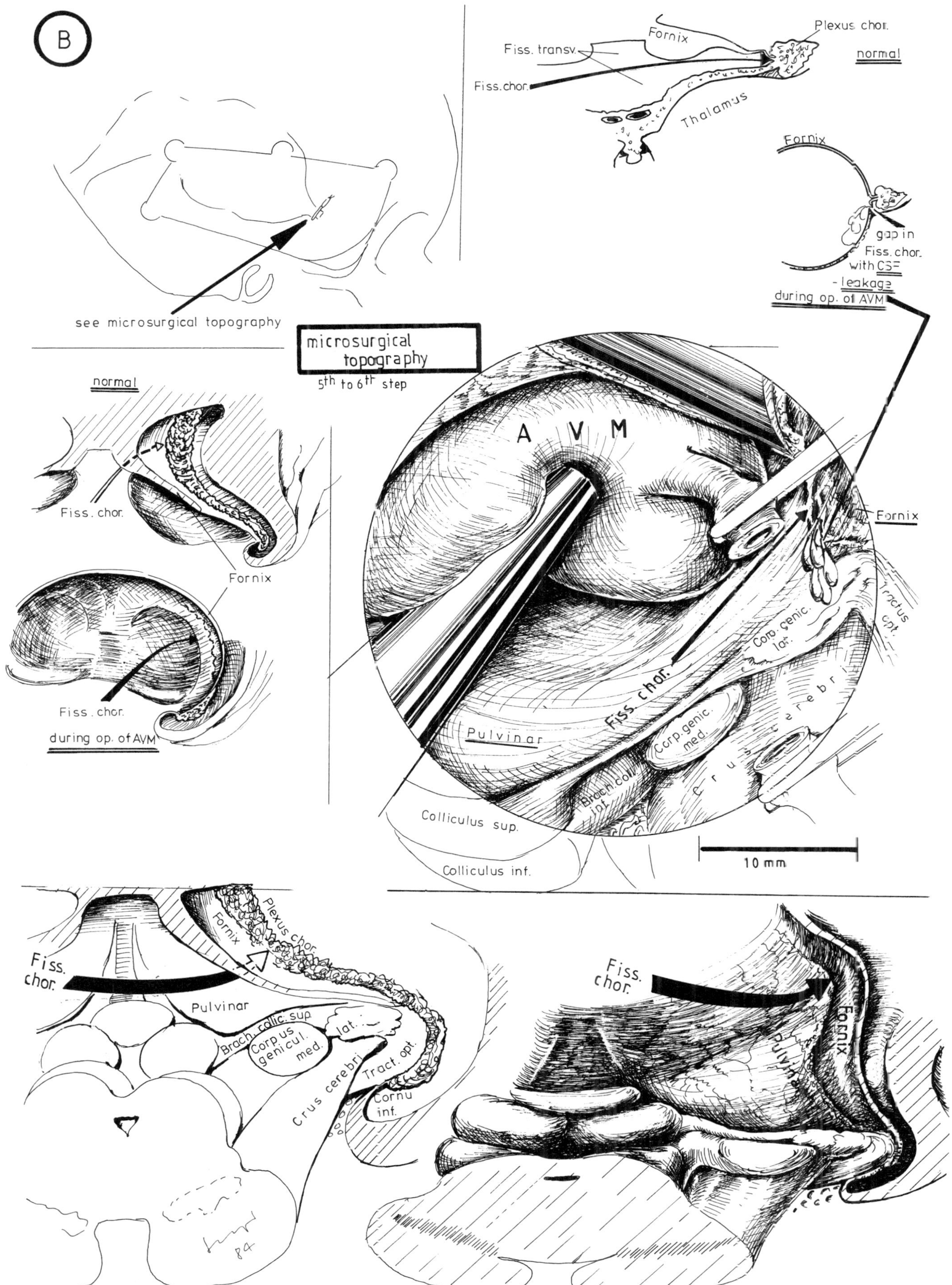
B
see microsurgical topography
Fornix
Plexus chor.
Fiss. transv.
normal
Fiss. chor.
Thalamus
Fornix
gap in
Fiss. chor.
with CSF
- leakage
during op. of AVM
microsurgical
topography
5th to 6th step
normal
Fiss. chor.
Fornix
Fiss. chor.
during op. of AVM
A V M
Fornix
Tractus opt.
Corp. genic. lat.
Fiss. chor.
Pulvinar
Corp. genic. med.
Crus cerebri
Brach. coll. inf.
Colliculus sup.
Colliculus inf.
10 mm
Fiss. chor.
Fornix
Plexus chor.
Pulvinar
Brach. collic. sup.
Corpus genicul.
lat.
med.
Crus cerebri
Tract. opt.
Cornu inf.
Fiss. chor.
Fornix
Pulv.

Fig. 69. **6th step:** the small accessory feeding arteries can come from the contralateral side. In order to reach them the angioma should be considerably shrunk. The approach should be come as far dorsal as possible and when possible not through a window in the Falx and without separation of the Corpus callosum or Fornix

B

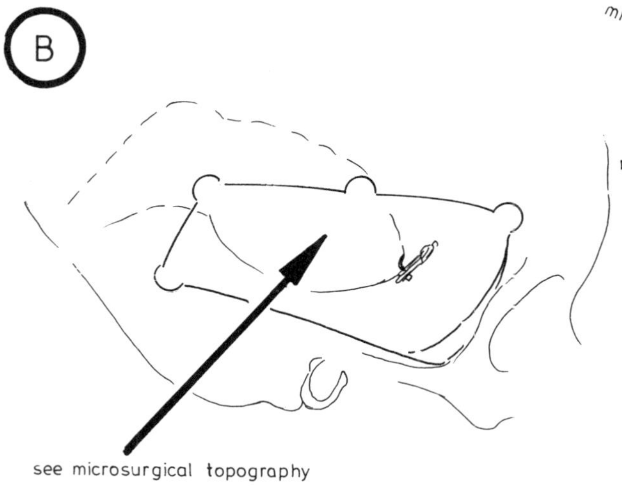

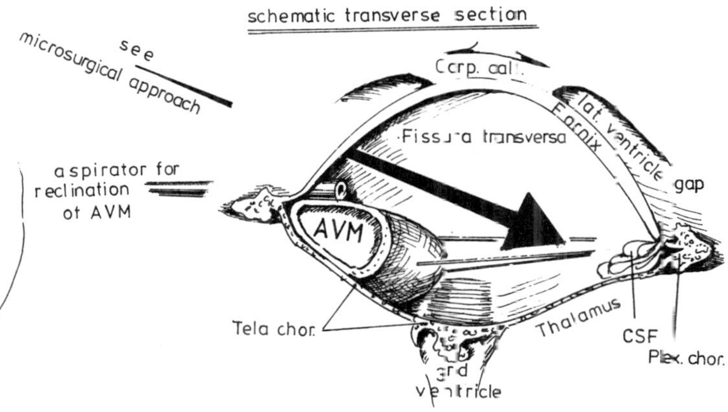

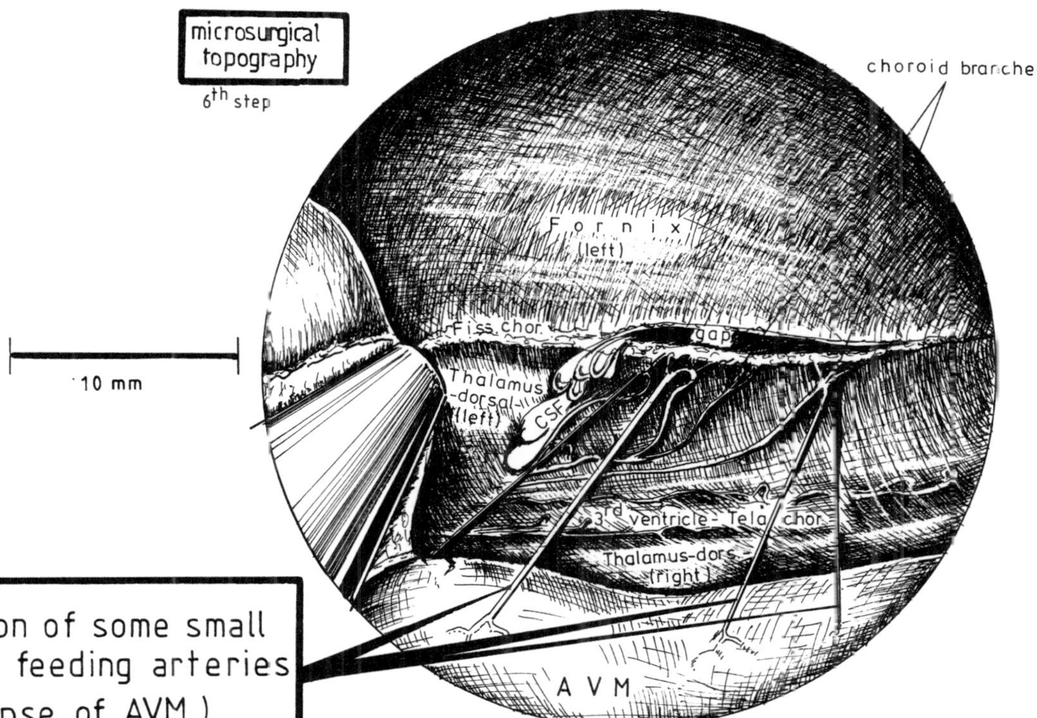

elimination of some small accessory feeding arteries (⟶ collapse of AVM)

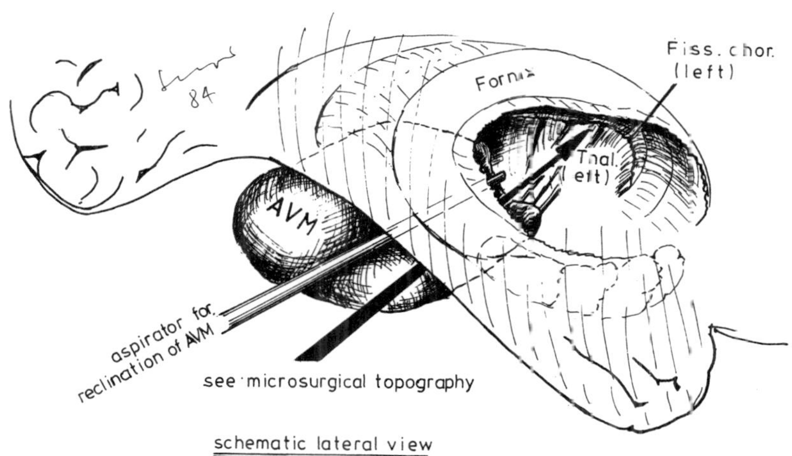

Fig. 70. **7th and 8th steps:** the interruption of the vein of Galen at the pass-over to the Sinus rectus requires patience due to its large cross-section. It must be carefully freed so that at the end of the operation considerable venous haemorrhaging is not provoked

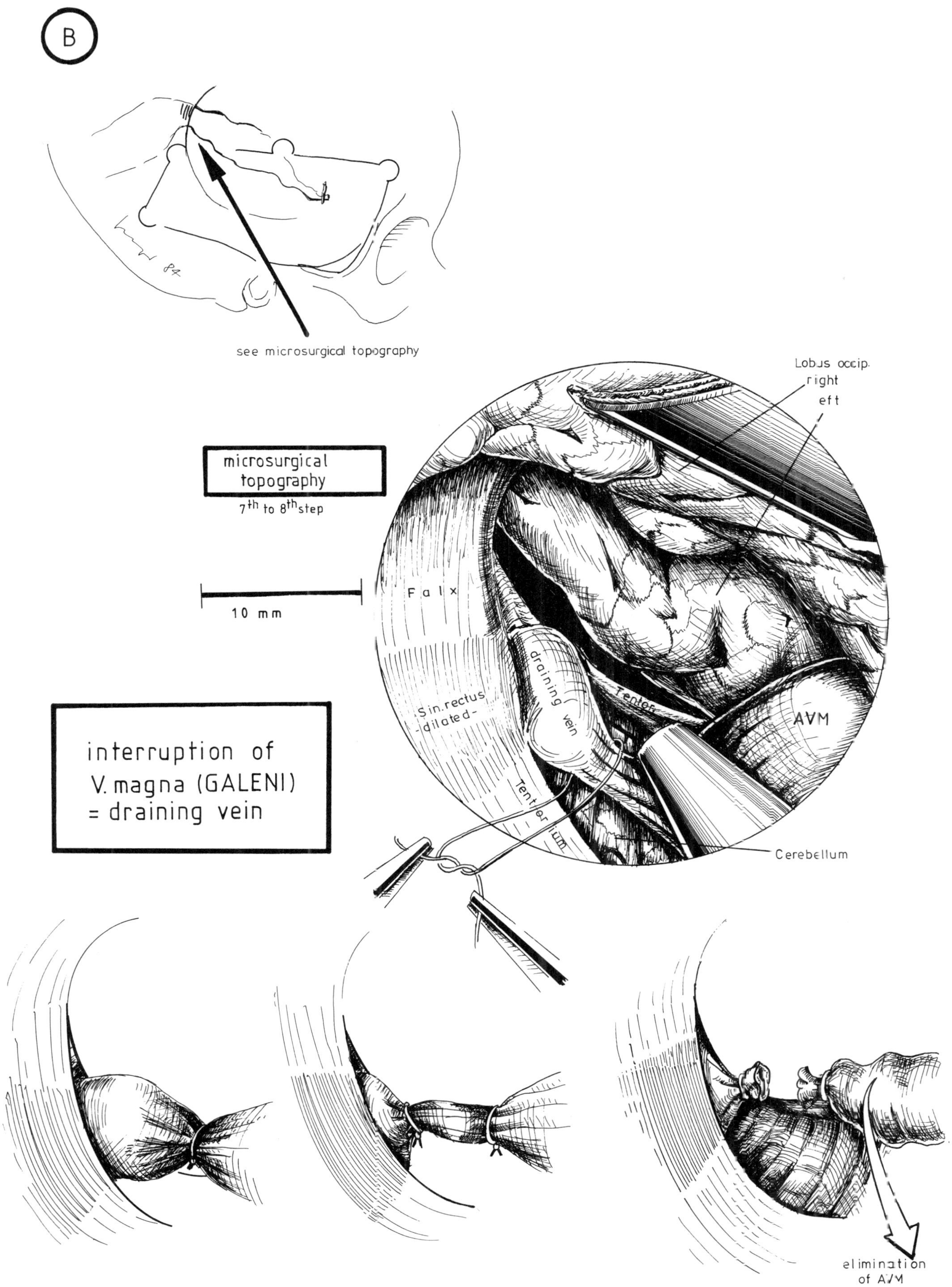
B
see microsurgical topography
microsurgical topography
7th to 8th step
10 mm
interruption of
V. magna (GALENI)
= draining vein
Lobus occip.
right
eft
Falx
draining vein
Sin. rectus
-dilated-
Tentor
Tentorium
AVM
Cerebellum
elimination
of AVM

Fig. 71. Tumor location in the Cisterna tecti and the posterior part of the 3rd ventricle. Regarding the best location, of top priority is the preservation of the limbic system and thereby the prevention of postoperative psychic disturbances. Therefore both the publications of Fedor Krause in the 20s and Yaşargil on microsurgical techniques recommend the improved infratentorial approach (approach **A**)

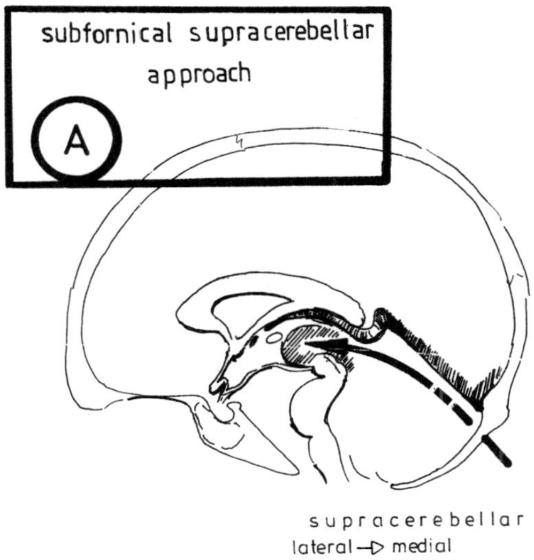

favorable

- limbic system not endangered
- galenic vein not endangered
- choroid branches not endangered
- sufficient reclination of Cerebellum

unfavorable

- tumor extension into 3rd ventricle

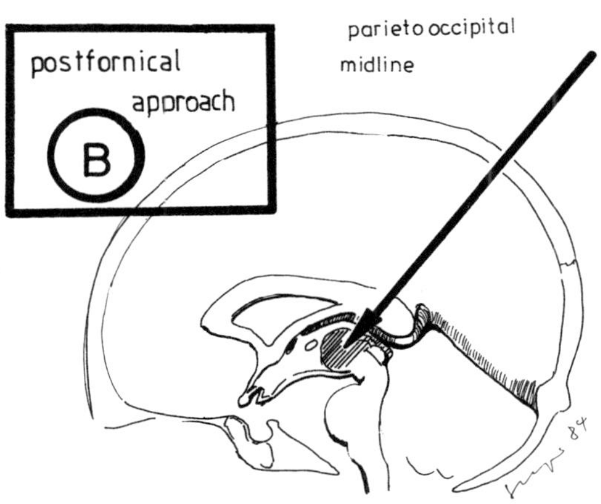

favorable

- tumor extension into 3rd ventricle

unfavorable

- galenic vein endangered
- limbic system (Gyrus cinguli, Induseum griseum corporis callosi, Crus fornicis, Commissura hippocampi) endangered respective split
- Splenium corp. call. split
- Area opt. (Praecuneus) endangered

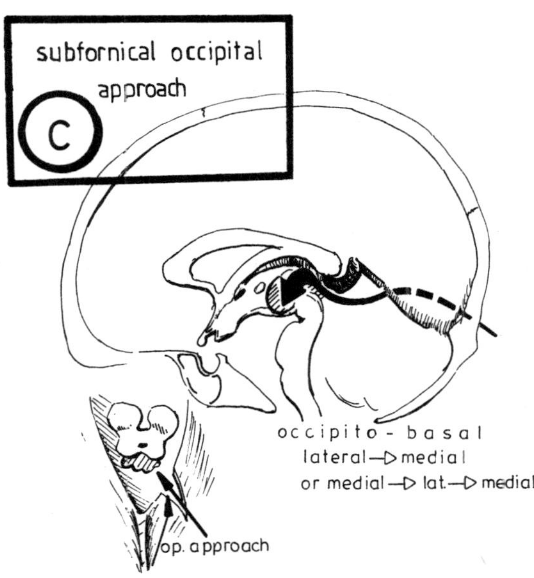

favorable

- Fornix not split (but endangered by spatula)

unfavorable

- op. approach smaller than (A) or (B)
- medial occipito-basal veins endangered
- galenic vein endangered
- limbic system (Isthmus gyri cinguli, Gyrus occipitotemp.med./parahippocampalis, Fasciola cinerea/Induseum griseum, Crus fornicis, Commissura hippocampi) endangered
- Area optica (Cuneus, Fiss. calcarina) endangered
- Splenium corp. call. endangered

Fig. 72. Large tumors of the Cisterna tecti including the neighbouring cisterns*

B Inclusion of the Fissura transversa cerebri and Fissura horizontalis cerebelli.

C Inclusion of the Fissura transversa cerebri.
In both cases the size of the tumors and the displacement of the limbic system allow a supratentorial approach without risk to the limbic system. By the approach type **C** the occipital subfornical approach can be hindered by the basal veins. This danger is, however, minimal with respect to the size of the tumor, since after hollowing of the tumor there is enough space for the radical dissection of the tumor

---

* These two cases were described in detail in Seeger, W., Microsurgery of Cerebral Veins. Wien–New York: Springer. 1984.

(B) postfornical approach

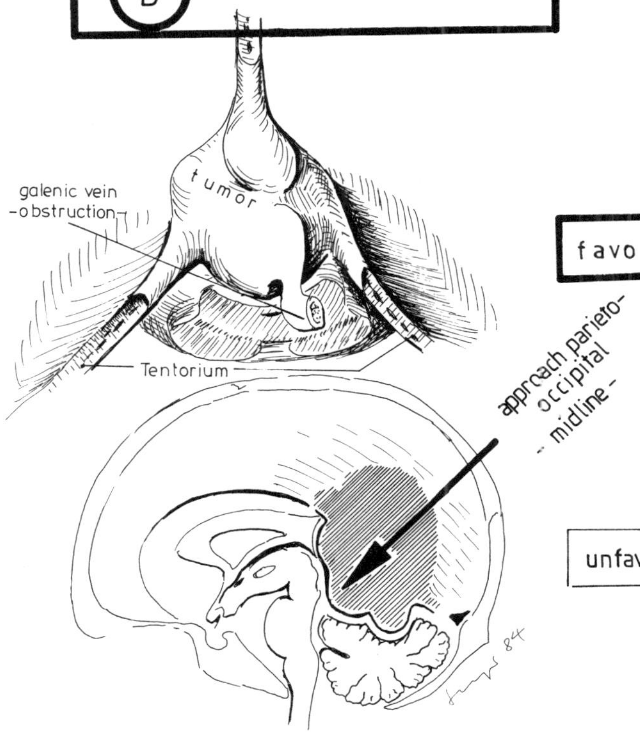

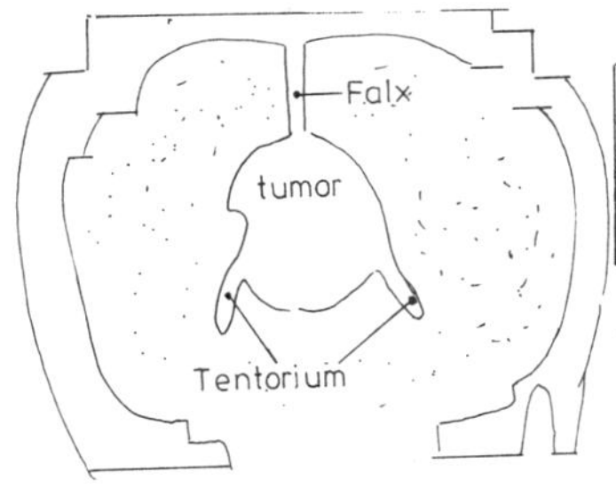

H. H., ♀, 9/15-23
CT reconstruction 11/9-81
op. 11/17-81

favorable

- tumor originates from Falx + Tentorium
- limbic system shifted aside + rostrally
- op. approach short and wide (during tumor-hollowing)
- galenic vein obstructed → venous collaterals
- choroid branches shifted → basal
- Corpus callosum shifted → rostral
- medial occipito-basal veins not endangered

unfavorable

- bilateral location
- Area optica (Praecuneus) bilateral endangered

(C) subfornical occipital approach

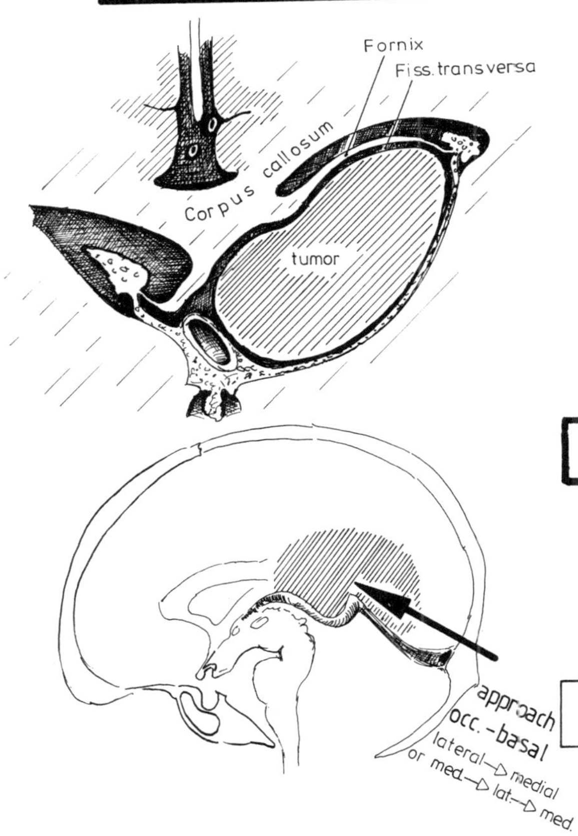

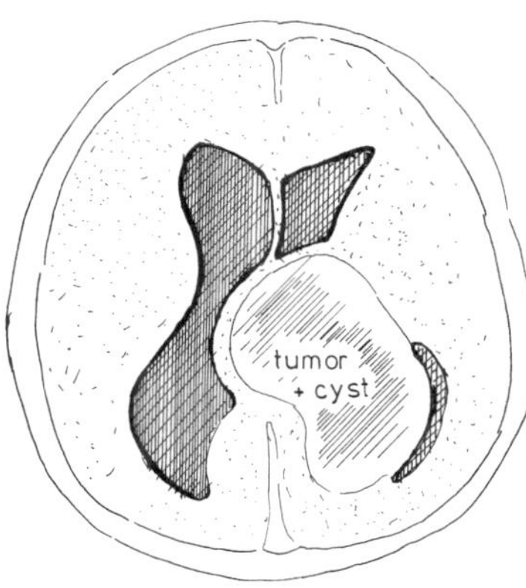

Sch. B., ♂, 1/26-60
CT 1/27-84
op. 1/31-84

favorable

- unilateral location – shift of galenic vein aside -
- location in Fissura transversa - basal from Fornix
- shift of choroid branches
- Splenium corporis callosi not endangered
- op. approach wide and short

unfavorable

- medial occipito-basal veins endangered
- Area optica (Cuneus, Fiss. calcarina) endangered

Fig. 73. Process of the Cisterna tecti spreading to the Fissura horizontalis cerebelli and, as the operation later showed, the 4th ventricle. The angioma had damaged the roof of the 4th ventricle – Velum medullare ant. – and had therefore broken into the 4th ventricle.

D (D1, D2): Thereby the supracerebellar (see type **A**) as well as the transventricular approach is possible

FIG. 73

D supracerebellar + transventricular combined approaches

D1

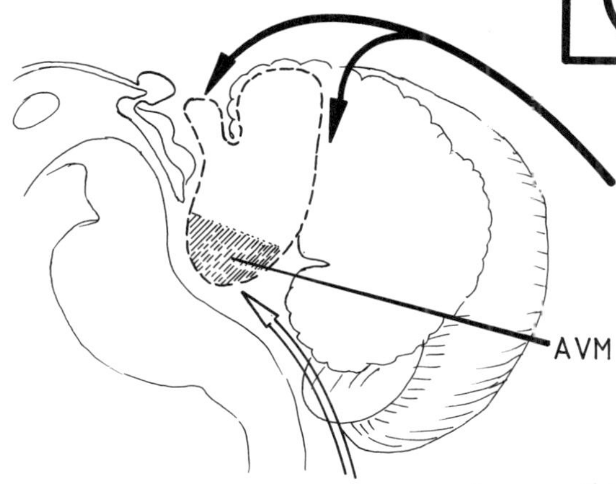

favorable	small residual AVM after first operation
unfavorable	during first operation danger of uncontrolled bleeding into ventricular system

D2

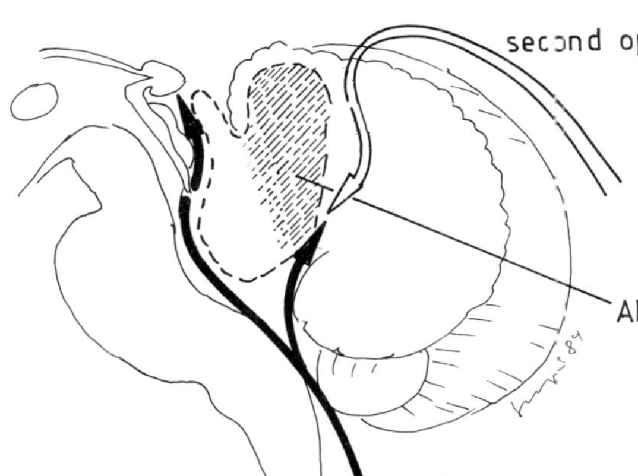

favorable	intraventricular bleeding during first operation under control
unfavorable	residual AVM may be more extensive

Fig. 74. A clinical example of a teratoma of the Cisterna tecti with bulging into the 3rd ventricle.
In November 1978 and later repeated attacks of headache with vomiting. Hospital admission April 29, 1981. Exaggerated Achilles tendon reflex bilaterally. Babinski signs positive more right than left, dysdiadochokinesis left. Gait with closed eyes atactic. There was no pupillary defect, and the ocular motility was regular. Immediate application of an atrioventricular shunt because of occlusive hydrocephalus. After removal of the tumor on June 4, 1981 Parinaud syndrome and gaze-evoked nystagmus, tonic pupils, preserved near convergence reaction. Visual acuity 0.6 both sides (optic atrophy). Deficits quickly improving and disappearing after 3 years follow-up period

FIG. 74

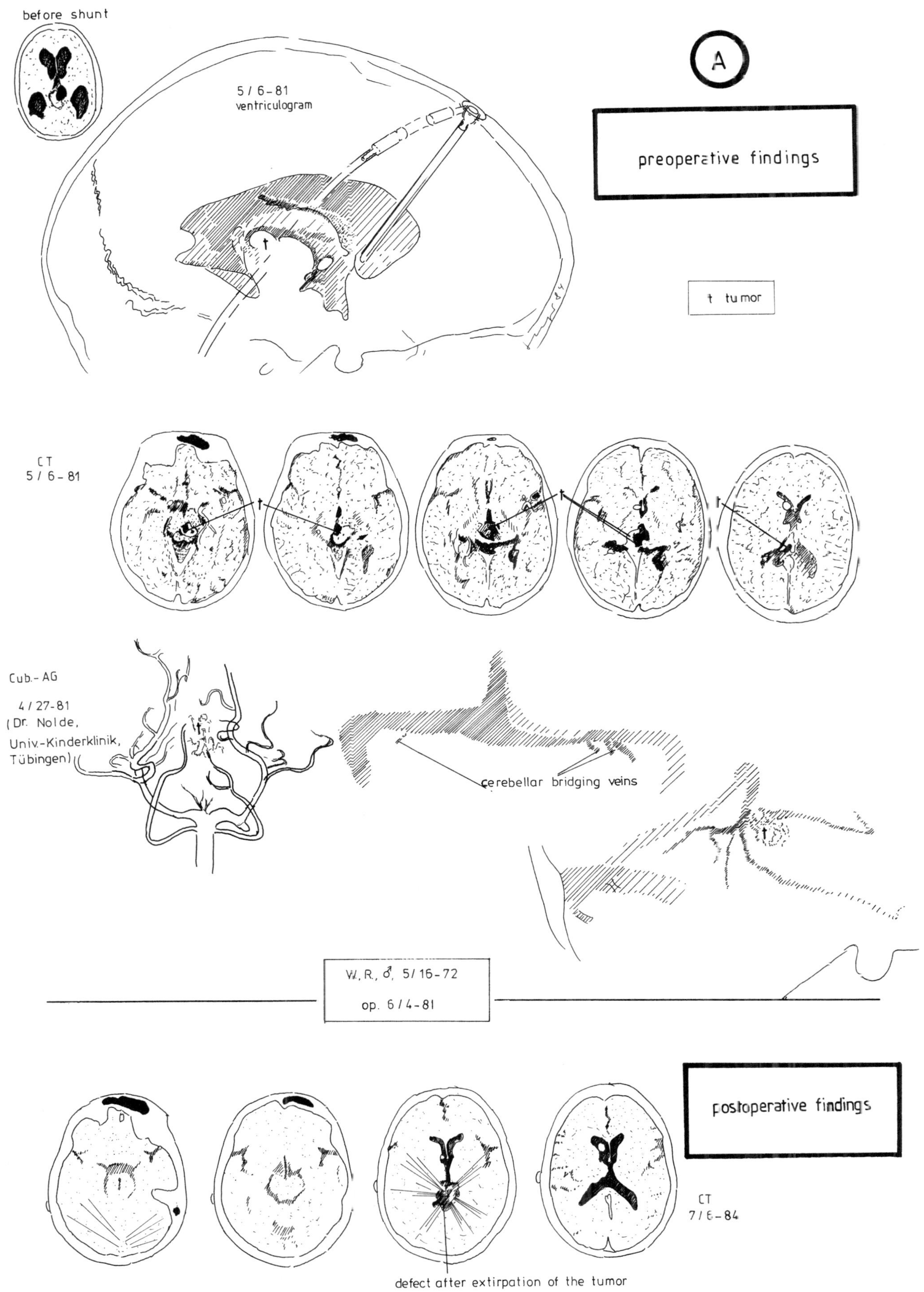
before shunt
5 / 6-81
ventriculogram
A
preoperative findings
t tumor
CT
5 / 6 - 81
Cub.- AG
4 / 27-81
(Dr. Nolde,
Univ.-Kinderklinik,
Tübingen)
cerebellar bridging veins
W.R., ♂, 5/16-72
op. 6 / 4-81
postoperative findings
CT
7/ 6-84
defect after extirpation of the tumor

Fig. 75. By means of a thorough arachnoid incision the Culmen cerebelli sinks down to revealing the Tectum *

---

* This method was presented in detail in Seeger, W., Microsurgery of the Brain, Vol. 2, and Seeger, W., Microsurgery of Cerebral Veins. Wien–New York: Springer. 1980 and 1984.

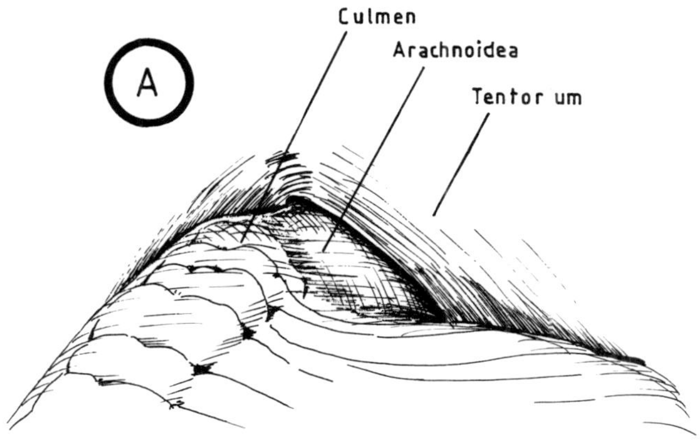

1st step

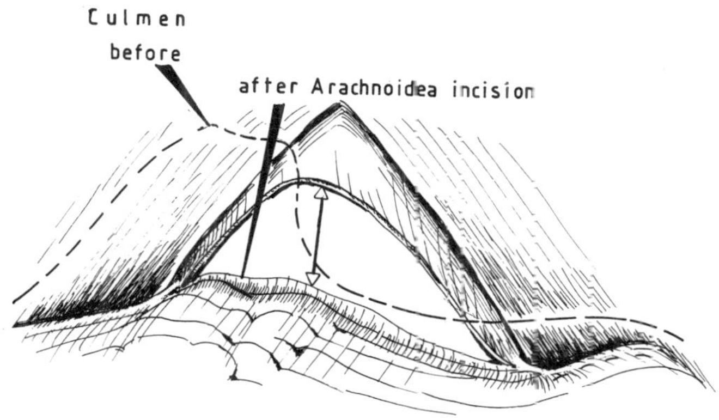

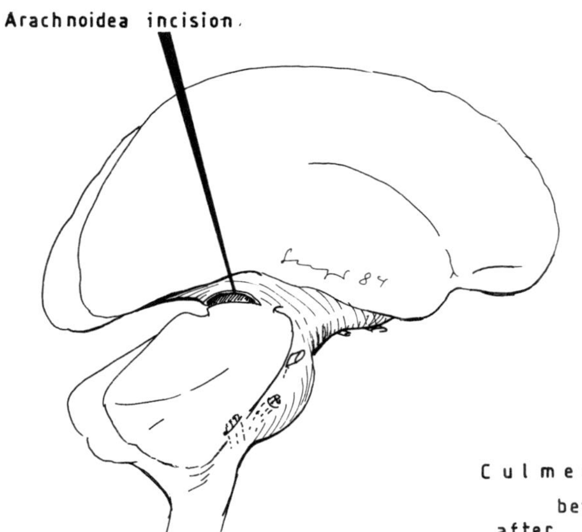

principles of operation

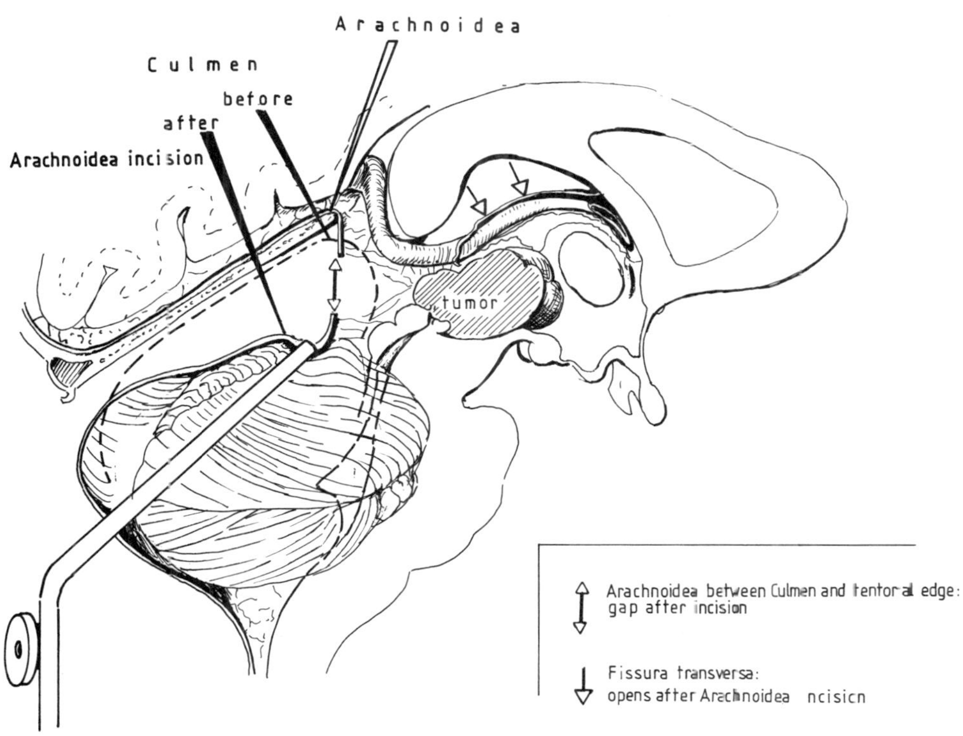

Fig. 76. The nature of the tumor is very variable. Despite the small size of the tumor, various techniques for its reduction are necessary

FIG. 76

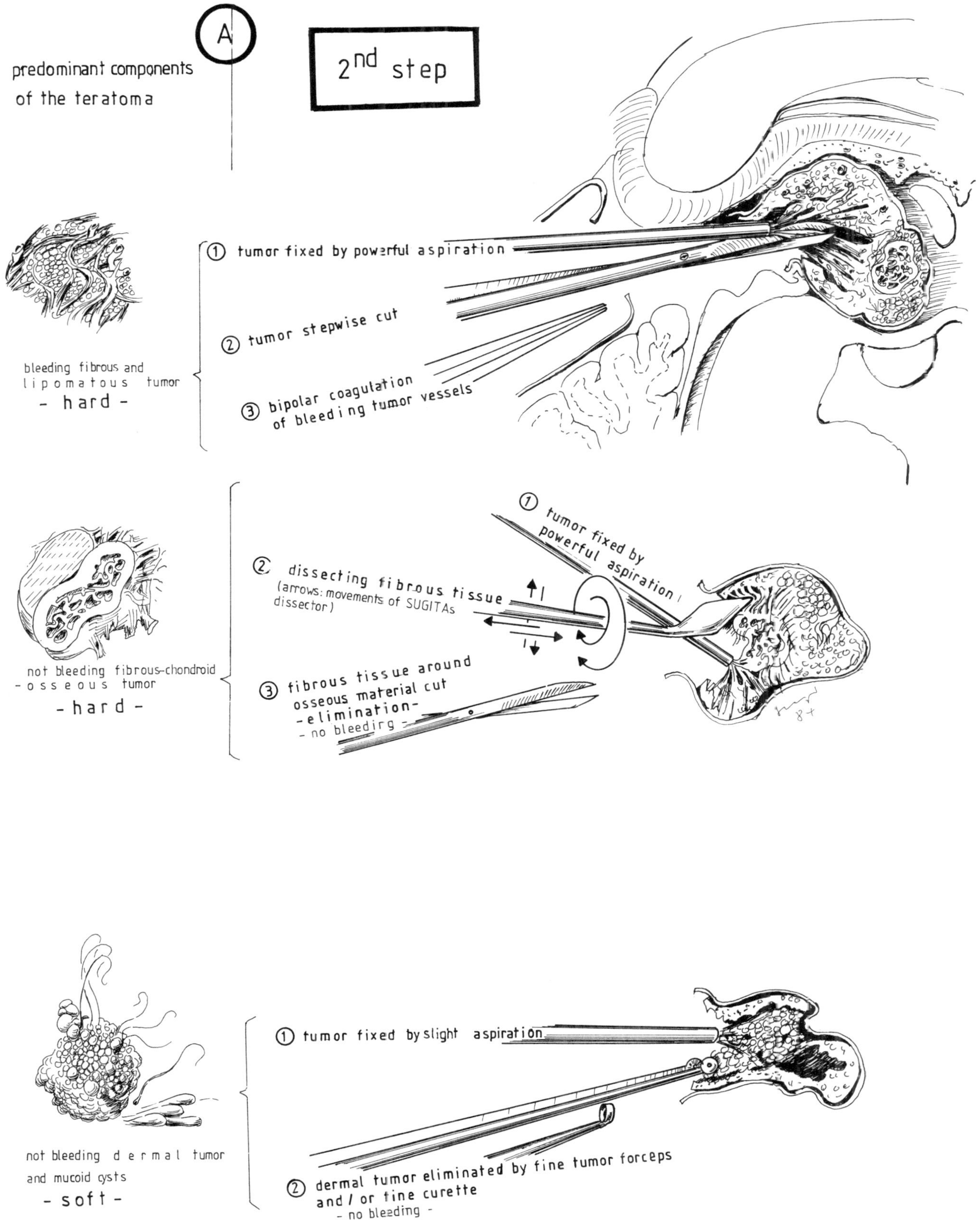
A
predominant components
of the teratoma
2nd step
① tumor fixed by powerful aspiration
② tumor stepwise cut
③ bipolar coagulation
of bleeding tumor vessels
bleeding fibrous and
lipomatous tumor
- hard -
① tumor fixed by
powerful aspiration
② dissecting fibrous tissue
(arrows: movements of SUGITAs
dissector)
③ fibrous tissue around
osseous material cut
-elimination-
- no bleeding -
not bleeding fibrous-chondroid
- osseous tumor
- hard -
① tumor fixed by slight aspiration
② dermal tumor eliminated by fine tumor forceps
and / or fine curette
- no bleeding -
not bleeding dermal tumor
and mucoid cysts
- soft -

Fig. 77. The tumor is removed from the cisternal arachnoidal capsule. Since, however, residual tumor could be seen on the arachnoidea, the arachnoidea was as far as possible removed whilst preserving the vessels in the area. During removal of the tumor from Tectum, the 3rd ventricle was always opened, resulting in a wide connection between the ventricular system and, following the tumor removal, considerable widening of the Cisterna tecti

3rd step:

(A)

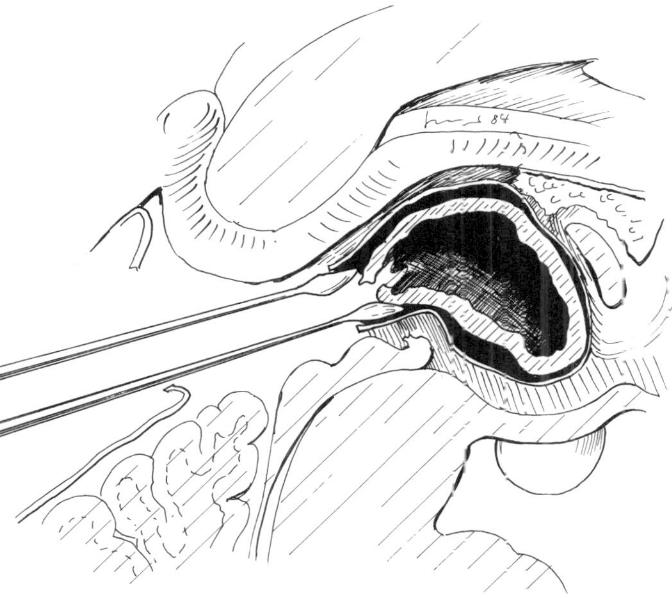

dissection from Arachnoidea

① dorsal

② basal

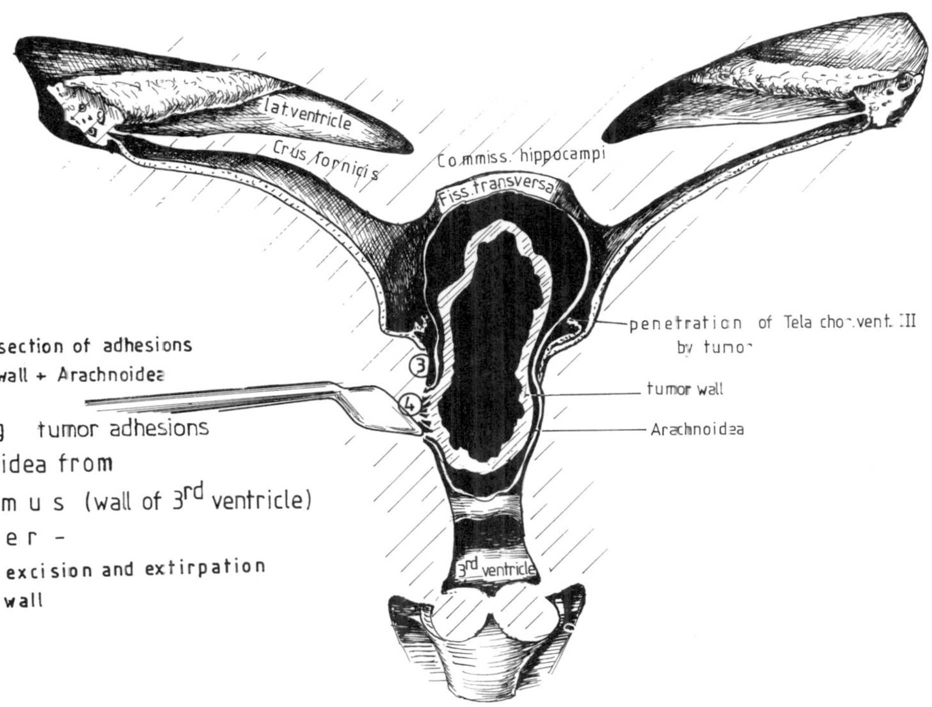

penetration of Tela cho·.vent. III by tumo·

tumor wall

Arachnoidea

③ lateral dissection of adhesions from tumor wall + Arachnoidea

④ dissecting tumor adhesions +Arachnoidea from Thalamus (wall of 3rd ventricle) - danger -

⑤ stepwise excision and extirpation of tumor wall

4th step

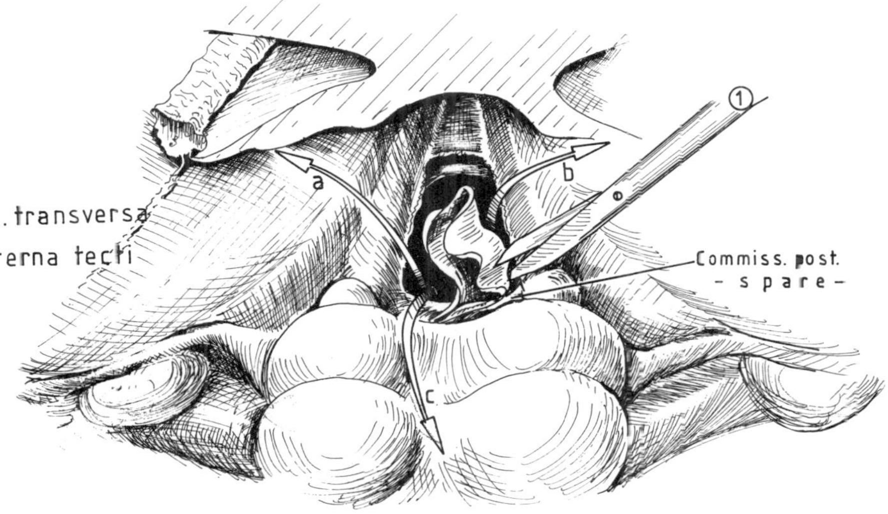

CSF of 3rd ventricle { a, b → Fiss. transversa; c → Cisterna tecti }

Commiss. post. - spare -

① elimination of tumor infiltrated Arachnoidea

Fig. 78. Various techniques of reducing the tumor in the microsurgical site (complemented by anatomical sketches)

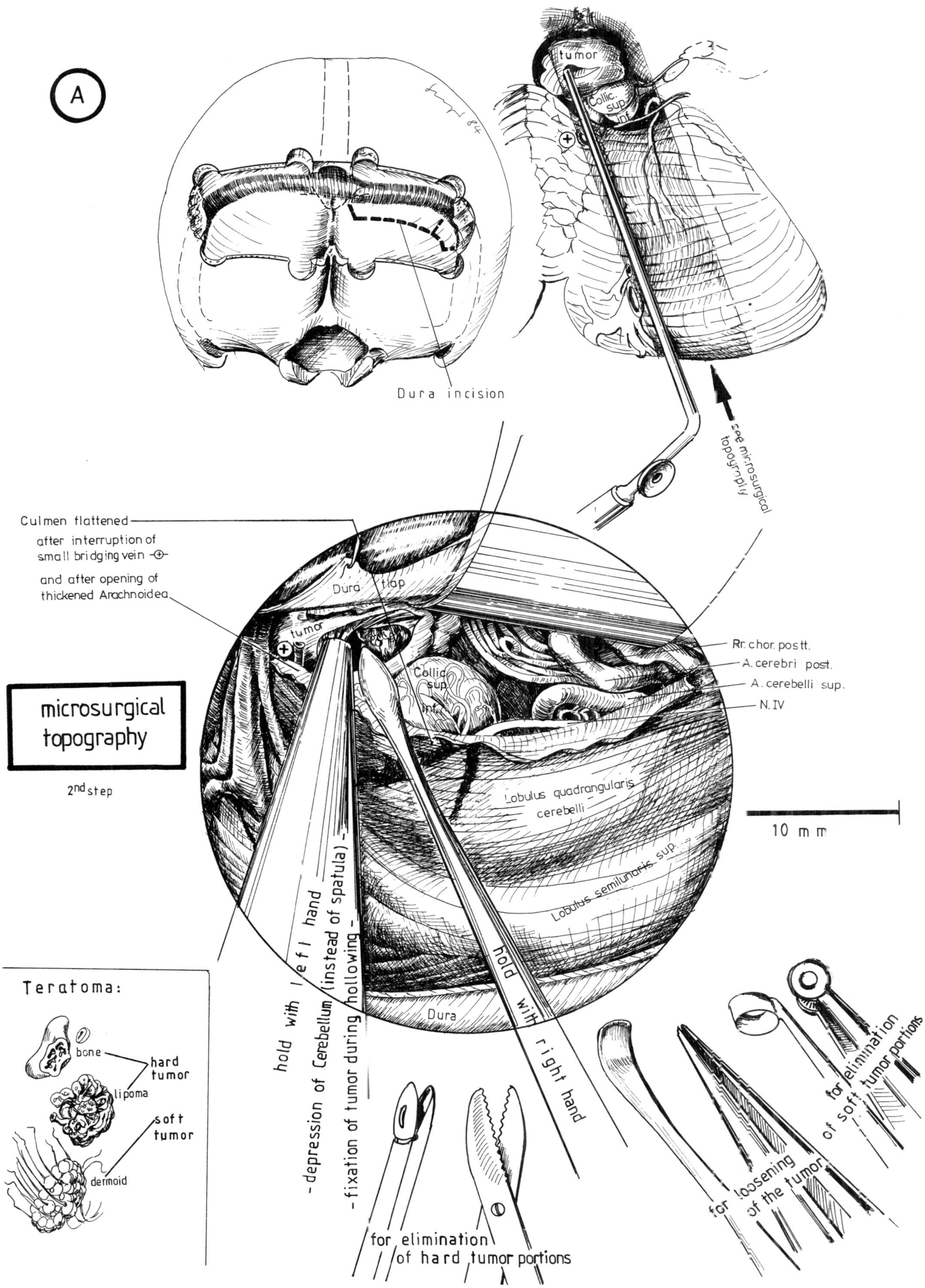
A
tumor
Collic.
sup.
inf.
Dura incision
see mirrosurgical topogrmply
Culmen flattened
after interruption of small bridging vein
and after opening of thickened Arachnoidea
Dura flap
tumor
Collic
sup.
inf.
Rr. chor. postt.
A. cerebri post.
A. cerebelli sup.
N. IV
microsurgical topography
2nd step
Lobulus quadrangularis cerebelli
10 mm
Lobulus semilunaris sup.
Dura
hold with left hand
- depression of Cerebellum (instead of spatula) -
- fixation of tumor during hollowing -
hold with right hand
Teratoma:
bone
hard tumor
lipoma
soft tumor
dermoid
for elimination of hard tumor portions
for loosening of the tumor
for elimination of soft tumor portions

Fig. 79. Site at the end of the operation

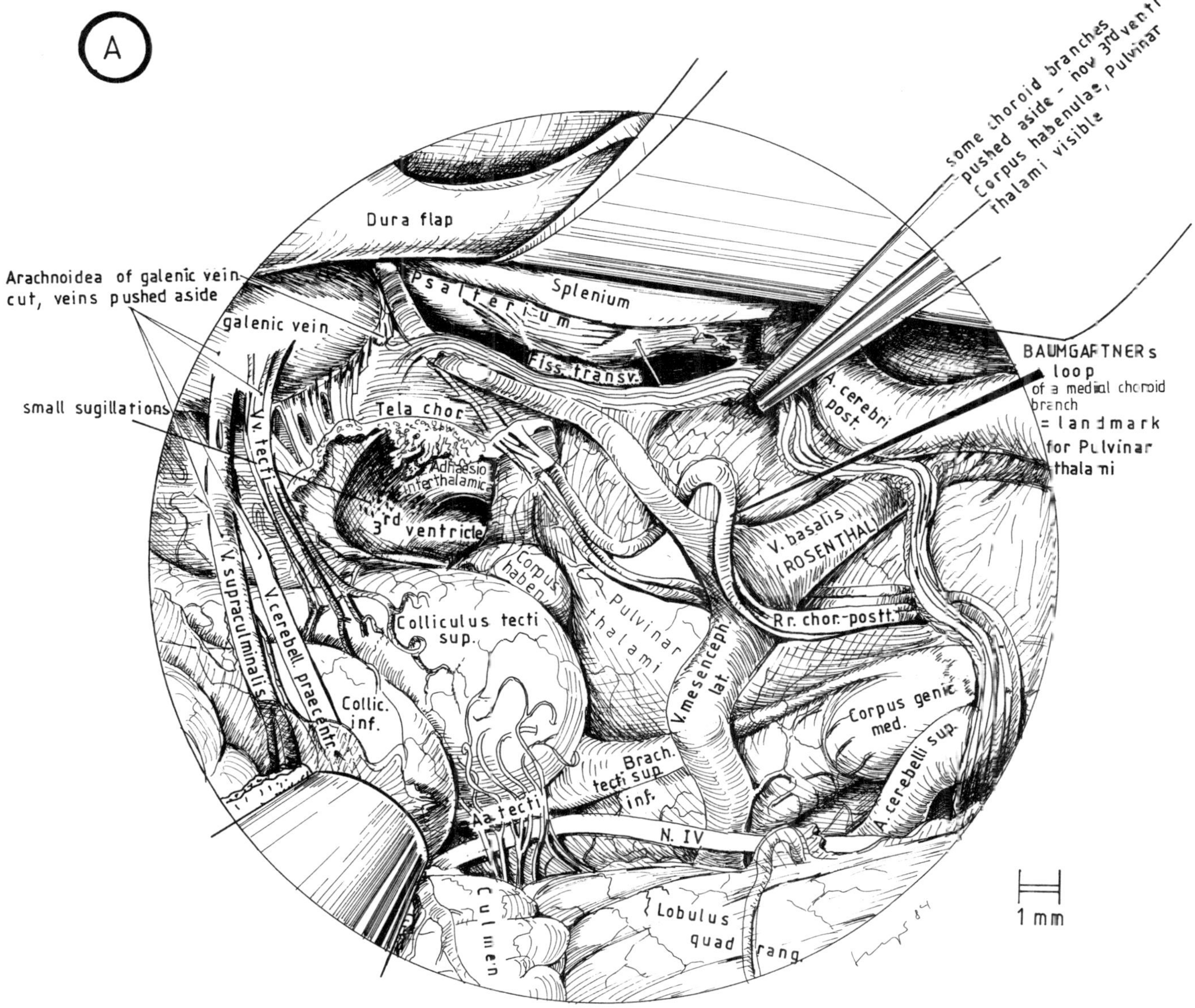

microsurgical topography

4th step

Figs. 80 and 81. Removal of a Falx/Tentorium meningioma with displacing of the Corpus callosum and Fornix forwards*

* The case was presented in detail in Seeger, W., Microsurgery of Cerebral Veins. Wien–New York: Springer. 1984.

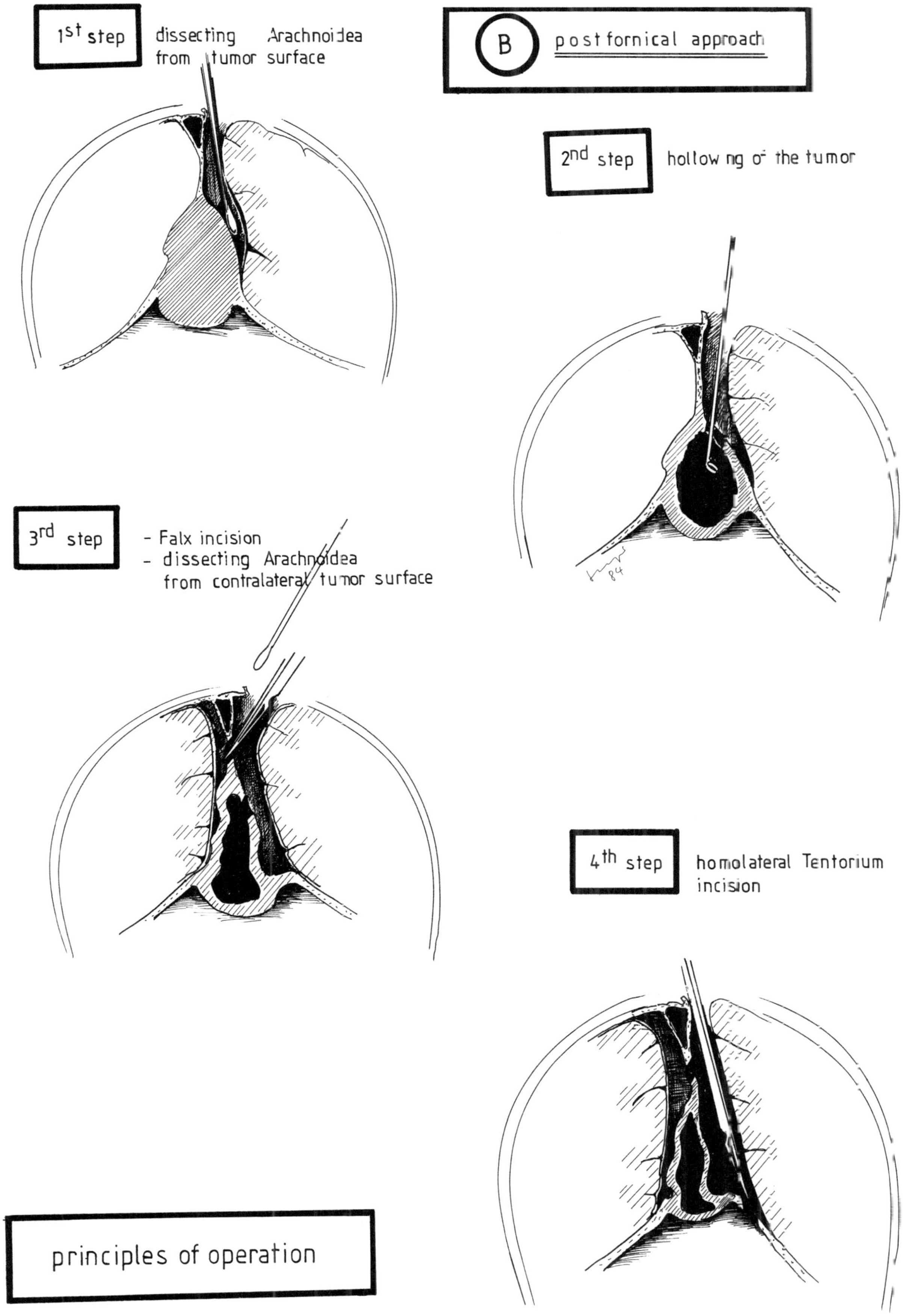
1st step
dissecting Arachnoidea from tumor surface
B
postfornical approach
2nd step
hollowing of the tumor
3rd step
- Falx incision
- dissecting Arachnoidea from contralateral tumor surface
4th step
homolateral Tentorium incision
principles of operation

Fig. 81

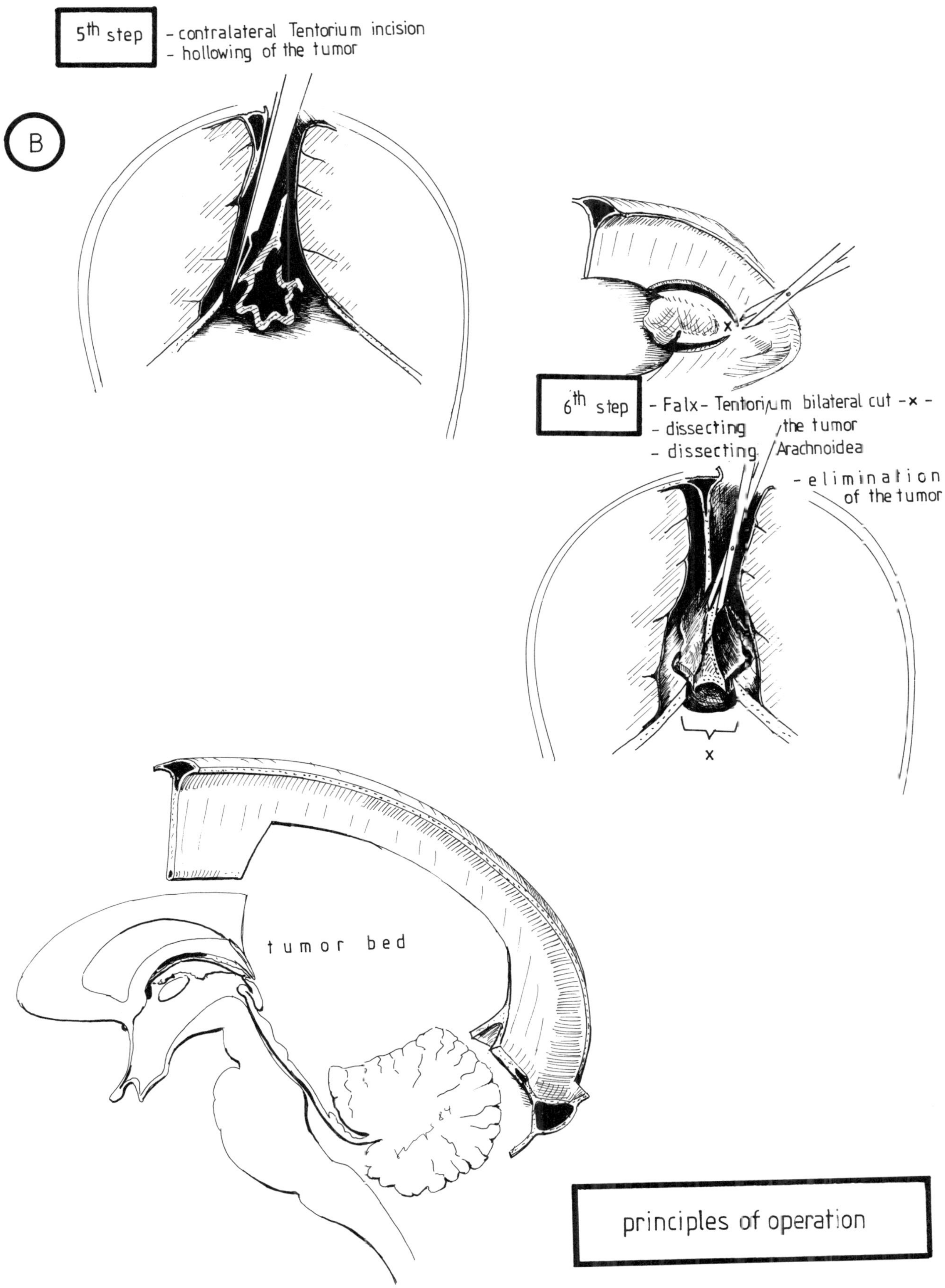
5th step
- contralateral Tentorium incision
- hollowing of the tumor
B
6th step
- Falx - Tentorium bilateral cut - x -
- dissecting the tumor
- dissecting Arachnoidea
- elimination of the tumor
x
tumor bed
principles of operation

Fig. 82. Type **C:** occipito-medial and occipito-basal approach*

* The case was presented in detail in Seeger, W., Microsurgery of Cerebral Veins. Wien–New York: Springer. 1984.

C subfornical occipital approach

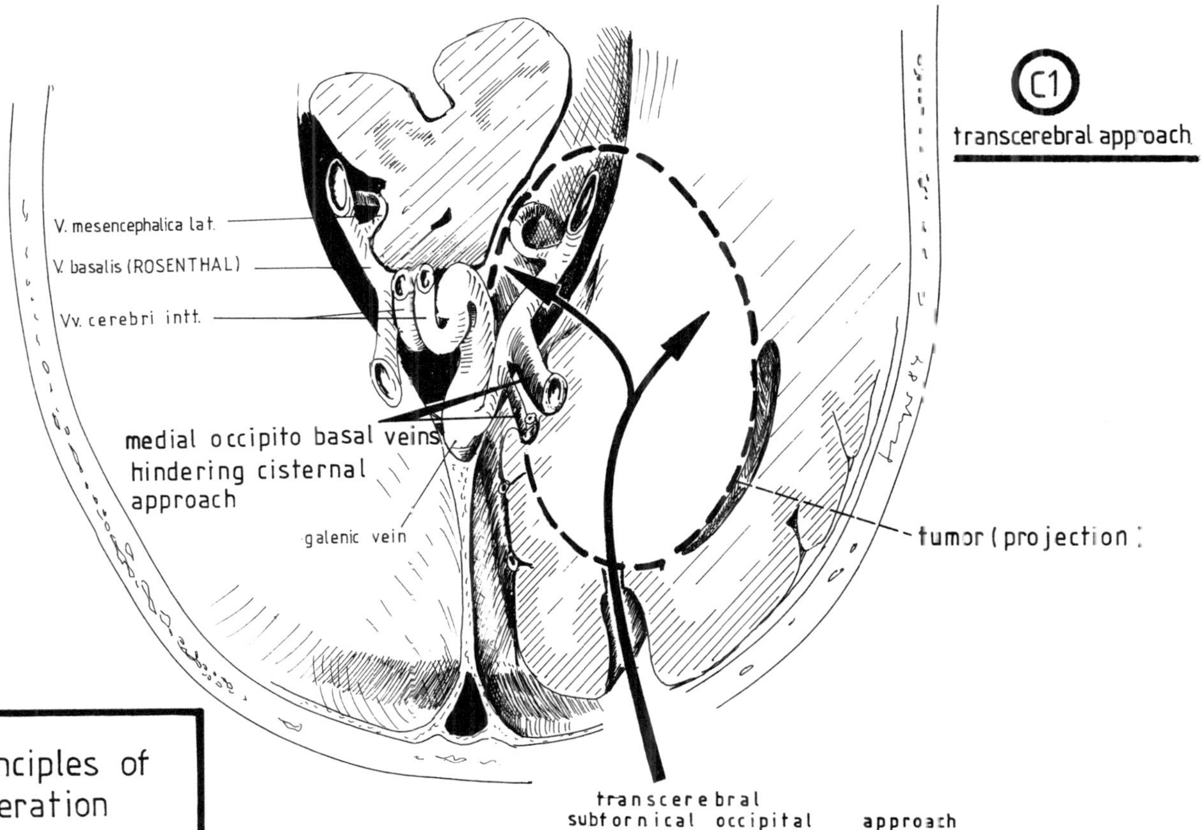

principles of operation

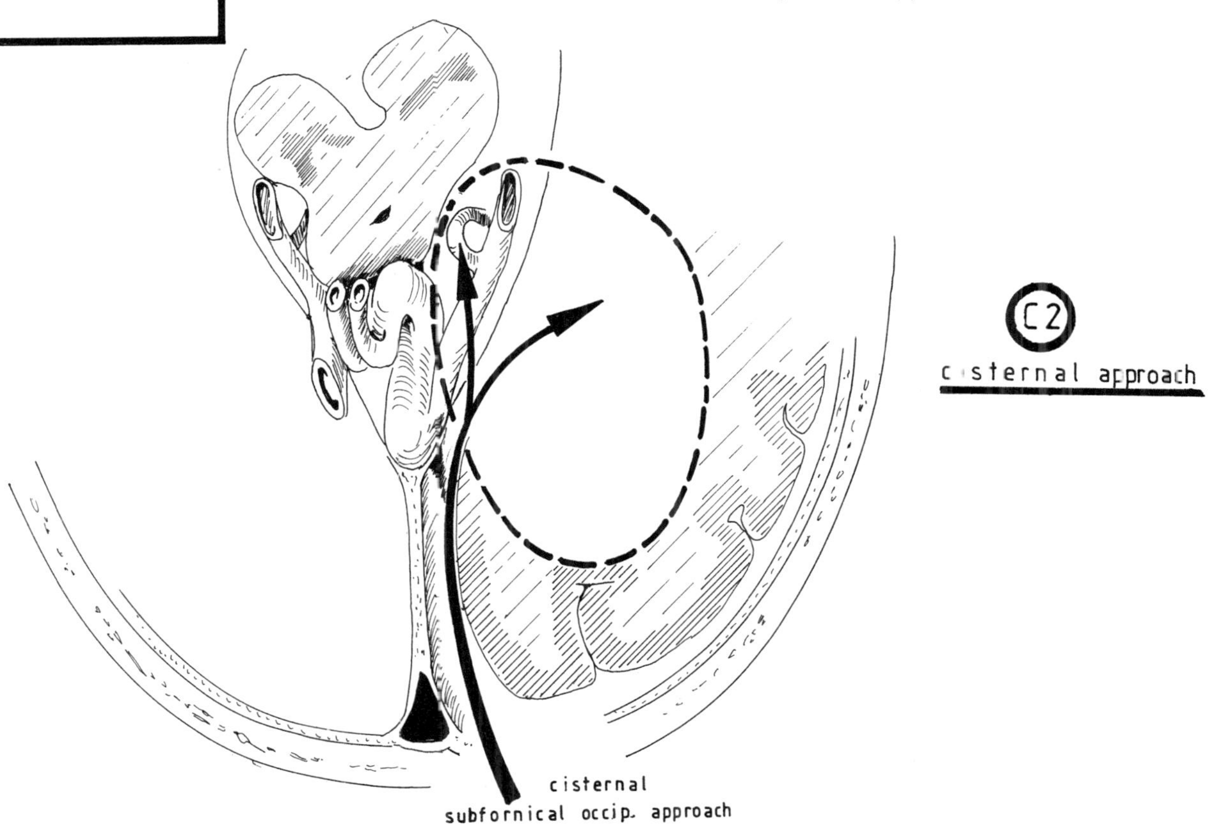

Fig. 83. Clinical example of an angioma of the Cisterna tecti* with extension towards Fissura horizontalis cerebelli, penetration of the 4th ventricle and affection of the surrounding cerebellar structures. Preoperative ataxia. Postoperatively rapid normalization

* Both operations were carried out by Dr. W. Hassler, coworker of the author, and the author together.

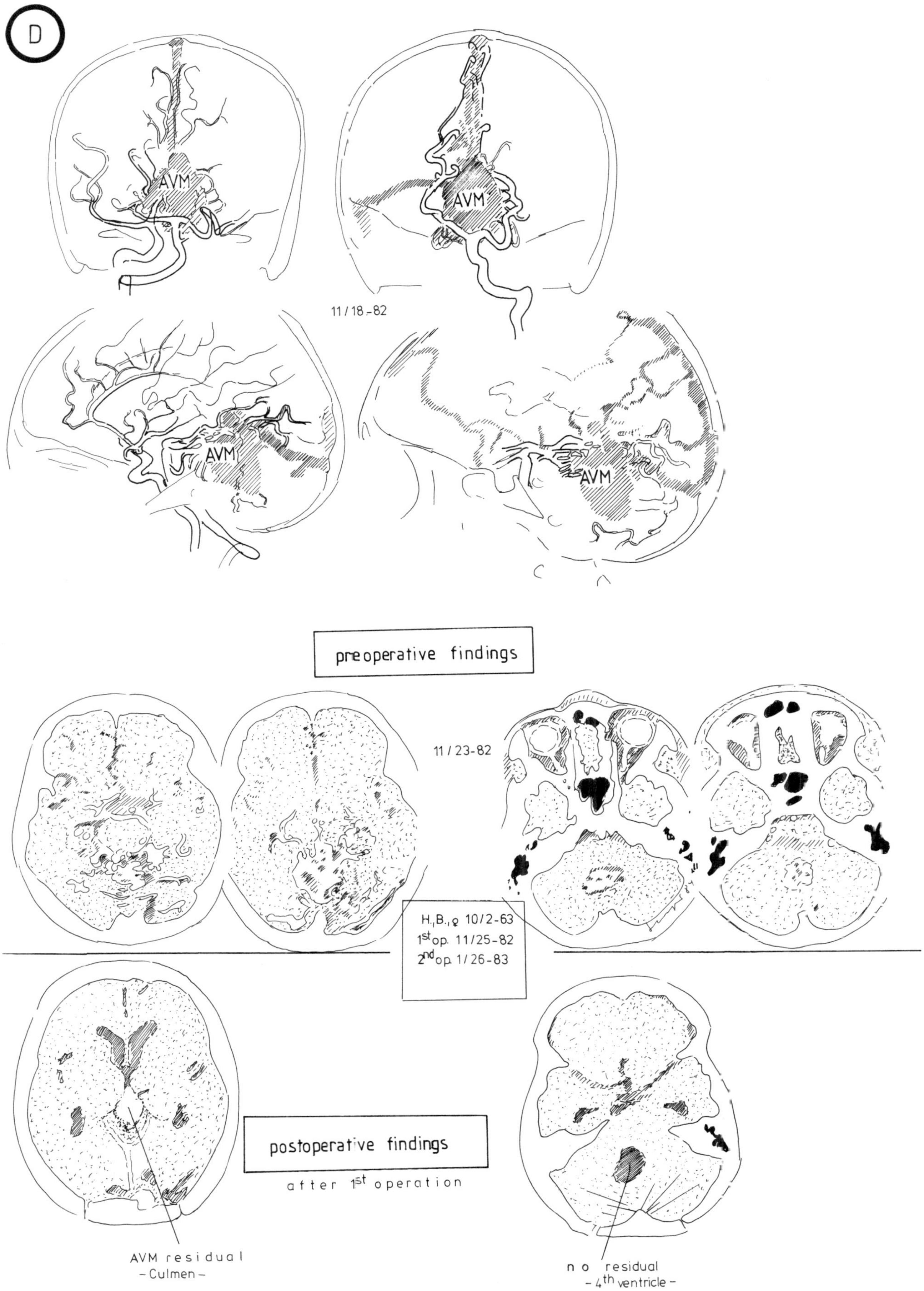
D
AVM
AVM
11/18-82
AVM
AVM
preoperative findings
11/23-82
H, B., ♀ 10/2-63
1st op. 11/25-82
2nd op. 1/26-83
postoperative findings
after 1st operation
AVM residual
- Culmen -
no residual
- 4th ventricle -

Fig. 84. After the first operation residuals of the angioma is recognizable in the area of the Culmen cerebelli. After the second operation there are no angioma remains anymore

D

immediately after 1st operation:
AVM residual of Culmen

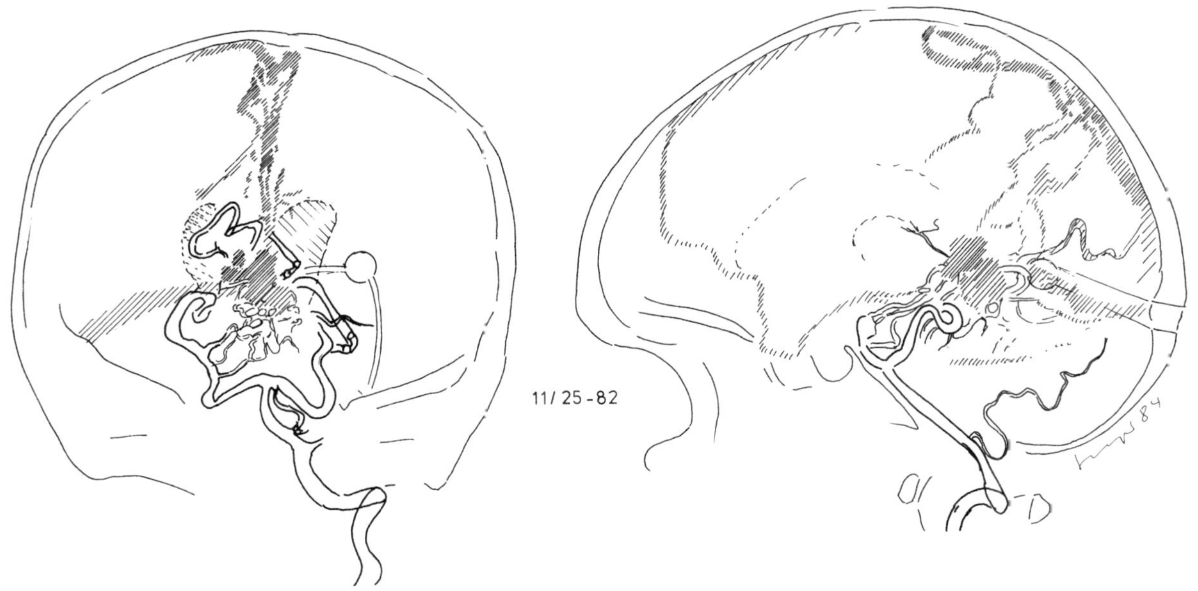

immediately after 2nd operation:
no residual

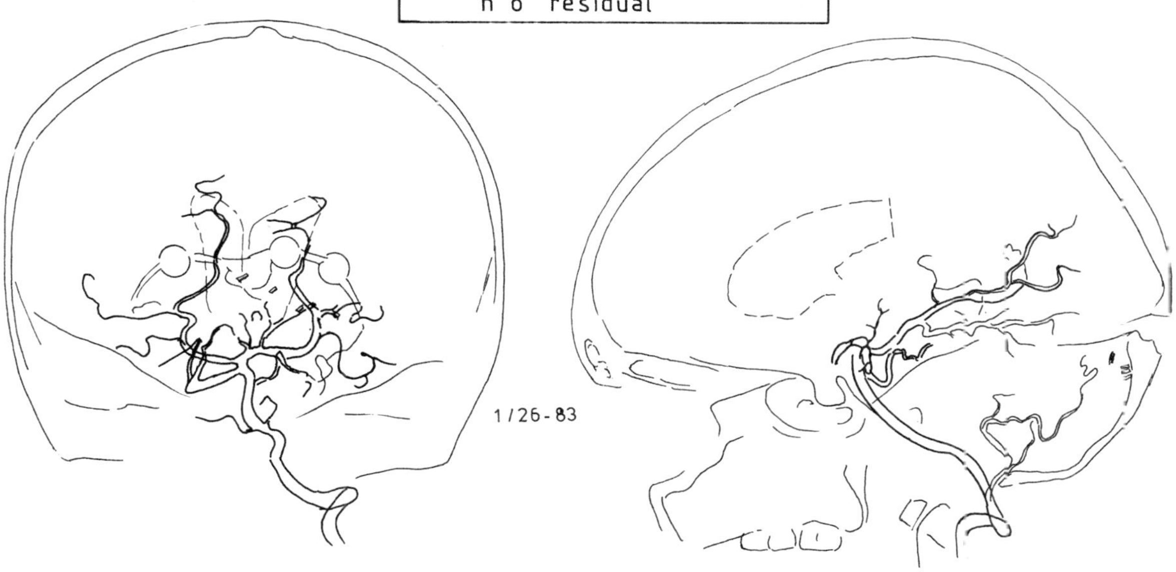

Figs. 85 and 86. Schematic anatomical presentation of both approaches

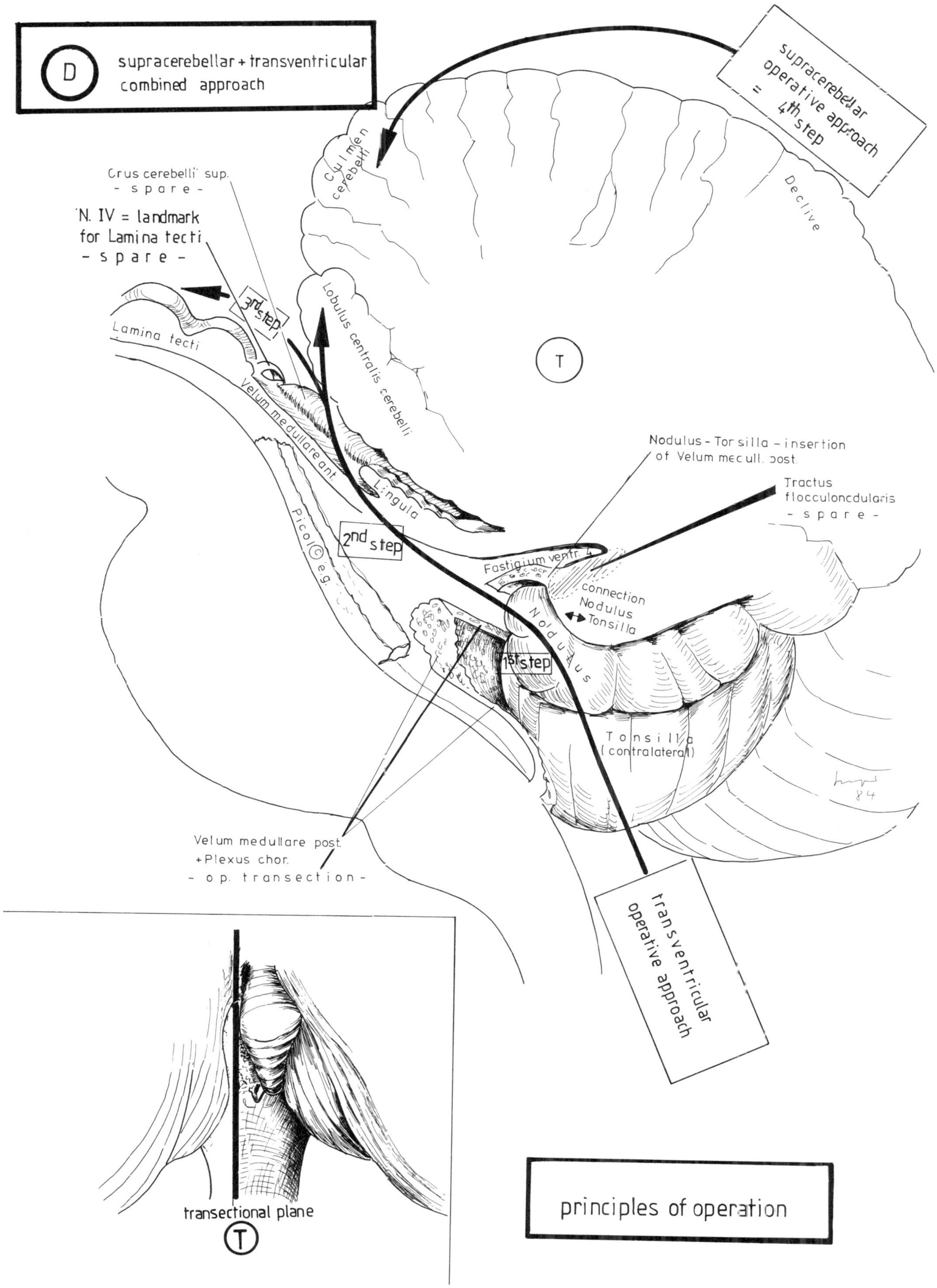

principles of operation

Fig. 86

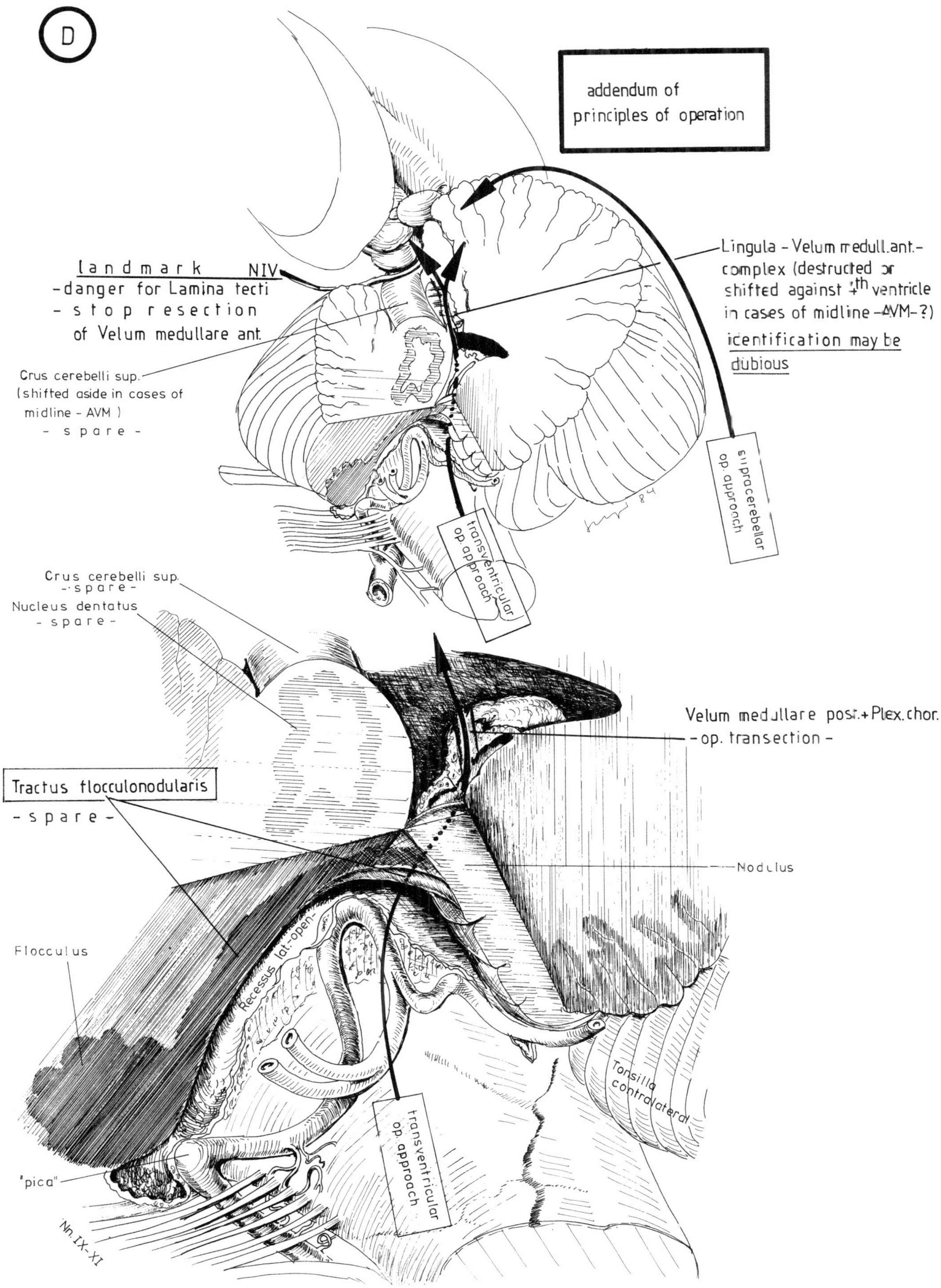
D
addendum of principles of operation
landmark NIV
-danger for Lamina tecti
- stop resection of Velum medullare ant.
Crus cerebelli sup. (shifted aside in cases of midline - AVM) - spare -
Lingula - Velum medull.ant.-complex (destructed or shifted against 4th ventricle in cases of midline -AVM-?)
identification may be dubious
supracerebellar op. approach
transventricular op. approach
Crus cerebelli sup. - spare -
Nucleus dentatus - spare -
Velum medullare post.+Plex.chor. - op. transection -
Tractus flocculonodularis
- spare -
Nodulus
Flocculus
Recessus lat. open-
Tonsilla contralateral
"pica"
Nn.IX-XI
transventricular op. approach

Fig. 87. Microsurgical (above) and macrosurgical (below) presentation of the start of the operation

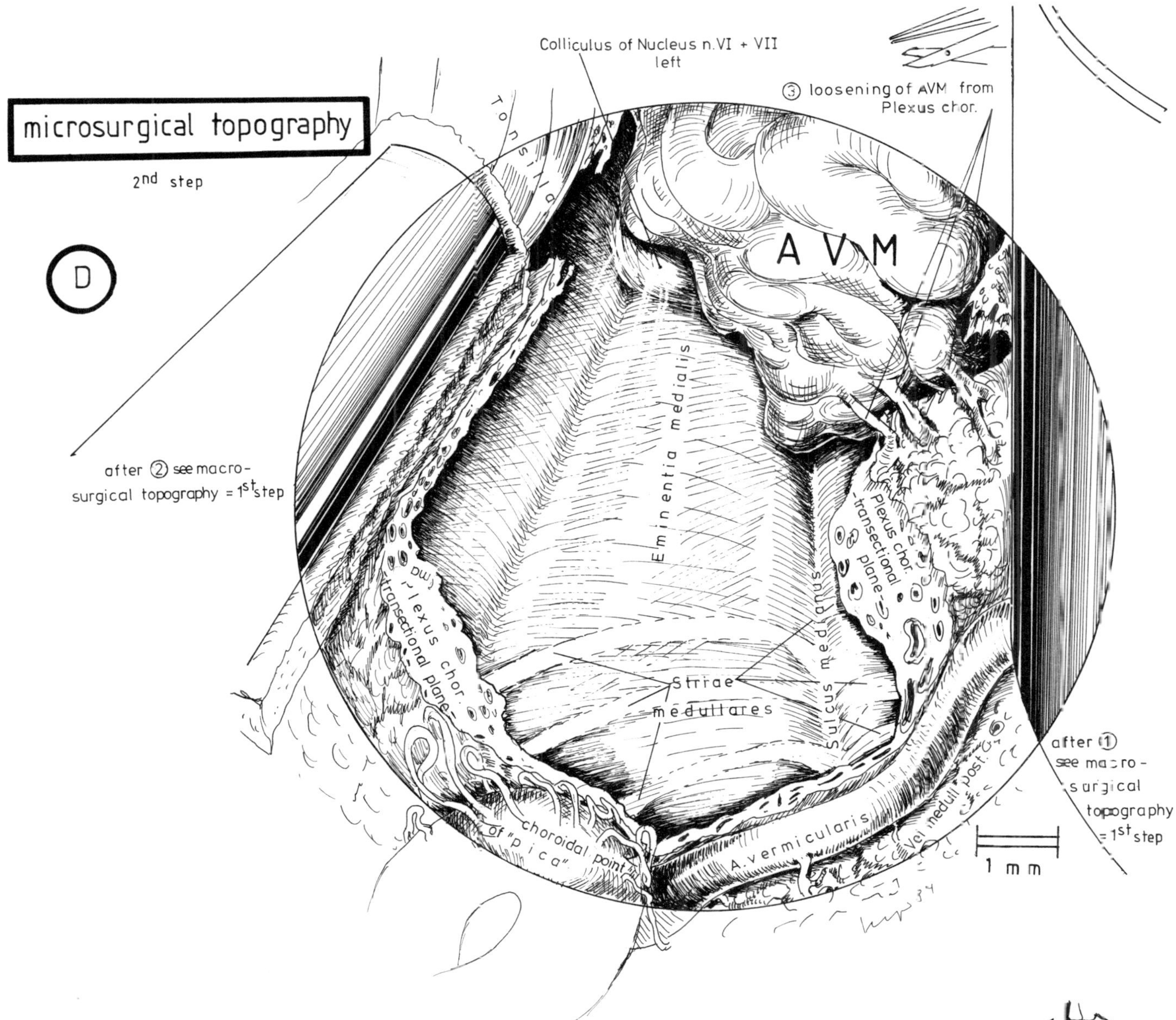

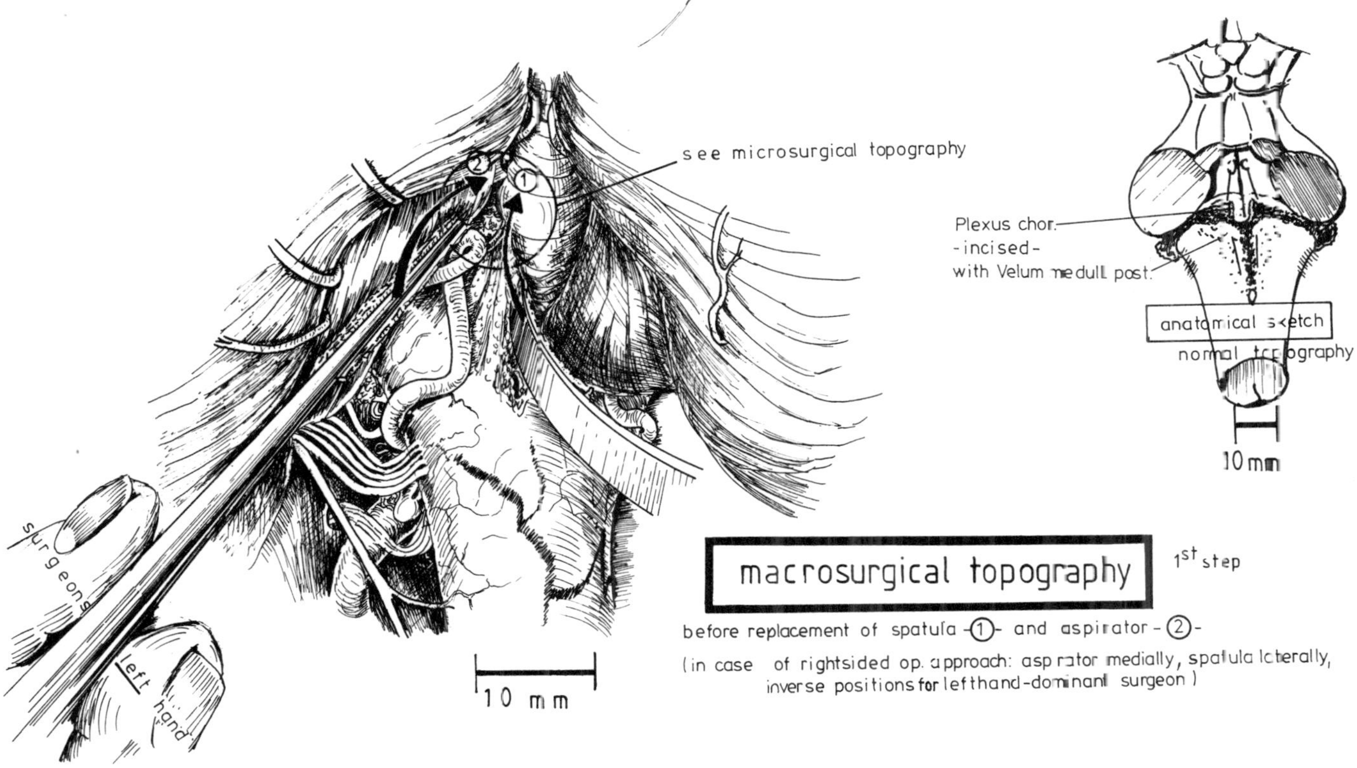

before replacement of spatula -①- and aspirator -②-

(in case of rightsided op. approach: aspirator medially, spatula laterally, inverse positions for lefthand-dominant surgeon)

Fig. 88. Transventricular reduction of the angioma

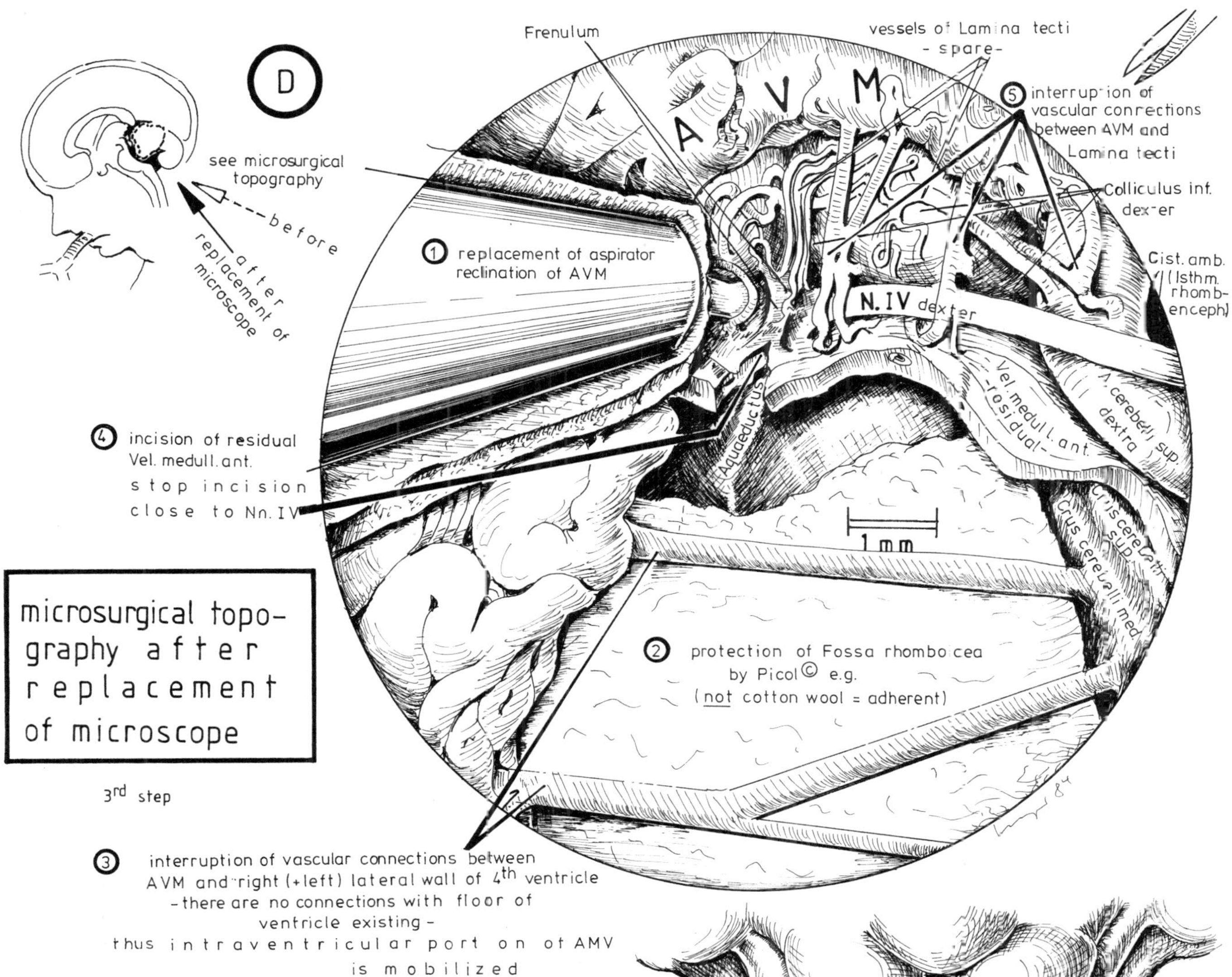
D
see microsurgical topography
before
after replacement of microscope
Frenulum
vessels of Lamina tecti - spare -
AVM
5 interruption of vascular connections between AVM and Lamina tecti
Colliculus inf. dexter
Cist. amb. (Isthm. rhomb-enceph)
1 replacement of aspirator reclination of AVM
N. IV dexter
Aqueductus
Vel. medull. ant. - residual -
A. cerebelli sup. dextra
Crus cerebelli sup.
Crus cerebelli med.
4 incision of residual Vel. medull. ant.
stop incision close to Nn. IV
1 mm
microsurgical topography after replacement of microscope
2 protection of Fossa rhomboidea by Picol© e.g. (not cotton wool = adherent)
3rd step
3 interruption of vascular connections between AVM and right (+left) lateral wall of 4th ventricle - there are no connections with floor of ventricle existing - thus intraventricular portion of AMV is mobilized

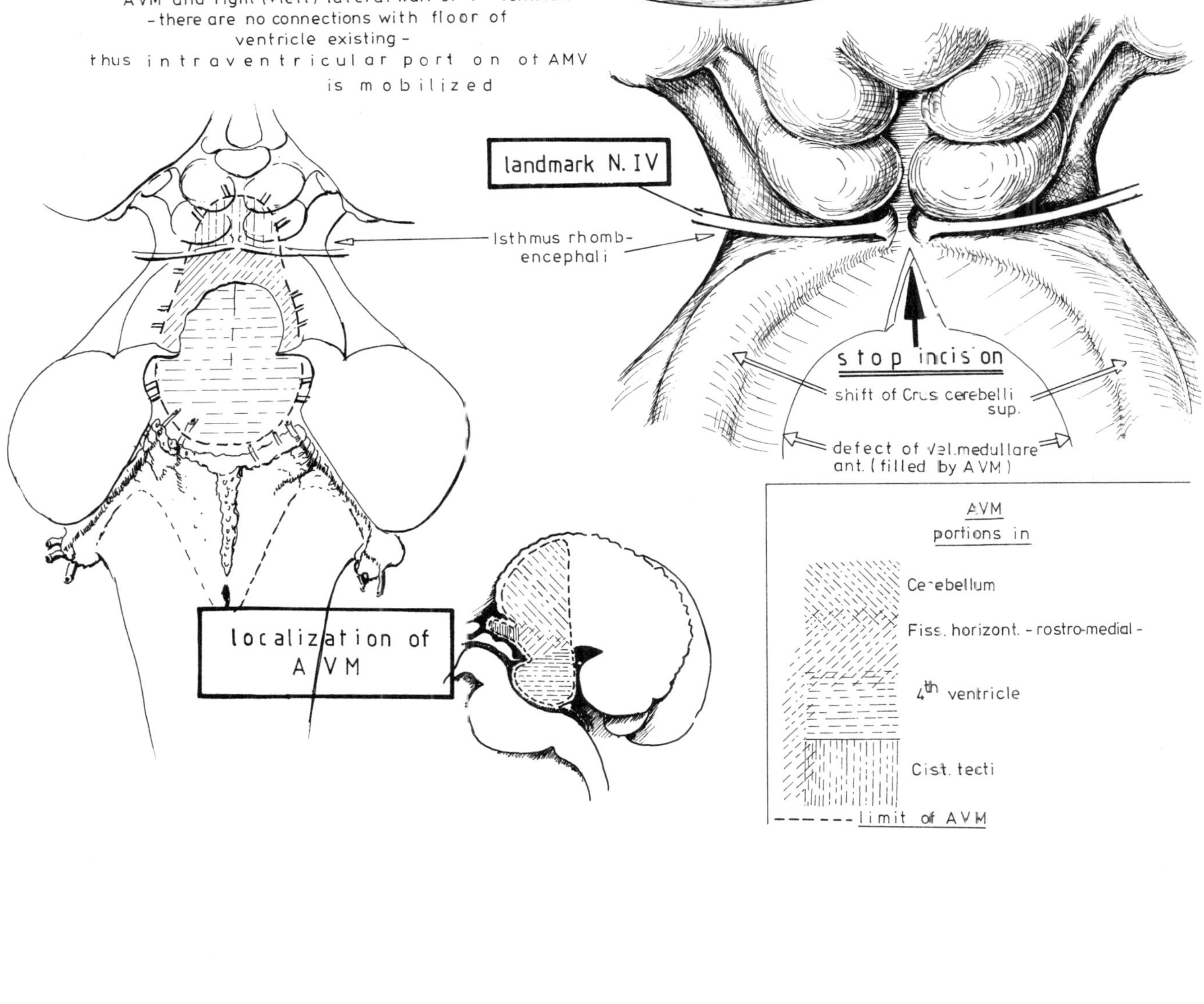
landmark N. IV
Isthmus rhomb-encephali
stop incision
shift of Crus cerebelli sup.
defect of Vel. medullare ant. (filled by AVM)
localization of AVM
AVM portions in
Cerebellum
Fiss. horizont. - rostro-medial -
4th ventricle
Cist. tecti
limit of AVM

Fig. 89. Topography after removal of the angioma. The remains of the AVM in the area of the Culmen (see anatomical sketch) is not visible in the microsurgical site

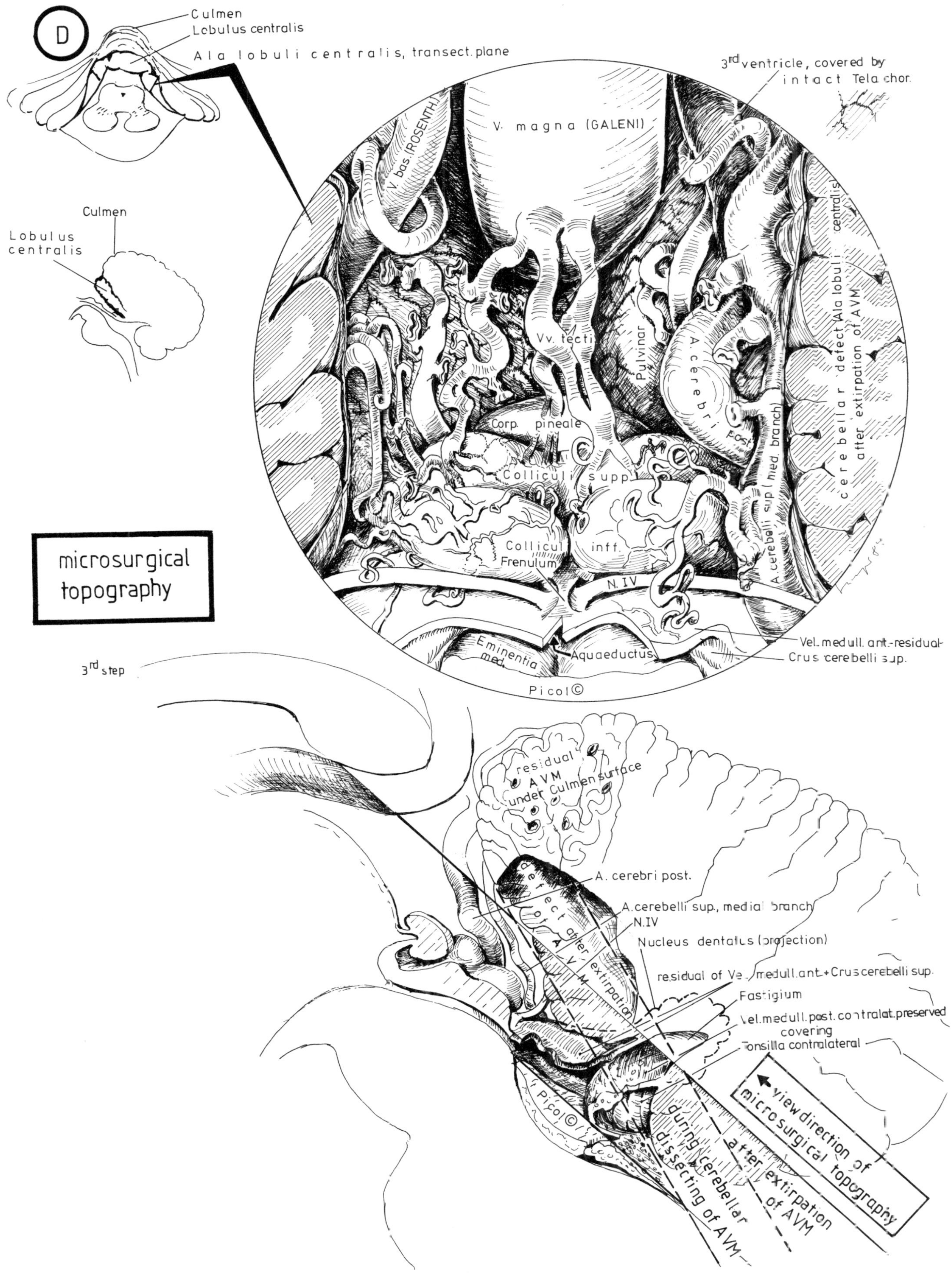
D
Culmen
Lobulus centralis
Ala lobuli centralis, transect. plane
Culmen
Lobulus centralis
3rd ventricle, covered by intact Tela chor.
V. magna (GALENI)
V. bas. (ROSENTH.)
Vv. tecti
Pulvinar
A. cerebri post.
cerebellar defect (Ala lobuli centralis) after extirpation of AVM
A. cerebelli sup. (med. branch)
Corp. pineale
Colliculi supp.
Colliculi inff.
Frenulum
N. IV
Vel. medull. ant.-residual-
Crus cerebelli sup.
Eminentia med.
Aquaeductus
Picol©
microsurgical topography
3rd step
residual AVM under Culmen surface
A. cerebri post.
A. cerebelli sup., medial branch
N.IV
Nucleus dentatus (projection)
residual of Vel. medull. ant.+Crus cerebelli sup.
Fastigium
Vel. medull. post. contralat. preserved covering
Tonsilla contralateral
defect after extirpation of AVM
Picol©
view direction of microsurgical topography
after extirpation of AVM
during cerebellar dissecting of AVM

Fig. 90. Site of the reoperation with removal of the AVM remains

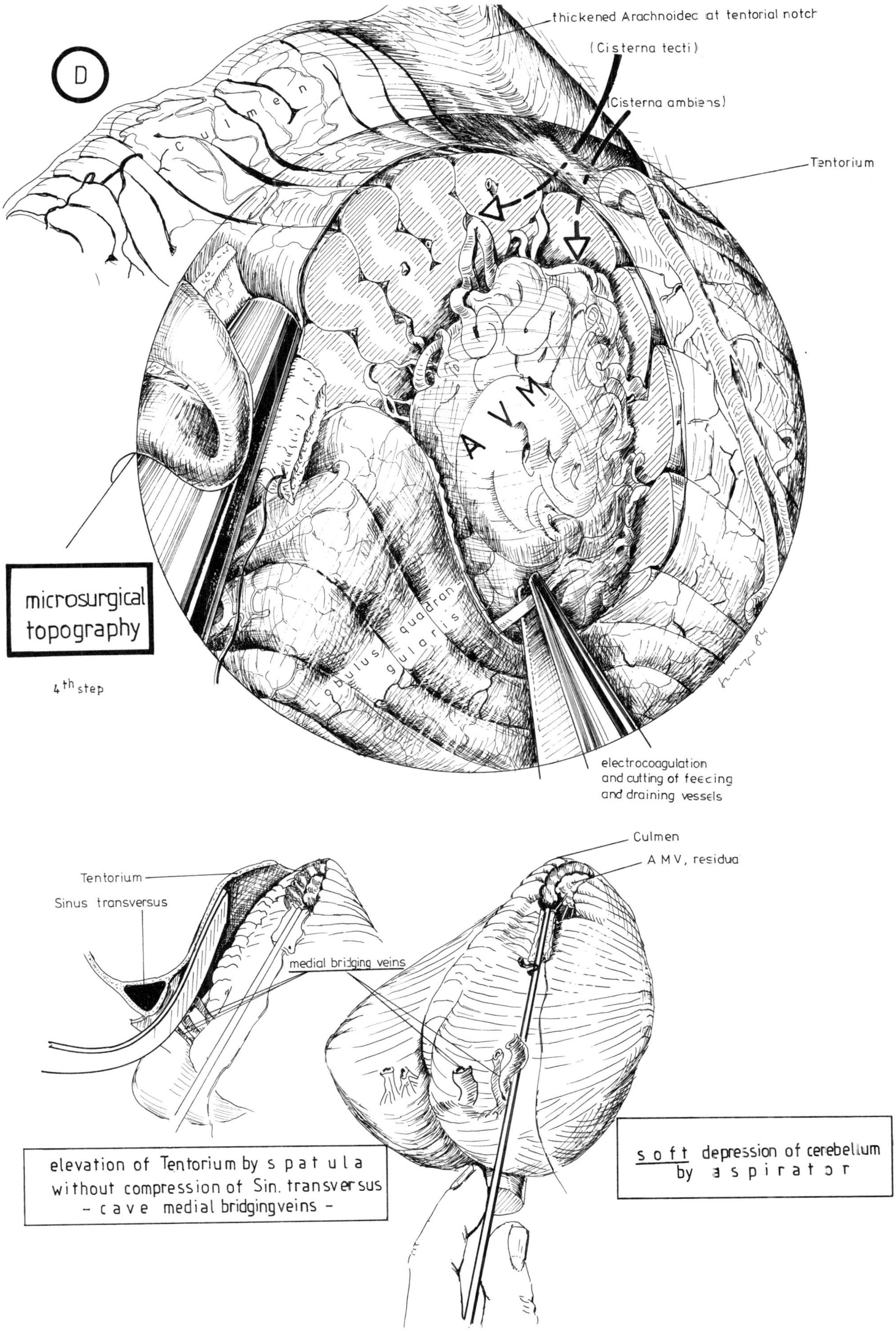

D
thickened Arachnoidea at tentorial notch
(Cisterna tecti)
(Cisterna ambiens)
Tentorium
Culmen
AVM
Lobulus quadrangularis
microsurgical topography
4th step
electrocoagulation and cutting of feeding and draining vessels
Culmen
A M V, residua
Tentorium
Sinus transversus
medial bridging veins
elevation of Tentorium by spatula without compression of Sin. transversus - cave medial bridgingveins -
soft depression of cerebellum by aspirator

Fig. 91. Lateral tumor localization in the Fissura horizontalis cerebelli
Floor of the Fissura: Brachium pontis
Roof of the Fissura: Lobulus quadrangularis cerebelli
Landmark of lateral limit: root of N. V. and lateral limit of Lobulus quadrangularis. Approach favorable for processes extending further medially as far as the Cisterna tecti (approach type **A**). The further lateral and caudal the process lies in the fissura, the more favorable is the infratentorial approach **(B)**. Example of an AVM close to the Cisterna tecti, located in the medial area of the Pedunculus cerebelli medius (Brachium pontis)

(A) temporobasal approach

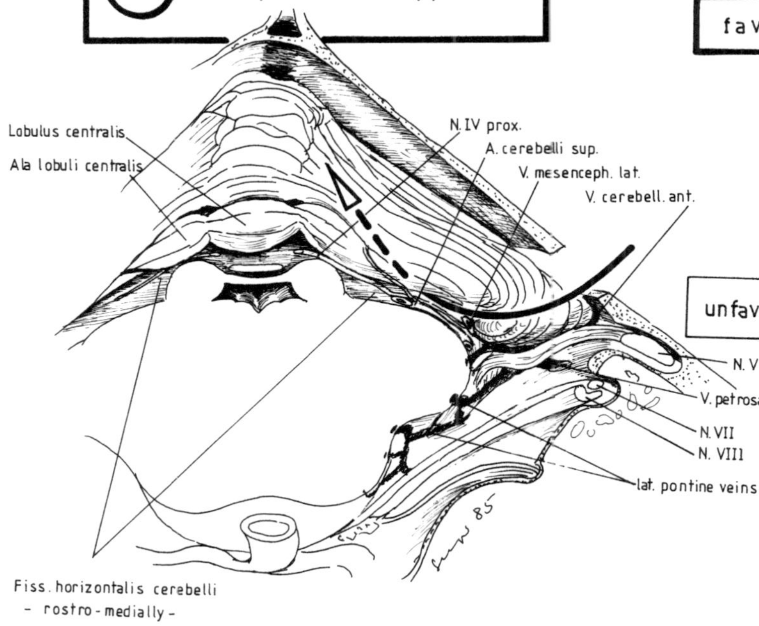

favorable

- rostro-medial location of Fiss. horizontalis
- A. cerebelli sup.
- V. mesencephalica lat.
- N.IV prox. (close to midbrain) + dist. (close to dura penetration and crossing over N.V)

unfavorable

- caudo-lateral location of Fiss. horizontalis
- N.V, Nn. VII/VIII
  (exception: combined with drilling of Apex ossis petrosi - SAMII, personal communication -)
- A. cerebelli inf. ant. ("AICA")
- V. cerebell. ant.
- lat. pontine veins
- V. petrosa sup.
- approach may be hindered by temporobasal veins

(B) infratentorial approach

favorable

- caudo-lateral location of Fiss. horizontalis
- N.IV prox., N.V, N.VII / VIII
- "AICA"
- V. cerebellaris ant.
- lat. pontine veins
- approach dorsal from V. petrosa sup. to Fiss. horiz.

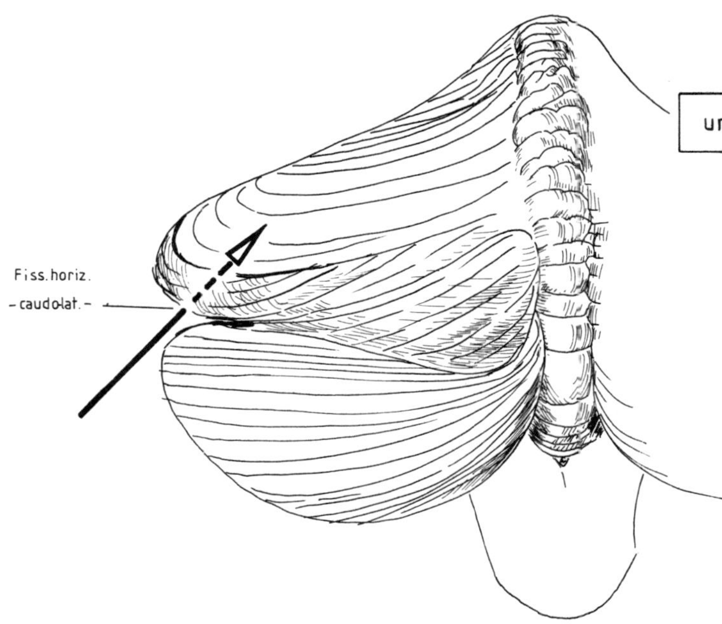

unfavorable

- rostromedial location of Fiss. horiz.
  (except large lesions)
- A. cerebelli sup.
- V. mesencephalica lat.
- N. IV dist.
- intrapontine portion of the lesion

see addendum

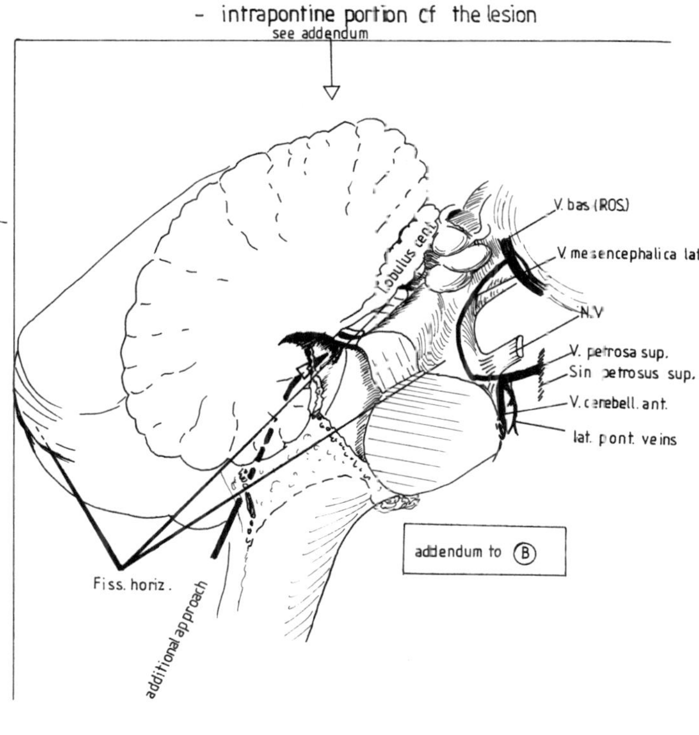

addendum to (B)

Fig. 92. Clinical example of a small AV-angioma of the Pedunculus cerebelli medius (Brachium pontis), located in the bottom of the lateral portion of the Fissura horizontalis cerebelli. Minimal temporary neurological deficits following a minor spontaneous haemorrhage. No additional deficits postoperatively *

* A picture of this case not included here is shown in Seeger, W., Atlas of Topographical Anatomy of the Brain and Surrounding Structures. Wien–New York: Springer. 1978.

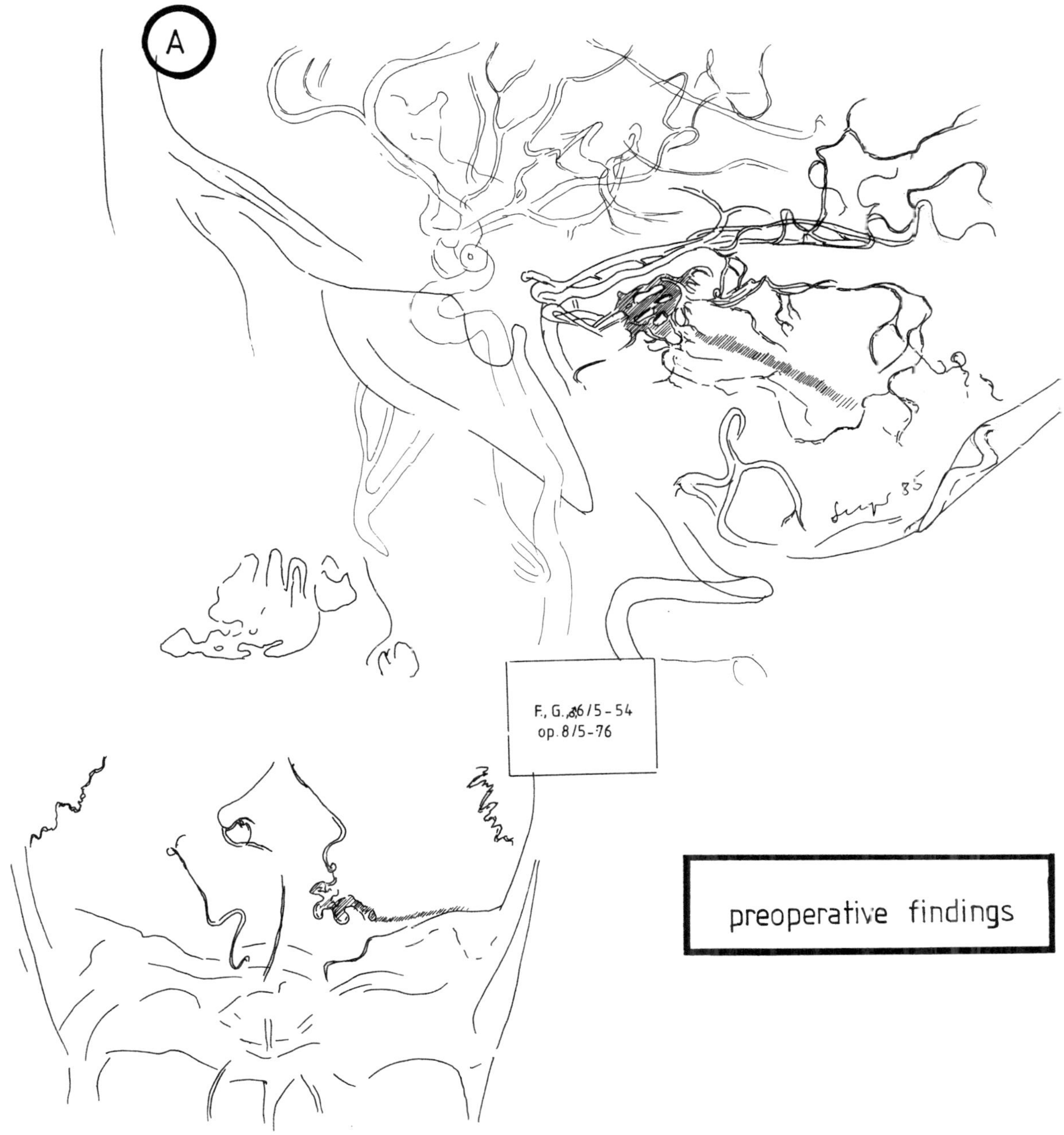

preoperative findings

A

principles of operation

1st step	temporobasal trepanation, Dura opening, reclination of temp. lobe
2nd step	incision of Tentorium + opening Cisterna ambiens
3rd step	opening Fiss. horizontalis cerebelli + dissecting AVM.

Fig. 93. Copy of a photo of the operation, accompanied by an anatomical sketch

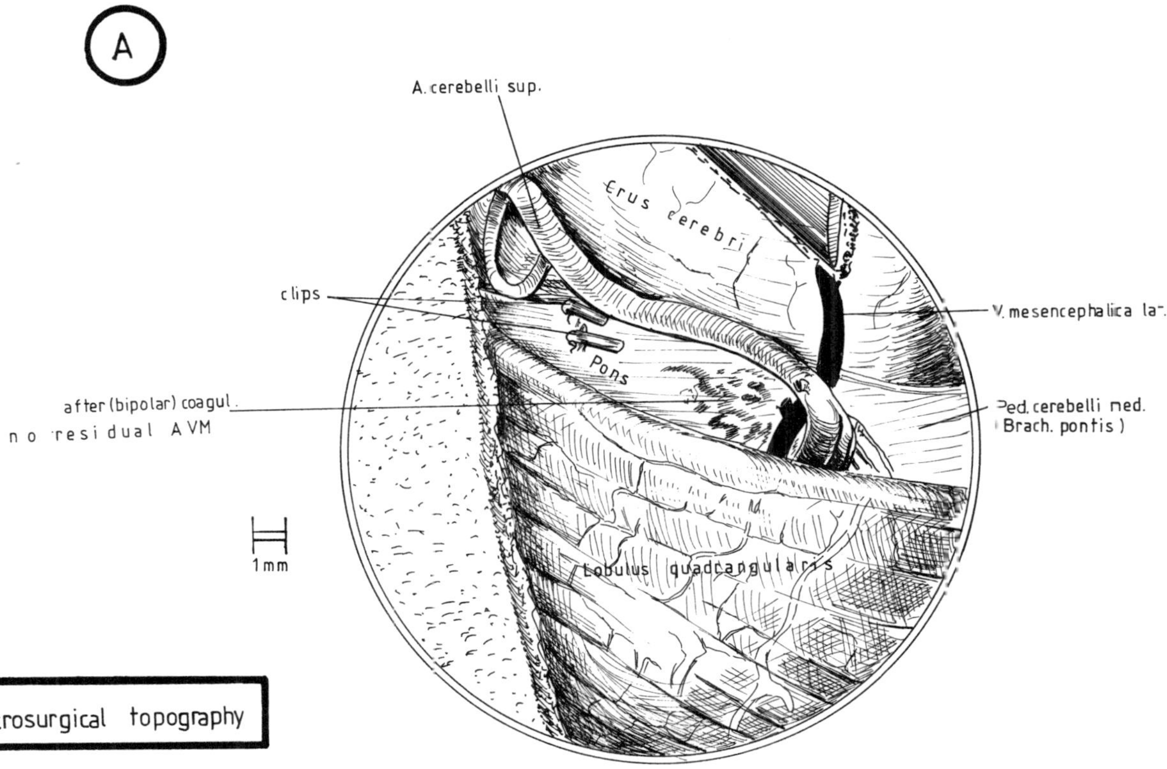

microsurgical topography

3rd step

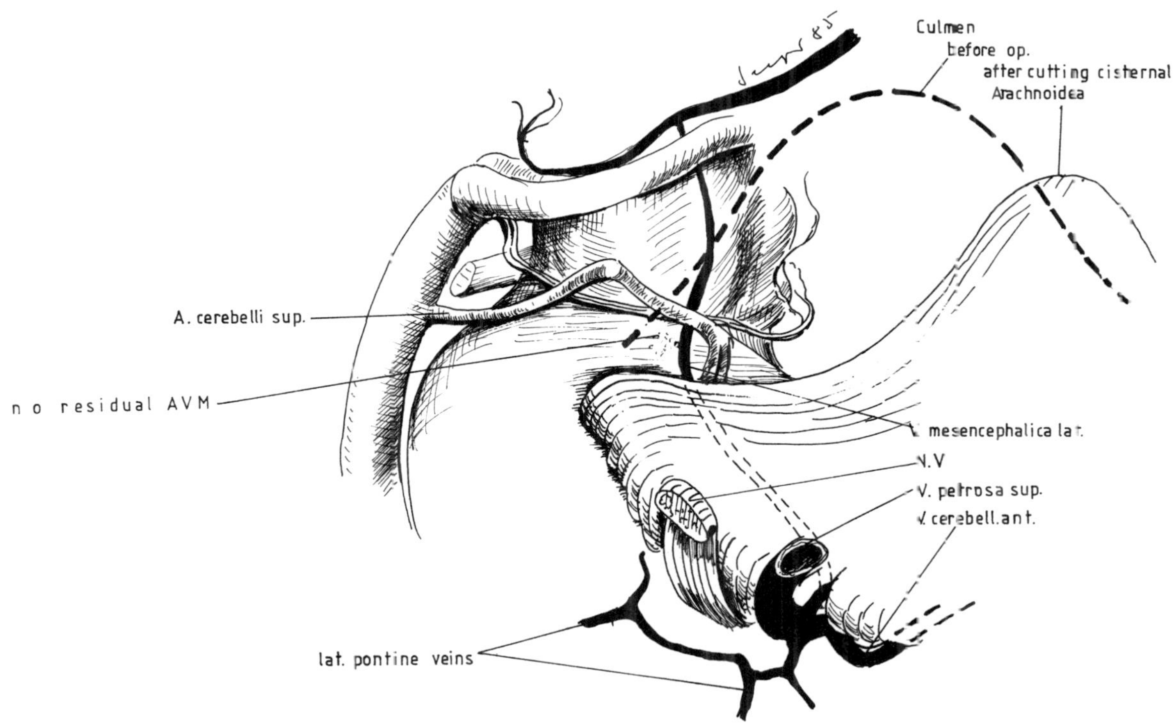

Fig. 94. Further copies of the photos during the operation of the same case

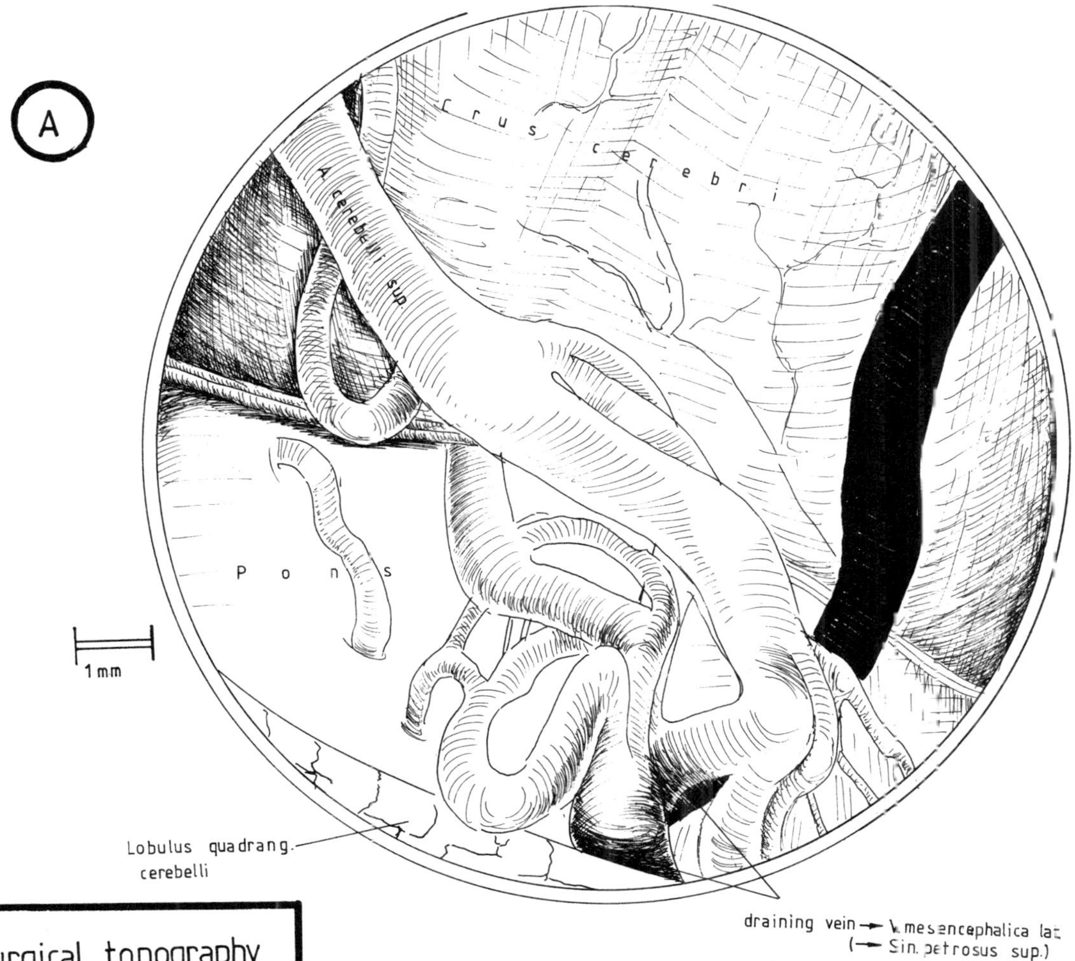

microsurgical topography

3rd step

magnification >
before extirpation of AVM

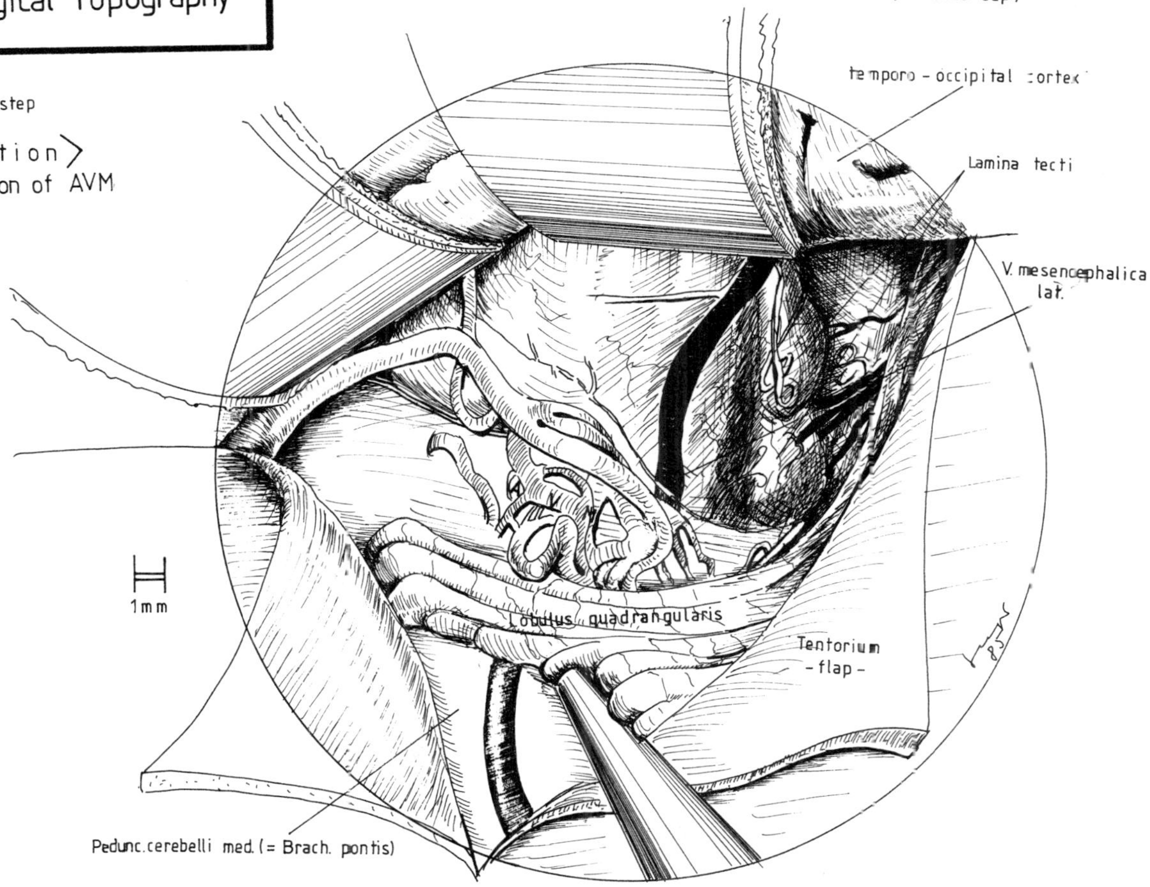

Fig. 95. Clinical example of a venous angioma in the lateral region of the Brachium pontis; operative approach infratentorially (approach **B**). Two years previously acute trigeminal deficits, then speech disturbances, left hemiparesis, paresis of the right leg, slowly progressing. The angioma was removed from the Pedunculus cerebelli medius (Brachium pontis). Since via Fissura horizontalis cerebelli the intrapontine part could not be reached, a second operation through the 4th ventricle was carried out. Here only the remains of the intrapontine haemorrhage was found, and no angioma*

* Both operations were carried out by Priv.-Doz. Dr. H. R. Eggert, coworker of the author.

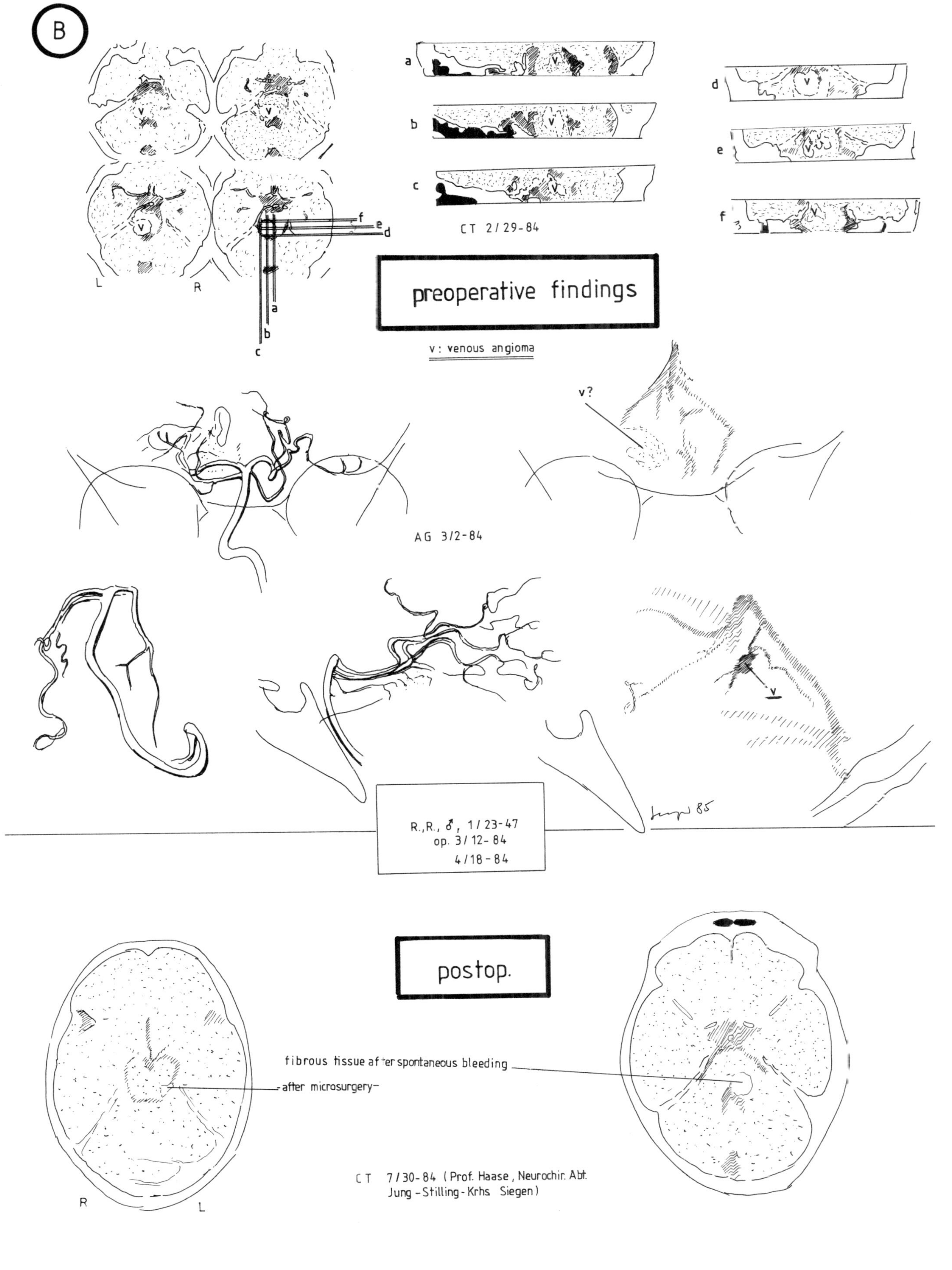
B
preoperative findings
v: venous angioma
CT 2/29-84
AG 3/2-84
v?
R.,R., ♂, 1/23-47
op. 3/12-84
4/18-84
postop.
fibrous tissue after spontaneous bleeding
- after microsurgery -
CT 7/30-84 (Prof. Haase, Neurochir. Abt.
Jung-Stilling-Krhs Siegen)
R
L

Fig. 96. First operation (1st to 3rd steps): Exposure of the lateral portions of the Fissura horizontalis cerebelli. Second operation (4th step): Transventricular approach to the Pons

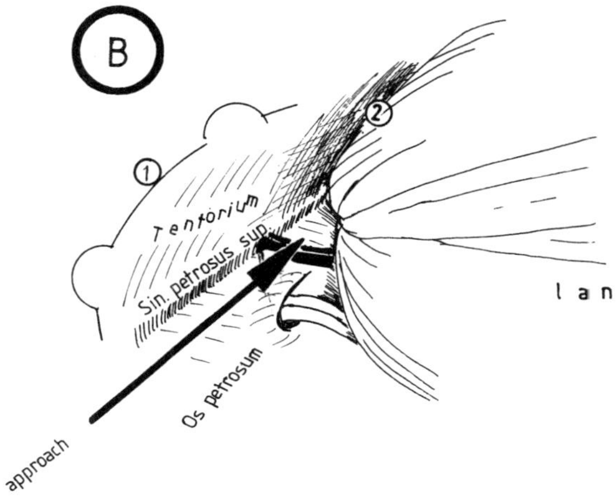

1st step

① suboccipital trepanation

② reclining Lobulus quadrangularis

landmarks for approach
- Sin. petrosus sup.: Tentorium / Os petrosum
- Nn. VII + VIII + Porus acusticus int.: Os petrosum (hard)
- N. V: Tentorium (elastic)

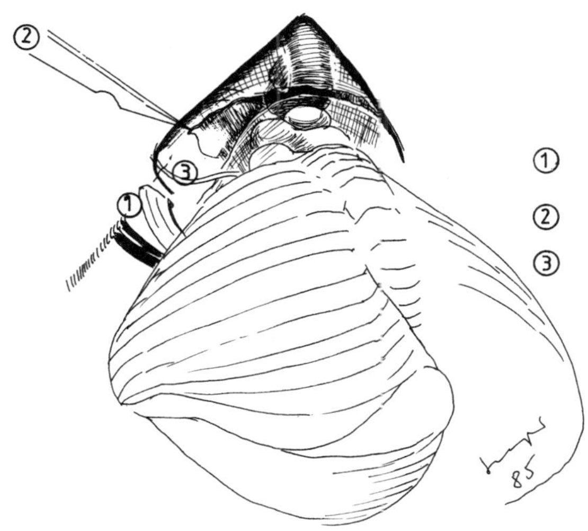

2nd step

① dissection of V. petrosa sup. + N. V

② opening Arachnoidea of Cisterna ambiens

③ dissecting N. IV

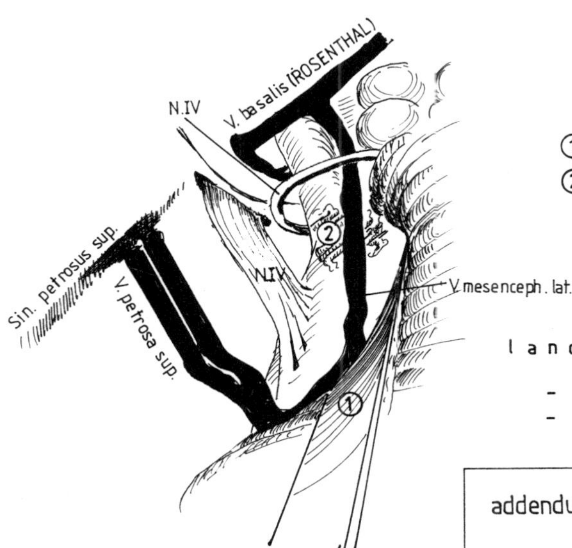

3rd step

① reclining ant. portion of Lobulus quadrangularis

② dissection of AVM in Isthmus rhombencephali

landmarks:
- N. IV : Isthmus rhombencephali (Pons – Mesencephalon)
- V. mesencephalica lat. (rostrally between Crus and Tectum mesenceph. caudally on Crus cerbelli sup.= Brach. pontis)

addendum: 4th step 2nd operation: midline approach to Fossa rhomboidea

Fig. 97. Copy of a microsurgical photograph of the same case*. Below: anatomical sketch

* The author thanks Priv.-Doz. Dr. H. R. Eggert, his coworker for the microsurgical photograph.

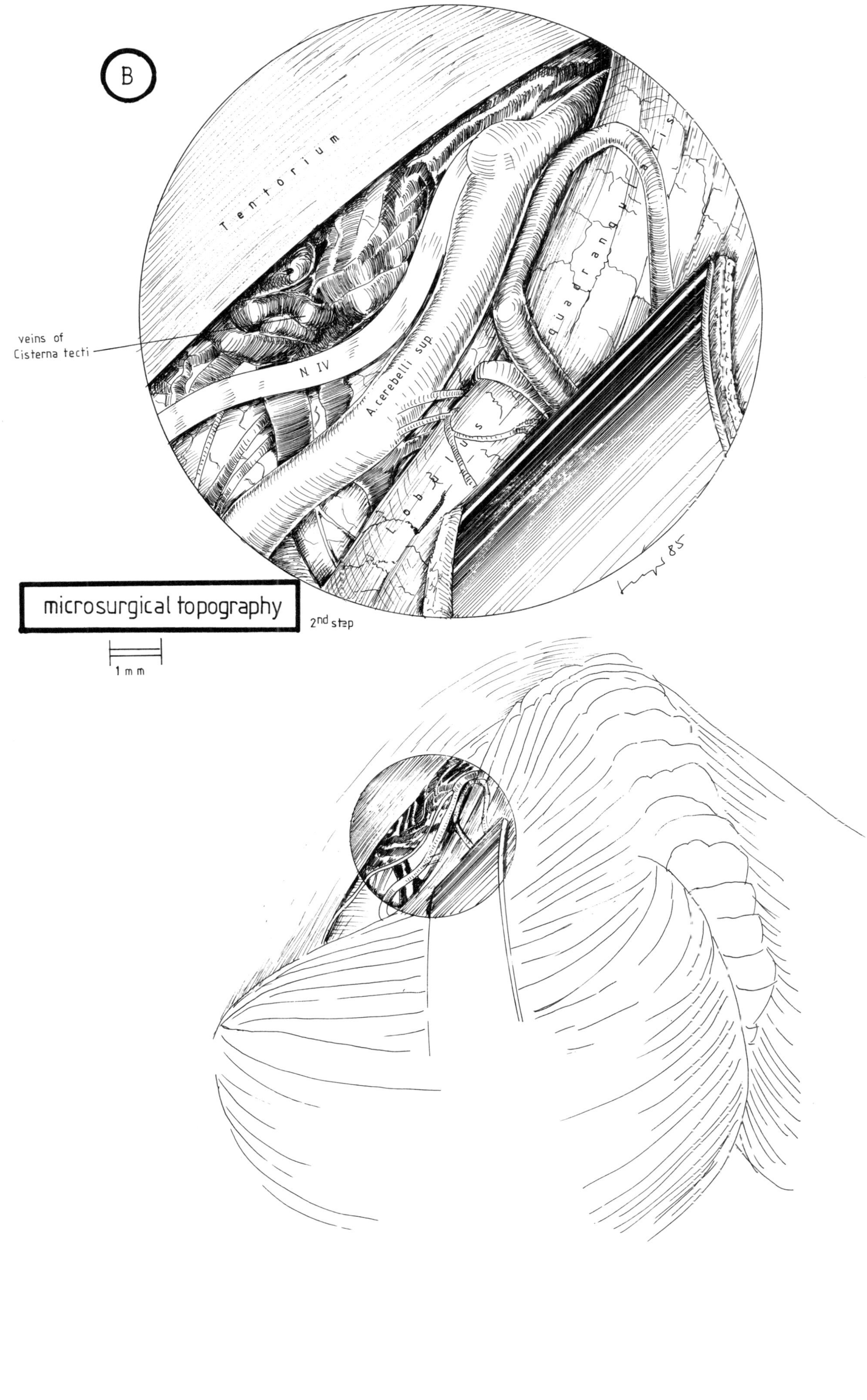
B
Tentorium
veins of Cisterna tecti
N IV
A. cerebelli sup.
quadrangularis
Lobulus
microsurgical topography
2nd step
1 mm

Fig. 98. Copy of a microsurgical photograph of the same case*. Below: anatomical sketch

---

* The author thanks Priv.-Doz. Dr. H. R. Eggert, his coworker for the microsurgical photograph.

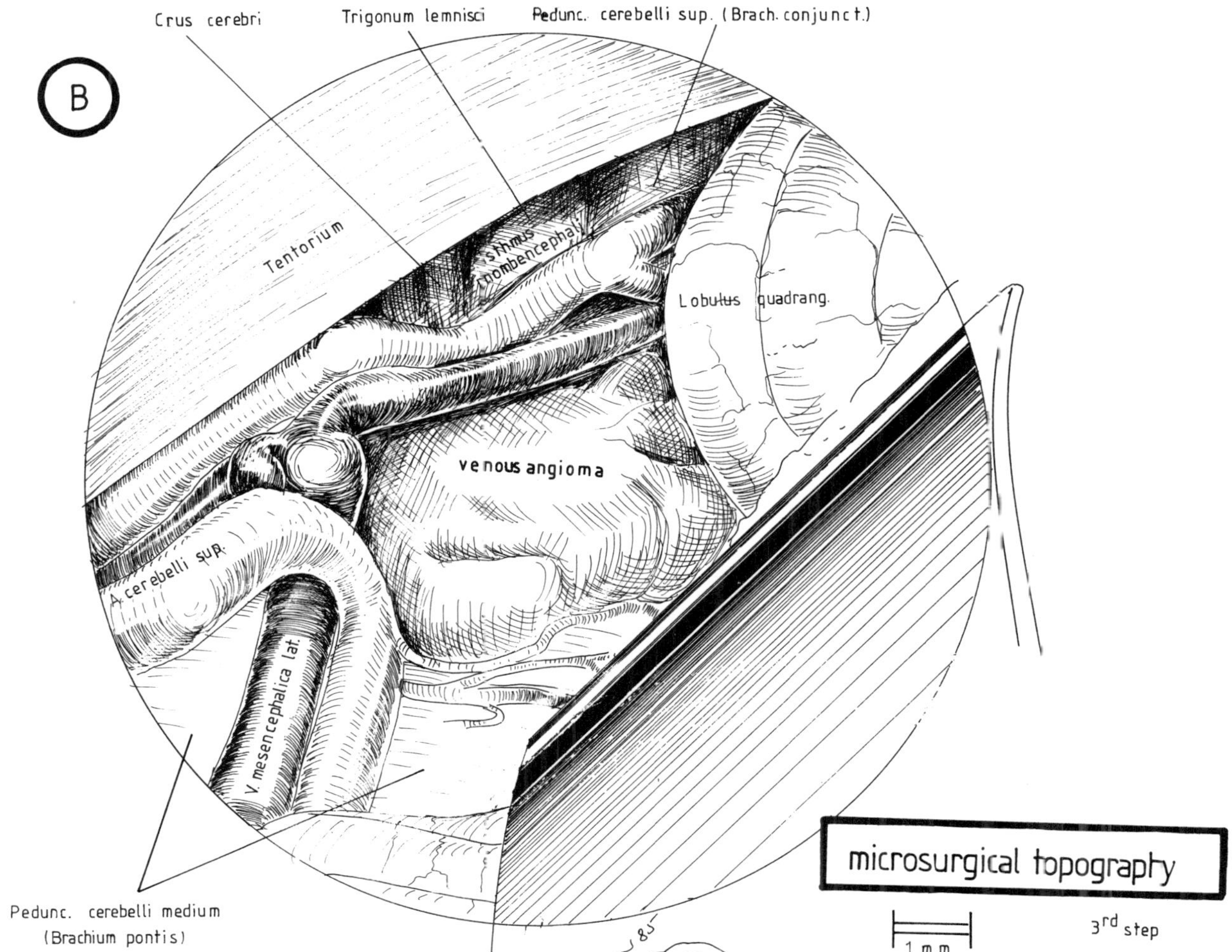
Crus cerebri
Trigonum lemnisci
Pedunc. cerebelli sup. (Brach. conjunct.)
B
Tentorium
Isthmus rhombencephali
Lobulus quadrang.
venous angioma
A. cerebelli sup.
V. mesencephalica lat.
Pedunc. cerebelli medium
(Brachium pontis)
microsurgical topography
1 mm
3rd step

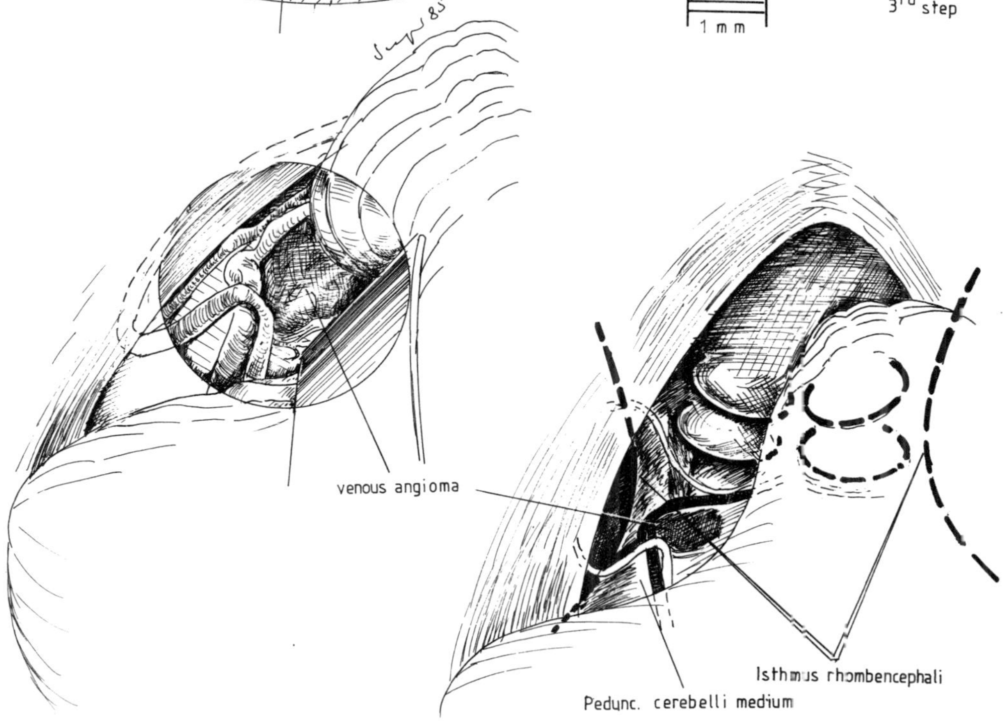
venous angioma
Isthmus rhombencephali
Pedunc. cerebelli medium

Fig. 99. Second operation * (4th step): Incision of the Fossa rhomboidea. No angioma. A yellow stain and fibrous tissue was found after bleeding of the angioma. Wound closure

* The here demonstrated method of arachnoid splitting between the Tonsille and Vermis cerebelli was described in more detail in Seeger, W., Microsurgery of the Brain, Vol. 2, and Seeger, W., Microsurgery of the Cerebral Veins. Wien–New York: Springer. 1980 and 1984, and in the following chapter. It is completely different from the typical approach to the fourth ventricle.

FIG. 99

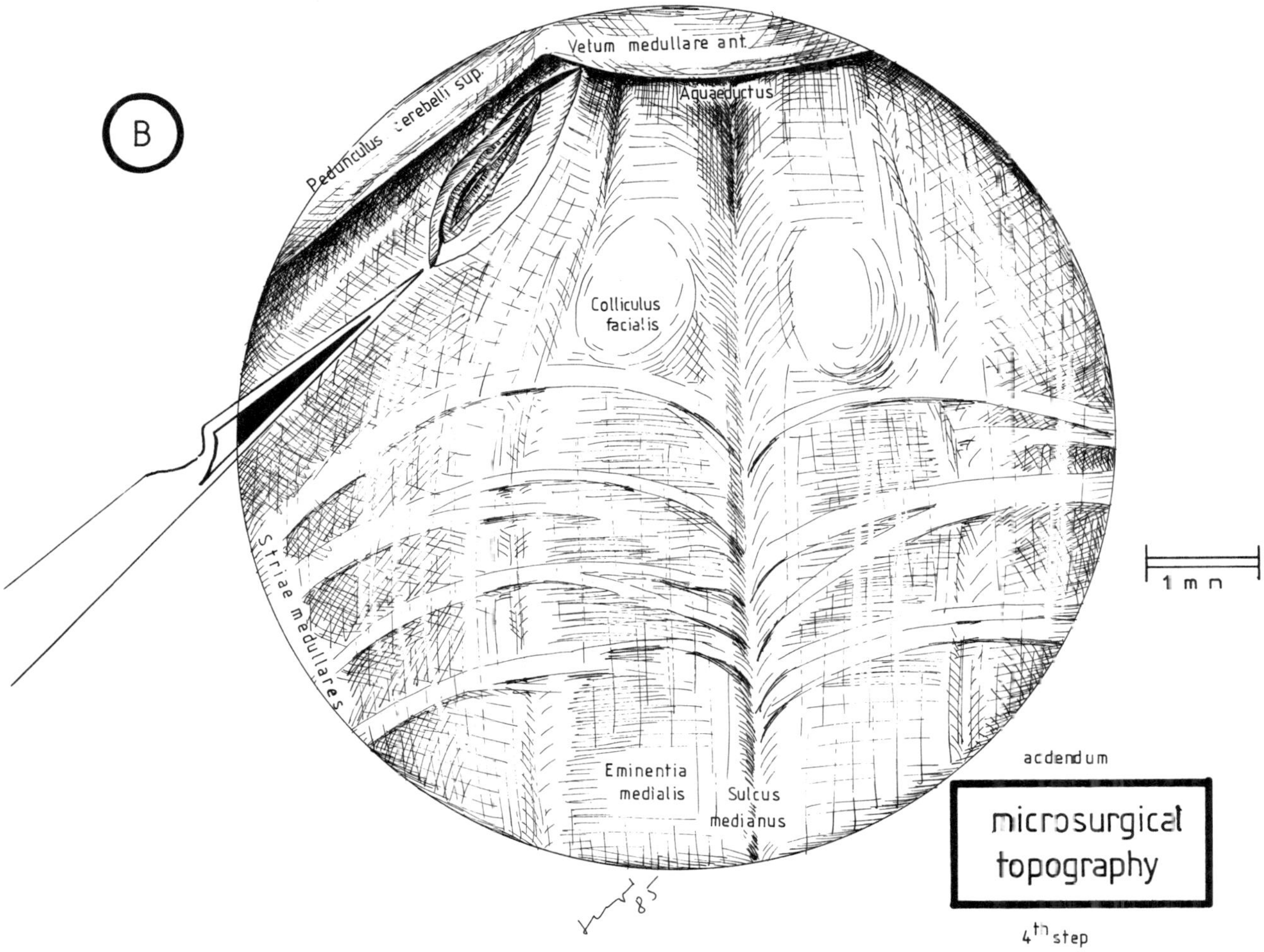
B
Velum medullare ant.
Aquaeductus
Pedunculus cerebelli sup.
Colliculus facialis
Striae medullares
Eminentia medialis
Sulcus medianus
1 mm
addendum
microsurgical topography
4th step

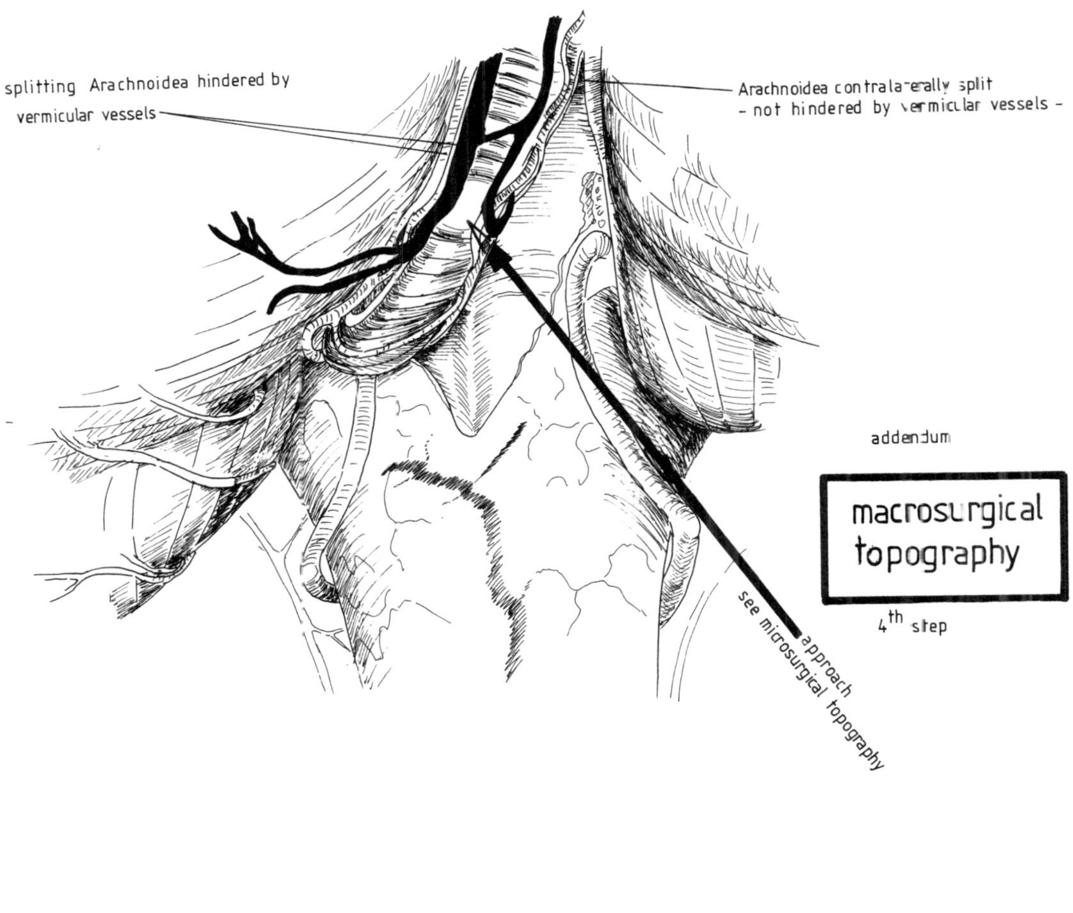
splitting Arachnoidea hindered by vermicular vessels
Arachnoidea contralaterally split
- not hindered by vermicular vessels -
approach
see microsurgical topography
addendum
macrosurgical topography
4th step

Chapter 4

Dorsal Cisterns and Fissures, Posterior Segment (Figs. 100 to 101)

Fig. 100. Conventional approach **A:** splitting the Vermis cerebelli. Personal approach **B:** nodular-tonsillar approach *

* This approach was described in detail in the previous volumes. Therefore one can limit oneself here to the principle.

lesions in 4th ventricle

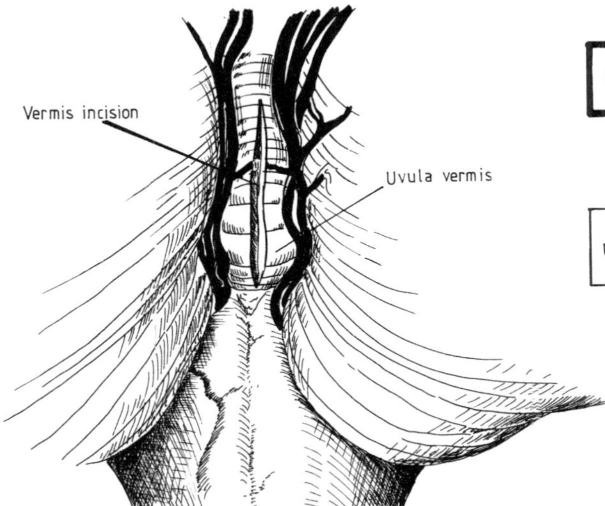

A median approach (split vermis)

favorable
- Vv. vermiculares

unfavorable
- Archicerebellum (Nodulus/Uvula - Flocculus-complex) split
- Velum medullare post. and its relationships to Fossa rhomboidea + Recessus lat. + choroid point of "pica" + Plexus chor.

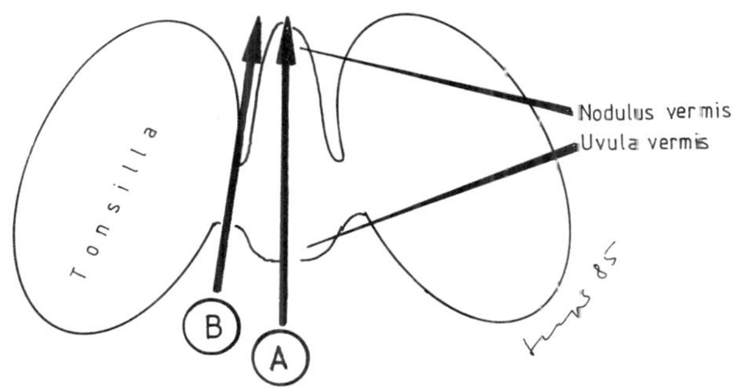

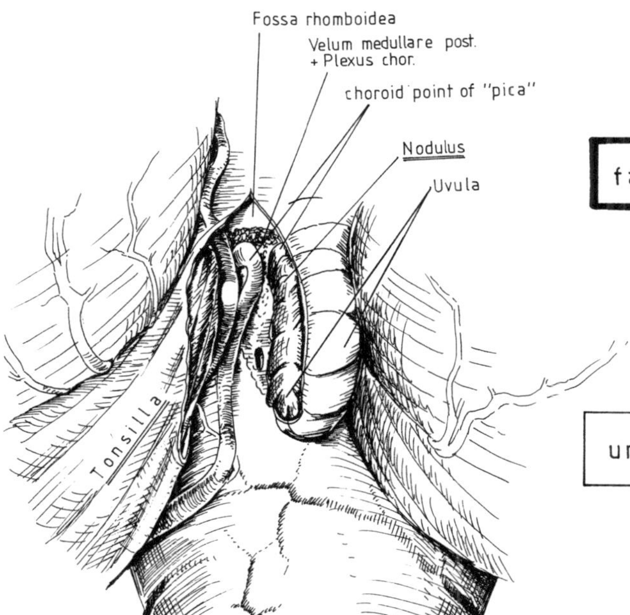

B nodulo - tonsillar approach (split Arachnoidea)

favorable
- Archicerebellum less endangered (cave Tractus flocculo-nodularis)
- Velum medullare post. and its relationships to Fossa rhomboidea + Recessus lat. + choroid point of "pica" + Plexus chor

unfavorable
- in some cases A.+V. vermicularis

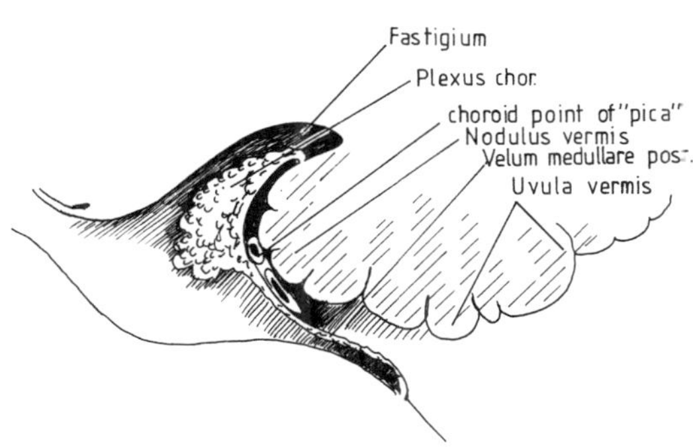

Fig. 101. Typical reduction of one of the tumors of the Fossa rhomboidea *

* Here again one can limit oneself to the presentation of the principle. For completion this approach should be mentioned again.

FIG. 101

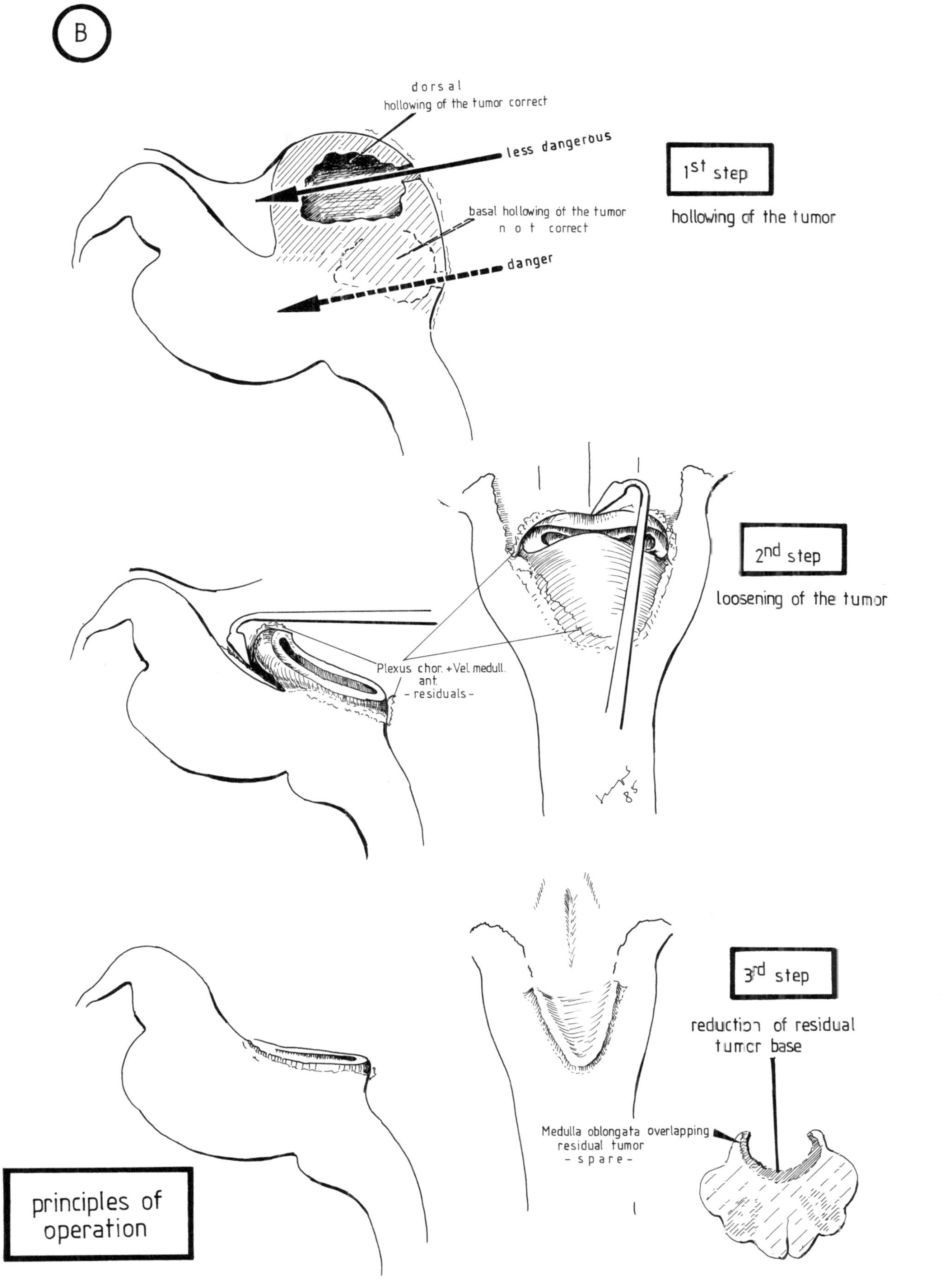
B
dorsal
hollowing of the tumor correct
less dangerous
basal hollowing of the tumor
not correct
danger
1st step
hollowing of the tumor
2nd step
loosening of the tumor
Plexus chor. + Vel. medull. ant.
- residuals -
3rd step
reduction of residual tumor base
Medulla oblongata overlapping residual tumor
- spare -
principles of operation

Chapter 5
Lateral Cisterns and Fissures, Middle Segment* (Figs. 102 to 137)

Fig. 102. Processes in the anterior region of the Putamen and Caudatum with connection to the ventricular system and to the basal cisterns can either be operated from basally **(A)** or transventricularly **(B).** The choice of the approach – **A** or **B** – depends on whether the basis of the process lies in the posterior fronto-basal region, that is the area of the Substantia perforata ant., or whether the process is more closely connected with the Nucleus caudatus, that is, the floor of the frontal horn

* One can designate the Cisterna fissurae Sylvii as the "anterior" segment of the lateral cisternal area. However, here there is no other approach due to its superficial position. The special problems of this area of the cisterns have been sufficiently covered in the previous volumes.

(A) pterional approach

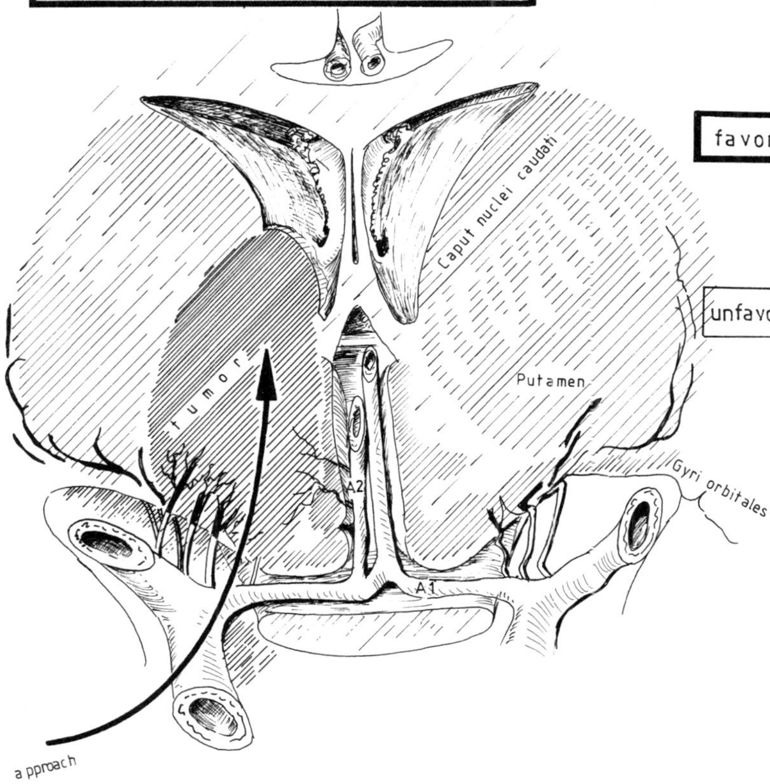

favorable
- cisternal tumor portion
- Putamen + Subst. perforata ant. + Rr. perforantes } tumor base
- Gyri orbitales

unfavorable
- dorsolateral (intraventricular) tumor portions
- midline/feeding arteries originating from A2
- no landmark for Capsula int.

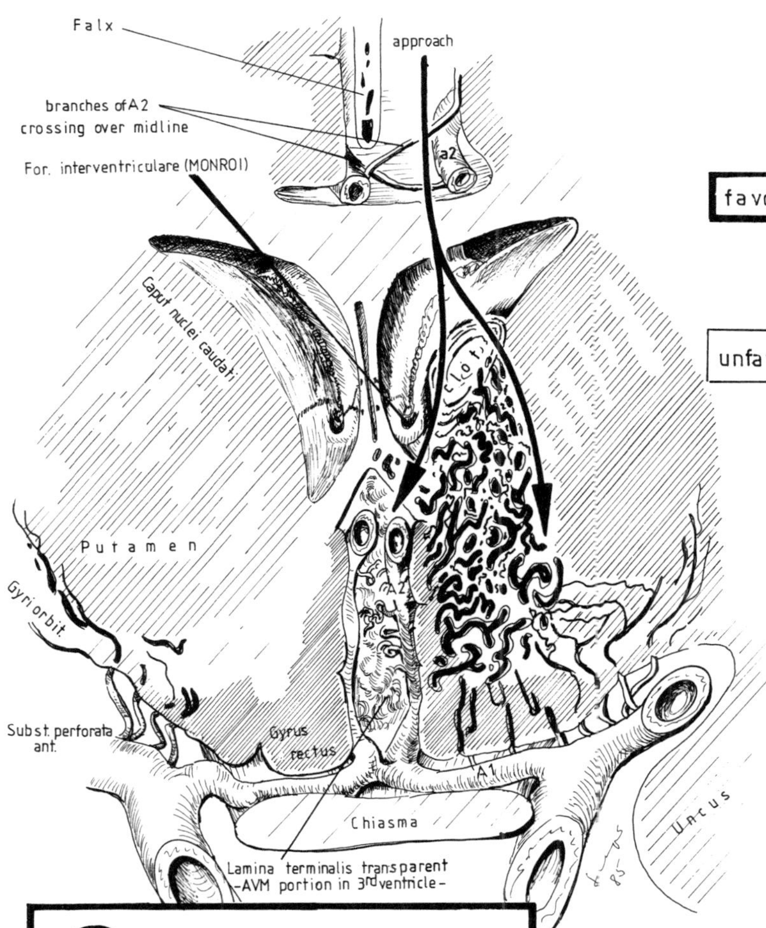

favorable
- dorsal (intraventricular) portions of AVM
- 3rd ventricle
- midline/feeding arteries originating from A2
- landmark for Capsula int.: For. interventric. (MONROI)

unfavorable
- feeding arteries in Subst. perforata ant. (from Rr. perforantes)
- Putamen
- in some cases branches of A2 (crossing over midline)

(B) midline-transventricular approach

Fig. 103. Clinical example of a dermoid between the Substantia perforata ant. and the frontal horn, relationships to the Caput nuclei caudati and the Putamen. Apoplectic right hemiparesis on June 7, 1984 due to infarction of the left basal ganglia (retrotumoral). No aphasia, slight right-sided hemihypaesthesia. Stereotactic puncture*. After stereotaxy and radical removal of the tumor no additional deficits. Pre- and postoperatively psychologically intact**

---

* Department of Stereotaxy, Freiburg (Director: Prof. Dr. F. Mundinger).

** Operation performed by Dr. W. Hassler, coworker of the author.

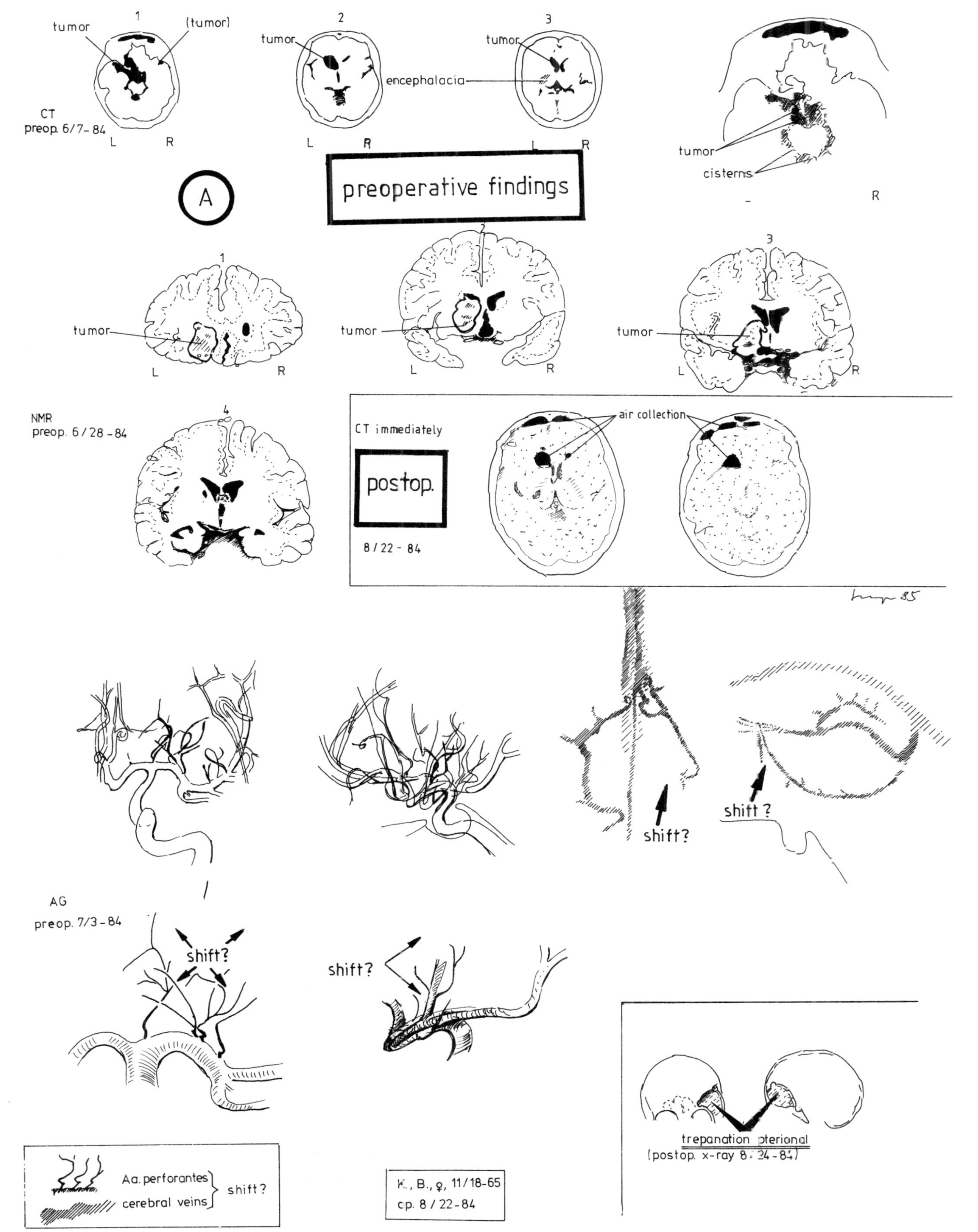
tumor
(tumor)
tumor
tumor
encephalacia
CT
preop. 6/7-84
L R
L R
L R
tumor
cisterns
R
A
preoperative findings
tumor
tumor
tumor
L R
L R
L R
NMR
preop. 6/28-84
CT immediately
postop.
8/22-84
air collection
shift?
shift ?
AG
preop. 7/3-84
shift?
shift?
Aa. perforantes
cerebral veins
shift?
K., B., ♀, 11/18-65
cp. 8/22-84
trepanation pterional
(postop. x-ray 8/24-84)

Fig. 104. Anatomical relationships of the process to the brain as shown by the computer-tomographic and nuclear magnetic resonance results

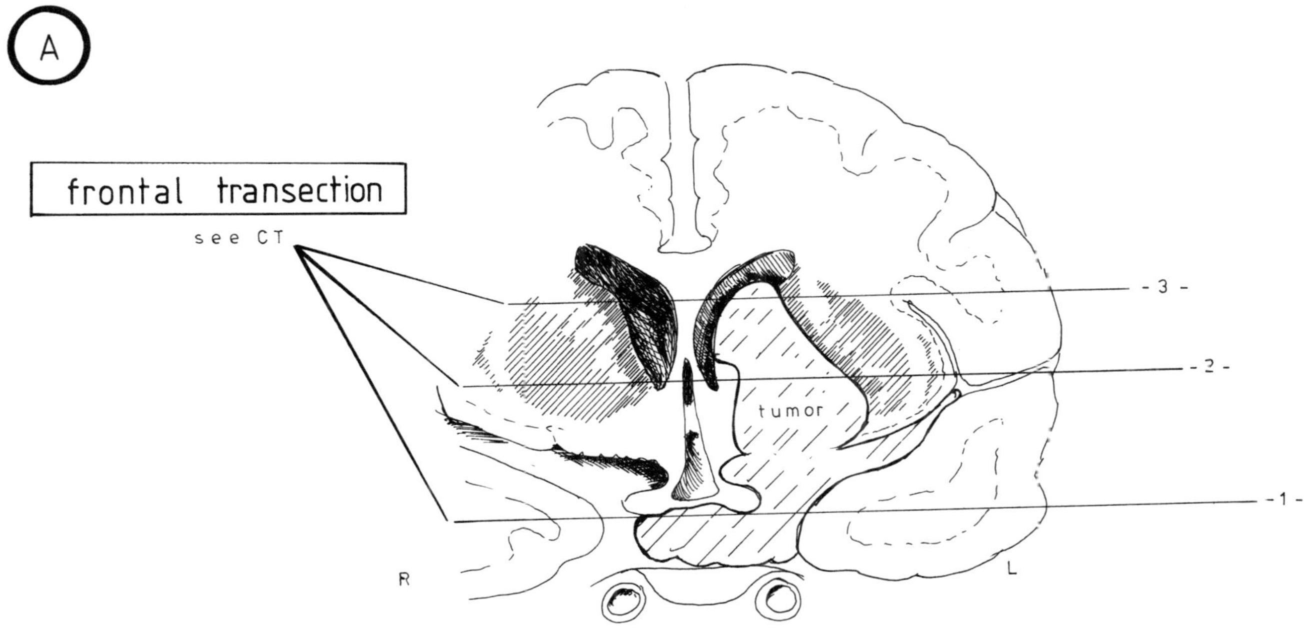
A
frontal transection
see CT
- 3 -
- 2 -
- 1 -
tumor
R
L

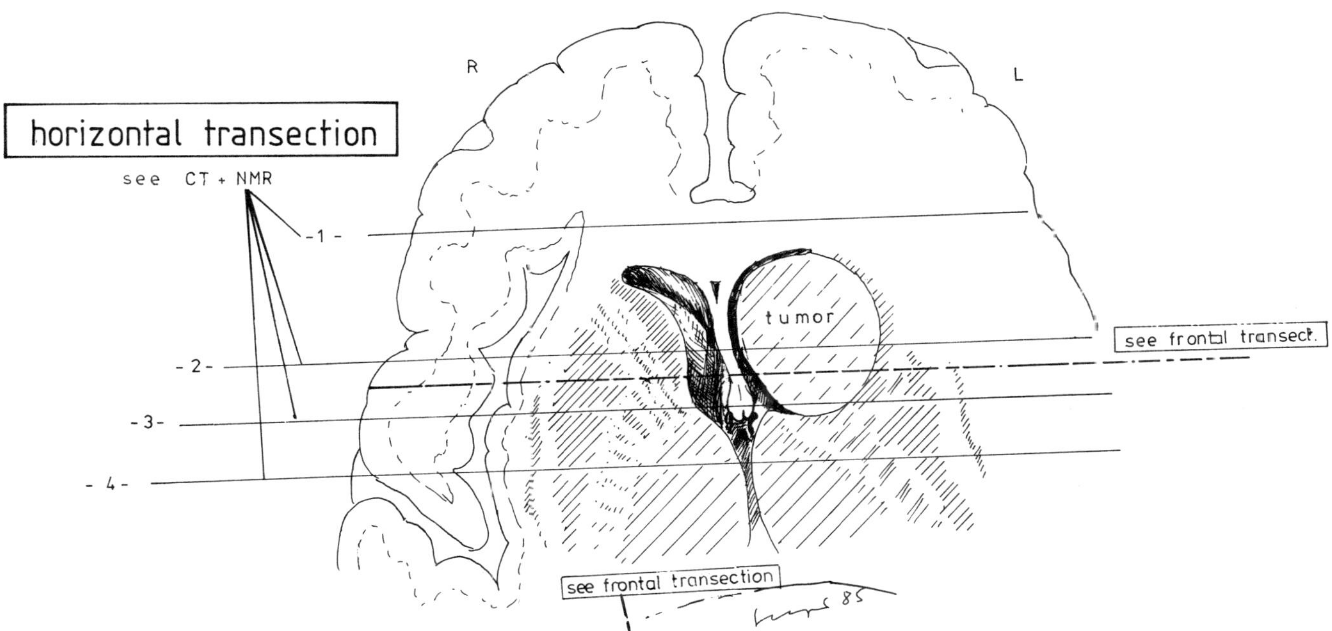
horizontal transection
see CT + NMR
R
L
-1 -
tumor
see frontal transect.
- 2 -
-3-
- 4 -

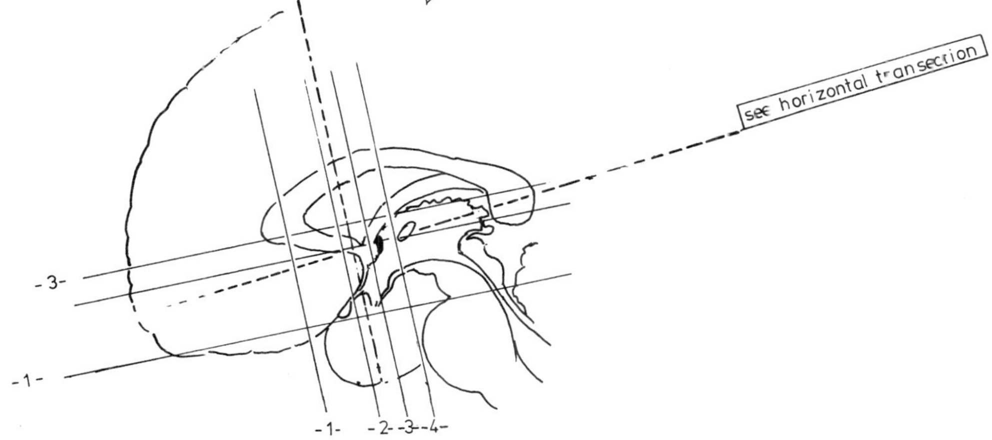
see frontal transection
see horizontal transecrion
-3-
-1-
-1- -2- -3- -4-

Fig. 105. The angiogram does not show the spatial relationships between the Aa. perforantes of the Substantia perforata anterior and the tumor well enough. By displacement of the vessels in a posterior direction the basal approach **A** would be more favorable. By freeing of the vessels in the whole tumor area would the transventricular approach **B** be more favorable than the approach **A** which was chosen in this example of a dermoid

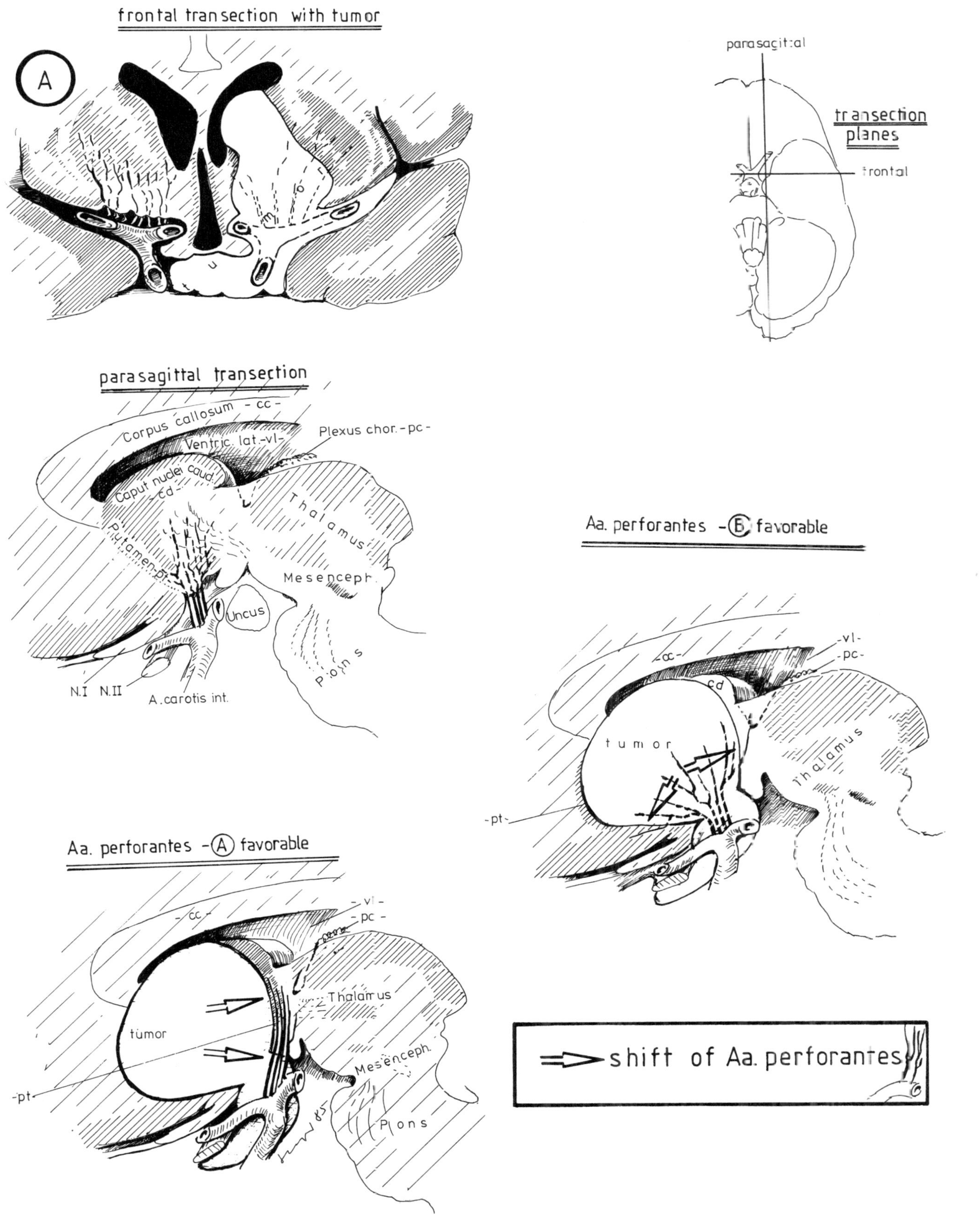
frontal transection with tumor
A
parasagital
transection planes
frontal
parasagittal transection
Corpus callosum - cc -
Ventric. lat.-vl-
Plexus chor.-pc-
Caput nuclei caud.
-cd-
Thalamus
Putamen-pt-
Mesenceph.
Uncus
Pons
N.I
N.II
A.carotis int.
Aa. perforantes -Ⓑ favorable
-vl-
-pc-
-cc-
cd
tumor
Thalamus
-pt-
Aa. perforantes -Ⓐ favorable
-vl-
-pc-
-cc-
Thalamus
tumor
Mesenceph.
Pons
-pt-
shift of Aa. perforantes

Fig. 106. Since it is not known how the Aa. perforantes are in relation to the tumor, the possibility should be considered of stopping approach **A** and completing via approach **B**. In a posteriorly placed Aa. perforantes is the approach **A** sufficient

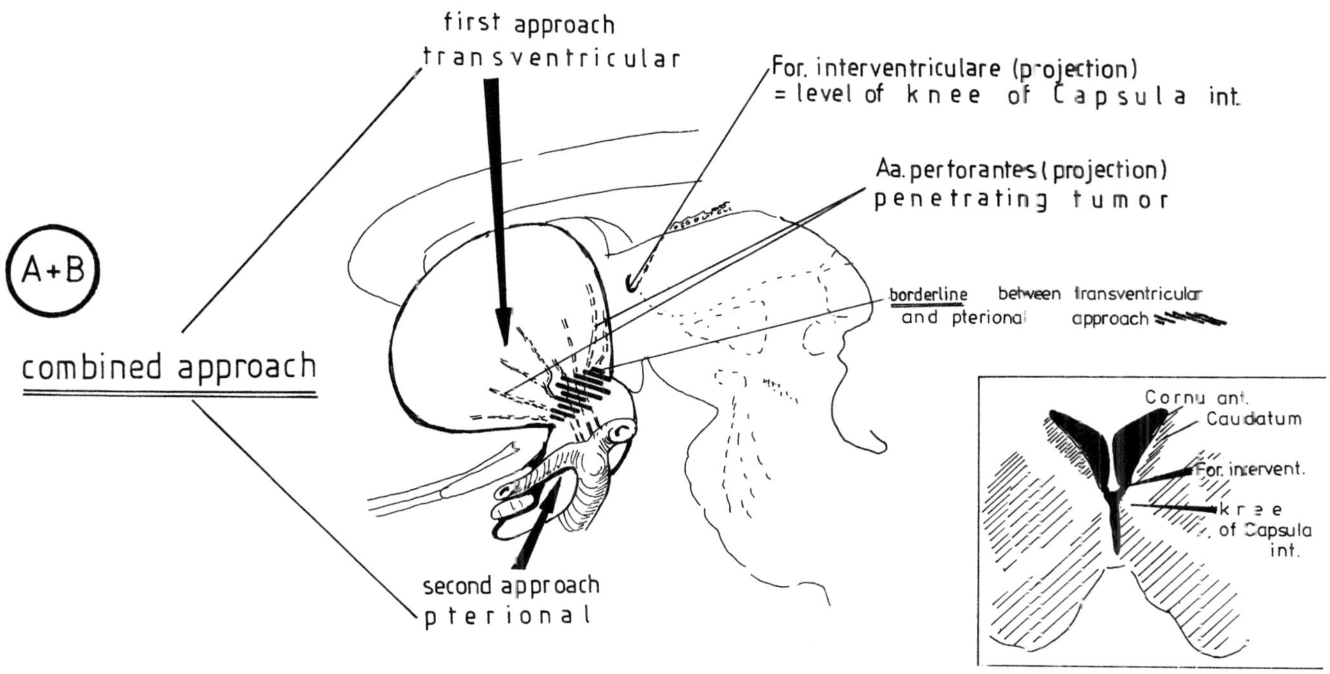

operative approach
modification?

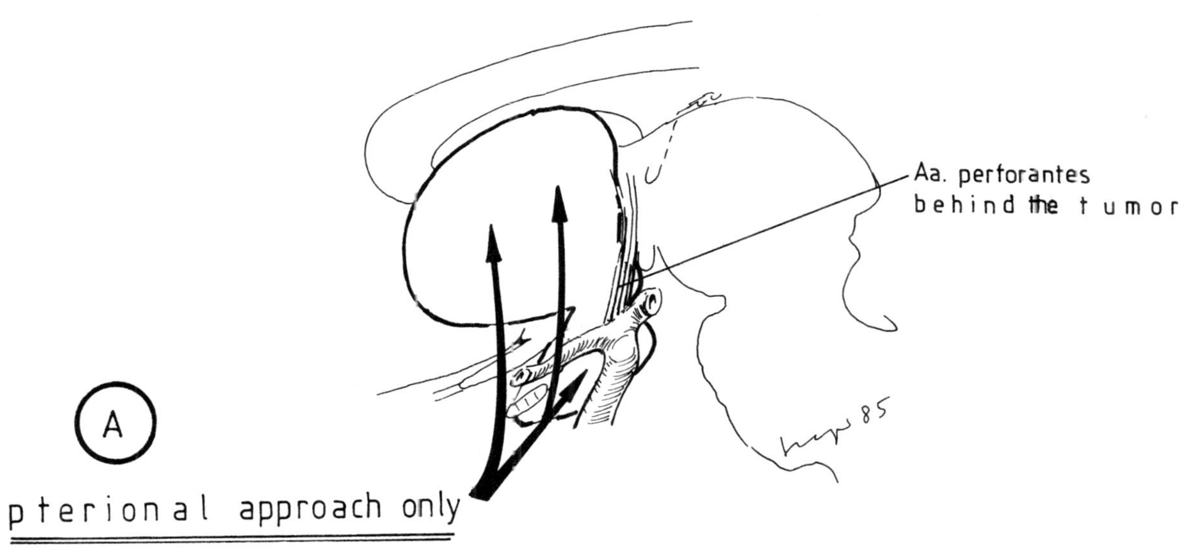

Fig. 107. Stepwise reduction of the tumor which showed no tendency of bleeding, was soft and well delineated

FIG. 107

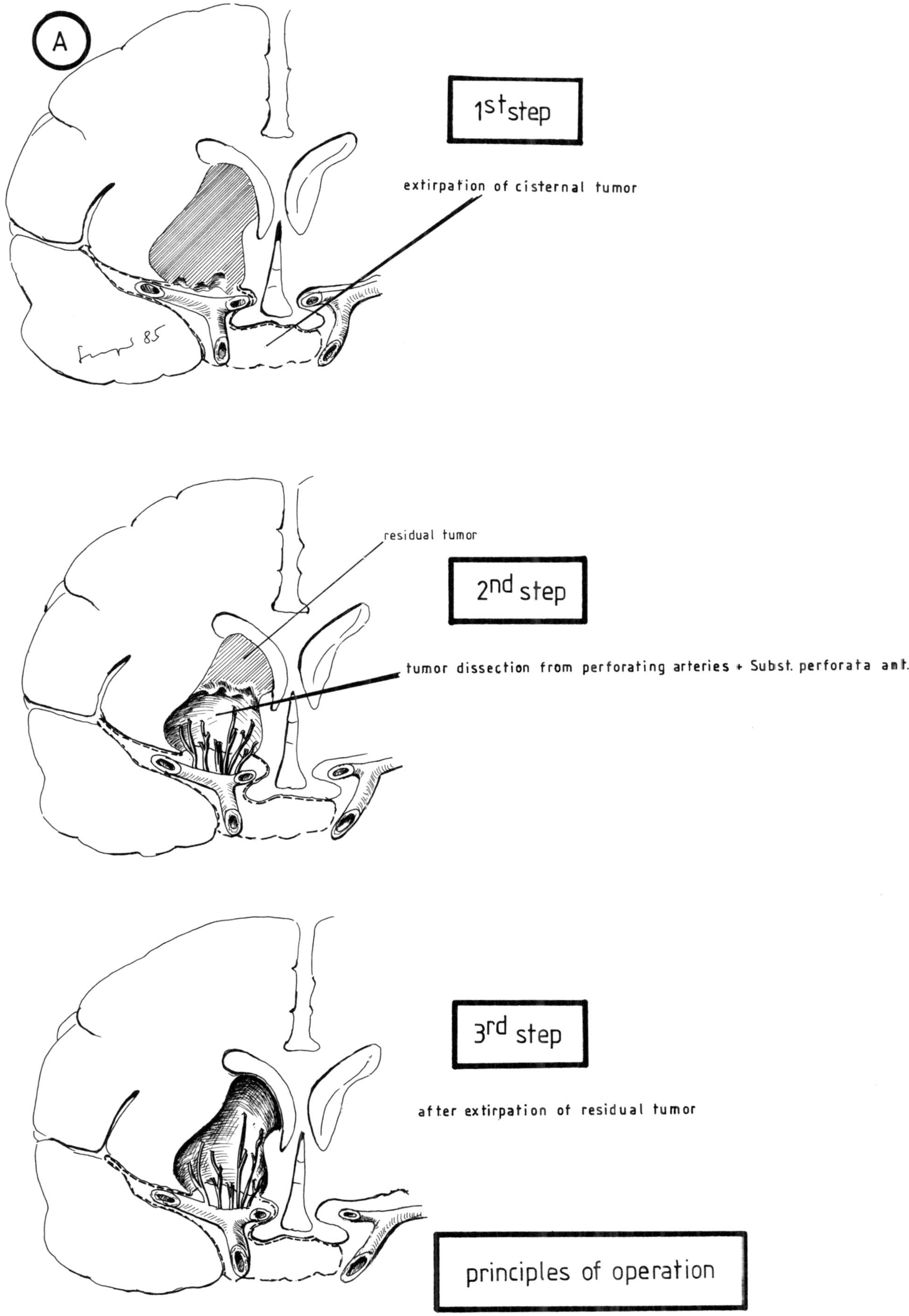
A
1st step
extirpation of cisternal tumor
residual tumor
2nd step
tumor dissection from perforating arteries + Subst. perforata ant.
3rd step
after extirpation of residual tumor
principles of operation

Fig. 108. Presentation of the operation with accompanying anatomical sketches

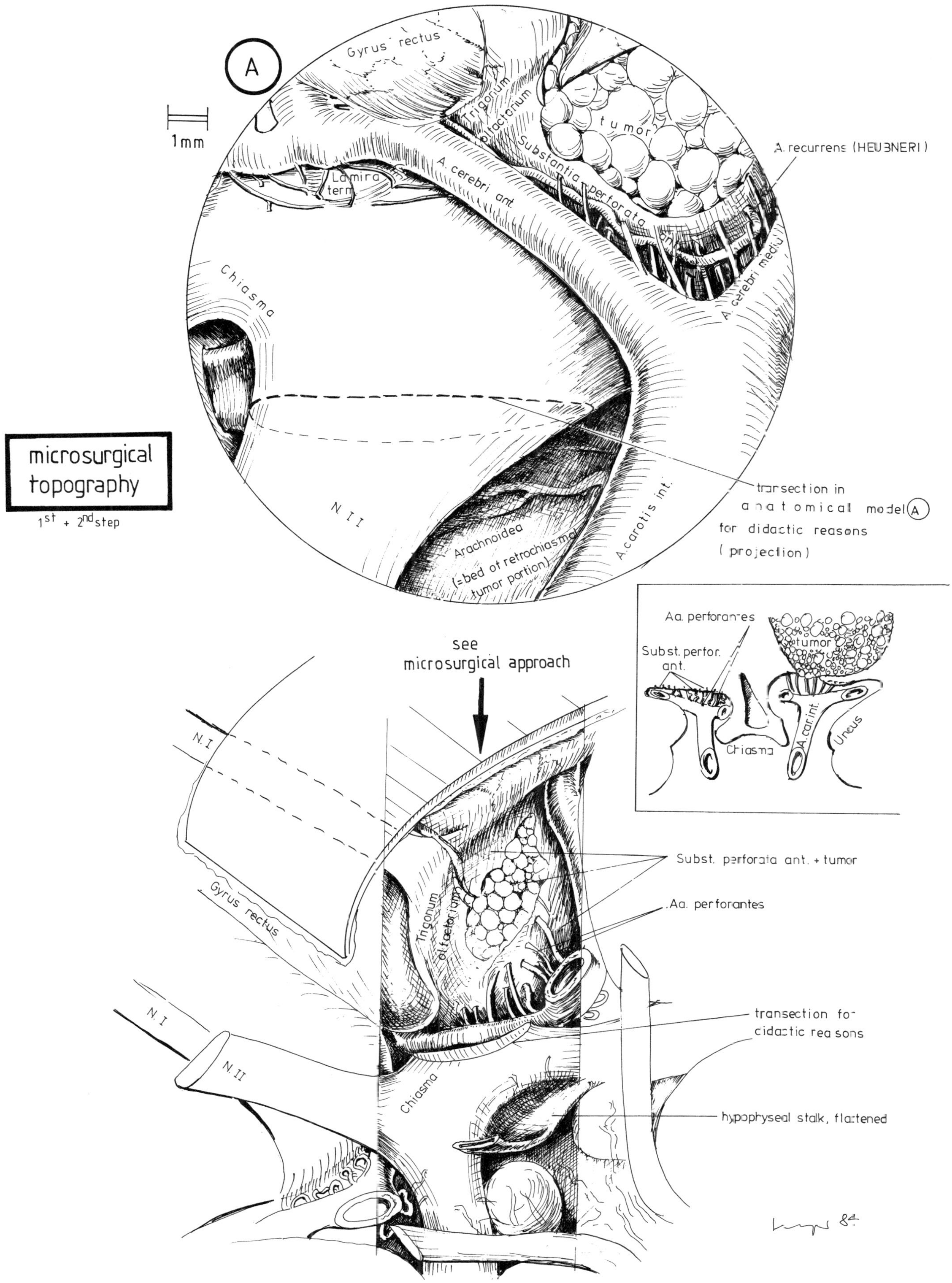
A
1mm
Gyrus rectus
Trigonum olfactorium
tumor
Substantia perforata ant.
A. recurrens (HEUBNERI)
Lamina term.
A. cerebri ant.
A. cerebri media
Chiasma
microsurgical topography
1st + 2nd step
N. II
Arachnoidea
(=bed of retrochiasmal tumor portion)
A. carotis int.
transection in anatomical model (A) for didactic reasons (projection)
Aa. perforantes
Subst. perfor. ant.
tumor
Chiasma
A. car. int.
Uncus
see microsurgical approach
N. I
Gyrus rectus
Trigonum olfactorium
Subst. perforata ant. + tumor
Aa. perforantes
N. I
N. II
Chiasma
transection for didactic reasons
hypophyseal stalk, flattened

Fig. 109. Continuation from Fig. 108. Favorable position of the Aa. perforantes laterally and behind the tumor. Thereby it was possible to carry out the surgical intervention exclusively from pterionally (type **A**)

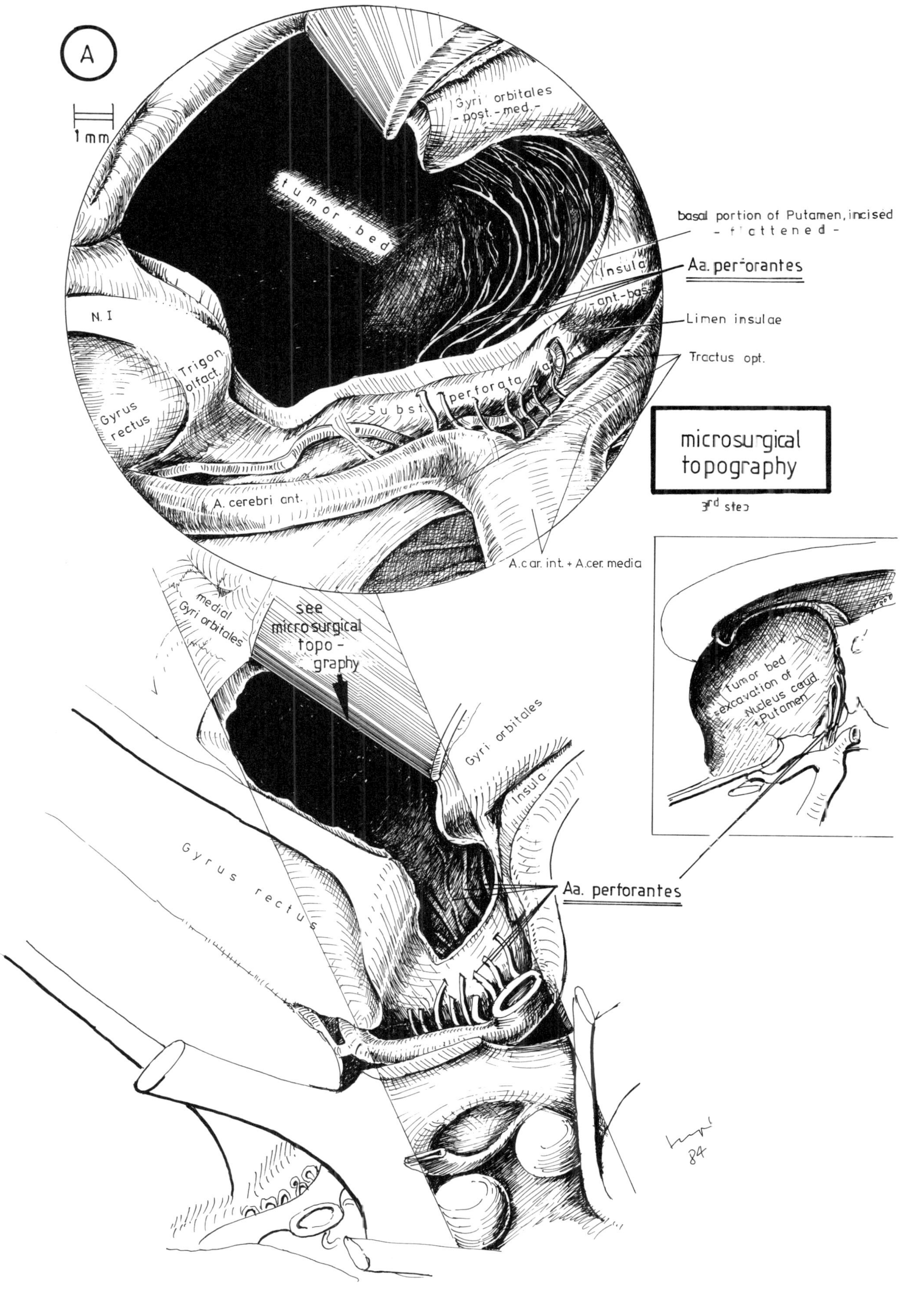
A
1 mm
Gyri orbitales
- post.-med. -
tumor bed
basal portion of Putamen, incised
- flattened -
Insula
Aa. perforantes
ant.-basal
Limen insulae
Tractus opt.
N. I
Trigon. olfact.
Gyrus rectus
Subst. perforata ant.
A. cerebri ant.
microsurgical topography
3rd step
A.car. int. + A.cer. media
medial Gyri orbitales
see microsurgical topography
Gyri orbitales
Insula
Gyrus rectus
Aa. perforantes
tumor bed
excavation of Nucleus caud. + Putamen
84

Fig. 110. Clinical example of an angioma of the 3rd ventricle, of the Rostrum corporis callosi, partially of the Columna fornicis, the frontal commissure, and the subcallosal area, and the medial portions of the Putamen inclusively. Psycho-organic changes in character following bleeding of the angioma, first increasing psychological changes after the operation, shunt problems, then gradual recovery. Neurologically intact*. The anatomical sketches of the angioma were based on the pre- and postoperative angiogram and the operative findings

* This case was presented in detail in Seeger, W., Microsurgery of the Brain, Vol. 1. Wien–New York: Springer. 1980. The pictures shown then have been replaced by other pictures which should show the principle of the intervention.

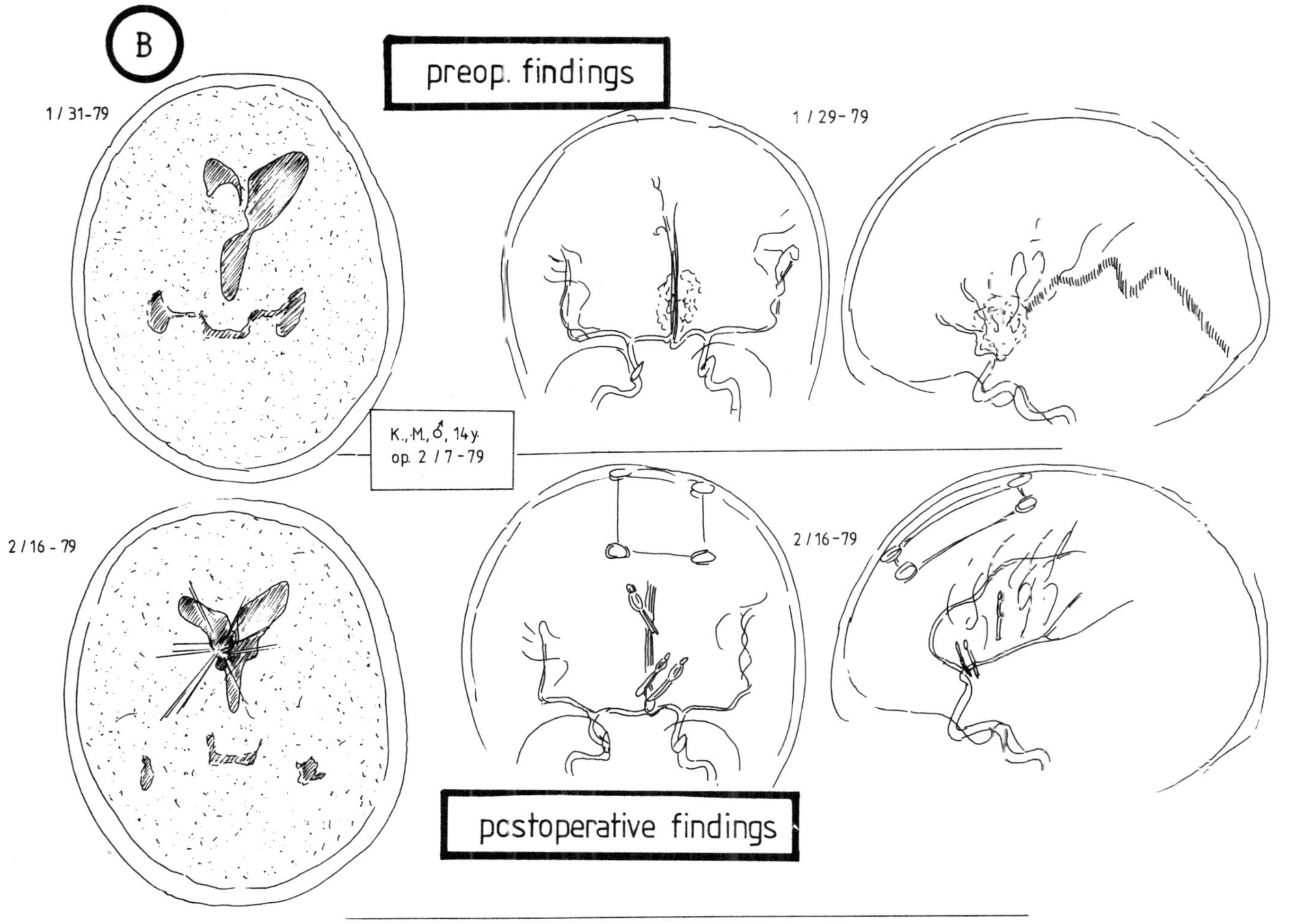
B
preop. findings
1/31-79
1/29-79
K., M., ♂, 14y
op. 2/7-79
2/16-79
2/16-79
postoperative findings

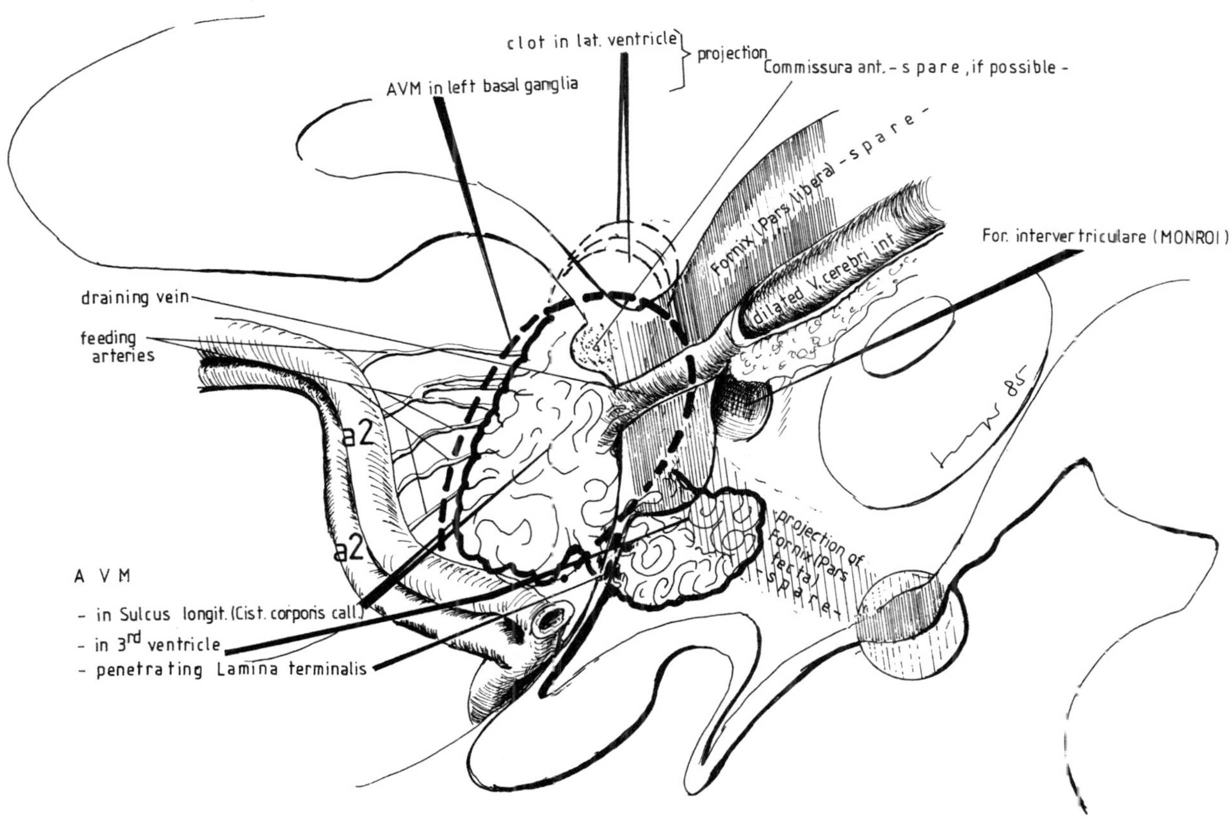
clot in lat. ventricle
projection
Commissura ant. - s p a r e , if possible -
AVM in left basal ganglia
Fornix (Pars libera) - s p a r e -
dilated V. cerebri int.
For. interventriculare (MONROI)
draining vein
feeding arteries
a2
a2
projection of Fornix (Pars tecta) s p a r e
A V M
- in Sulcus longit. (Cist. corporis call.)
- in 3rd ventricle
- penetrating Lamina terminalis

Fig. 111. When the transventricular approach (type **B**) is used the roof (Corpus callosum) must be split. By using the transcerebral approach the roof fibers would also be split, but further laterally. But in addition damage of the Cortex and white matter would have to be accepted. In the Freiburg Clinic the intervention is made in principle via the longitudinal fissure. Thereby variants of the Aa. pericallosae must be considered during the preparation of the callosal surface. **In any case, despite the numerous variants of the Aa. pericallosae, an approach via the longitudinal fissure with splitting Corpus callosum is possible.** Thereby the transcerebral approach, which always causes, at least a temporary, psychosyndrome, can be avoided

B

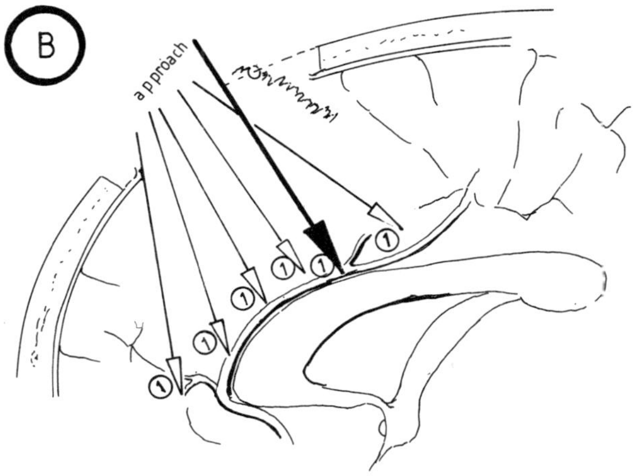

1st step

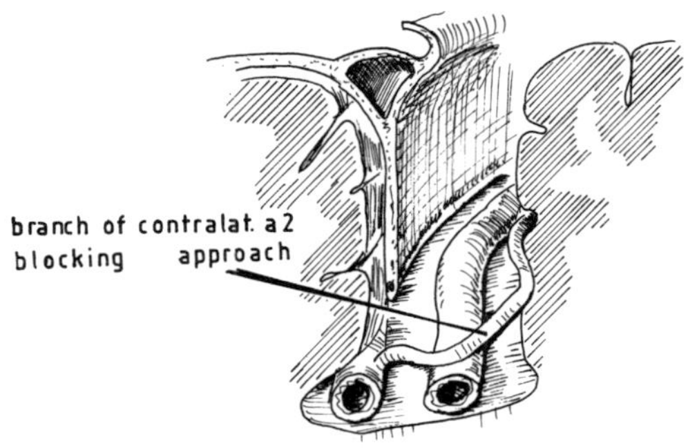

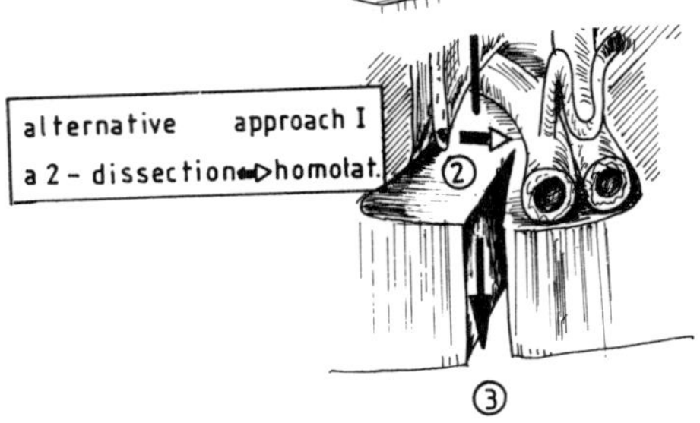

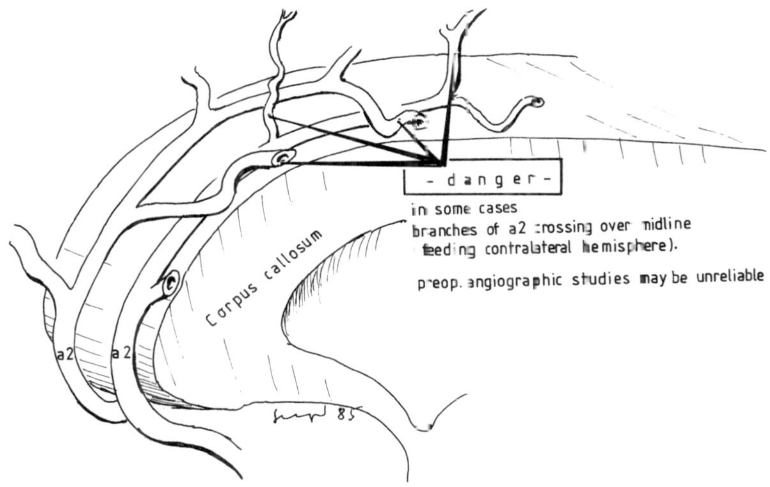

① loosening of adhesions between hemisphere and Falx

② preservation of a2 + branches (e.g. alternative I or II)

③ incision of Corpus callosum

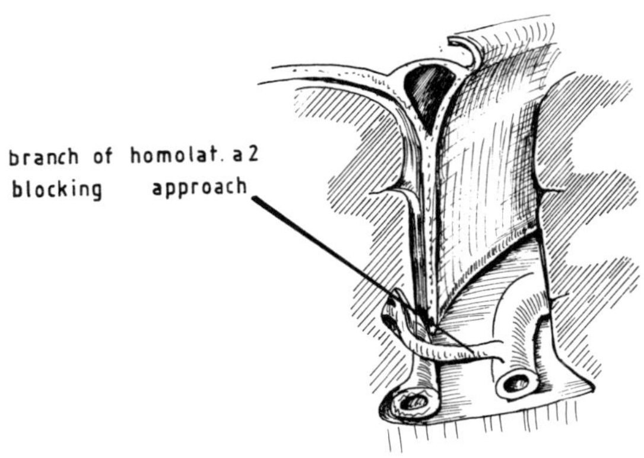

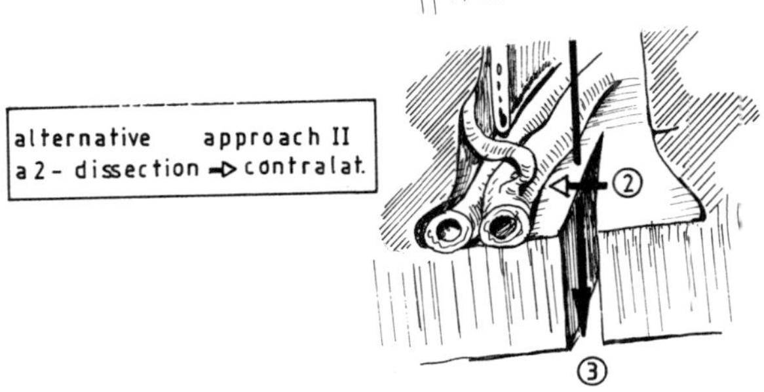

principles of operation

Fig. 112. Prevention of damage to the Columna fornicis also on one side, as far as is possible

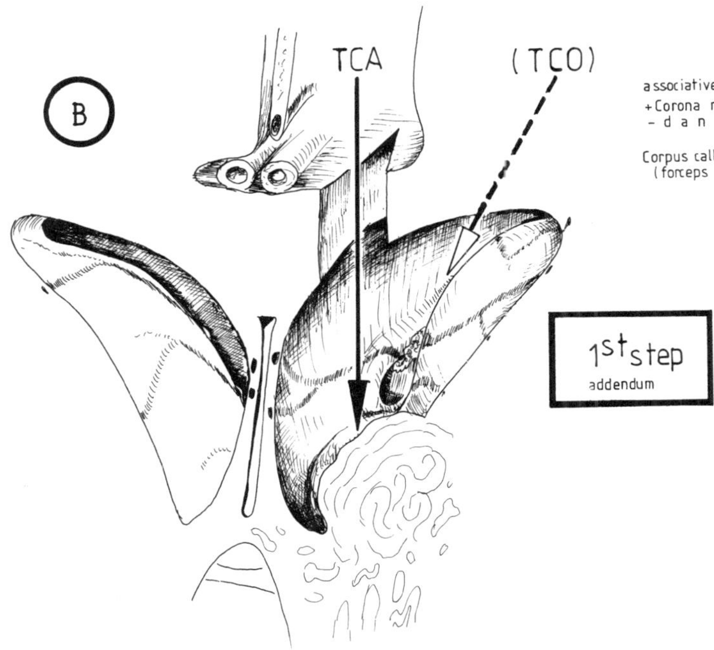

1st step
addendum

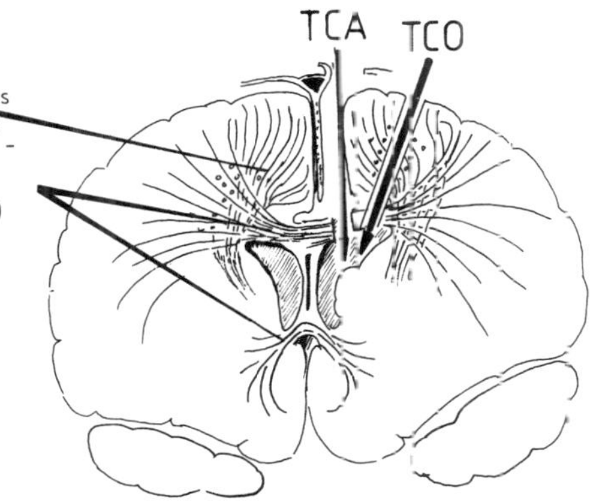

op. approach transcallosa -TCA-
or
transcortical -TCO-
?

TCA: Corpus callosum cut - recommendable
TCO Radiatio corp.call. = Corp.call.cut
in addition associative fibers (+ant. Corona radiata) cut } not correct

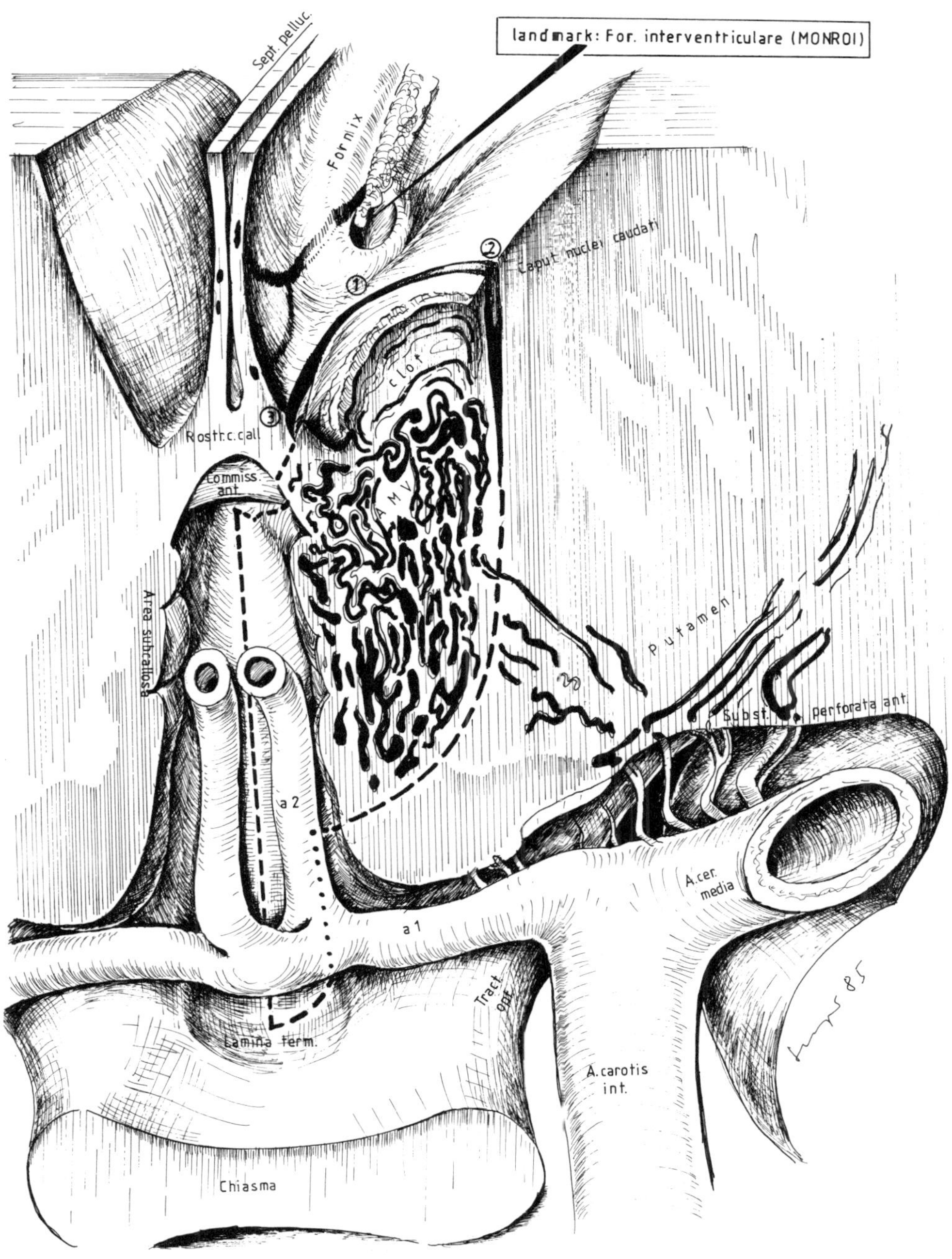

2nd step

circumcision of AVM

① anterior from For. interventricul. (MONROI)
② lateral basal ganglia
③ medial < post. → 3rd ventricle; ant. → Cist. corp. callosi

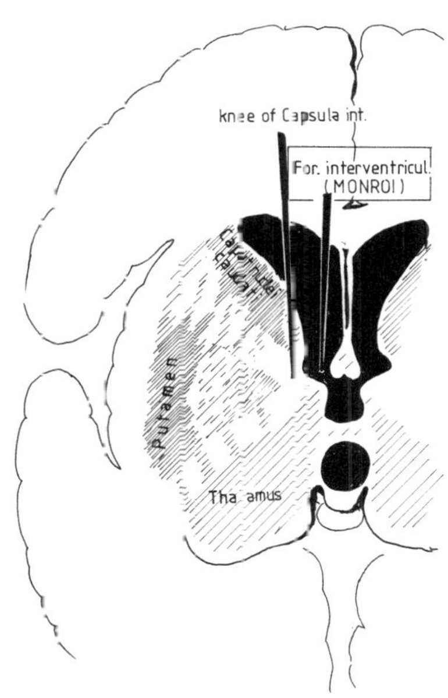

Fig. 113. After bipolar coagulation shrinkage of the angioma. Only those parts of the Rostrum corporis callosi, the Commissura ant., the Area subcallosa and the Putamen affected by the angioma were resected. In contrast, those parts of the Lamina terminalis not affected by the angioma were also resected in order to achieve a better view of the intraventricular parts of the angioma

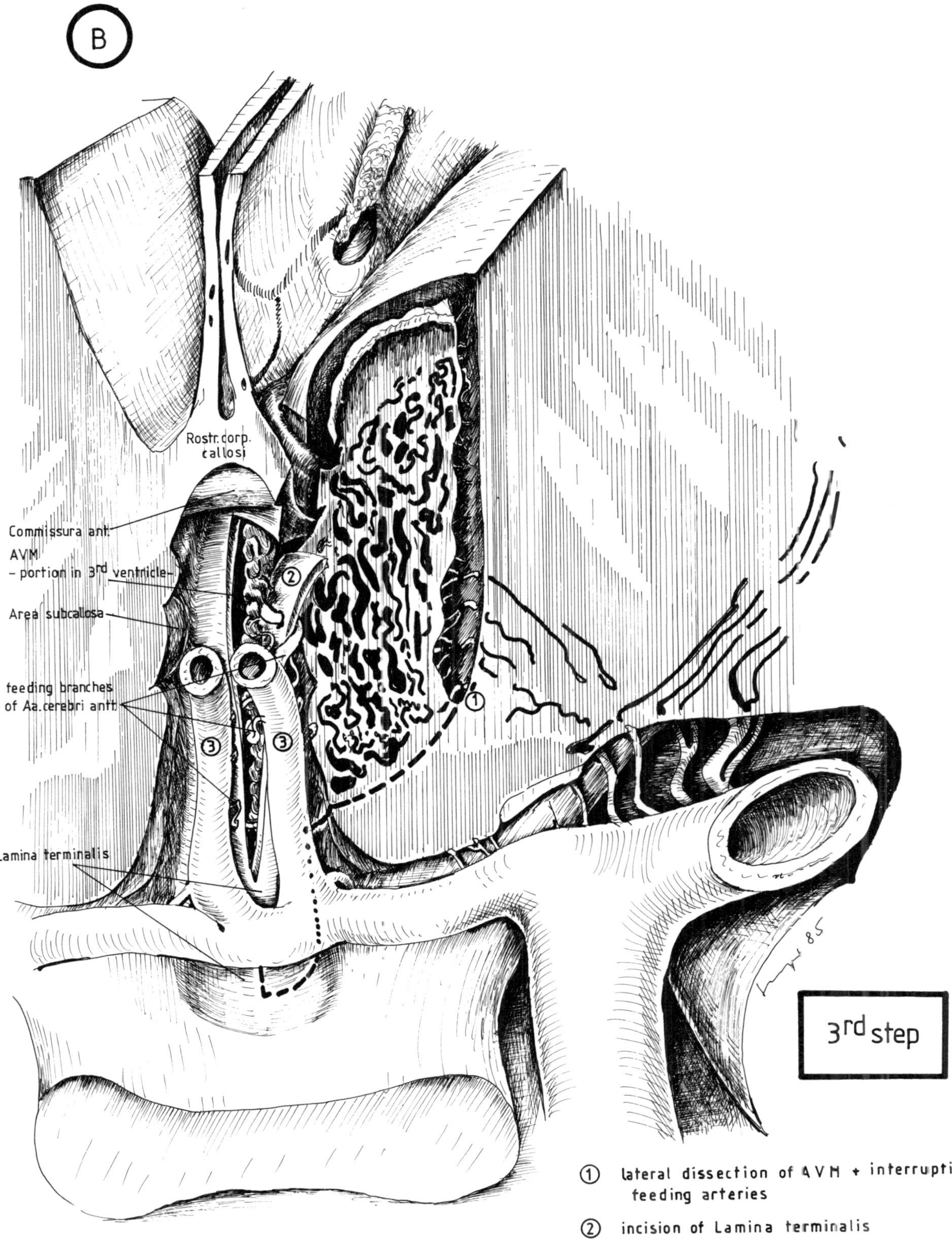

① lateral dissection of AVM + interruption of feeding arteries

② incision of Lamina terminalis

③ dissection of Aa.cerebri antt. and feeding branches

Fig. 114. Feeding arteries and draining veins were interrupted only when the entire angioma was isolated and by means of coagulation markedly shrunk

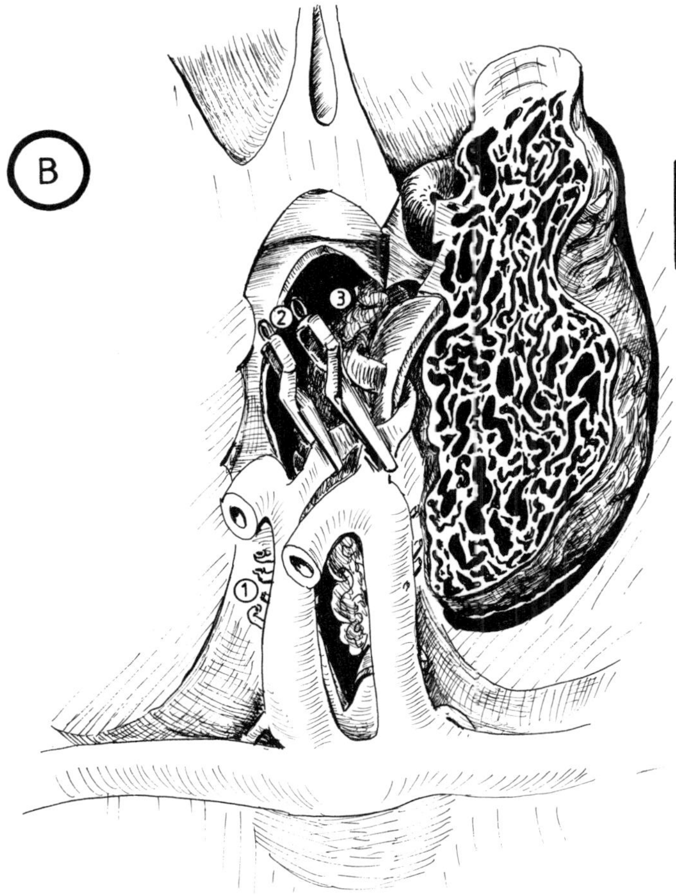

4th step

① small feeding arteries cut

② large feeding arteries clipped

③ dissection of AVM in 3rc ventricle

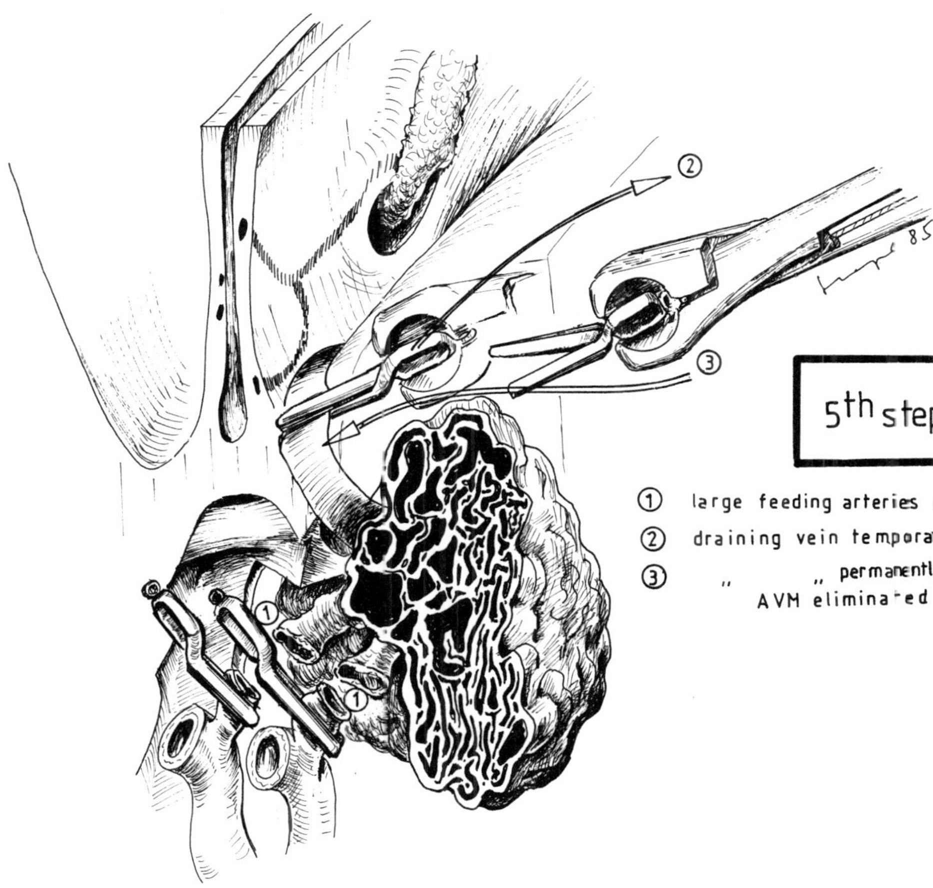

5th step

① large feeding arteries cut

② draining vein temporarily clipped

③ " " permanently clipped and cu-
AVM eliminated

Fig. 115. At the end of the surgical intervention the 3rd ventricle, the angioma bed in the region of the frontal basal ganglia area and Area subcallosa comprise a combined cavity. The defect was separated from the Foramen interventriculare (Monroi) by the preserved Columna fornicis. Thereby was the damage to the area of the limbic system minimalized

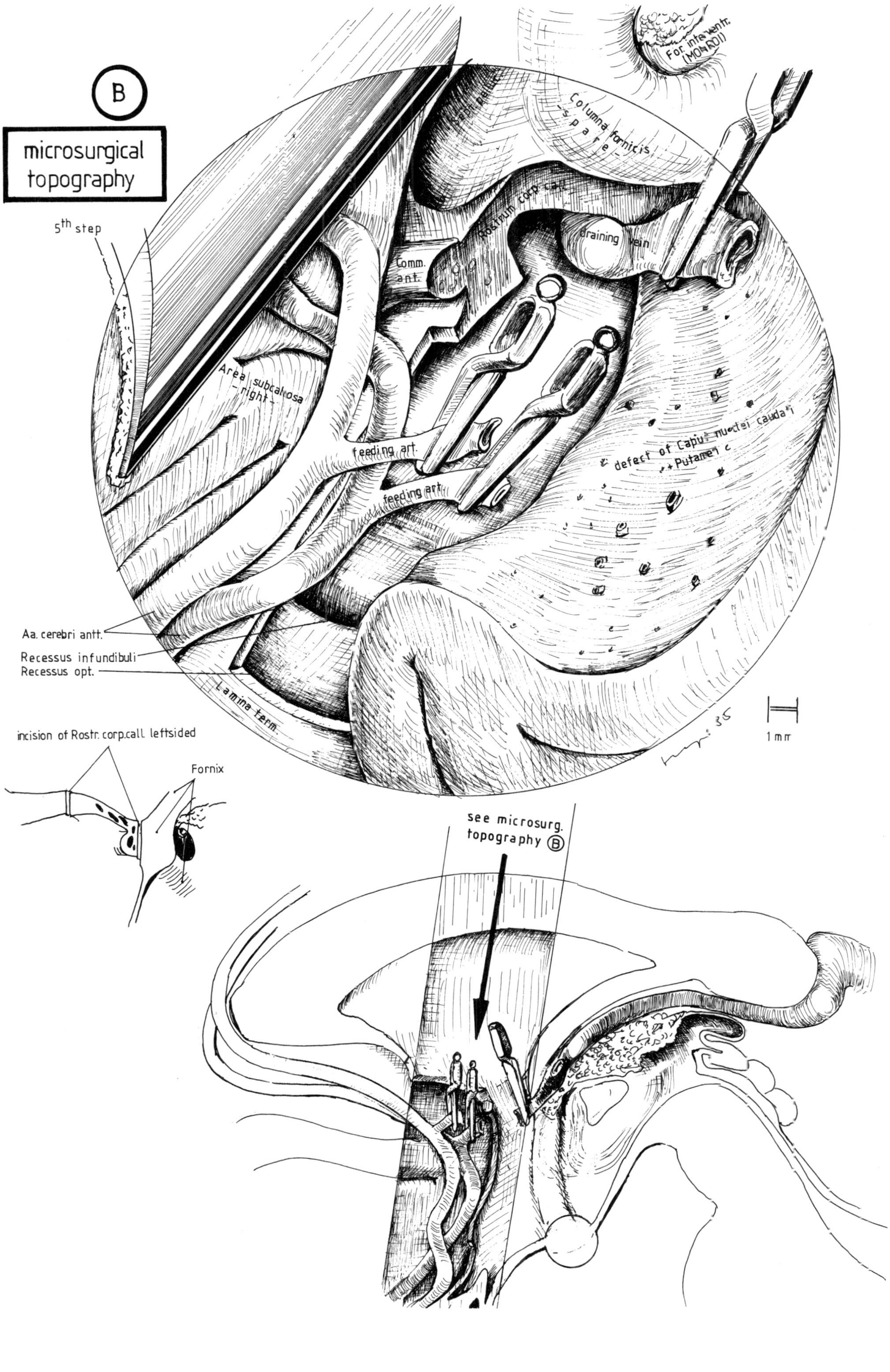
B
microsurgical topography
5th step
For. interventr. (MONROI)
Columna fornicis -spare-
Rostrum corp.call.
draining vein
Comm. ant.
Area subcallosa -right-
feeding art.
feeding art.
defect of Capu nuclei caudati
+ Putamen
Aa. cerebri antt.
Recessus infundibuli
Recessus opt.
Lamina term.
1 mm
incision of Rostr. corp.call. leftsided
Fornix
see microsurg. topography B

Fig. 116. Small basal processes in the area of the Cisterna ambiens, e. g. aneurysms of the posterior cerebral artery, or the bifurcation of the basilar artery, are directly attainable through a temporo-basal approach, and less favorably pterionally*

* Yaşargil and the author both are afraid of venous softening of the temporal lobe resulting from the interruption of the temporo-basilar veins, which Drake described while approaching the basilar artery (personal communication).

(A) temporobasal approach

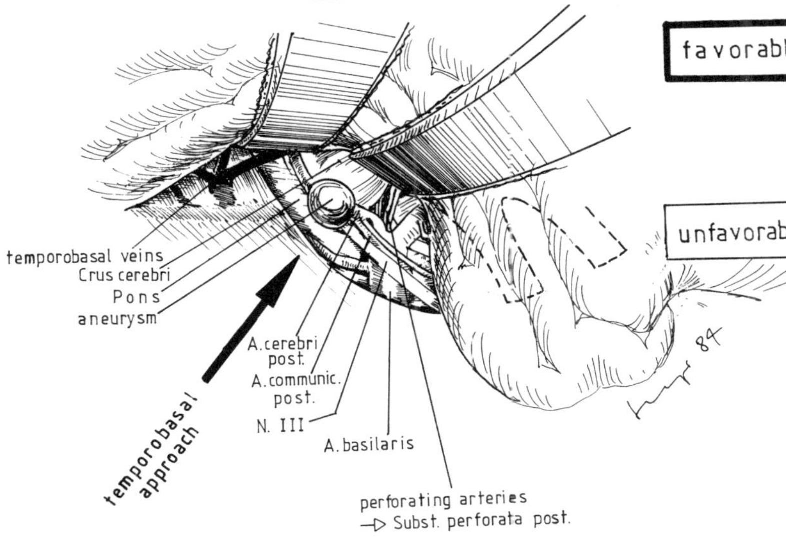

favorable

- dissection of aneurysm not hindered by Uncus, Tractus opt., A.carotis int.
- no brain damage by spatula

unfavorable

- temporobasal veins

(B) pterional approach

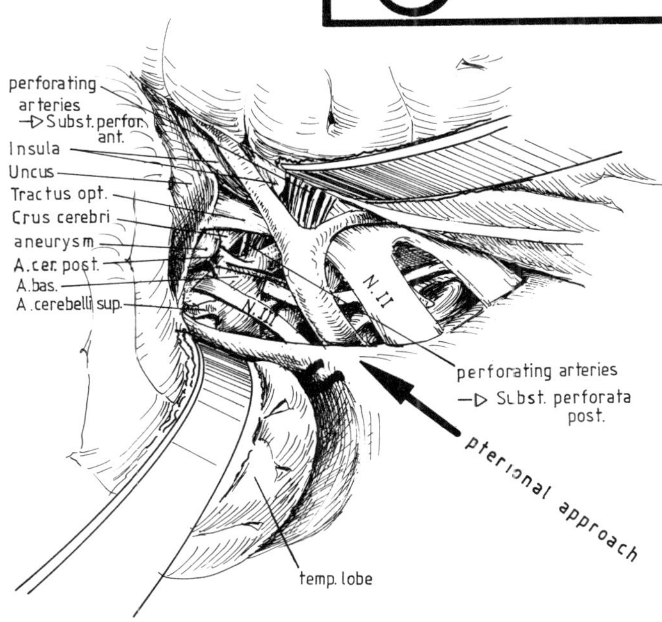

favorable

- temporobasal veins preserved

unfavorable

- even in extreme reclination of the brain dissection of aneurysm is hindered by
  - Uncus
  - Tractus opt
  - A. carotis int.
- brain damage by extreme reclination of the brain

Fig. 117. Larger processes in the basal part of the Cisterna ambiens are more securely reached pterionally than temporo-basally

(A) temporobasal approach

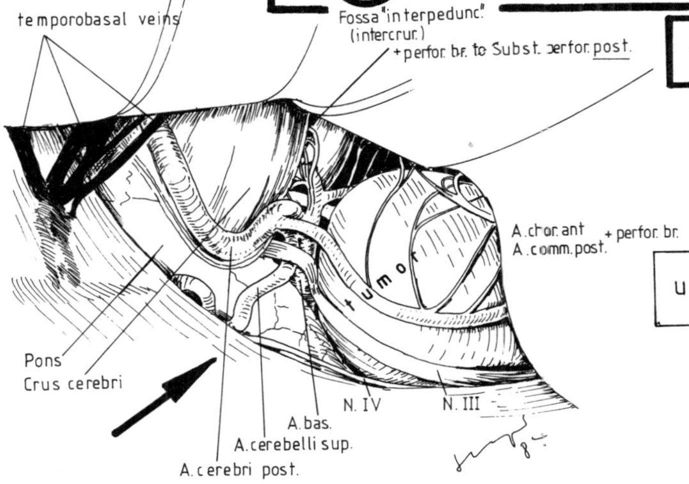

favorable

- A. bas. + A. comm. post. + A. cer. post. + perfor. br.
- N. III close to brainstem
- Tractus opt. + A. chor. ant. far from cranial base

unfavorable

- narrow approach
- temporobasal veins
- tumor base (Dorsum + Diaphragma sellae)
- Cist. optica, N. II, A. car. int.
- hypophyseal stalk
- N. III, segment close to Dura penetration
- Hypothalamus, Corpora mam.

(B) pterional approach*

- good reclination of the frontal lobe after extensive splitting of Arachnoidea of sylvian fissure

favorable

- 4 different ways (arrows):
  - 1st — N. II
  - 2nd — N. II
  - 3rd — A. carotis int. / Uncus
  - 4th — bifurcation of A. carotis int. / Subst. perforata ant.
- tumor base (Diaphragma + Dors. sellae)
- Cisterna opt., N. II
- N. III, segment close to Dura penetration
- A. car. int. + perfor. branches (except way No. 4)
- A. chor. ant. + A. comm. post. + perfor. branches
- hypophyseal stalk
- temporopolar veins (only slight reclination by aspirator or without any reclination)

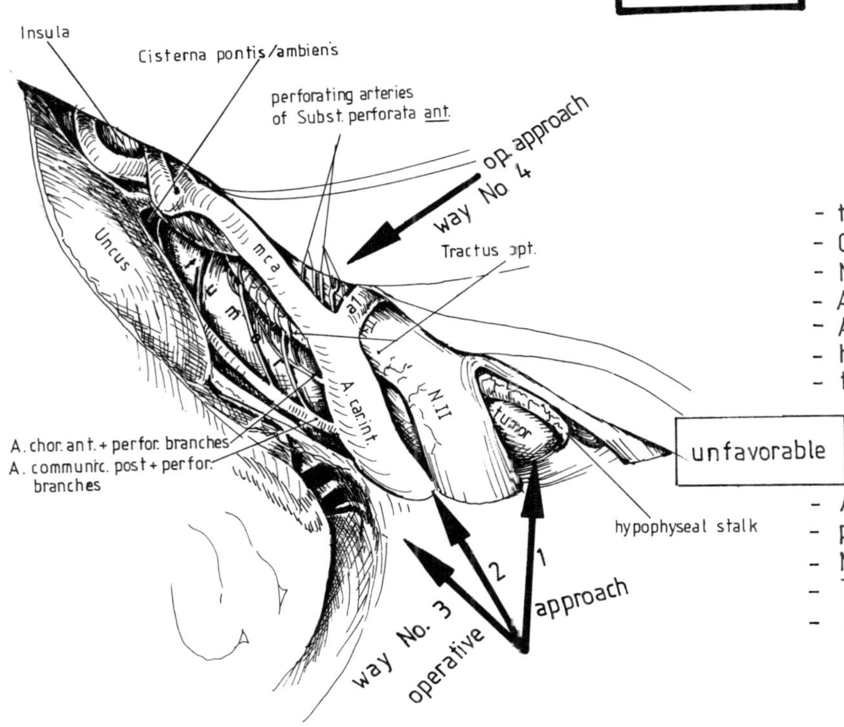

unfavorable

- A. bas. + A. cer. post
- perfor. branches of Subst. perfor. post. + Hypothal.
- N. III close to the brainstem
- Tractus opt. close to Chiasma and cranial base
- Hypothalamus + Corpora mam.

Fig. 118. Clinical example of a small aneurysm lying basally in the Cisterna ambiens (posterior cerebral artery, proximal segment). Situation after partial thrombosis of the aneurysm with temporary midbrain symptoms. Operative exclusion was not possible without narrowing of the A. cerebri post. Therefore, the present day very rare wall-in technique had to be used. No additional deficits postoperatively*. The aneurysm is clearly smaller in the angiogram than that demonstrated in the CT

* Operation performed by Prof. Dr. J. Gilsbach, coworker of the author.

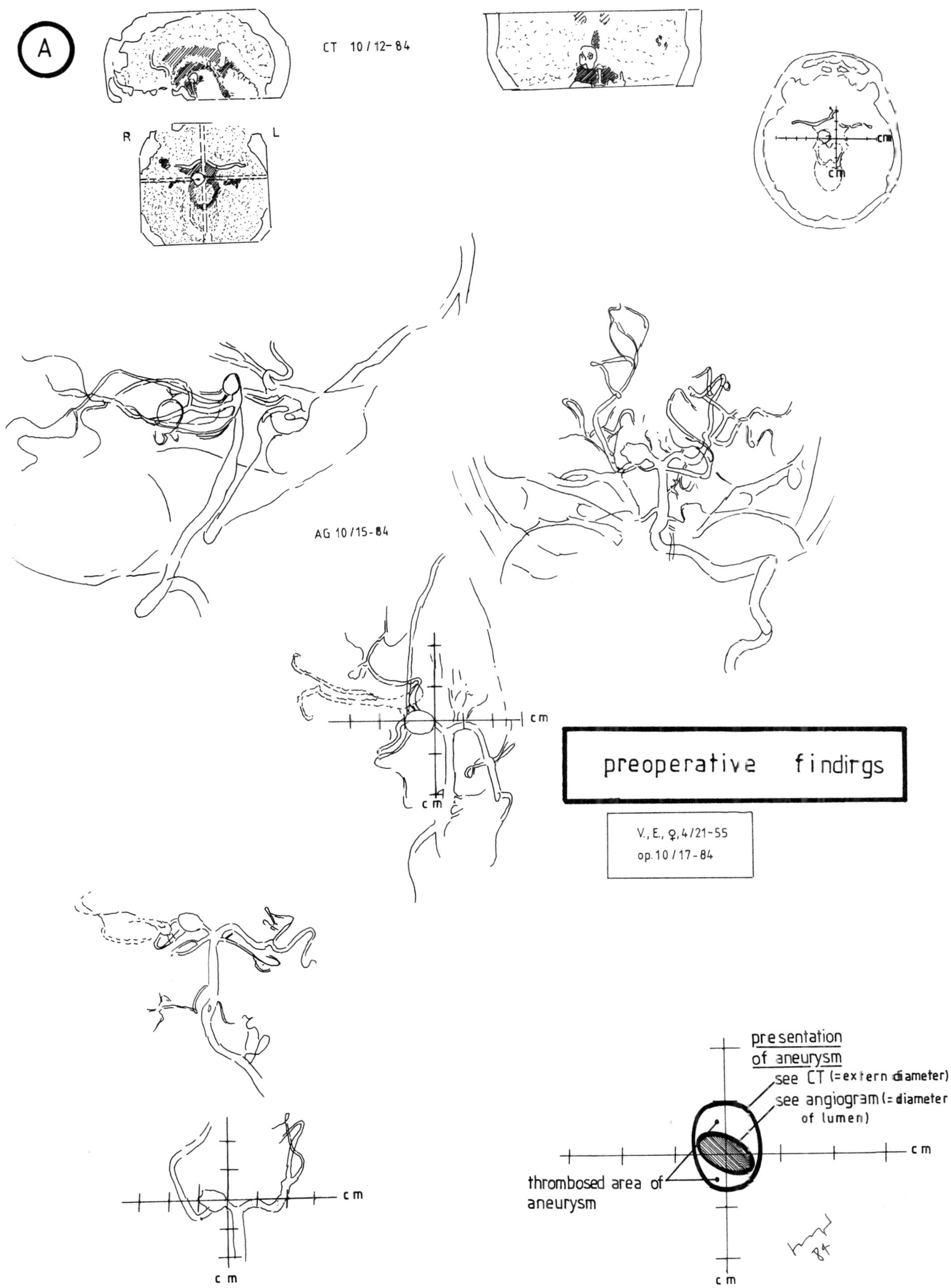
A
CT 10/12-84
R
L
cm
cm
AG 10/15-84
cm
cm
preoperative findirgs
V., E., ♀, 4/21-55
op. 10/17-84
presentation of aneurysm
see CT (=extern diameter)
see angiogram (= diameter of lumen)
thrombosed area of aneurysm
cm
cm
cm
cm
84

Fig. 119. Anatomical sketches, prepared on the basis of the discrepancy between the angiographic and CT findings. A partial thrombosis was expected with corresponding stiffening of the wall, which made clipping problematical. From the anamnesis it could in any case be assumed that the aneurysm had never bled. The midbrain symptoms may be explained by the closure of peripheral arteries during the thrombosis procedure. The mesencephalic symptoms may be explained by thrombosis of perforating arteries

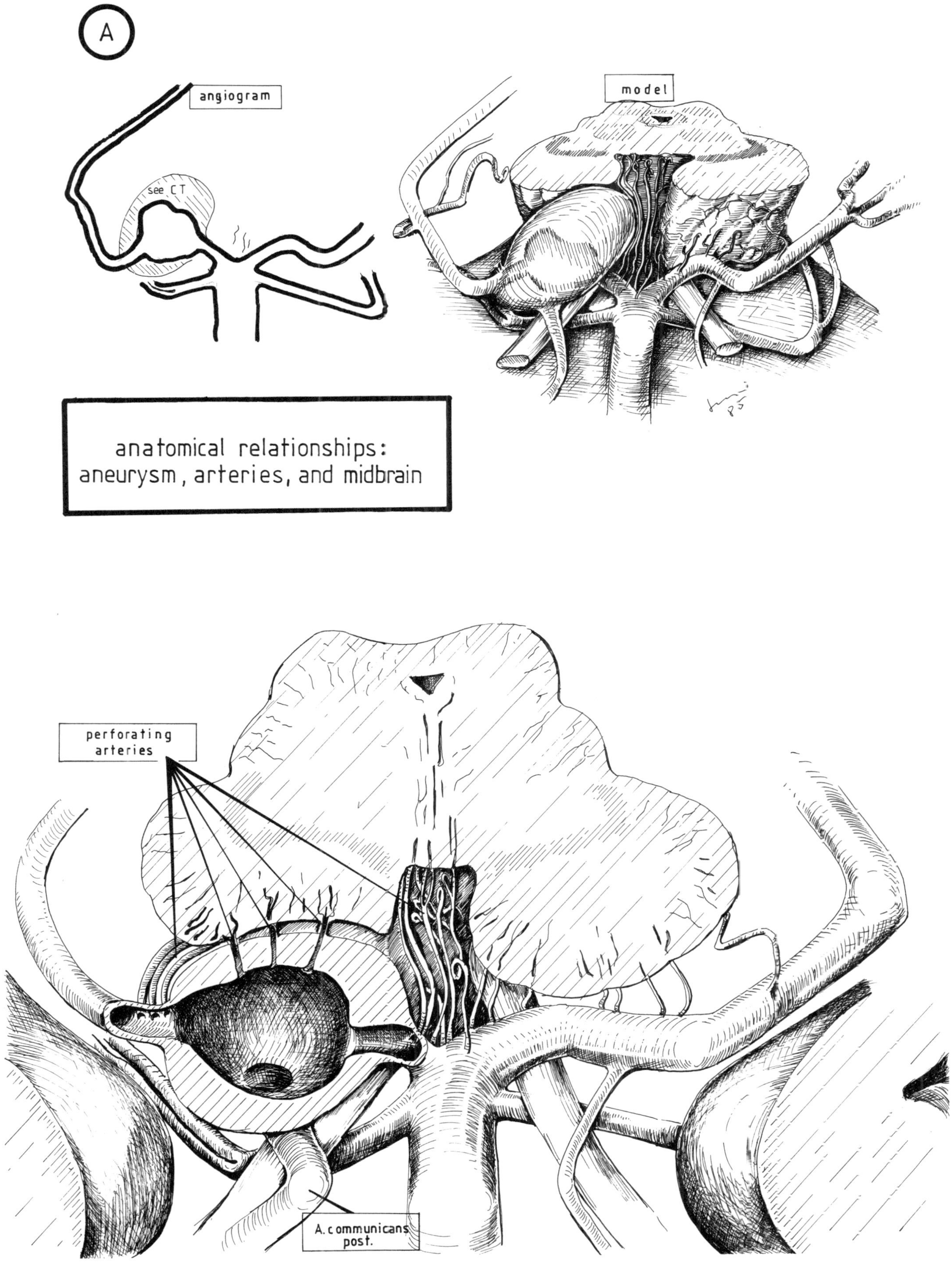
A
angiogram
see CT
model
anatomical relationships:
aneurysm, arteries, and midbrain
perforating
arteries
A. communicans
post.

Fig. 120

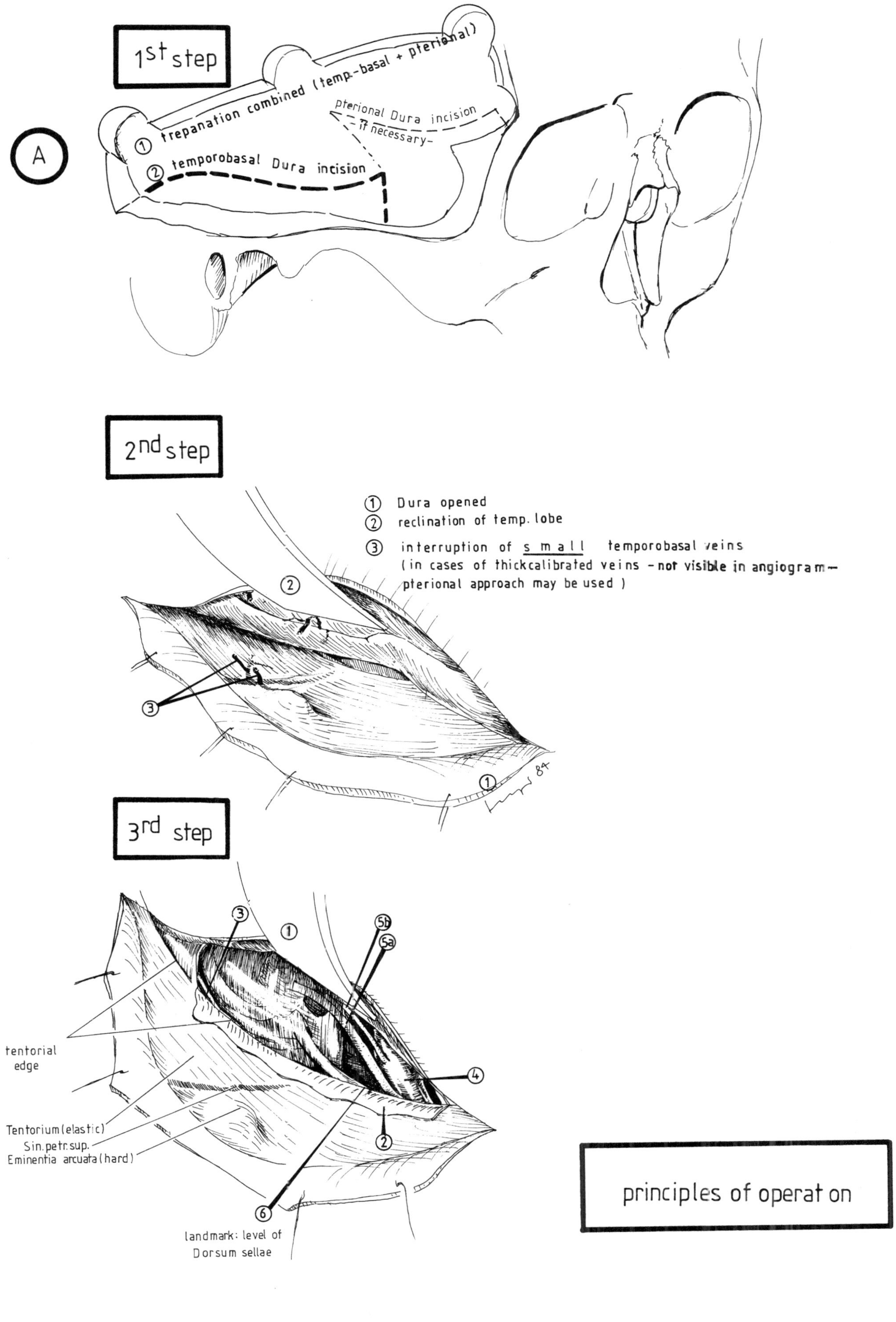
1st step
A
① trepanation combined (temp.-basal + pterional)
② temporobasal Dura incision
pterional Dura incision
- if necessary -
2nd step
① Dura opened
② reclination of temp. lobe
③ interruption of small temporobasal veins
(in cases of thickcalibrated veins - not visible in angiogram -
pterional approach may be used)
3rd step
tentorial
edge
Tentorium (elastic)
Sin. petr. sup.
Eminentia arcuata (hard)
landmark: level of
Dorsum sellae
principles of operat on

Fig. 121

4th step

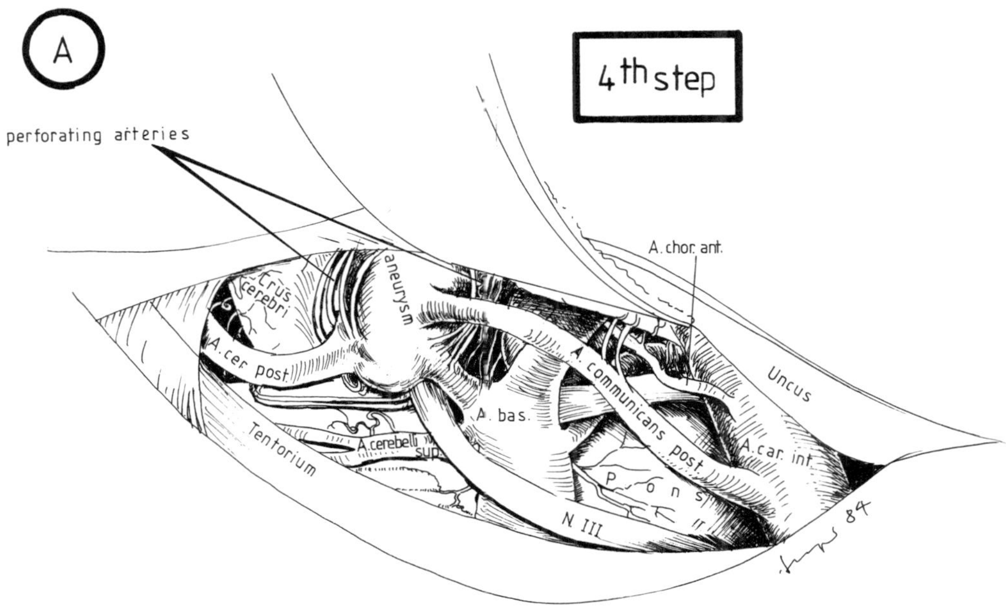

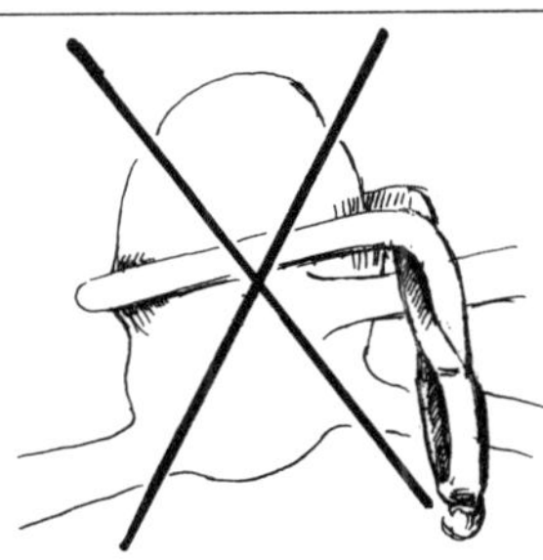

clipping not possible:
- wall of aneurysm thickened and calcareous

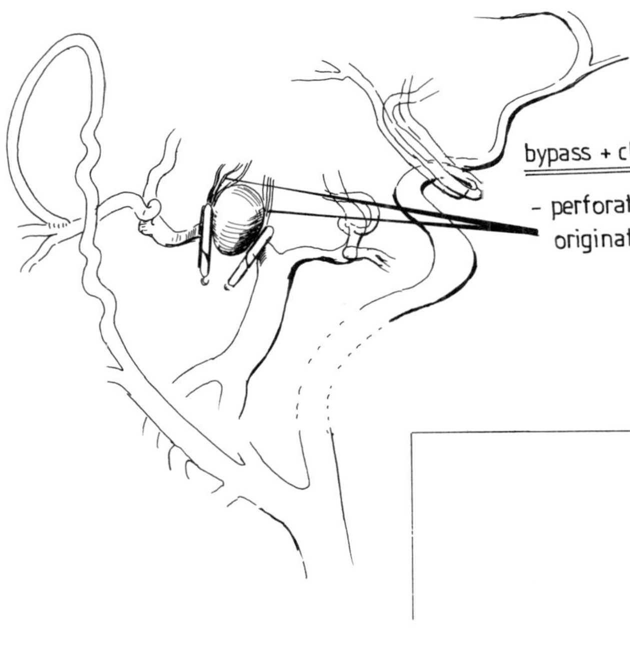

bypass + clipping not possible:
- perforating branches originating from aneurysm

5th step

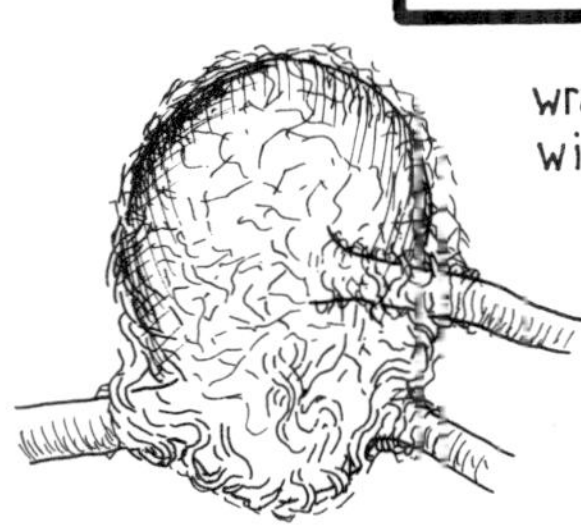

wrapping aneurysm with cotton wool

Fig. 122. Clinical example of a larger process between the Cisterna ambiens and the basal cisterns. Since six months intermittent disturbances of vision on the left, rapid reduction in visual field left for 14 days, poorer motivation, no hormonal disturbances. Neurologically an incomplete homonimous hemianopsia of the left, bilateral with emphasis on left damage of the Opticus. The operation revealed a meningioma, confirmed histologically. No additional deficits postoperatively apart from temporary polyurea and polydipsia. Improvement in the visual field deficits

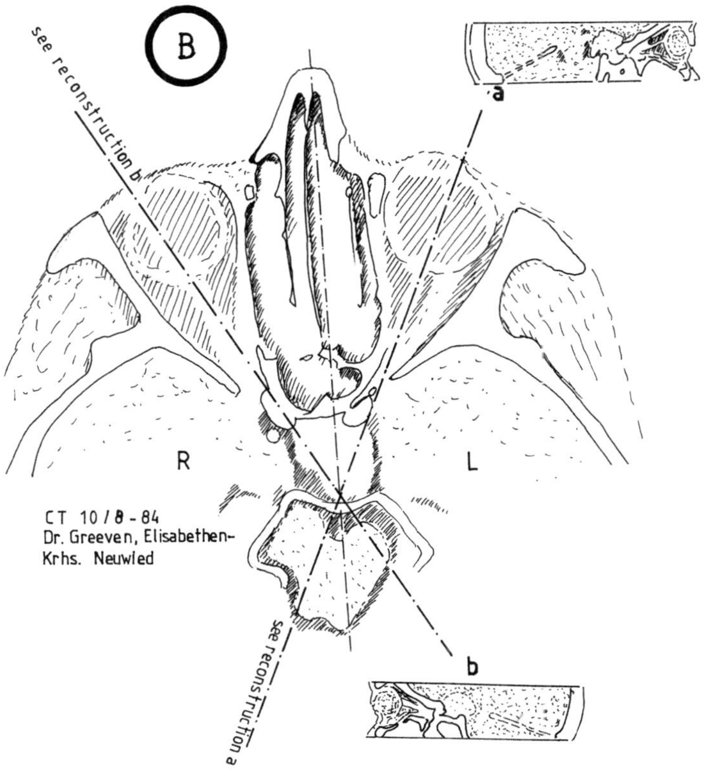

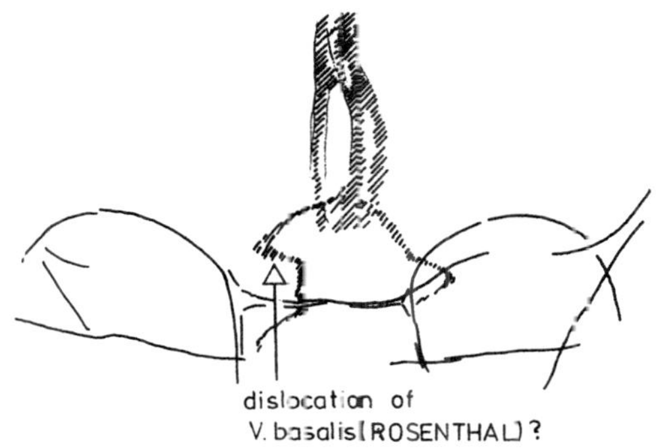

preoperative findings

H., M., 9/23-45
op. 10/18-84

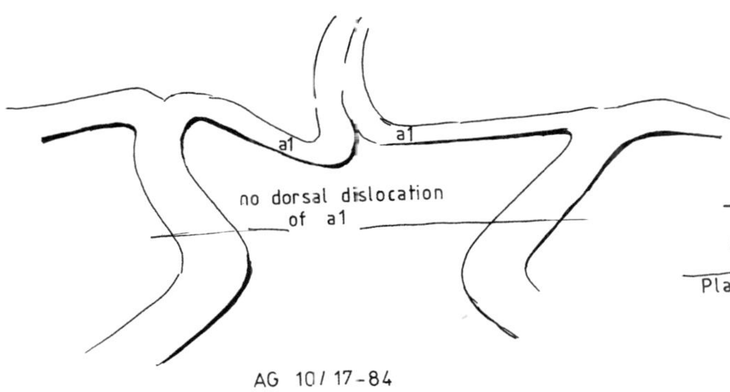

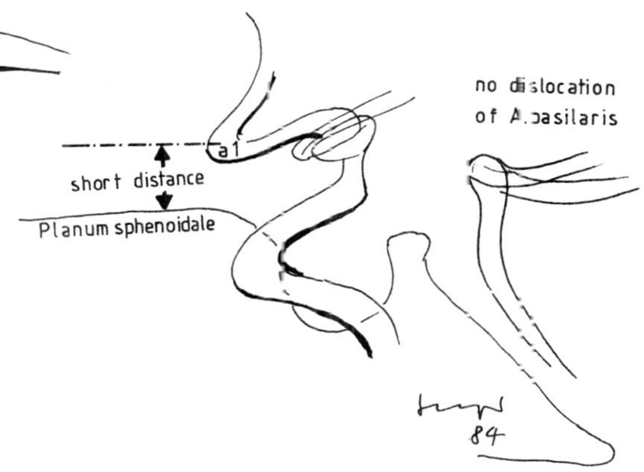

postop. CT

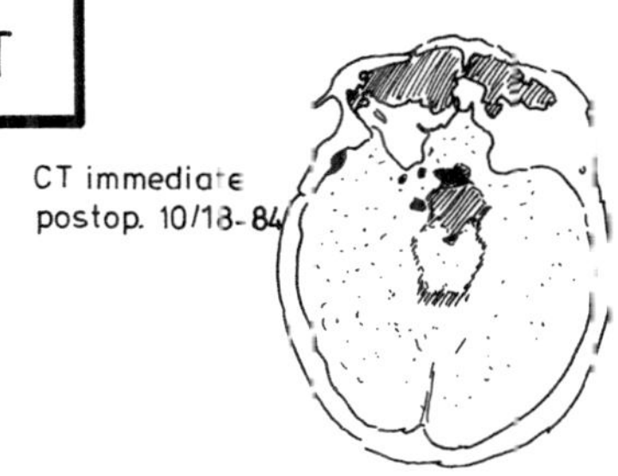

Fig. 123. Possible anatomical variants which had to be considered before the surgical intervention

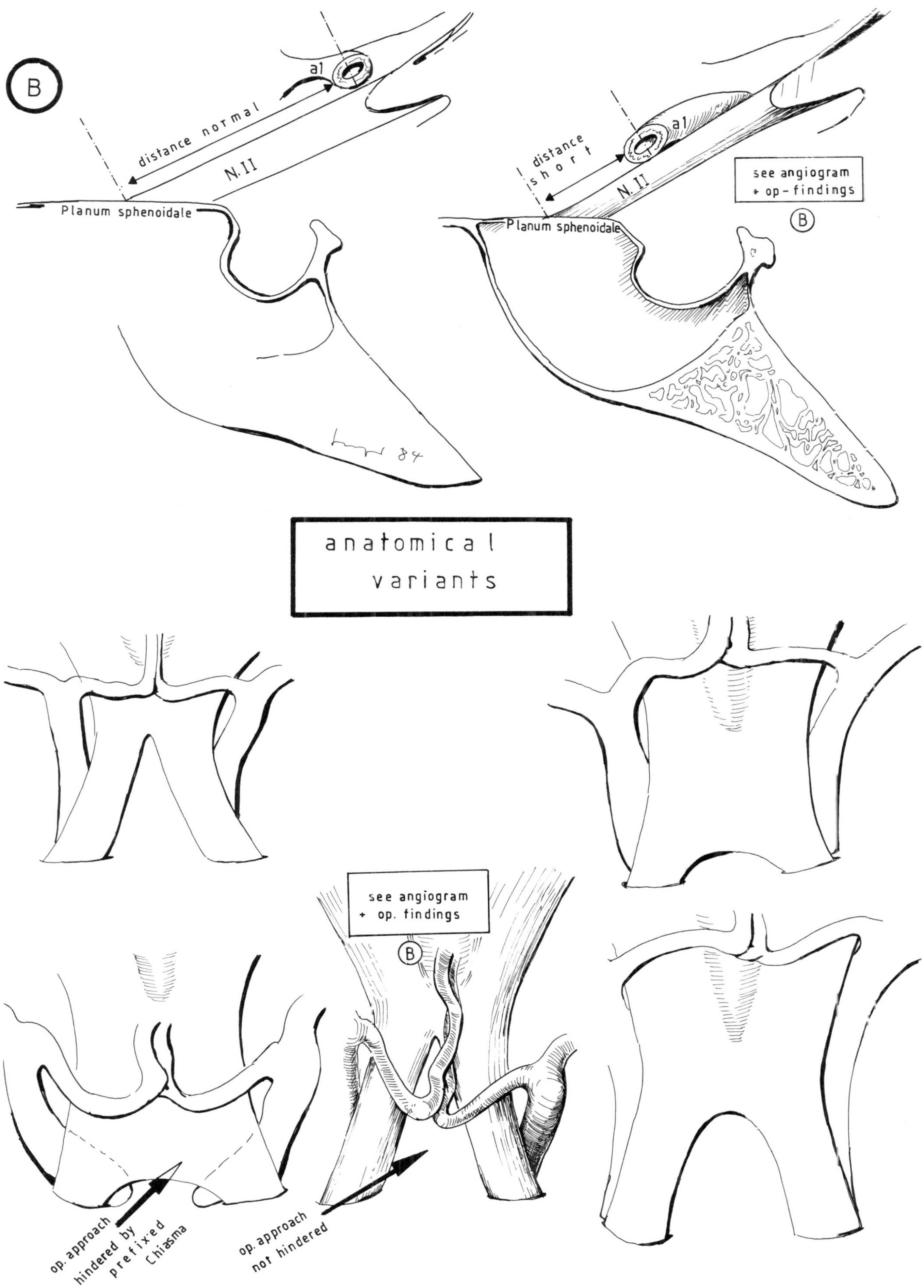
B
a1
distance normal
N. II
Planum sphenoidale
a1
distance short
N. II
see angiogram + op-findings
B
Planum sphenoidale
anatomical variants
see angiogram + op. findings
B
op. approach hindered by prefixed Chiasma
op. approach not hindered

Fig. 124

B

1st step

① dissection of cisternal arachnoicea
② incision + hollowing of the tumor

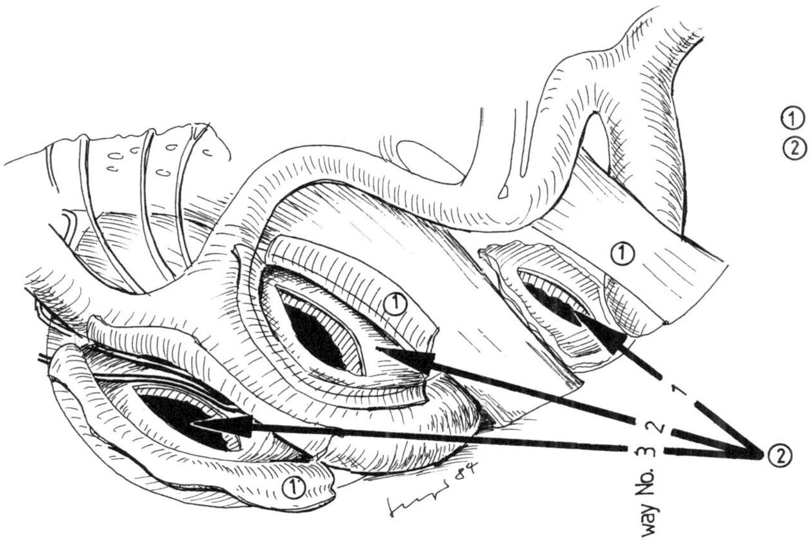

2nd step

① + ② see first step

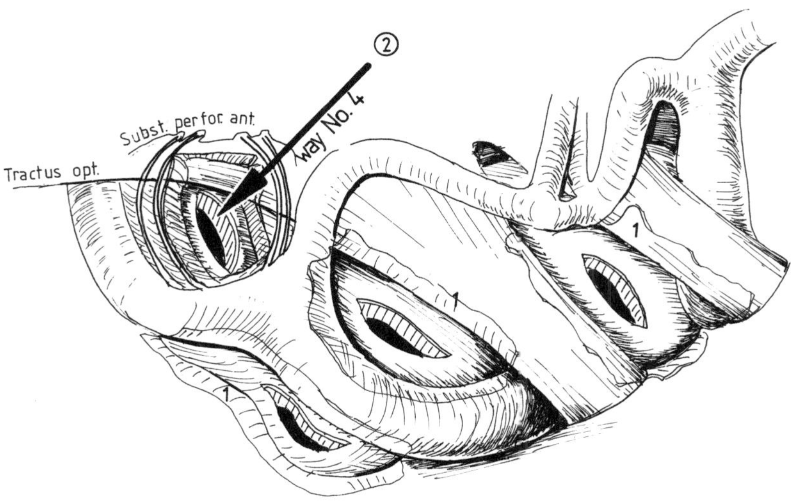

3rd step

① further dissection of cisternal arachnoidea from arachnoid layer of the tumor
② hollowing
③a transection of the tumor
③b elimination of the tumor exept for portion covered by homolateral N. II

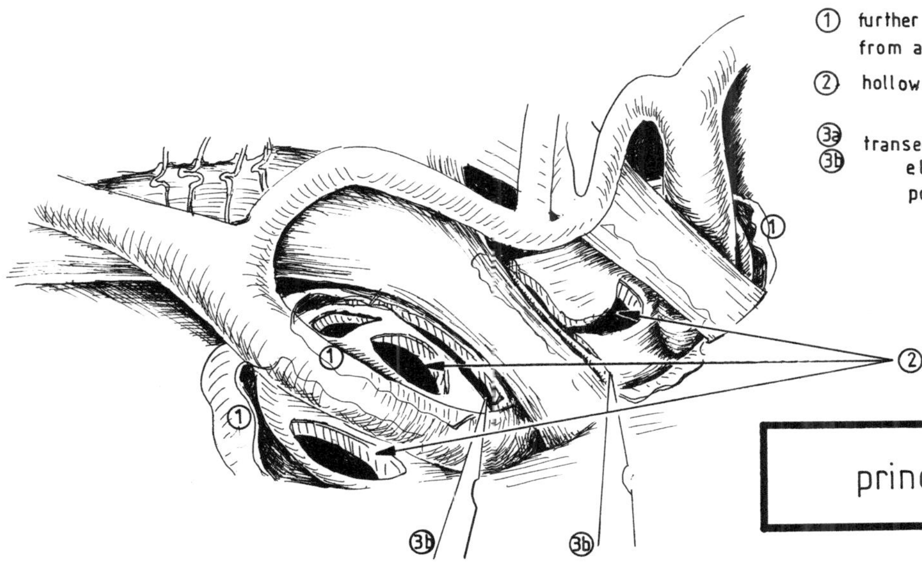

principles of operation

Fig. 125

(B)

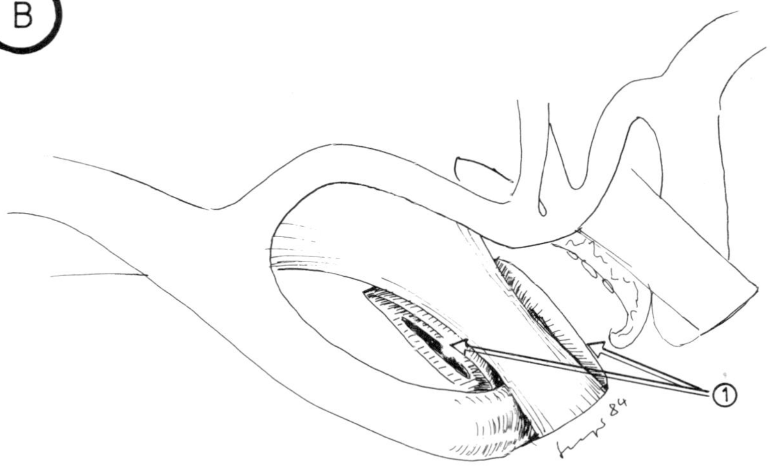

4th step

① hollowing and elimination of residual tumor covered by homolateral N.II

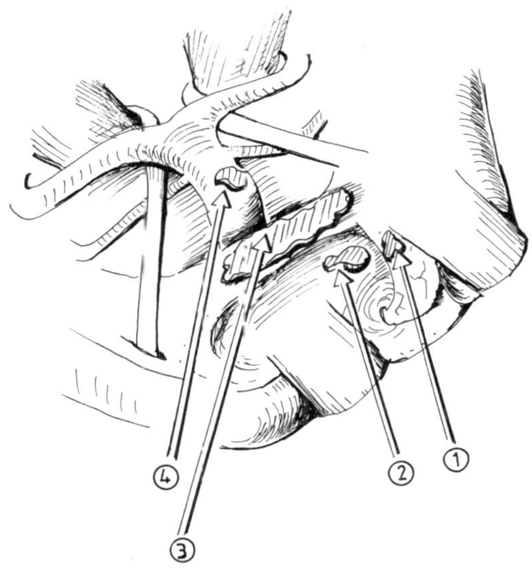

5th step

①②④ elimination of small residual tumor of Arachnoidea

③ elimination of residual tumor base at Dorsum sellae

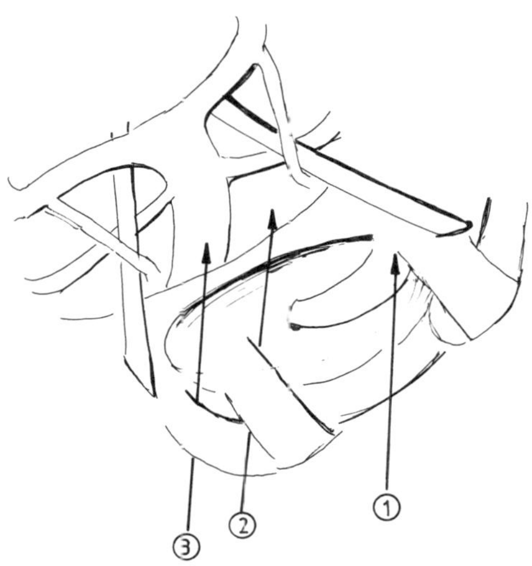

6th step

①②③ control of <u>different</u> areas of the tumor bed

Fig. 126. The removal of the tumor was achieved at four different locations. By means of which it was possible to remove the tumor so thoroughly, even in less visible regions, so that it could be radically removed with only limited danger

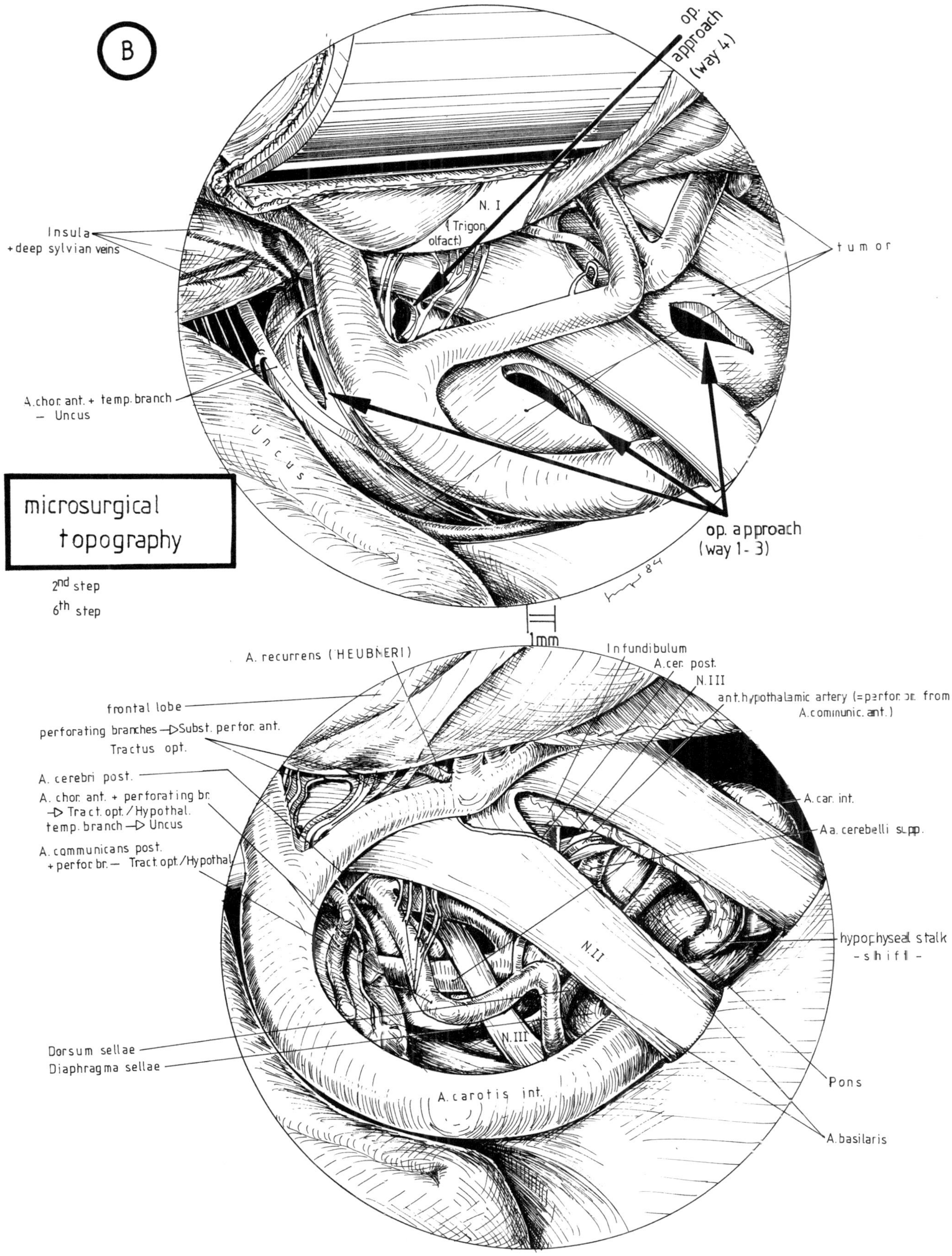
B
op. approach (way 4)
Insula + deep sylvian veins
N. I (Trigon. olfact.)
tumor
A. chor. ant. + temp. branch – Uncus
Uncus
microsurgical topography
op. approach (way 1-3)
2nd step
6th step
1mm
A. recurrens (HEUBNERI)
Infundibulum
A. cer. post.
N. III
ant. hypothalamic artery (=perfor. br. from A. communic. ant.)
frontal lobe
perforating branches –▷ Subst. perfor. ant.
Tractus opt.
A. cerebri post.
A. chor. ant. + perforating br. –▷ Tract. opt. / Hypothal. temp. branch –▷ Uncus
A. communicans post. + perfor. br. – Tract. opt. / Hypothal.
A. car. int.
Aa. cerebelli sup.
N. II
hypophyseal stalk - shift -
N. III
Dorsum sellae
Diaphragma sellae
A. carotis int.
Pons
A. basilaris

Fig. 127. Large tumor of the Cisterna ambiens (anterior meningioma of the tentorium with a portion of the tumor in the posterior cranial fossa). **The problem with such tumors lies in whether they should be primarily operated supratentorially or infratentorially**

(A) combined approach 1.) pterional 2.) suboccipital

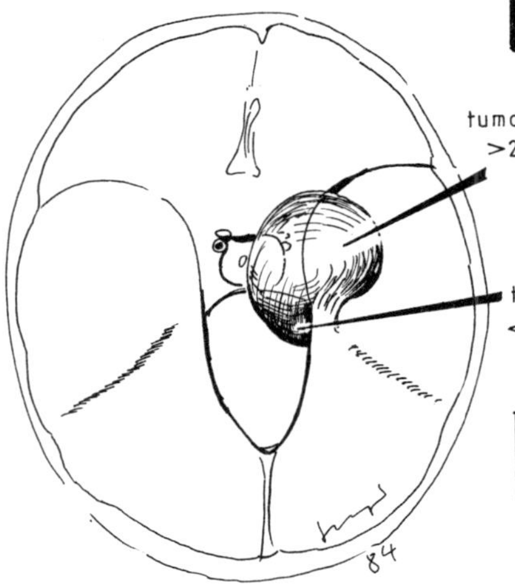

favorable

- in Fossa cranii post. s m a l l residual tumor after 1st op.
- N. II, A. carotis int. + Aa. perforantes
- A. communicans post. + " " "
- A. chorioidea ant. + " " "
- N. III, N. IV (dist.)
- bifurcation of A. basil. + " " "
- A. cerebri post. + " " "
- A. cerebelli sup. (prox.)$^{x)}$ + " " "

unfavorable

- N. V, N. VI, N. VII / N. VIII
- A. basilaris, caudal segment + Rr. ad pontem
- "AICA" + " "
- Vv. pontis
- A. cerebelli sup. (dist.)$^{x)}$
- approach to Fossa cranii post (1st op.)
  - more favorable after drilling Apex ossis petrosi during 1st operation (SAMII 1984 personal communication)

(B) combined approach 1.) suboccipital 2.) pterional – temporobasal

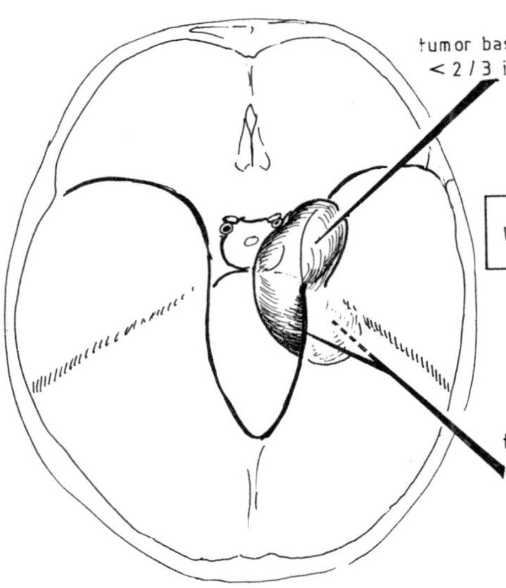

favorable

- N. VIII, N. VII, N. VI, N. V, N. IV (prox.)$^{x)}$
- in Fossa cranii media s m a l l residual tumor after 1st op.
- A. basil., caudal segment + Rr. ad pontem
- "aica" + " "
- Vv. pontis
- A. cerebelli sup. (dist.)$^{x)}$

unfavorable

- A. cerebelli sup. (prox.)$^{x)}$
- N. IV (dist.)$^{x)}$
- A. cerebri post. + Aa. perforantes
- bifurcation of A. basil. + " " "
- N. III
- A. communicans post. + " " "
- A. chorioidea ant. + " " "
- N. II, A. carotis int. + " " "
- approach to Fossa cranii media (1st op.)

$^{x)}$ during 1st operation

Fig. 128. Clinical example of a tumor primarily operated supratentorially (meningioma of the Dorsum sellae with extension into the prepontine region, the Cisterna interpeduncularis and the Cisterna cerebello-pontina). Since 4 to 5 years relapsing dizziness and vomiting. Ventriculo-atrial shunt operation on July 4, 1983 in another clinic due to hydrocephalus occlusus. Since then increasing tetraspasticity and indistinct speach, psychological slowing, orientated in time and place. Postoperatively a partial oculomotor paresis, rapid reversal of the preoperatively present speech disturbance and the tetraspasticity. The oculomotor paresis also reduced. After the second operation on December 12, 1983 hypaesthesia of the right half of the face, Abducens and facial paresis, as well as a right hypacusis and a light cerebellar ataxia, rapid improvement in the postoperative deficits with corresponding considerable reversal*

* Both operations were performed by Dr. W. Hassler, coworker of the author.

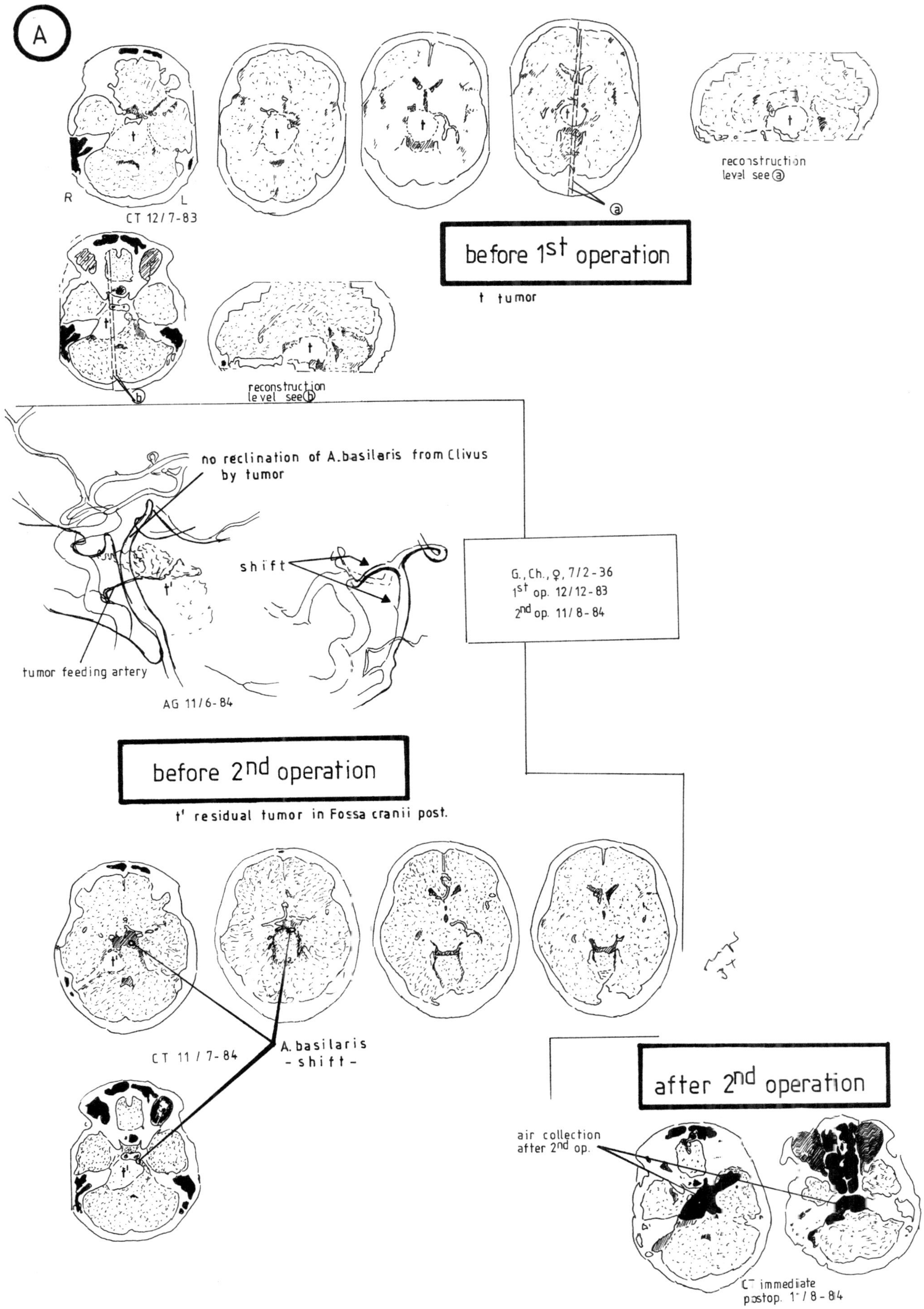
A
R
L
CT 12/7-83
reconstruction
level see ⓐ
ⓐ
before 1st operation
t tumor
reconstruction
level see ⓑ
ⓑ
no reclination of A.basilaris from Clivus
by tumor
shift
t'
tumor feeding artery
AG 11/6-84
G., Ch., ♀, 7/2-36
1st op. 12/12-83
2nd op. 11/8-84
before 2nd operation
t' residual tumor in Fossa cranii post.
CT 11/7-84
A. basilaris
- shift -
after 2nd operation
air collection
after 2nd op.
CT immediate
postop.

Fig. 129. First operation supratentorially

Ⓐ

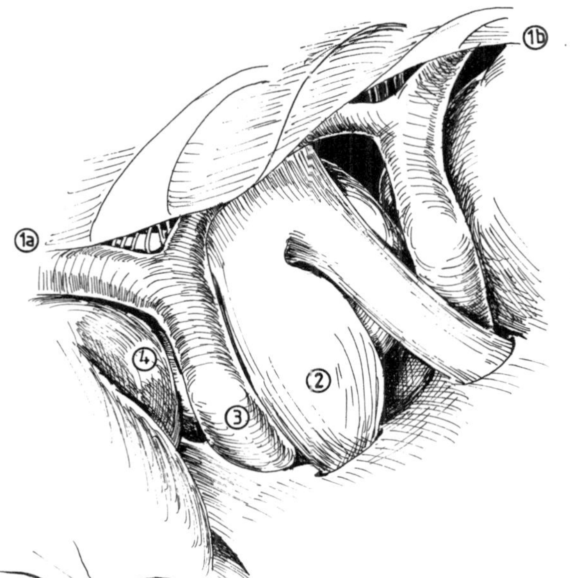

1st step

1a medial arachnoid splitting of sylvian fissure
1b " " " " " ,-contra-lat.-
2 N. II -dissection-
3 A. carotis int. - dissection-
4 Uncus -dissection-

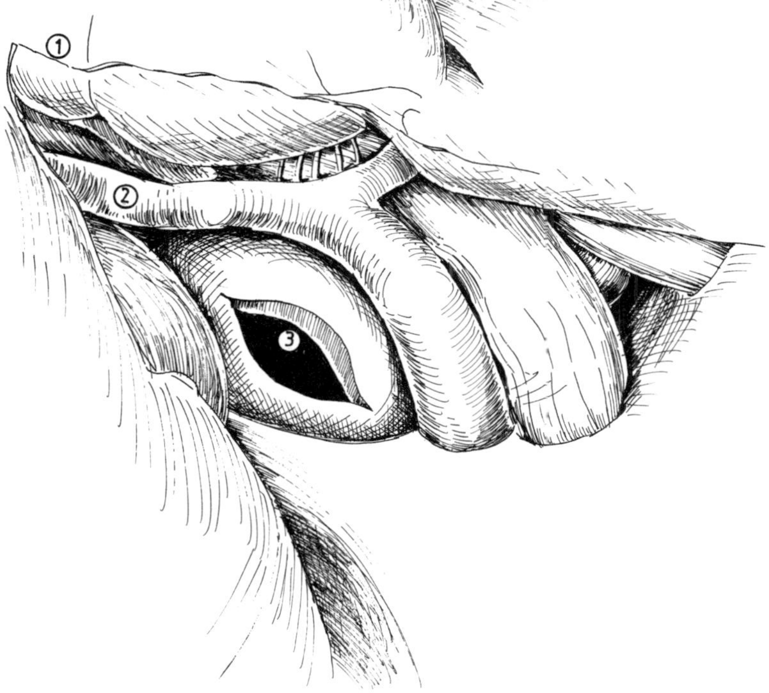

2nd step

1 lateral arachnoid splitting of sylvian fissure
2 A. cerebri media - dissection-
3 hollowing of the tumor

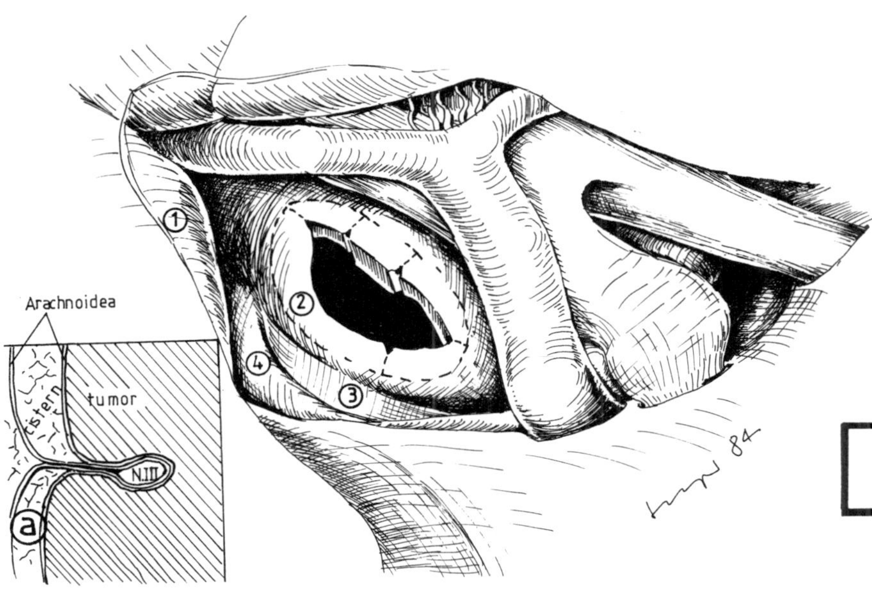

3rd step

1 Uncus dissection
2 tumor - hollowing + resection -
3 N. III - dissection-
relationships to tumor + Arachnoidea see sketch (a)
4 tumor - hollowing + resection

principles of 1st operation

Fig. 130

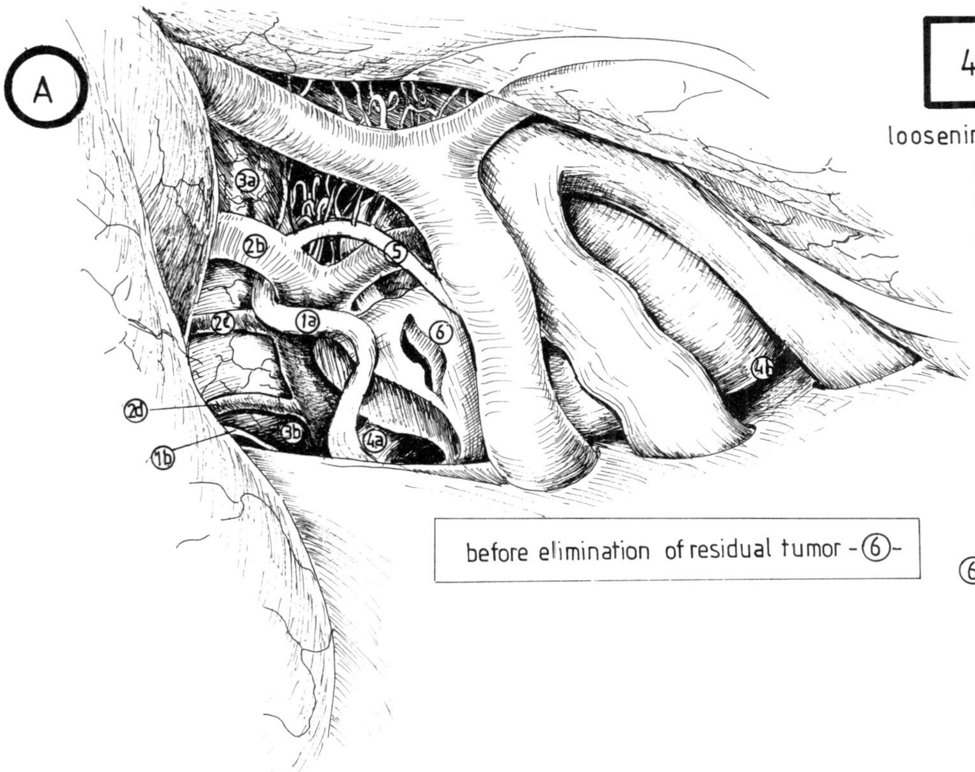

before elimination of residual tumor -⑥-

4th step

loosening of the tumor from

- 1a N. III
- 1b N. IV
- 2a A. basilaris
- 2b A. cerebri post.
- 2c A. cerebelli sup.
- 2d "AICA"
- 3a Crus cerebri
- 3b Pons
- 4a Dors. sellae -tumor base-
- 4b Diaphragma sellae-tumor base-
- 5 A. communicans post.
- 6 extirpation of supratentorial residual tumor

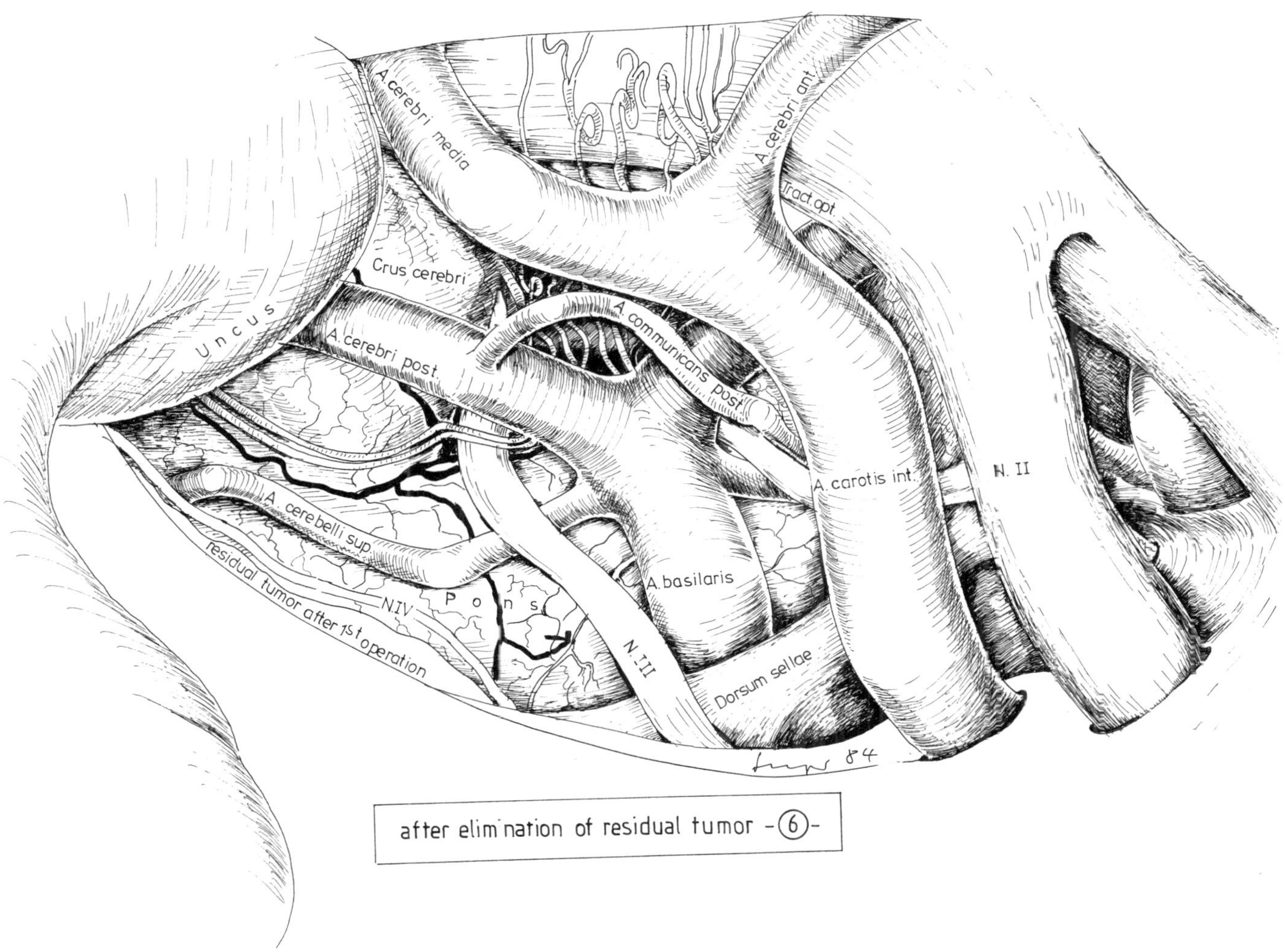

after elimination of residual tumor -⑥-

Fig. 131. Second operation infratentorially

Ⓐ second operation

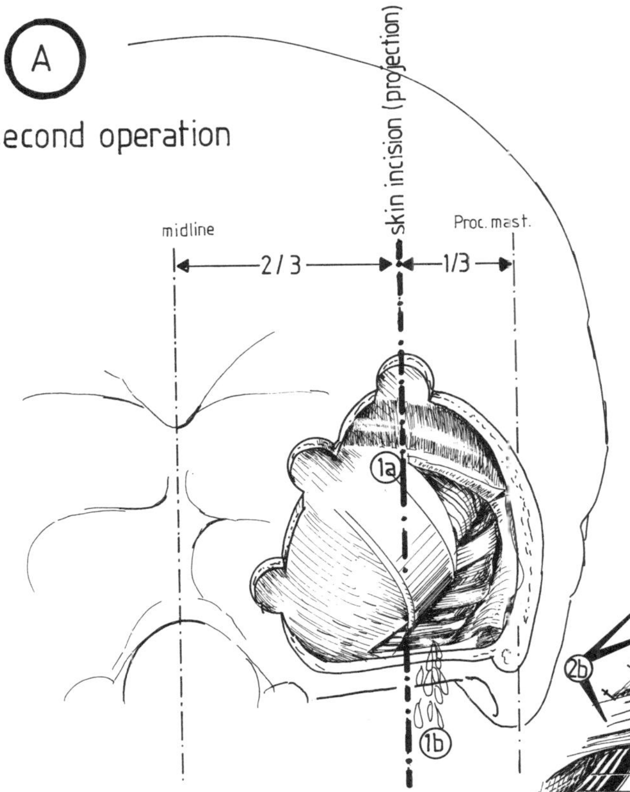

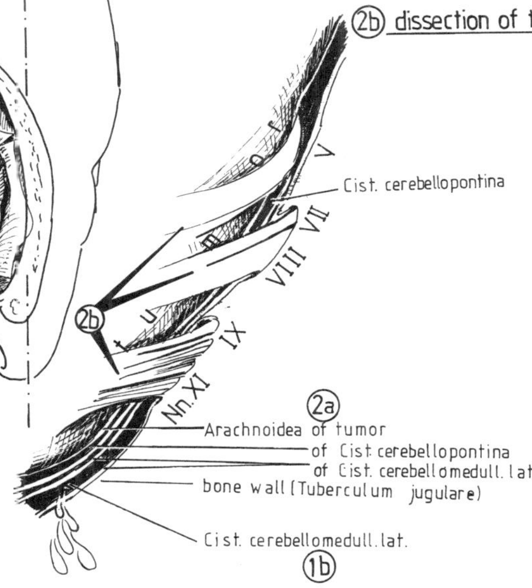

1st step

(1a) skin incision, trepanation, Dura incision

(1b) CSF-aspiration after incision of Arachnoidea below Nn. XI-IX (Cist. cerebellomed. lat.)

(2a) dissection of tumor Arachnoidea after incision and dissect. of arachnoid wall of Cisterna cerebellopontina

(2b) dissection of tumor involved Nn. XI-X-IX-VIII-VII -V

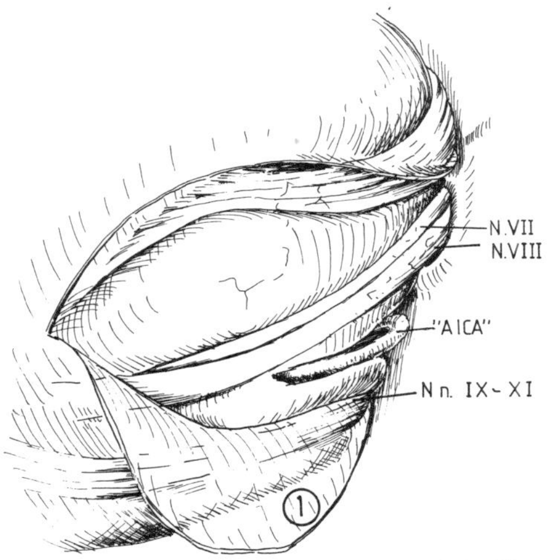

2nd step

① further dissection of arachnoid wall of Cist. cerebellopontina

② further dissection of tumor Arachnoidea enclosing Nn. XI-X-IX-VIII-VII-V and "AICA" + small branches → Nn. XI-IX and Nn. VIII-VII

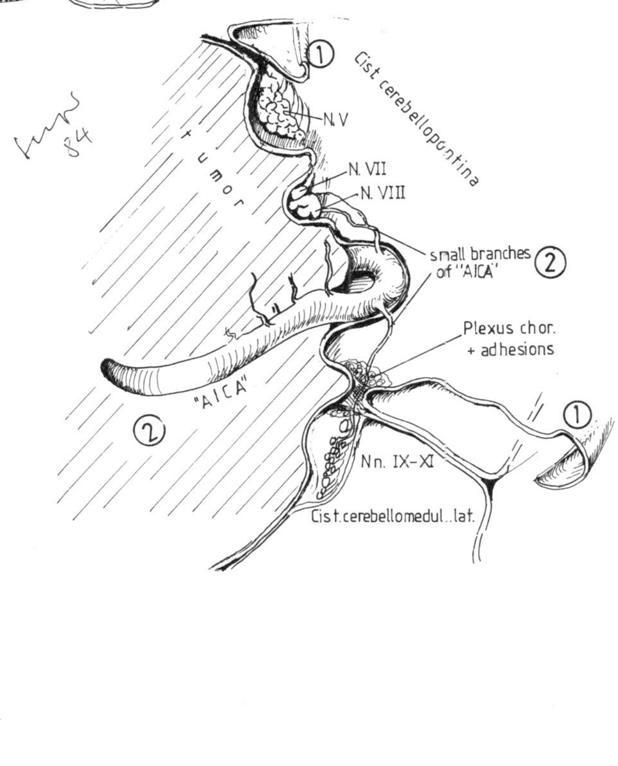

principles of operation

Fig. 132

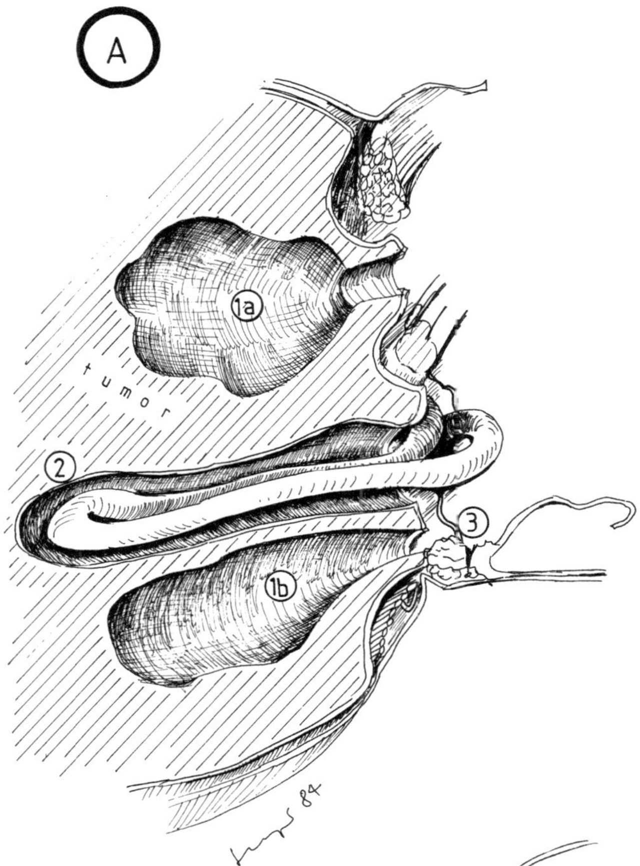

3rd step

(1a)(1b) hollowing of the tumor

(2) further dissection of "AICA"

(3) transection of adhesions

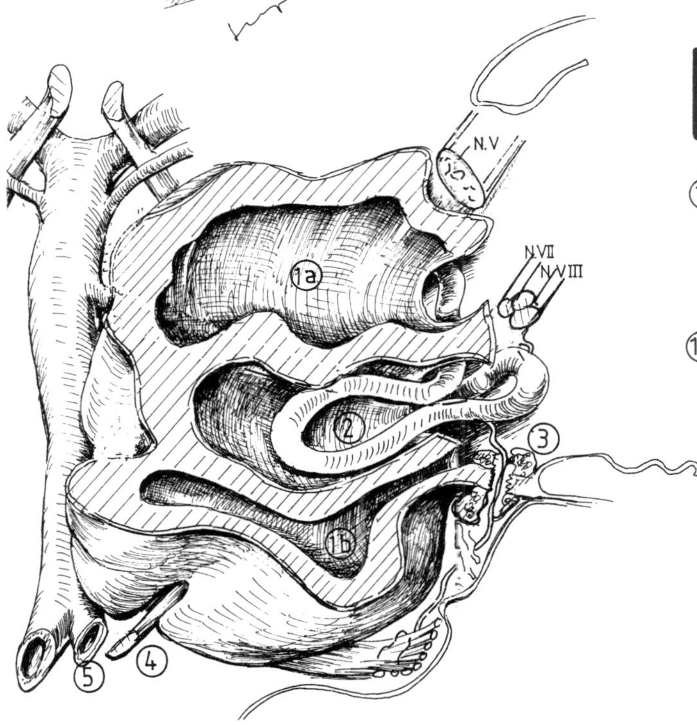

4th step

(1a) to (3) as 3rd step

(4) dissection of N.VI

(5) dissection of A. vertebralis / basilaris (+ perforating branches - be careful -)

(1a) to (5) repeat

Fig. 133

(A)

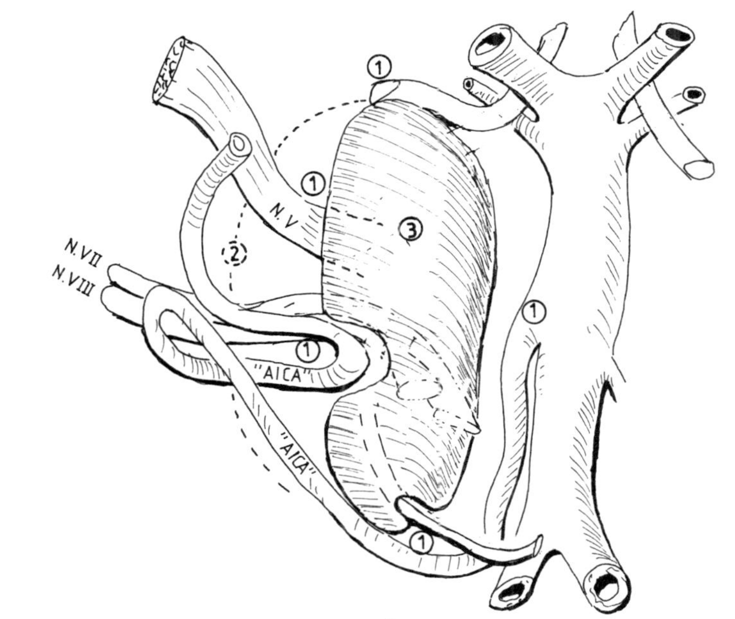

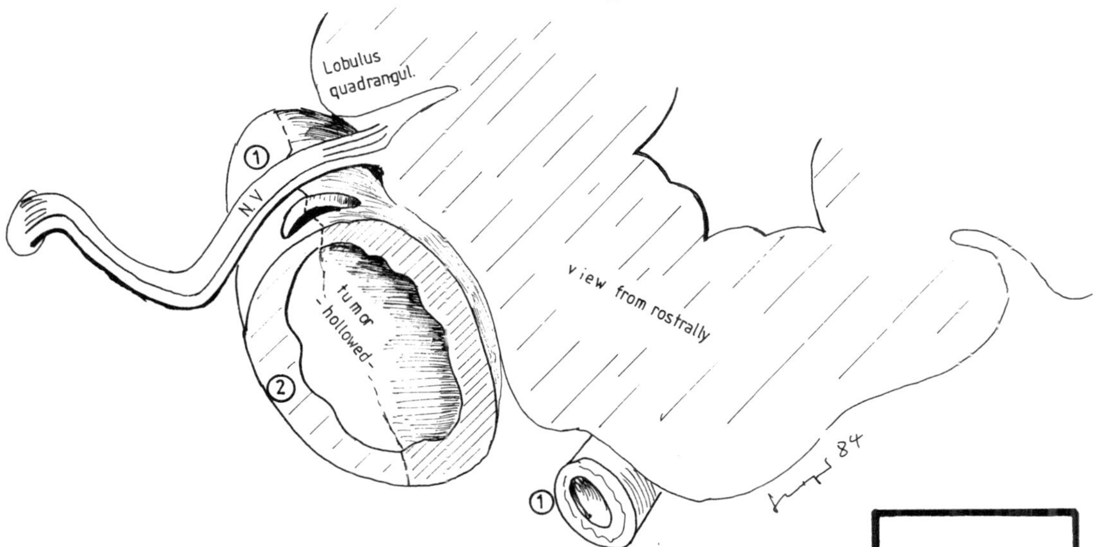

5th step

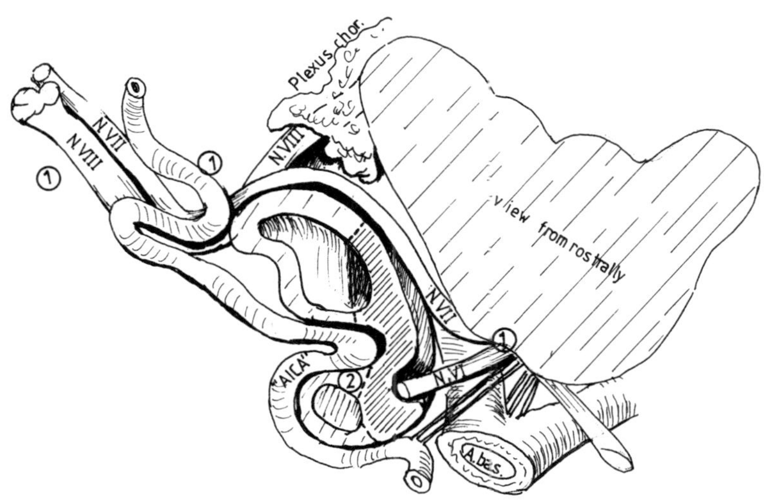

① further dissection of cranial nerves, "AICA," A. basil. and brainstem

② extirpation of lateral tumor portion

③ extirpation of residual (medial) tumor

Fig. 134. As with an acoustic neurinoma is the preparation of the arachnoidea of the cisterns the most important presupposition for the considerate radical removal. The V. petrosa superior, which can be thrombosed due to the tumor pressure, as an exception does not need to be preserved in this case

(A)

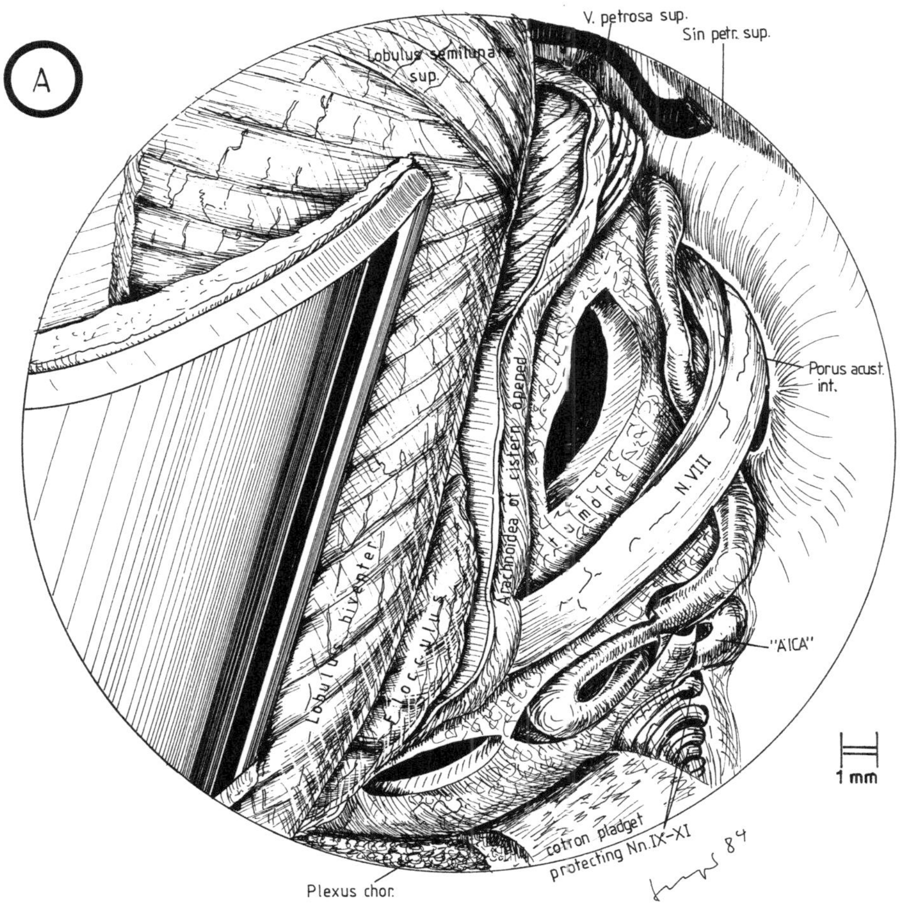

microsurgical topography

5th step

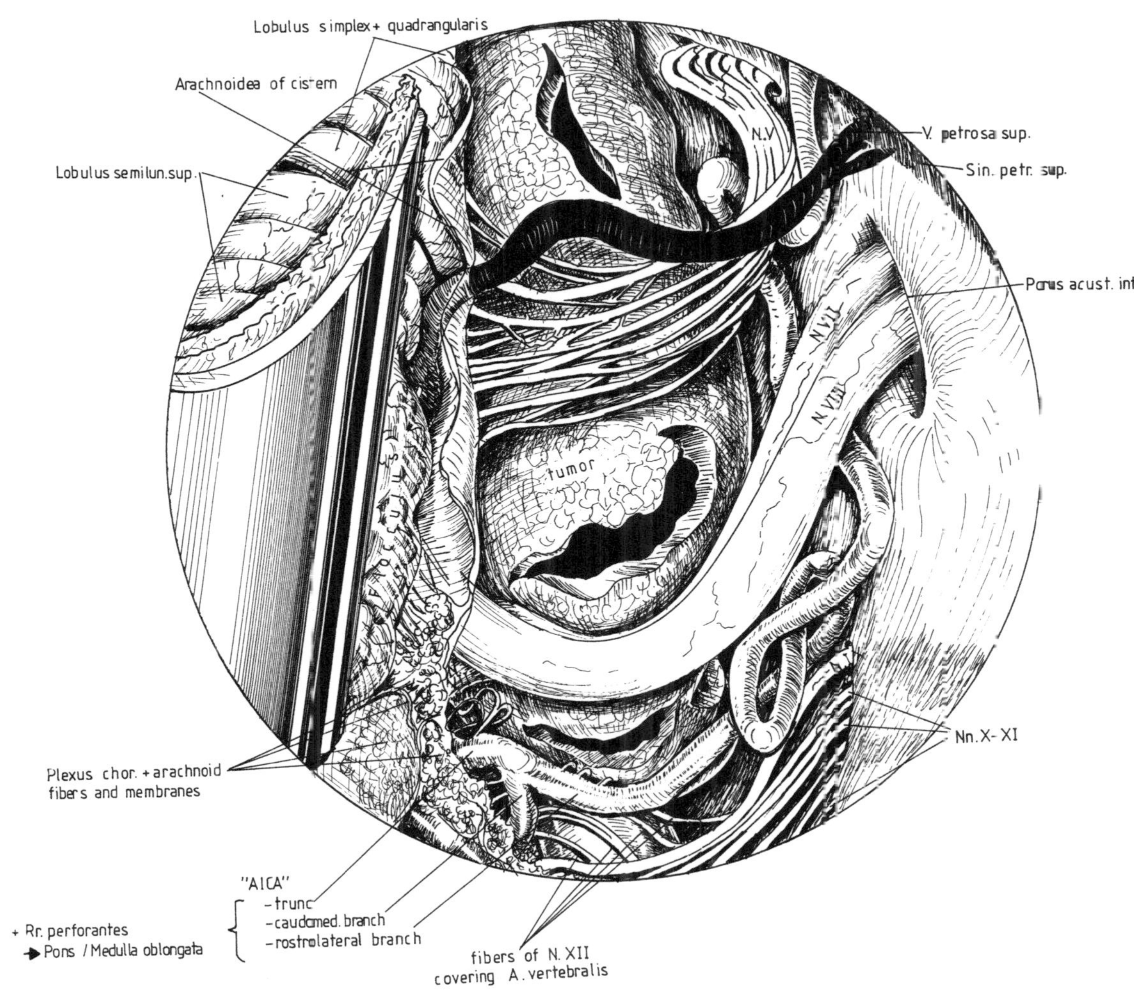

Fig. 135. Site of operation after removal of the tumor. The preservation of the vessels, particularly of the perforating arteries, was of importance for the exceptionally favorable course. Therefore a schematic view of the relevant vessels in the area of the operative vascular bed is included

(A)

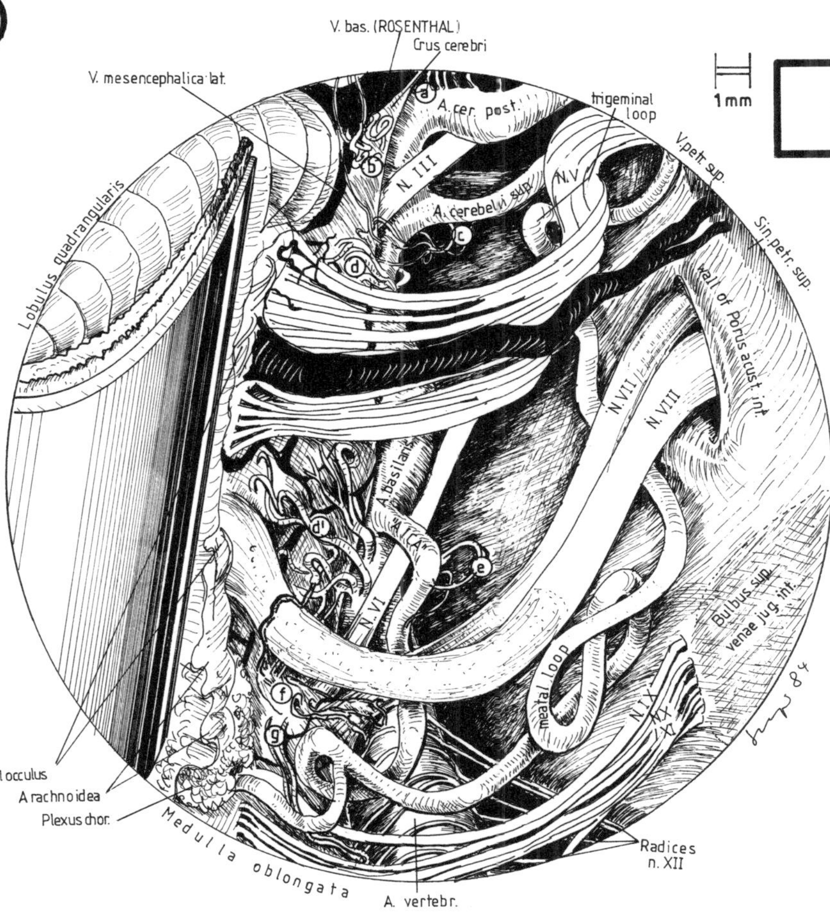

1 mm

microsurgical topography

after 5th step

(a) to (g) perforating arteries of brainstem

	originating from	running to
(a)	A. cerebri post. -prox segment-	Subst. perfor. post., Infund., Chiasma + Tractus opt.
(b)	A. cerebri post. -prox.+dist.segm.-	Crus cerebri, Tract. cpt., Tegmentum
(c)	A. cerebelli sup.	Pons /Mesenceph. (Isthmus rhombencephali)
(d) (d')	A. basilaris	Pons (Rr. ad pontem, -Rr. longi et breves-) Pons-Med. oblong.
(e)	"AICA"	Pons-Med. oblong. - Fossa supraolivaris -
(f)	A. vertebralis	
(g)	"PICA"	

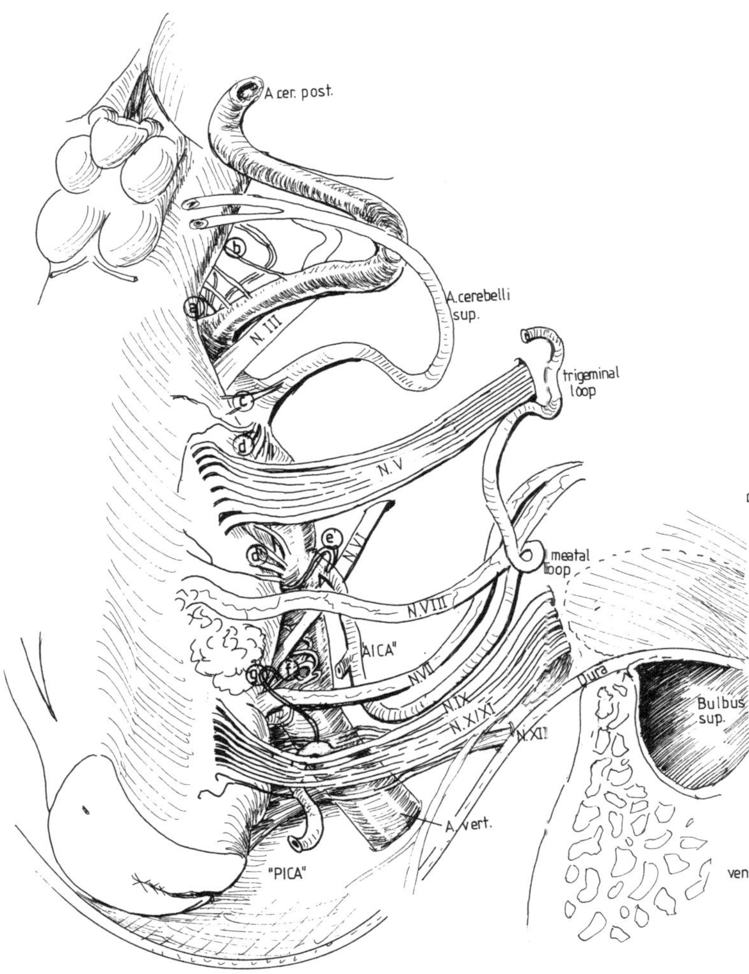

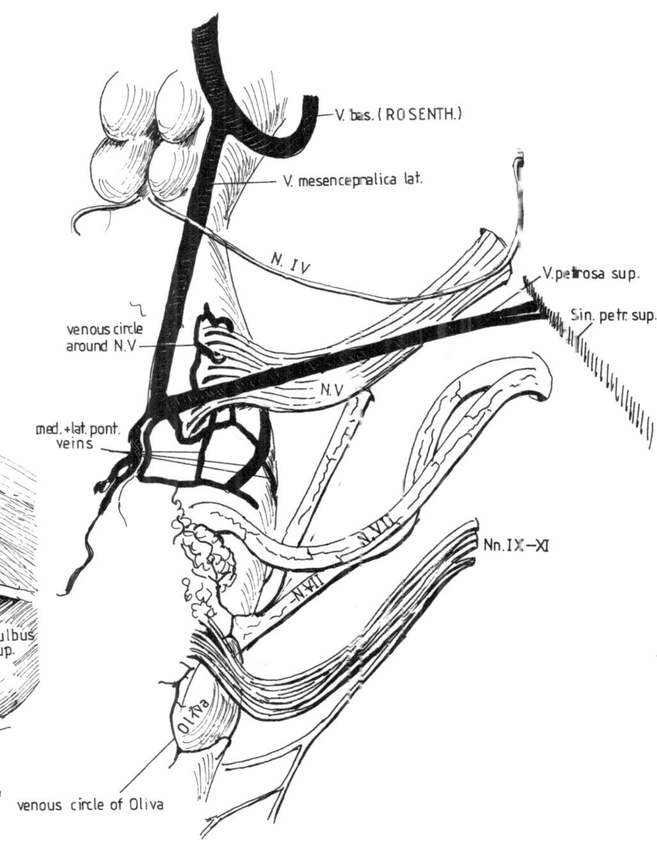

Fig. 136. Clinical example of a petroclival meningioma. In contrast to type **A** it was operated first from an infratentorial approach and following recurrence the small supratentorial remainder from a supratentorial approach. Marked deficits of the caudal cerebral nerves with disturbances in standing and walking, which improved markedly after the first intervention, so that the patient could take care of her household again. The worsening before the second intervention was not noticeably improved by the intervention

* Both interventions were performed by Prof. Dr. J. Gilsbach, coworker of the author. The first operation alternately with Priv.-Doz. Dr. H. Friedrich (now at the Neurosurgical University Clinic in Hannover, Director: Prof. Dr. H. Dietz). The second intervention was made alternately with Dr. W. Hassler, coworker of the author.

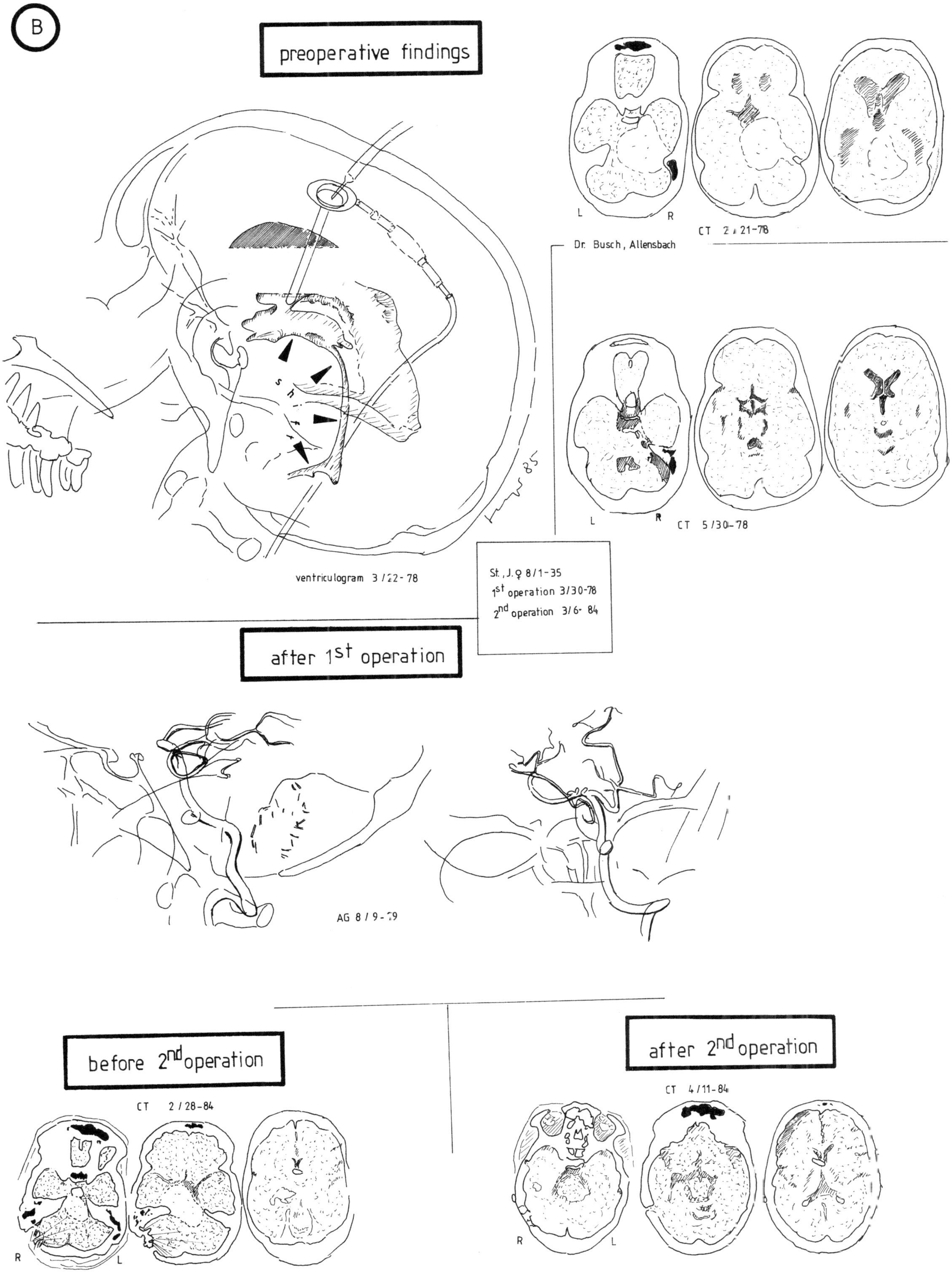
B
preoperative findings
L
R
CT 2/21-78
Dr. Busch, Allensbach
shift
L
R
CT 5/30-78
ventriculogram 3/22-78
St., J. ♀ 8/1-35
1st operation 3/30-78
2nd operation 3/6-84
after 1st operation
AG 8/9-79
before 2nd operation
CT 2/28-84
R
L
after 2nd operation
CT 4/11-84
R
L

Fig. 137. Microsurgical site at the end of the second intervention. The large tumor left a cavity, which enabled visualization caudally as far as the ventral rim of the Foramen occipitale magnum

(A)

microsurgical topography

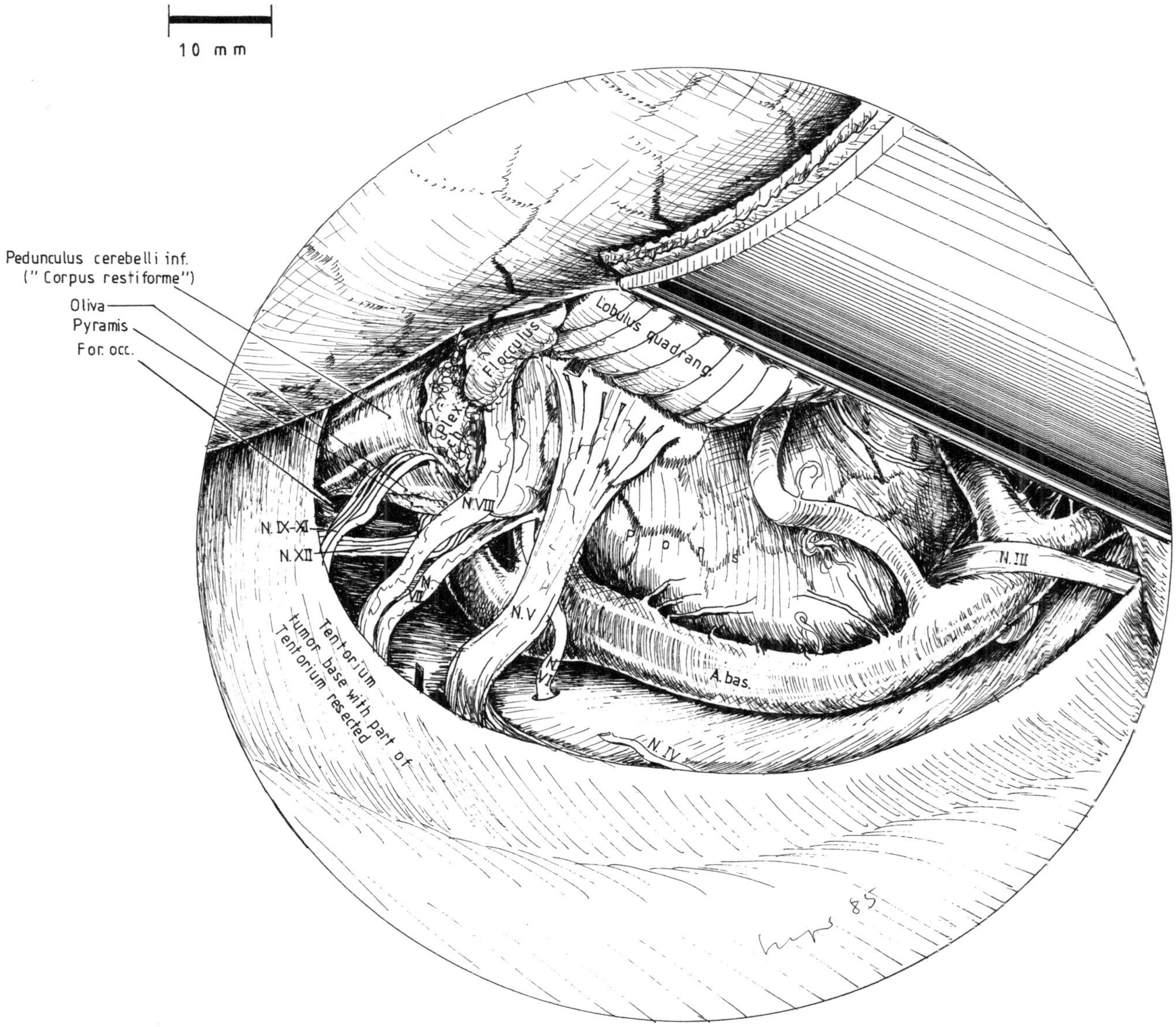

Chapter 6
Lateral Cisterns and Fissures, Posterior Segment (Figs. 138 to 160)

The following descriptions of petroclival interventions concern tumors which were localized not only in the cisterns of the cerebellopontine angle, but also in the petrous portion of the temporal bone

Fig. 138. The neurosurgical intervention has priority when a large intradural tumor is present which threatens vital functions (type **A**). In all other cases (type **B** and type **C**) is the priority of the neurosurgical intervention at least controversial, in that the extensive otosurgical exposure makes a clear visualization and removal of the intradural portion of the tumor

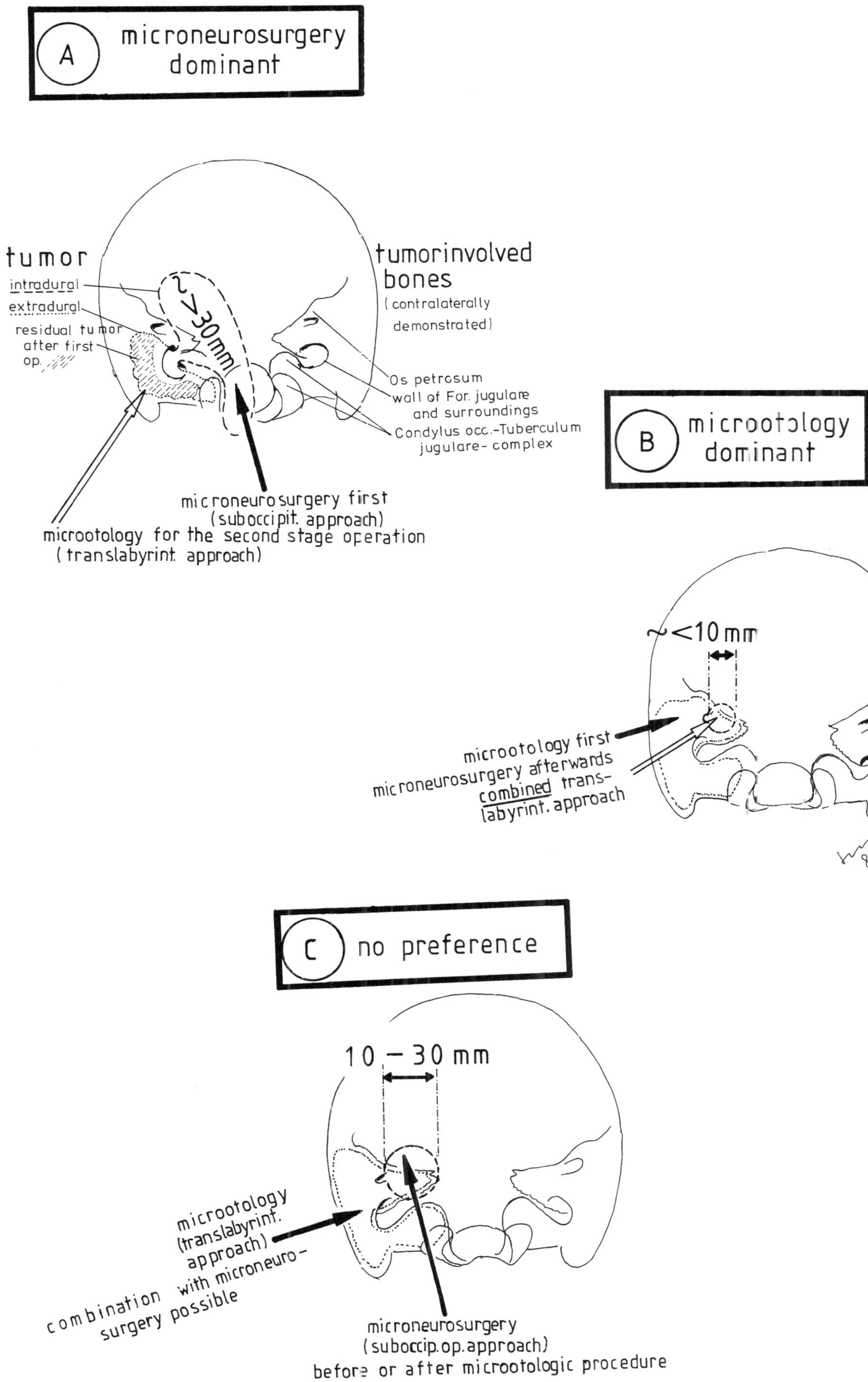
A microneurosurgery dominant
tumor
intradural
extradural
residual tumor after first op.
~>30mm
tumorinvolved bones
(contralaterally demonstrated)
Os petrosum
wall of For. jugulare and surroundings
Condylus occ.-Tuberculum jugulare-complex
microneurosurgery first
(suboccipit. approach)
microotology for the second stage operation
(translabyrint. approach)
B microotology dominant
~<10mm
microotology first
microneurosurgery afterwards
combined trans-
labyrint. approach
C no preference
10 – 30 mm
microotology
(translabyrint.
approach)
combination with microneuro-
surgery possible
microneurosurgery
(suboccip.op.approach)
before or after microotologic procedure

Fig. 139. Clinical example of an extra- and intradural growing neurinoma of the cerebellopontine angle, of the petrous portion of the temporal bone, including the condyl area. Disturbances in balance since six months due to obstruction of the aqueduct. Atrioventricular shunt introduced and neurologically afterwards a right torticollis, horizontal gaze nystagmus of both sides, right papilledema hypaesthesia of the left cornea, left-sided pyramidal signs, left hypacusis. First operation: suboccipital, typical approach from the cerebello-pontine angle *

* The operation was performed by Dr. W. Hassler, coworker of the author. Thereby was the dorso-caudal part of the tumor in the area of the Condylus occipitalis neurosurgically reduced. Postoperatively no additional deficits.

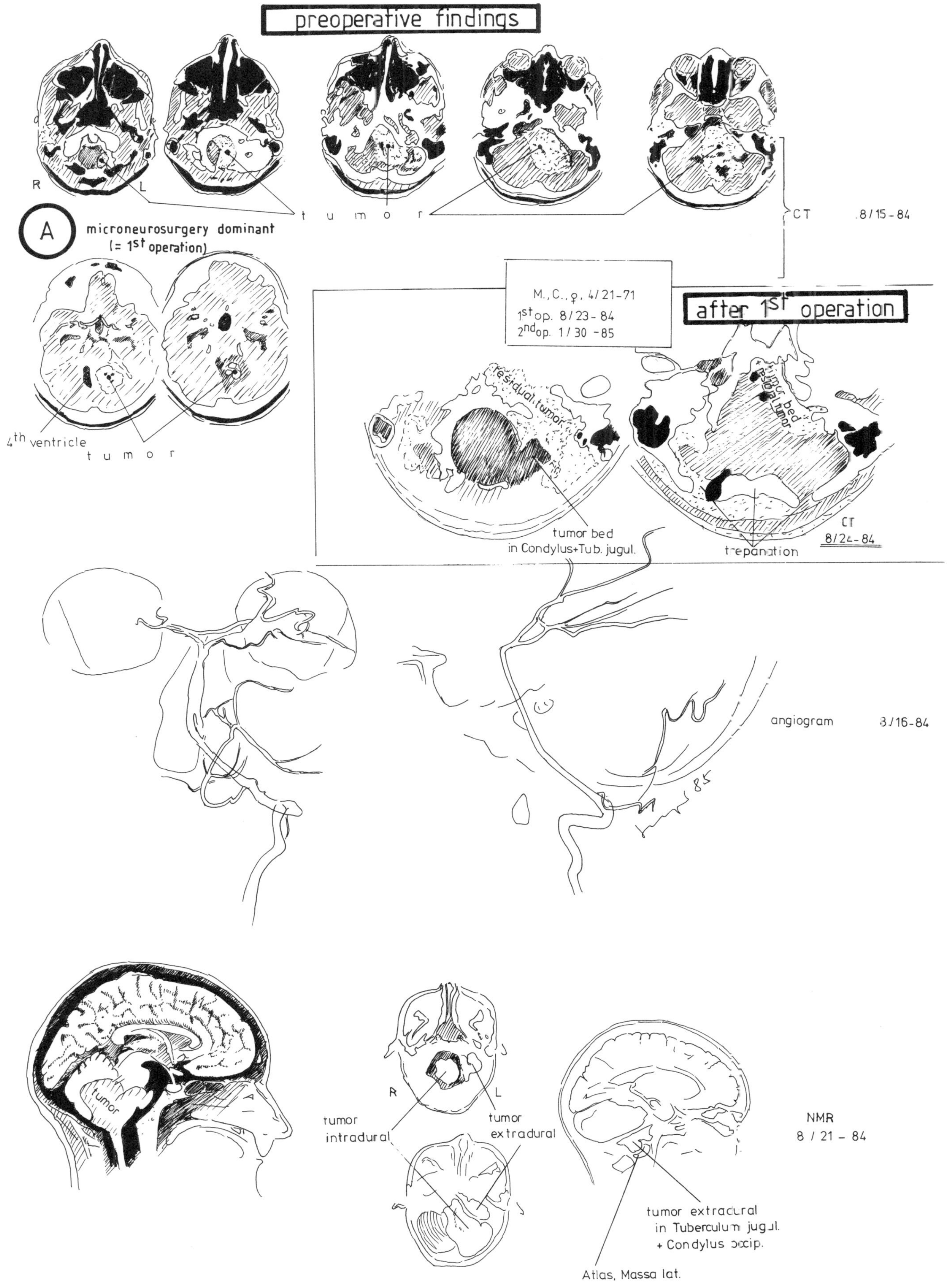
preoperative findings
R
L
t u m o r
CT .8/15-84
A
microneurosurgery dominant
(= 1st operation)
4th ventricle
t u m o r
M., C., ♀, 4/21-71
1st op. 8/23-84
2nd op. 1/30-85
after 1st operation
residual tumor
tumor bed
in Condylus+Tub. jugul.
CT
8/24-84
trepanation
angiogram 8/16-84
tumor
R
L
tumor
intradural
tumor
extradural
NMR
8 / 21 - 84
tumor extradural
in Tuberculum jugul.
+ Condylus occip.
Atlas, Massa lat.

Fig. 140. Computertomographical results after otorhinological intervention. Indication of the localization of the tumor on the basis of the results from the second intervention*

* Operation performed by Prof. Dr. W. Mann (Ear, Nose and Throat Clinic of Freiburg University, Director: Prof. Dr. Chl. Beck), together with Prof. Dr. J. Gilsbach, coworker of the author.

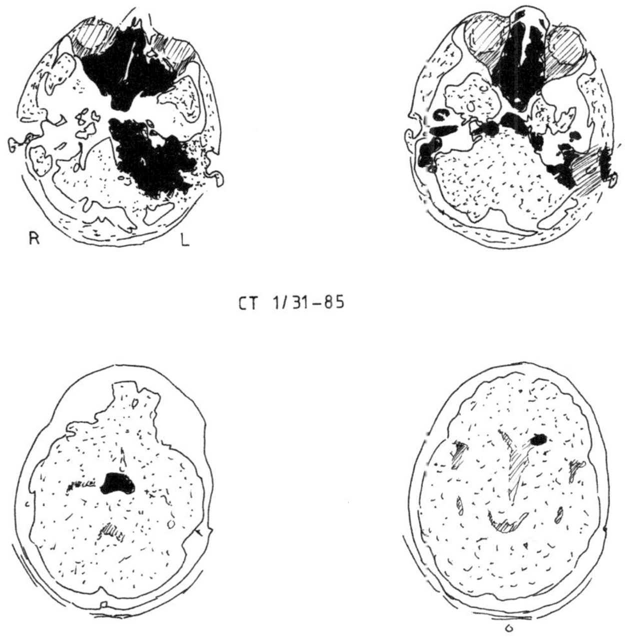

after 2nd operation

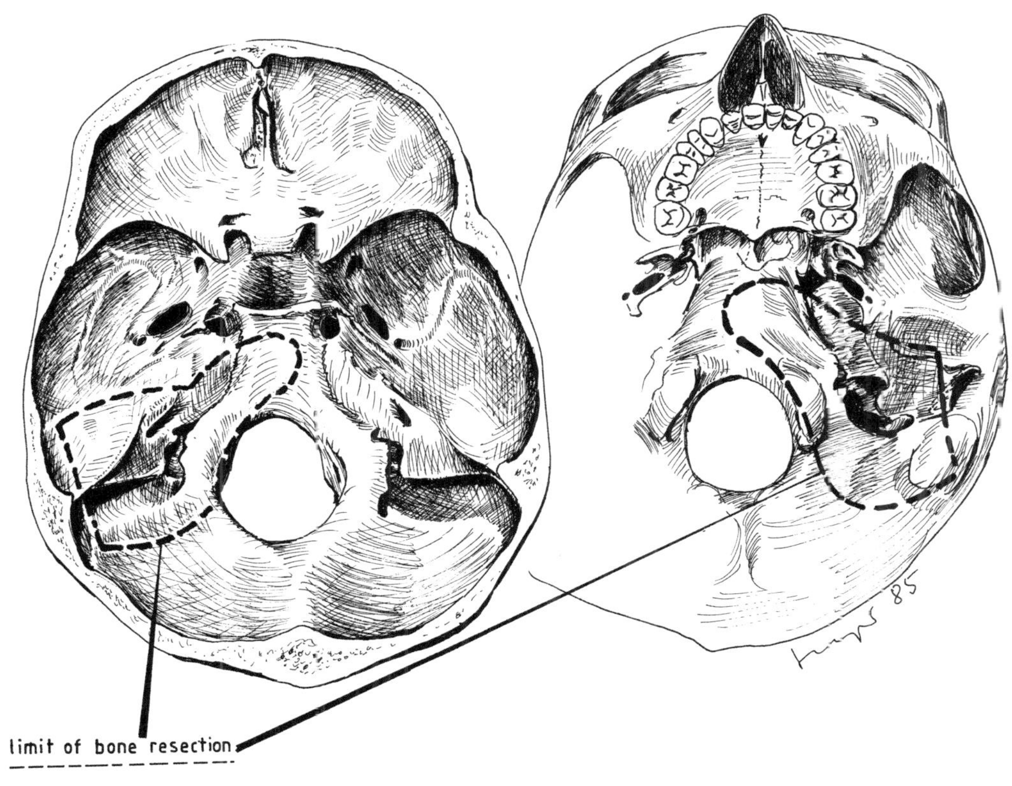

Fig. 141. Development and relationships of the tumor to the brain, as assumed from the result of the first intervention

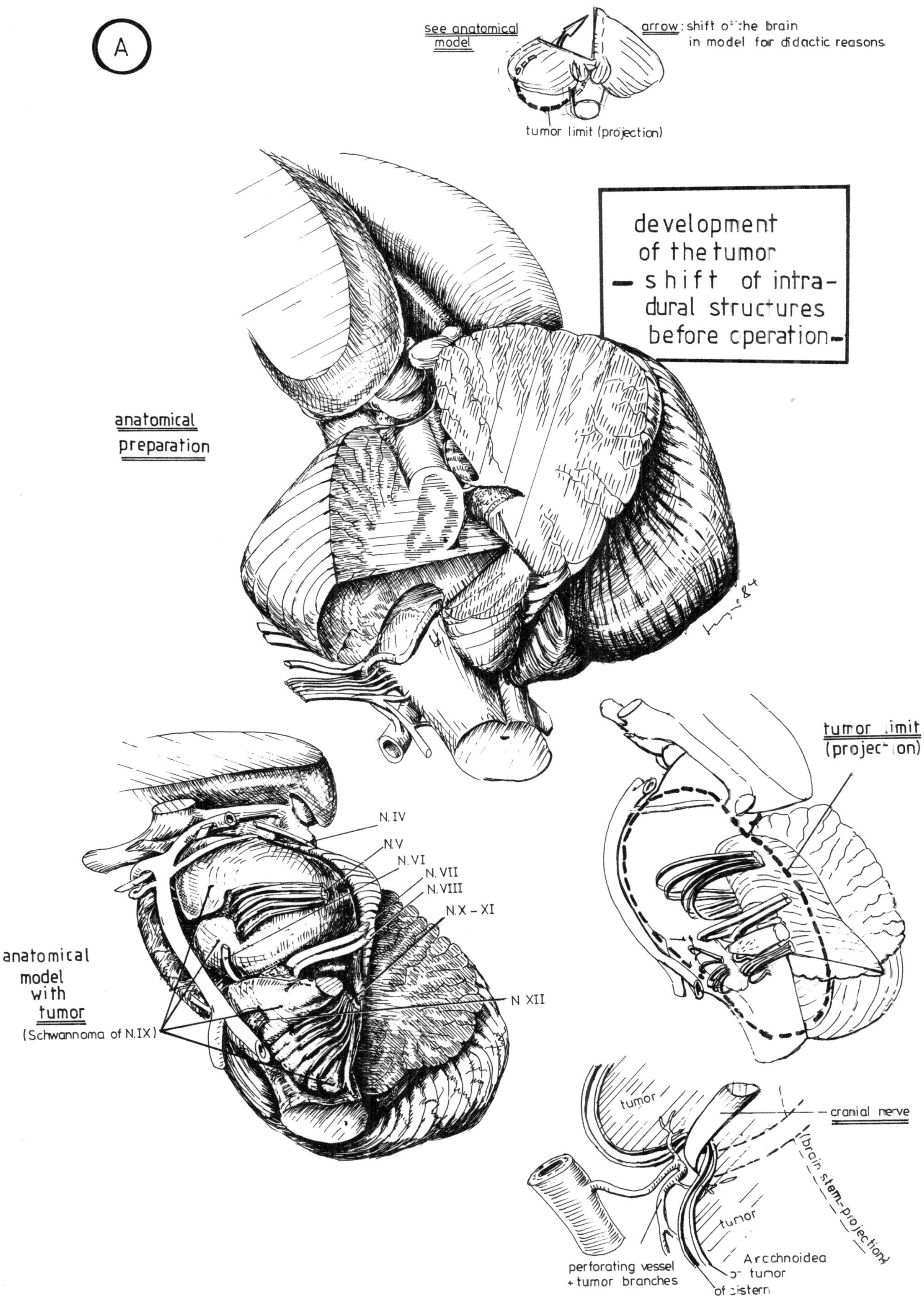
A
see anatomical model
arrow: shift o the brain
in model for didactic reasons
tumor limit (projection)
development
of the tumor
– shift of intra-
dural structures
before operation –
anatomical
preparation
N. IV
N. V
N. VI
N. VII
N. VIII
N. X – XI
N XII
anatomical
model
with
tumor
(Schwannoma of N. IX)
tumor limit
(projec on)
tumor
cranial nerve
(brain stem-projection)
tumor
perforating vessel
+ tumor branches
Arachnoidea
of tumor
of cistern

Fig. 142. Development and relationships of the tumor to the extradural structures, as assumed from the second (otorhinological) intervention

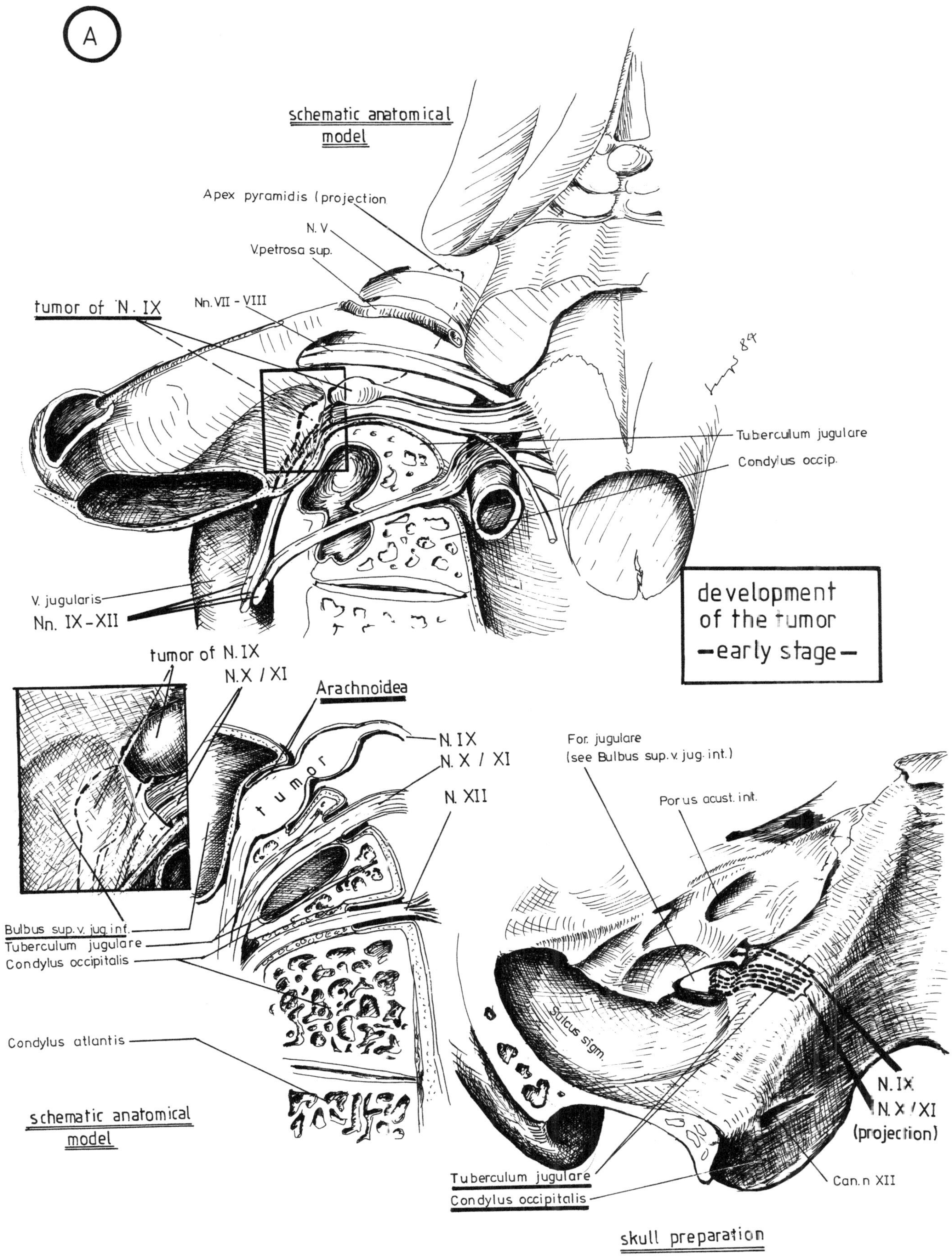
A
schematic anatomical model
Apex pyramidis (projection
N. V
V.petrosa sup.
tumor of N. IX
Nn. VII - VIII
Tuberculum jugulare
Condylus occip.
V. jugularis
Nn. IX-XII
development of the tumor
-early stage-
tumor of N. IX
N.X / XI
Arachnoidea
N. IX
N. X / XI
N. XII
tumor
Bulbus sup. v. jug. inf.
Tuberculum jugulare
Condylus occipitalis
Condylus atlantis
schematic anatomical model
For. jugulare
(see Bulbus sup. v. jug. int.)
Porus acust. int.
Sulcus sigm.
N. IX
N. X / XI
(projection)
Tuberculum jugulare
Condylus occipitalis
Can. n XII
skull preparation

Fig. 143. Relationships of the intra- and extradural portions of the tumor, as assumed from both operations

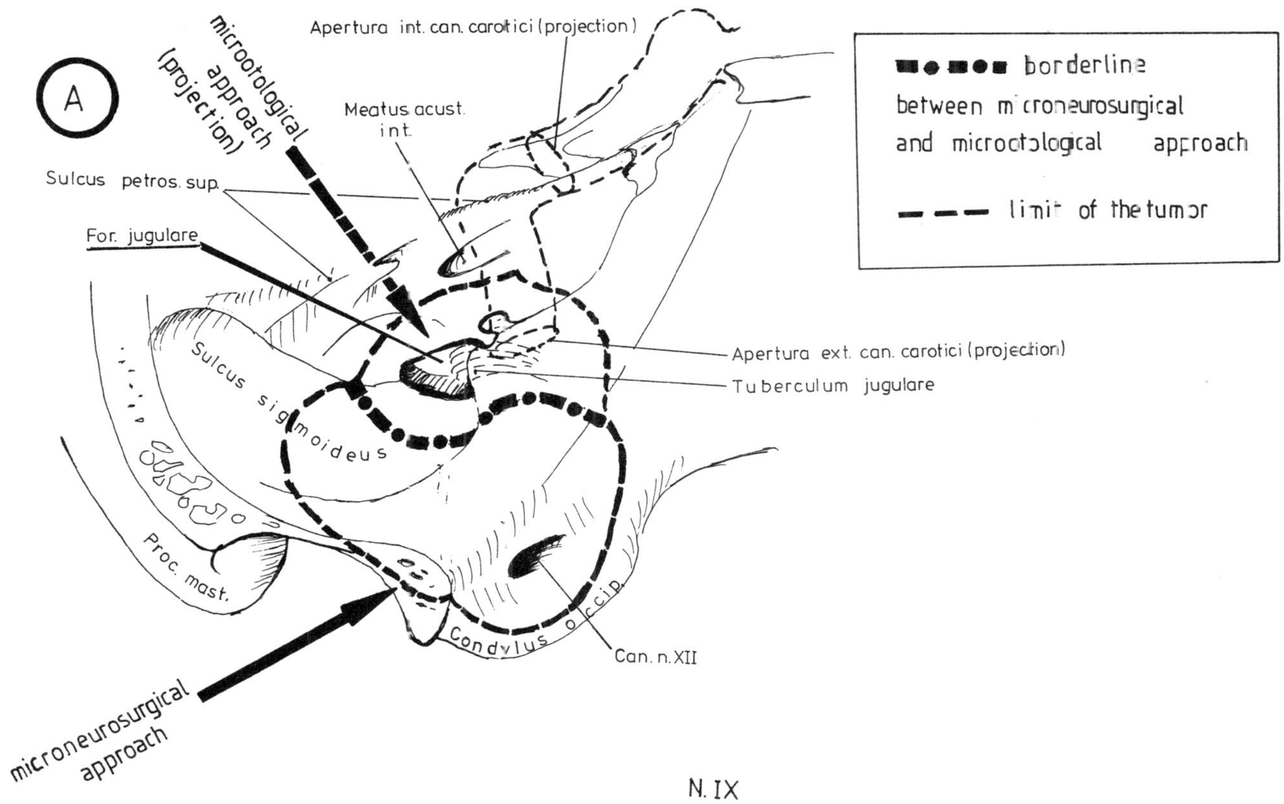
A
microotological approach (projection)
Apertura int. can. carotici (projection)
Meatus acust. int.
Sulcus petros. sup.
For. jugulare
Sulcus sigmoideus
Apertura ext. can. carotici (projection)
Tuberculum jugulare
Proc. mast.
Condylus occip.
Can. n. XII
microneurosurgical approach
borderline between microneurosurgical and microotological approach
limit of the tumor

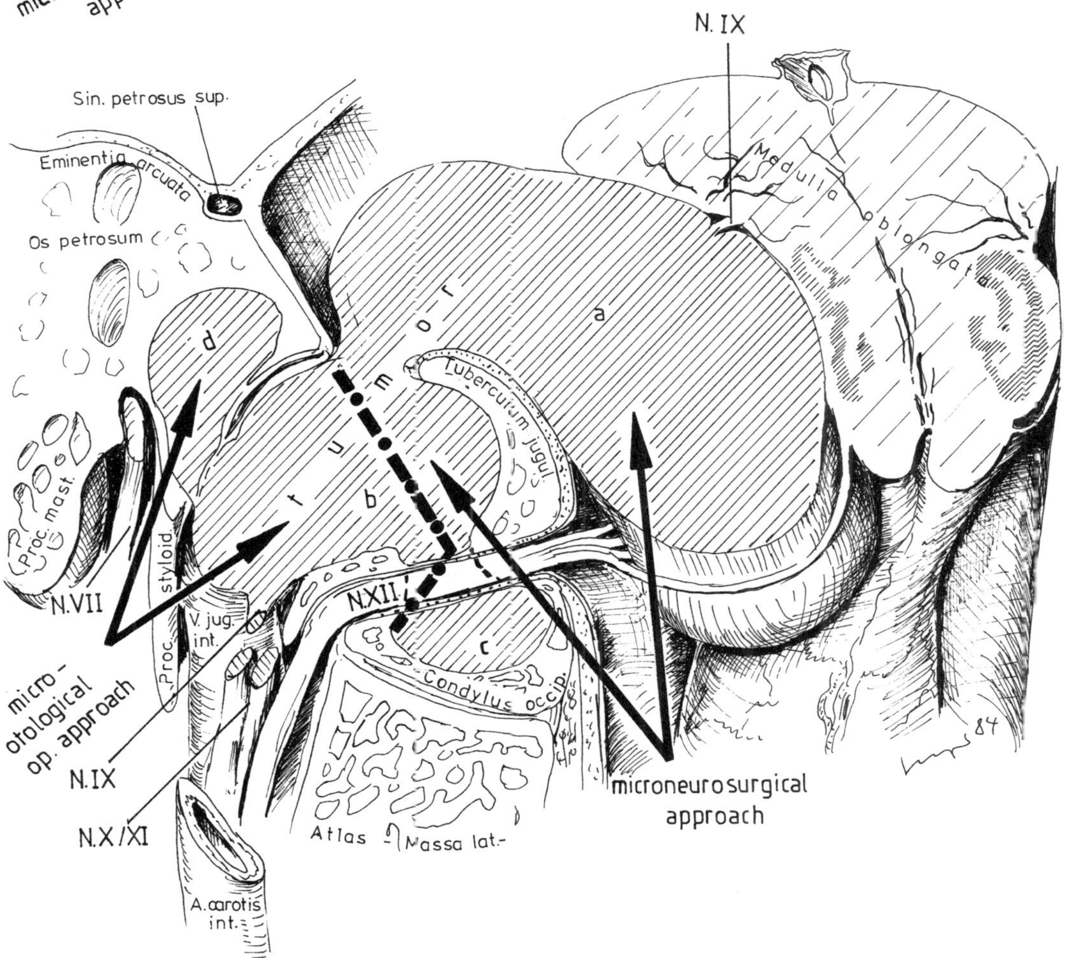
N. IX
Sin. petrosus sup.
Eminentia arcuata
Os petrosum
Medulla oblongata
d
a
tumor
Tuberculum jugul.
b
Proc. mast.
Proc. styloid.
N. VII
V. jug. int.
N XII
c
Condylus occip.
micro-otological op. approach
N. IX
N. X/XI
Atlas
Massa lat.
A. carotis int.
microneurosurgical approach

Fig. 144. Start of the neurosurgical intervention: extirpation of the portions of the tumor from the Condylus occipitalis with visualization of the extradural course of the XIIth nerve-Tuberculum jugulare-Condylus complex

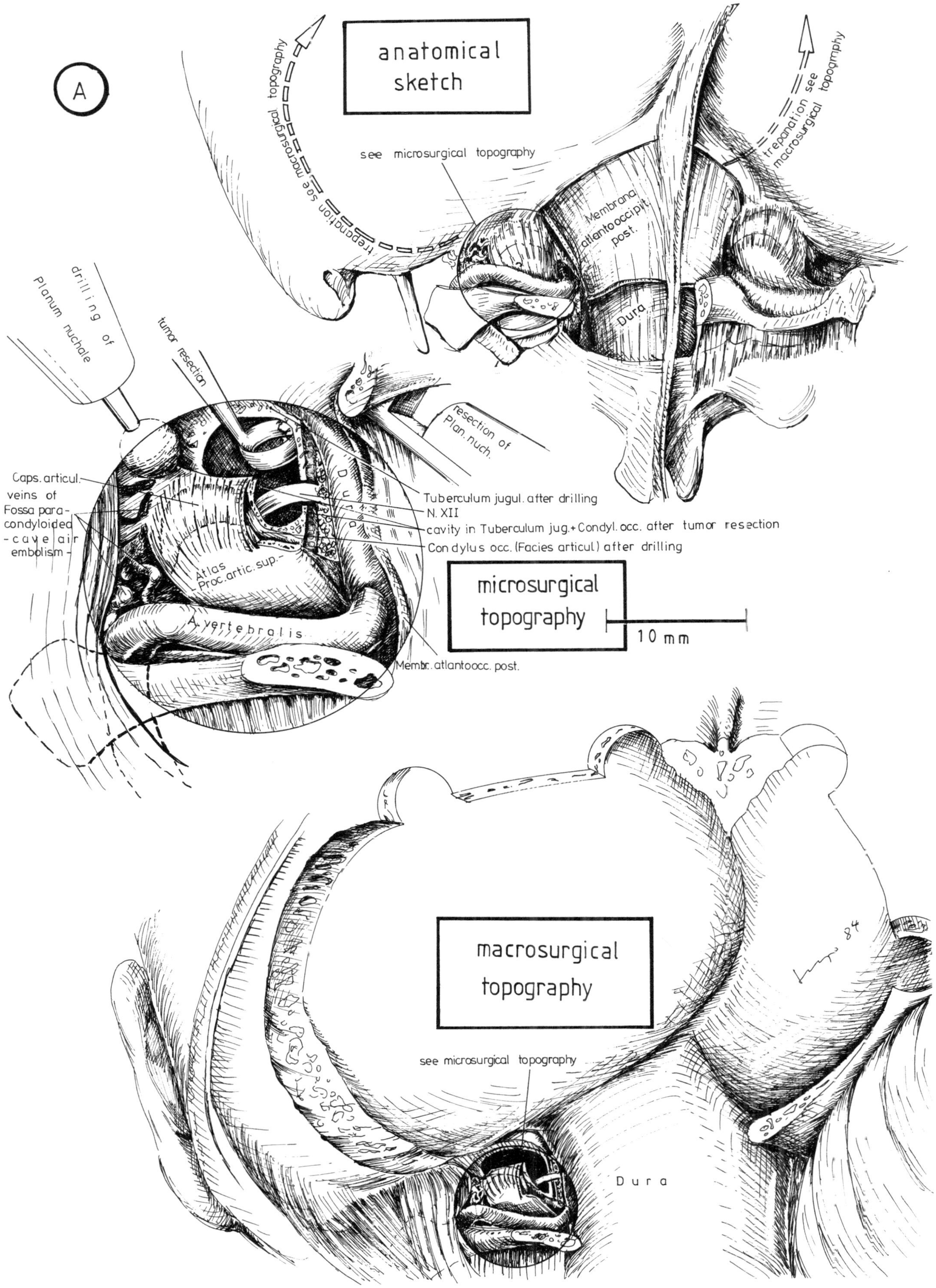
A
anatomical sketch
see macrosurgical topography
trepanation see macrosurgical topography
see microsurgical topography
Membrana atlantooccipit. post.
Dura
drilling of Planum nuchale
tumor resection
resection of Plan. nuch.
Caps. articul.
veins of Fossa paracondyloidea - cave air embolism -
Tuberculum jugul. after drilling
N. XII
cavity in Tuberculum jug.+ Condyl. occ. after tumor resection
Condylus occ. (Facies articul.) after drilling
Dura
Atlas Proc. artic. sup.
A. vertebralis
Membr. atlantoocc. post.
microsurgical topography
10 mm
macrosurgical topography
see microsurgical topography
Dura

Fig. 145. Opening of the Dura. Relationships among the cerebral nerves, vessels, and tumor. Caution while shrinking the tumor!

FIG. 145

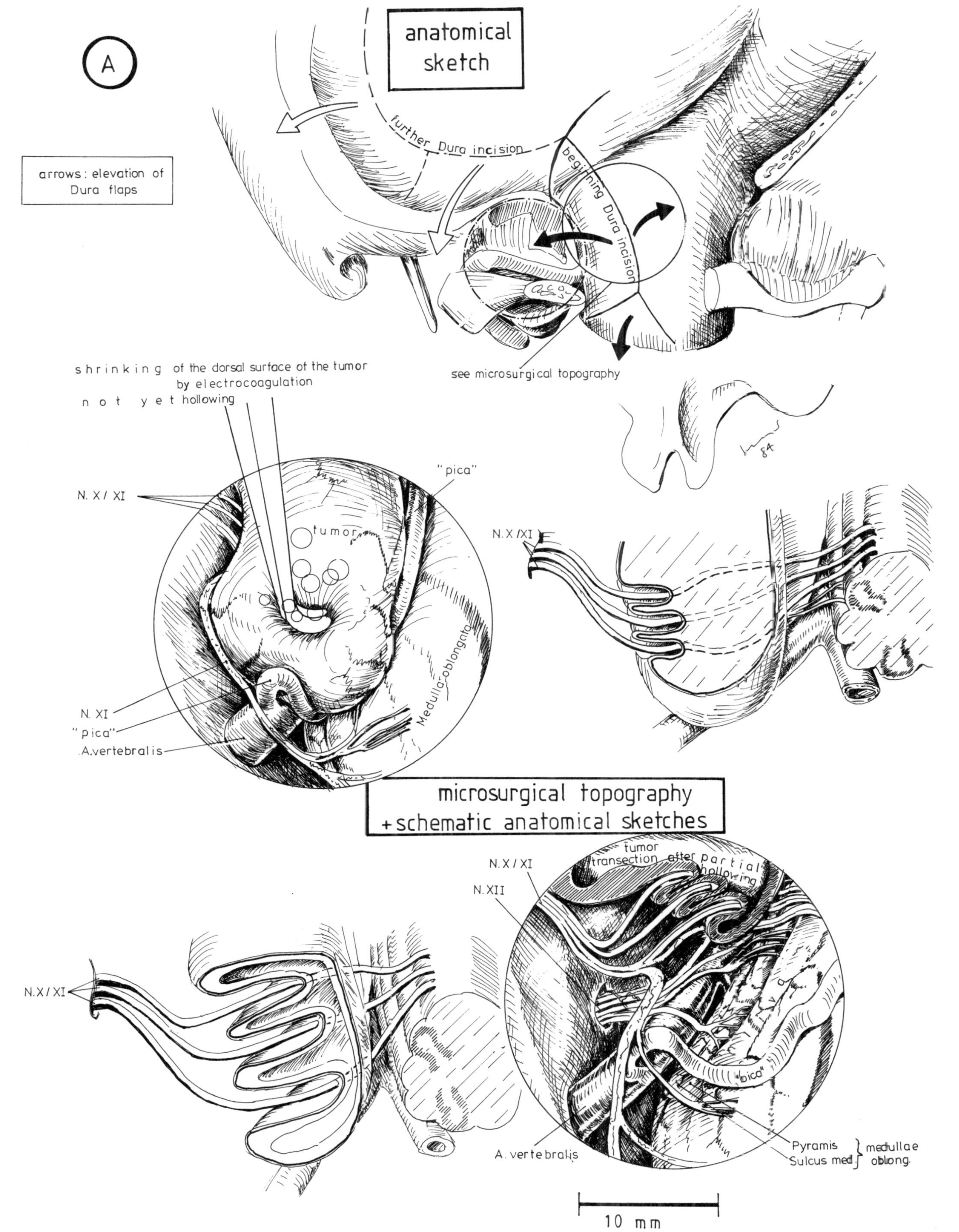
A
anatomical sketch
arrows: elevation of Dura flaps
further Dura incision
beginning Dura incision
shrinking of the dorsal surface of the tumor by electrocoagulation
not yet hollowing
see microsurgical topography
N. X / XI
"pica"
tumor
N. XI
"pica"
A.vertebralis
Medulla oblongata
N.X/XI
microsurgical topography
+schematic anatomical sketches
N.X/XI
N.XII
tumor transection after partial hollowing
"pica"
N.X/XI
A. vertebralis
Pyramis
Sulcus med
medullae oblong.
10 mm

Fig. 146. Start of the tumor preparation caudally at the level of the Medulla oblongata. Hollowing of the tumor in small steps. Between each step the cerebral nerves and vessels must be detached as far as possible from the tumor

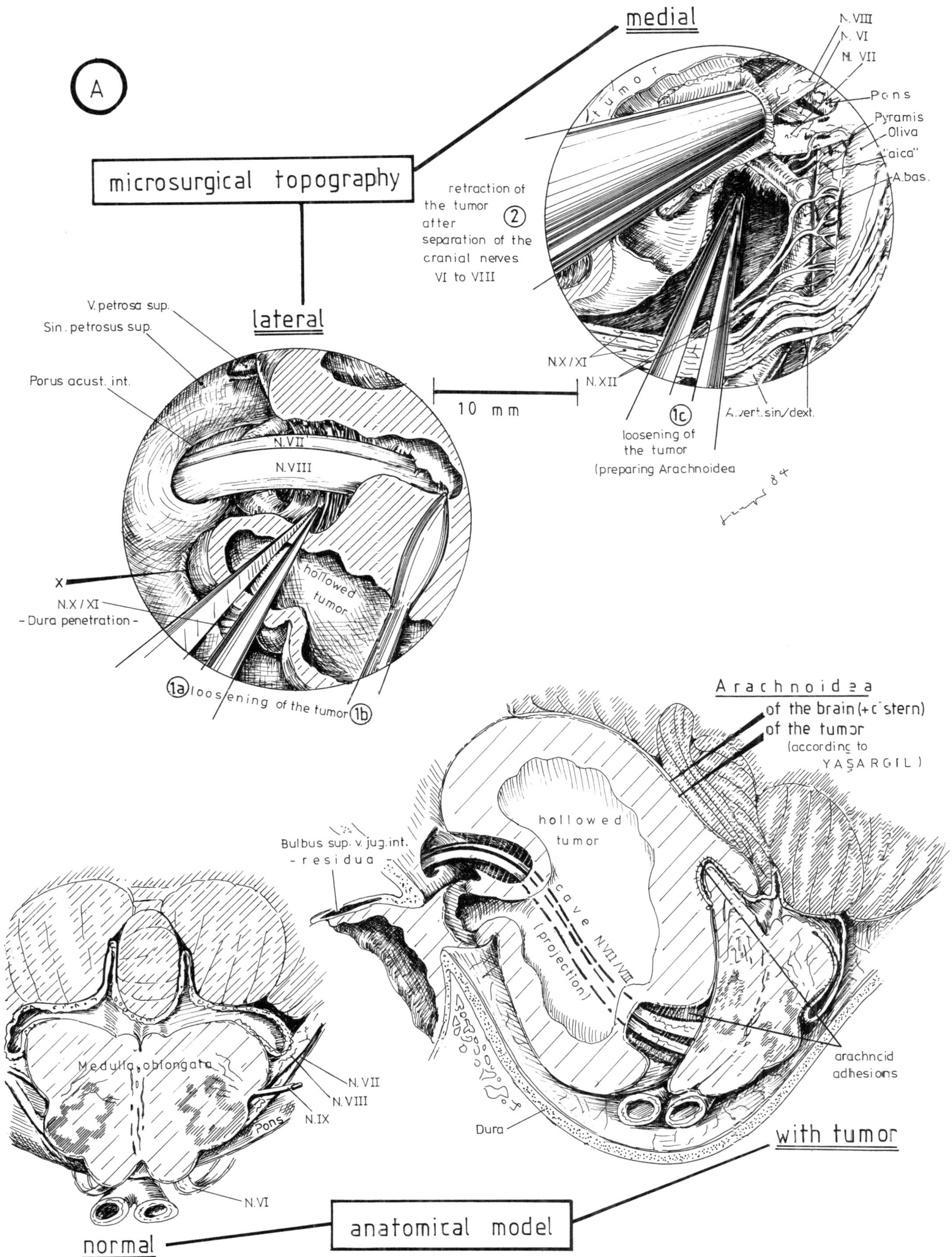

A
microsurgical topography
medial
lateral
N. VIII
N. VI
N. VII
Pons
Pyramis
Oliva
"aica"
A.bas.
tumor
retraction of the tumor after separation of the cranial nerves VI to VIII
2
N.X / XI
N.XII
1c
loosening of the tumor
(preparing Arachnoidea
A.vert.sin/dext.
10 mm
V. petrosa sup.
Sin. petrosus sup.
Porus acust. int.
N.VII
N.VIII
hollowed tumor
x
N.X / XI
- Dura penetration -
1a
loosening of the tumor
1b
Arachnoidea
of the brain (+cistern)
of the tumor
(according to YAŞARGIL)
hollowed tumor
cave N.VII/VIII (projection)
Bulbus sup. v. jug. int.
- residua
arachnoid adhesions
Dura
with tumor
Medulla oblongata
N. VII
N. VIII
N. IX
Pons
N. VI
normal
anatomical model

Fig. 147. Continuation of the preparation at the level of the Pons. The principles of the preparation are the same as close to the Medulla oblongata

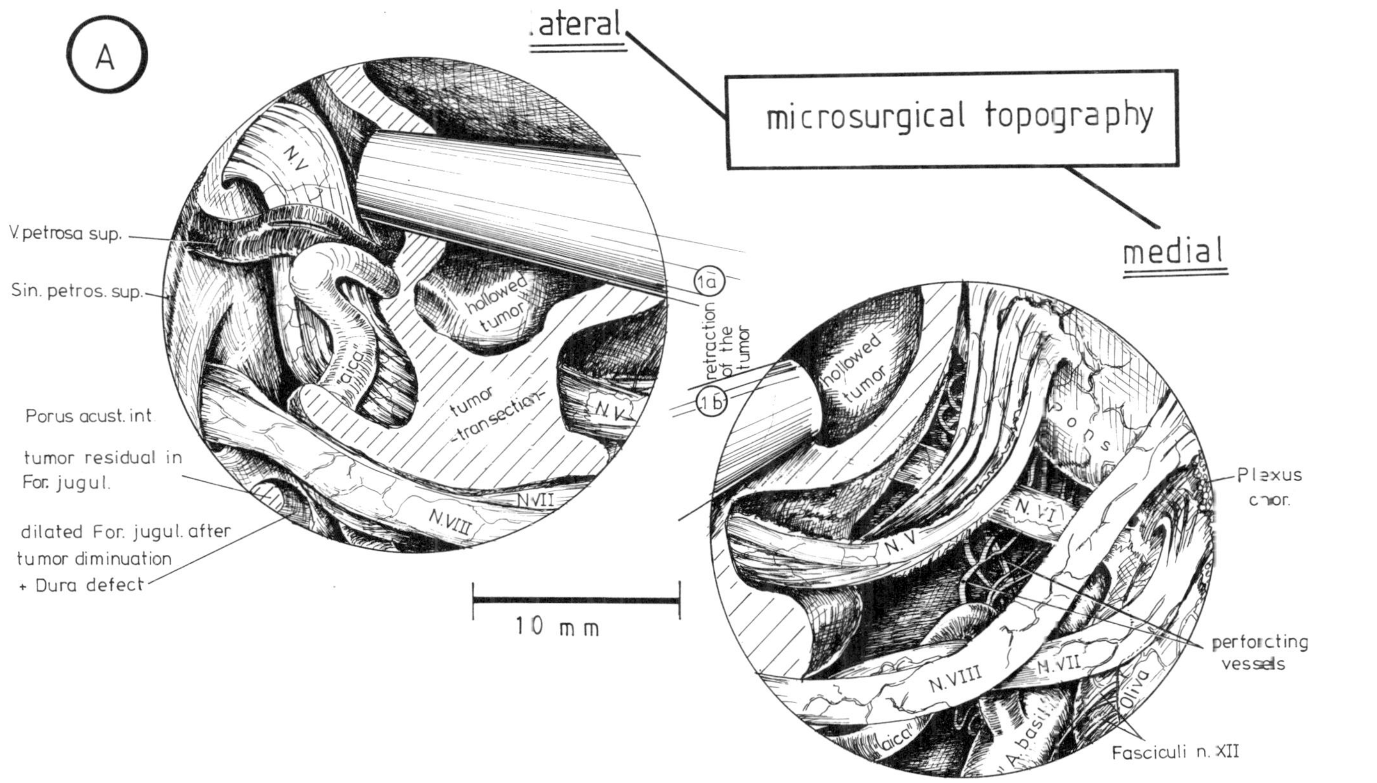
A
lateral
microsurgical topography
medial
V.petrosa sup.
Sin. petros. sup.
Porus acust. int
tumor residual in For. jugul.
dilated For. jugul. after tumor diminuation + Dura defect
N.V
"aica"
hollowed tumor
tumor -transection-
N.VII
N.VIII
1a
1b
retraction of the tumor
10 mm
Plexus chor.
perforcting vessels
Fasciculi n. XII
Oliva
A. basil.
N.VI

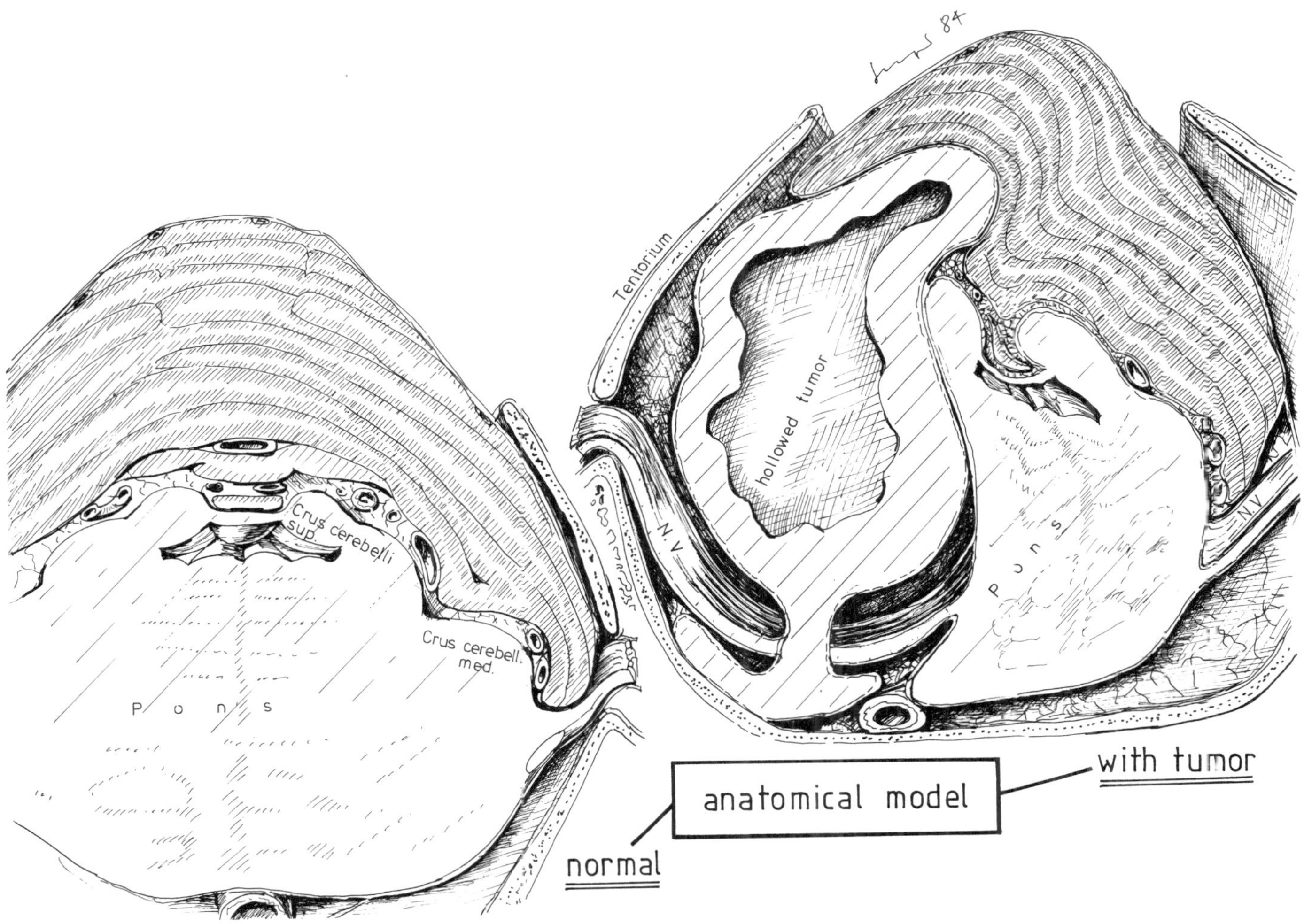
Tentorium
hollowed tumor
N.V
Pons
Crus cerebelli sup.
Crus cerebell. med.
anatomical model
normal
with tumor

Fig. 148. Preparation of the tumor at the level of the Mesencephalon. The principles are the same as at the level of the Pons and Medulla oblongata

FIG. 148

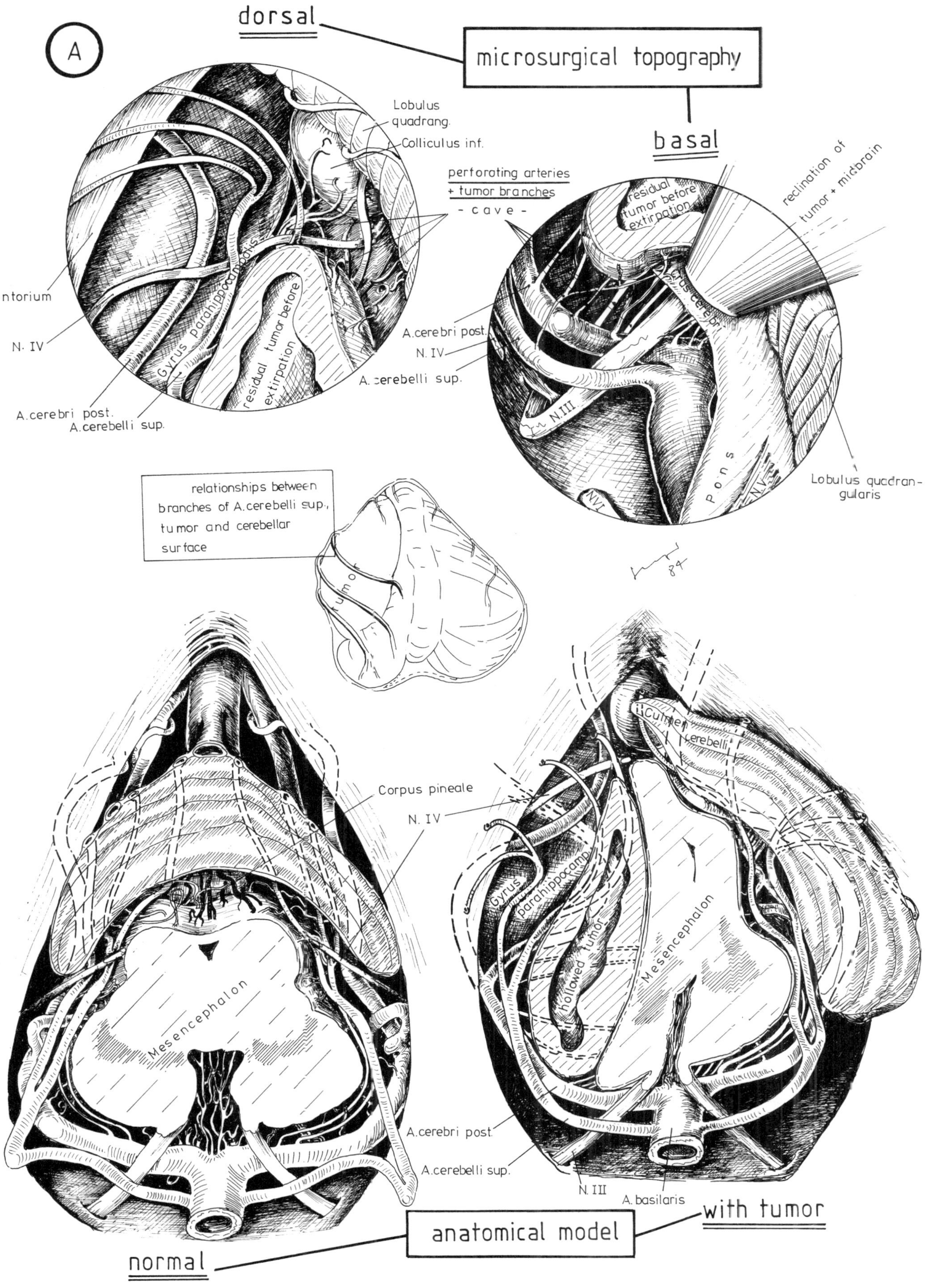
A
dorsal
microsurgical topography
basal
Lobulus quadrang.
Colliculus inf.
perforating arteries + tumor branches
- cave -
Tentorium
N. IV
Gyrus parahippocampalis
residual tumor before extirpation
A. cerebri post.
A. cerebelli sup.
reclination of tumor + midbrain
residual tumor before extirpation
Crus cerebri
A. cerebri post.
N. IV
A. cerebelli sup.
N. III
Pons
Lobulus quadrangularis
relationships between branches of A. cerebelli sup., tumor and cerebellar surface
Corpus pineale
N. IV
Mesencephalon
Culmen cerebelli
Gyrus parahippocamp.
hollowed tumor
A. cerebri post.
A. cerebelli sup.
N. III
A. basilaris
with tumor
anatomical model
normal

Fig. 149. Projection of the structures lying in the petrous portion of the temporal bone to the outer surface of the temporal bone. Labyrinth not taken into consideration, as it must not be preserved during the operation. Tube particularly important as a landmark

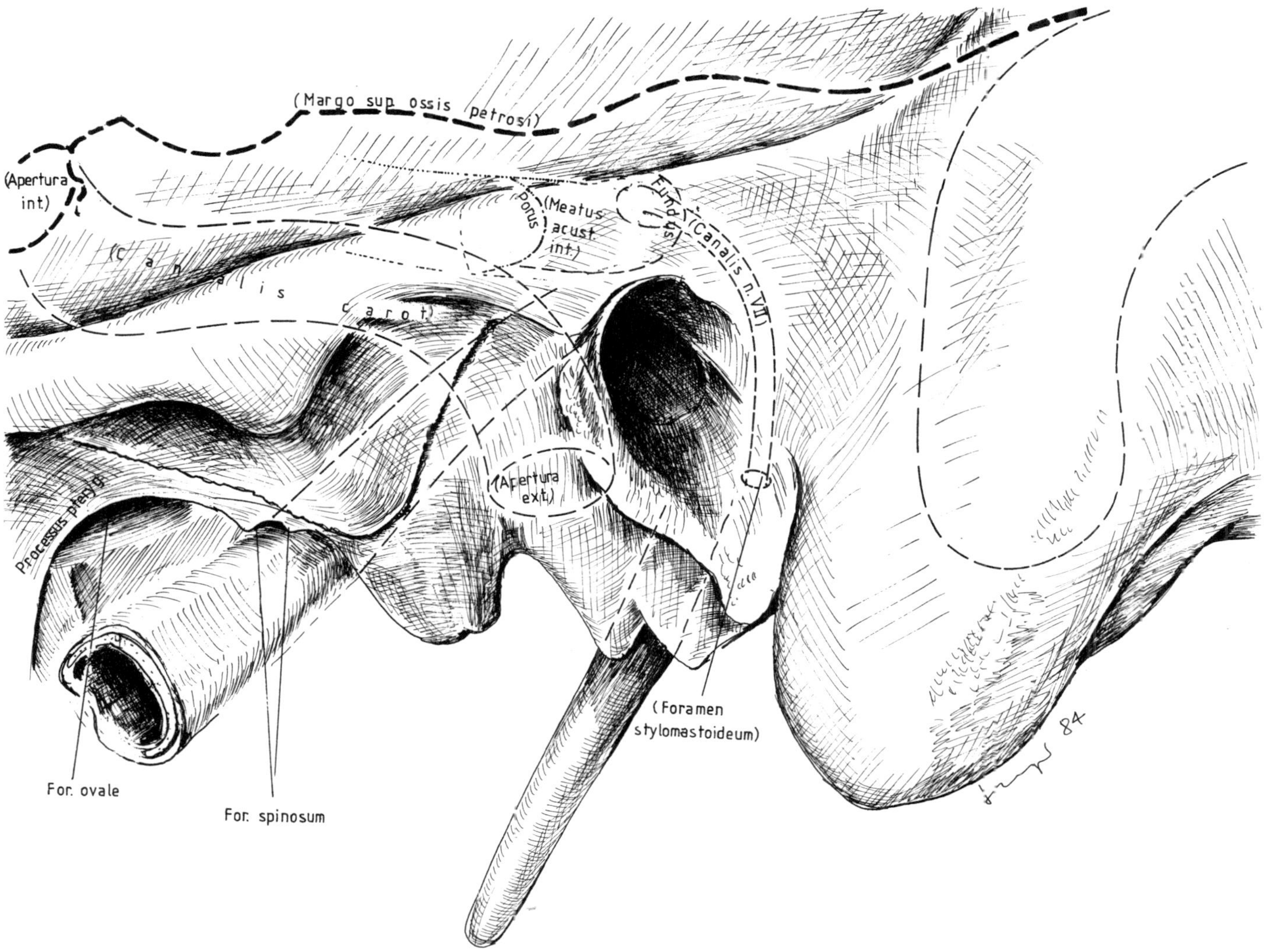

(Margo sup. ossis petrosi)
(Apertura int.)
(Canalis carot.)
Porus
(Meatus acust. int.)
Fundus
(Canalis n. VII)
(Apertura ext.)
Processus pterygo
(Foramen stylomastoideum)
For. ovale
For. spinosum
84

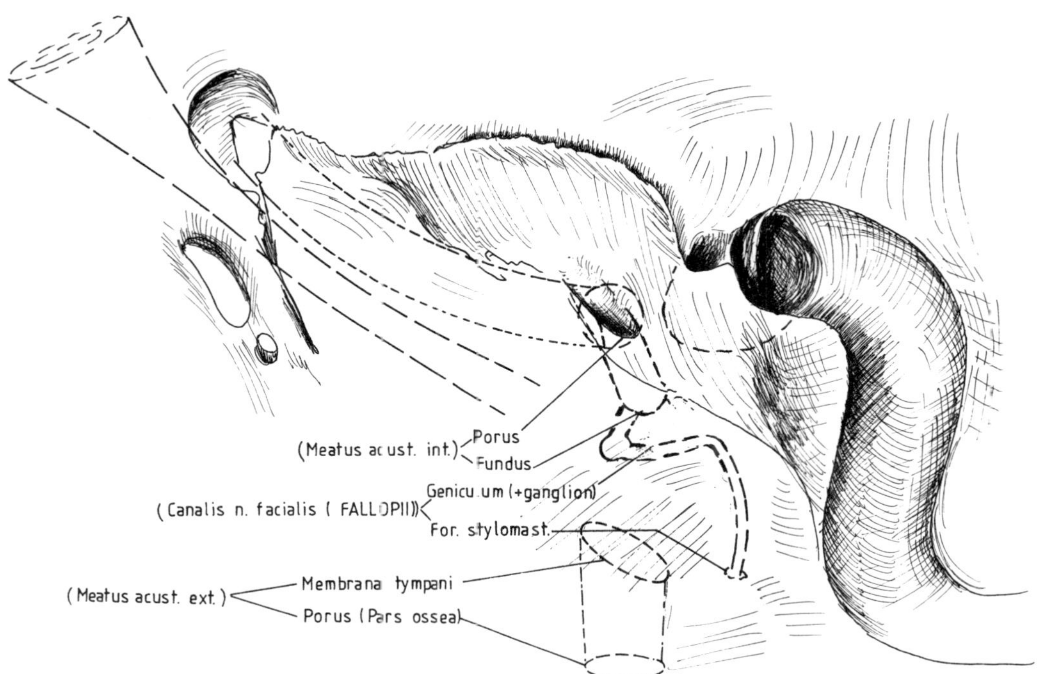

(Meatus acust. int.) Porus
Fundus
(Canalis n. facialis (FALLOPII)) Geniculum (+ganglion)
For. stylomast.
(Meatus acust. ext.) Membrana tympani
Porus (Pars ossea)

Fig. 150

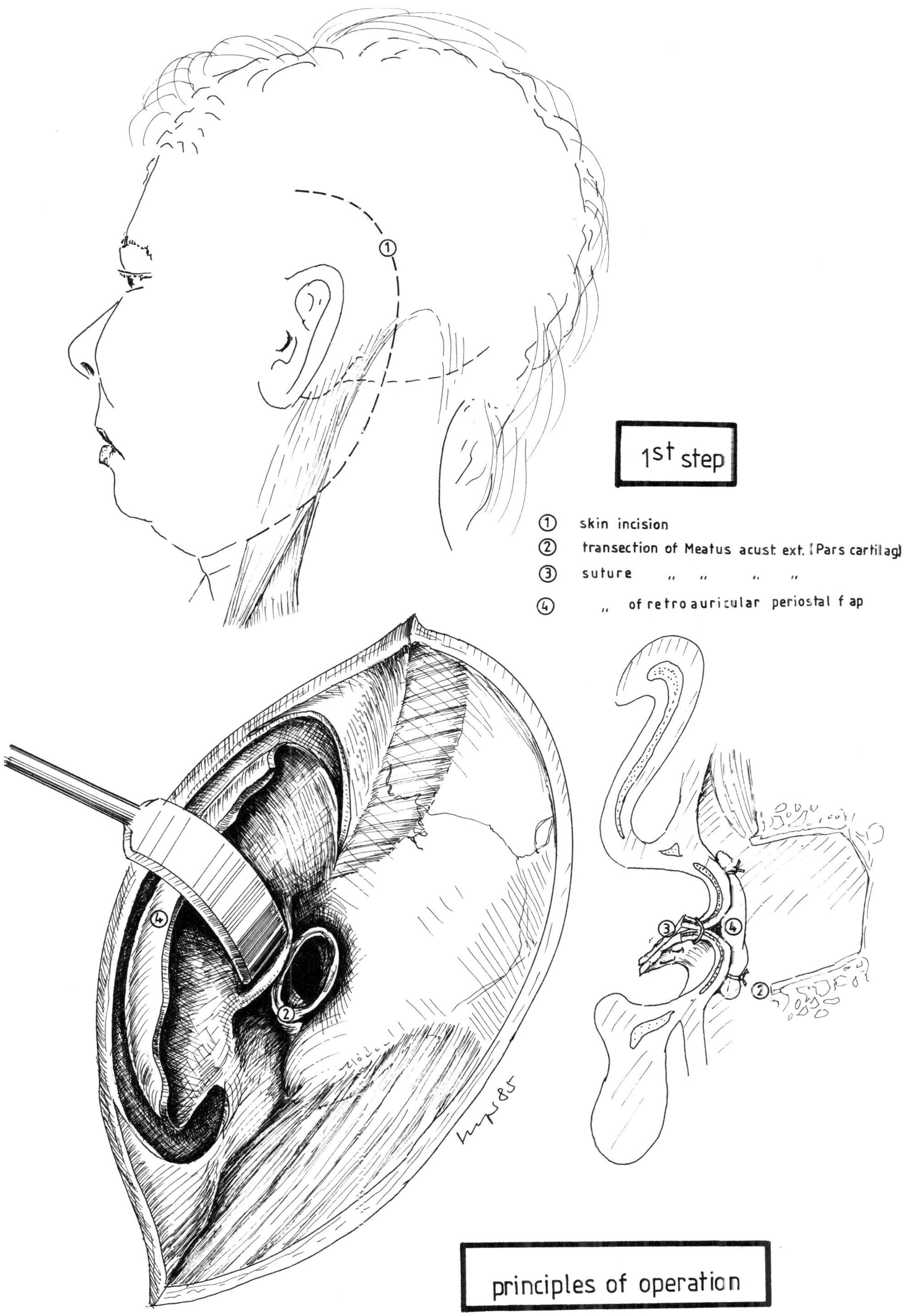
1st step
① skin incision
② transection of Meatus acust. ext. (Pars cartilag)
③ suture " " " "
④ " of retro auricular periostal f ap
principles of operation

Fig. 151

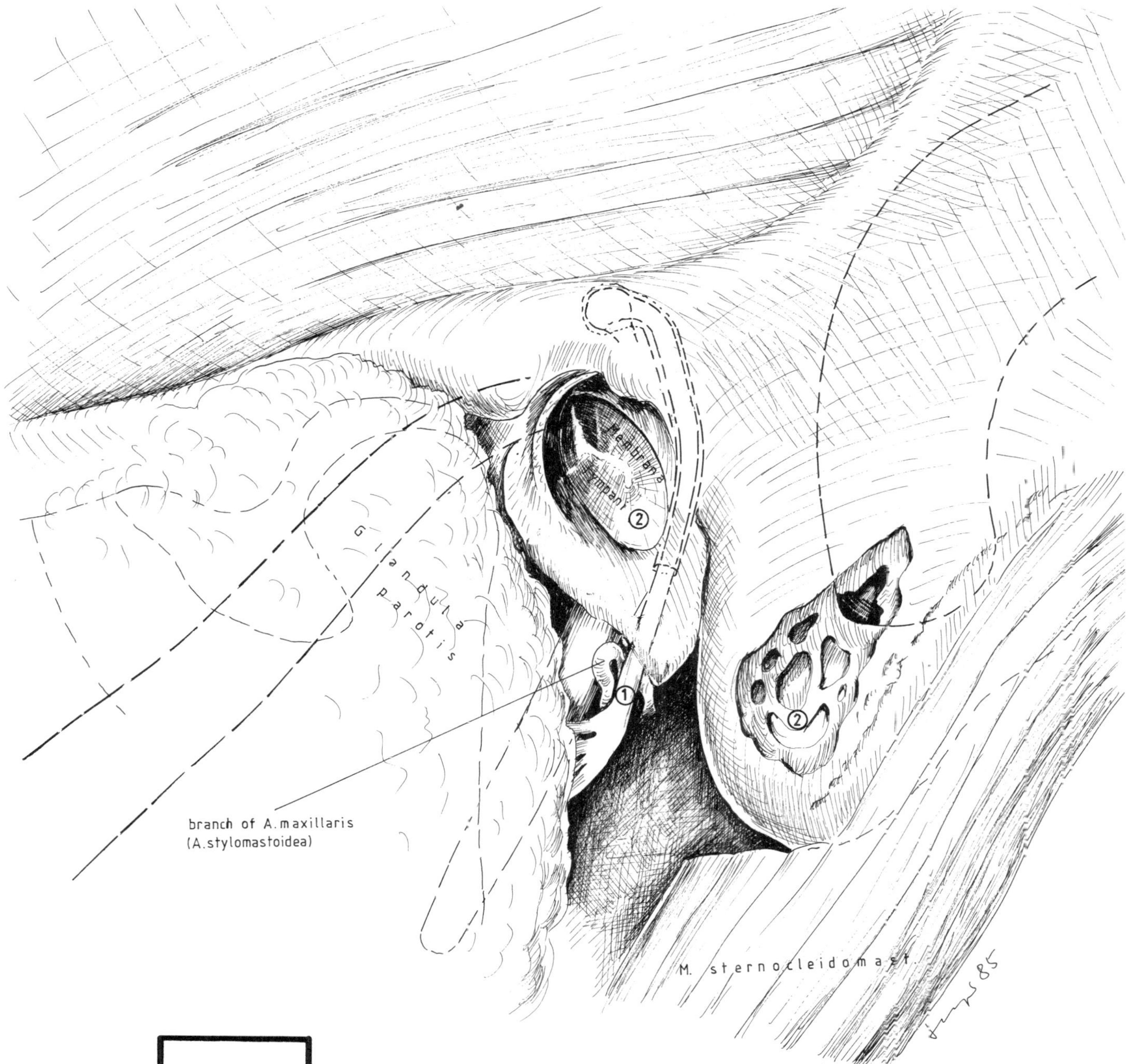

2nd step (after preparation of Glandula parotis)

① dissection of N.VII between For. stylomast. and trifurcation)

② drilling of mastoid (and removal of Membrana tympani + ossicles)

ad ① :
For. stylomastoideum
- lateral view -
overlapped by Pars tympanica of petrous bone

it becomes visible with changed position of microscope (view direction see arrow)

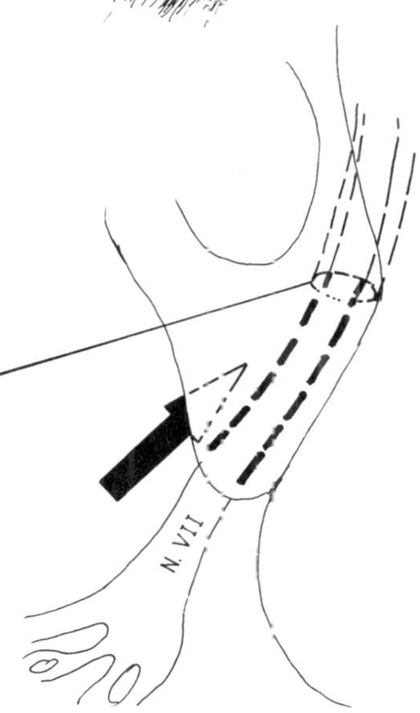

Fig. 152

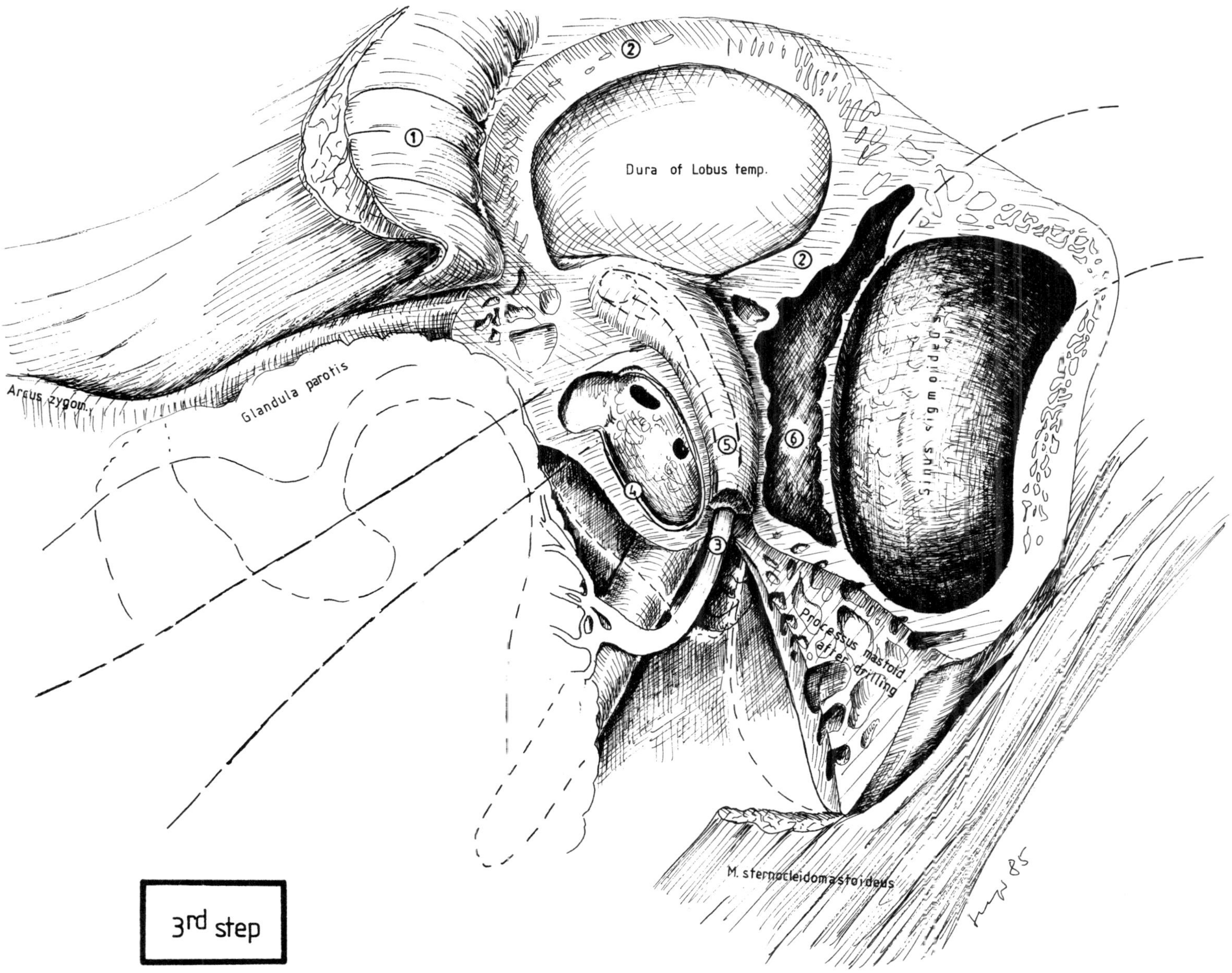

3rd step

① dissection of M. temporalis
② temporal trepanation

③ resection of Os tympanicum (wall of Meatus acust. ext.) between Porus and For. stylomastoideum
④ " " " " - remnants -
⑤ wall of Canalis n. VII - initially preserved -

⑥ revision of deeper mastoid cells

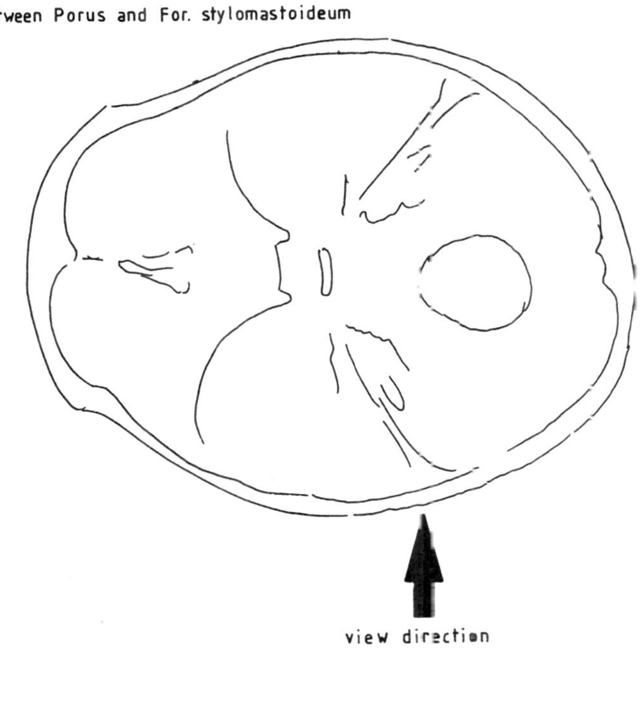

Fig. 153

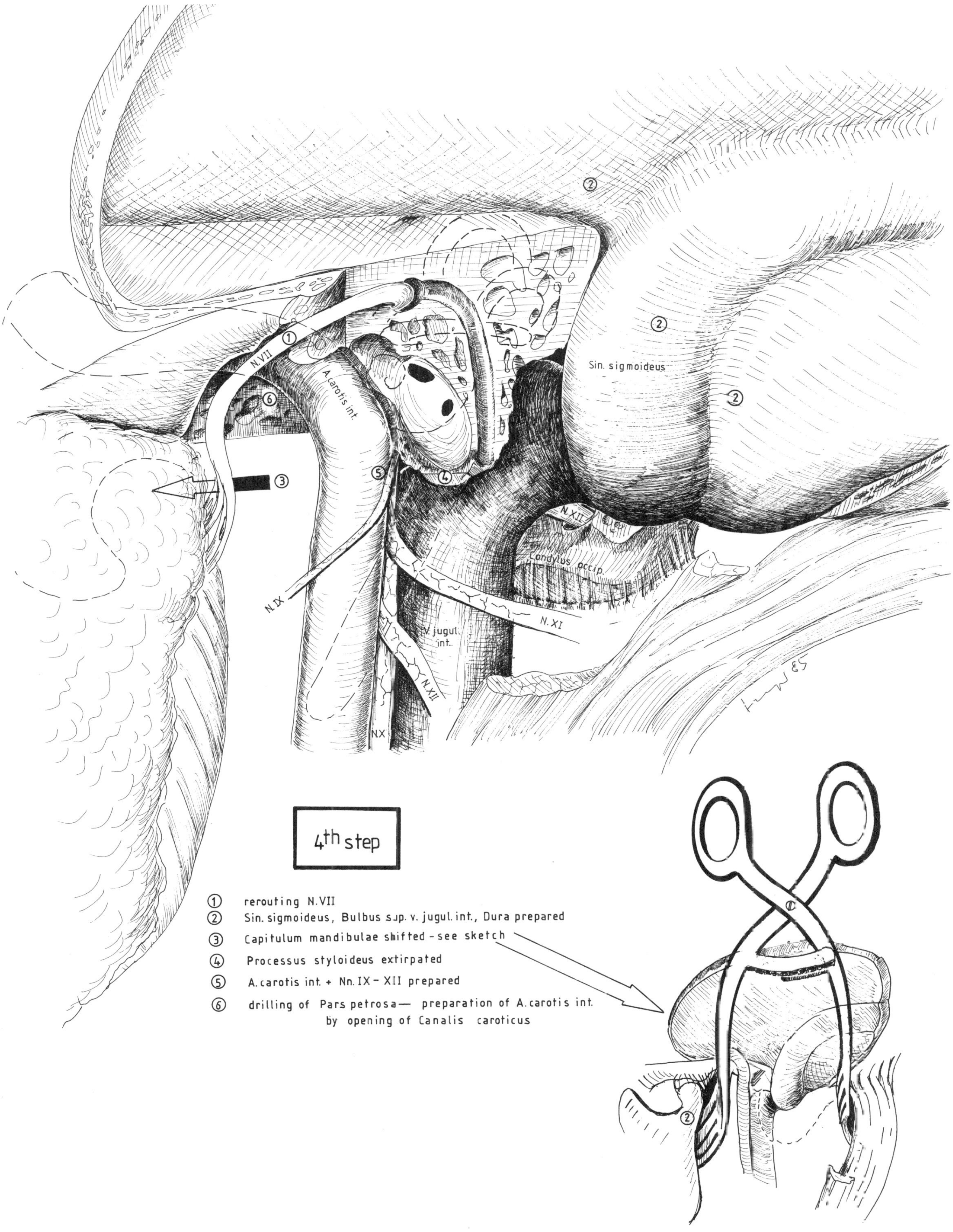

②
②
Sin. sigmoideus
②
①
N.VII
A.carotis int.
⑥
⑤
④
③
N.XII
Condylus occip.
N.IX
N.XI
V. jugul. int.
N.XII
N.X
4th step
① rerouting N.VII
② Sin. sigmoideus, Bulbus sup. v. jugul. int., Dura prepared
③ Capitulum mandibulae shifted - see sketch
④ Processus styloideus extirpated
⑤ A. carotis int. + Nn. IX - XII prepared
⑥ drilling of Pars petrosa— preparation of A. carotis int. by opening of Canalis caroticus
②

Fig. 154

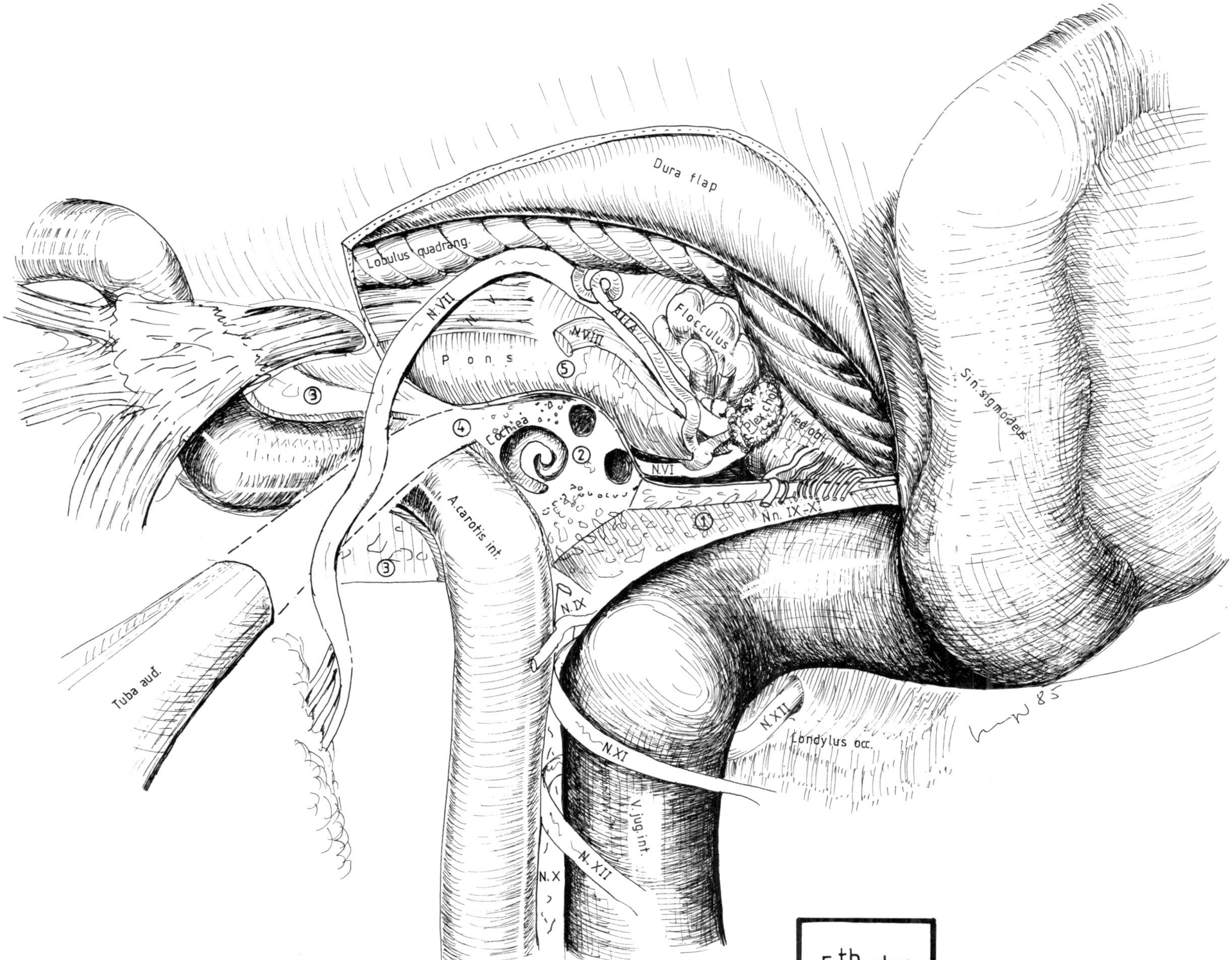

5th step

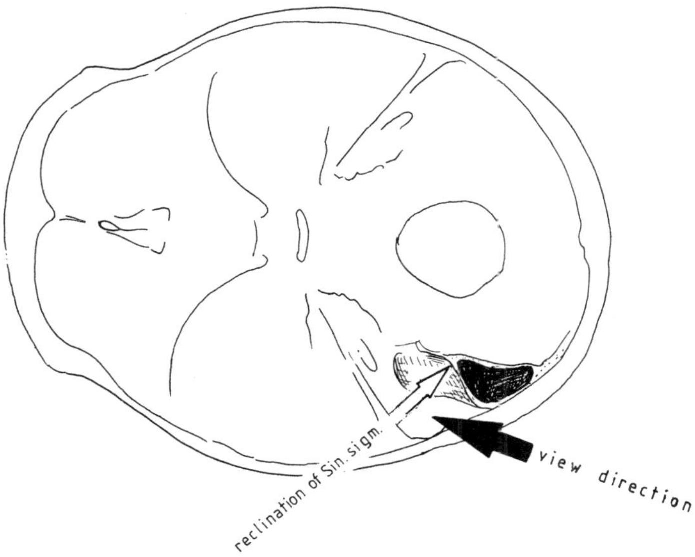

① drilling Tuberculum jugulare-Condylus occipitalis-complex

② drilling labyrinth-complex

③ opening of Can. caroticus

④ proximal resection of Tuba auditiva

⑤ opening of the dura (+ removal of intradural residual tumor from cerebellopontine angle)

Fig. 155

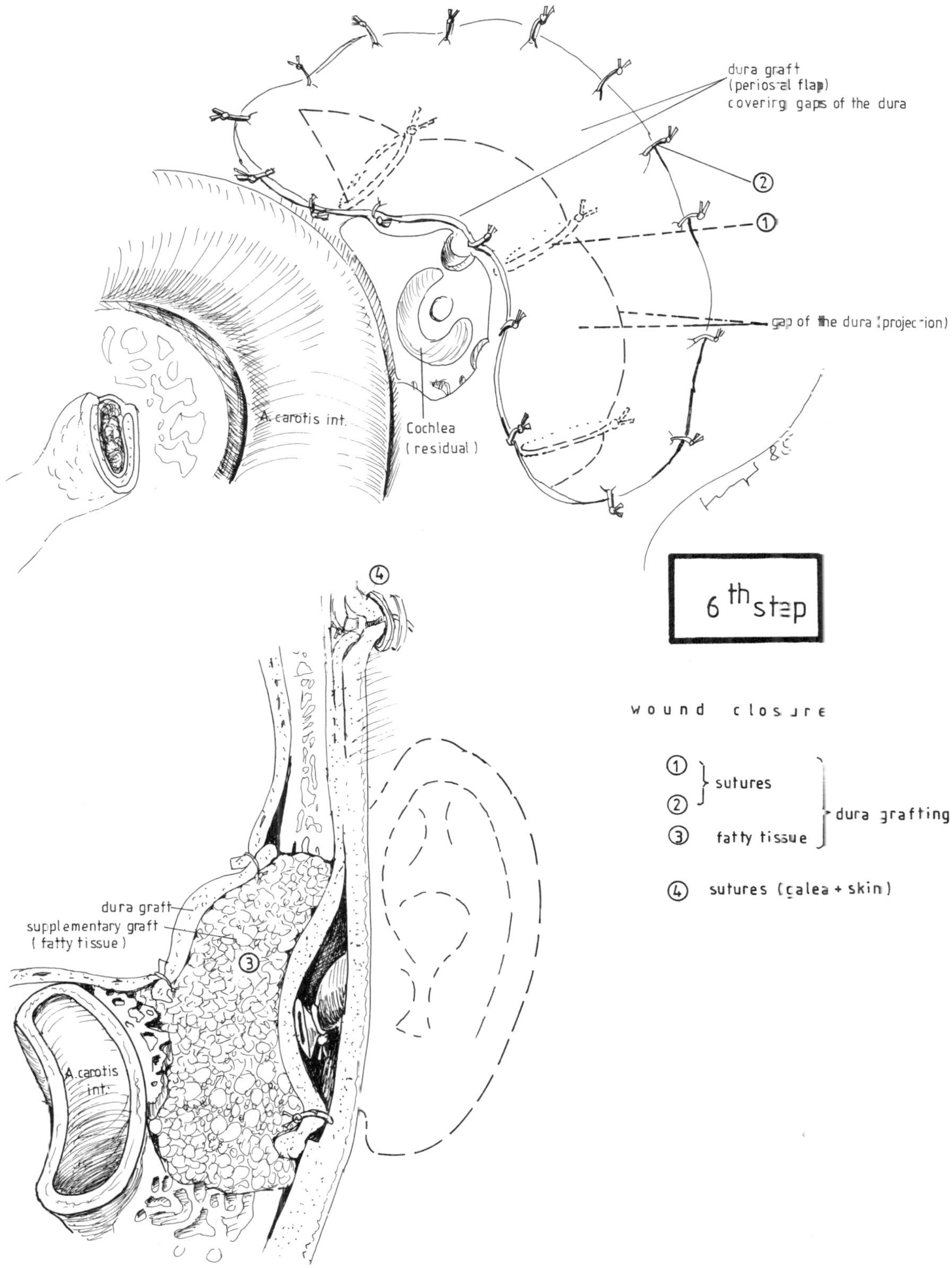
dura graft
(periostal flap)
covering gaps of the dura
②
①
gap of the dura (projection)
A. carotis int.
Cochlea
(residual)
④
6th step
wound closure
① } sutures
② }
③ fatty tissue
dura grafting
④ sutures (galea + skin)
dura graft
supplementary graft
(fatty tissue)
③
A. carotis
int.

Fig. 156. Three clinical examples*

B1: Meningioma of the cerebellopontine angle with infiltration of the petrous portion of the temporal bone and mastoid. Since five years noises in the left ear; since two years reduction in hearing; incomplete functional disturbances in the IXth and Xth left cerebral nerves. Postoperatively temporary horizontal gaze nystagmus more on the right, left corneal reflex expired, hypaesthesia in nerves V 1–3, left incomplete peripheral facial paresis, left anacusis, nerves IX to XI nonfunctional, light left hypoglossus paresis, unstable gait; pointing test competent, later improvement in deficits.

B2: Since 1976 operations in other clinics for a glomus tumor confirmed histologically. In 1982 ligation and resection of the internal jugular vein, superselective embolisation of the recurred glomus tumor, after which difficulties in swallowing and bleeding from the left ear. Now, preoperatively a light weakness of the glossopharyngeus on the left. Postoperatively a partial left peripheral facial paresis, a weak left corneal reflex, and glosso-pharyngeal paresis on the left.

C: Glomus tumor with a larger intradural part of the tumor in the cerebellopontine angle. Since 1976 worsening hearing on the left, 1977 first otosurgical operation, diagnosis histologically confirmed. Second and third operations 1979. Now preoperatively deaf on the left, incomplete non-function of nerves IX to XII. Postoperatively left facial paresis. One day after the operation secondary haemorrhage removed, after which additional hypaesthesia of the left side of the face and left abducens paresis, slight left hemiparesis which improved rapidly. Postoperative apathy, at first persistent, after introduction of shunt for hydrocephalus aresorptivus (January 29, 1985) rapid improvement with swallowing again possible.

In all cases a total petrosectomy with removal of tumorous parts adjacent to the petrous portion of the temporal bone was performed. In case **C** the large intradural part of the tumor was also removed translabyrinthally

---

* All operations were performed alternately by Prof. Dr. W. Mann (Ear, Nose and Throat Clinic of Freiburg University, Director: Prof. Dr. Chl. Beck) and Prof. Dr. J. Gilsbach, coworker of the author.

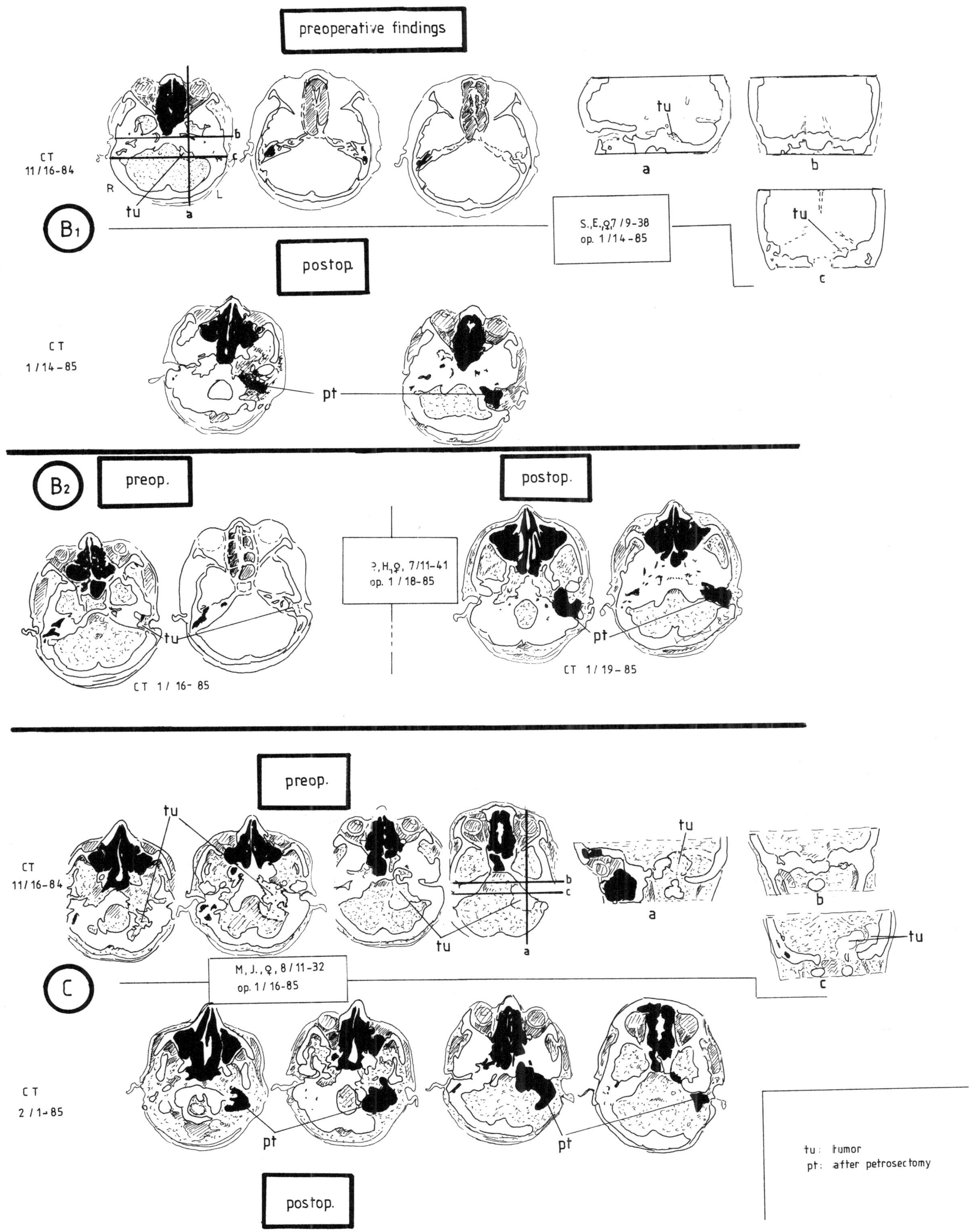
preoperative findings
CT
11/16-84
R
L
tu
a
b
c
B1
S.,E.,♀,7/9-38
op. 1/14-85
postop.
CT
1/14-85
pt
B2
preop.
postop.
op. 1/18-85
tu
CT 1/16-85
pt
CT 1/19-85
preop.
CT
11/16-84
tu
a
b
c
C
M, J., ♀, 8/11-32
op. 1/16-85
CT
2/1-85
pt
postop.
tu: tumor
pt: after petrosectomy

Fig. 157. The angiograms show the marked vascularization in the area of the petrous portion of the temporal bone affected by the tumor in all three cases

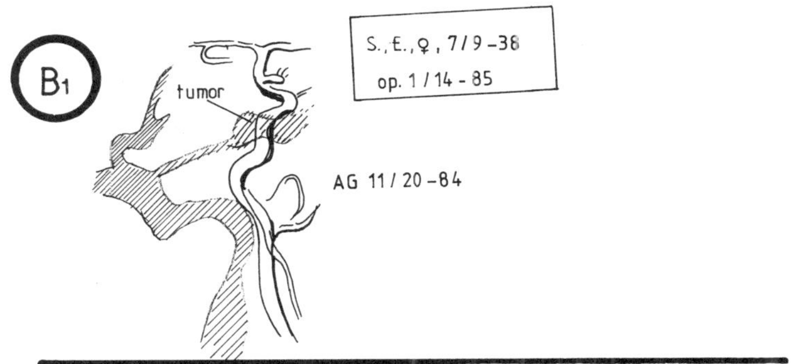

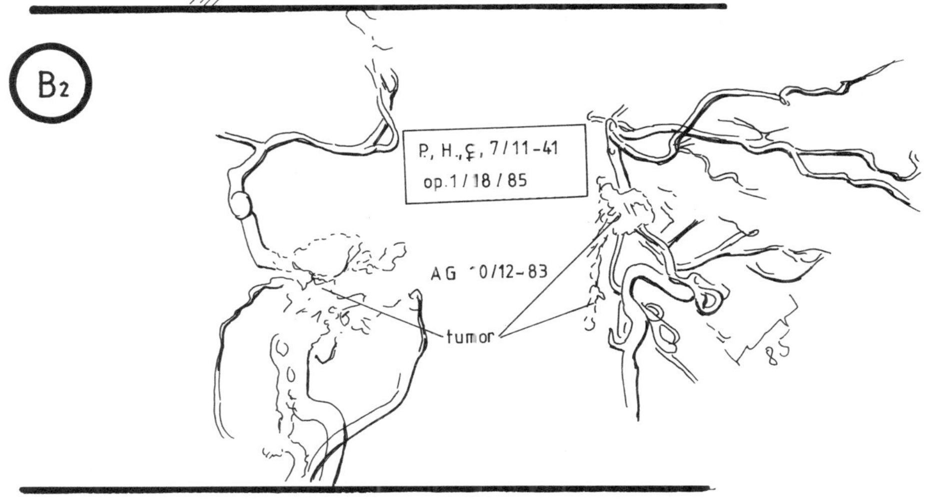

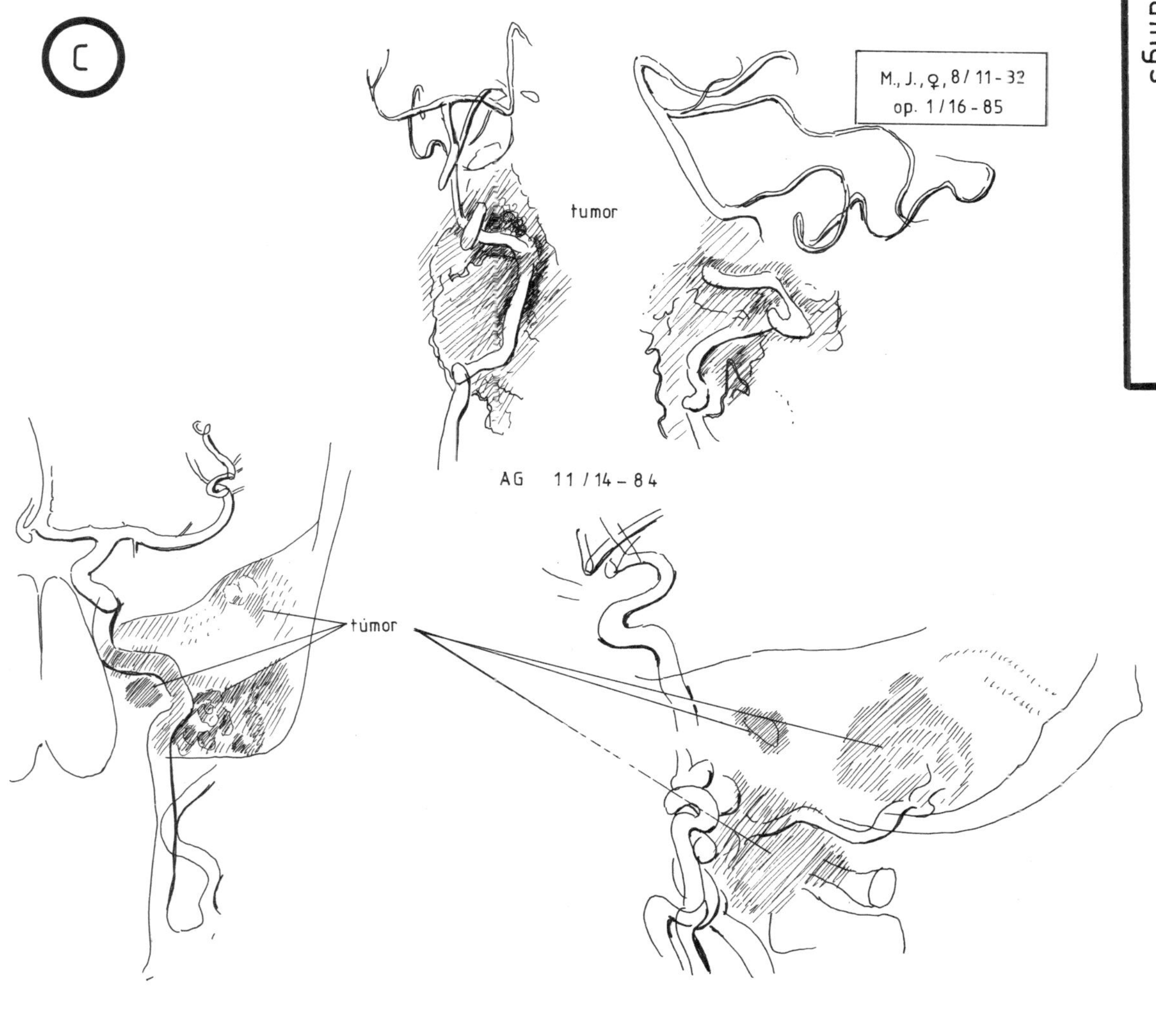

preoperative findings

Fig. 158. Copies of two photos* during operation of case **B1.** The facial nerve is freed from the Canalis Fallopii and displaced forward. The medial wall of the middle ear is intact. Landmarks: Foramen ovale and Foramen rotundum. The tube can be sounded (arrow)

---

* Photos taken by Prof. Dr. W. Mann.

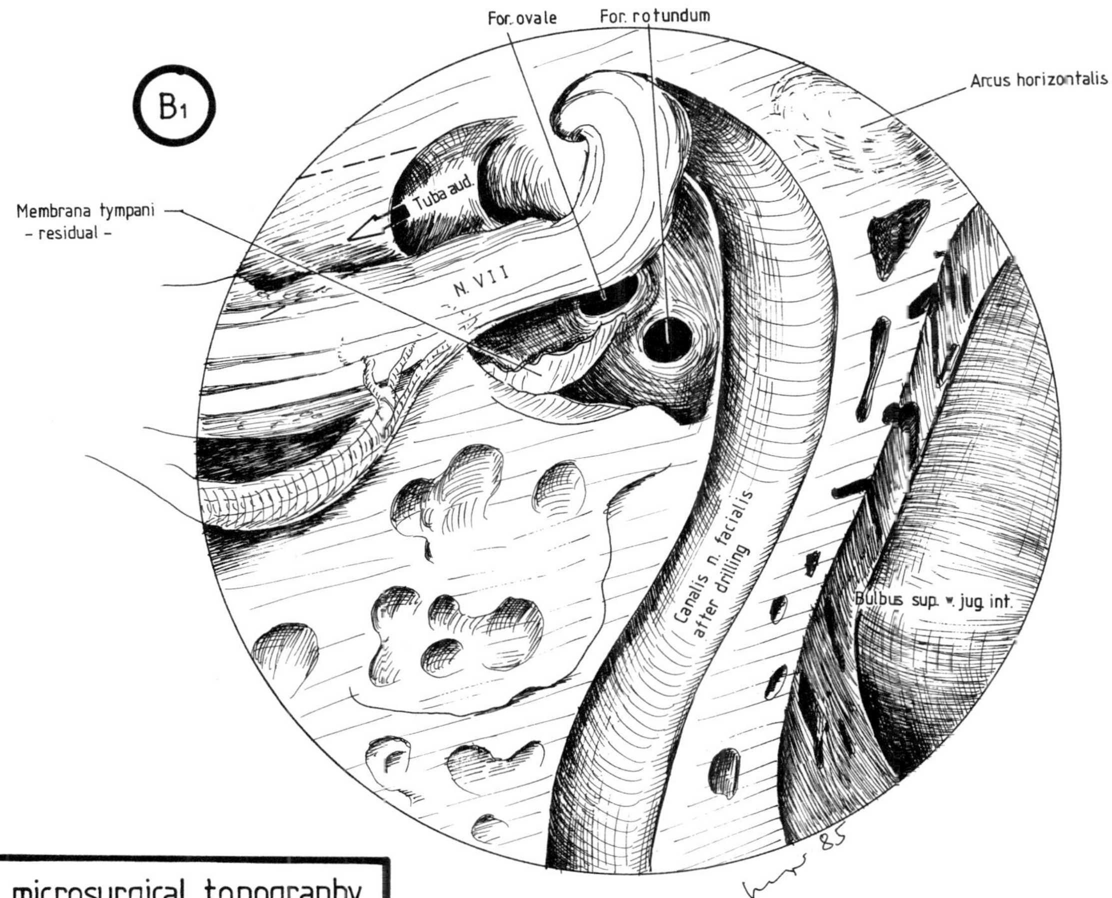

microsurgical topography

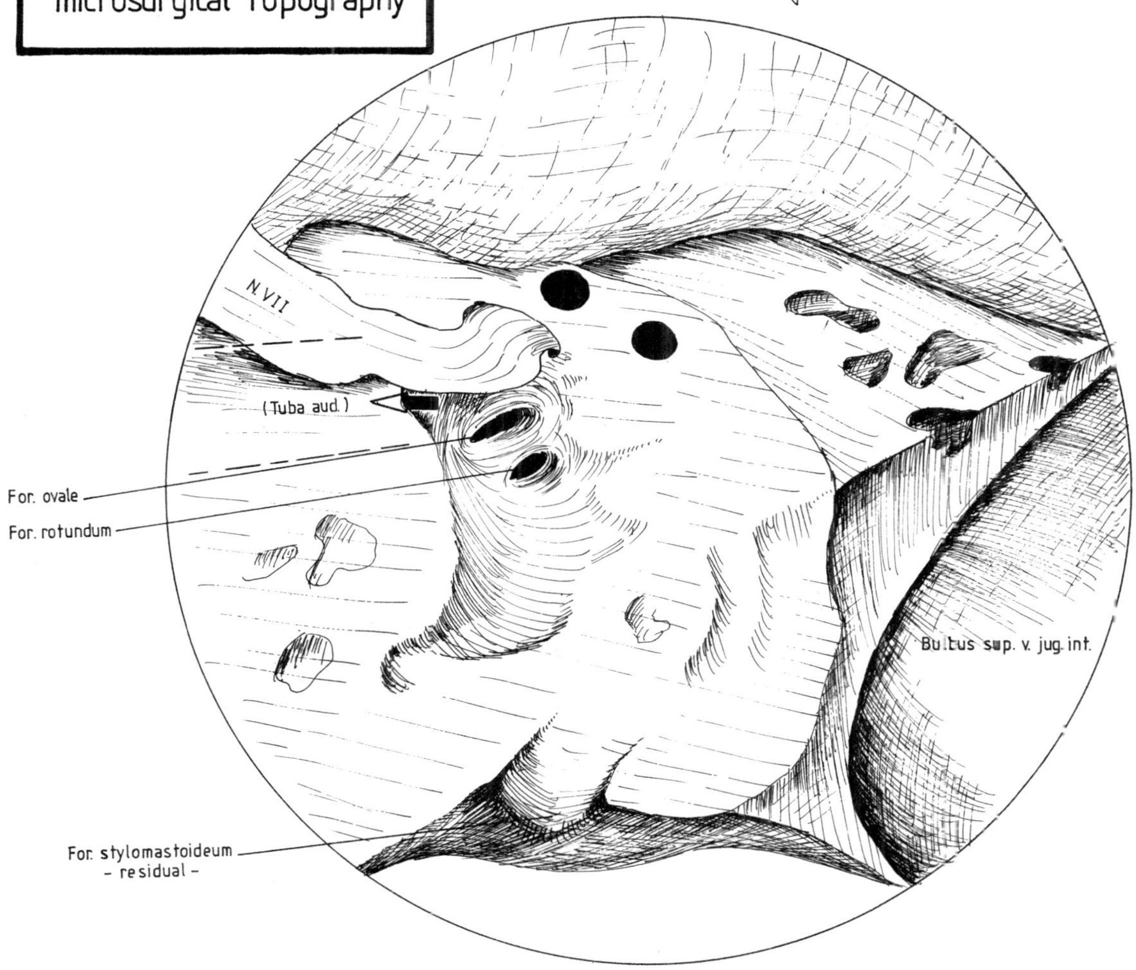

Fig. 159. Copies of microsurgical photos* from case **B1**

---

* Photos taken by Prof. Dr. W. Mann.

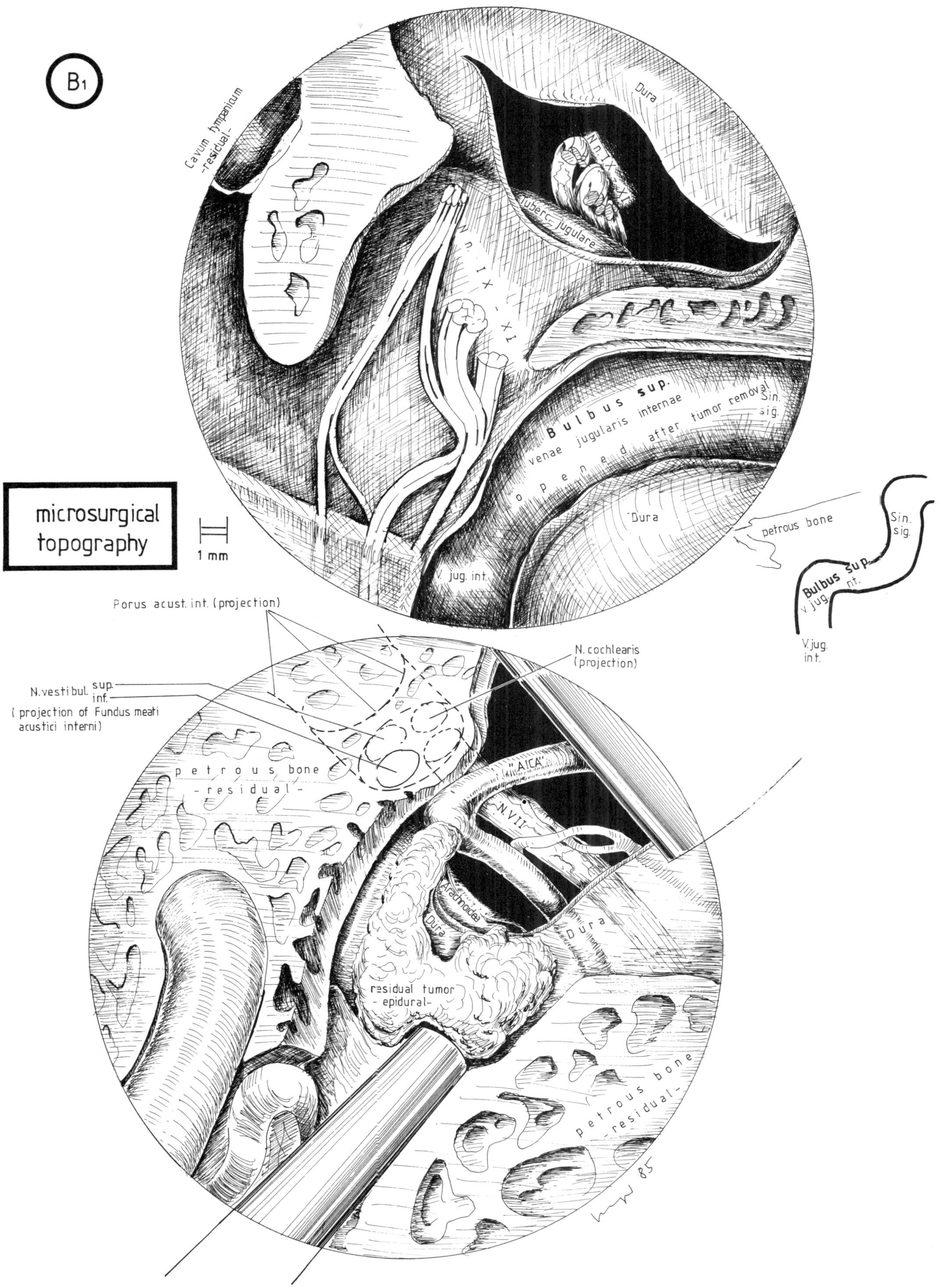
B1
Cavum tympanicum
-residual-
Dura
Nn. X - XI
Tuberc. jugulare
N. IX - XI
Bulbus sup.
venae jugularis internae
opened after tumor removal
Sin. sig.
Dura
V. jug. int.
microsurgical
topography
1 mm
petrous bone
Sin. sig.
Bulbus sup.
V. jug. int.
V. jug. int.
Porus acust. int. (projection)
N. cochlearis
(projection)
N. vestibul. sup.
inf.
(projection of Fundus meati
acustici interni)
petrous bone
-residual-
"AICA"
N. VII
Arachnoidea
Dura
Dura
residual tumor
- epidural-
petrous bone
-residual-

Fig. 160. Copies of microsurgical photos from cases **B2** and **C** *

* Photos taken by Prof. Dr. W. Mann.

B2

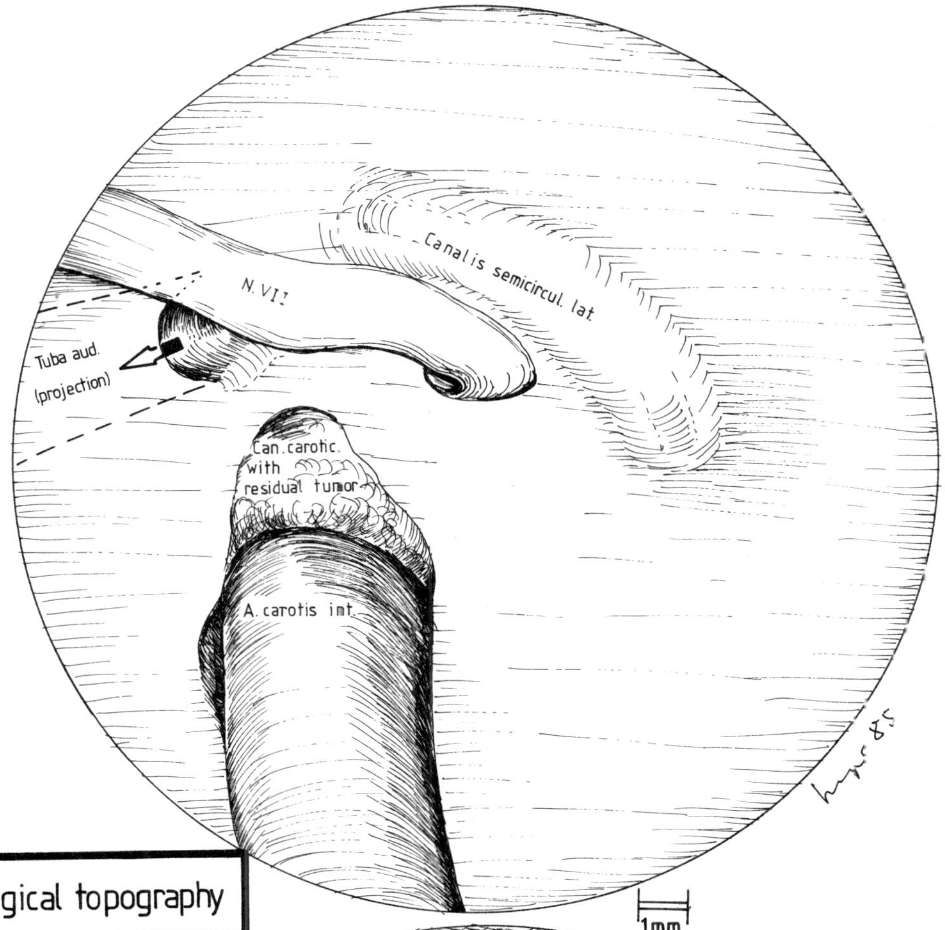

microsurgical topography

C

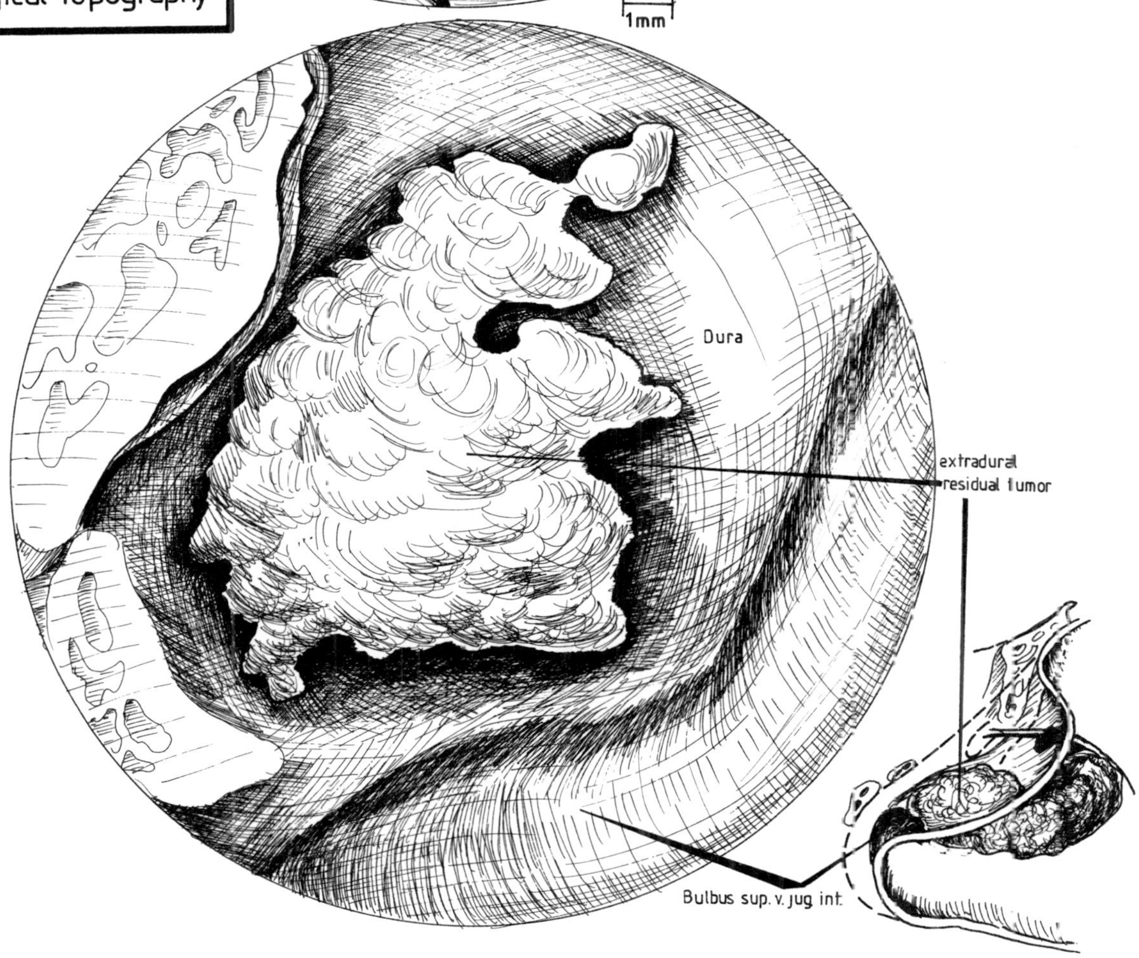

Chapter 7
Basal Cisterns, Anterior Segment
(Figs. 161 to 176)

Fig. 161. Fronto-basal tumors with infiltrations of the nasoethmoidal area

(A) transdural–transfacial combined approach

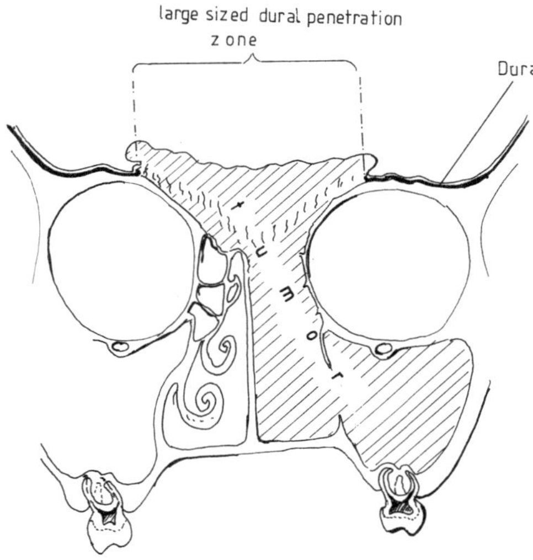

favorable
- no bone defect in the midface
- no uncontrolled bleeding ⟶ CSF-space
- no liquor fistula after grafting dura defect
- branches of A. facialis + Vasa infraorbitalia + N. V_{1-3} preserved
- cosmetic result (skin incision frontoparietal; wall of Sin. max. - Os zyg. + Os maxill. - Os nasale preserved

unfavorable
- risk of infection

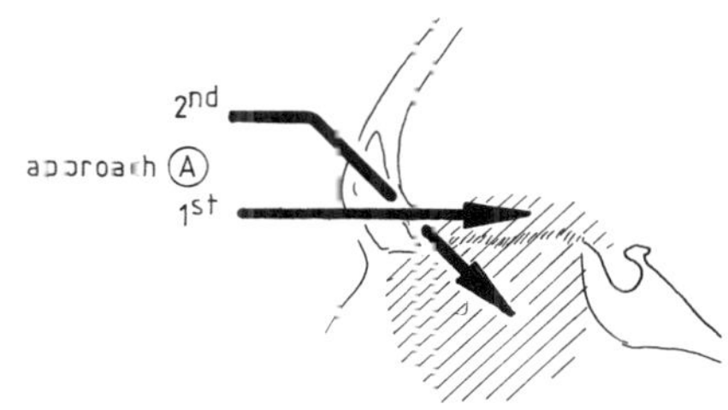

(B) transfacial–transdural combined approach

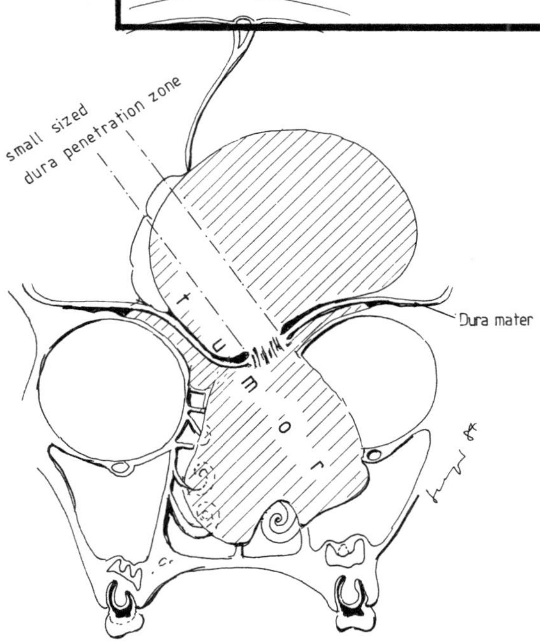

favorable
- improved approach to intradural tumor portion from below after removal of extradural (epidural + intranasal - intraorbital) tumor portions
- no liquor fistula after grafting dura defect
- branches of A. facialis + Vasa infraorbitalia + N. V_{1-3} preserved
- cosmetic result (see (A))

unfavorable
- uncontrolled bleeding ⟶ CSF-space possible
- risk of infection

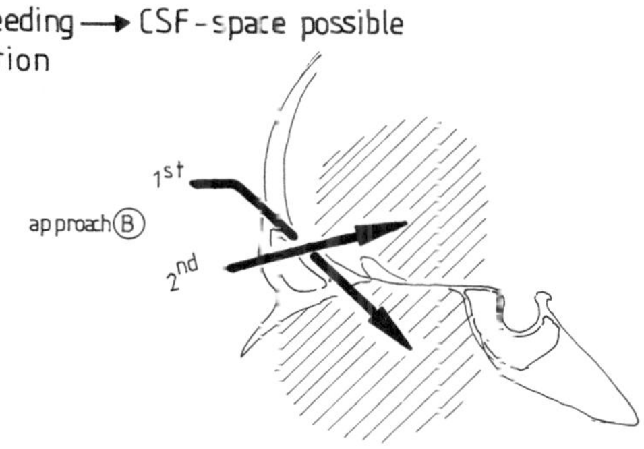

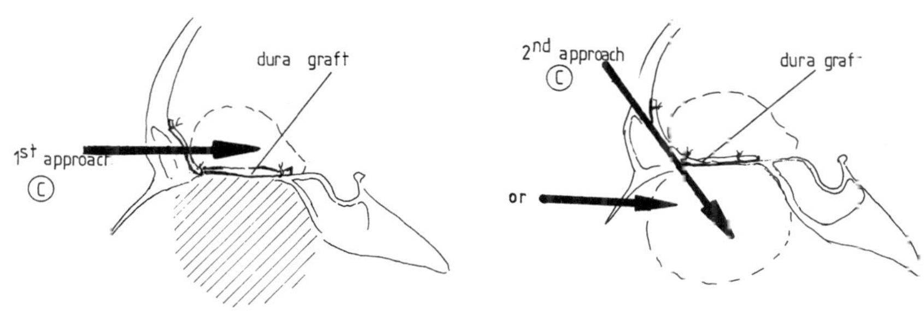

(C) 2 operations

no personal experience

favorable
- see (A)
- reduced risk of meningitis

unfavorable
- malignant tumor would grow between 1st and 2nd op. approach

Fig. 162. Clinical example of a recurrent meningioma. In 1978 first operated transcranially in another clinic. Now increasing exophthalmus on both sides, hindered breathing through the nose, increasing left peripheral facial paresis. Removal of craniofacial tumor*. A small meningioma in the cerebellopontine angle area which was visualized in the CT was not exposed

* Operation performed alternately by Prof. Dr. W. Mann (Ear, Nose and Throat Clinic of Freiburg University, Director: Prof. Dr. Chl. Beck) and Prof. Dr. J. Gilsbach, coworker of the author.

FIG. 162

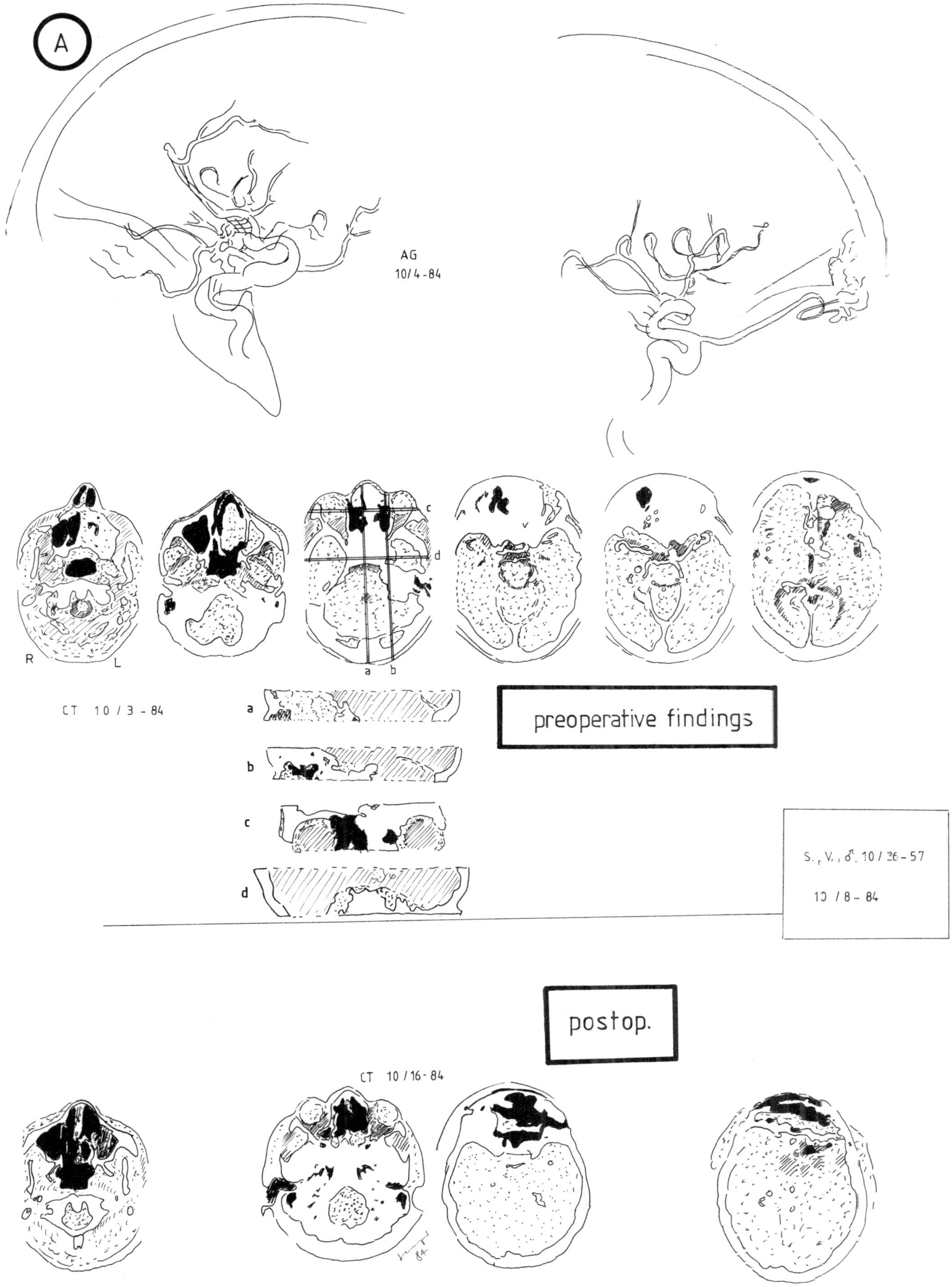
A
AG
10/4-84
R
L
a
b
c
d
CT 10/3-84
preoperative findings
S., V., ♂, 10/26-57
10/8-84
postop.
CT 10/16-84

Fig. 163

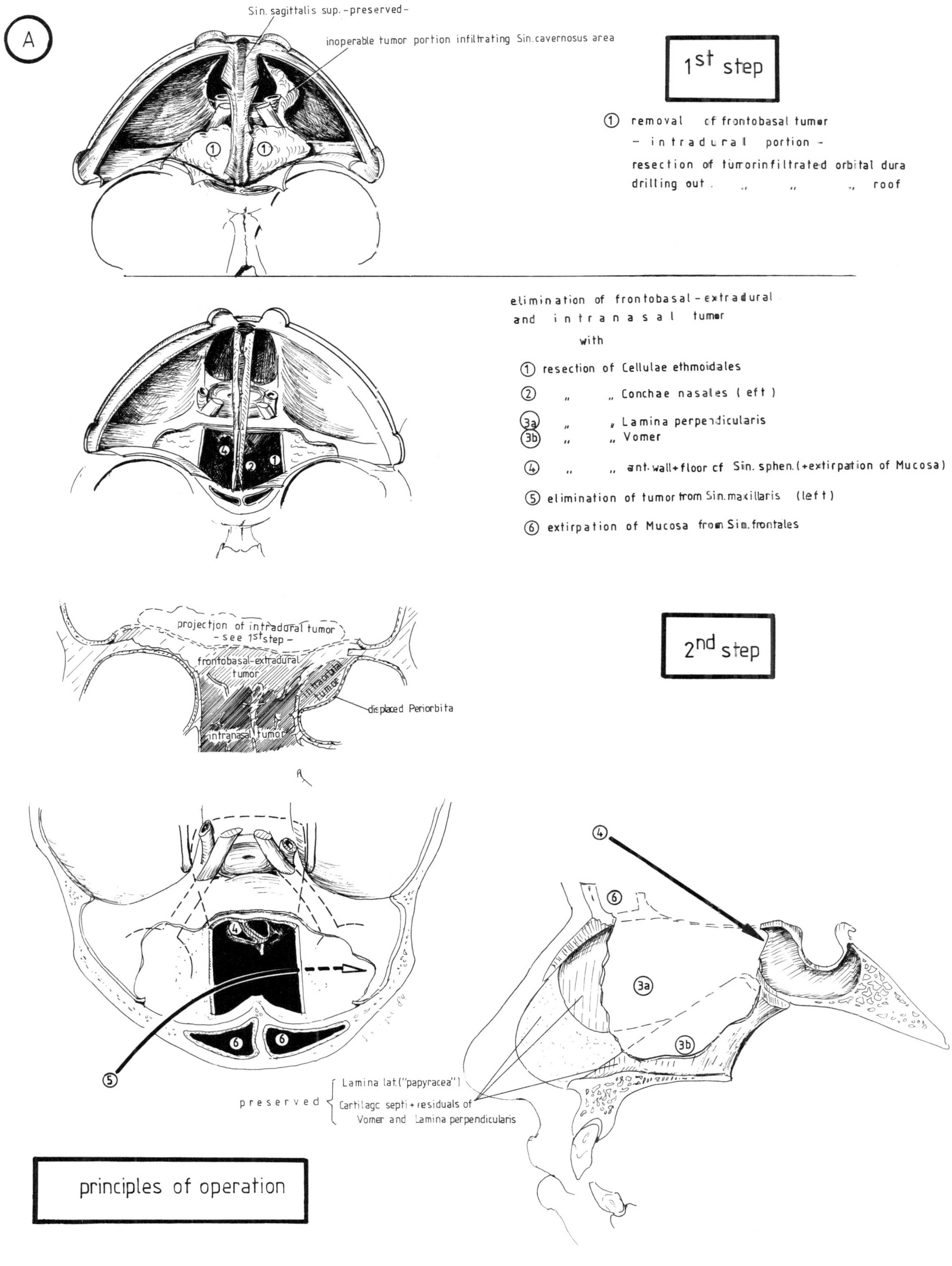
A
Sin. sagittalis sup. -preserved-
inoperable tumor portion infiltrating Sin. cavernosus area
1st step
① removal of frontobasal tumor
- intradural portion -
resection of tumorinfiltrated orbital dura
drilling out . ,, ,, ,, roof
elimination of frontobasal - extradural
and intranasal tumor
with
① resection of Cellulae ethmoidales
② ,, ,, Conchae nasales (eft)
3a ,, ,, Lamina perpendicularis
3b ,, ,, Vomer
④ ,, ,, ant. wall + floor of Sin. sphen. (+ extirpation of Mucosa)
⑤ elimination of tumor from Sin. maxillaris (left)
⑥ extirpation of Mucosa from Sin. frontales
projection of intradural tumor
- see 1st step -
frontobasal-extradural tumor
intraorbital tumor
displaced Periorbita
intranasal tumor
2nd step
preserved
Lamina lat. ("papyracea")
Cartilago septi + residuals of
Vomer and Lamina perpendicularis
principles of operation

Fig. 164

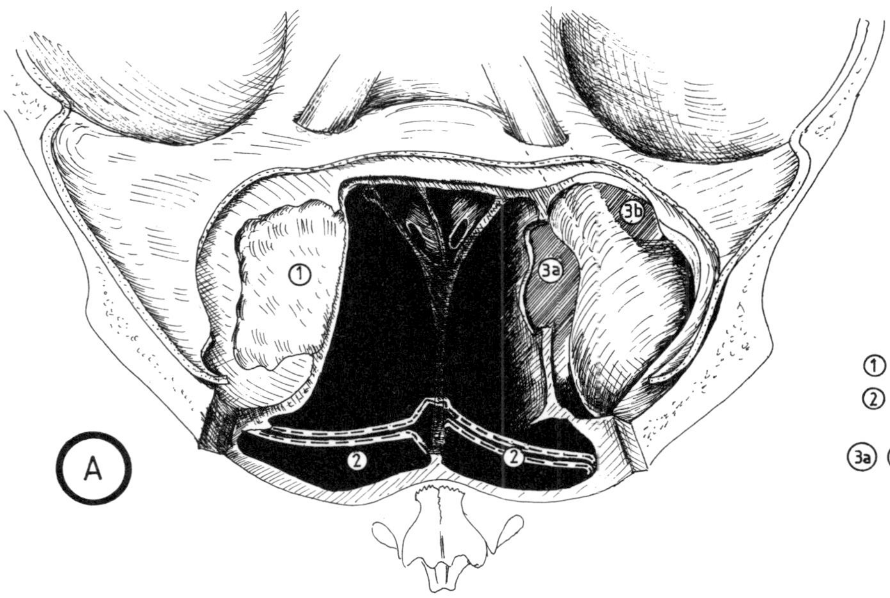

3rd step

① right orbital roof after drilling
② Sinus frontales after resection of post wall (dotted lines) and after elimination of further residual tumor
(3a) (3b) elimination of residual tumor in left Orbita

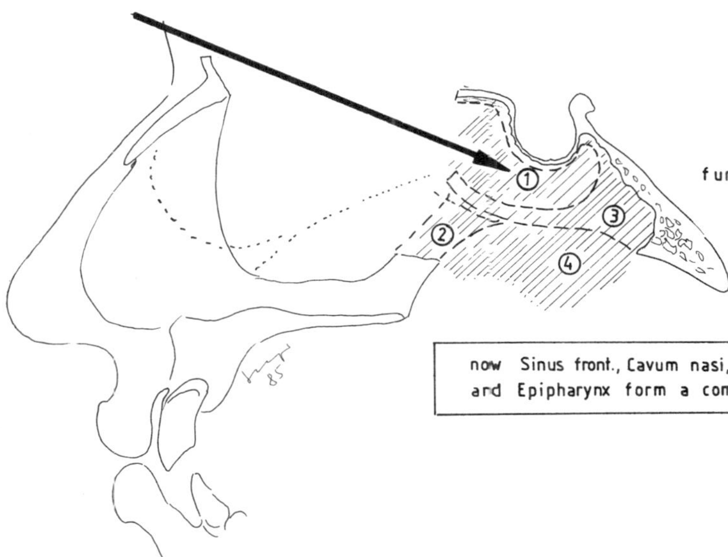

4th step

further elimination of residual tumor in
① Sin. sphenoidalis
② Choanae
③ Pars basilaris of Os occipitale
④ Epipharynx

now Sinus front., Cavum nasi, Cellulae ethmoidales, left Orbita, Sin. sphenoidal., defect of Pars basilaris and Epipharynx form a common space. Anterior and basal portions of Septum nasi preserved

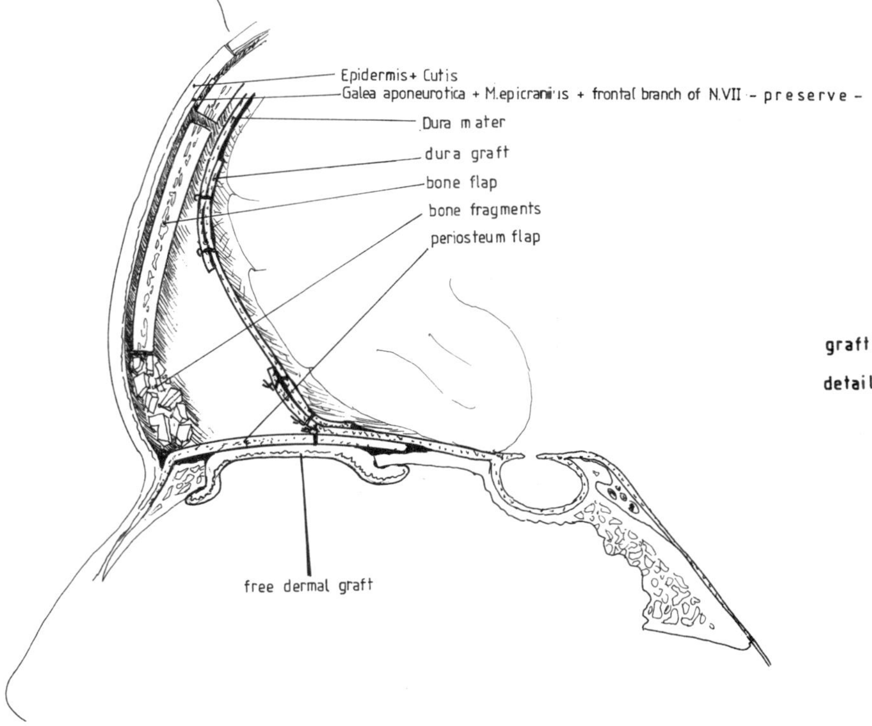

5th step

grafting / wound closure
details see principles of operation (B)

Fig. 165

FIG. 165

Ⓐ

*) Periorbita = Periosteum of Orbita

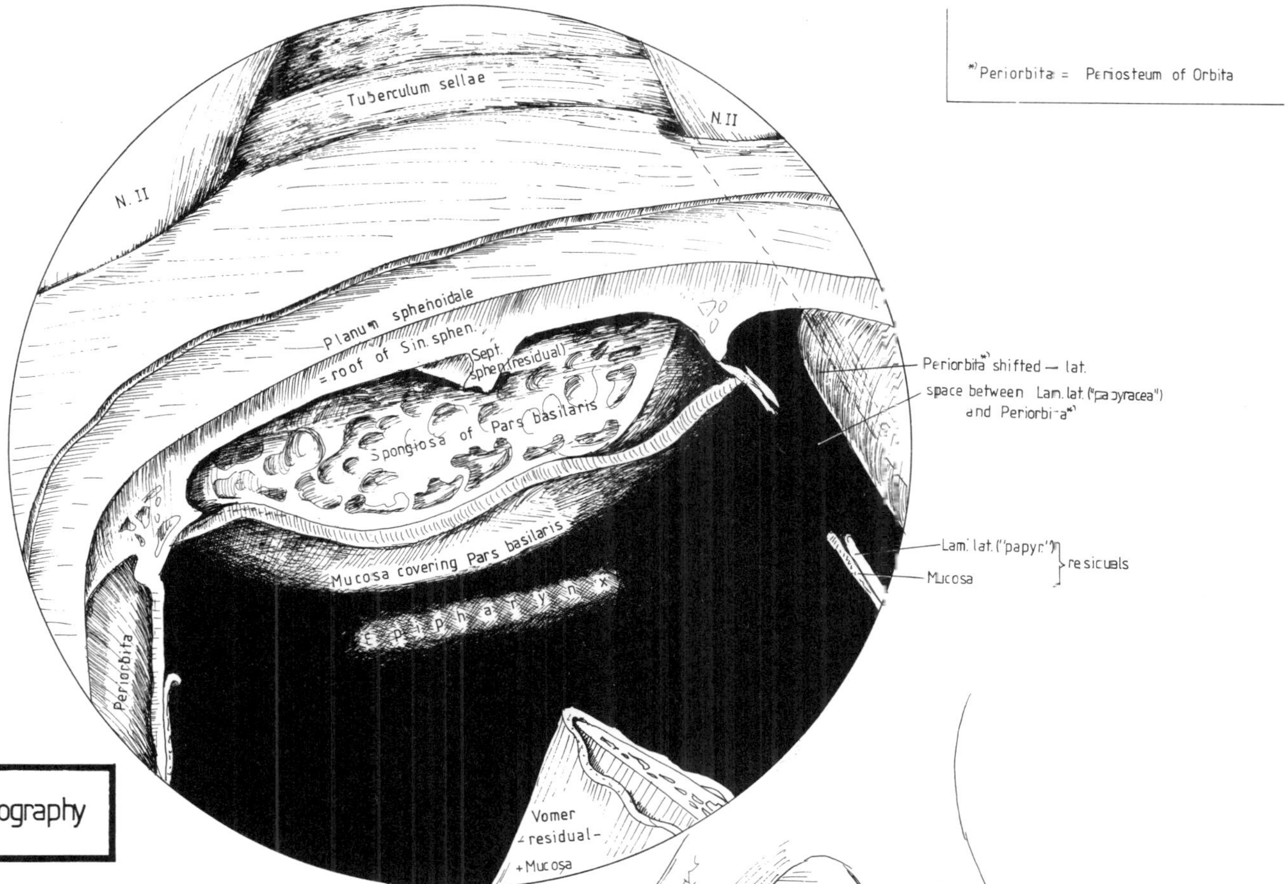

microsurgical topography

after extirpation of the tumor

see principles of operation Ⓐ after 4th step

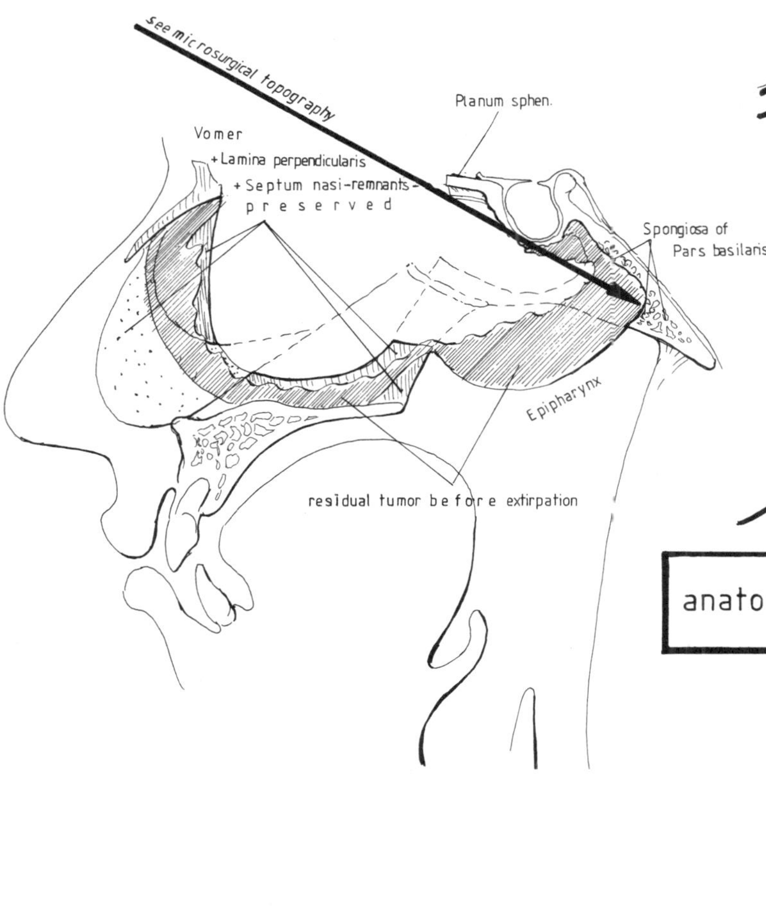

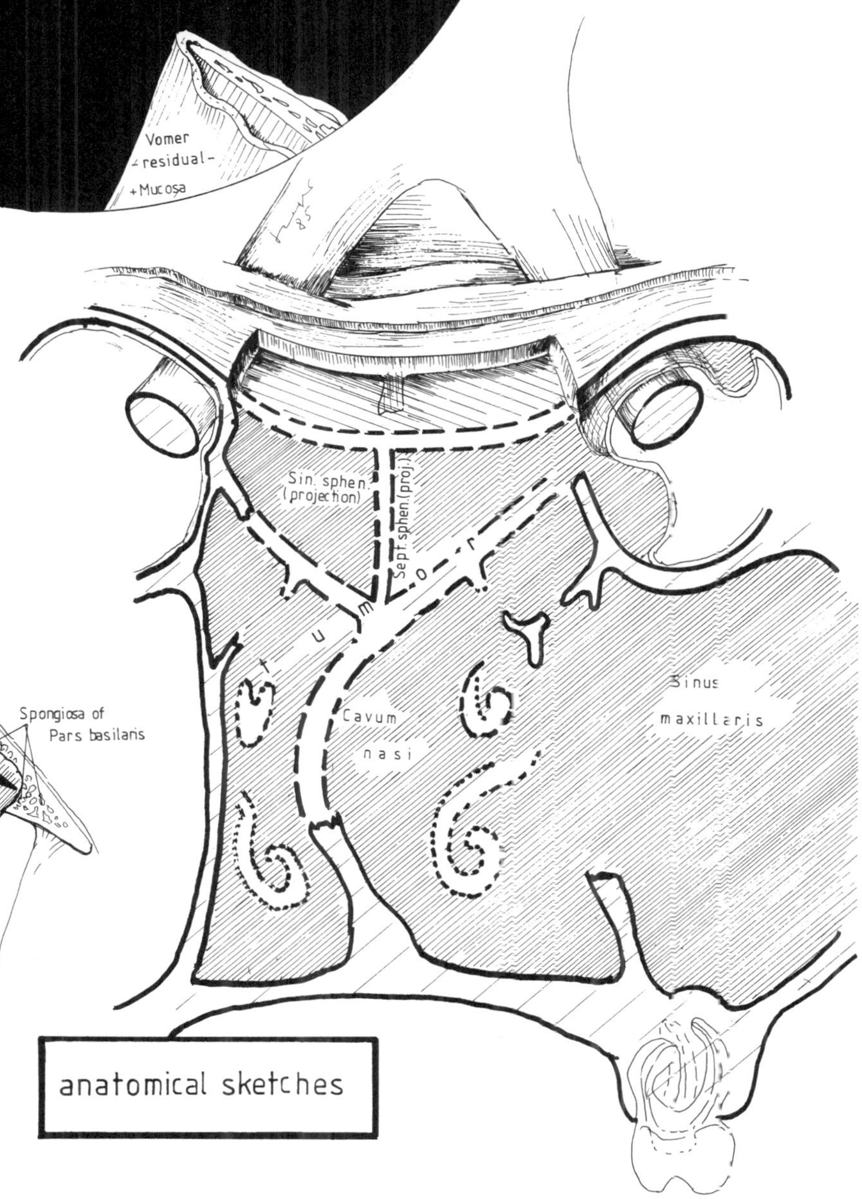

anatomical sketches

Fig. 166. Clinical example of an aggressively growing fronto-basal and nasoethmoidal Rhabdomyosarcoma, also in the area of both sphenoidal sinuses, emphasized on the left. Preoperatively threatening intracranial pressure symptoms, tumor growth recognizable in the area of the outer nasal openings. Postoperatively rapid reversal of intracranial pressure symptoms, psychological recovery, visus stable, ability to smell still absent *

* Operation performed alternately by Prof. Dr. W. Mann (Ear, Nose and Throat Clinic of Freiburg University, Director: Prof. Dr. Chl. Beck) and Prof. Dr. J. Gilsbach, coworker of the author.

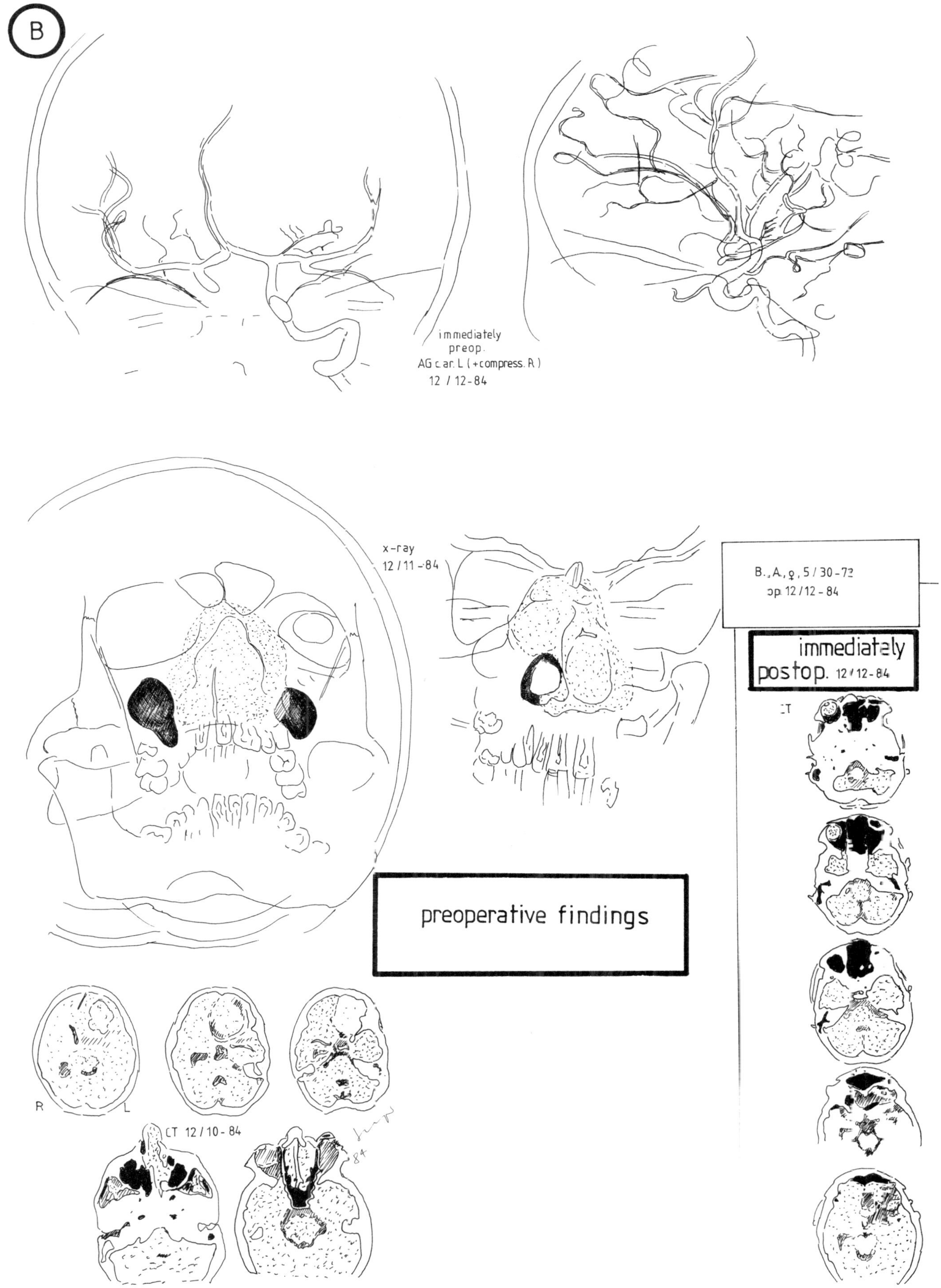
B
immediately
preop.
AG c.ar. L (+compress. R)
12 / 12-84
x-ray
12 / 11-84
B., A., ♀, 5 / 30-72
op. 12 / 12-84
immediately
postop. 12 / 12-84
CT
preoperative findings
R
L
CT 12 / 10-84

Fig. 167

B

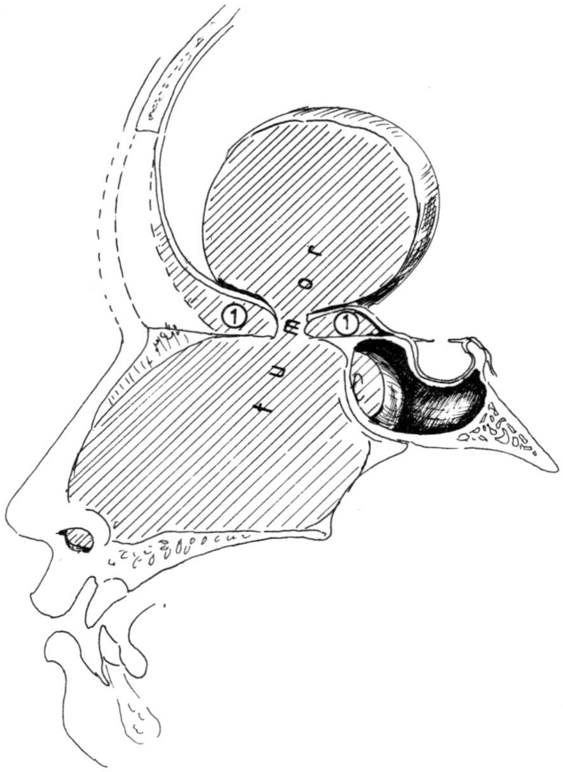

1st step

① elimination of epidural tumo-

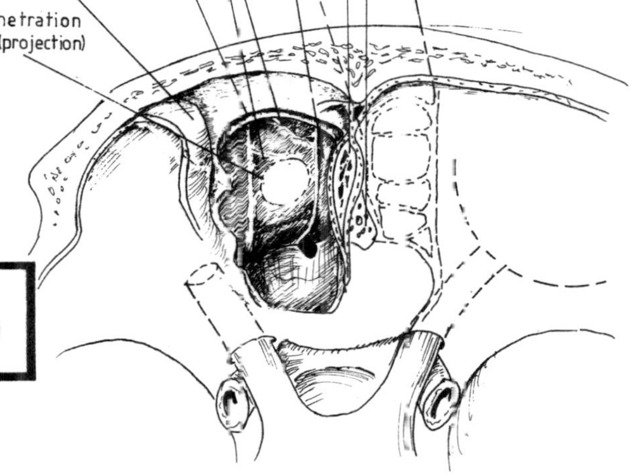

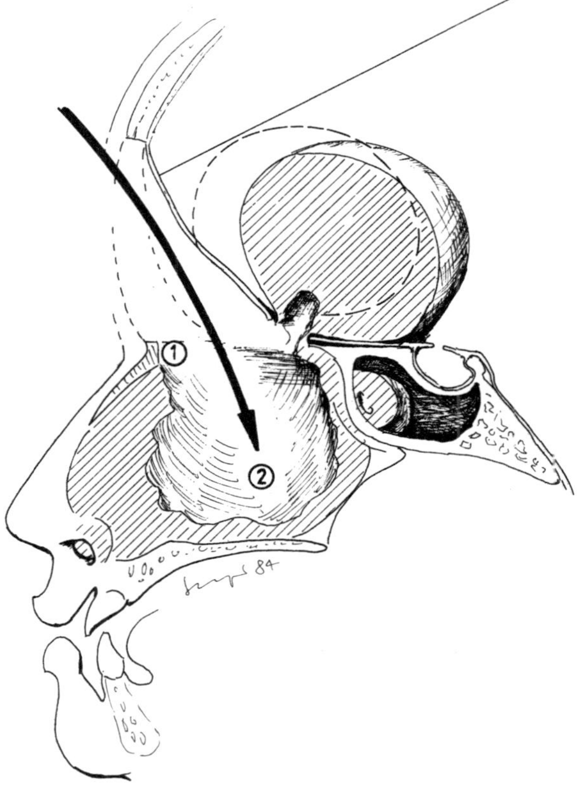

2nd step

① resection of Lamina cribrosa + Planum sphenoidale left
② dissection and removal of intranasal tumor portion left

principles of operation

Fig. 168

B

3rd step

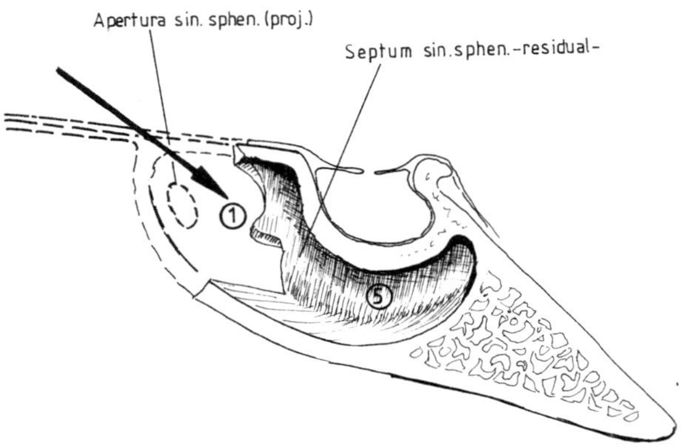

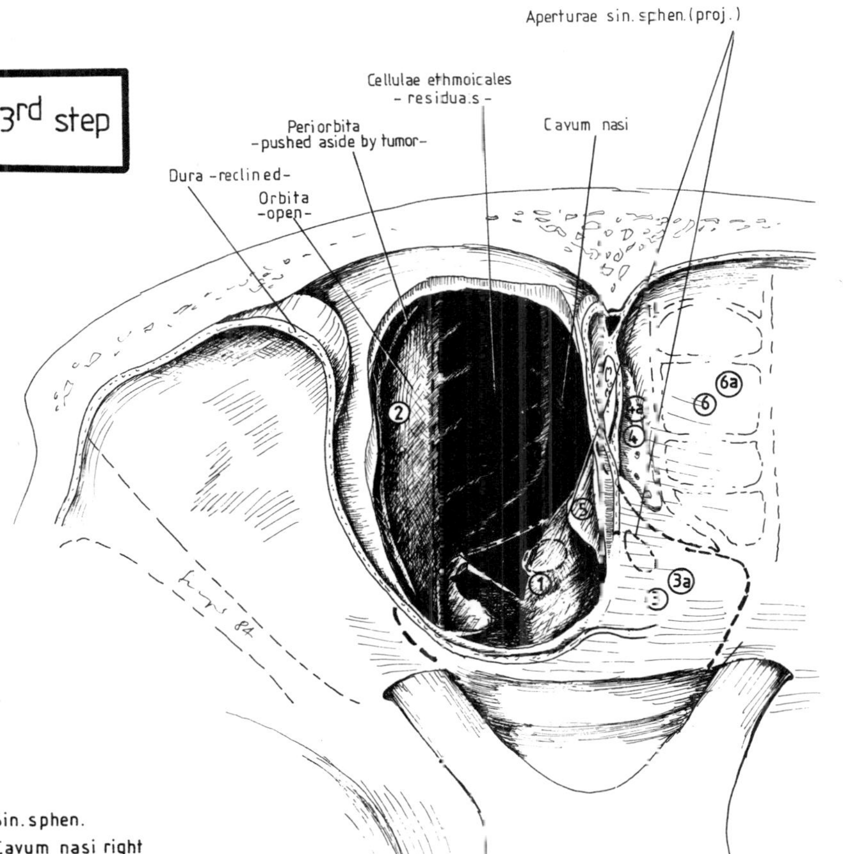

① opening of left Sin. sphenoidalis, extirpation of residual tumor + Mucosa

② opening of left Orbita, extirpation of the tumor

③ resection of Planum sphen. right = opening of right Sin. sphen.

④ „ „ Lamina cribrosa „ = „ „ „ Cavum nasi right

⑤ „ „ Sept. sin. sphen.

⑥ „ „ roof of Cellulae ethmoidales right

③a + ⑥a + ④a extirpation of residual tumor right

4th step

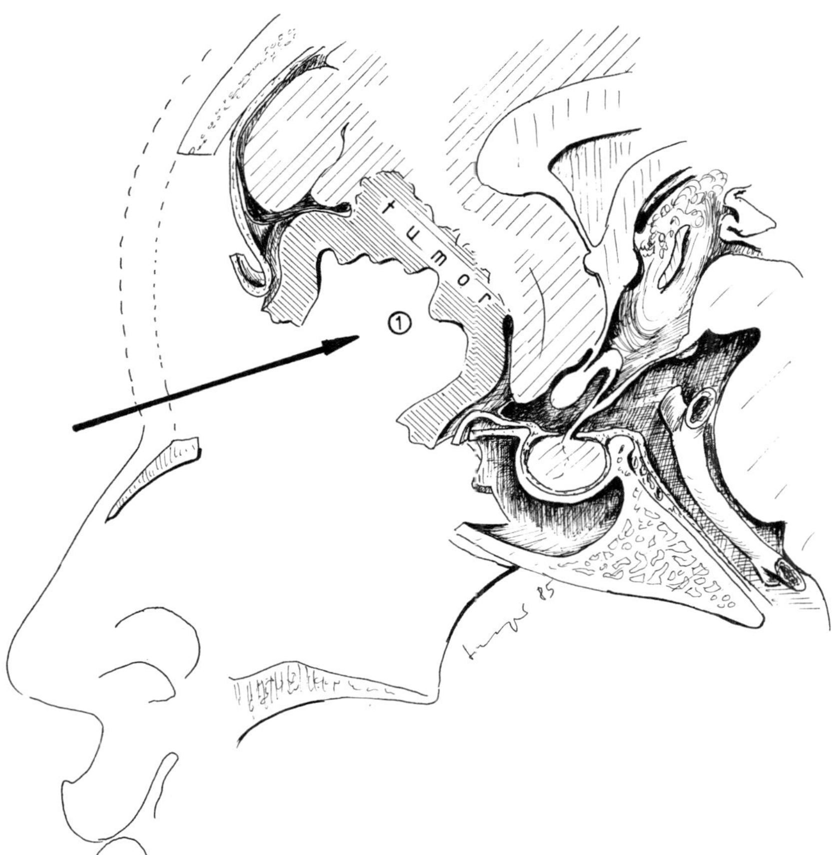

① hollowing and extirpation of intradural residual tumor

Fig. 169

Ⓑ

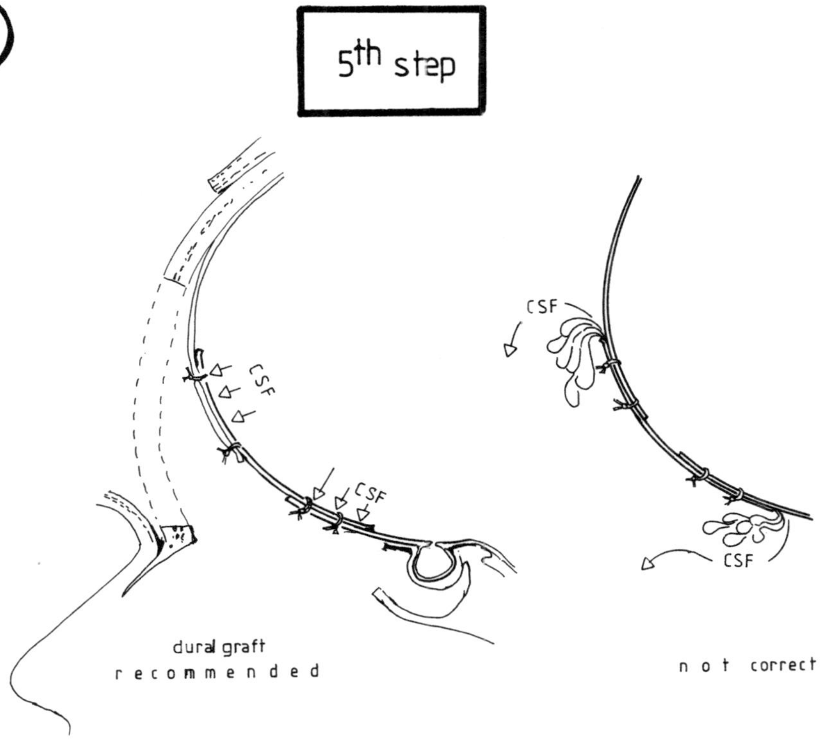

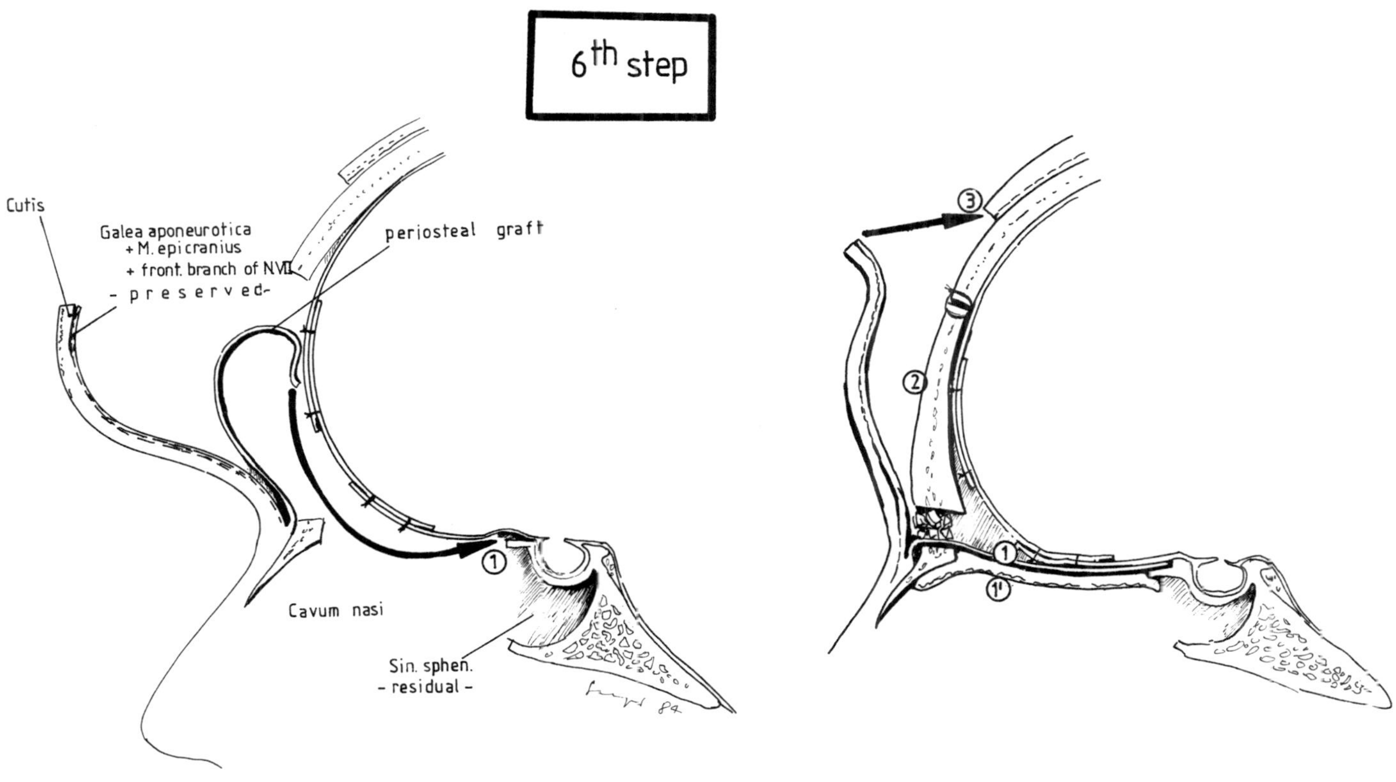

① periosteal graft covering Cavum nasi + Cell. ethmoidales + Sin. sphen. (+ -in adults- Sin. front.)

② reimplantation of bone flap

③ wound closure

①' free dermal graft, if necessary

Fig. 170. The wide opening of the nasal cavity and paranasal cavities required an extensive plastic covering at the end of the intervention. No postoperative liquor fistula

Ⓑ

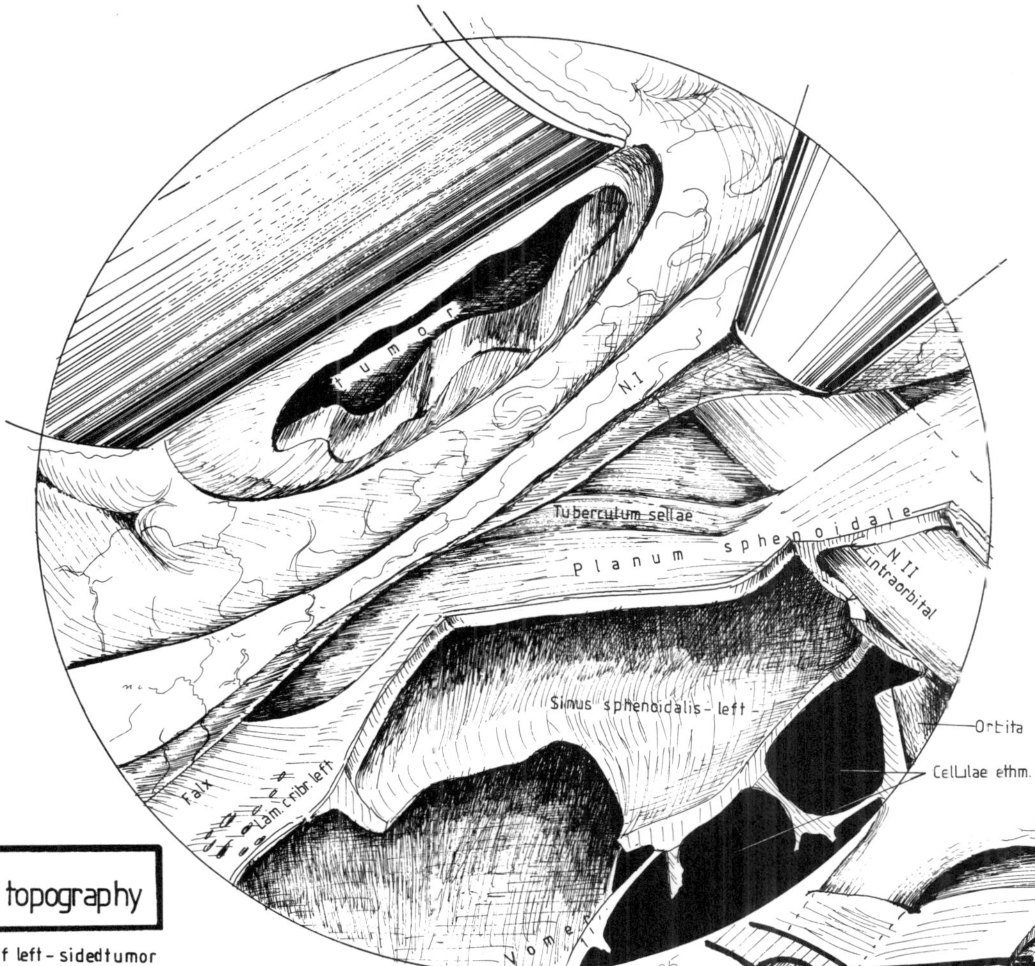

microsurgical topography

after extirpation of left-sided tumor
before resection of Planum sphen. right, Sept. sin. sphen. and Sept. nasi

see principles of operation Ⓑ 3rd step

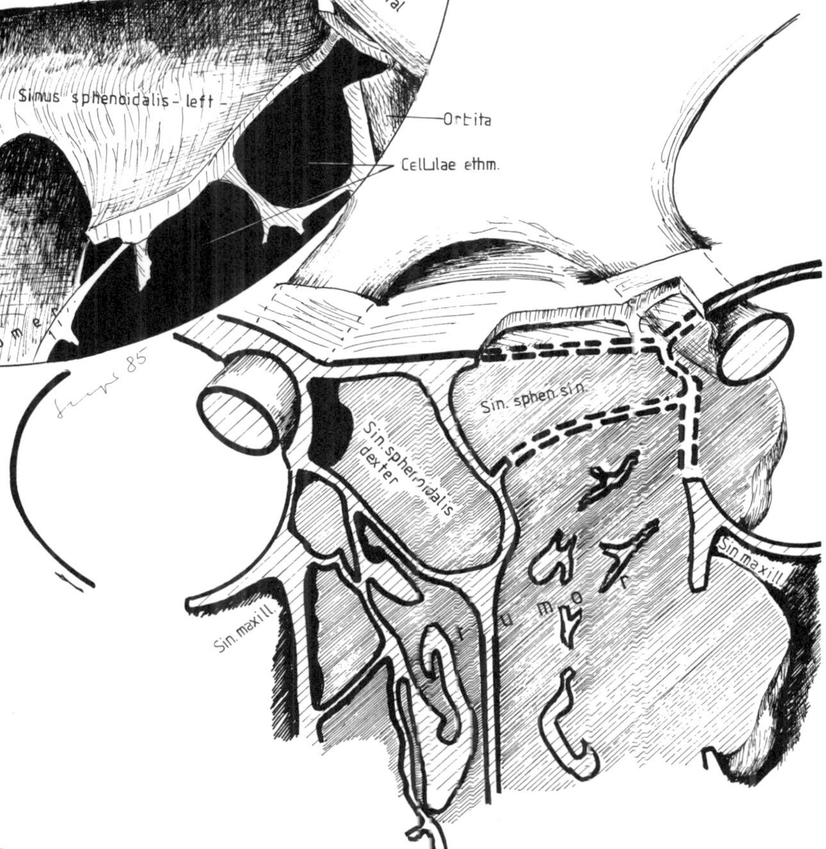

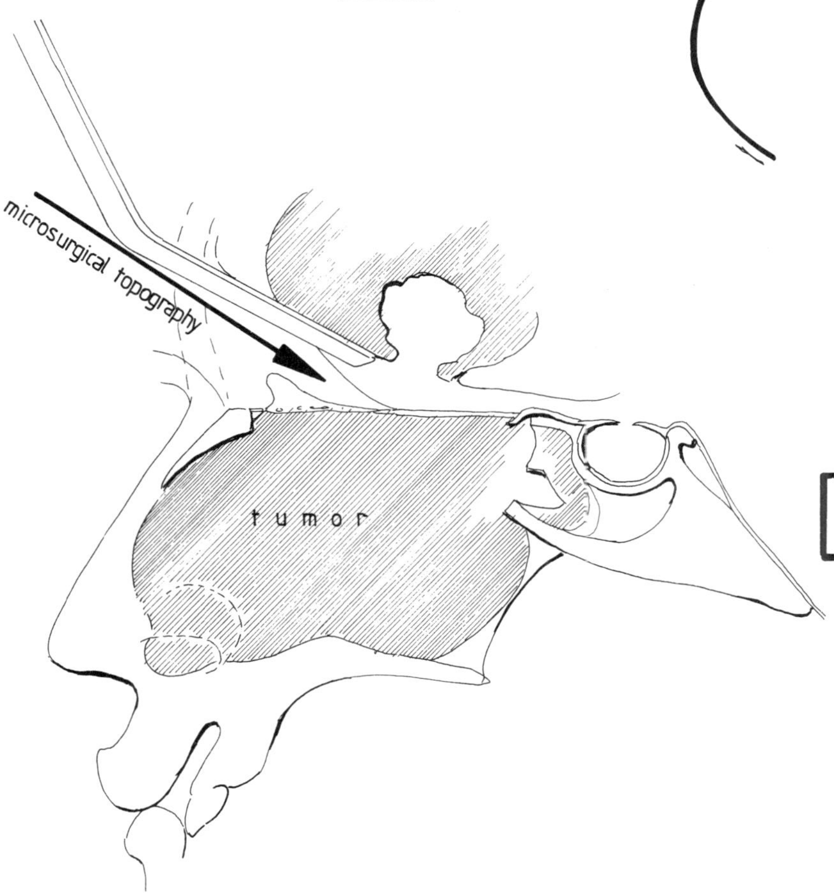

anatomical sketches

before extirpation of the tumor

see principles of operation Ⓔ 2nd step

Fig. 171. Patient, an Ear, Nose and Throat Specialist and since 1979 twice operated in another clinic because of a fronto-basal meningioma originating from the Falx. Liquor fistula and meningitis present. Grafting of the liquor fistula. Now at admission a new liquor fistula, an organic psychosyndrome, loss of smell. Postoperatively no additional deficits, no more liquorrhea

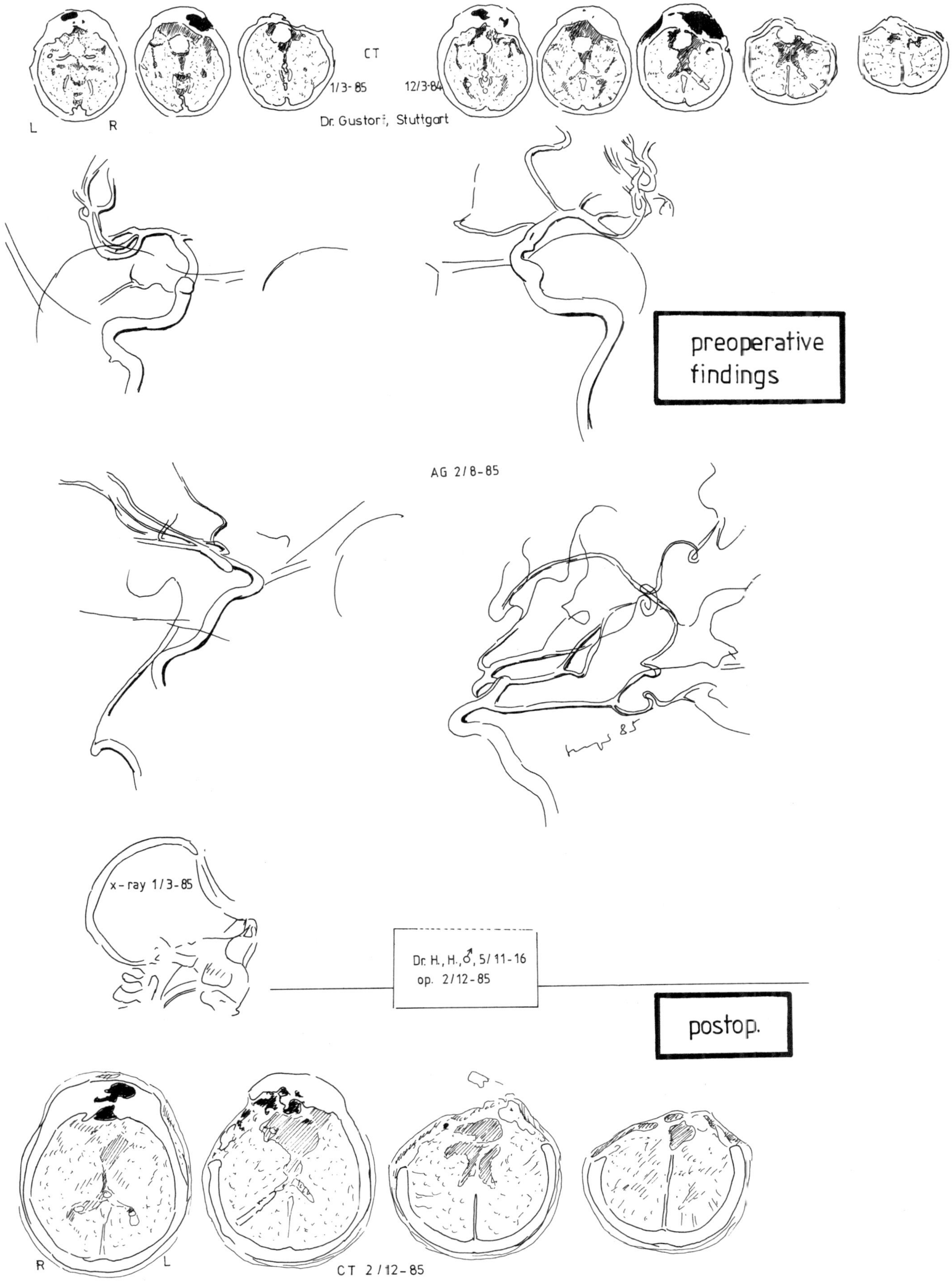
L
R
CT
1/3-85
12/3-84
Dr. Gustorf, Stuttgart
preoperative findings
AG 2/8-85
x-ray 1/3-85
Dr. H., H., ♂, 5/11-16
op. 2/12-85
postop.
R
L
CT 2/12-85

Fig. 172. Anatomical relationships of the recurrent tumor on the basis of observations made during the operation

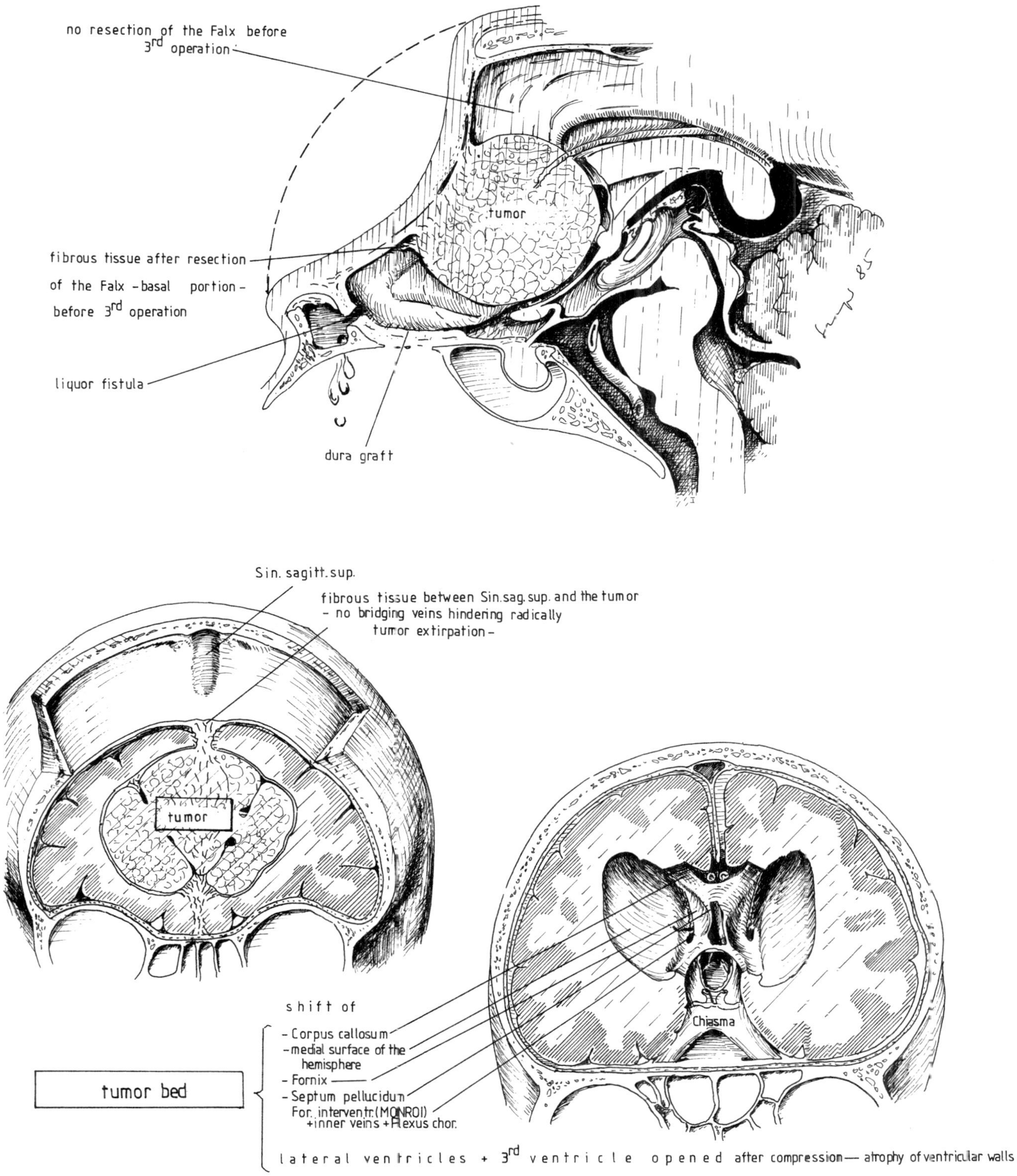

no resection of the Falx before 3rd operation
tumor
fibrous tissue after resection of the Falx - basal portion - before 3rd operation
liquor fistula
dura graft
Sin. sagitt. sup.
fibrous tissue between Sin. sag. sup. and the tumor - no bridging veins hindering radically tumor extirpation -
tumor
tumor bed
shift of
- Corpus callosum
- medial surface of the hemisphere
- Fornix
- Septum pellucidum
For. interventr. (MONROI) + inner veins + Plexus chor.
lateral ventricles + 3rd ventricle opened after compression — atrophy of ventricular walls
Chiasma

Fig. 173

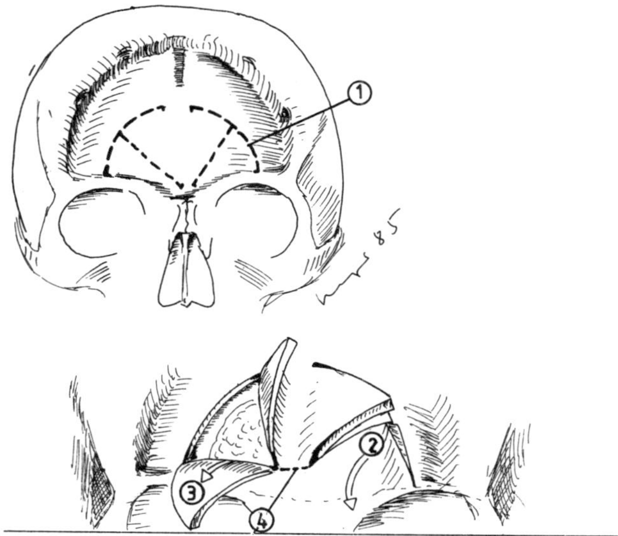

1st step

① Dura incision
② ③ eversion of lateral Dura flaps
④ Dura incision

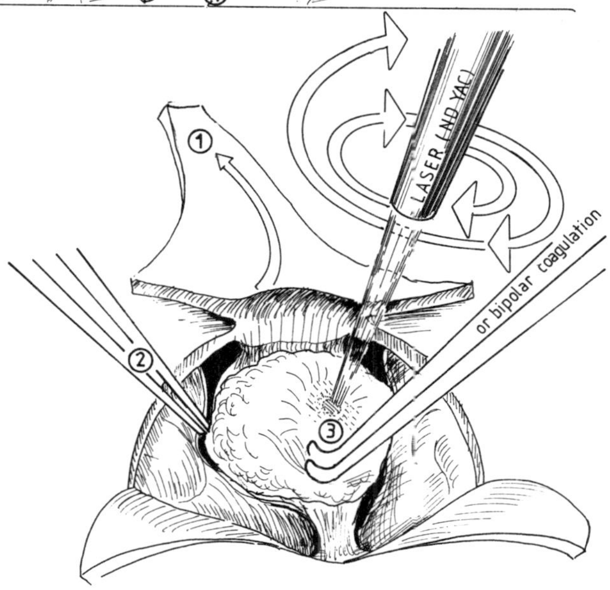

2nd step

① eversion of medial Dura flap
② dissecting Arachnoidea
③ shrinking of the tumor

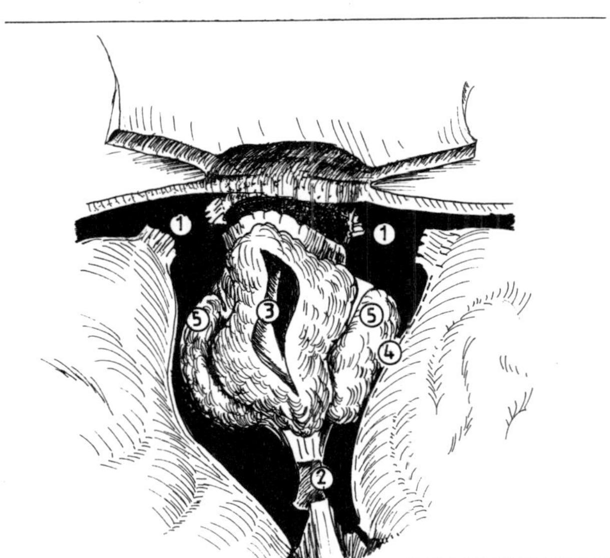

3rd step

① ② transecting adhesions
③ hollowing the tumor
④ dissecting Arachnoidea
⑤ repeated shrinking

principles of operation

Fig. 174

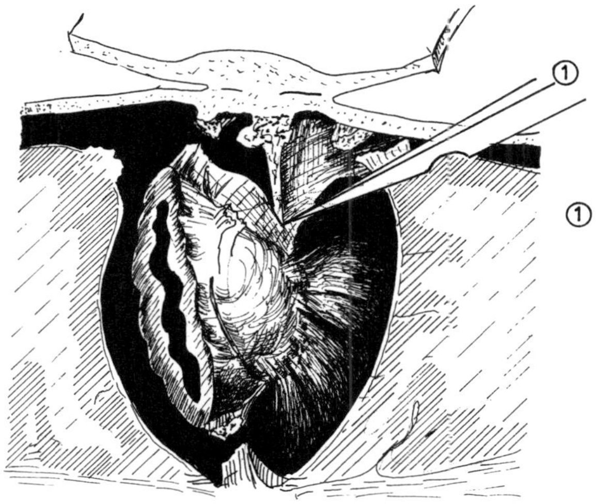

4th step

① Falx resection

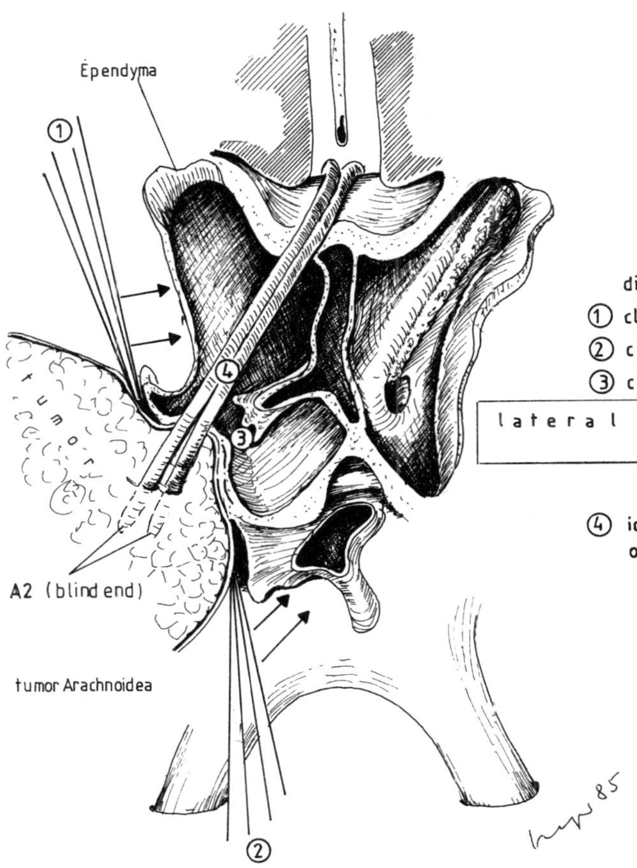

5th step

dissecting flattened Ependyma from tumor Arachnoidea

① close to the lateral wall of Ventriculus lat.

② close to Lamina terminalis (c a v e Hypothalamus)

③ close to Septum pellucidum

l a t e r a l ventricles, 3rd ventricle – Cavum septi pellucidi widened

④ identification and cutting of blind end (proof preop. angiogram) of both A2 close to the tumor

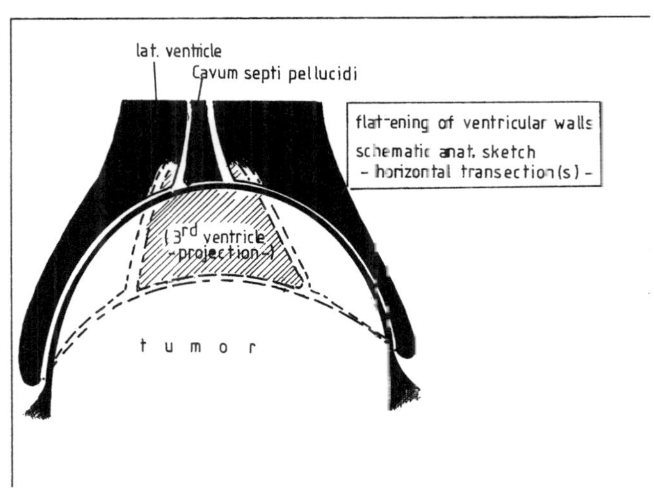

Fig. 175

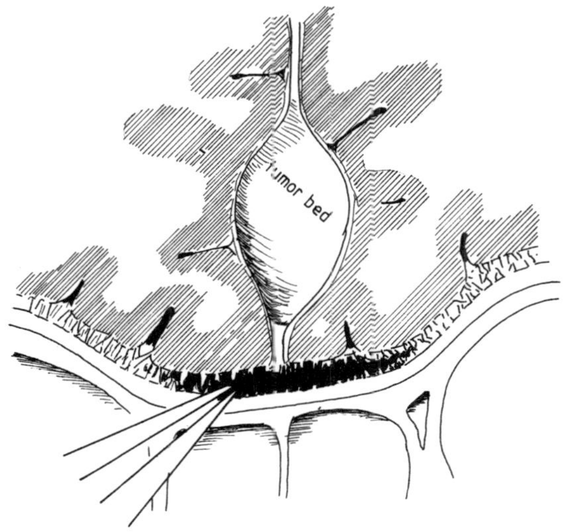

6th step

① dissecting frontobasal adhesions

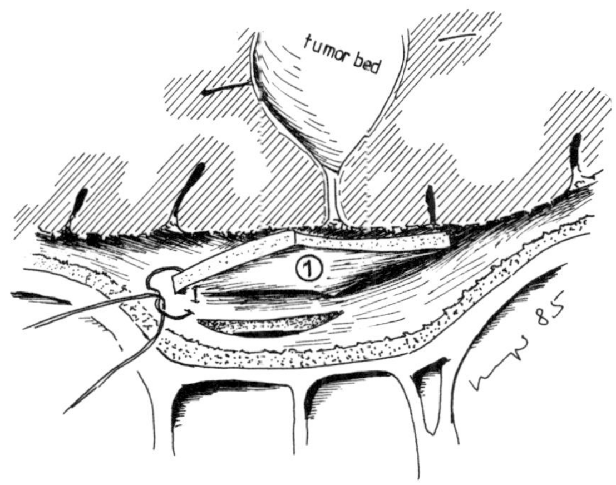

7th step

① grafting of liquor fistula

Fig. 176. The presumed interruption of the anterior cerebral artery seen in the preoperative angiogram was confirmed at operation. When isolating the tumor in the area of the limbic system, particularly in the area of the Fornices, one must pay particular attention to the exact preparation of the correct tissue layer, otherwise one can expect an increase in the organic psychosyndrome

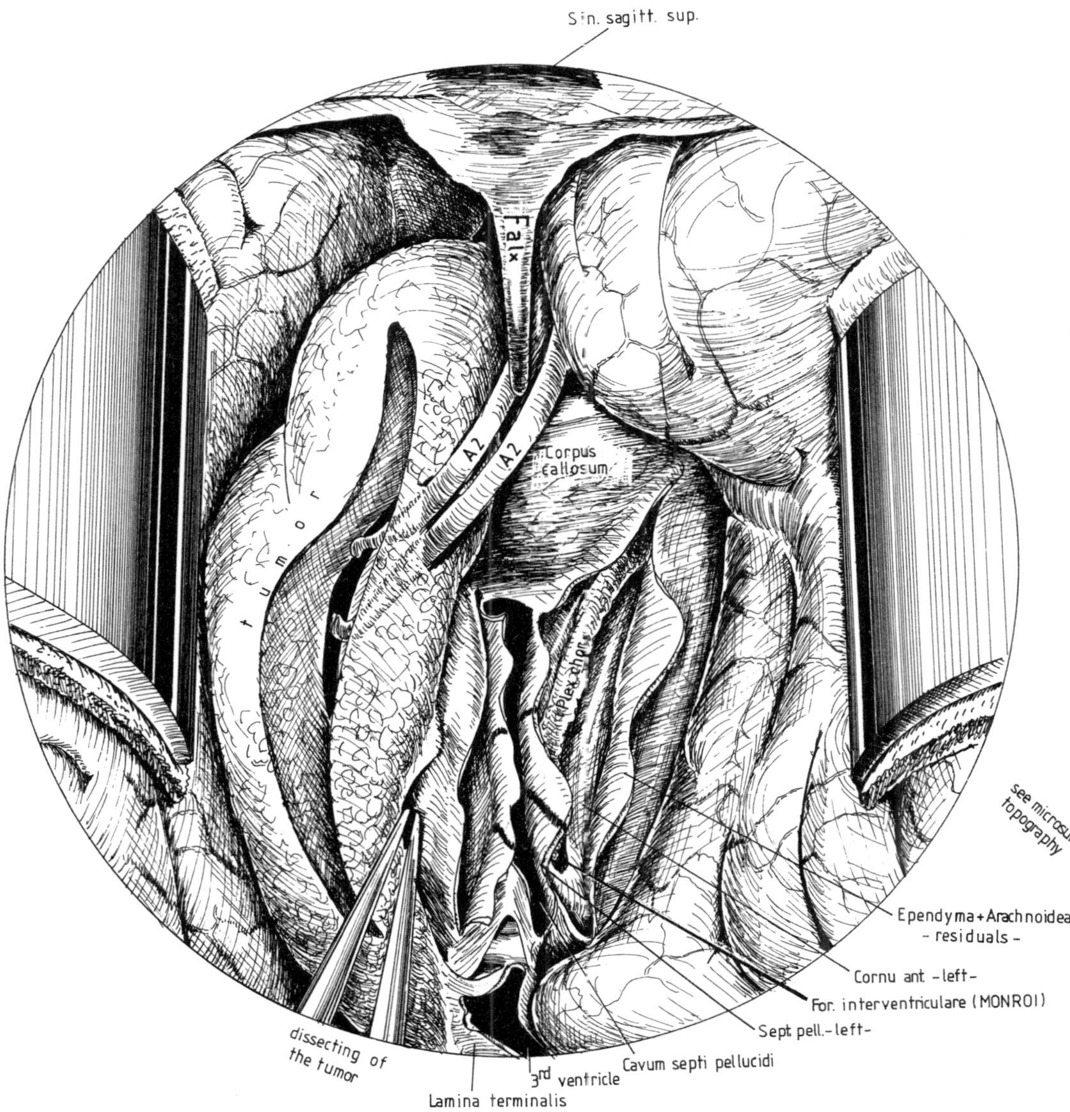

microsurgical topography

5th step

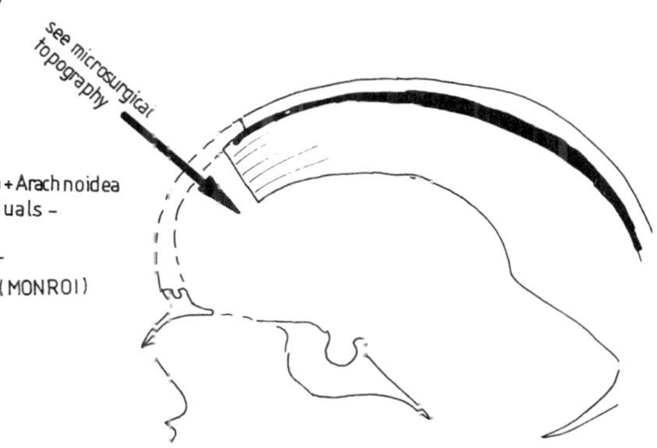

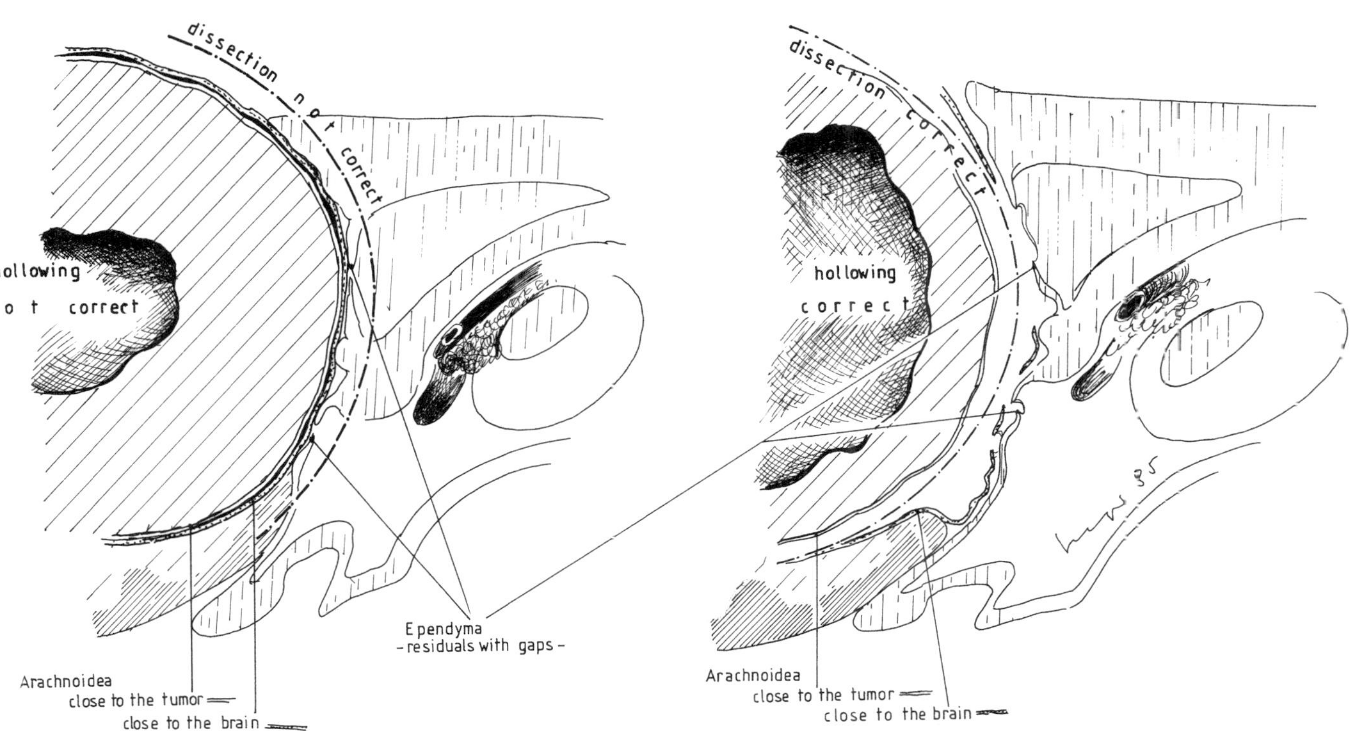

Chapter 8
Basal Cisterns, Middle Segment
(Figs. 177 to 198)

Fig. 177. Marked juvenile angiofibroma of the nasal passages without preoperative deficits*. Postoperatively Facialis intact, apart from disturbances in the 3rd branch of the Trigeminus no deficits. No tumor remains visualized in postoperative CT

* Operation performed alternately by Prof. Dr. W. Mann (Ear, Nose and Throat Clinic of Freiburg University, Director: Prof. Dr. Chl. Beck) and Prof. Dr. J. Gilsbach, coworker of the author.

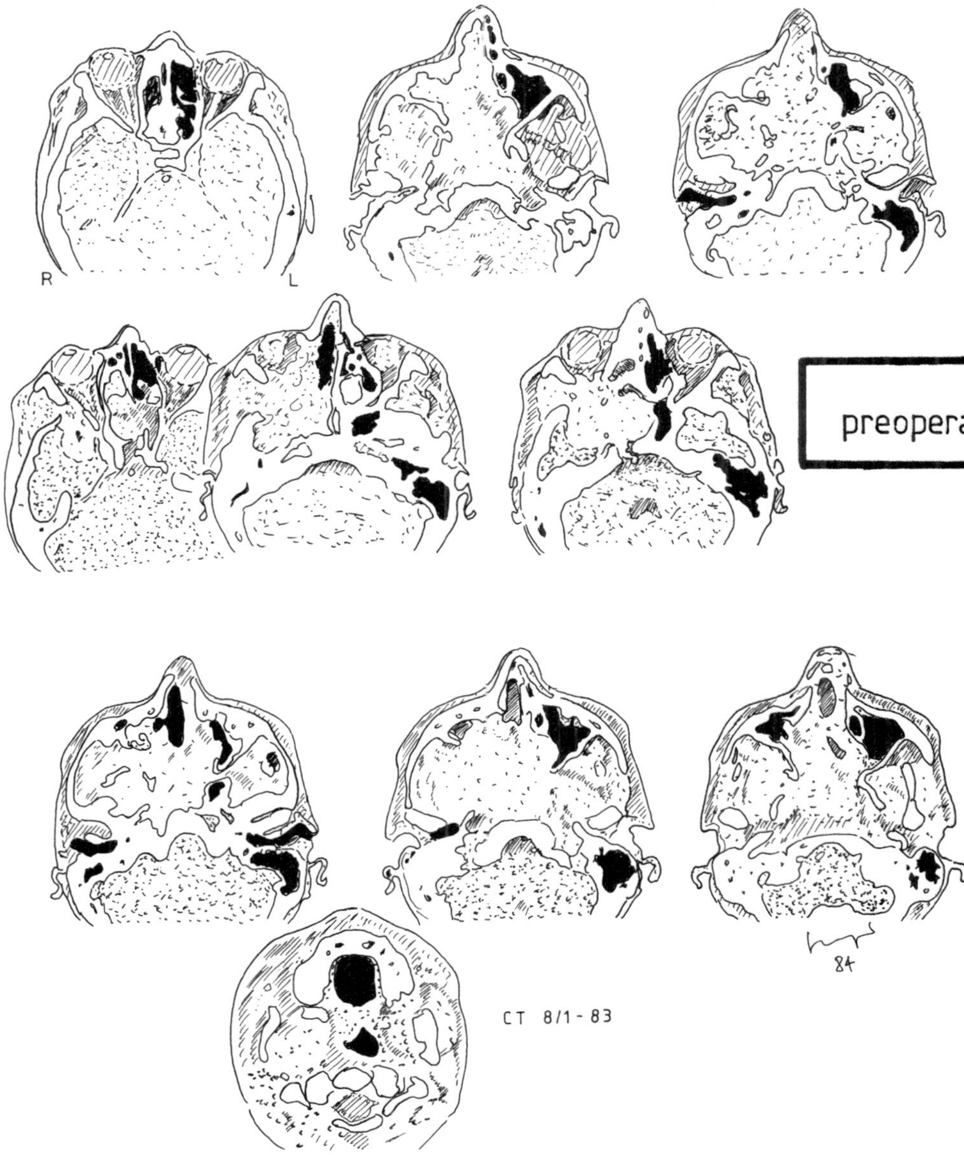

preoperative findings

CT 8/1-83

M.,N., ♂, 2/13-67
op. 8/9-83

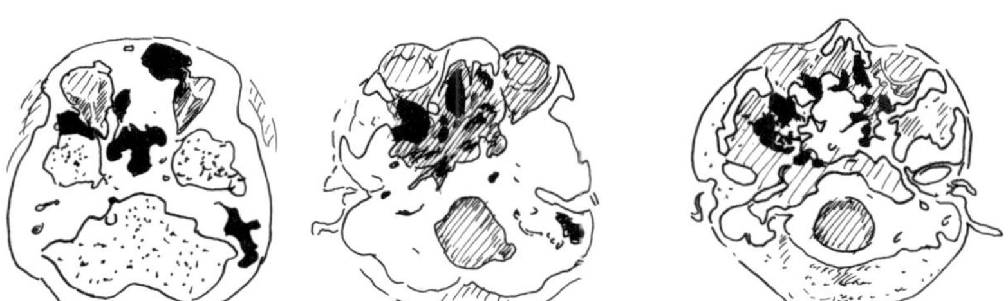

CT 8/9-83

postop.

Fig. 178. Postoperative angiogram showed no tumor remains

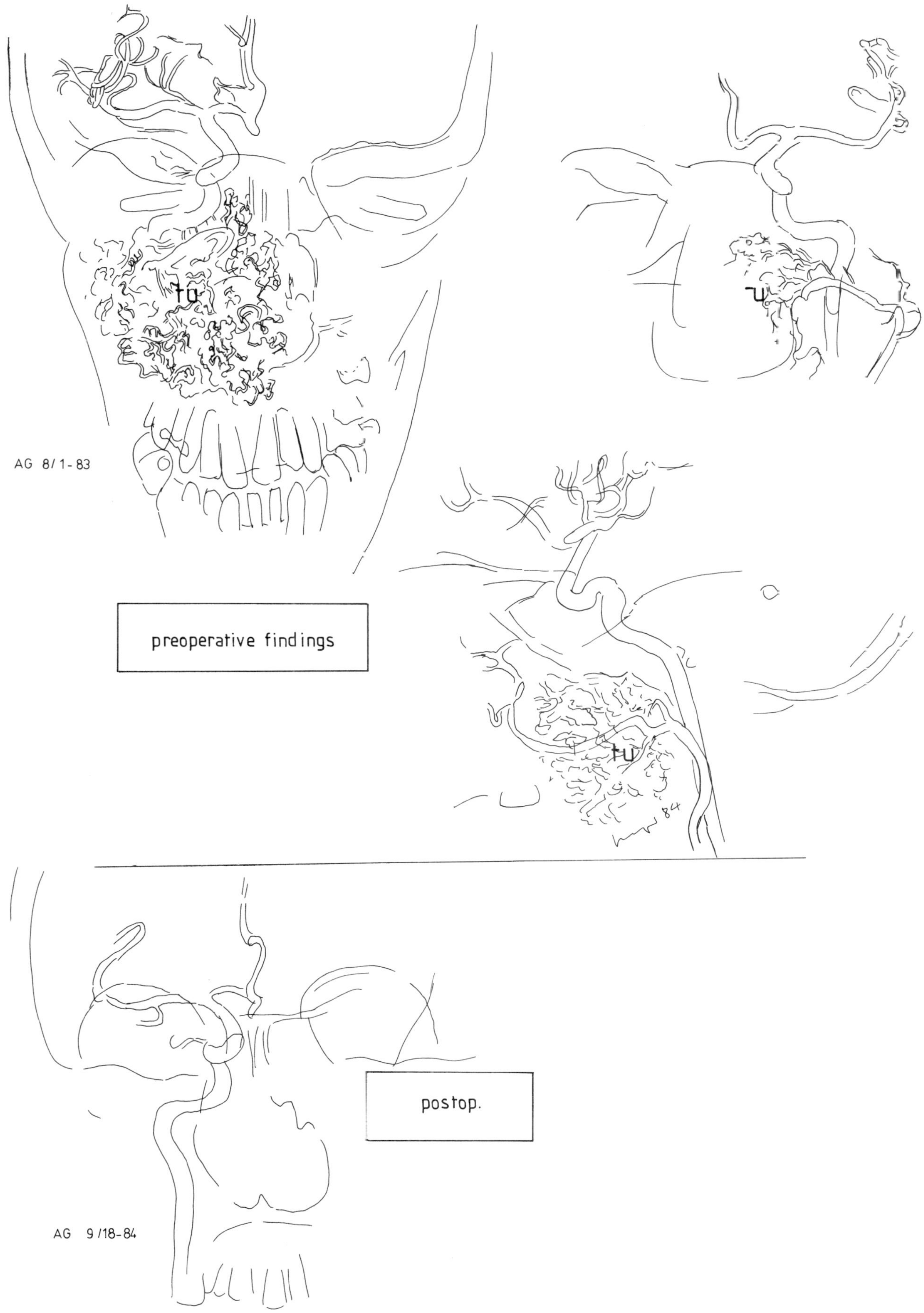
tu
AG 8/1-83
preoperative findings
tu
84
postop.
AG 9/18-84

Fig. 179

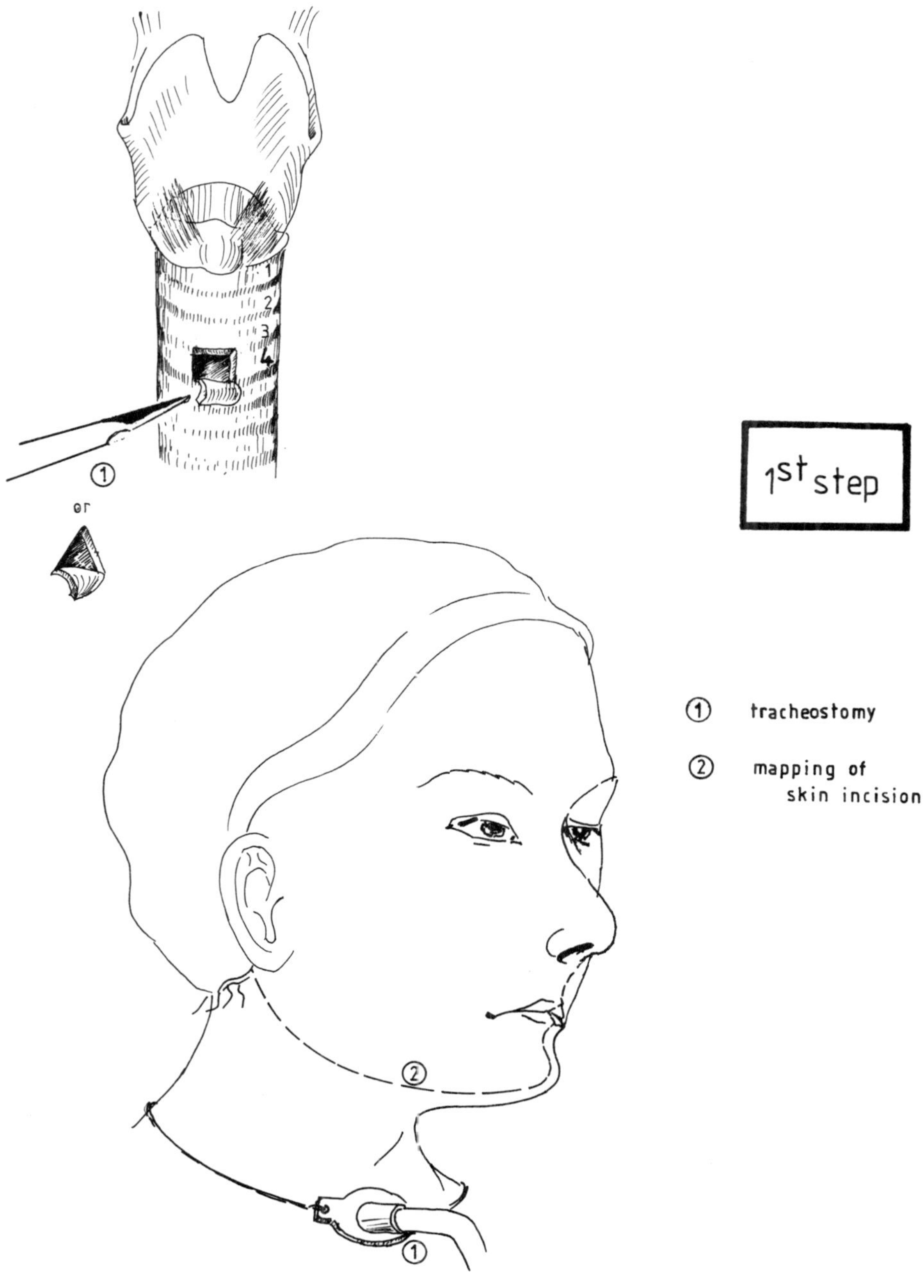

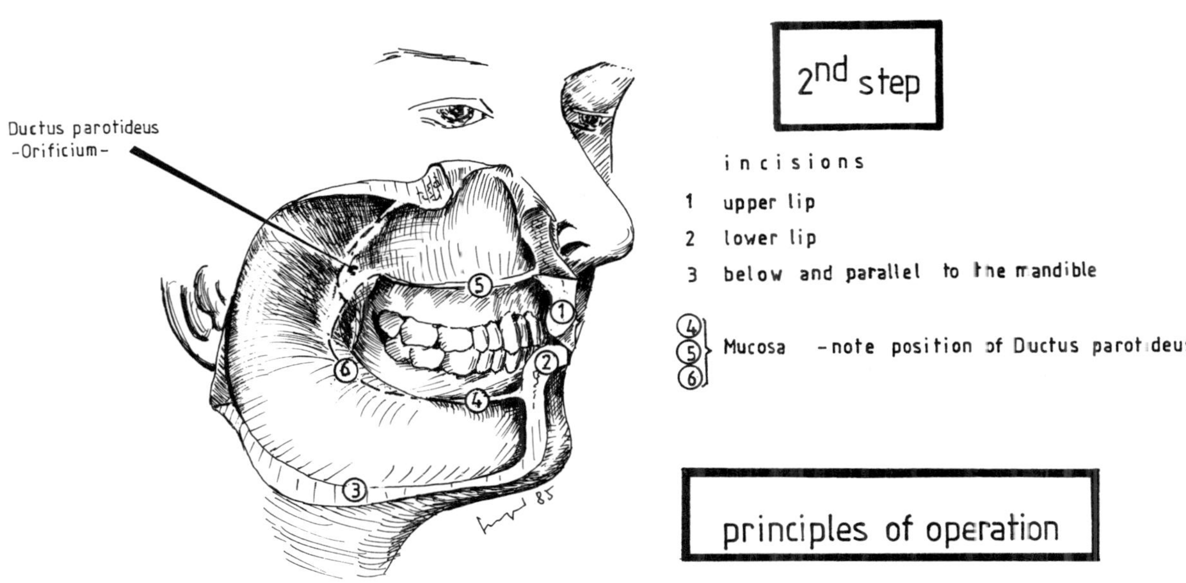

principles of operation

Fig. 180

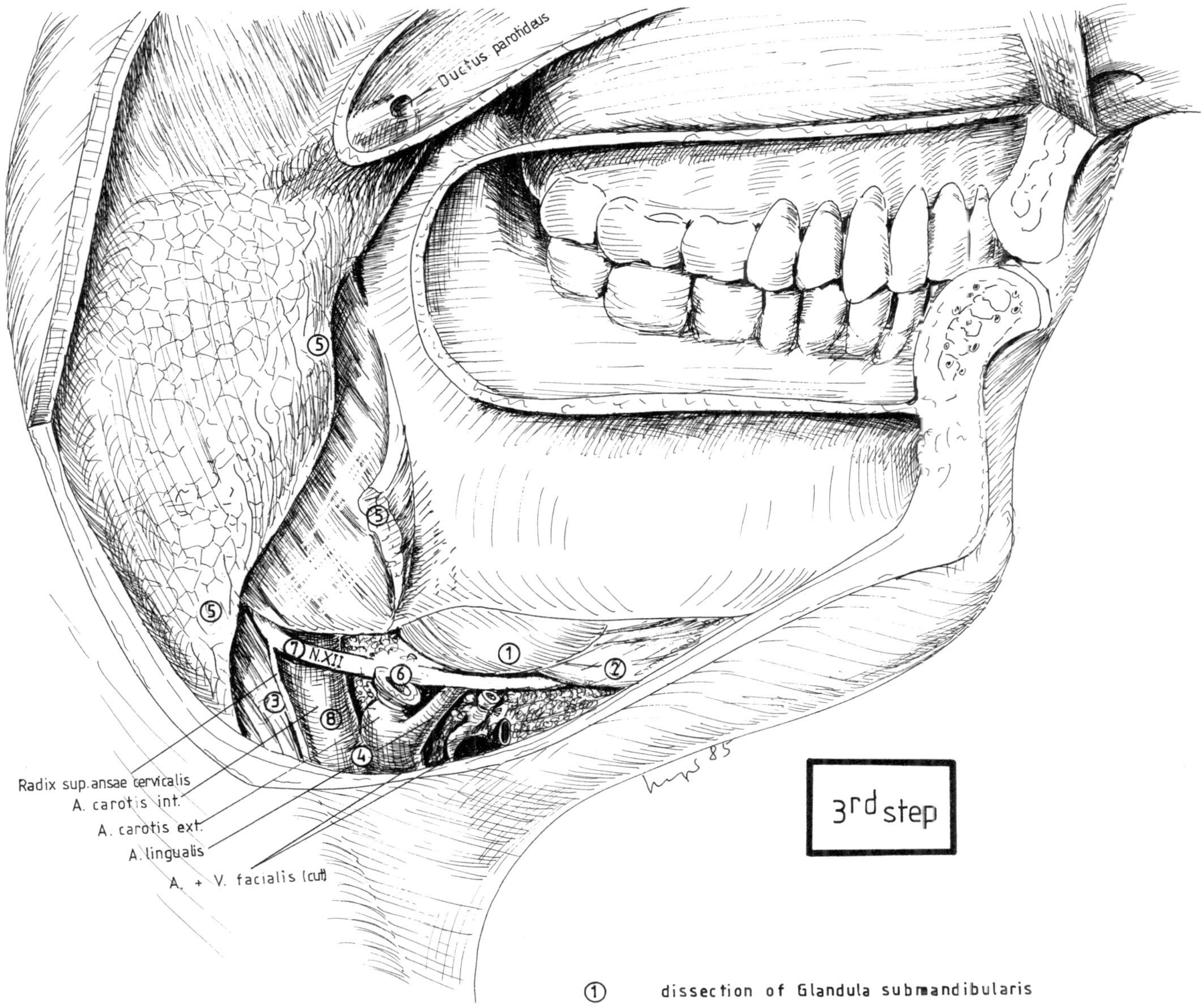

① dissection of Glandula submandibularis

② " " M. biventer

③ " " M. sternocleidomast. (ant. margin) from Glandula parotis

④ " " bifurcation of A. carotis comm.

⑤ detachment of Glandula parotis + M. masseter from Mandibula

⑥ ligation of A. carotis ext. distal to the origin of A. lingualis

⑦ dissection of N. XII

⑧ " " A. carotis int.

Fig. 181

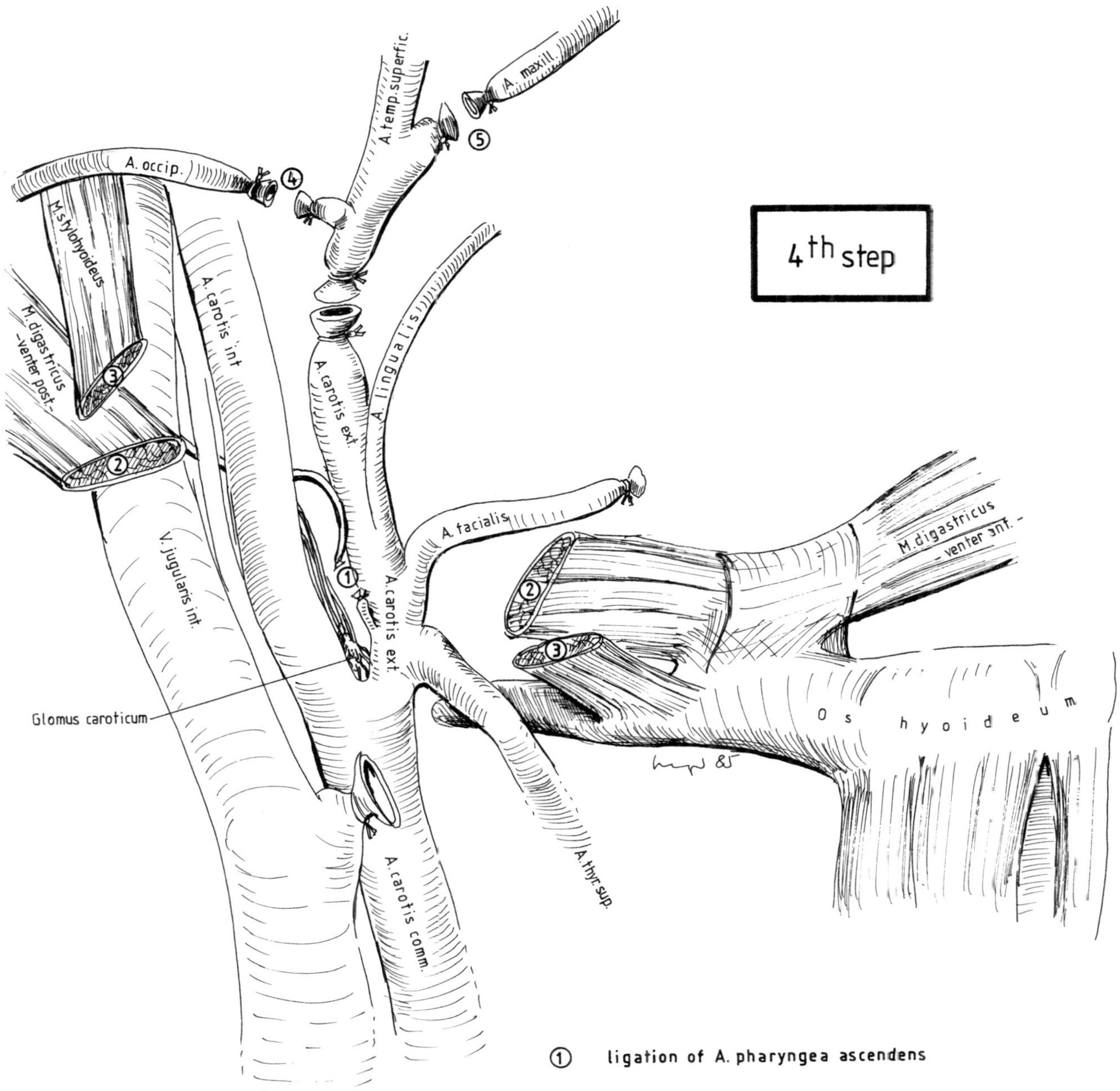

① ligation of A. pharyngea ascendens

② M. digastricus cut

③ M. stylohyoideus cut

④ A. occipitalis } ligation

⑤ A. maxillaris } ligation

Fig. 182

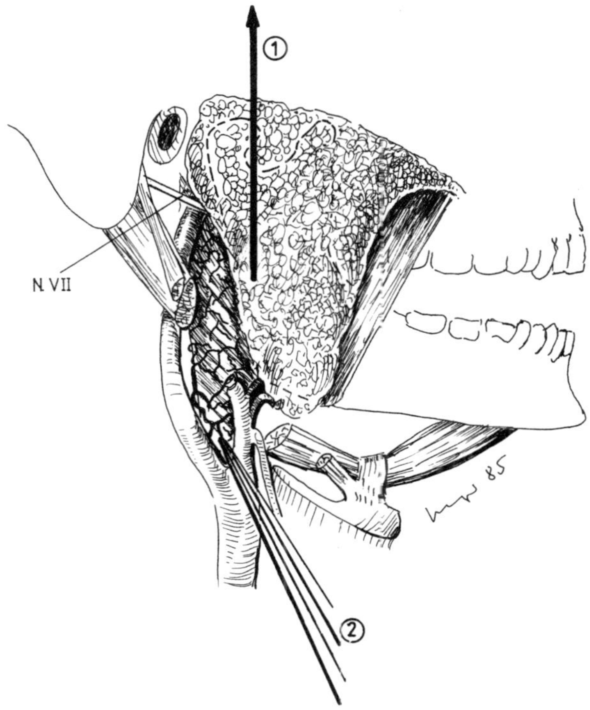

5th step

① elevation of skin-parotis-muscle-flap as 6th step①
- cave traction N.VII -

② coagulation of retropharyngeal plexus
(arteries and veins)

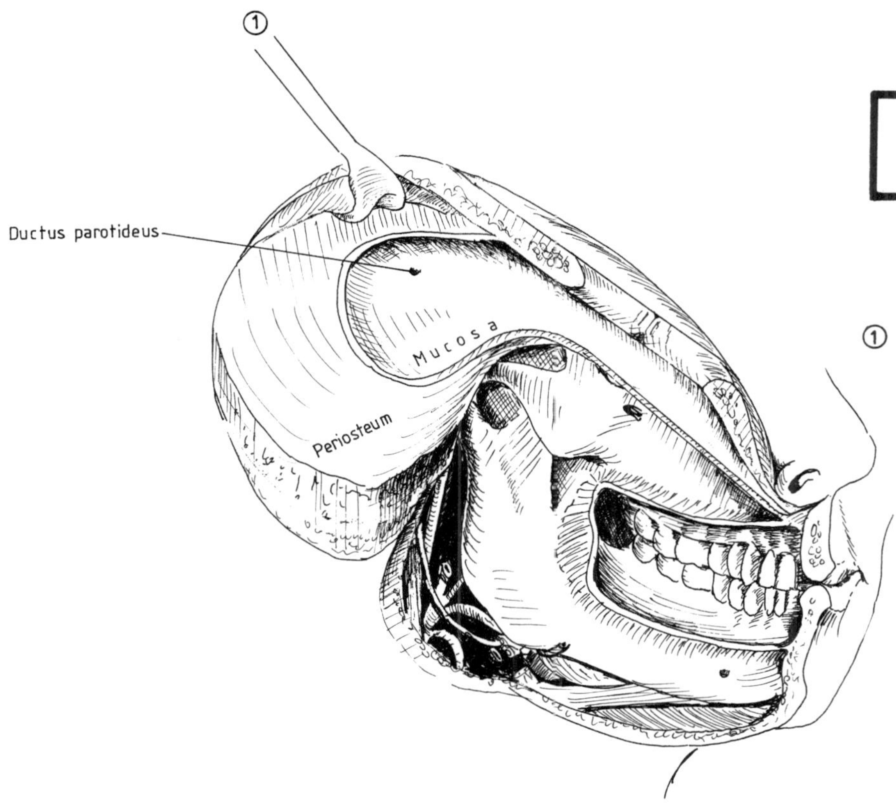

6th step

① elevation of flap as 5th step①.
(Glandula parotis + facial nerve
+ facial muscle + M. masseter
+ Mucosa)
flap mobilized

Fig. 183

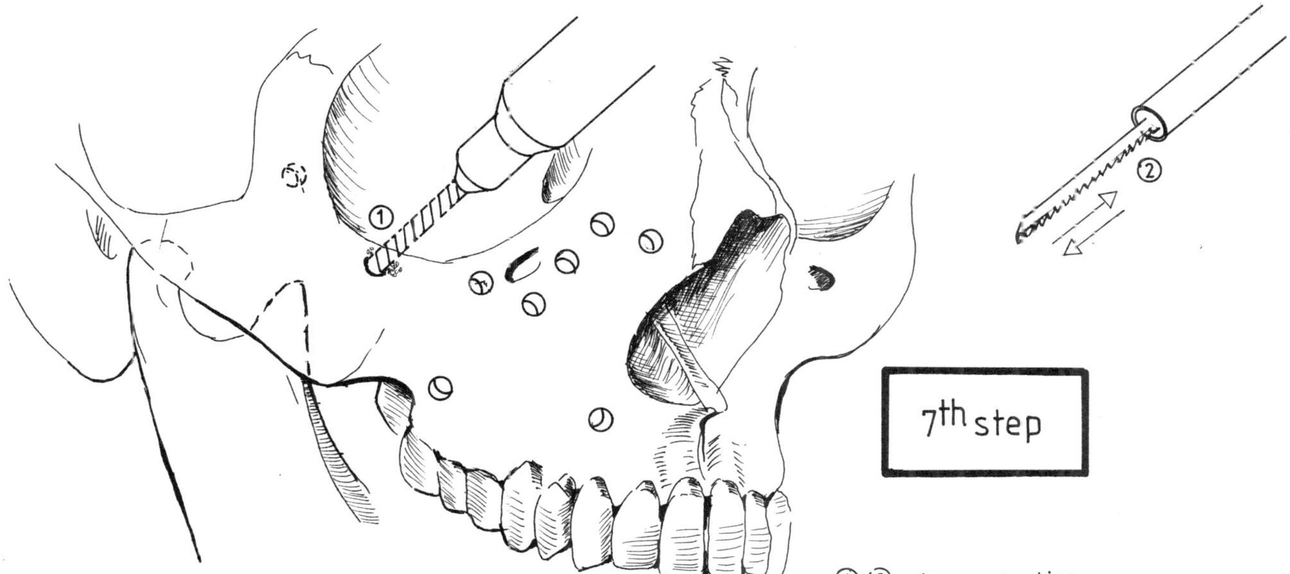

7th step

①+② bone resection

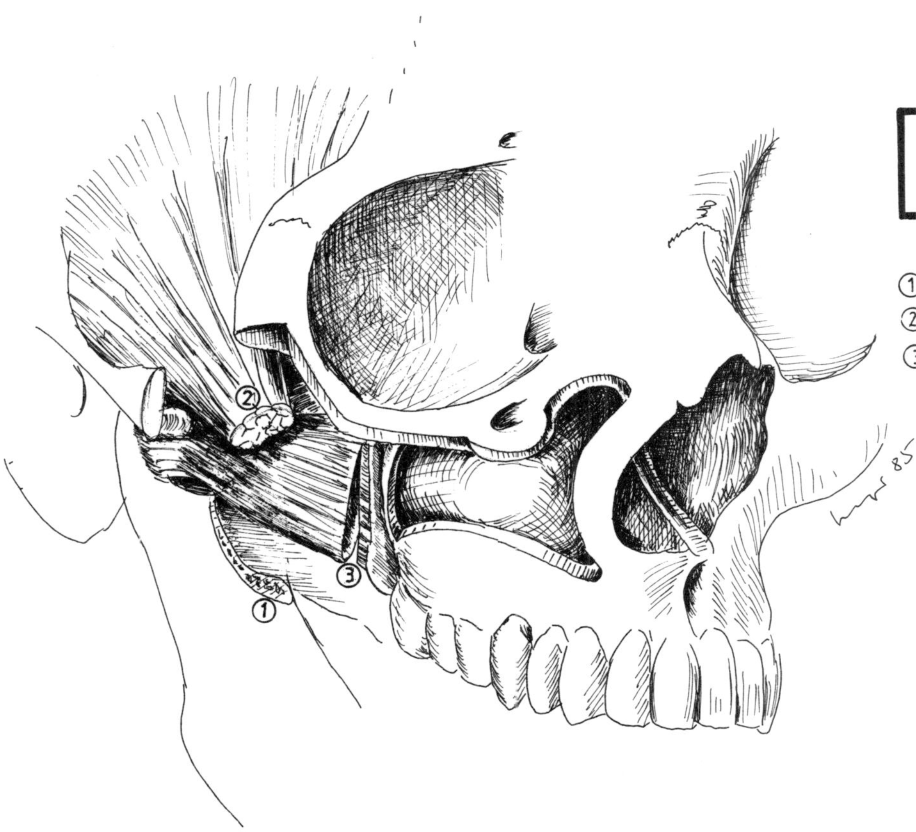

8th step

① Proc. coron. mandibulae cut
② M. temp. cut
③ M. pterygoid. lat. cut

Fig. 184

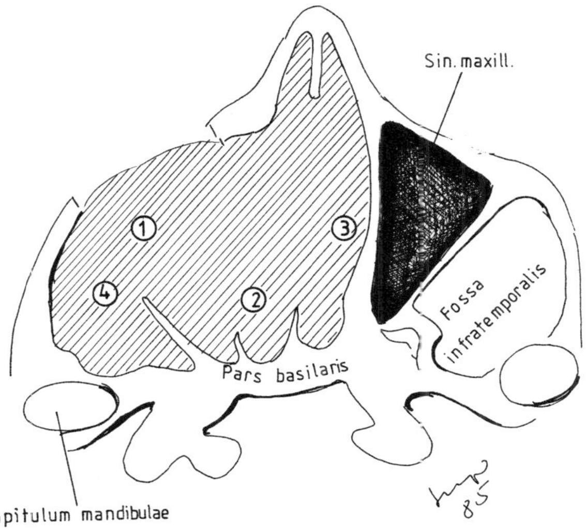

9th step

tumor removal from

1. Sin. maxillaris
2. 3. Cavum nasi bilaterally
4. Fossa infratemporalis = retromaxill.

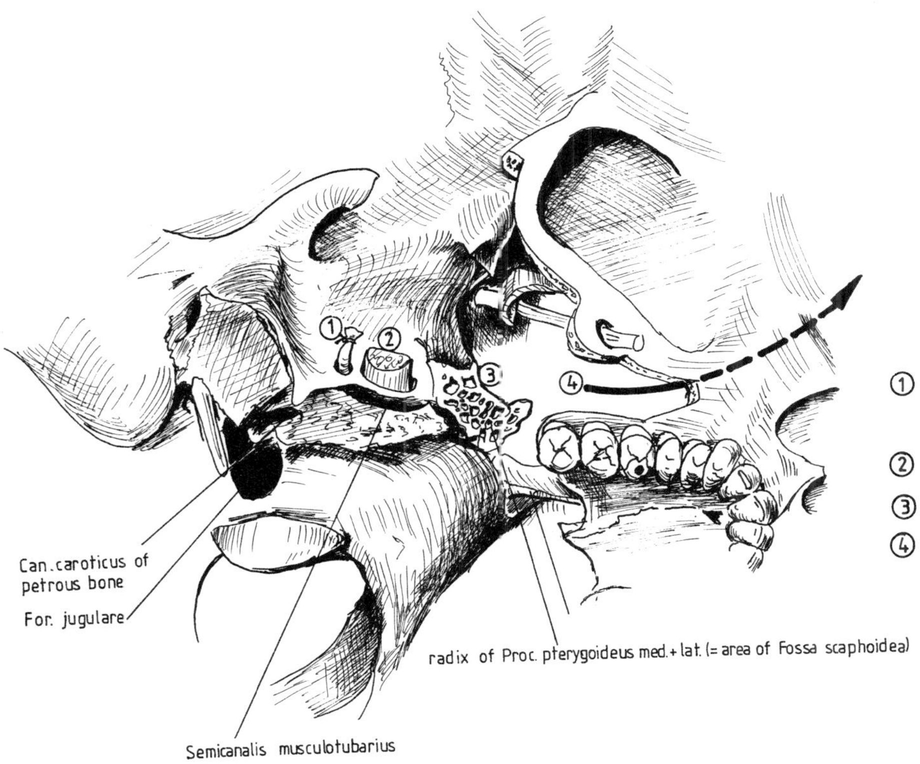

10th step

1. ligation and cutting of A. menirgea media
2. cutting of N. mandibularis
3. tumor removal in Fossa retromaxill.
4. " " from ethmoid

Fig. 185

FIG. 185

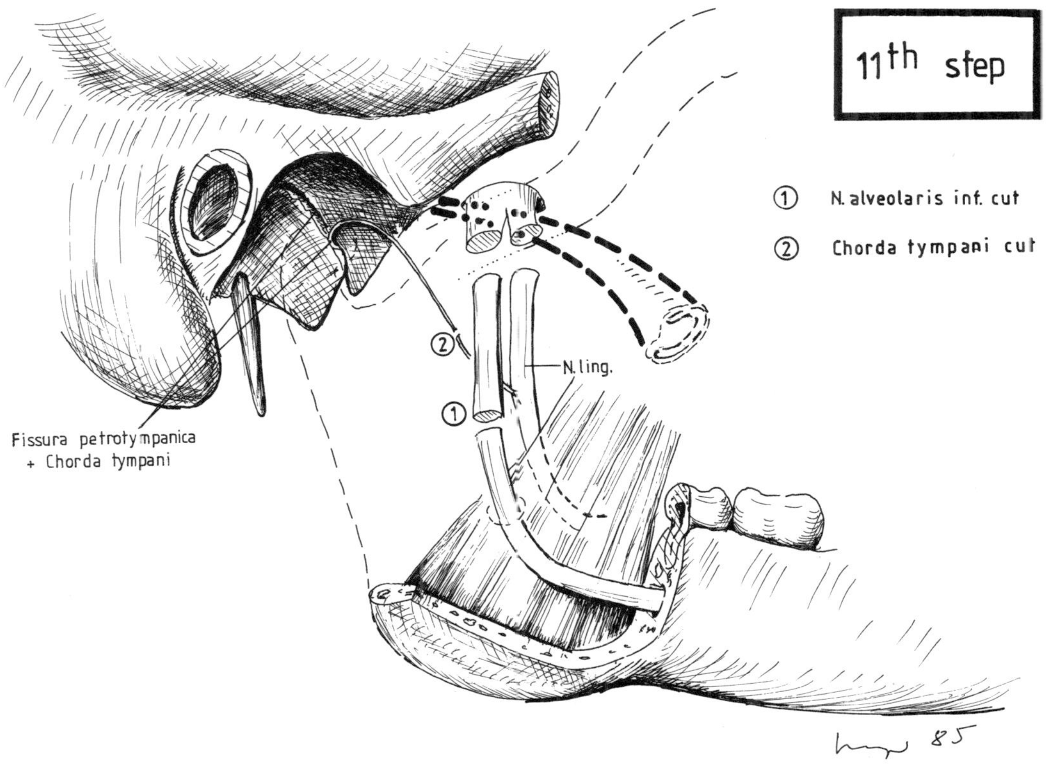
11th step
① N. alveolaris inf. cut
② Chorda tympani cut
N. ling.
Fissura petrotympanica
+ Chorda tympani

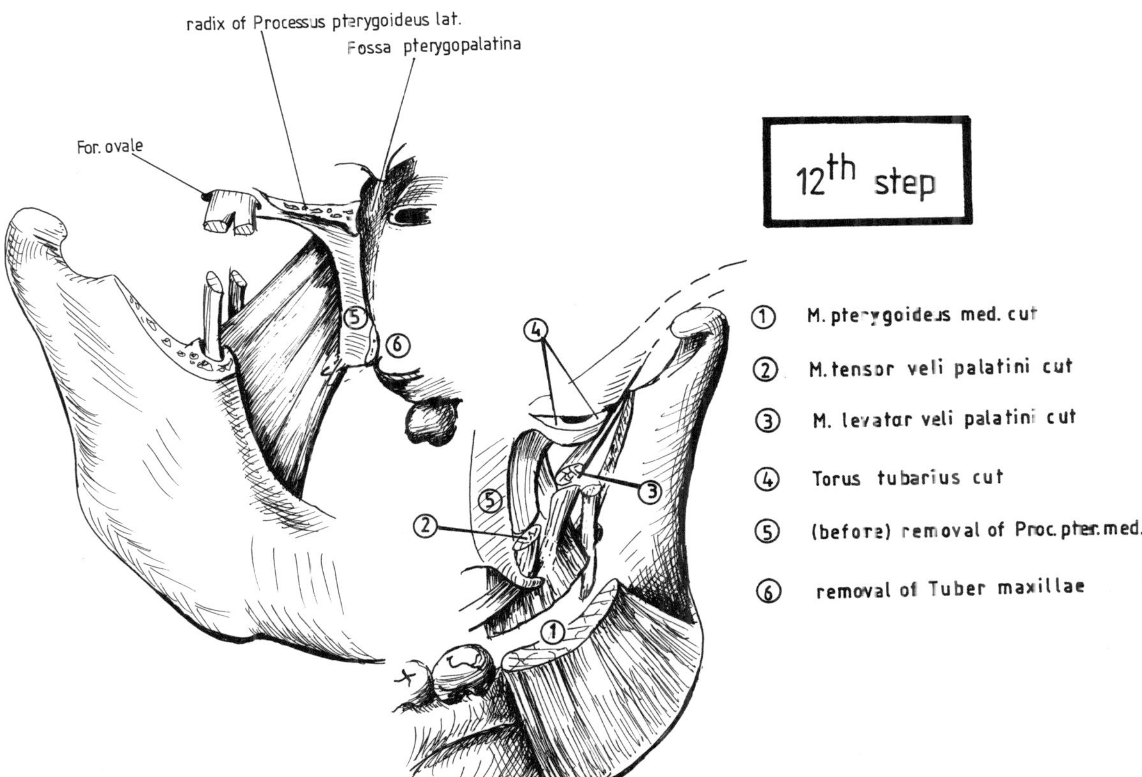
radix of Processus pterygoideus lat.
Fossa pterygopalatina
For. ovale
12th step
① M. pterygoideus med. cut
② M. tensor veli palatini cut
③ M. levator veli palatini cut
④ Torus tubarius cut
⑤ (before) removal of Proc. pter. med.
⑥ removal of Tuber maxillae

Fig. 186

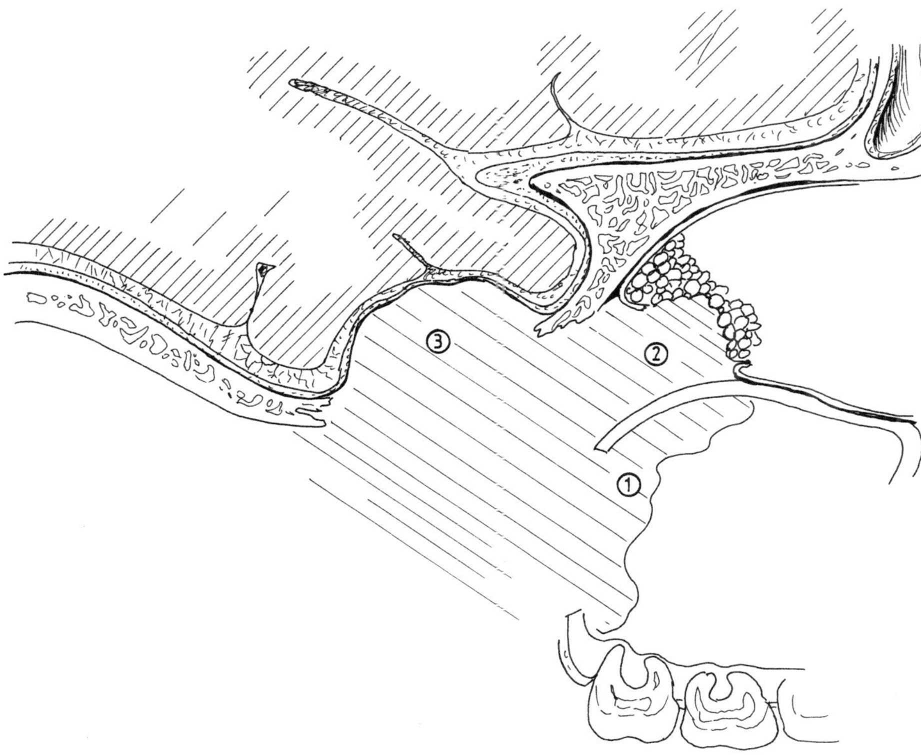

13th step

removal of tumor from

① Sinus maxillaris (residual tumor)

② Orbita

③ epidural space

④ Sinus sphenoidalis

⑤ Cavum nasi

⑥ Cellulae ethmoidales

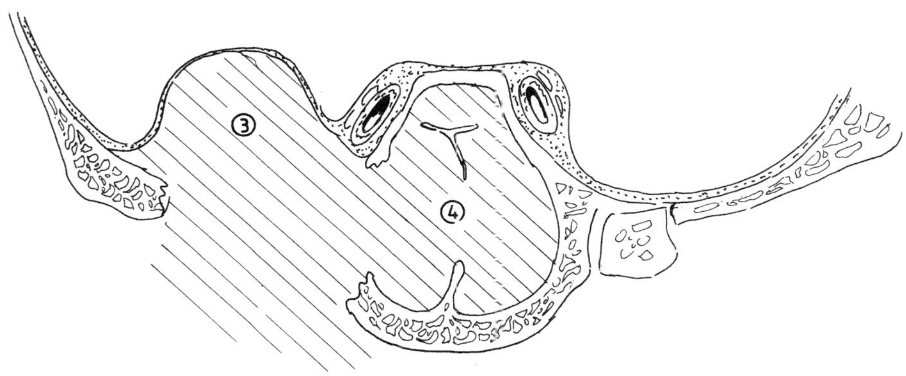

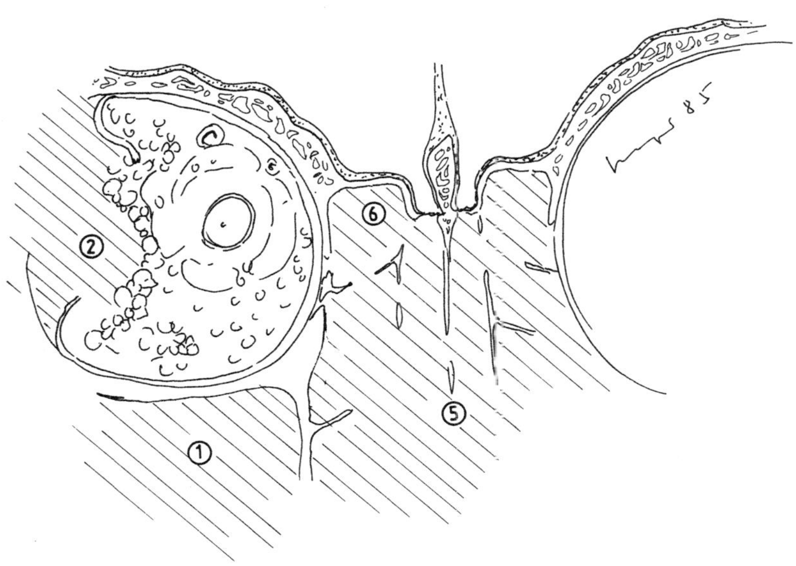

Fig. 187

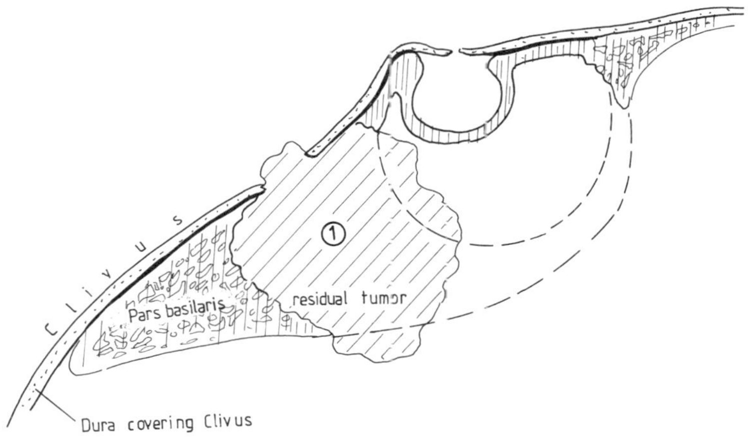

14th step

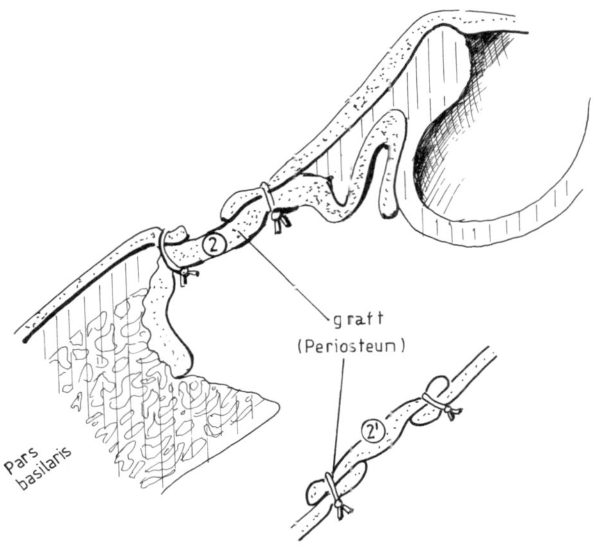

① removal of residual tumor

② closure of dura defect after tumor removal

②' preferable, but only in few cases practicable

③ additional closure of dura defect

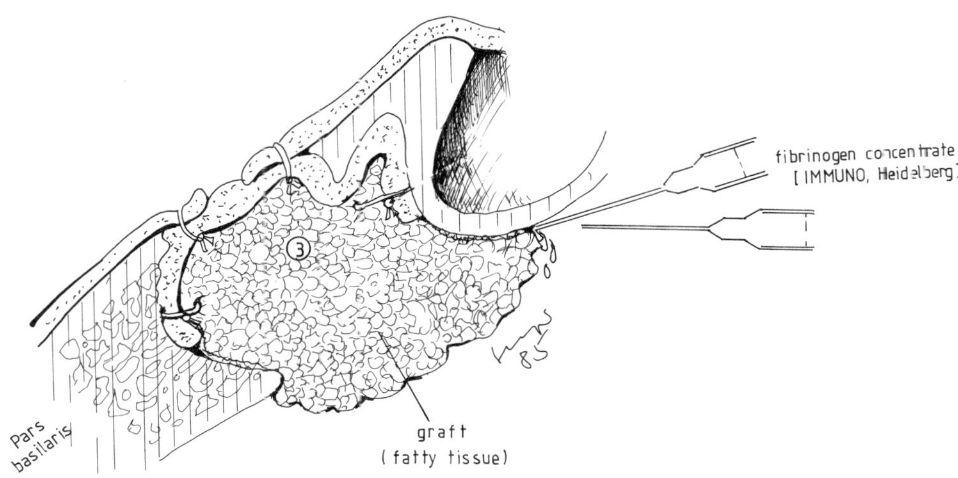

Fig. 188

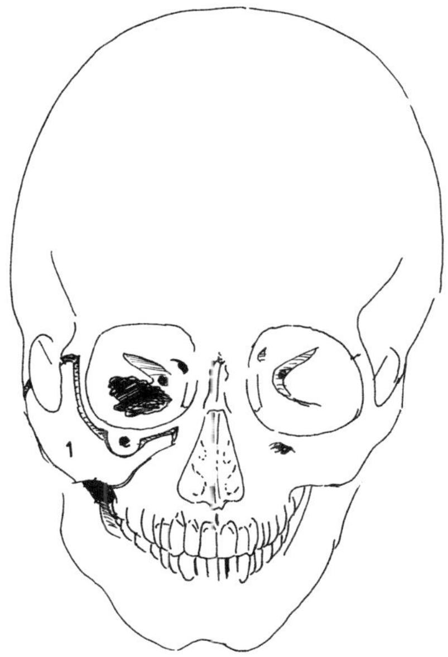

15th step

wound closure

① reimplantation of bone graft

② suture of Mucosa

③ suture of Subcutis / Cutis

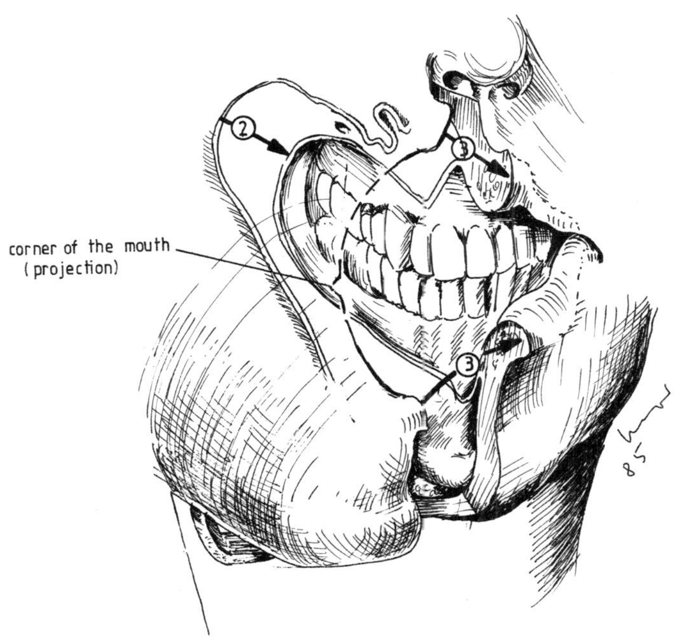

Fig. 189. The example below of the skin cut is preferable. Here the skin-muscle-flap can be pulled up almost to the level of Orbita

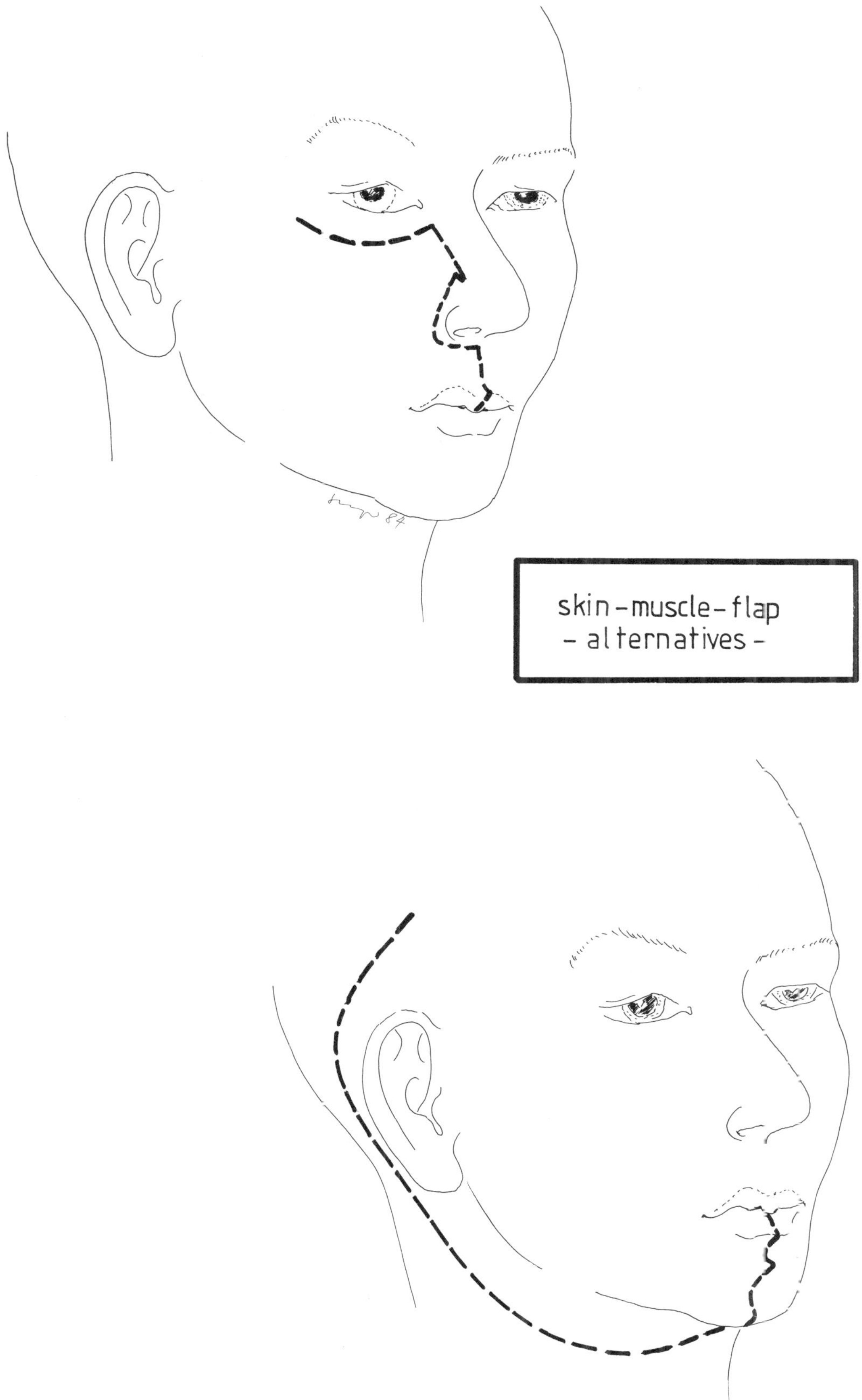
skin-muscle-flap
- alternatives -

Fig. 190. In the present case a larger skin-muscle-flap was chosen because of the expansion of the tumor

FIG. 190

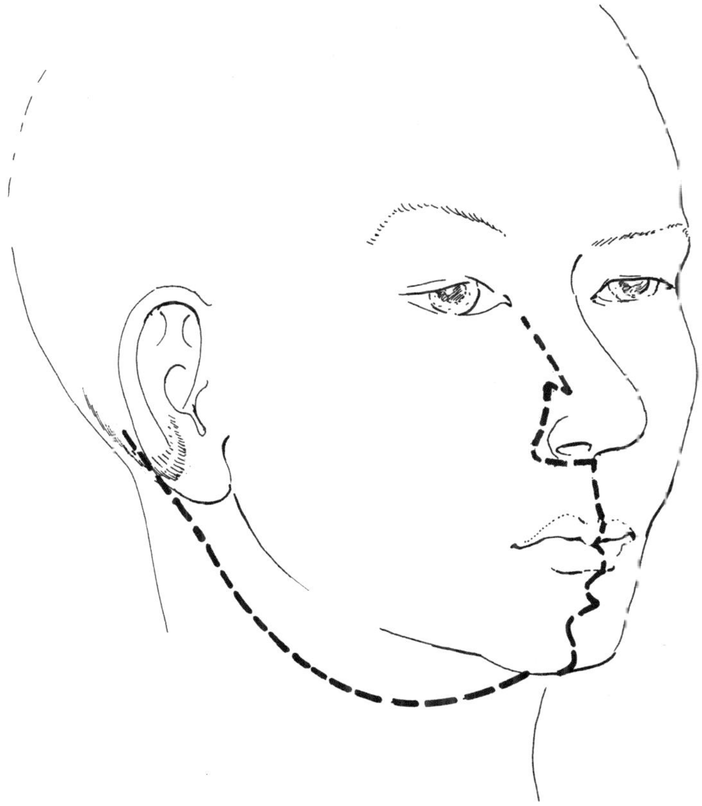

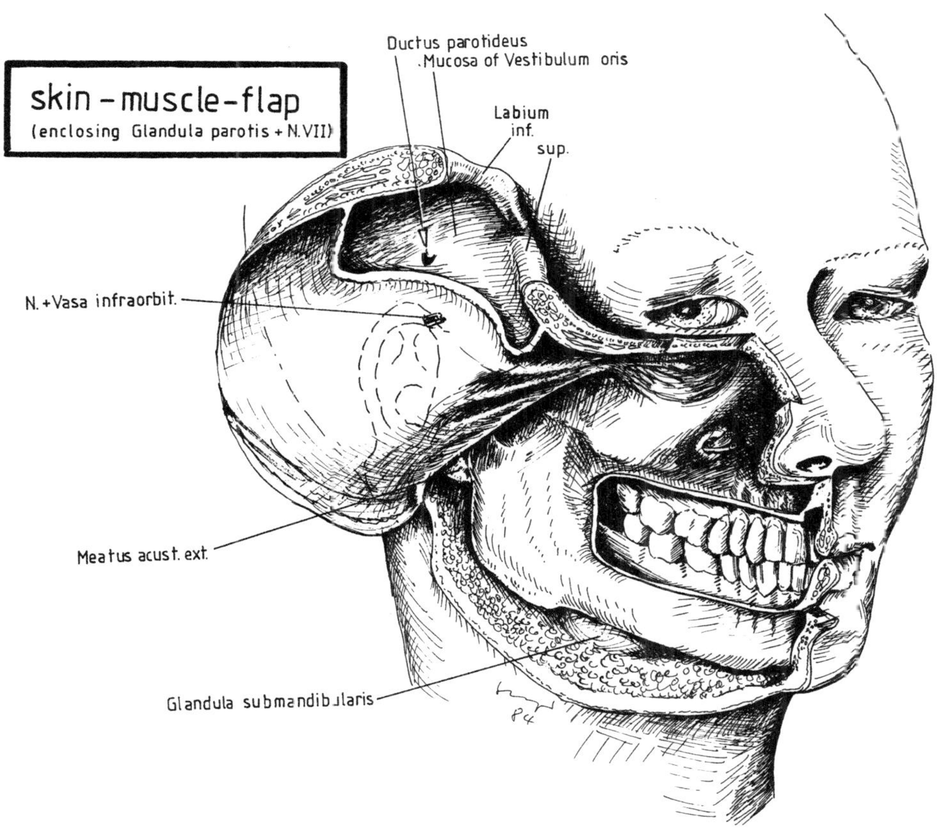
skin - muscle - flap
(enclosing Glandula parotis + N. VII)
Ductus parotideus
Mucosa of Vestibulum oris
Labium
inf.
sup.
N. + Vasa infraorbit.
Meatus acust. ext.
Glandula submandibularis

Fig. 191

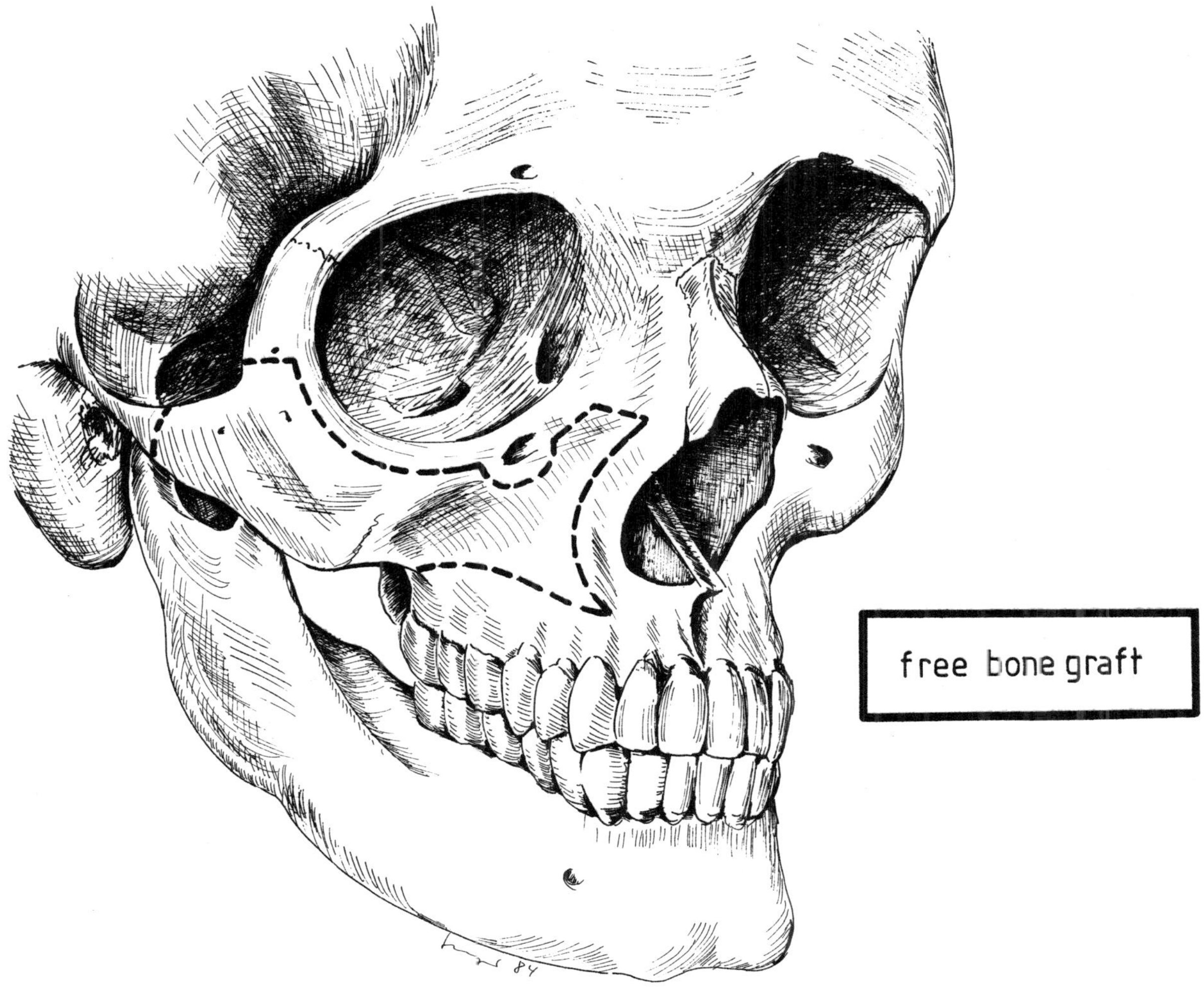
free bone graft

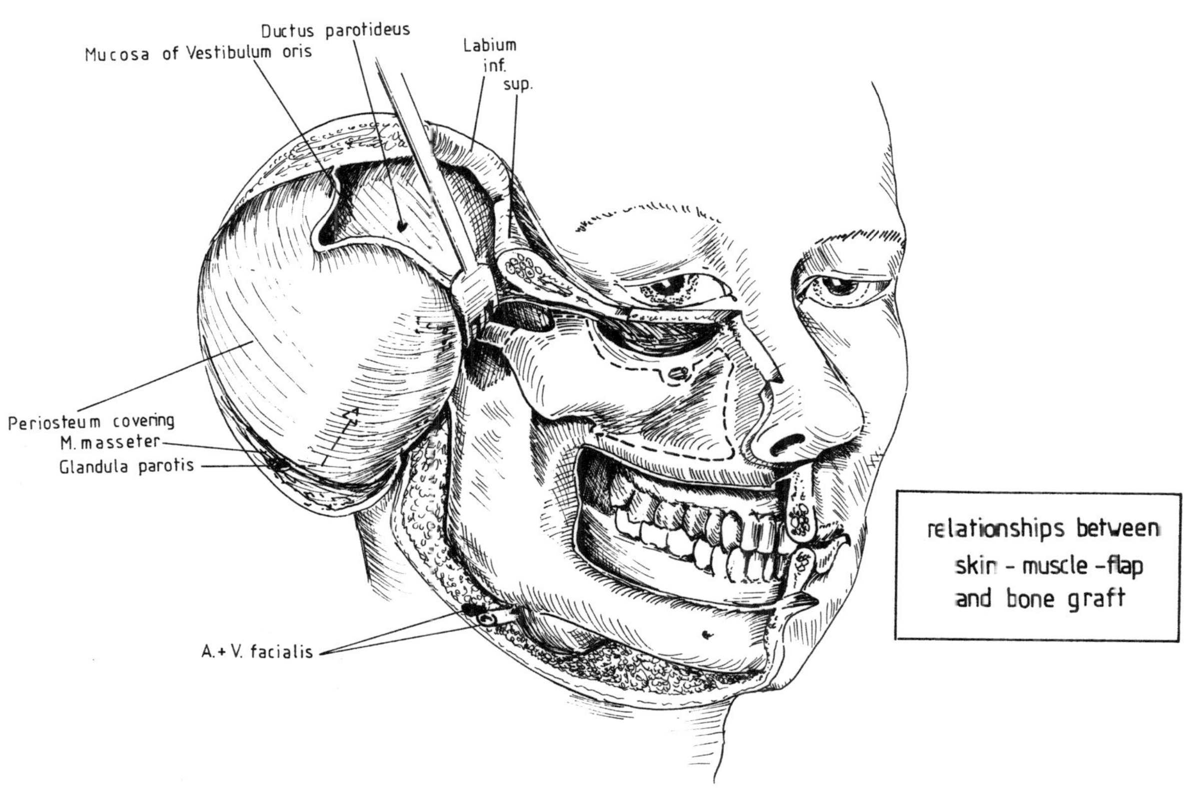
Ductus parotideus
Mucosa of Vestibulum oris
Labium
inf.
sup.
Periosteum covering
M. masseter
Glandula parotis
A.+V. facialis
relationships between
skin - muscle -flap
and bone graft

Fig. 192

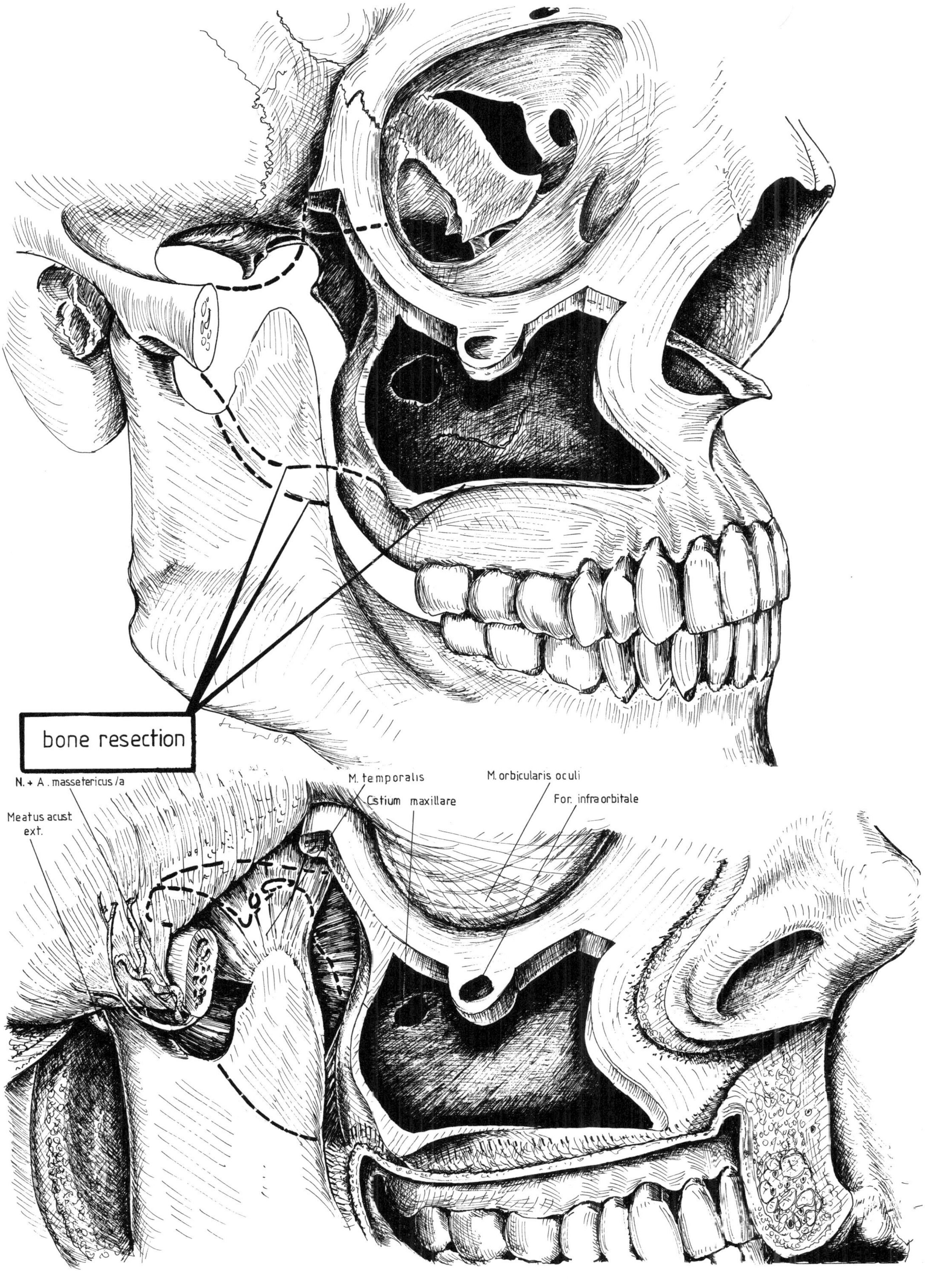
bone resection
N. + A. massetericus /a
Meatus acust. ext.
M. temporalis
Ostium maxillare
M. orbicularis oculi
For. infraorbitale

Fig. 193

microsurgical topography

after resection of

- lateral wall of Sinus maxillaris (Os zygomaticum + Os maxillare)
- Processus coronoideus mandibulae
- Arcus zygomaticus

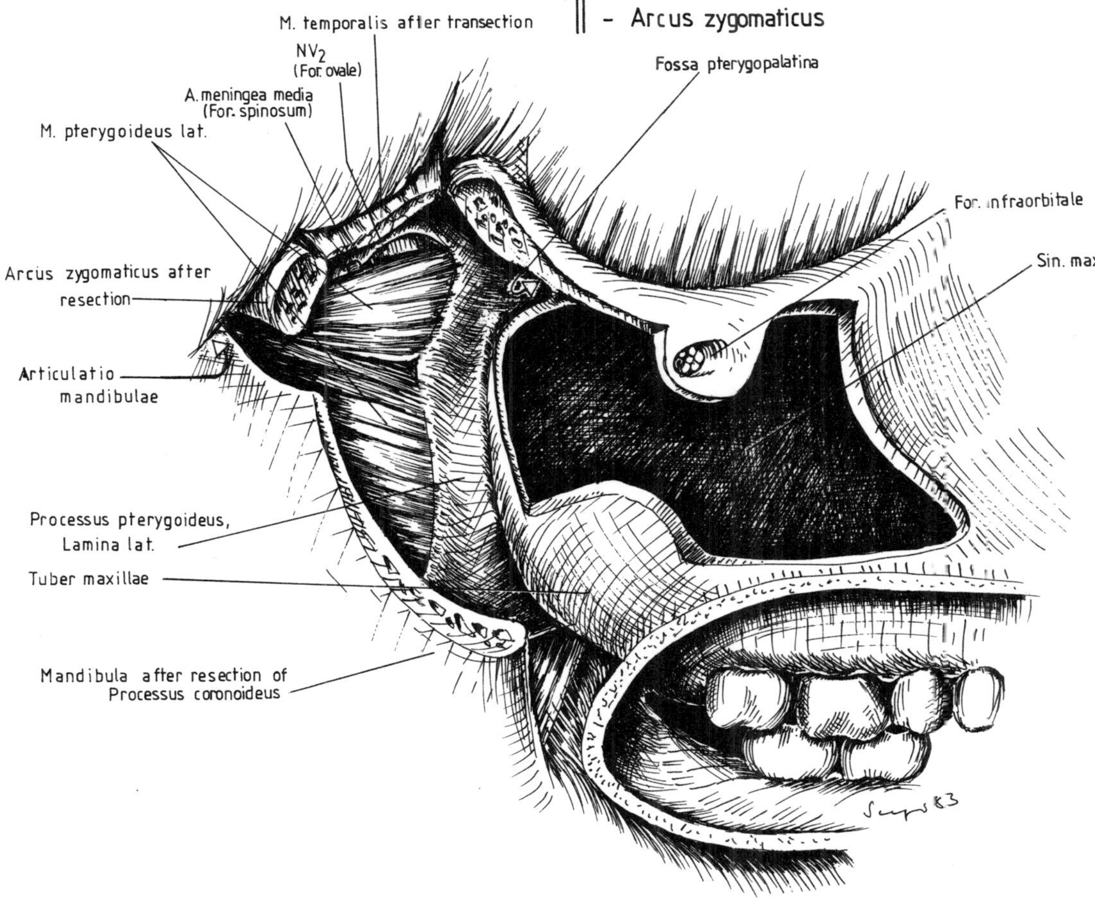

Fig. 194

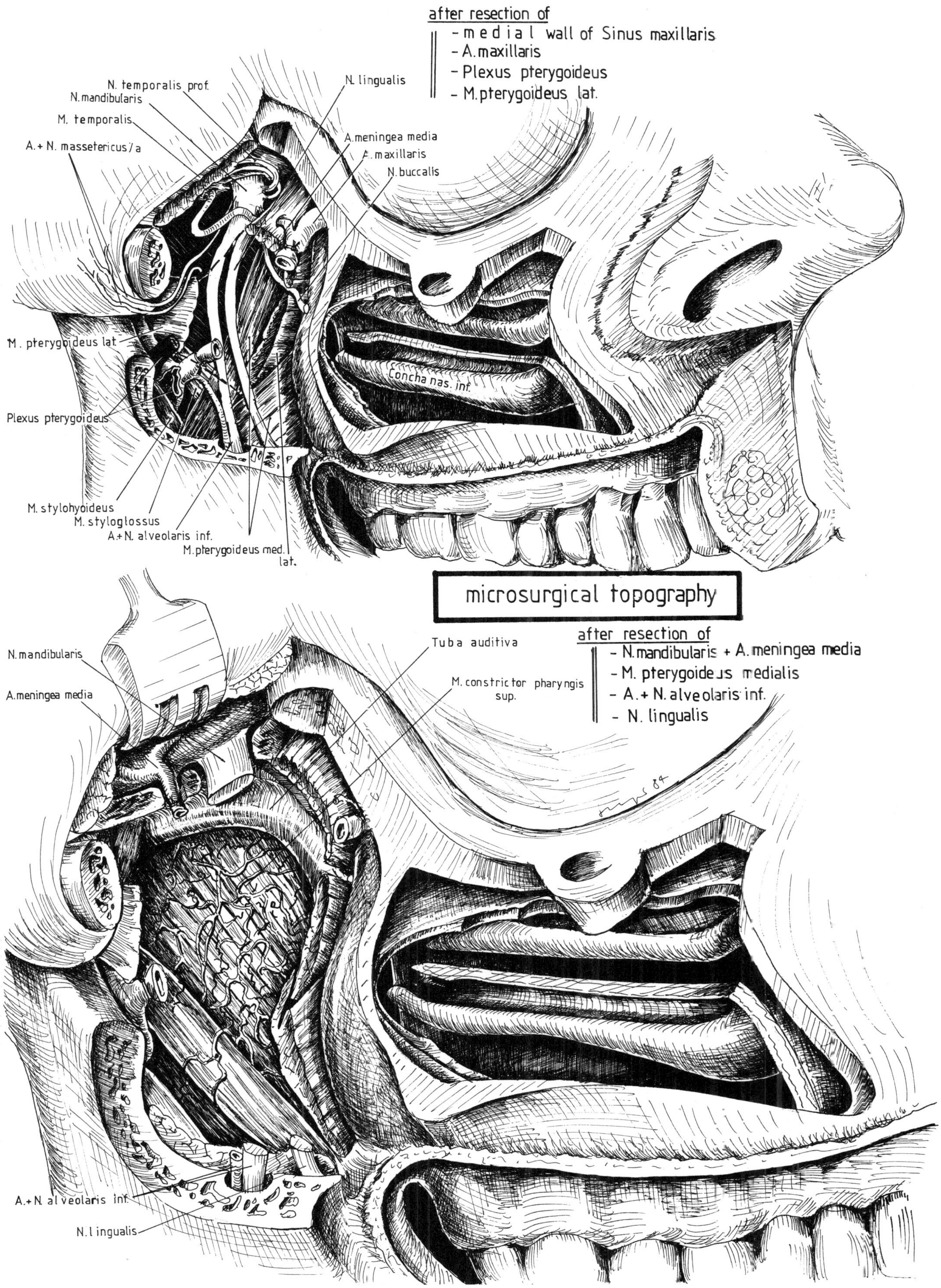
after resection of
- m e d i a l wall of Sinus maxillaris
- A. maxillaris
- Plexus pterygoideus
- M. pterygoideus lat.
N. temporalis prof.
N. mandibularis
M. temporalis
A.+N. massetericus/a
N. lingualis
A. meningea media
A. maxillaris
N. buccalis
M. pterygoideus lat.
Concha nas. inf.
Plexus pterygoideus
M. stylohyoideus
M. styloglossus
A.+N. alveolaris inf.
M. pterygoideus med.
lat.
microsurgical topography
after resection of
- N. mandibularis + A. meningea media
- M. pterygoideus medialis
- A.+N. alveolaris inf.
- N. lingualis
Tuba auditiva
M. constrictor pharyngis sup.
N. mandibularis
A. meningea media
A.+N. alveolaris inf.
N. lingualis

Fig. 195

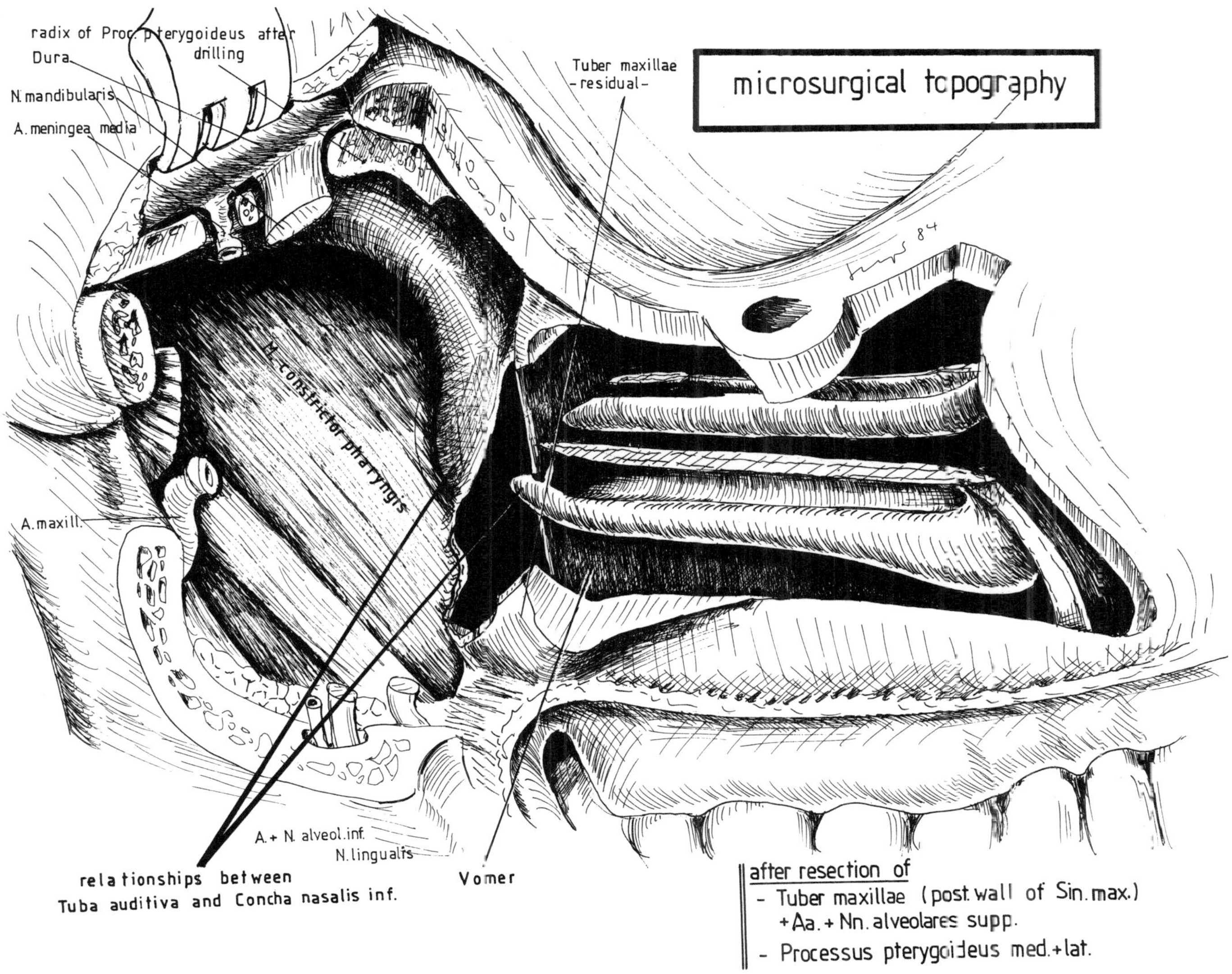
radix of Proc. pterygoideus after drilling
Dura
N. mandibularis
A. meningea media
Tuber maxillae -residual-
microsurgical topography
M. constrictor pharyngis
A. maxill.
A. + N. alveol. inf.
N. lingualis
relationships between Tuba auditiva and Concha nasalis inf.
Vomer
after resection of
- Tuber maxillae (post. wall of Sin. max.) + Aa. + Nn. alveolares supp.
- Processus pterygoideus med. + lat.

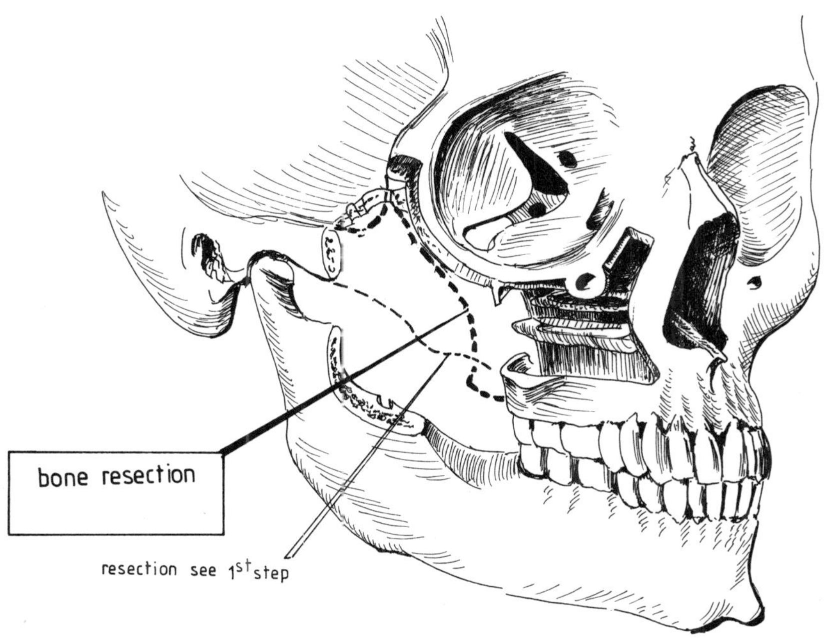
bone resection
resection see 1st step

Fig. 196. Microsurgical topography after removal of the tumor, supplemented by anatomical sketches of the resection in the area of the bony base

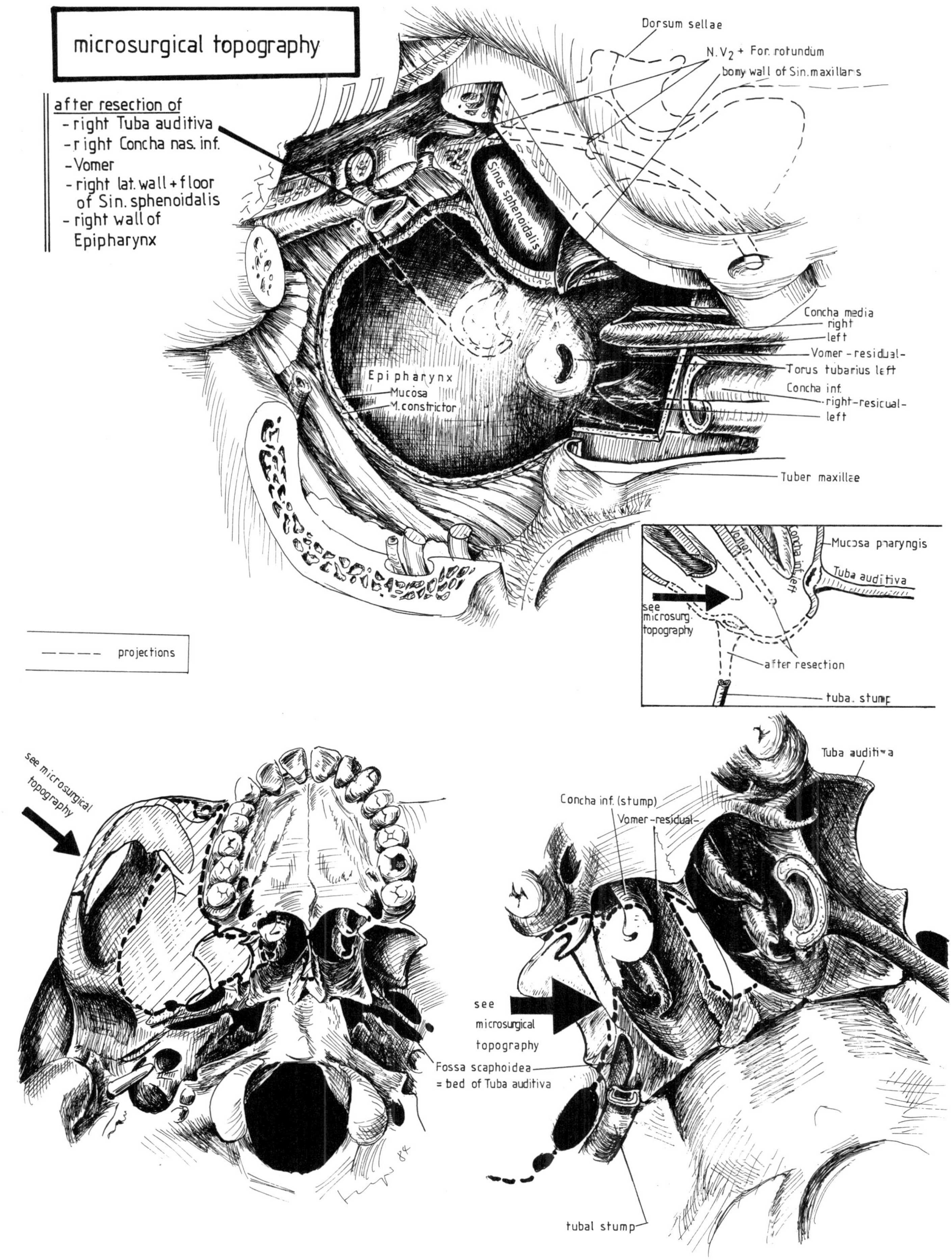

microsurgical topography
after resection of
- right Tuba auditiva
- right Concha nas. inf.
- Vomer
- right lat. wall + floor of Sin. sphenoidalis
- right wall of Epipharynx
Dorsum sellae
N. V2 + For. rotundum
bony wall of Sin. maxillaris
Sinus sphenoidalis
Concha media
right
left
Vomer -residual-
Torus tubarius left
Concha inf.
right -residual-
left
Epipharynx
Mucosa
M. constrictor
Tuber maxillae
projections
Vomer
Concha inf. left
Mucosa pharyngis
Tuba auditiva
see microsurg. topography
after resection
tubal stump
see microsurgical topography
Tuba auditiva
Concha inf. (stump)
Vomer -residual-
see microsurgical topography
Fossa scaphoidea = bed of Tuba auditiva
tubal stump

Fig. 197. Greatly magnified microsurgical site* of another clinical case**. In 1983 radiation therapy for an epithelial carcinoma of the left nasal passage (total dose 60 Gy). Since four months stabbing pain in the left ear and one-sided headache with poor hearing on the left since four weeks. Reduction in sensitivity of the left border of the tongue, vomiting reflex absent on both sides, reduction in movement of the left half of the soft palate. CT: tumor of the Epipharynx and Fossa infratemporalis extending to the Tuber maxillare and hard palate. Postoperatively bleeding from nose and mouth, nasal tamponade, temporary bleeding also from the left ear. Awake, orientated, apart from facial paresis and non-function of the mandibular nerve, no additional neurological deficits as compared with preoperatively

* From a photo made by Prof. Dr. W. Mann.

** Operation performed alternately by Prof. Dr. W. Mann (Ear, Nose and Throat Clinic of Freiburg University, Director: Prof. Dr. Chl. Beck) and Prof. Dr. J. Gilsbach, coworker of the author.

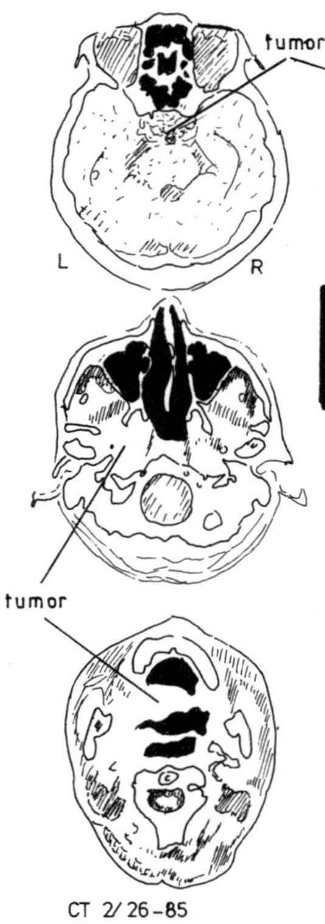

preoperative findings

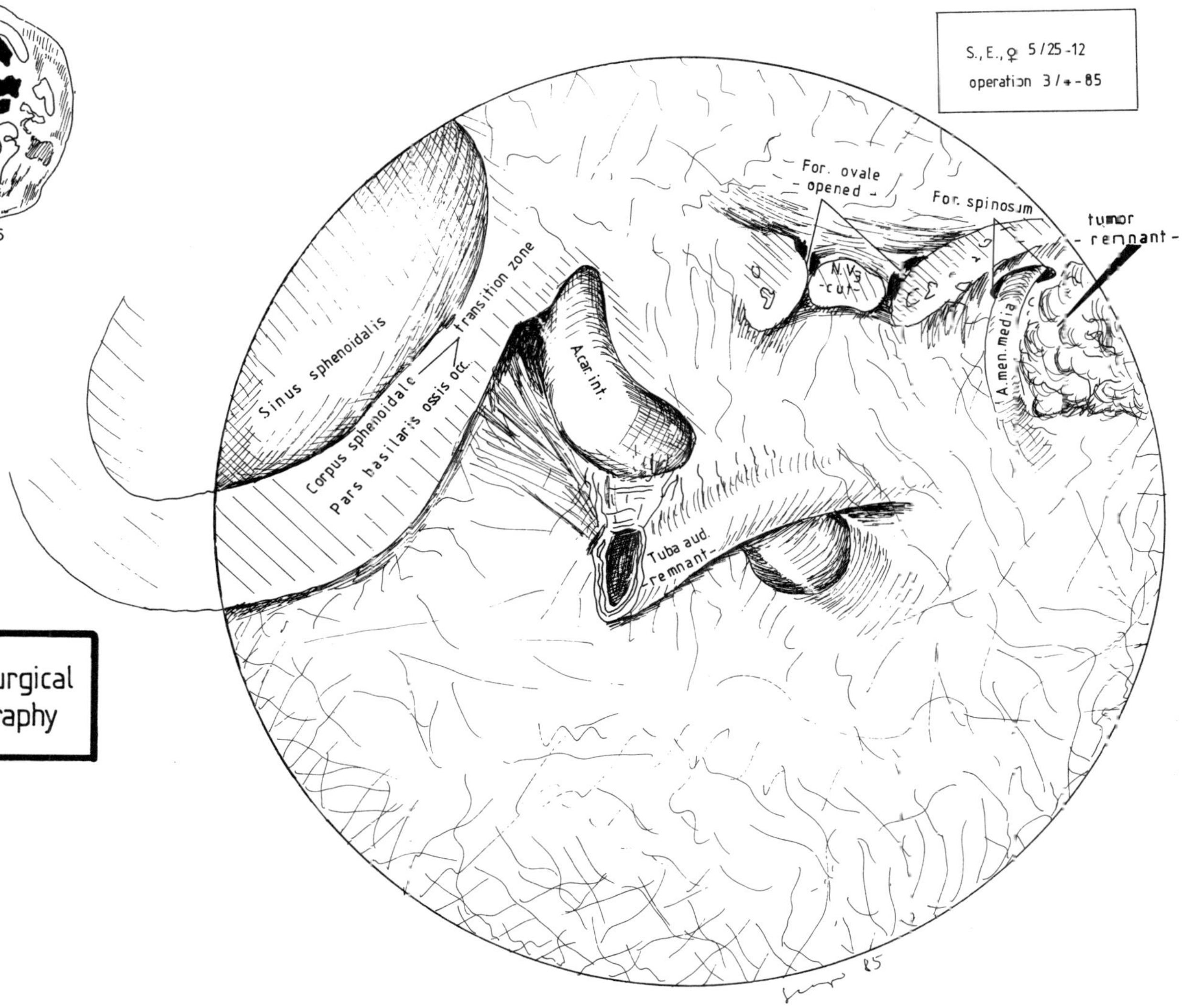

microsurgical topography

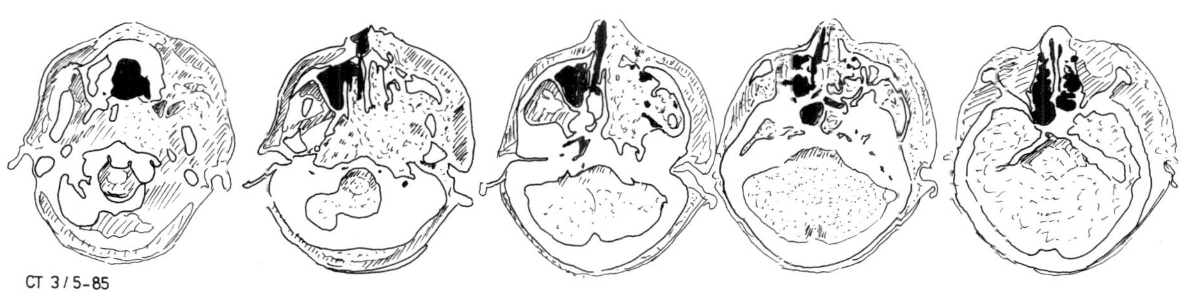

postop.

Fig. 198

reimplantation of bone graft

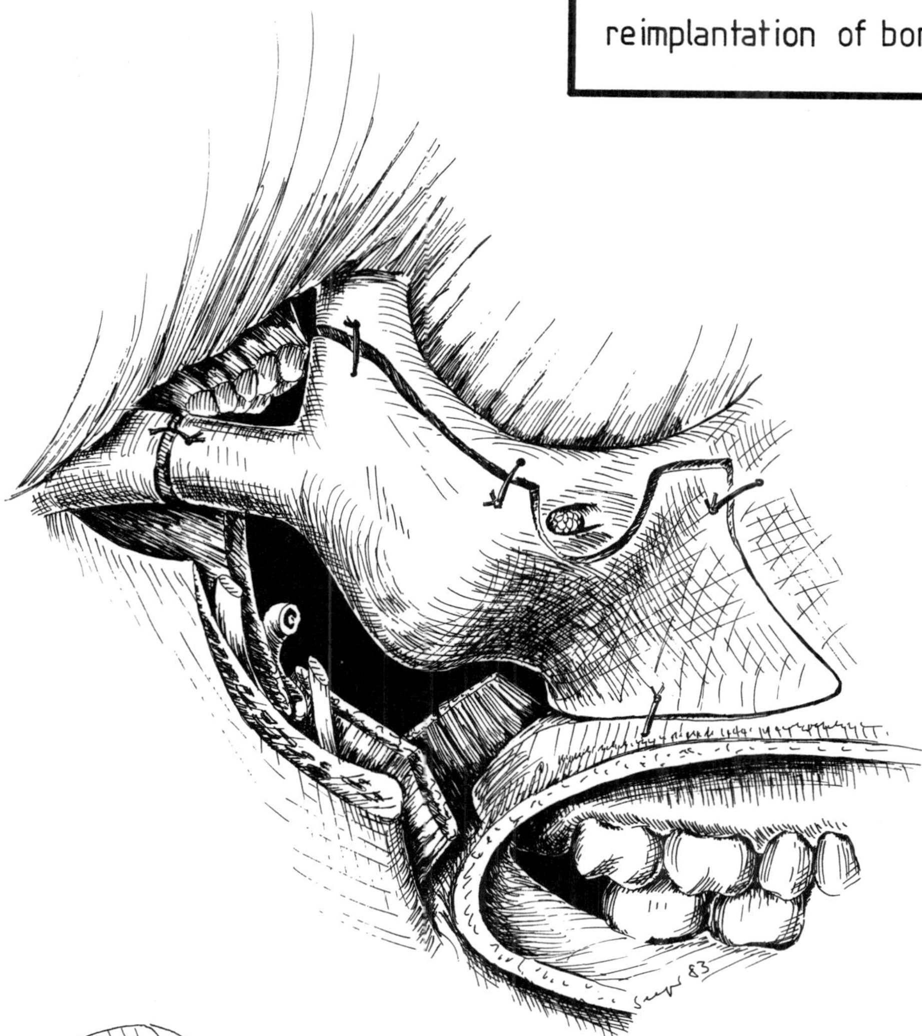

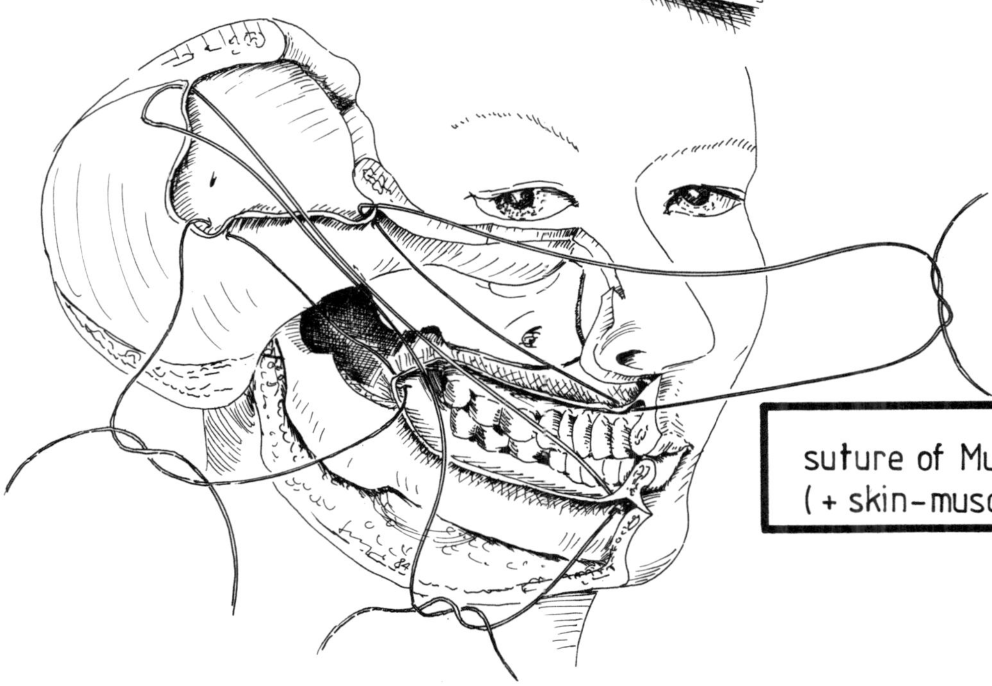

suture of Mucosa of Vestibulum oris
(+ skin-muscle-flap)

Chapter 9
Basal Cisterns, Posterior Segment
(Figs. 199–201)

Fig. 199
A Typical approach
B Dorso-lateral approach with resection of the Condylus occipitalis and the Tuberculum jugulare *

* The following indicates the principle only briefly. The method was developed by the author in 1976 and presented in Seeger, W., Topographical Anatomy of the Brain and Surrounding Structures, and Seeger, W., Microsurgery of Cerebral Veins. Wien–New York: Springer. 1978 and 1984.

ventrolateral aneurysm of "pica" ⊙

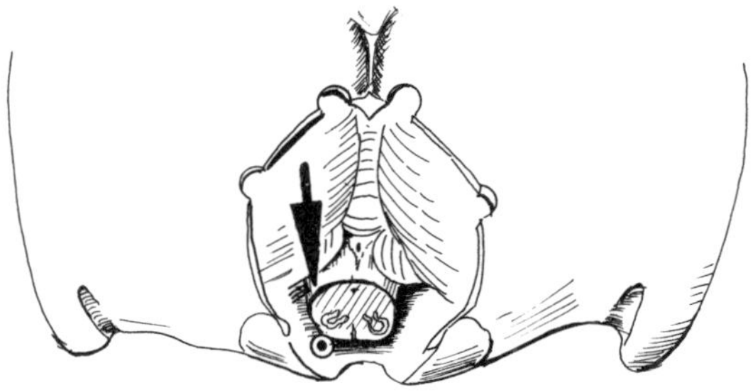

favorable: well known approach

unfavorable: approach hindered by Medulla oblongata + cranial nerves

Ⓐ midline approach

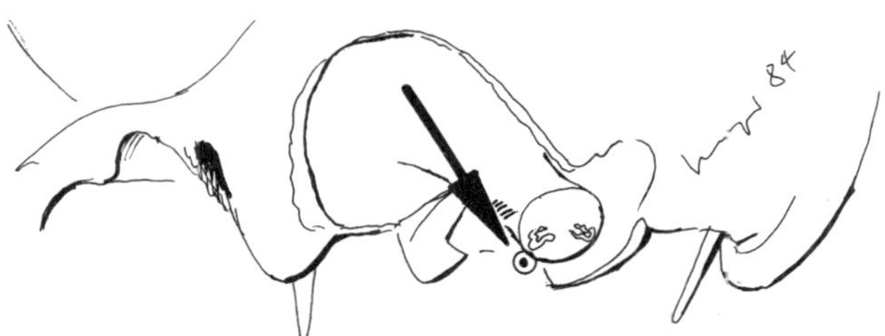

favorable: approach not hindered by Medulla oblongata

unfavorable: approach hindered by cranial nerves

Ⓑ dorsolateral approach

Fig. 200. Clinical case of a "PICA" aneurysm with subarachnoid haemorrhage on November 19, 1984, and operated at the acute stage. Preoperatively grade II to III. Postoperatively no deficits, rapid recovery *

* Operation performed by Dr. W. Hassler, coworker of the author.

(B)

preoperative findings

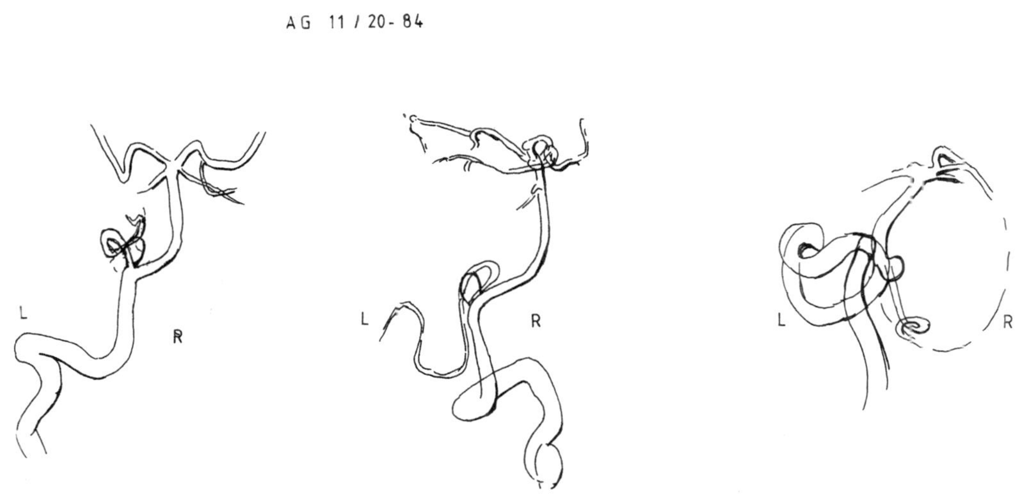

B., O., ♀, 6/30 - 44
op. 11 / 20 - 84

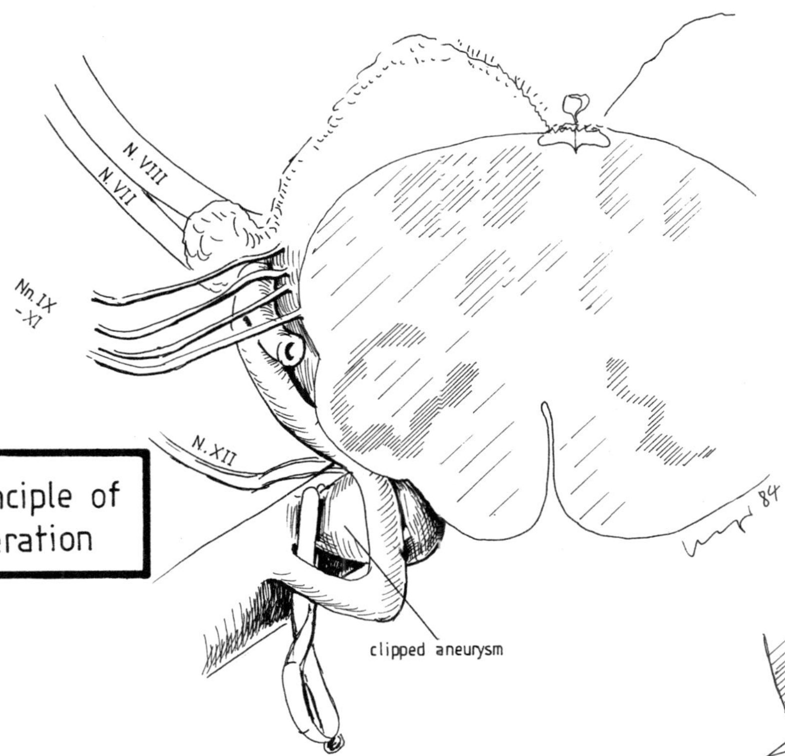

principle of operation

pcstop. findi-gs

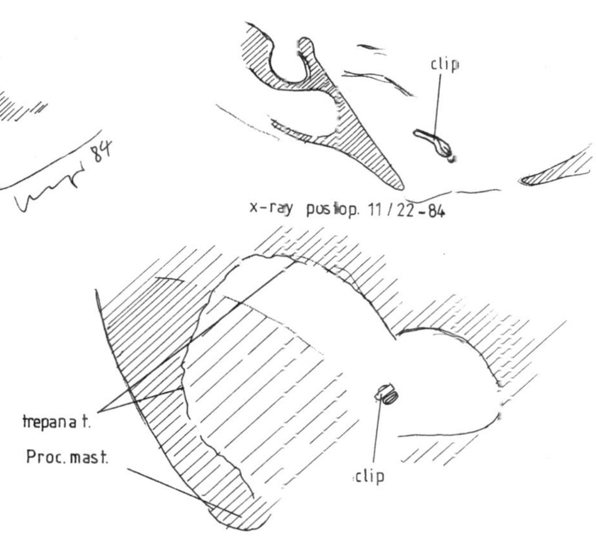

Fig. 201. Clinical case from Fig. 200

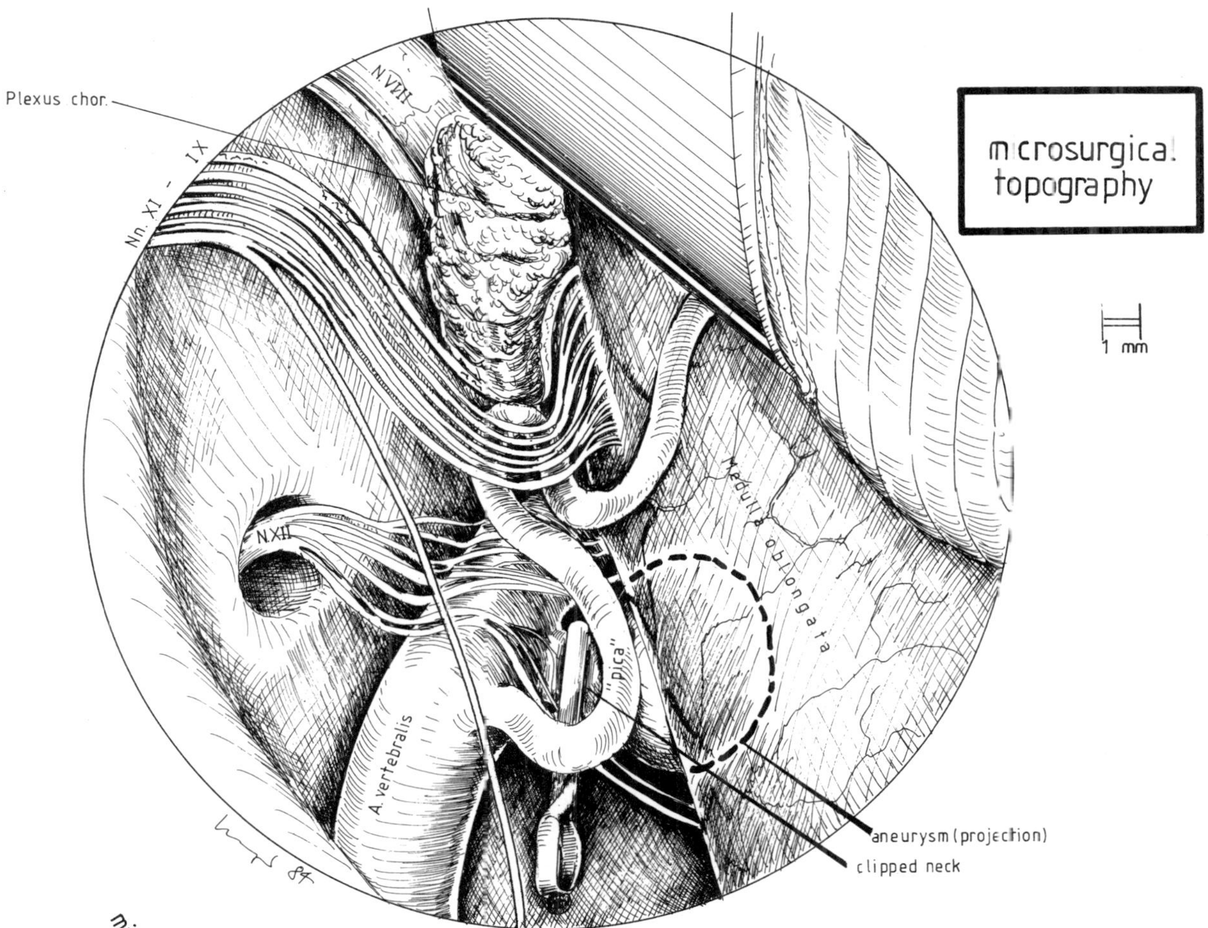
Plexus chor.
N.VIII
Nn.XI - IX
N.XII
A. vertebralis
"pica"
Medulla oblongata
aneurysm (projection)
clipped neck
microsurgical topography
1 mm

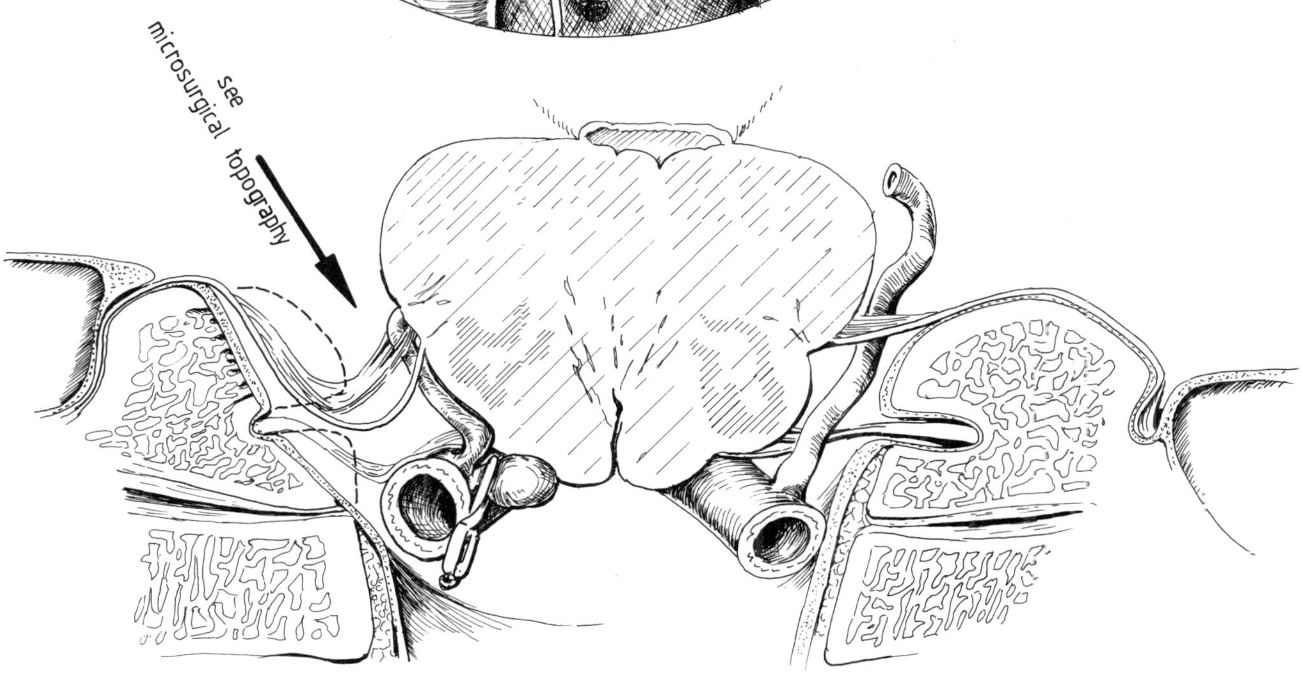
see microsurgical topography

References

Chapter 1

Becker, H.: Die Bedeutung der arteriellen Grenzzonen für die Pathologie der Hirndurchblutung. Dtsch. Z. Nervenheilk. **164,** 560 (1950).

Cushing, H.: Intracranial Tumours. Notes upon a series of two thousand verified cases with surgical-mortality percentages pertaining thereto. Springfield, Ill.: Ch. C Thomas. 1932.

Guleke, N.: Die Eingriffe am Gehirnschädel, Gehirn, an der Wirbelsäule und am Rückenmark. In: Allgemeine und spezielle Operationslehre (Guleke, N., Zenker, R., eds.), Vol. 2, 2nd ed., pp. 335–343. Berlin–Göttingen–Heidelberg: Springer. 1950.

Kempe, L. G.: Operative Neurosurgery, Vol. 1. Berlin–Heidelberg–New York: Springer. 1968.

Key, A., Retzius: Studien in der Anatomie des Nervensystems und des Bindegewebes. Stockholm: Norstad. 1875.

Krayenbühl, H. A., Yaşargil, M. G.: Die zerebrale Angiographie. Lehrbuch für Klinik und Praxis. Stuttgart: Thieme. 1965.

Krayenbühl, H., Yaşargil, M. G., Hrsg. Peter Huber: Cerebrale Angiographie in Klinik und Praxis. Stuttgart: Thieme. 1979.

Nomina anatomica, fourth edition. Amsterdam–Oxford: Excerpta Medica. 1977.

Seeger, W.: Microsurgery of the Brain. Anatomical and Technical Principles, Vol. 1 + 2. Wien–New York: Springer. 1980.

Wilkins, R. H., Odom, G. L.: General operative technique. In: Neurological Surgery (Youmans, J. R., ed.), Vol. 5, pp. 527–550. Philadelphia–London–Toronto: Saunders. 1973.

Yaşargil, M. G., Microsurgical anatomy of the basal cisterns and vessels of the brain, diagnostic studies, general operative techniques and pathological considerations of the intracranial aneurysms. In: Microneurosurgery (Yaşargil, M. G., ed.), Vol. 1. Stuttgart–New York: Thieme. New York: Thieme Stratton. 1984.

Youmans, J. R.: Neurological Surgery, Vol. 6, 2nd Ed. A comprehensive Reference Guide to the Diagnoses and Management of Neurosurgical Problems. Philadelphia: W. B. Saunders Company. 1982.

Chapter 2

Benninghoff, A., Goerttler, K.: Lehrbuch der Anatomie des Menschen, Bd. III, 9. Aufl. (Ferner, H., Staubesand, J. eds.). München–Berlin–Wien: Urban und Schwarzenberg. 1975.

Chan, R. C., Thompson, G. B.: Third ventricular colloid cysts presenting with acute neurological deterioration. Surg. Neurol. **19,** 358–362 (1983).

McCormick, W. F., Hardmann, J. M., Boulter, T. B.: Vascular malformations ("Angiomas") of the brain with specific reference to those occurring in the posterior fossa. J. Neurosurg. **28,** 241–251 (1968).

Delmas, A., Pertuiset, B., Bertrand, G.: Les veines du lobe temporal. C. R. Ass. Anat. **57,** 185 (1949).

Fischer, E.: Röntgenologische Untersuchungen zur Lageabhängigkeit der tiefen Hirnvenen, insbesondere des Angulus venosus, von der Form des Schädels. Acta Neurochir. (Wien) **14,** 25–52 (1966).

Gray, H.: Anatomy of the Human Body, 28th ed. Philadelphia: Lea and Febiger. 1966.

King, T. T.: Removal of intraventricular craniopharyngiomas through the lamina terminalis. Acta Neurochir. (Wien) **45,** 277–286 (1979).

Krause, F.: Die spezielle Chirurgie der Gehirnkrankheiten, Bd. 2 b u. 3. In: Neue Deutsche Chirurgie, Bd. 49 b u. 50. Stuttgart: F. Enke. 1941, 1932.

Lang, J.: Klinische Anatomie des Kopfes, Neurokranium, Orbita, kraniozervikaler Übergang. Berlin–Heidelberg–New York: Springer. 1981.

Lanz, T. v., Wachsmuth, W. (Eds. Lang, J., Wachsmuth, W.): Praktische Anatomie, Bd. I. Teil 1 B. Lang, J.: Gehirn- und Augenschädel. Berlin–Heidelberg–New York: Springer. 1979.

Logue, V.: Surgery of meningiomas. In: Operative Surgery Fundamental International Techniques Neurosurgery (Symon, L., ed.), pp. 128–173. London – Boston – Sydney – Wellington – Durban – Toronto: Butterworths. 1979.

Long, D. M., Leibrock, L.: The transcallosal approach to the anterior ventricular system and its application in the therapy of craniopharyngioma. Clin. Neurosurg. C. N. S. **27,** 160–168 (1980).

Milhorat, T. H., Baldwin, M.: A technique for surgical exposure of the cerebral midline. Experimental transcallosal microdissection. J. Neurosurg. **24,** 687–691 (1966).

Newton, T. H., Potts, D. G.: Radiology of the skull and brain. Angiography, Vol. 2, Bd. 3, 128–155, 1853–2227 (1974).

Nomura, T.: Atlas of Cerebral Angiography. Berlin–Heidelberg–New York: Springer. 1970.

Okonek, G.: Beitrag zur Erkennung und Behandlung basaler Meningeome. Zbl. Chir. **22,** 1912–1025 (1941).

Olivecrona, H.: The surgical treatment of intracranial tumors. In: Neurochirurgie (Olivecrona, H., Tönnis, W., eds.) Vol. 4, part 4, pp. 228–301. Berlin–Heidelberg–New York: Springer. 1967.

Pernkopf, E. (Ed. Ferner, H.): Atlas der topographischen und angewandten Anatomie des Menschen, 1. Bd.: Kopf und Hals. München–Berlin: Urban und Schwarzenberg. 1980.

Pia, H. W.: Die Schädigung des Hirnstammes bei den raumfordernden Prozessen des Gehirns. Wien: Springer. 1957.

Poppen, J. L.: An Atlas of Neurosurgical Techniques. Philadelphia–London: W. B. Saunders Company. 1960.

Potts, D. G., Newton, T. H.: Radiology of the Skull and Brain, Angiography. Saint Louis: The C. V. Mosby Company. 1974.

McRae, D. L., Castorina, G.: Variations in corpus callosum, septum pellucidum and fornix, and their effect on the encephalogram and cerebral angiography. Acta radiol. **1**, 872–880 (1963).

Rand, R. W.: Microneurosurgery, 2nd ed. St. Louis: Mosby. 1978.

Rhoton, A. L., Jr.: Micro-operative techniques. In: Neurological Surgery (Youman, J. R., ed.) ed. 2., Vol. 1, pp. 1160–1194. Philadelphia: Saunders. 1982.

Rhoton, A. L., Jr., Yamamoto, I., Peace, D. A.: Microsurgery of the third ventricle, Part 2. Operative approaches. Neurosurgery **8**, 357–373 (1981).

Ring, B. A.: Variations in the striate and other cerebral veins affecting measurements of the "venous angle". Acta radiol. (Stockh.) **52**, 433–447 (1959).

Risse, G. L., LeDoux, J., Springer, S. P., Wilson, D. H., Gazzaniga, M. S.: The anterior commissure in man: Functional variation in a multi-sensory system. Neuropsychologia **16**, 23–31 (1978).

Rubinstein, L. J.: Tumors of the central nervous system. In: Atlas of Tumors Pathology, 2nd series, fascicle 6. Washington, D. C.: Armed Forces Institute of Pathology. 1972.

Scheremet, R.: Zur Topographie der Brückenvenen im Bereich des Temporallappens. Inaug. Diss. Freiburg i. Br. 1984.

Shucart, W. A., Stein, B. M.: Transcallosal approach to the anterior ventricular system. Neurosurgery **3**, 339–343 (1978).

Sobotta, J., Becher, H. (Hrsg. Ferner, H., Staubesand, J.): Atlas der Anatomie des Menschen, Bd. 3, 17. Auflage, München–Berlin–Wien: Urban und Schwarzenberg. 1973.

Sperry, R. W., Gazzaniga, M. S., Bogen, J. E.: Interhemispheric relationships. The neocortical commissures; syndromes of hemisphere disconnection. In: Handbook of Clinical Neurology, Vol. 4, Disorders of Speech, Perception, and Symbolic Behaviour (Vinken, P. J., Bruyn, G. W., eds.), pp. 273–290. Amsterdam: North-Holland. 1969.

Stephens, R. B., Stillwell, D. L.: Arteries and Veins of the Human Brain. Springfield, Ill.: Ch. C Thomas. 1969.

Sweet, W. H., Talland, G. A., Ervin, F. R.: Loss of recent memory following section of the fornix. Trans. Am. Neurol. Assoc. **84**, 76–82 (1959).

Wendling, L. R., Moore, J. S., Kieffer, S. A., Goldberg, H. I., Latchaw, R. E.: Intracerebral venous angiomas. Radiology **119**, 141–147 (1976).

Winston, K. R., Cavazzuti, V., Arkins, T.: Absence of neurological and behavioral abnormalities after anterior transcallosal operation for third ventricular lesions. Neurosurgery **4**, 386–393 (1979).

Woolsey, R. M., Nelson, J. S.: Asymptomatic destruction of the fornix in man. Arch. Neurol. **32**, 556–568 (1975).

Yamamoto, I., Rhoton, A. L., Peace, D. A.: Microsurgery of the third ventricle: Part 1. Microsurgical anatomy. Neurosurgery **3**, 334–356 (1981).

Yaşargil, M. G.: Clinical considerations, surgery of the intracranial aneurysms and results. In: Microneurosurgery (Yaşargil, M. G., ed.). Vol. 2. Stuttgart–New York: Thieme. New York: Thieme Stratton. 1984.

Yaşargil, M. G., Fox, J. L., Ray, M. W.: The microtechnical "pterional" approach. In: Advances and Technical Standards in Neurosurgery (Krayenbühl, H., et al., eds.), Vol. 2, pp. 113–170. Wien–New York: Springer. 1975.

Yaşargil, M. G., Jain, K. K., Antic, J., Laciga, R.: Arteriovenous malformations of the splenium of the corpus callosum: microsurgical treatment. Surg. Neurol. **5**, 5–14 (1976).

Chapter 3

Abbie, A. A.: The clinical significance of the anterior choroidal artery. Brain **56**, 233–246 (1933).

Abe, H., Tsuru, M., Ito, T., et al.: Temporal lobe damage as pitfalls at subtemporal transtentorial approach. No Shinkei Geka **9**, 819–827 (1981) (Jpn.).

Appuzzo, M. L. J.: Transcallosal interfornicial exposure of lesions of the third ventricle. In: Operative Neurological Techniques: Indications and Methods (Schmidek, H. H., ed.). New York: Grune and Stratton. 1982.

Appuzzo, M. L. J., Chikovani, O. K., Gott, P. S., Teng, E. L. Zee, C. S., Giannotta, S. L., Weiss, M. H.: Transcallosal, interfornicial approaches for lesions affecting the third ventricle: Surgical considerations and consequences. Neurosurgery **5**, 547–554 (1982).

Baldwin, M., Ommaya, A. K., Farrier, R., MacDonald, F.: Mesial cerebral incision. J. Neurosurg. **20**, 679–686 (1963).

Baumgartner, J., Tournadel, A., Plas, J. Y.: Étude anatomochirurgicale de la voie d'abord de la toile choroidienne supérieure du 3ᵉ ventricule. A propos d'un anévrysme artério-veineux choroidien postérieur. Neurochirurgie **27**, 97–102 (1981).

Ben-Amor, M., Marion, C. H., Heldt, N.: Normal and pathological radioanatomy of the superior choroid vein. Neuroradiology **3**, 16–19 (1971).

Benes, V.: Sequelae of transcallosal surgery. Child's Brain **9**, 69–72 (1982).

Bergh, R., Van den Brucher, J. M.: L'abord transventriculaire dans les crânio-pharyngiomes du troisième ventricule: Aspects neurochirurgiaux et neuropathologiques. Neurochirurgie **16**, 51–65 (1970).

Busch, E.: A new surgical approach for the removal of tumors of the third ventricle. Acta Psychiat. (Kbh.) **19**, 57–60 (1944).

Cambria, S.: Thrombosis of the veins of Labbé with haemorrhagic cerebral infarction. Rev. Neurol. (Paris) **136**, 321–326 (1980).

Diamond, S. J., Scammell, R. E., Browers, E. Y. M., Weeks, R.: Functions of the centre section (trunk) of the corpus callosum in man. Brain **100**, 543–562 (1977).

Dandy, W. E.: An operation for the removal of pineal tumors. Surg. Gynec. Obstet. **33**, 113–119 (1921).

Dandy, W. E.: Diagnosis, localization and removal of tumours of the third ventricle. Bull. Johns Hopkins Hosp. **33**, 188–189 (1922).

Dandy, W. E.: Benign Tumours in the Third Ventricle of the Brain; Diagnosis and Treatment. Springfield Ill.: Ch. C Thomas. 1933.

Dandy, W. E.: Operative experience in cases of pineal tumor. Arch. Surg. **33**, 19–46 (1936).

Ehni, G.: Transcallosal removal of brain tumors, movie avaliable from American College of Surgeons and Baylor College of Medicine. 1969.

Ferry, D. J., Mylander, K., Hardman, J.: Radiographic identification and surgical removal of a teratoid tumor of the roof of the third ventricle. J. Neurosurg. **36**, 231–234 (1972).

Fischer, E.: Eine neue Methode zur Lokalisation des Angulus venosus der tiefen Hirnvenen unter Berücksichtigung der Form des Schädels. Acta Neurochir. (Wien) **14**, 53–68 (1966).

Fortuna, A., Celli, P., Ferrante, L., Turano, C.: A review of paillomas of the third ventricle. J. Neurosurg. Sci. **23**, 61–72 (1979).

Gazzaniga, M. S., Freedman, H.: Observations on visual processes after posterior callosal section. Neurology (Minneap.) **23,** 1126–1130 (1973).

Gazzaniga, M. S., Risse, G. L., Springer, S. P., Clark, E., Wilson, D. H.: Psychologic and neurologic consequences of partial and complete cerebral commissurotomy. Neurology (Minneap.) **25,** 10–15 (1975).

Geffen, G., Walsh, A., Simpson, D., Jeeves, M.: Comparison of the effects of transcortical and transcallosal removal of intraventricular tumours. Brain **103,** 773–788 (1980).

Gerber, S. S., Plotkin, R.: Lipoma of the Corpus callosum. J. Neurosurg. **57** (1982), 281–285.

Geschwind, N.: Disconnexion syndromes in animals and man, Part. 1. Brain **88,** 237–294 (1965).

Giudicelli, G., Salamon, G.: The veins of the thalamus. Neuroradiology **1,** 92–98 (1970).

Glasauer, F. E.: An operative approach to pineal tumors. Acta Neurochir. (Wien) **22,** 177–180 (1970).

Gordon, H. W., Bogen, J. E., Sperry, R. W.: Absence of deconnexion syndrome in two patients with partial section of the neocommissures. Brain **94,** 327–336 (1971).

Greenwood, J., Jr.: Radical surgery of tumors of the thalamus, hypothalamus, and third ventricle area. Surg. Neurol. **1,** 29–33 (1973).

Hawkins, J. C.: Treatment of choroid plexus papillomas in children. A brief analysis of twenty years' experience. Neurosurgery **6,** 380–384 (1980).

Heilman, K. M., Sypert, G. W.: Korsakoff's syndrome resulting from bilateral fornix lesions. Neurology (NY) **27,** 490–493 (1977).

Hitchon, P. W., Abu-Yousef, M. M., Graf, C. J., Turner, D. M., Van Gilder, J. C.: Management and outcome of pineal region tumors. Neurosurgery **3,** 248–253 (1983).

Jamieson, K. G.: Excision of pineal tumors. J. Neurosurg. **35,** 550–553 (1971).

Jeeves, M. A., Simpson, D. A., Geffen, G.: Functional consequences of the transcallosal removal of intraventricular tumours. J. Neurol. Neurosurg. Psychiat. **42,** 134–142 (1979).

Kobayashi, S., Sugita, K., Tanaka, Y., Kyoshima, K.: Infratentorial approach to the pineal region in the prone position: Concorde position. J. Neurosurg. **58,** 141–143 (1983).

Krause, F.: Die spezielle Chirurgie der Gehirnkrankheiten, Bd. 2b u. 3. In: Neue Deutsche Chirurgie, Bd. 49b u. 50. Stuttgart: F. Enke. 1941, 1932.

Kunicki, A.: Operative experiences in 8 cases of pineal tumor. J. Neurosurg. **17,** 815–823 (1960).

Lapras, Cl., Dechaume, J. P., Deruty, R., et al.: Traitement des tumeurs de la région pinéale. Lyon Chir. **69,** 196–198 (1973).

Lavyne, H. M., Patterson, R. H., Jr.: Subchoroidal trans-velum interpositum approach to mid-third ventricular tumors. Neurosurgery **1,** 86–94 (1983).

Long, D. M., Chou, S. N.: Transcallosal removal of craniopharyngiomas within the third ventricle. J. Neurosurg. **39,** 563–567 (1973).

Neuwelt, E. A., Batjar, H.: Surgical management of pineal region tumors. Contemp. Neurosurg. **4,** 1–5 (1982).

Nieuwenhuys, R., Voogd, J., von Juijzen, Chr.: The Human Central Nervous System. A Synopsis and Atlas. Berlin–Heidelberg–New York: Springer. 1978.

Palacios, E., Fine, M., Haughton, V. M.: Multiplanar Anatomy of the Head and Neck for Computed Tomography. New York: John Wiley & Sons. 1980.

Pendl, G.: Infratentorial approach to mesencephalic tumors. In: Clinical Microneurosurgery (Koos, W. T., Böck, F. W., Spetzler, R. F., eds.), pp. 143–150. Stuttgart: Thieme. 1976.

Poppen, J. L.: The right occipital approach to a pinealoma. J. Neurosurg. **25,** 706–710 (1966).

Poppen, J. L., Marion, R., Jr.: Pinealomas and tumors of the posterior portion of the third ventricle. J. Neurosurg. **28,** 357–364 (1968).

Rand, R. W., Lemmen, L. J.: Tumors of the posterior portion of the third ventricle. J. Neurosurg. **10,** 1–18 (1953).

Reid, W. S., Clark, W. K.: Comparison of the infratentorial and transtentorial approaches to the pineal region. Neurosurgery **3,** 1–8 (1978).

Rhoton, A. L., Jr., Yamamoto, I., Peace, D. A.: Microsurgery of the third ventricle: Part II. Operative approaches. Neurosurgery **8,** 357–377 (1981).

Rozario, R., Adelman, L., Prager, R. J., Stein, B. M.: Meningiomas of the pineal region and third ventricle. Neurosurgery **5,** 489–495 (1979).

Stein, B. M.: The infratentorial supracerebellar approach to pineal lesions. J. Neurosurg. **35,** 197–202 (1971).

Stein, B. M.: Transcallosal approach to third ventricular tumors. In: Current Techniques in Operative Neurosurgery (Schmidek, H. H., Sweet, W. H., eds.), pp. 247–255. New York: Grune and Stratton. 1977.

Stein, B. M.: Supracerebellar approach for pineal region neoplasms. In: Current Techniques in Operative Neurosurgery. (Schmidek, H. H., Sweet, W. H., eds.), pp. 257–264. New York: Grune and Stratton. 1977.

Stein, B. M.: Supracerebellar-infratentorial approach to pineal tumors. Surg. Neurol. **11,** 331–337 (1979).

Suzuki, J., Iwabuchi, T.: Surgical removal of pineal tumors (pinealomas and teratomas): Experience in a series of 19 cases. J. Neurosurg. **23,** 565–571 (1965).

Tamaki, N., Taomoto, K., Fujiwara, K., Yamashita, H., Matsumoto, S., Takeda, H.: The venous drainage fo the tectum mesencephali. Neuroradiology **11,** 151–157 (1976).

Viale, G. L., Turtas, S.: The subchoroid approach to the third ventricle. Surg. Neurol. **14,** 71–76 (1980).

Wagenen, W. P. Van: A surgical approach for the removal of certain pineal tumors. Surg. Gynec. Obstet. **53,** 216–220 (1931).

Yamamoto, I., Kageyama, N.: Microsurgical anatomy of the pineal region. J. Neurosurg. **53,** 205–221 (1980).

Yamamoto, I., Rhoton, A. L., Jr., Peace, D. A.: Microsurgery of the third ventricle: Part I. Microsurgical anatomy. Neurosurgery **8,** 334–356 (1981).

Chapter 4

Beau, A., Rabischong, P.: Les veines internes du cerveau. C. R. Ass. anat. **102,** 175–181 (1959).

Browder, J., Browder, A., Kaplan, H. A.: Benign tumors of the cerebral dural sinuses. J. Neurosurg. **37,** 576–579 (1972).

Browder, J., Browder, A., Kaplan, H. A.: Anatomical relationships of the cerebral and dural venous systems in the parasagittal area. Anat. Rec. **176,** 329–332 (1973).

Hermann, E., Seeger, W.: Die diagnostische Bedeutung des Verlaufs der Arteria basalis und deren großen Endäste im Vertebralis-Angiogramm. Deutsch. Z. Nervenheilk. **187,** 531 (1965)

Markowski, J.: Über die Entwicklung der Sinus durae matris und der Hirnvenen bei Embryonen von 15,5–49 mm Scheitel-

Steißlänge. Bull. d. l'Acad. d. Sci. de Cracovie, Cl. d. Sci. math.-nat. Serie B (1911).

Mokrohisky, J. F., Paul, R. E., Lin, P. M., Stauffer, H. M.: The diagnostic importance of normal variants in deep cerebral phlebography. Radiology **67,** 34–47 (1956).

Nieuwenhuys, R., Voogd, J., van Juijzen, Ch.: The Human Central Nervous System. A Synopsis and Atlas. Berlin–Heidelberg–New York: Springer. 1978.

Schlesinger, B.: The venous drainage of the brain, with special reference to the Galenic system. Brain **62,** 274–291 (1939).

Chapter 5

Bernstein, M., Hoffmann, H. J., Halliday, W. C., Hendrick, E. B., Humphreys, R. P.: Thalamic tumors in children. Long-term follow-up and treatment guidelines. J. Neurosurg. **61,** 649–656 (1984).

Diamond, C., Torvik, A., Amundsen, P.: Angiographic diagnosis of telangiectasias with cavernous angioma of the posterior fossa. Acta radiol./Diag. (Stockh.) **17,** 281–288 (1976).

Fierstein, S. B., Pribram, H. W., Hieshima, G.: Angiography and computer tomography in the evaluation of cerebral venous malformations. Neuroradiology **17,** 137–148 (1979).

Hardy, D. G., Rhoton, A. L.: Microsurgical relationships of the superior cerebellar artery and the trigeminal nerve. J. Neurosurg. **49,** 669–678 (1978).

Hochstetter, F.: Über eine Varietät der Vena cerebralis basalis des Menschen nebst Bemerkungen über die Entwicklung bestimmter Hirnnerven. Z. Anat. Entwickl.-Gesch. **108,** 311–336 (1938).

Hölzel, G.: Die lateralen subependymalen Ventrikelvenen. Inaug. Diss. Freiburg i. Br. 1977.

Huang, Y. P., Wolf, B. S.: The basal cerebral vein and its tributaries. In: Radiology of the Skull and Brain, Vol. 2, Book 3 (Newton, T. H., Potts, D. G., eds.), pp. 2111–2154. Saint Louis: Mosby. 1974.

Liliequist, B.: The subarachnoid cisterns. Anatomic and roentgenologic study. Acta radiol. (Stockh.) Suppl. 185 (1959).

Maehara, T., Tasaka, A.: Cerebral venous angioma: computerized tomography and angiographic diagnosis. Neuroradiology **16,** 296–298 (1978).

Michels, L. G., Bentson, J. R., Winter, J.: Computed tomography of cerebral venous angiomas. J. Comput. Assist. Tomog. **1,** 149–154 (1977).

Pia, H. W.: Die Schädigung des Hirnstammes bei den raumfordernden Prozessen des Gehirns. Wien: Springer. 1957.

Preissig, R. S., Preissig, S. H., Goree, J. A.: Angiographic demonstration of a cerebral venous angioma. J. Neurosurg. **44,** 628–631 (1976).

Saito, Y., Kobayashi, N.: Cerebral venous angiomas. Radiology **139,** 87–94 (1981).

Scotti, L. N., Goldman, R. L., Rao, G. R., Heinz, E. R.: Cerebral venous angiomas. Neuroradiology **9,** 125–128 (1975).

Chapter 6

Barbosa, J. F.: Surgery of extensive cancer of the paranasal sinuses. Arch. Otolaryngol. **73,** 129–138 (1961).

Bébéar, J. P.: Apport des techniques récentes dans le diagnostic et le traitement du neurinome de l'acoustique. Thèse Bordeaux **71,** 10 (1973).

Bourguet, J., Bourdinière, J., Carsin, J., et al.: A propos de 30 fibromes nasopharyngiens. Ann. Otolaryngol. Chir. Cervicofac. **97,** 295–303 (1980).

Bull, J.: The angiographic pattern of the petrosal veins in the normal and pathological. Neuroradiology **1,** 20 (1971).

Casson, P. R., Bonanno, P. C., Converse, J. M.: The midface degloving procedure. Plast. Reconstr. Surg. **53,** 102–103 (1974).

Charachon, R.: Anatomie de l'aftère auditive interne chez l'homme. Thèse, Lyon 1961.

Crockett, D. J.: Surgical approach to the back of the maxilla. Br. J. Surg. **50,** 819–821 (1963).

Economos, D., Prosalentis, A.: L'artère cérébelleuse supérieure dans les tumeurs de la fosse postérieure. Acta Radiol. **1,** 267 (1963).

Fay, T.: The management of tumors of the posterior fossa by the transtentorial approach. Surg. Clin. N. Amer. **10,** 14 (1931).

Fisch, U.: L'anatomie chirurgicale du système artériel du conduit auditif interne chez l'homme. Rev. Laryng. (Bordeaux) **89,** 659 (1968).

Fisch, U.: The surgical anatomy of the so-called internal auditory artery. In: Disorders of the Skull Base Region; Proceedings: Nobel Symposium, 10th, Stockholm, 1968 (Hamberger, C.-A., Wersäll, J., eds.), pp. 121–130. Stockholm: Almqvist and Wiksell, New York: Wiley. 1968.

Fisch, U.: The infratemporal fossa approach for nasopharyngeal tumors. Laryngoscope **93,** 36–44 (1983).

Fisch, U., Yaşargil, M. G.: Abord translabyrinthine du neurinome de l'acoustique. Méd. Hyg. **26,** 1190 (1968a).

Fisch, U., Yaşargil, M. G.: Approche transtemporale, extradurale du conduit auditif interne. Pract. Otorhinolaryng. **30,** 377 (1968b).

Hitselberger, W. E., House, W. F.: A combined approach to the cerebellopontine angle: a suboccipital-petrosal approach. Arch. Otolaryng. (Chic.) **84,** 267 (1966).

Hitselberger, W. E., Gardner, G.: Other tumors of the cerebellopontine angle. Arch. Otolaryng. (Chic.) **88,** 712 (1968).

Hermann, E., Seeger, W.: Die diagnostische Bedeutung des Verlaufs der Arteria basalis und deren großen Endäste im Vertebralis-Angiogramm. Deutsch. Z. Nervenheilk. **187,** 531 (1965)

House, W. F.: Surgical exposure of the internal auditory canal and its contents through the middle cranial fossa. Laryngoscope (St. Louis) **11,** 1363 (1961).

Kraus, H., Böck, F., Grunert, V., Koos, W.: Advances in surgery for acustic neurinoma (a synopsis). Advances Neurosurg. **1,** 248 (1973).

Krause, C. J., Baker, S. R.: Extended transantral approach to pterygomaxillary tumors. Ann. Otol. Rhinol. Laryngol. **91,** 395–398 (1982).

Mann, W. F., Gilsbach, J., Seeger, W., Flöel, H.: Use of a malar bone graft to augment skull-base access. Arch. Otolaryngol. **111,** 30–33 (1985).

Mazzoni, A.: Internal auditory canal: Arterial relations at the porus acusticus. Ann. Otol. Rhinol. Laryngol. **78,** 797–814 (1969).

Mündnich, K.: Zur Röntgendiagnostik und Operation maligner Oberkiefer- und Flügelgaumengrubentumoren. Z. Laryng. Rhinol. Otol. **33,** 125–127 (1954).

Nager, G. T.: Origins and relations of the internal auditory artery and the subarcuate artery. Ann. Otol. Rhinol. Laryngol. **63,** 51–61 (1954).

Naidich, T. P., Kricheff, I. I., George, A. E., Lin, J. P.: The

anterior inferior cerebellar artery in mass lesions: Preliminary findings with emphasis on the lateral projection. Radiology **119,** 375–383 (1976).
Rhoton, A. L.: Microsurgical removal of acoustic neuromas. Surg. Neurol. **6,** 211–219 (1976).
Schramm, V. L., Myers, E. N., Maroon, J. C.: Anterior skull base surgery for benign and malignant disease. Laryngoscope **89,** 1077–1091 (1979).
Som, P. M., Biller, H. F., Lawson, W.: Tumors of the parapharyngeal space preoperative evaluation, diagnostic and surgical approaches. Ann. Otol. Rhinol. Laryngol. **90,** 3–15 (1981).
Ward, P. H., Thompson, R., Calcaterra, T., et al.: Juvenile angiofibroma: A more rational therapeutic approach based upon clinical and experimental evidence. Laryngoscope **84,** 2181–2194 (1974).
Watt, J. C., McKillip, A. N.: Relation of arteries to roots of nerves in posterior fossa in man. Arch. Surg. **30,** 336–345 (1935).
Yaşargil, M. G., Subokzipitale-transmeatale mikrotechnische Exstirpation des Akustikusneurinoms. In: Naumann, Kopf- u. Hals-Chirurgie, Bd. III Ohrregion, S. 545. Stuttgart: Thieme. 1976.
Yaşargil, M. G., Fox, J. L.: The microsurgical approach to acoustic neuromas. Surg. Neurol. **2,** 393–398 (1974).
Zehm, S.: Die Grenzen der Operabilität der Geschwülste des Nasenrachens. Stuttgart: Thieme. 1970.

Chapter 7

Balèiaux-Wada, D., Mortelmans, L. L., Dupont, M. G., et al.: The use of coronal scans for computed tomography of the orbits. Neuroradiolgy **14,** 89 (1977).
Barbosa, J. F.: Surgery of extensive cancer of the paranasal sinuses. Arch. otolaryngol. **73,** 129–138 (1961).
Bostroem, A., Spatz, H.: Über die von der Olfactoriusrinne ausgehenden Meningeome und über die Meningeome im allgemeinen. Nervenarzt **2,** 505–521 (1929).
Chiari, O.: Über eine Modifikation der Schloffer'schen Operation von Tumoren der Hypophyse. Wien. klin. Wschr. **25,** 5–6 (1912).
Collins, W. F., Jr.: Transsphenoidal surgery in pituitary adenomas. In: The Pituitary–a Current Review (Allen, M. B., Mahesh, V. B., eds.), pp. 431–442. New York–San Francisco–London: Academic Press. 1977.
Cope, V. Z.: Surgery of the pituitary fossa. Brit. J. Surg. **4,** 107–144 (1916).
Cummings, C. W., Johnson, J.: Transsphenoidal approach to the pituitary adenomas. In: Current Techniques in Operative Neurosurgery (Schmidek, H. H., Sweet, W. H., eds.), pp. 173–180. New York: Grune and Stratton. 1977.
Cushing, H.: Surgical experiences with pituitary disorders. J. A. M. A. **63,** 1515–1525 (1914).
Duvernoy, H. M.: The Superficial Veins of the Human Brain. Veins of the Brain Stem and of the Base of the Brain. Berlin–Heidelberg–New York: Springer. 1975.
Ehlers, N., Malmros, R.: The suprasellar meningioma. Acta Ophthalmol. (Copenhagen) Suppl. 121 (1973).
Hacker, H.: Normal supratentorial veins and dural sinuses. In: Radiology of the Skull and Brain (Newton, T. H., Potts, D. G., eds.), Vol. 2, pp. 1851–1877. Saint Louis: Mosby. 1974.
Hamberger, C. A., Hammer, G.: Der transnasale Weg der Hypophysektomie. In: Hals-Nasen-Ohren-Heilkunde (Berendes, J., Link, R., Zöllner, F., eds.), Vol. 1, pp. 795–818, Stuttgart: Thieme. 1964.
Hardy, J.: Transsphenoidal Hypophysectomy. J. Neurosurg. **34,** 582–594 (1971).
Karduck, A., Bock, W. J.: Rhinological findings following transantrosphenoidal surgery of the pituitary gland. Acta Otolaryngol. **85,** 449–452 (1978).
Liliequist, B.: The subarachnoid cisterns. Anatomic and roentgenologic study. Acta radiol. (Stockh.) Suppl. 185 (1959).
Loewe, L.: Über die Freilegung der Sehnervenkreuzung und der Hypophysis und über die Beteiligung des Siebbeinlabyrinthes am Aufbau der Supraorbitalplatte. Z. Augenheilk. **19,** 456–464 (1908).
Renn, W. H., Rhoton, A. L., Jr.: Microsurgical anatomy of the sellar region. J. Neurosurg. **43,** 288–298 (1975).
Rhoton, A. L., Jr., Hardy, D. G., Chambers, S. M.: Microsurgical anatomy and dissection of the sphenoid bone, Cavernous sinus and sellar region. Surg. Neurol. **12,** 63–104 (1979).
Samii, M., Draf, W.: Course on Surgery of the Skull Base. Hannover, West-Germany. 1979.
Samii, M., Jannetta, P. J.: Symposium on Cranial Nerves. Hannover, West-Germany. 1980.
Schramm, V. L., Myers, E. N., Maroon, J. C.: Anterior skull base surgery for benign and malignant disease. Laryngoscope **89,** 1077–1091 (1979).
Stein, B. M.: Third ventricular tumors. Clin. Neurosurg. C. N. S. **27,** 315–331 (1980).
Tadmor, R. R., New, F. J.: Computed tomography of the orbit with special emphasis on coronal sections: Part 1. Normal anatomy. J. Comput. Assist Tomogr. **2,** 24 (1978).
Unsöld, R., Newton, T. H., Berninger, W.: The value and clinical application of multiplanar computer reformations in orbital diagnosis. In: Diagnostic Radiology 1980. Proceedings of the Annual Postgraduate Course in Diagnostic Radiology, San Francisco, Mar 3–7, 1980 (Margulis, A. R., Gooding, C. A., eds.) San Francisco: University of California, Department of Radiology. 1980.
Zehm, S.: Die Grenzen der Operabilität der Geschwülste des Nasenrachens. Stuttgart: Thieme. 1970.

Chapter 8

Barbosa, J. F.: Surgery of extensive cancer of the paranasal sinuses. Arch. Otolaryngol. **73,** 129–138 (1961).
Bonnal, J., Thibaut, A., Brotchi, J., et al.: Invading meningiomas of the sphenoid ridge. J. Neurosurg. **53,** 587–599 (1980).
Bourguet, J., Bourdinière, J., Carsin, J., et al.: A propos de 30 fibromes nasopharyngiens. Ann. Otolaryngol. Chir. Cerviofac. **97,** 295–303 (1980).
Calcaterra, T. C., Rand, R. W.: Current adjuncts for surgery of the sphenoid sinus and pituitary gland. Laryngoscope **86,** 1692–1698 (1976).
Carlsson, B., Lodin, H.: Size of interpeduncular, pontine, pontocerebellar cisterns and cisterna magna in childhood. Acta radiol. (Stockh.) **8,** 65–73 (1969).
Casson, P. R., Bonanno, P. C., Converse, J. M.: The midface degloving procedure. Plast. Reconstr Surg. **53,** 102–103 (1974).

Crockett, D. J.: Surgical approach to the back of the maxilla. Br. J. Surg. **50,** 819–821 (1963).

Ferner, H.: Anatomische und phlebographische Studien der inneren Hirnvenen des Menschen. Z. Anat. Entwickl.-Gesch. **120,** 481–491 (1958).

Fisch, U.: The infratemporal fossa approach for nasopharyngeal tumors. Laryngoscope **93,** 36–44 (1983).

Krause, C. J., Baker, S. R.: Extended transantral approach to pterygomaxillary tumors. Ann. Otol. Rhinol. Laryngol. **91,** 395–398 (1982).

Krogius, A.: Neue Methode, den Nasopharyngealraum für die Operation von Basalfibromen und Hypophysengeschwülsten freizulegen. Zbl. Chir. **36,** 1420 (1909).

Lindgren, E.: Handbuch der Neurochirurgie, Bd. II: Roentgenologie. Berlin–Göttingen–Heidelberg: Springer. 1954.

Mann, W. F., Gilsbach, J., Seeger, W., Flöel, H.: Use of malar bone graft to augment skull-base access. Arch. Otolaryngol. **111,** 30–33 (1985).

Mündnich, K.: Zur Röntgendiagnostik und Operation maligner Oberkiefer- und Flügelgaumengrubentumoren. Z. Laryng. Rhinol. Otol. **33,** 125–127 (1954).

Perese, D. M.: Superficial veins of the brain from a surgical point of view. J. Neurosurg. **17,** 402–412 (1960).

Rauber, A., Kopsch, F.: Lehrbuch und Atlas der Anatomie des Menschen, Bd. I, 20. Aufl. neu bearbeitet von W. Bargmann. Stuttgart: G. Thieme. 1968.

Rhoton, A. L., Jr., Hardy, D. G., Chambers, S. M.: Microsurgical anatomy and dissection of the sphenoid bone, cavernous sinus and sellar region. Surg. Neurol. **12,** 63–104 (1979).

Russell, D. S., Rubinstein, L. J.: Pathology of Tumours of the Nervous System, 4th ed. Edinburgh: E. Arnold. 1977.

Seeger, W.: Atlas of Topographical Anatomy of the Brain and Surrounding Structures. Wien–New York: Springer. 1978.

Som, P. M., Biller, H. F., Lawson, W.: Tumors of the parapharyngeal space preoperative evaluation, diagnostis and surgical approaches. Ann. Otol. Rhinol. Laryngol. **90,** 3–15 (1981).

Schramm, V. L., Myers, E. N., Maroon, J. C.: Anterior skull base surgery for benign and malignant disease. Laryngoscope **89,** 1077–1091 (1979).

Ward, P. H., Thompson, R., Calcaterra, T., et al.: Juvenile angiofibroma: A more rational therapeutic approach based upon clinical and experimental evidence. Laryngoscope **84,** 2181–2194 (1974).

Zehm, S.: Die Grenzen der Operabilität der Geschwülste des Nasenrachens. Stuttgart: G. Thieme. 1970.

Chapter 9

Atkinson, W. J.: The anterior inferior cerebellar artery: Its variations, pontine distributions, and significance in the surgery of cerebello-pontine angle tumors. J. Neurol. Neurosurg. Psychiat. **12,** 137–151 (1949).

Pia, H. W.: Die Schädigung des Hirnstammes bei den raumfordernden Prozessen des Gehirns. Wien: Springer. 1957.

Seeger, W.: Atlas of Topographical Anatomy of the Brain and Surrounding Structures. Wien–New York: Springer. 1978.

Seeger, W.: Microsurgery of the Brain, Anatomical and Technical Principles, Vol. 1. Wien–New York: Springer. 1980.

Subject Index

Printed by Ferdinand Berger & Söhne Gesellschaft m.b.H., A-3580 Horn

By the same author:

Atlas of Topographical Anatomy of the Brain and Surrounding Structures

for Neurosurgeons, Neuroradiologists, and Neuropathologists

1985. 258 figures. IX, 544 pages.
Format: 17 cm × 24,5 cm
ISBN 3-211-81851-0

Soft Cover Edition

Distribution rights for Japan: Eastern Book Service, Tokyo

Also available in Format 23,7 cm × 32 cm
ISBN 3-211-81447-7

Distribution rights for Japan: Nankodo Co. Ltd., Tokyo
Distribution rights for Socialist Countries: J. A. Barth, Leipzig

Micro-neurosurgical techniques demand an enlarged representation of the anatomy under conditions that correspond to the microsurgical site. Anatomical drawings (made by the author himself) are used throughout the work to illustrate brain structures and separate arterial and venous structures, as well as their positions in relation to each other. This outstanding presentation immediately distinguishes itself from the usual anatomical atlases and surgical textbooks by its unique approach to questions and techniques. After the great success of the original edition we now make this outstanding work also available as a low price paperback edition.

Microsurgery of the Cranial Base

1983. 200 figures. VII, 416 pages.
Format: 23,7 cm× 32 cm
ISBN 3-211-81769-7

Distribution rights for Japan: Nankodo Co. Ltd., Tokyo

This book helps you to *minimize the risks* inherent in most microsurgical maneuvers in the cranial base. At the same time, it helps you to *maximize the scope of your microsurgical skills* there. It does this by offering you lucid technical presentations in conjunction with *precise anatomic models.* The techniques are designed to help you avoid common pitfalls. The models help to enhance your three-dimensional orientation to an operation by illustrating important neighboring structures not ordinarily visible during surgery.

Microsurgery of the Spinal Cord and Surrounding Structures

Anatomical and Technical Principles

1982. 201 figures. VII, 410 pages.
Format: 23,7 cm× 32 cm
ISBN 3-211-81648-8

Distribution rights for Japan: Nankodo Co. Ltd., Tokyo

Here is information about operative interventions in extra-and intra-dural tumors, angiomas, and malformations of the spinal canal (including some typical lesions occurring there). Precise anatomic models are provided to help you see the principles of the procedures and to show neighboring structures generally not visible from the surgeon's perspective, but which nevertheless can play an important role. Also included are typical computer tomography sections illustrating possible sources of diagnostic error.

Microsurgery of the Brain

Anatomical and Technical Principles

1980. 351 figures. XI, IV, 727 pages.
In two volumes, not sold separately.
Format: 23,7 cm × 32 cm
ISBN 3-211-81573-2

Distribution rights for Japan: Nankodo Co. Ltd., Tokyo

Thoralf M. Sundt Jr. in *Journal of Neurosurgery:*
"Seldom does one have the opportunity to review a book of this quality. It is indeed a solid contribution to the neurosurgical literature and one that should be in all department libraries and readily available for the resident staff. Experienced neurosurgeons will also find it most interesting and probably would find it useful for their own personal library as well.
The book is prepared by a master anatomist and artist. The drawings are oriented according to surgical exposures and if the term 'practical or surgical anatomy' really deserves a separate category, this book would certainly qualify as a classic in that field ... It is well worth the asking price."

Springer-Verlag
Wien New York